Sarah Newbery RFHSM

Applied Pharmacology

Applied Pharmacology

H. O. Schild

MD, PhD, DSc, FRS
Professor Emeritus of Pharmacology in the University of London
at University College London;
Honorary Member of the British Pharmacological Society

TWELFTH EDITION

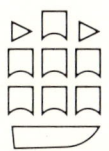

CHURCHILL LIVINGSTONE
EDINBURGH LONDON MELBOURNE AND NEW YORK 1980

CHURCHILL LIVINGSTONE
Medical Division of the Longman Group Limited

Distributed in the United States of America by Churchill Livingstone Inc., 19 West 44th Street, New York, N.Y. 10036, and by associated companies, branches and representatives throughout the world.

© J. & A. Churchill Limited 1959, 1968
© Longman Group Limited 1975, 1980

All rights reserved. No part of this publication may be reproduced, stored in a retrieval system, or transmitted in any form or by any means, electronic, mechanical, photocopying, recording or otherwise, without the prior permission of the publishers (Churchill Livingstone, Robert Stevenson House, 1-3 Baxter's Place, Leith Walk, Edinburgh, EH1 3AF).

First edition 1923
Second edition 1927
Third edition 1929
   Spanish translation 1929
Fourth edition 1932
Fifth edition 1933
   Chinese translation 1935
Sixth edition 1937
Seventh edition 1940
Eighth edition 1952
Ninth edition 1959
Tenth edition 1968
ELBS edition of first published 1968
   Italian translation 1972
Eleventh edition 1975
ELBS edition of eleventh edition 1975
   Italian translation 1980
Twelfth edition 1980

ISBN 0 443 02199 6

British Library Cataloguing in Publication Data
Schild, Heinz Otto
   Applied pharmacology. — 12th ed.
   1. Drugs — Physiological effects
   I. Title II. Wilson, Andrew, b. *1909*
   615'.7 RM300 80-40315

Printed in Singapore by Singapore Offset Printing Pte Ltd

Preface

Following the untimely death of my old friend and co-author Andrew Wilson it fell to me to prepare the 12th edition of *Applied Pharmacology*. My own retirement provided the opportunity and leisure for a thorough revision of the text which continues to follow the intention of its original author, A. J. Clark, of presenting an account of the subject of pharmacology within the framework of the cognate disciplines of physiology, biochemistry, pathology and clinical medicine. A principal aim of this book has been to demonstrate to students of pharmacology the essential unity of the subject which is best understood if its fundamental and clinical aspects are considered together.

The text of this edition is organised in seven main sections dealing respectively with general principles of drug action, neurohumoral transmission and local hormones, pharmacology of the central nervous system and local anaesthetics, hormones and vitamins, chemotherapy of tumours and infections and finally environmental pharmacology. An attempt has been made to include in the 12th edition important new developments in pharmacology including amongst others: radioimmunoassay, bioavailability, Hansch analysis, cytochrome P450, presynaptic receptors, membrane noise, thromboxanes, plasma digoxin measurement, calcium current, chenodeoxycholic acid, transferrin, fibrinolysis, sedative-hypnotic drug dependence, lithium, carbamazepine, amine mechanisms in manic depressive disease, dopamine hypothesis of schizophrenia, opiate receptors, oestrogen receptors, chemical character of LH and FSH, cortisol binding, metabolic activation of vitamin D, antiviral agents, protein-calorie malnutrition and male contraception. Two new chapters deal with pharmacology of the skin and fundamental aspects of hormone action.

I am most grateful to Dr T. D. Whittet, former Chief Pharmacist, Department of Health and Social Security, for having agreed to prepare the pharmacy addenda which should help to make more concrete the pharmacology discussions by providing the doses and modalities of administration of drug preparations.

London, 1980   H.O.S.

Contents

Section 1. General principles of drug action
1. Introduction — 3
2. Drug-receptor interactions — 9
3. Measurement of drug action — 19
4. Absorption, distribution and fate of drugs — 34

Section 2. Neurohumoral transmission and local hormones
5. Cholinergic transmission — 53
6. Adrenergic mechanisms — 73
7. Autonomic control of intrinsic muscles of the eye — 86
8. Local hormones and allergy — 90

Section 3. Pharmacology of organ systems
9. The circulation — 109
10. The heart — 131
11. The kidneys — 151
12. Respiration and bronchi — 167
13. The alimentary canal — 184
14. The haemopoietic system — 202
15. The uterus — 217
16. The skin — 227

Section 4. Pharmacology of the central nervous system and local anaesthetics
17. Basic neurohumoral and electrophysiological mechanisms — 235
18. Central depressants: hypnotics and tranquillisers — 243
19. Antidepressants and stimulants of mental activity — 257
20. Central depressants of motor function — 268
21. Analgesic drugs — 278
22. Anaesthetics — 295
23. Local anaesthetics — 308

Section 5. Hormones and vitamins
24. Fundamental aspects of hormone action — 319
25. Pituitary, thyroid and parathyroid hormones — 324
26. Insulin and corticosteroids — 337
27. Sex hormones — 351
28. The vitamins — 360

Section 6. Chemotherapy of tumours and infections
29. Cytotoxic drugs in the treatment of cancer — 375
30. Basic aspects of antibacterial chemotherapy — 385
31. Synthetic compounds for the chemotherapy of infections — 392
32. Penicillin and cephalosporin antibiotics — 398
33. Other antibiotics for the chemotherapy of infections — 408
34. Tuberculosis and leprosy — 418
35. Trypanosomiasis, leishmaniasis and spirochaetal infections — 430
36. Malaria and amoebiasis — 438
37. Anthelmintics — 448
38. Disinfectants — 456

Section 7. Environmental pharmacology
39. Ecology and environmental health — 465
40. Control of population growth — 476
41. Drug dependence — 481

Index — 493

SECTION ONE

General principles of drug action

1. Introduction

Systems of medicine 3; Development of pharmacology 5; Pharmacopoeas 5; Voluntary schemes for the control of drugs 6; Mandatory schemes 7; Commercial influences in therapeutics 7.

Pharmacology may be defined as the study of the manner in which the functions of living organisms can be modified by chemical substances. The scope of this treatise of Applied Pharmacology may be defined as the application of pharmacology in the treatment of disease in man.

SYSTEMS OF MEDICINE

Mankind applies its powers of reason in a curiously erratic manner. In some subjects, such as pure chemistry and physics, the implications of the existing knowledge are explored promptly and confidently, but in other subjects, of which therapeutics is an outstanding example, there has been extreme hesitation to apply scientific methods. This difference often results in contrasts that are glaring and absurd. For example, Robert Boyle's work *The Sceptical Chemist* (1661) provided the foundation for modern chemistry and was particularly characterised by the bold and critical reasoning it contained. The same author, however, when dealing with therapeutics (*A Collection of Choice Remedies* 1692) was content to describe and recommend a hotchpotch of messes with ingredients such as worms, horse dung, human urine and moss from a dead man's skull. The great scientist, when he approached therapeutics, ceased to think, and was content to be a collector of semi-magical folklore.

It may be said, indeed, that therapeutics was scarcely influenced by scientific progress until the middle of the nineteenth century, at which date it was possible for Virchow to dismiss the subject with the contemptuous phrase: 'Therapy is in an empirical stage cared for by practical doctors and clinicians, and it is by means of a combination with physiology that it must rise to be a science, which today it is not'.

The late development of the science of therapeutics was partly due to the fact that in order to understand the effects produced by remedies on the functions of the diseased body, it was necessary to know something about the normal functions of the body (physiology), and also something of the manner in which these functions were deranged by disease (pathology of function).

The effects of this lack of knowledge were undoubtedly accentuated by a subconscious feeling that disease and death were semi-sacred subjects which should be dealt with by authoritarian rather than rationalist methods. This attitude was strengthened by the accident that authority and tradition, based on very poor translations of Galen, reigned supreme in European medicine from the time of Galen until the Renaissance. For example, the use of antimony was opposed in the sixteenth century, not because it was thought to be harmful or useless, but because its use lacked the authority of Galen. This reliance on tradition and authority sometimes produced extraordinary results, because anyone who succeeded in establishing himself as an authority was followed in a completely uncritical manner.

The history of the treatment of malaria provides a striking example of the manner in which clinical practice and tradition can vary in obedience to authority and in defiance of what appear to be the most obvious and easily ascertainable facts. Cinchona bark, on its introduction in the seventeenth century, was quickly recognised to be a specific cure for remittent fevers, and as early as 1765 Lind laid down the correct treatment for malaria, namely, the administration of cinchona bark in full doses as soon as the disease was diagnosed.

In 1804, however, James Johnson stated that it was unsafe to give cinchona bark until the fever had subsided, and recommended instead the employment of large doses of calomel. This treatment was based on the experience of a visit of a few weeks to India, but it accorded with the general clinical tradition of the period, and in spite of the fact that the results were murderous this form of treatment was continued in India until 1847, when Hare, in face of the bitterest opposition, succeeded in re-introducing the rational use of quinine.

Allopathy

Repeated attempts were made to construct so-called 'rational' systems of therapeutics, but there was no adequate knowledge of physiology or pathology to provide a proper basis for such systems, and in practice they led to even worse results than did pure empiricism. The dominating personality of James Gregory (1753-1821) helped greatly to spread over the world the system of heroic symptomatic treatment which was termed allopathy. The favourite remedies were blood-letting, emetics and purgatives, and these were used until the dominant symptoms of the disease were suppressed. The scale on which these procedures were practised is illustrated by the following examples. Malaria and dysentry were treated by purging with 20-grain doses of calomel until collapse was induced. In the year 1827, 32 million leeches were used in France, and since bloodletting was practised on a corresponding scale, opponents of the system dubbed it 'vampirism'. In a large proportion of cases the suppression of the symptoms by collapse was followed shortly by death, and it was in connection with such an event that the phrase was used '*il est mort guéri*'.

Homoeopathy

Hahnemann revolted against this unsatisfactory system at the commencement of the nineteenth century. It is his merit to have conceived the idea of an experimental science of pharmacology based upon observations of the actions of drugs upon normal individuals. Unfortunately, he combined this excellent idea with two erroneous principles — firstly, that like cures like; and secondly, that the actions of drugs are potentiated by dilution. Lauder Brunton states that Hahnemann's first principle was a sweeping generalisation based on the fact that a large dose of cinchona bark induced in him a malarial paroxysm; the reason for this occurrence being that he had previously suffered from malaria and the gastric irritation excited the paroxysm. His second principle was based on the fact that trituration of mercury increased its pharmacological action. This effect was due to the oxidation of the mercury, first to mercurous and, later, to mercuric oxide. Hahnemann's system of homoeopathy rapidly drifted into absurdities. From 1829 onwards he recommended the administration of all drugs at the thirtieth potency, which corresponds to a concentration of 1 part in 10^{60} parts. This works out at a content of 1 molecule of drug in a sphere with a circumference equal to the orbit of Neptune. Homoeopathy and allopathy were equally devoid of any scientific basis, and it must be admitted that the former did much less damage in practice. Homoeopathic methods at least gave a chance to the natural defence mechanisms possessed by the body, whereas the classical allopathic methods used during the period of heroic treatment were sufficient to produce death without the aid of the disease.

Modern therapeutics has inherited from allopathy the knowledge of certain useful drugs and from homoeopathy the knowledge of the remarkable powers the body possesses of healing itself, if given a chance, but as regards its basic principle it owes nothing to these or to any other of the numerous systems that once flourished and are now forgotten.

Experimental medicine

Claude Bernard in 1865 defined the attitude of modern medicine: 'La médecine expérimentale, par sa nature même de science expérimentale, n'a pas de système et ne repousse rien en fait de traitement ou de guérison de maladies: elle croit et admet tout, pourvu que cela soit fondé sur l'observation et prouvé par l'expérience'. This great principle laid down so clearly by Claude Bernard has never been understood by the general public and is sometimes in danger of being forgotten by the profession. Since modern therapeutics is an inductive science based on observation it has nothing in common with any of the past or present systems of medicine based on authority. The best known of such systems which survive today are homoeopathy, osteopathy, chiropraxis and Ayurvedic medicine. These bear much the same relation to medical science as astrology does to astronomy.

It is, however, a commonplace of science that an accurate observer working on a fallacious hypothesis may make valuable new discoveries. Although the astrologers were devout believers in a complex system of absurdities, yet they made observations of considerable practical value and interest. Therefore medical science should always be ready to investigate claims that can be confirmed or disproved by observation, irrespective of the question as to the possibility of the truth of the theory which led to their discovery. This argument works in two ways, and it is equally true that there is no necessity to accept an improbable theory merely because it has led to the discovery of facts of value.

The science of therapeutics is more encumbered than any other science with pseudo-scientific rivals. There are several reasons for this. In the first place, therapeutics was placed on a scientific basis only relatively recently, and popular beliefs are usually about one generation behind scientific knowledge. Secondly, it is more difficult to make adequate controlled observations in therapeutics than in any other science, and hence it is very difficult to provide rigid proof or disproof of any statement. Finally, serious disease always tends to arouse superstition. The sufferer wants immediate relief from suffering and fear, and if science cannot promise this he turns eagerly to anyone who promises to work a miracle on his behalf. The popularity of the numerous systems of faith healing is striking testimony of the strength of this impulse.

Therapeutic nihilism

Medical science began its rapid development in the middle of last century. The first twenty-five years were dominated by the rise of morbid pathology. The last quarter of the nineteenth century was dominated by the rise of the science of bacteriology, which made possible the sensational development of surgery and preventive medicine that occurred in that period. Physiology had developed steadily during this half-century, but had produced few results of practical importance, and the same was true of pharmacology. Consequently, therapeutics advanced relatively little and the philosophy of therapeutic nihilism which predominated in the early years of the twentieth century found particularly clear expression in the early editions of Osler's *Principles of Medicine*. This book dealt almost exclusively with the morbid anatomy and diagnosis of disease, and less than 10 per cent of the space was given to treatment. This attitude unfortunately led to the attention of physicians being focused on the post-mortem room rather than on the ward, and the term 'a complete case', which was commonly in use, indicated that the latter was regarded as the ante-room of the former. The rapid development of pharmacological knowledge and its application to the prevention and treatment of disease has now deprived therapeutic nihilism of any rational basis.

DEVELOPMENT OF PHARMACOLOGY

Rational therapeutics commenced during the second half of the nineteenth century, when the foundation of modern pharmacology was laid by the critical experimental analysis of the mode of action of drugs on the functions of the body. During this same period, the rise of the science of organic chemistry profoundly influenced the development of pharmacology.

The first synthetic organic drugs introduced into medicine were the anaesthetics; these were followed by the antiseptics; and in 1860 chloral hydrate was introduced. The synthesis of chemotherapeutic agents, of which salvarsan was the first, was one of the greatest services that organic chemistry has rendered to medicine, and it has continued to exert a profound influence in many other ways. Prior to the nineteenth century the only substances available for use as drugs were those that happened to occur in nature, but today the number of organic compounds known is almost unlimited, and systematic searches are proceeding continuously to discover new compounds which will meet special therapeutic needs. The production of chemotherapeutic substances for the control of protozoal and bacterial infections has made extremely rapid progress during the present century. Less spectacular but equally important has been the development of remedies to control or modify symptoms, by depressing or stimulating natural activities of the body. The variety of drugs acting on the central nervous system as well as the large selection of drugs acting on the autonomic, respiratory and cardio-vascular system now available are in marked contrast to the meagre and often inefficient drugs of 50 years ago.

The services rendered by biochemistry are equal in importance to those rendered by synthetic organic chemistry, for to it we owe our knowledge of endocrine secretions and of vitamins. Endocrinology has gradually revealed a system by means of which all the functions of the body are regulated by drugs synthesised therein. Successful endocrine therapy commenced in 1891, when Murray treated cases of myxoedema and cretinism by administration of thyroid gland. In the next thirty years many other endocrine secretions were identified, but none of these was of a therapeutic importance comparable with thyroid. The discovery of insulin by Banting and Best in 1921, and its use in the treatment of diabetes mellitus was, however, an advance at least equal in importance to the discovery of thyroid therapy. The isolation of cortisone in 1935 by Kendall and his colleagues and its introduction into clinical practice has revolutionised the treatment of previously intractable collagen diseases.

The discovery of vitamins was an advance of equal practical importance for it revealed a means of preventing and curing some of the commonest diseases that afflict mankind. A new field of preventive medicine was opened up, and pellagra, beriberi and rickets have joined scurvy in the class of easily preventable diseases.

The introduction of the sulphonamides in 1935 marked the beginning of effective antibacterial chemotherapy and was rapidly followed by the isolation and identification of penicillin. These developments have been of the utmost importance and have led to the extensive range of powerful antibiotics with antibacterial actions now available for the treatment of many infections. The scourge of tuberculosis has virtually been eradicated in many communities by the use of streptomycin and other antituberculosis drugs such as isoniazid.

The critical analysis of the mode of action of drugs has made it possible to study more exactly the nature of disease processes. Some of the most widespread ailments affecting mankind can be relieved by drugs, for example, hypertension can now be effectively controlled by the use of drugs.

PHARMACOPOEIAS

The collection of medicinal formulae has been a favourite occupation of medical writers since the time of Galen. The first national book of drugs with directions for their preparation, however, was published as the London Pharmacopoeia in 1618. It was compiled by the College of Physicians, now the Royal College of Physicians, exactly a hundred years after the College was incorporated by Charter in the reign of Henry VIII. A corresponding type of book, the first French Codex, was published in 1639; and in Scotland and Ireland respectively, the first editions of the Edinburgh Pharmacopoeia appeared in 1699 and of the Dublin Pharmacopoeia in 1807.

The pharmacopoeias of the seventeenth and eighteenth centuries were veritable museums containing relics of all the superstitions that had flourished and died in Europe. The flesh and excrements of animals constituted nearly half their contents. This rubbish was slowly eliminated during the eighteenth and nineteenth centuries, and in the latter period the alkaloids were discovered and synthetic drugs were introduced.

In most countries a pharmacopoeia consists of a list of

drugs for each of which a complete group of standards and assays is set; this is intended to provide a guarantee of the activity and purity of these drugs. The selection of drugs might reasonably be expected to be based on evidence of the pharmacological activity and clinical usefulness of a drug but recognition is also made of drugs, which, though they have no well-defined pharmacological activity, are frequently used in medical practice. Thus in company with very potent drugs such as cyanocobalamin, frusemide, morphine, penicillin and prednisolone, other substances such as quillaia, tragacanth and tolu balsam are described. The justification for the inclusion of the latter substances is that since they are frequently incorporated in medicinal preparations as emulsifying, flavouring or colouring agents, it is better to ensure their purity and consistency by describing appropriate standards for them in the pharmacopoeia.

The British Pharmacopoeia. The Medical Act of 1858, which authorised the publication of the British Pharmacopoeia (B.P.) assigned the task of carrying out this work to the General Medical Council and the first edition was published in 1864. Successive editions of the B.P. were issued at various intervals throughout the intervening years and after publication of the eleventh edition in 1968, responsibility for this work was transferred to the Medicines Commission, established in accordance with the Medicines Act of 1968.

In compiling the list of drugs in the B.P., the British Pharmacopoeia Commission, appointed by authority of the Medicines Act, consult medical and pharmaceutical authorities throughout the Commonwealth; there is also considerable liaison with corresponding committees of the European Pharmacopoeia (E.P.), the United States Pharmacopoeia (U.S.P.) and the World Health Organisation.

The European Pharmacopoeia (E.P.), published under a convention signed by the governments of Belgium, France, West Germany, Italy, Luxembourg, Netherlands, Switzerland and the United Kingdom, is intended to provide the standards in its monographs for any article used in medical practice in these respective countries. Volume I of the European Pharmacopoeia was published in 1969 and by a resolution of a Committee of the Council of Europe, the monographs described in it were agreed to be adopted by these countries in 1972. For articles described in the B.P. which are also in the E.P., the standards will be those of the latter.

The British Pharmaceutical Codex (B.P.C.), the Extra Pharmacopoeia (Martindale) and the United States Dispensatory (U.S.D.) contain in addition to the drugs listed in the pharmacopoeias of the respective countries, a description of the action and uses of other drugs.

The British National Formulary (B.N.F.) is compiled by a committee representative of the medical and pharmaceutical professions and contains a description of the properties, actions and uses of most of the preparations of drugs which are currently used in medical practice. It provides useful information on the relative therapeutic value of different remedies and is more frequently consulted by medical practitioners than is the British Pharmacopoeia which is chiefly concerned with descriptions of the standards for the purity and activity of drugs. The Prescribers' Journal provides brief authoritative statements on the current use of drugs in the treatment of disease. It is published every two months and is distributed without charge to medical practitioners in the National Health Service and to all clinical medical students in the United Kingdom.

AMA Drug Evaluations is a compilation produced jointly by the American Medical Association and the American Society for Clinical Pharmacology and Therapeutics. It is organised into sections based on therapeutic classifications.

VOLUNTARY SCHEMES FOR THE CONTROL OF DRUGS

Prior to 1962, all that was demanded of a compound was proof of its safety and these demands were not very stringent, for they relied mainly upon the results of animal tests. Proof of its efficacy rested almost entirely on the subsequent experience of its widespread use in therapeutic practice. A dramatic change occurred in 1961, when convincing evidence was disclosed of the teratogenicity of thalidomide, an apparently harmless sedative and hypnotic drug. The impact on most civilised communities of these tragic events led to a drastic revision of the conditions required for marketing new drugs. Some of the provisions introduced in Great Britain for the control of drugs are described below.

The Safety of Drugs Committee was established in 1963 as a more or less independent body, under the Chairmanship of Sir Derrick Dunlop. Within the framework of a voluntary scheme, pharmaceutical manufacturers agreed to submit details of tests on new drugs and formulations for the consideration, advice and approval of the Committee before the products were given clinical trials or marketed as human medicines. The primary purpose of this arrangement was the assessment of relative safety, and not necessarily of efficacy; clearance of a product for marketing did not imply a recommendation of it by the Committee as a therapeutic remedy, but only its reasonable safety for its intended purpose. A register of adverse reactions has enabled the Committee to ensure that an early warning was issued to doctors when a medicine was found to give rise to undue or unexpected toxic effects. For example, there was an increase in the number of sudden and unexplained deaths in asthmatic patients between 1961 and 1967 and in the latter years the Safety of Drugs Committee issued a warning to all doctors about the potential dangers of overdosage of bronchodilator drugs administered by pressurised aerosols. Since then, the number of deaths had fallen by 1970 to about the level of 1961. The rise and subsequent fall in deaths from asthma was accompanied by an increase and subsequent decrease in the sales of these pressurised aerosols.

Two other voluntary schemes for controlling the use of pesticides and of veterinary products had previously been arranged between manufacturers of these substances and Government Departments under the aegis of the The Advisory Committee on Pesticides and Other Toxic Chemicals, an independent body of experts. The Pesticides Safety Precautions Scheme was introduced in 1957 to safeguard the human population, livestock, domestic animals and wild life against risks from the use of pesticides. A few years later a similar scheme was introduced for the control of veterinary products.

MANDATORY SCHEME FOR THE CONTROL OF DRUGS

The Medicines Act 1968

Despite the satisfactory nature of the voluntary scheme, there were a number of severe limitations on its effectiveness in securing adequate supervision of the conditions for the manufacture, storage and distribution of medicines. Satisfactory methods were lacking to ensure quality control of preparations according to B.P. specifications; this was particularly evident in respect of medicines imported from abroad. It was considered that the introduction of a licensing scheme for all medicines for human and veterinary purposes and also medicated animal feeding stuffs would ensure proper control of manufacture, safety and quality; moreover it would involve more adequate standards for the advertisement and promotion of these substances. Substances used for medicinal purposes are defined in the Medicines Act as those used for

1. Treating or preventing disease.
2. Diagnosing disease.
3. Contraception.
4. Inducing anaesthesia.

The Medicines Act included provisions for the establishment of a Licensing Authority for which the Health and Agriculture Ministers are responsible, to issue licences governing the manufacture, importation and marketing of new medicines for human and veterinary use. For medicinal products already on the market, Licences of Right are issued for a temporary period until their safety and quality can be reviewed. Expert committees such as the Committee on Safety of Medicines and the Veterinary Products Committee are appointed to give advice directly to the Licensing Authority on matters relating to the safety and quality of medicinal products.

The Medicines Commission, which is quite distinct from the Licensing Authority, consists of members of the medical, veterinary and pharmaceutical professions and related disciplines. It is responsible for advising the Minister on many important matters relating to the execution of the Medicines Act, for example it gives advice on the number, functions and constitution of Committees, such as the Committee on Safety of Medicines, the Veterinary Products Committee and the British Pharmacopoeia Commission. Another duty of the Medicines Commission is to direct the preparation and publication of any information it considers necessary about substances or articles used in human and veterinary medicine. The Commission has also an important appellate function: it will act as an appeal tribunal should an appeal be made by an applicant who has been refused a licence or has been prohibited from engaging in the sale, supply or importation of medicinal products or medicated animal feeding stuffs.

COMMERCIAL INFLUENCES IN THERAPEUTICS

The introduction of active biological products and potent synthetic drugs has had many consequences. It has involved the development of complex technical methods for the formulation of medicines to ensure their stability and efficiency when administered for appropriate therapeutic purposes. Even more important is the fact that the scientific expertise and equipment necessary to foster the discovery and development of new drugs involves the outlay of considerable financial resources. It is not surprising, therefore, that much of this work is undertaken in the research laboratories of the pharmaceutical industry, which is now the main source of supply of the most valuable drugs used in medical practice.

Proprietary names. Since the development of a new medicinal compound and the elaboration of methods for producing it on a commercial scale are expensive processes, the manufacturer endeavours to recoup this initial expense partly by the protection given by patents covering the methods of manufacture and also by introducing the new drug under a proprietary name which is registered as a trade mark. If the new substance is a therapeutic success, alternative methods of manufacture or of formulation are usually developed and very soon the new compound is promoted under several different proprietary names. The use of proprietary or brand names for medicines is a legitimate method of commerce and has the advantage that the names are short, and easy to remember. Since there are over 3000 of these products on the market, however, this has led to much confusion amongst prescribers.

Approved names. When a new drug has been shown to have some likely application in medicine, it is given an approved name. Approved or non-proprietary names are devised or selected by the British Pharmacopoeia Commission and lists of these names are published at intervals by the Medicines Commission. The approved name is usually based on a contraction of the full chemical nomenclature; it is often unwieldy to write and difficult to remember. Since there is no monopoly associated with its sale under this name, the drug continues to be promoted under its various proprietary names. Consequently it is difficult to establish the popular use of an approved name. Although many medicinal compounds are less expensive when prescribed by their approved instead of by proprietary name, this is not always so because the manufacture and supply of a new compound may be entirely controlled by one firm.

Drug advertisements provide an important method of promoting the prescribing and sale of medicinal products. Sometimes in these advertisements the claims made for some products outrun the bounds of legitimate commercial optimism for they bear no relation to the established facts or probabilities. There are considerable difficulties in defining the limits of ethical advertisements of drugs and opinions on this matter differ in different countries. In the United Kingdom considerable progress has been effected by the control of such advertisements under the Medicines Act. The sending or delivery of an advertisement for a medicinal product to a doctor, dentist or veterinarian is prohibited, unless a *data sheet* accompanies it or has recently been sent or delivered. The data sheet is required to set out the essential information about the product, in respect to its name together with the approved name (if any), a description of the form, composition and quantitative list of active ingredients, the therapeutic indications, dosage and methods of administration, contra-indications and precautions, main side-effects and adverse reactions. Additional information may also be required in respect to storage precautions, legal or other restrictions on its availability and the name and address of the holder of the product licence.

Various legislative measures in different countries for controlling the manufacture and distribution of medicinal products have been designed to ensure their safety, quality and efficacy. The extent to which this control is successful will depend on the responsibility exercised by those who prescribe and use these products in the management of human and animal diseases. A thorough knowledge and understanding of pharmacology is one of the most reliable methods of achieving this aim.

FURTHER READING

British Pharmacopoeia 1975. Add. 1977. Add. 1978. H.M.S.O., London
European Pharmacopoeia. Vol. I 1969. Vol. II 1971. Vol. III 1975. Suppl 1977
British Pharmaceutical Codex (1979)
Martindale 1977 The extra pharmacopoeia. The Pharmaceutical Press, London
British National Formulary (1976–78)
Prescribers Journal 1979 Blackburn, Leeds
United States Pharmacopoeia 1975
AMA Drug Evaluations 1977
Osol A, Pratt R 1973 United States Dispensatory. Lippincott, Philadelphia
Dunlop D 1970 Legislation on medicines. Br. med. J: 3: 760.

2. Drug-receptor interactions

Mode of action of drugs 9; Chemical constitution and drug action 9; Drug receptors 10; Competitive drug antagonism 11; Classification of drug receptors 13; Other types of drug antagonism 15; Specific and non-specific drug action 16; Isolation of drug receptors 17; Membrane noise 17.

MODE OF ACTION OF DRUGS

The brief notes on the history of pharmacology given in the last chapter show that its development has been empirical, and that the numerous theoretical systems of therapeutics which have been evolved in the past have hindered rather than advanced science. Nevertheless, the vast mass of experimental data accumulated during the last half-century suffices to permit of certain cautious generalisations regarding the mode of action of drugs. This subject is difficult and in many ways still obscure, but since it seems logical to deal with general principles before discussing detailed evidence, certain problems will be dealt with briefly in this chapter.

Empirical knowledge of the mode of action of drugs and poisons is of great antiquity and, indeed, the most primitive savages frequently showed a surprising skill in the use of poisons. On the other hand, our knowledge of the manner in which opium produces its sedative action although it can now be expressed in terms of drug receptor interactions is not fundamentally advanced beyond the stage represented by the classical response of the candidate:

'Quid est in eo
Virtus dormitiva.'

Many drugs produce actions in doses so small and in such low concentrations that the dimensions almost resemble those used in astronomy. For example some substances produce obvious effects on isolated tissues at dilutions of 1 part in 1000 million. There are, however, 6×10^{23} molecules in a gram molecule of a chemical compound; one drop of a solution of adrenaline at a dilution of 10 000 million contains about 10 000 million molecules. Pharmacological actions therefore do not involve the assumption of vital forces other than those already known in physics and chemistry.

As a general rule the action of drugs on patients can be interpreted on the assumption that administration of the drug results in a certain concentration being attained in the blood and tissue fluids, and that a chemical reaction occurs between the drug and the cells. The simplest assumption regarding the nature of this reaction is that the drug combines with specific receptors in the cells. Modern biochemistry is revealing the cell as a complex system of enzymes whose activities are organised and correlated in a precise manner. In such a system it is easy to conceive of the cell organisation being deranged by the activation or inactivation of a comparatively small number of enzymes or of other forms of active groups. Drugs, therefore, must be regarded, not as mysterious charms, but as chemical agents which produce their effect provided that an adequate concentration is attained at their site of action.

At the same time it must be recognised that we can only provide a partial explanation for a few of the simpler effects produced by drugs. Our present knowledge does not provide a satisfactory explanation for the highly selective action which is the special characteristic of the most important drugs, e.g. the depressant action of morphine on the cough centre or the excitant action of apomorphine on the vomiting centre. The severe limitations of our present knowledge are only too obvious, but it is important to recognise that the fundamental problems of drug action are beginning to reveal themselves as examples of selective chemical action upon a very complex biological system.

CHEMICAL CONSTITUTION AND DRUG ACTION

Nearly half a million organic compounds are already known and the number of new compounds which can be synthesised by the organic chemist is practically unlimited. Hence, if it were possible to establish laws relating chemical constitution and drug action it would be possible to make drugs which would produce almost any action that was desired.

Enormous numbers of drugs have been made and tested for all kinds of purposes, and a limited number of relations between constitution and action have been discovered. One of the most striking of these is the curariform action possessed by nearly all quaternary ammonium salts which was discovered by Crum-Brown and Fraser in 1896, but since that date few other discoveries have been made in this field, comparable with this remarkable piece of pioneer work.

The limitations of present knowledge in this subject are indicated by the fact that drugs have sometimes been developed for one purpose and have been found to produce valuable actions of a kind totally different from that originally intended. For example, the synthetic analgesic drug pethidine was originally synthesised in an attempt to find new anti-spasmodic drugs with atropine-like properties. The search for new remedies at present is therefore forced to proceed along the laborious lines of trial and error, and thousands of compounds are often tested before one is found which is worth clinical trial.

Structural specificity
Pharmacologically active molecules can be broadly classified into those which are structurally specific, e.g. atropine, and those which are structurally unspecific, e.g. ether. The former are believed to exert their effects as the result of interaction with specific receptors with which they form complexes which are generally reversible. The dissociation constants of the complexes will be influenced by the closeness of fit of the molecules and their receptors and will thus depend on the stereochemical structure of drugs.

The importance of stereochemical features in drug action is shown by the differential pharmacological effects of optical isomers or enantiomorphs. Optical isomers differ from one another as an object differs from its mirror image; they rotate the plane of polarised light by equal and opposite amounts but otherwise have identical physical properties. Their chemical properties are identical except when reactions with other asymmetric molecules are involved. The fact that enantiomorphs often have vastly different pharmacological activities — the bronchodilator activity of the laevo-form of adrenaline is 45 times as great as the dextro-form and in the case of isoprenaline it is 800 times as great — is strong evidence that the receptor surface itself has a specific stereochemical structure. A three-point alignment between drug and receptor may be required for pharmacological activity. It would then be expected that if this can be achieved with one of the isomers it will not be achieved with the other since they are geometrically not superimposable.

PHYSICO-CHEMICAL ACTIVITY RELATIONSHIPS. HANSCH ANALYSIS

Apart from highly specific interactions with drug receptors, it has long been appreciated that the physico-chemical properties of drugs are related to their biological activities. Hansch has emphasised that certain parameters of molecules such as their size, degree of ionisation and partition coefficient between lipid and water phase may be derived from their chemical structure by the application of semi-empirical rules. By adding together contributions from each part of the molecule the physicochemical properties of compounds can thus be tentatively predicted. Next, correlations are made by the method of regression analysis in which equations are established relating the biological activities of each drug to its physicochemical properties. Finally these results may be used to design more effective drugs.

This type of approach relies largely on computers because of the complex statistical calculations involved. Although this approach has not, so far, yielded spectacular results in the discovery of new drugs, it can be readily mechanised and will undoubtedly be increasingly employed and improved.

DRUG RECEPTORS

Drug receptor is a convenient term to describe those constituents of a cell with which drugs react when they produce their effects. Receptors are thought to be of molecular size and probably form part of the lipo-protein structure of the cell, particularly the cell membrane. Receptor theory is at present in a rapidly progressing phase and is likely in future to provide a more rational approach to the study of drug action.

The concept of receptors was introduced by Paul Ehrlich who considered that 'substances can only be anchored at any particular part of the organism if they fit into the molecule of the recipient complex like a piece of mosaic finds its place in a pattern'. A more modern writer some 60 years later, defined receptors in terms of interacting forces as follows: 'The drug receptor is in general a pattern R of forces of diverse origin forming a part of some biological system, and having roughly the same dimensions as a certain pattern M of forces presented by the drug molecule, such that between patterns M and R a relationship of complementarity for interaction exists' (Schueler, 1960). A variety of forces may act between drug and receptor including ionic and dipole interactions, hydrogen bonds, hydrophobic interactions, van der Waals forces and in rare cases covalent bonds. Of special importance are the charge distributions and steric configurations of both drug and receptor. Stereoisomers may have widely differing activities and steric hindrance by a methyl group in a strategic position may prevent the close apposition of drug and receptor.

The characteristic property of receptors like that of enzymes is their specificity; acetylcholine, adrenaline, histamine and morphine each is believed to act on a different receptor. Our ideas of drug receptors are patterned on those of active centres of enzymes. The active centre of an enzyme is the region where reactants are bound, interact and are chemically altered; the receptor is the region where drugs are bound, interact and induce a pharmacological effect. The analogy can be extended to antagonists: competitive enzyme inhibitors compete with substrate for attachment to the active centre, whilst competitive drug antagonists compete with agonists for attachment to the receptor.

It is generally assumed that the initial process in drug action is the formation of a reversible complex between receptor R and drug D and that this leads to a pharmacological response probably through several intermediate stages. If the law of mass action applies to the combination between the drug and the receptor

$$R + D \rightleftharpoons RD \quad (1)$$

then the proportion, y, of the receptors affected by the drug should be given by the expression

$$y = \frac{K_1 A}{K_1 A + 1} \quad (2)$$

where A is the concentration of drug and K_1 is the affinity constant (i.e. the reciprocal of the dissociation constant) of the drug-receptor complex.

COMPETITIVE DRUG ANTAGONISM

The above treatment refers to the situation in which one drug interacts with a receptor. This can be extended to the situation where an agonist and an antagonist are competing for the same receptor, and the following equations (first derived by Gaddum) are obtained

$$y = \frac{K_1 A}{K_1 A + 1} = \frac{K_1 A x}{K_1 A x + K_2 B + 1} \quad (3a)$$

$$K_2 = \frac{x - 1}{B} \quad (3b)$$

where y is the proportion of receptors occupied by agonist, A and B are the concentrations of agonist and antagonist in solution; K_1 and K_2 are affinity constants of agonist-receptor and antagonist-receptor complex respectively and x is the dose ratio. The *dose ratio* is the factor by which the concentration of agonist must be multiplied to maintain a given response in the presence of antagonist.

Equation (2) is formally identical with Langmuir's adsorption isotherm, and its application to the action of drugs was first explored by A. J. Clark. An immediate difficulty was that it is difficult to measure y directly, and so establish the relationship between receptor occupancy and final response. At first Clark considered the fraction of receptors occupied to be directly proportional to the pharmacological response and a 100% response to mean 100% receptor occupation, but this assumption has now been abandoned by most workers. On the other hand a more restricted assumption is widely accepted and is indeed implicitly assumed in equation (3a), namely that equal effects produced in the absence and presence of a competitive antagonist involve equal numbers of activated receptors.

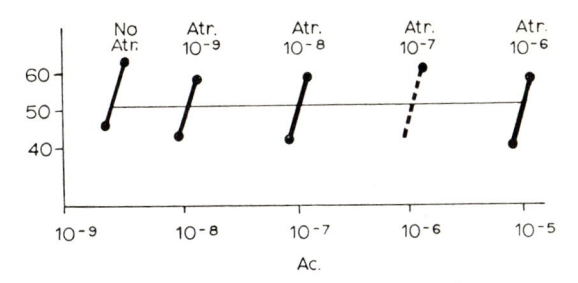

Fig. 2.1(a) Parallel log dose-response curves (denoting competitive antagonism) over 1000-fold range. Acetylcholine and atropine on guinea pig ileum. Ordinate: contraction (%). (After Arunlakshana and Schild, 1959, *Brit. J. Pharmacol.*)

An example of the measurements and calculations required to establish a case of simple competitive antagonism is shown in Figure 2.1(a) and 2.1(b). By simple competitive antagonism is meant the case where one molecule of antagonist reacts with one receptor molecule, as is implied in equation (3a).

Figure 2.1(a) is a plot of the responses of isolated guinea pig ileum to acetylcholine in the absence and presence of atropine on a logarithmic dose axis. The log dose-response curves are parallel which is *prima facie* evidence for competitive antagonism. In order to establish whether this is a simple competitive antagonism a regression line is drawn as shown in Figure 2.1(b). This is based on a logarithmic transformation of equation (3b) by plotting log $(x - 1)$ as ordinate and $-\log$ molar concentration of B, atropine in this case, as abscissa. The regression line is linear with slope approximately 1 (actually 1.04) as expected for simple competitive antagonism. The affinity constant of atropine may now be determined graphically from the point of intersection of the regression line with the abscissa, corresponding to $\log K_2 = pA_2$.

pA_2 is an expression frequently used as a measure of drug antagonism. It is defined as 'the negative logarithm of the molar concentration of antagonist which reduces the effect of a double dose of agonist to that of a single dose'. Figure 2.2 shows examples of representative pA_2 measurements. Although pA_2 is an empirical measure it has theoretical significance in the special case where the antagonism is of a simple competitive type when $pA_2 = \log K_2$.

Some general principles

Quantitative aspects are of prime importance in discussing drug antagonism. For example, atropine in high concentration is a competitive antagonist not only of acetylcholine but also of histamine. It does not follow, however, that acetylcholine and histamine act on the same receptor because both are antagonised by atropine. It is more reasonable to assume that atropine has affinity for both receptors; high affinity for acetylcholine receptors and an independent, 1000 times lower affinity for

ACETYLCHOLINE—ATROPINE

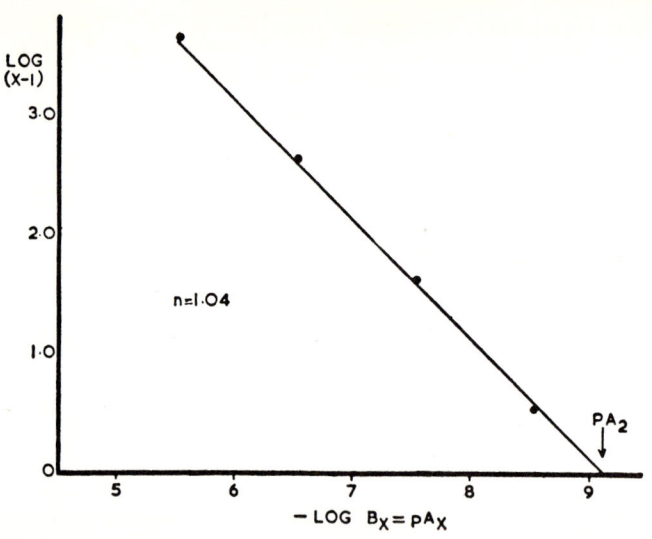

Fig. 2.1(b) Using data from Fig. 2.1(a): $x = $ (conc. Ach in presence of atropine)/(conc. Ach in absence of atropine). Slope of regression line (≈ 1) denotes simple competitive antagonism. $B_x = $ conc. of atropine.

histamine receptors. Antagonists are seldom, if ever, completely receptor-specific. The degree of specificity of antagonists can be conveniently assessed by comparing their pA_2 values. Figure 2.2 shows that, contrary to atropine, mepyramine is a strong histamine antagonist with low anti-acetylcholine activity.

A general principle of receptor theory is that drugs acting on the same receptor can be expected to be antagonised by the same antagonist. If the antagonist is competitive the drugs can be expected to be antagonised by the same concentration of antagonist and produce with it the same dose ratios and also the same pA_2 values. This is illustrated in Figure 2.3 which shows that histamine and pyridylethylamine both stimulate guinea pig ileum but

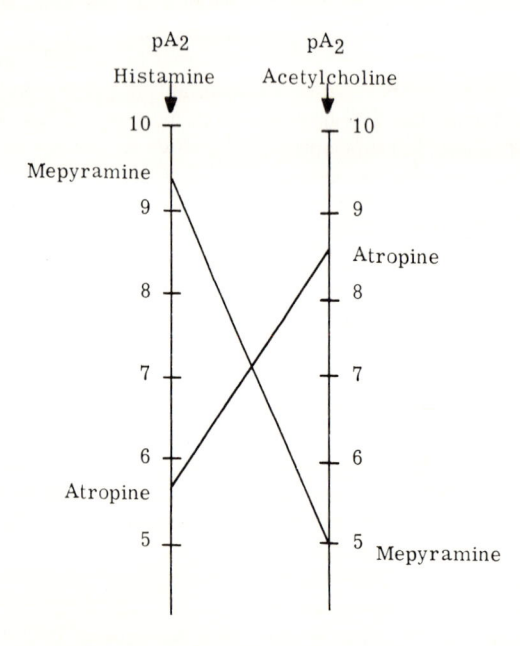

Fig. 2.2 The activities of mepyramine and atropine against histamine and acetylcholine as measured on the guinea-pig ileum. pA_2 is the negative logarithm of the molar concentration of antagonist which reduces the effect of a dose of histamine or of acetylcholine to that of half the dose. Points on the two scales referring to the same antagonist are joined. (After Schild, 1947. *Br. J. Pharmac.*)

differ in activity about 30-fold. The two drugs nevertheless presumably act on the same receptor since their log-dose response curves are equally displaced by a particular concentration of the antihistamine diphenhydramine. This type of evidence for a common receptor is suggestive rather than conclusive; but if the outcome had been the opposite, namely a differential antagonism by diphenhydramine of the two agonists, then the hypothesis of a common receptor would be refuted.

Criteria for competitive antagonism can be summarised as follows:

1. Parallelism of log dose-response curves in the absence and presence of antagonist. This is a necessary but not sufficient condition. To support the notion of *simple* competitive antagonism (1:1 relationship between receptor and antagonist) a more detailed analysis with several concentrations of antagonist is needed.
2. Linear regression with slope 1 when log (x − 1) is plotted against log B. The locus of intersection with the abscissa (y = 0) represents the pA_2 of the competitive antagonist.

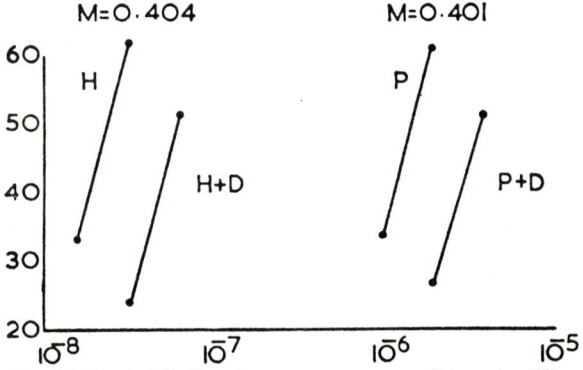

Fig. 2.3 Equal shift of log dose-response curves of histamine (H) and pyridylethylamine (P) by an antihistamine (D) (3×10^{-9} diphenhydramine), suggesting that the two agonists act on the same receptor. Guinea pig ileum. Ordinate: contraction (%). M = log dose-ratio. (After Arunlakshana and Schild, 1959, *Brit. J. Pharmacol.*)

CLASSIFICATION OF DRUG RECEPTORS

Establishing the affinity (or dissociation) constants of competitive antagonists has provided a simple, but surprisingly powerful, tool for the classification of receptors. Two principles are involved which are consequences of receptor theory: (1) when different agonists acting on the same receptor are tested with the same competitive antagonist the affinity constant of the latter should be the same; (2) identical receptors in different preparations should produce the same affinity constants with the same competitive antagonists.

Data for drug classification have frequently been obtained by simple pA_2 measurements but this may lead to erroneous conclusions unless the antagonism is of a simple competitive type in which case $pA_2 = \log K_2$. It is preferable to measure $\log K_2$ values from series of parallel log concentration-effect curves applying the calculations outlined in relation to Figure 2.1(b). No valid data suitable for receptor classification can be derived unless this type of plot is linear with slope = 1.

Examples of receptor definition by competitive antagonists

Muscarinic acetylcholine receptors can be quantitatively defined in terms of their affinities for atropine. Table 2.1 shows that muscarinic receptors in tissues as different as chick amnion, frog heart and mammalian intestine have closely similar affinities for atropine. This provides evidence that they are all similar in nature and it implicitly supports the notion that these receptors are definite chemical entities. The table shows that acetylcholine receptors of frog rectus have much less affinity for atropine than the rest. This agrees with Dale's views that acetylcholine has two types of actions, muscarinic and nicotinic (p. 58). The frog rectus, being a striated muscle, has nicotinic receptors which can be activated by acetylcholine but have only small affinity for atropine.

Table 2.1 Affinity of receptors in different tissues for atropine (After Schild, 1968). The first four are muscarinic receptors, the last nicotinic receptors.

	$\log K_2 (pA_2)$ Acetylcholine-atropine
Guinea pig ileum	9.0
Guinea pig lung (perfused)	8.8
Chick amnion	8.8
Frog auricle	8.8
Frog rectus	5.2

Histamine receptors provide another example of definition of receptors by antagonists. One type of histamine receptor referred to as H_1 receptor, can be identified by its affinity for typical antihistamines such as mepyramine. Table 2.2 shows different pharmacological preparations possessing this receptor. It has now become apparent that a second histamine receptor (H_2 receptor) can be identified by means of a new group of antagonists. The H_2 antagonists do not antagonise effectively the H_1 effects of histamine on intestinal and tracheal smooth muscle, but they antagonise certain other effects of histamine including stimulation of acid gastric secretion.

Table 2.2 Affinity of H_1 receptors in different tissue preparations for mepyramine.

	$\log K_2 (pA_2)$ Histamine-mepyramine
Guinea pig ileum	9.3
Guinea pig trachea	9.1
Guinea pig lung (perfused)	9.4
Human bronchi	9.3

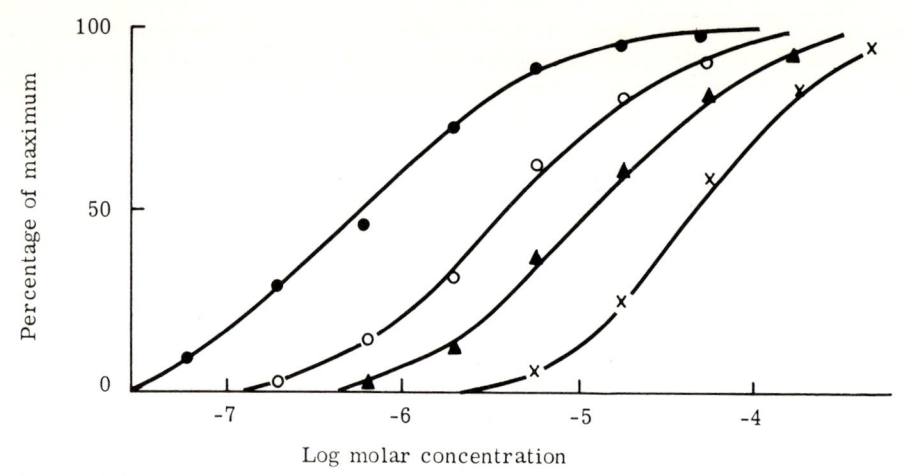

Fig. 2.4 Histamine cumulative log-dose response curves from guinea-pig atrium: without antagonist (●) and after equilibration with burimamide 2×10^{-5} M (O), 4×10^{-5} M (▲) and 2.7×10^{-4} M (x). (After Black et al., 1972, *Nature*.)

The histamine H_2 receptor was identified by Black et al who used three test preparations which responded to histamine but were apparently not endowed with H_1 receptors since their histamine effects were not antagonised by mepyramine. Their test systems were (1) stimulation of acid secretion in rat stomach, (2) heart rate stimulation in isolated guinea pig atrium and (3) inhibition of longitudinal muscle of rat uterus. Their aim was to discover substances which antagonised histamine in the three test preparations showing similar receptor affinities in each (principle 2 above). It was found that a structural analogue of histamine, lacking intrinsic histamine-like activity, burimamide (Fig. 13.7) behaved as a competitive antagonist of histamine in each preparation. It produced a parallel shift of log dose-response curves (Fig. 2.4) and a slope of approximately unity on plotting $\log(x-1)$ v. log B. A common pA_2 of 5.1 suggested that a second histamine receptor had been identified.

Attempts have been made to define the alpha and beta receptors for catecholamines (p. 78) by means of antagonists. Alpha receptors can be defined by their affinities for typical competitive alpha blockers such as phentolamine. By contrast it has proved difficult to define the beta receptors quantitatively in terms of a common affinity constant applicable to the various beta effects of catecholamines. There is evidence based on experiments with both agonists and competitive antagonists of more than one type of ß adrenoceptor. Typical evidence from competitive antagonists is illustrated in Figure 2.5 which shows that practolol, has differential affinity, higher for ß-receptors in heart than in smooth muscle, whilst the more powerful ß-blocker propranolol shows similar affinity for receptors in both tissues. Both drugs are shown to be competitive antagonists of isoprenaline with 'slope' 1 (Fig. 2.5). These findings indicate that in contrast to propranolol, practolol is a cardioselective ß-blocker

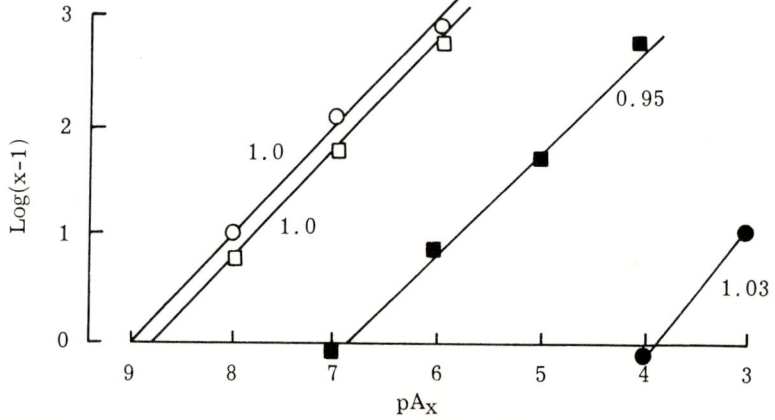

Fig. 2.5 A–S plots for propranolol (open symbols) and practolol (closed symbols), with isoprenaline as agonist. Tests were carried out on the relaxant effect on the rabbit aorta (O,●) and on the increased rate of beating of rabbit atria (□,■). (From Bristow, Sherrod & Green, redrawn in Rang, 1973. *Drug Receptors*, MacMillan.) (Numbers indicate 'slope'.)

reacting with a subgroup of ß receptors called ß₁. Evidence from agonists for ß subtypes includes the finding that the ß-agonist salbutamol (p. 179) acts selectively on ß-receptors in tracheal smooth muscle, called ß₂-receptors, whilst having relatively little activity on the heart (Fig. 12.6). The subject of subtypes of ß-receptors has considerable clinical implications as discussed in later chapters.

FURTHER DEVELOPMENTS OF RECEPTOR THEORY

Receptor theory was initially concerned with defining the relationship between drug concentration and receptor occupation expressed by equation (2).

An important development has been the distinction between the affinity of a drug and its intrinsic activity (Ariens) or efficacy (Stephenson), the affinity being a measure of the tendency of the drug to combine with its receptor and the efficacy a measure of the tendency of the drug-receptor complex to elicit a pharmacological response. According to one theory the response (R) is a function f of the product of the fraction of receptors occupied (y) and the efficacy (e) as expressed by the equation

$$R = f(ey) = f\left(e\frac{K_1 A}{K_1 A + 1}\right) \qquad (4)$$

Thus the response is considered to be dependent on the affinity and the efficacy of the drug. A drug with high efficacy will have a steeper log dose-response curve and frequently a higher maximum than a drug with low efficacy. The physical meaning of efficacy (e) is undefined. One interpretation of e is in terms of ion channels. The interaction of agonist and receptor may result in a conformational change which leads to the opening of ion channels and drugs may differ in their ability to open ion channels. Drugs with high efficacy may open a greater abundance of ion channels than those with low efficacy.

A simple two state allosteric receptor model is based on the assumption that ion channels exist in only two conformations, open or closed. A somewhat analogous model can be applied to the interaction at receptor level of agonists and antagonists, the former increasing the proportion of open channels, the latter that of closed channels; the two states are assumed to be in equilibrium.

The concept of efficacy has been fruitful and has clarified thinking in relation to new drugs. In terms of this concept, antagonists are drugs which have affinity but lack efficacy; a competitive antagonist combines with the same receptors as the agonist but for unknown reasons it is incapable of activating the receptor. Partial agonists are drugs which have less efficacy than full agonists; they produce flatter log dose-response curves than full agonists whilst capable of antagonising them by occupying the same receptors. Nalorphine (p. 285) could be considered a partial morphine-like agonist capable of producing weak morphine-like effects whilst at the same time antagonising morphine.

The rate theory (Paton) postulates that the activation of receptors is proportional not to the number of occupied receptors but to the frequency of collision between drug and receptor. It follows that if a drug occupies the receptor for a relatively long time, the opportunity for collisions between free drug and unoccupied receptors becomes limited, so that the drug has little stimulant action. According to this theory the rate of dissociation from the receptor determines whether a drug is an agonist or an antagonist. Drugs which dissociate rapidly from receptors are considered to be agonists and drugs which dissociate slowly antagonists.

Although the various receptor theories, classical 'occupation' theory, 'rate' theory and 'allosteric' theory postulate different drug-receptor mechanisms, it has been found that their quantitative consequences in the analysis of interaction between agonists and competitive antagonists at equilibrium are remarkably similar. Thus the quantitative predictions of occupation and rate theory at equilibrium are identical, and, as shown by Colquhoun, the results predicted by allosteric models are very similar to the classical predictions.

OTHER TYPES OF DRUG ANTAGONISM

Competitive antagonism is by no means the only or even the most frequently occurring type of drug antagonism, but it is the only type of drug antagonism that has been explored quantitatively with some success.

In view of the similarities between drug-receptor interactions and substrate-enzyme interactions it is tempting to transfer to drug antagonism, concepts which have been found useful in enzyme kinetics; for example by analysing drug response curves by means of double reciprocal (Lineweaver-Burk) plots. It is doubtful whether this manner of treatment is legitimate since it presupposes that the pharmacological response is linearly related to receptor occupation which is not generally warranted. It also seems unwarranted to deduce from Lineweaver-Burk plots that a case of drug antagonism is *noncompetitive* or *uncompetitive* in the sense used in enzyme kinetics. In view of these analytical difficulties pharmacologists have tended to adopt descriptive criteria, not necessarily based on mechanism, for most types of drug antagonism other than simple competitive antagonism.

Unsurmountable antagonism

This is a term introduced by Gaddum to describe antagonists which produce log dose-response curves which become increasingly flatter with increasing antagonist concentration and in the end cannot be 'surmounted' by any concentration of agonist. They contrast with competitive antagonists which produce parallel log dose-response curves in the absence and presence of antagonist.

Whilst classical receptor theory has been highly successful in analysing competitive antagonism leading to the development of new drugs (H_2-antagonists), analysis of nonparallel (unsurmountable) log dose-response curves has been a good deal less successful. One explanation is that in competitive antagonism it is a fair assumption that equal responses without and with antagonist are due to activation of the same number of receptors whilst in unsurmountable antagonism this assumption may not apply. The following mechanisms have been invoked in cases of non-parallel log dose-response curves.

True non-competitive antagonism

It is assumed that the antagonist reacts reversibly with a different receptor site from the agonist thereby blocking its effect. The resulting theoretical curves are as follows (symbols as in eq. 3)

$$Y = \frac{K_1 A}{K_1 A + 1} = \frac{K_1 A x}{K_1 A x + 1} \quad \frac{1}{K_2 B + 1} \quad (5)$$

This results in a series of log dose-response curves which have a common origin and become progressively flatter. A series of experimental curves which obey qualitatively this type of relationship is shown in Figure 2.6.

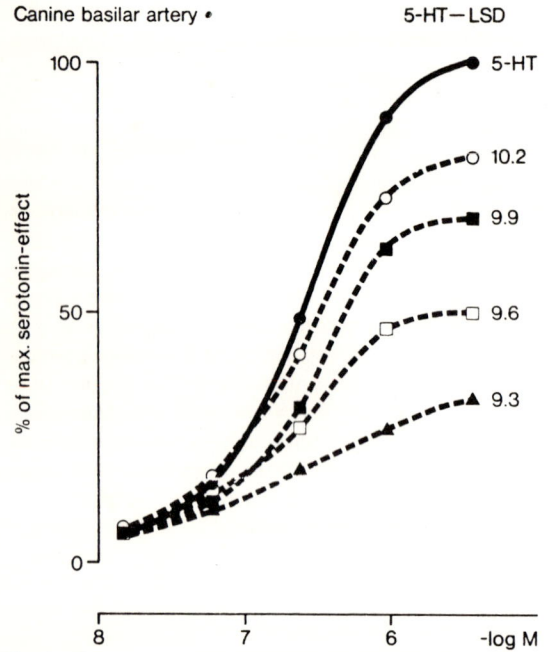

Fig. 2.6 Cumulative dose-response curves of 5HT alone and together with LSD $10^{-10.2}$ to $10^{-9.3}$ M. Spiral strips of canine basilary arteries. (Data kindly supplied by Dr. Müller-Schweinitzer.)

Non-equilibrium antagonism

Certain unsurmountable antagonists equilibrate slowly with receptors, so that response to agonist depends on duration of exposure to antagonist, as shown in the example of Figure 2.7.

Phenoxybenzamine, an α-adrenergic blocking drug reacts in two stages. At first the drug is in mass action equilibrium with receptors and can be washed out. In a second stage the haloalkylamine drug gives rise to an ethyleneiminium intermediate which reacts covalently with receptors inactivating them progressively.

Physiological antagonism

Drugs may antagonise each other by producing opposite effects, for example, histamine produces a contraction and adrenaline a relaxation of bronchial muscle. The two drugs act on different receptors but their ultimate effects are antagonistic. Similarly picrotoxin stimulates respiration and morphine depresses it but they do not act on the same receptors. This type of antagonism has also been called independent because the primary receptors on which the antagonistic drugs act are different.

Chemical antagonism

This is a rare type of antagonism in which the antagonist combines chemically with the agonist to form an inactive compound. A classical example is the neutralisation of heavy metals such as mercury and arsenic by the sulphydryl compound dimercaprol (p. 473).

SPECIFIC AND NON-SPECIFIC DRUG ACTION

Not all drug effects can be explained by interactions with specific receptors. Some drugs are characterised by a lack of specificity; their effects do not depend on polar groups which can react with receptors, but rather on physical

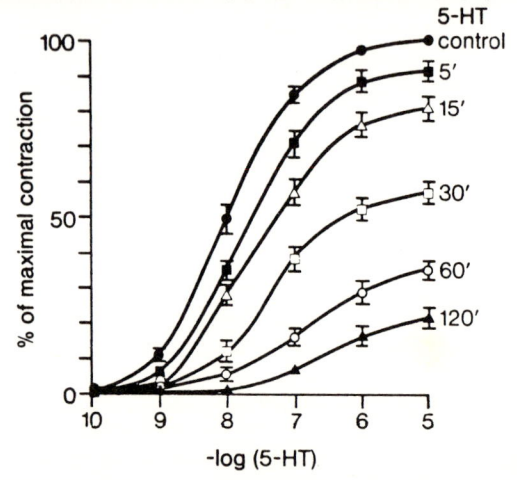

Fig. 2.7 Dose-response curves of 5-HT alone and with 1nM methysergide after different incubation times of rat fundus strip. (After Frankhujsen and Bonta 1974, *Eur. J. Pharmacol.*)

properties such as fat solubility which may allow their accumulation in the lipid phases of the cell. These non-specific drugs are often depressant and many are general anaesthetics. Their effectiveness is related to their solubility in lipid rather than in water as shown in Table 2.3.

Table 2.3 Concentrations in water of various substances required to produce a given degree of narcosis in tadpoles and the corresponding equilibrium concentration of the substances in a lipoid (after Meyer & Hemmi, 1935, *Biochem. Z.*)

Compound	Conc. in water (moles/litre)	Distribution coefficient oleinalcohol water	Conc. in oleinalcohol (moles/litre)
Ethyl alcohol	0.33	0.1	0.033
Phenazone	0.07	0.3	0.021
Amidopyrine	0.03	1.3	0.039
Salicylamide	0.0033	5.9	0.021
Phenobarbitone	0.008	5.9	0.048
Thymol	0.000047	950	0.045

There is, however, no absolute distinction between specific and non-specific drug action. Some drugs, notably the local anaesthetics, possess polar groups suitable for interaction with receptors, but at the same time their activities are bound up largely with their physical properties. Thus it has been shown that local anaesthetic activity is closely related to the ability of drugs to penetrate monolayers of lipids, particularly lipids derived from nervous tissue. Drugs producing equal local anaesthetic effects produce equal increases in the spreading force of lipid monolayers. Local anaesthetic drugs are considered to act by 'stabilising' the membrane potential thereby reducing the ability of the nerve membrane to respond to a slight depolarisation by a large transient increase of its permeability to sodium ions which underlies the action potential (p. 308).

NEW APPROACHES TO THE MECHANISM OF DRUG ACTION

Two recent approaches have aroused great interest: attempts at isolating drug receptors and the analysis of 'membrane noise'.

The identification and isolation of receptors

Receptors and enzymes can both be considered as proteins with characteristic prosthetic groups, but the problems involved in their isolation are different and they are particularly formidable in the receptor case. Enzymes can be identified and monitored through all the stages of purification by their catalytic activities. Isolated receptor proteins, however, cannot be identified by their characteristic receptor *activities* which are lost when the cell structure is destroyed. They are generally identified by their binding properties making use of receptor 'probes' such as specific antagonists or agonists binding to the particular receptor. Irreversible or semi-irreversible antagonists are amongst the most useful receptor probes.

The identification of receptors by their binding characteristics can be a source of serious error, for example a cholinergic receptor probe may bind to cholinesterase. Another possibility is binding to 'silent' drug uptake sites. Both agonists and antagonists can bind to drug receptors and their interactions may be investigated by binding studies as well as by the classical pharmacological approach based on drug action. Although a completely satisfactory integration of the two approaches has not been achieved as yet, this remains a challenging task for the future.

Identification of particular receptors

ACh receptors
Some of the earliest studies in this field have dealt with the identification of the nicotinic acetylcholine (ACh) receptor present in the frog motor endplate and in the electric organ of *Torpedo*. The snake venom α-bungarotoxin (BuTX) has been the chief receptor probe used. BuTX binds selectively and practically irreversibly to nicotinic ACh receptors and it has been shown that when labelled BuTX is applied to the motor endplate up to 20 per cent of its surface appears to be occupied by receptors.

The isolated receptor material may be solubilised with detergents and purified and a large molecular protein isolated from it. After saturation of the endplate receptors with BuTX the access of low-molecular ligands such as d-tubocurarine is impeded.

Other receptors
Several attempts have been made to identify the ß-*adrenergic receptor* by its ability to bind ^{3}H-isoprenaline or labelled pindolol. Since ß-adrenergic action is closely linked to adenylcyclase activation the latter has also been used in investigations of ß-adrenergic receptors present in isolated cells such as turkey erythrocytes.

Attempts have been made to identify receptors in the CNS by binding studies. Thus it has been suggested that the spinal cord may contain *glycine receptors* with which strychnine can combine. These studies are difficult and their interpretation is controversial, but they have undoubtedly opened up entirely new vistas for the investigation of receptors in the CNS.

Membrane noise

The analysis of membrane noise represents a new approach to drug-receptor interactions. Katz and Miledi showed that when acetylcholine (ACh) was applied by microionophoresis to frog motor endplate it produced increased fluctuations of the endplate potential. When the

ACh 'noise' is analysed statistically it can provide information about the molecular events when a 'packet' of ACh (p. 65) impinges on receptors causing transient opening of ionic channels. With certain assumptions a frequency analysis of noise variance can provide an indication of the average life span of an ACh-induced open ionic channel.

This approach, in spite of its technical novelty and formidable difficulties of interpretation seems capable of providing a deeper understanding of mechanisms underlying drug-receptor interactions. As an example, attempts are being made to distinguish by means of membrane noise analysis between competitive and noncompetitive drug antagonists. Preliminary results suggest that certain (competitive) antagonists reduce the occurrence of open ionic channels whilst leaving their average life span unchanged, whereas other (noncompetitive) antagonists have the effect of reducing the average life span of open channels.

Noise analysis has led to a re-examination of the relation between agonist and antagonist in certain cases. Thus the neuromuscular blocking action of tubocurarine has been regarded as a typical case of competitive antagonism attributed to a reversible attachment to endplate receptors, thereby blocking access to ACh and so preventing its depolarising action. This view was based on the parallel shift of the ACh log dose-response curve in frog striated muscle and it was supported by the finding that tubocurarine, like ACh itself, is capable of delaying the irreversible binding of α-bungarotoxin to the endplate receptors.

More recent evidence, based partly on noise analysis, suggests that tubocurarine has two distinct postsynaptic actions. It appears to form reversible bonds with ACh receptors but in addition it acts on another site which leads to 'plugging' of the opened ionic channels. This second action may be due to tubocurarine attaching itself to the activated receptor complex. It is interesting that α-bungarotoxin does not have these two actions, it reacts only with the normal receptor attachment sites of ACh.

Electrophysiological analysis of drug-receptor interactions
Recent studies based on membrane noise analysis and voltage clamp techniques are beginning to reveal an entirely new approach to drug-receptor interactions differing from classical receptor theory. New ideas are arising such as the notion of agonists opening ionic channels and antagonists blocking them. These notions will necessitate a revision of standard receptor theory to attune it to ideas arising from electrophysiological findings. It will be an important future task of theoretical pharmacology to incorporate the results of electrophysiological analysis and combine them with the fruitful notions derived from classical receptor theory.

REFERENCES AND FURTHER READING

Ariens E J ed 1964 Molecular pharmacology. Academic Press, New York
Arunlakshana O, Schild H O 1959 Some quantitative uses of drug antagonists. Br. J. Pharmac. 14: 48
Barlow R B 1964 Introduction to chemical pharmacology. Methuen, London
Clark A J 1937 General pharmacology. Handbuch der exp. Pharmakol. 4
Ehrlich P 1960 On partial functions of the cell (Nobel Lecture). Collected papers of Paul Ehrlich. Vol. 3. Pergamon, London
Furchgott R F 1972 The classification of adreno-receptors. Handb. exp. Pharmac. 33: 283–335
Gaddum J H 1937 The quantitative effects of antagonistic drugs. J. Physiol. 89: 7P
Goldstein A, Aronow L, Kalman S M 1974 Principles of drug action. Wiley, New York
Goodford P J 1973 Prediction of pharmacological activity by the method of physicochemical activity relationships. In: Advances in pharmacology. Vol. 11
Katz B, Miledi R 1978 A re-examination of curare action at the motor endplate. Proc. R. Soc. B 203: 119–133
Paton W D M 1961 A theory of drug action based on the rate of drug receptor combination. Proc. R. Soc. B 154: 21
Porter R, O'Connor M ed 1970 Molecular properties of drug receptors. Ciba Symposium. Churchill, London
Rang H P ed 1973 Drug receptors. Symposium. MacMillan, London
Schild H O 1968 A pharmacological approach to drug receptors. In: Tedeschi and Tedeschi eds, Importance of fundamental principles in drug evaluation. Raven Press, New York
Schueler F W 1960 Chemobiodynamies and drug design. McGraw-Hill, New York
Stephenson R P 1956 A modification of receptor theory. Br. J. Pharmac. 11: 379
Van Rossum J M 1963 Cumulative dose-response curves: evaluation of drug parameters. Arch. Int. Pharmacodyn. 143: 299
Verveen A A, DeFelice L J 1974 Membrane noise. Progress in biophysics 28: 189
Waud D R 1968 Pharmacological receptors. Pharm. Rev. 20: 49

3. Measurement of drug action

Biological assay 19; Radioimmunoassay 19; Biological standardisation 20; Design of bioassays 21; Analytical and comparative assays 22; Comparative bioassays in man 23; Ceiling effects 26; Individual variation in response to drugs 26; Pharmacogenetics 28; Therapeutic index 29; Assessment of therapeutic value of drug 30; Assessment of drug toxicity 30; Adverse effects of drugs in man 31; Classification of unwanted drug effects 31; Therapeutic trials 32; Statistics in drug trials 32.

BIOLOGICAL ASSAY

Chemical analysis was the only method used to estimate the strength of drugs until near the end of the last century. Biological assay was first introduced to measure the activity of drugs such as antitoxins, whose active principles could not be measured by chemical means. Biological assay methods have been of great importance for the development of pharmacology. In the first place the development of serum therapy has depended entirely on such methods. Secondly, these methods have made possible the remarkable development of endocrine therapy, since experience has shown that in almost every case before any new hormone can be used with success in therapeutics, it is necessary to find some biological test by means of which the activity of preparations can be measured. Thirdly, bioassays have played a crucial part in the study of humoral transmitters and other active substances present in tissue fluids. Fourthly, bioassays are indispensable in assessing the activity of new drugs.

Biological assay is essentially a method of measurement in which a biological reaction is used as the indicator. Although biological responses are inherently variable, bioassays can be devised to give almost any required degree of accuracy by repeating the tests and using statistical methods in the interpretation of the results. A well-planned assay should be so designed as to furnish evidence not only of the activity of the test preparation but also of the limits of error of the test. Bioassays usually depend on a comparison between the sample to be tested and a standard preparation. Such assays are of two kinds (*a*) those in which there is a qualitative difference between the two preparations, and (*b*) those in which there is only a quantitative difference, the test solution containing an unknown quantity of the standard. These two types are referred to as *comparative* and *analytical dilution* assay respectively.

Assays of the first type are used to assess the activity of new drugs. For example, a new analgesic drug may be compared with morphine or a local anaesthetic with procaine. In this type of assay, however, the result depends on the method and species used, and the relative activity of the drugs in animal experiments can give only a preliminary indication of their relative activity in man.

Assays of the second type have the same object as chemical determinations and they are used only where no adequate chemical methods are available. Such assays are used either for substances such as insulin which cannot be measured in any other way or for drugs such as acetylcholine which are commonly present in concentrations too low to be detected by other methods. Provided that standard and unknown have the same composition the final result of this type of assay does not depend on the method and species used.

A special form of analytical assay of high sensitivity is referred to as saturation analysis or by its most common variety, radioimmunoassay. This form of assay has been introduced relatively recently and is gaining increasing importance.

Radioimmunoassay

The extent to which unlabelled ligand competes with labelled ligand for a limited number of binding sites on a macromolecule, serves as a basis of quantitation in radioimmunoassays. These assays are extremely sensitive, picogram amounts of a particular compound can sometimes be estimated. Once the binding antibody and labelled ligand are available, the assays are relatively simple to perform: mixtures containing labelled ligand, antibody and an unknown quantity of unlabelled ligand are incubated; free labelled ligand is separated from antibody-bound ligand, and the extent of binding is determined.

Radioimmunoassays involving specific antibodies represent one particular type of 'saturation analysis'. Other macromolecules may be employed in place of antibodies such as enzymes or cell membranes containing drug receptors (receptor assays). Whilst radioactive labels are most convenient, they are not an essential requirement of immunoassays. Alternative techniques of marking may be used, e.g. fluorescent compounds, spin labelled compounds (detected by electron-spin-resonance spectrometry) and enzyme coupled compounds. Originally radioimmunoassays were based on ^{3}H or ^{14}C isotope labelling, but this had the disadvantage that liquid scintillation counting is required. For this reason the simpler technique of gamma ray counting by labelling compounds with ^{124}I or ^{131}I is now being increasingly employed whenever such labelling is feasible.

Clinical applications

New radioimmunoassays and radioligand receptor assays

are continuously being developed and many are now used routinely as diagnostic procedures. Some radio-immunoassays of proved clinical value are shown below (after Landon 1974 *Br. Med. Bull.*).

Table 3.1 Some clinically used radioimmunoassays

	Peptide and protein hormones
Anterior pituitary	Luteinizing hormone (LH); follicle-stimulating hormone (FSH); thyroid-stimulating hormone (TSH); human growth hormone (HGH); prolactin; corticotrophin (ACTH)
Posterior pituitary	Arginine-vasopressin (AVP)
Parathyroid	Parathyroid hormone (PTH)
Pancreas	Insulin
Placenta	Human placental lactogen (HPL); human chorionic gonadotrophin (HCG)
Others	Angiotensin I and II; renin; gastrin
	Other peptides and proteins
Plasma proteins	IgE; fibrinogen; other clotting factors
Microbiological antigens	Hepatitis-associated antigens
Specific tumour antigens	α Fetoprotein; carcino-embryonic antigen
	Hapten hormones
Thyroid	Thyroxine (T_4); tri-iodothyronine (T_3)
Adrenal	Cortisol; deoxycorticosterone; aldosterone
Gonadal	Testosterone; progesterone; various oestrogens
	Other haptens
Drugs	Digoxin; morphine; cannabis; diphenylhydantoin
Others	Folic acid; cyclic AMP; vitamin B_{12}; vitamin D

Usable radioimmunoassays for drugs are still scarce. They are needed to measure drug concentrations in tissue fluids both for pharmacokinetic studies and for monitoring treatment. The main problem in developing drug radioimmunoassays is the production of suitable antisera. Because of their low molecular weight, drugs and steroid hormones are not naturally immunogenic. It is first necessary to couple the drug covalently to a carrier protein, such as bovine serum albumin, before raising antibodies to it in rabbits and guinea pigs.

Cardiac glycosides. Radioimmunoassays have been developed for digoxin and digitoxin. They exhibit cross-reactivity but clinically this is unimportant if the individual drugs are used. Commercial kits are now available by which rapid measurements may be made to provide evidence of digitalis overdosage.

Morphine. There is no satisfactory method for measuring morphine in blood. Attempts are being made to develop radioimmunoassays for morphine. They are still at the laboratory stage and seem to show little specificity as between morphine, codeine and heroin.

Steroids. Analytical techniques based on protein binding are now widely used in the steroid field. Two types of methods are employed.

1. The use of naturally occurring steroid binding proteins such as transcortin for cortisol binding or a testosterone binding protein in human plasma.
2. The use of covalently linked steroid-protein conjugates for purposes of radioimmunoassay.

Gastro-intestinal hormones. Radioimmunoassays of several of these hormones have been developed including gastrin, enteroglucagon and secretin.

Thyroid hormones. Concentrations in blood of the thyroid hormones thyroxine (T_4) and tri-iodothyronine (T_3) (p. 331) can be measured by using human thyroxine-binding globulin in a competitive protein binding assay. More recently radioimmunoassays for both T_3 and T_4 have been described. The main problem in their clinical use is the presence, in serum samples, of several proteins which bind thyroid hormones with great avidity.

BIOLOGICAL STANDARDISATION

Voltaire defined therapeutics as the pouring of drugs, of which one knew nothing, into a patient, of whom one knew less. This comment expresses the general truth that there are two possible variables — the drug and the patient. Since patients cannot be standardised, drugs of uniform activity are essential for reliable therapeutic effects.

The purpose of biological standardisation is to ensure that drugs conform to a standard of uniform activity. The method used in biological standardisation is the comparison of the activity of the preparation under investigation with that of a standard preparation. In many cases international standard preparations are available. For example, the standard preparation of insulin is a quantity of purified insulin (ox, 52 per cent; pig, 48 per cent) 0.04 mg of which contains 1 unit of activity.

Biological standardisation involves difficult techniques, is consequently expensive, and therefore increases the cost of drugs. For this reason it is only employed when it is strictly necessary.

In general it may be said that the first step in the successful therapeutic use of a biological product such as an antitoxin, hormone or vitamin, is to discover some method by which its activity can be measured accurately. The final stage is the discovery of the chemical nature of the product, and when it can be obtained in a pure chemical form, either by extraction from natural sources or by synthesis, biological standardisation in most cases ceases to be necessary; the development of the penicillins is a good example.

DESIGN OF BIOASSAYS

Three main bioassay designs are used, each based on a comparison between standard and unknown. They are conveniently classified as direct, indirect quantitative, and indirect quantal assays.

Direct assays
The basis of a direct assay is that the dose of drug is adjusted until a desired effect is produced. For example for the biological standardisation of digitalis, a solution of the drug is infused slowly intravenously into an anaesthetised guinea pig until the heart stops. This procedure is repeated in several guinea pigs with solutions of the standard and unknown. The reciprocal of the ratio of the mean effective volumes of standard and unknown is then considered to be their activity ratio.

A frequent form of direct assay is the *matching assay* in which doses of standard and unknown are adjusted until the responses match. Acetylcholine released during nerve stimulation may thus be assayed by its effect in an isolated preparation against an acetylcholine standard. A further refinement is to test the unknown against standard in several different types of assay preparations. If they all show the same activity ratio with standard then the presumption that standard and unknown are identical is greatly strengthened. This procedure is called *parallel quantitative assay*.

Indirect assays
Direct assays have certain disadvantages, the most important being that they are not readily amenable to statistical analysis. By contrast, indirect assays, which are based on dose-response curves, can be analysed by precise statistical procedures. Indirect assays may be based either on graded or on all-or-none responses: in the latter case the proportion of positive responses is recorded and plotted on the dose-response curve employing an appropriate linearising transformation or *metameter* (p. 22). These two kinds of indirect assay are sometimes referred to as 'quantitative' and 'quantal' respectively.

Quantitative assays
Bioassays generally make use of the linear portion of the dose response curve. Experience has shown that in many graded-response assays linear relationships are obtained over part of the range when the response is plotted against the logarithm of the dose. Such assays give rise to parallel curves for standard and unknown and are therefore called *parallel-line assays*. In some cases linear relationships are obtained when responses are plotted against dose of drug; these are called *slope ratio assays*.

The simplest form of parallel-line assay is the *2 + 2 assay* (four point assay), in which two doses of standard and two of unknown, both in the same ratio, are used. Figure 3.1 illustrates a 2 + 2 assay of histamine on the isolated guinea pig ileum in which blocks of four doses were administered in successive randomised sequences. The 2 + 2 assay is based on a symmetrical design in which calculations are greatly simplified. The activity ratio in a 2 + 2 assay such as that illustrated in Figure 3.1 may be calculated from the formula

$$M = \frac{A}{B} d$$

where M = log activity ratio, d = log ratio of two doses of standard (or unknown), $A = U_L + U_S - S_L - S_S$, and $B = U_L + S_L - U_S - S_S$; the symbols U_L, U_S, S_L, S_S refer to the mean response to large and small doses of unknown and standard respectively. Perhaps the most important aspect of this kind of design is that the evidence for the validity and error limits of each experiment can be obtained from the data of the experiment itself. Evidence of validity is obtained by a procedure called *analysis of variance* which embodies *tests of significance*. These may show for example a significant regression of response on dose (without which the assay would be invalid) or a lack of significant deviation from parallelism between the two dose-response lines. The error limits of the estimated activity ratio (more precisely the *fiducial* or *confidence limits*) may be calculated by formulae which provide these limits in the form of probability statements.

Quantal assays
Trevan showed that when the effect of a drug is recorded as an all or none event, e.g. death or survival, and the percentage of affected individuals is plotted against dose of drug, regular S-shaped curves result. Gaddum later showed that these S-shaped curves become symmetrical if a logarithmic dose axis is used and that they may be linearised by a transformation of co-ordinates in which *normal equivalent deviations* or *probits* (Fig. 3.11) are plotted on the y axis instead of percentages. The linearised curves may then be used for the assay of unknown in terms of a standard.

Figures 3.2(a) and 3.2(b) illustrate the meaning of S-shaped quantal dose response curves. Figure 3.2(a) shows some data obtained by Behrens investigating the sensitivity of frogs to k-strophanthin. His apparatus enabled him to administer strophanthin by slow intravenous infusion into a frog lymph sac and thus determine the exact lethal dose for each frog. The frequency distribution of lethal doses is shown in Figure 3.2(a). Another way of presenting the same data is to plot for each dose the percentage of frogs killed by that dose

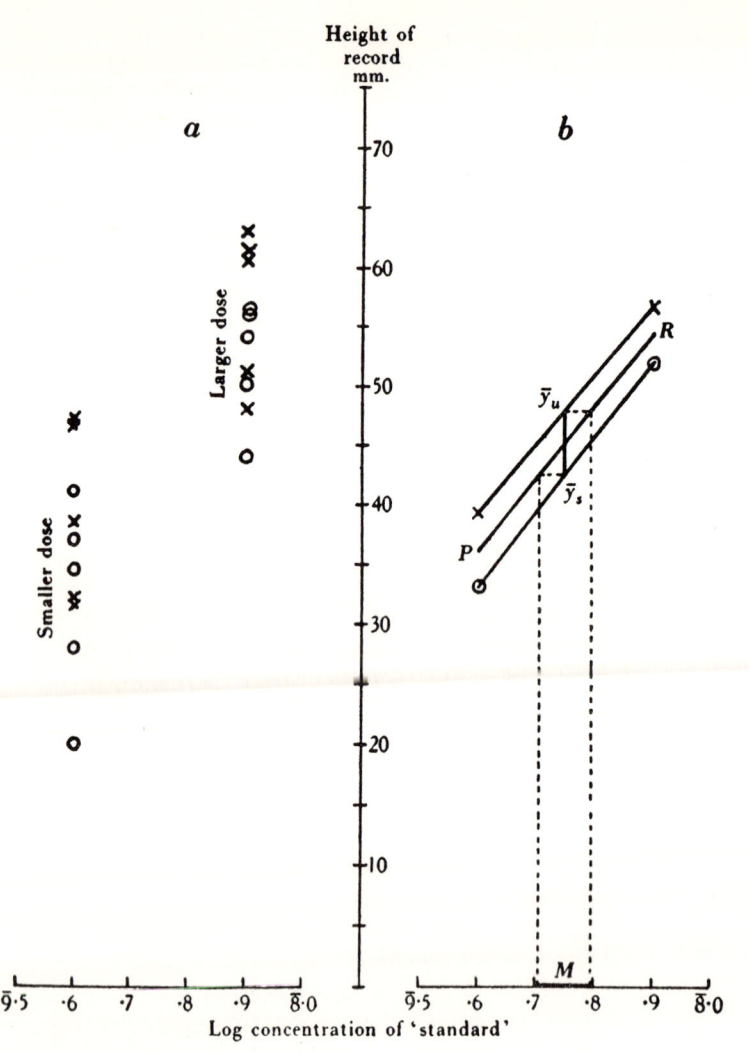

Fig. 3.1 Result of 2+2 assay of histamine of g.p. ileum. Two doses of 'standard' (0.1 and 0.2 μg) and two doses of 'unknown' (0.125 and 0.025 μg) were administered in five successive randomised blocks: (a) individual results; (b) mean results. The activity ratio determined experimentally was 1.23 (M = log activity ratio = 0.09). PR = mean regression line. (After Schild, 1942, *J. Physiol.*)

plus the percentage killed by all smaller doses obtaining thus the S-shaped *cumulative* frequency curve shown in Figure 3.2(b). If it is assumed that dose-mortality curves are approximations of normal or Gaussian curves then the continuous curve in Figure 3.2(b) can be considered as an approximation to the integrated form of a Gaussian curve.

Figure 3.2(b) also incorporates another set of data obtained independently by Trevan using a simpler procedure. Trevan injected graded doses of another cardiac glycoside (digitalis) into groups of frogs and determined the percentage killed by each dose. The similarity of Trevan's experimental curve and the curve computed from Behrens' results suggests that they both basically represent the same integrated frequency distribution.

Linearised dose mortality curves (probit curves) (p. 28) can be used for determinations of drug toxicity and of LD50 values. The LD50 is the dose of drug producing 50 per cent mortality in a group of animals. Toxicity determinations are often carried out in the form of comparisons with a known or standard drug in order to eliminate species and strain variability.

Analytical and comparative bioassays
Bioassays were originally used for the standardisation of drugs and the detection of minute quantities of biologically active substances. This type of analytical dilution assay has declined in importance as impure drugs have been replaced by pure drugs and as sensitive physico-chemical methods became available such as fluorescence and radioimmunoassays which are capable of detecting many (though not all) biologically active tissue products.

By contrast, the importance of comparative bioassays in

MEASUREMENT OF DRUG ACTION 23

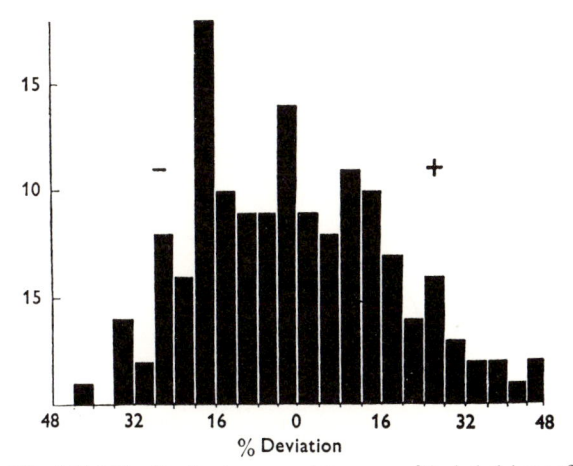

Fig. 3.2(a) The distribution around the mean of the lethal doses of strophanthin for different frogs. The ordinates are numbers of frogs. (Behrens, *Arch. exp. Path. Pharmak.*, 1929). The deviations extend from 44 per cent below the mean (shown on abscissa as 0) to 48 per cent above.

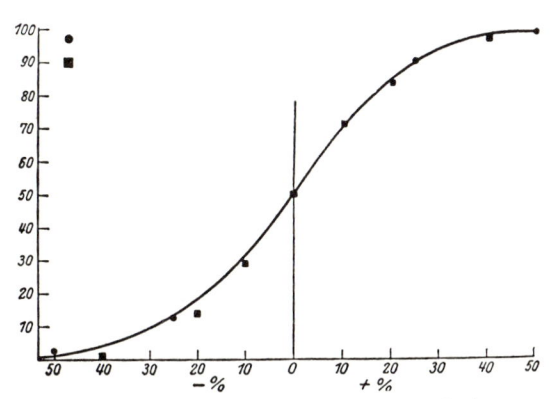

Fig. 3.2(b) Relation of dose to percentage mortality for frogs injected with ● digitalis (Trevan), ■ strophanthin (Behrens). (After Burn, Finney and Goodwin, 1950. *Biological Standardisation*, Oxford Univ. Press.)

which the effects of *different* drugs are compared has, if anything, increased over the years. Comparative bioassays have been criticised on the grounds that they do not conform to the fundamental criterion of similarity between standard and test and therefore cannot be considered to be rigorous bioassays. They are nevertheless extensively used and are indeed indispensable for the laboratory development of new drugs and their initial assessment in man.

COMPARATIVE BIOASSAYS IN MAN

Ideally, when a new drug is introduced into clinical medicine it should be compared with established drugs for its activity and time course. Such studies might involve the establishment of dose-response and time-response curves both in normal subjects and patients. In practice such detailed evaluation is seldom undertaken, partly because it is too laborious and 'wasteful' of human material and frequently also because suitable criteria for measuring the effects of drugs may simply not exist. Thus the effects of neuroleptic drugs on psychotic patients cannot at present be validly assessed by measurable parameters. Because of these difficulties only relatively few human comparative bioassays based on dose-response curves have been reported in the literature. Some example from different fields are discussed below.

Histamine antagonists

In the experiments described by Bain and his colleagues wheal areas after intradermal histamine injection were measured. The previous administration of an oral antihistamine produced a graded diminution of the wheal areas, the effect being linearly related to log dose of antihistamine. The activity of antihistamines was compared in this way as shown in Figure 3.3.

The authors concluded that the relative potencies of antihistamines could not be adequately expressed in terms of a single parameter and calculated three separate quotients by which the potencies of antihistamines could be assessed. They called these (a) 'mean potency quotient' based on the ratio of equiactive doses, (b) 'mean duration quotient' based on the times required for the maximum antihistamine effect of each drug to be reduced by half and (c) 'mean therapeutic quotient' based on the total amount of drug needed during 24 hours. The mean therapeutic quotient (not to be confused with therapeutic index, p. 29) was estimated clinically by determining the daily doses required to suppress chronic urticaria. The mean therapeutic quotient (which could not be determined as accurately as the other two ratios) seemed to be a function of both intensity and duration of effect.

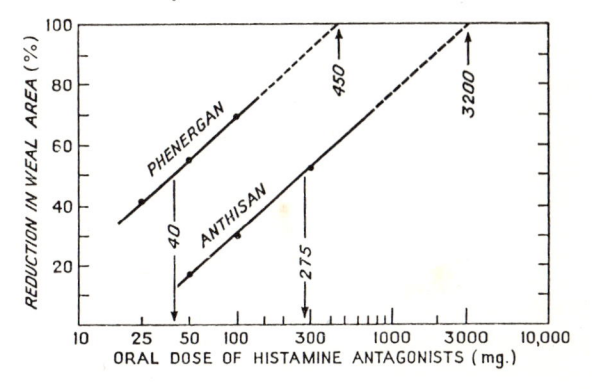

Fig. 3.3 Relationship between dose and maximum antihistamine response for phenergan (promethazine) and anthisan (mepyramine). Mean results from six people. Mean doses to give 50 per cent reduction of wheal area are shown on lower abscissa, and theoretical mean doses to produce 100 per cent reduction on upper abscissa. (After Bain, Broadbent and Warin, 1949, *Lancet*.)

Oxytocic drugs

Human assay methods for oxytocic drugs are needed because the drug responses of the human uterus differ profoundly from those of animal uteri. Methods of recording contractions of the human uterus fall into two main groups, intra-uterine and external (tocographic) methods; the latter involve less inconvenience and risk for the patient. Unfortunately, tocographic methods cannot be used except during pregnancy whilst the uterus is close to the abdominal wall and for a short time after parturition, when they involve no risk to the foetus. Clinical bioassays on the postpartum uterus are practically limited to two doses per patient given on the second and third day after delivery and this limitation determines their statistical design.

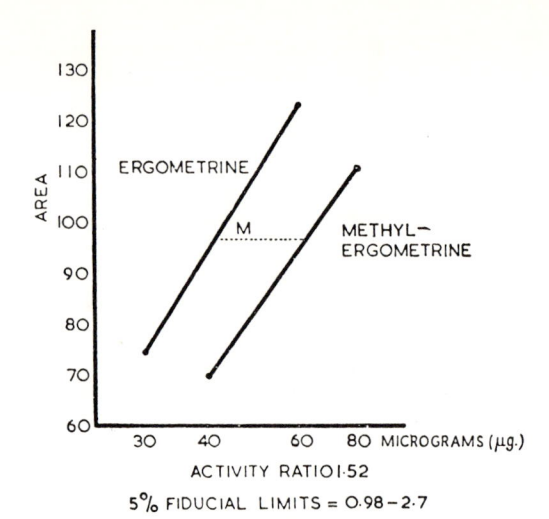

Fig. 3.4(b) Comparison of the effects of ergometrine and methylergometrine. The effects of two doses of each drug were measured in a number of patients and plotted as shown. From these results the activity ratio of the two drugs was calculated to be 1.52. (After Myerscough and Schild, 1958, Brit. J. Pharmacol.)

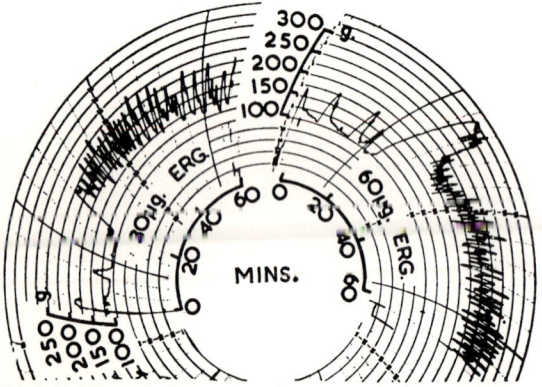

Fig. 3.4(a) Record of human uterine contractions in response to two doses of ergometrine administered intravenously to a patient on the second and third days after delivery. The contractions were recorded by a tocograph strapped to the abdominal wall. The response to the drug is measured by the area enclosed between the base line and the tracing during the first twenty minutes after injection.

A suitable design is that of balanced incomplete blocks of two. The design is basically a 2 + 2 assay but instead of giving all four doses to each subject, any one subject receives only two doses in various dose combinations (incomplete randomised block design). In the tocographic assay shown in Figures 3.4(a) and 3.4(b) this plan was applied to the comparison of the oxytocic effects of ergometrine and methylergometrine. This experiment showed, contrary to previous belief, that ergometrine was about 1.5 times as active as methylergometrine.

Sedative drugs

The psychogalvanic reflex (PGR) is a short lasting diminution in the skin resistance caused by an external stimulus such as a brief sound. The PGR shows a tendency to decrease with repetition of the auditory stimulus, i.e. it habituates. When a sedative drug such as a barbiturate is administered to a subject the rate of habituation of the PGR increases in a dose-dependent manner and this parameter may be used as an index of the activity of the sedative drug. The curves of Figure 3.5 show this effect. These curves can be linearised by a suitable transformation of coordinates, making it possible to obtain a linear relationship between dose of drug and response. Habituation of the PGR can thus be made the basis of a bioassay of sedative drugs in man. The assay is of the slope-ratio variety since dose, rather than log dose, is linearly related to response in this case.

This method of testing can be applied to patients with anxiety states. It was found that in anxious patients the PGR habituates more slowly than in normal controls (Fig. 18.6) but that their rate of habituation increases after receiving a sedative drug and approaches that of normals. A comparative bioassay of sedative drugs may thus be carried out. Figure 3.6 shows the outcome of a slope-ratio assay on 30 patients which showed 300 mg amylobarbitone to be equivalent to about 40 mg chlordiazepoxide. In an assay of this kind it is preferable to avoid single dose administration and to use instead long-term administration which corresponds better to the clinical usage of the drugs and has the further advantage of generating steadier blood levels of the drug.

Analgesic drugs

The measurement of subjective responses presents special difficulties. In the bioassays so far discussed, the response parameter has been a physical measurement or some combination of physical measurements, but pain is a subjective response which cannot be expressed by a physical measurement. Objective responses such as autonomic concomitants of pain could in theory be used

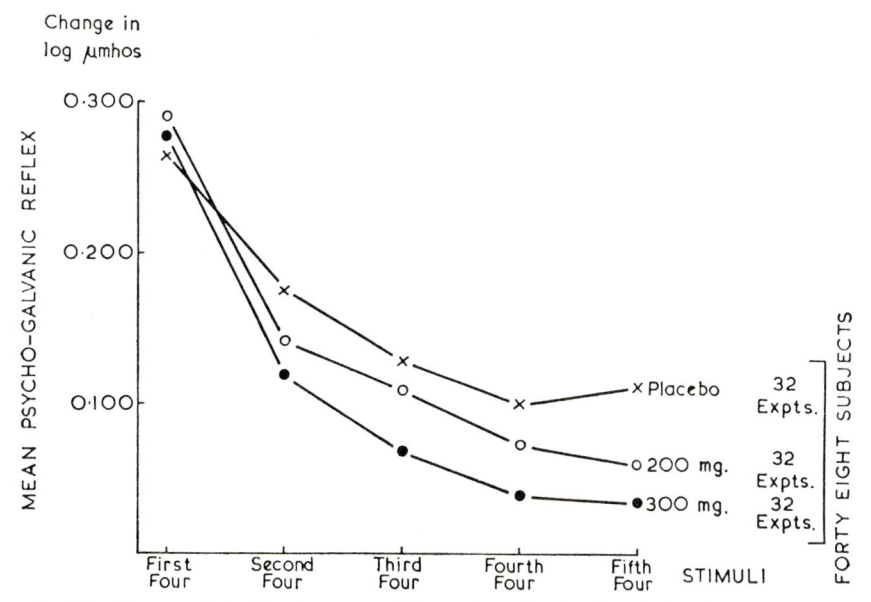

Fig. 3.5 The effect of cyclobarbitone on the habituation curve of the psycho-galvanic reflex. Each point represents the sum of four mean responses. Skin resistance was measured at intervals of approx. 1 min following a brief auditory stimulus; values were converted to log skin conductance. (After Lader, 1964, *Brain*.)

but they are not sufficiently reliable indices of pain and they may also be directly affected by drugs, independently of their analgesic action.

One method of measuring analgesic action in man is to employ some graded stimulus such as radiant heat (Fig. 21.3) and determine the threshold at which pain is felt. It is generally agreed, however, that this type of artificially induced superficial pain is different in quality and cannot provide an adequate model of clinical pain. Tests have therefore been developed in which the pain spontaneously occurring in disease is used to quantitate analgesic action. The pain of malignant disease, because of its chronic and persistent nature, is particularly appropriate for such tests.

One method of assessing analgesic drugs clinically is by *pain charts* in which the patient is asked to assess the degree of pain or of pain relief experienced during treatment and to express it on an agreed scale. It has been found, however, that patients' own assessments tend to be

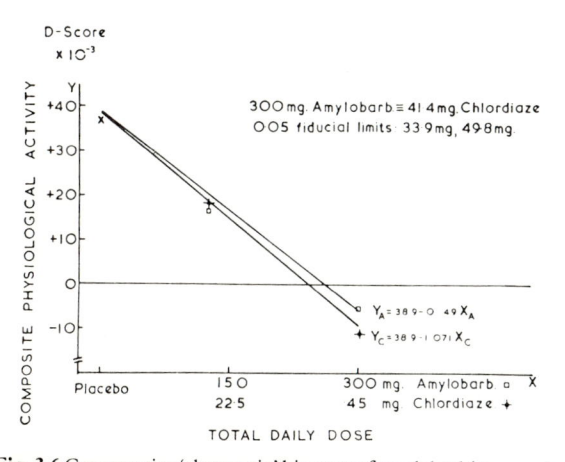

Fig. 3.6 Comparative 'slope ratio' bioassay of amylobarbitone and chlordiazepoxide using a composite score depending on various physiological parameters as index. Total daily doses of 300 mg amylobarbitone and 41 mg chlordiazepoxide produced equal effects. Measurements were performed after administering drugs to patients with anxiety states for periods of one week. (After Lader and Wing, 1965, *J. Neurol. Neurosurg. Psychiat.*)

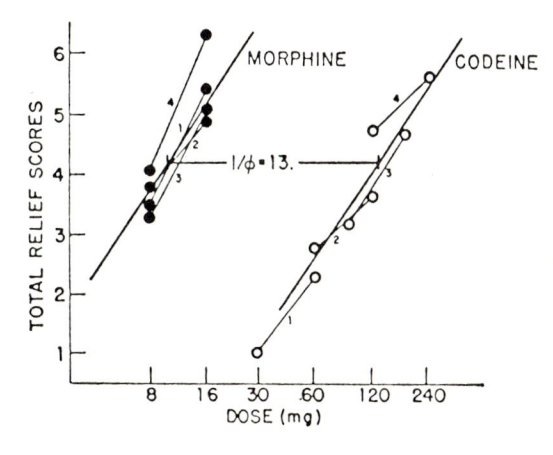

Fig. 3.7 Log-dose-effect curves for intramuscular codeine and morphine in man. The 'relief scores' represent mean scores obtained by trained observers who questioned the patients as to the pain relief experienced. About 13 times the dose of codeine was required to produce the same analgesic effect as morphine. (After Houde, Wallenstein and Beaver (1965), in *Analgetics*, Academic Press, N.Y.)

influenced by their preoccupation with the disease and their personal problems. A better approach is to use as an intermediary a trained observer who questions the patient and elicits from him an appraisal of pain relief. This is then quantified on some arbitrary scale such as complete, considerable, moderate, slight or no relief, and finally expressed numerically.

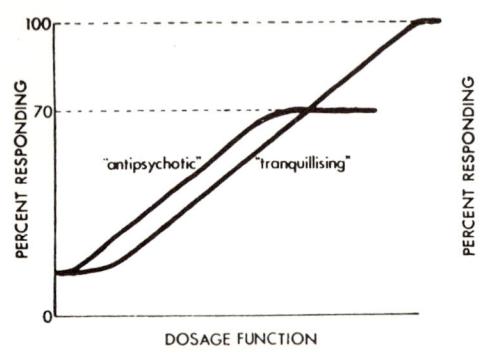

Fig. 3.8 Hypothetical quantal dose-response curves for chlorpromazine in schizophrenic and non-schizophrenic patients. (After Lader, 1971, *Psychological Medicine*.)

Analgesic test drugs may be given at fixed intervals, but more frequently they are given on demand and the degree of pain relief is then recorded for a period o, say, six hours. It is essential in such studies that patients should be cooperative and able to communicate with the observer. It is also essential that they should be informed of the study and agree to it, but that neither the patient nor the observer should know which drug has been given in a particular instance.

In the assay by Houde and colleagues shown in Figure 3.7 two analgesic drugs, morphine (the standard) and codeine (the test) were used in a 2 + 2 design, in which each patient received all four drug doses. Variation between patients, which is very important in analgesic assays, is thus eliminated from the comparison. The design was sequential in that codeine dosage was progressively changed until test and standard became equiactive. The activity ratio morphine/codeine worked out at 13.

Clearly, the fact that one analgesic drug is more active than another in a comparative asssay does not prove its superiority, it merely shows that a smaller dose is needed to produce the same effect. Determinations of activity ratios are, however, essential preliminaries for therapeutic assessment of the relative merits of two drugs. For example a comparison of their relative side effects, tolerances and addiction proneness can be meaningful only if carried out on the basis of equiactive doses.

Ceiling effects

An important though somewhat controversial point is whether it is possible to demonstrate ceiling effects of drugs and whether different drugs have different ceiling effects. It must be understood that the word ceiling in relation to a dose-response curve can have two distinct meanings.

Ceiling of a graded dose-response curve. Attempts to establish a graded response ceiling for drugs such as analgesics or diuretics have run into difficulties, largely because if sufficiently high doses of drug are given to produce a plateau effect the toxic symptoms in human subjects tend to become prohibitive. Thus, although it is widely believed that morphine has a higher analgesic ceiling than codeine, it has proved difficult to substantiate this view by adequate quantitative measurements because of the toxic effects produced by large doses. Differences in ceiling effects have, nevertheless, been clearly demonstrated with some drugs, e.g. in the field of diuretics (p. 158).

Ceiling of a quantal dose-response curve. The term *per cent effectiveness* (Lader) denotes the ceiling of a quantal curve in which a dose function is related to percentage of a population responding. The point is illustrated schematically in relation to chlorpromazine in Figure 3.8. Chlorpromazine can be considered to act as tranquilliser in almost all patients, i.e. its effectiveness in this respect approaches 100 per cent. It also has a specific antipsychotic or antischizophrenic effect in a proportion of such patients but there is an appreciable residue of patients in which the schizophrenic symptoms are not controlled. Thus in relation to the antischizophrenic effect the per cent effectiveness of chlorpromazine is less, probably only about 70 per cent.

There are bound to be considerable uncertainties in this type of assessment. The result could depend on the definition of schizophrenia adopted, which in turn would determine the type of patient included in the trial. Nevertheless this type of approach has been used in trying to assess the value of drugs, particularly psychotropic drugs.

INDIVIDUAL VARIATION IN RESPONSE TO DRUGS

It is important to realise that no two individuals respond to any drug in an identical manner. In the first place, a small minority of persons react to certain drugs in a wholly abnormal manner. Apart from these abnormal cases there is a wide individual variation in the dose of drug needed to produce an equal effect.

The extent of this variation is shown in Figure 3.9 which shows the doses of sodium salicylate needed to produce mild symptoms of intoxication in 300 male patients. Two-thirds of this population responded to doses between 100 and 200 grains, but the extreme limits of variation were 50 and 500 grains. These figures were obtained with diseased individuals, whose ages varied widely, and the doses were not calculated per unit of body weight.

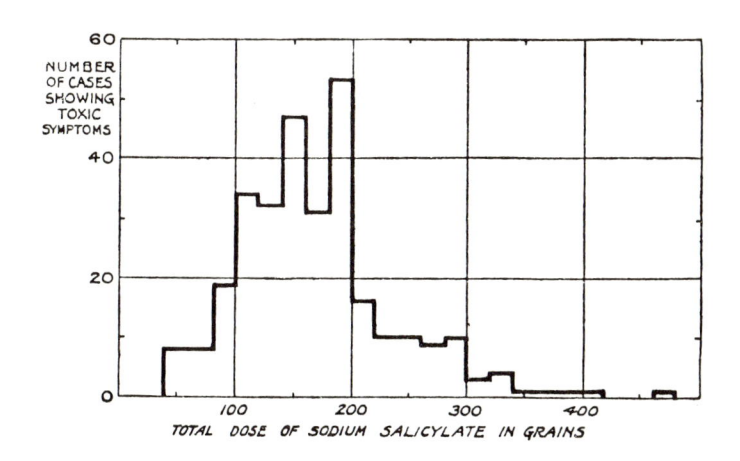

Fig. 3.9 The individual variation amongst 300 males in the amount of sodium salicylate taken before toxic symptoms appeared. (Hanzlik, 1913).

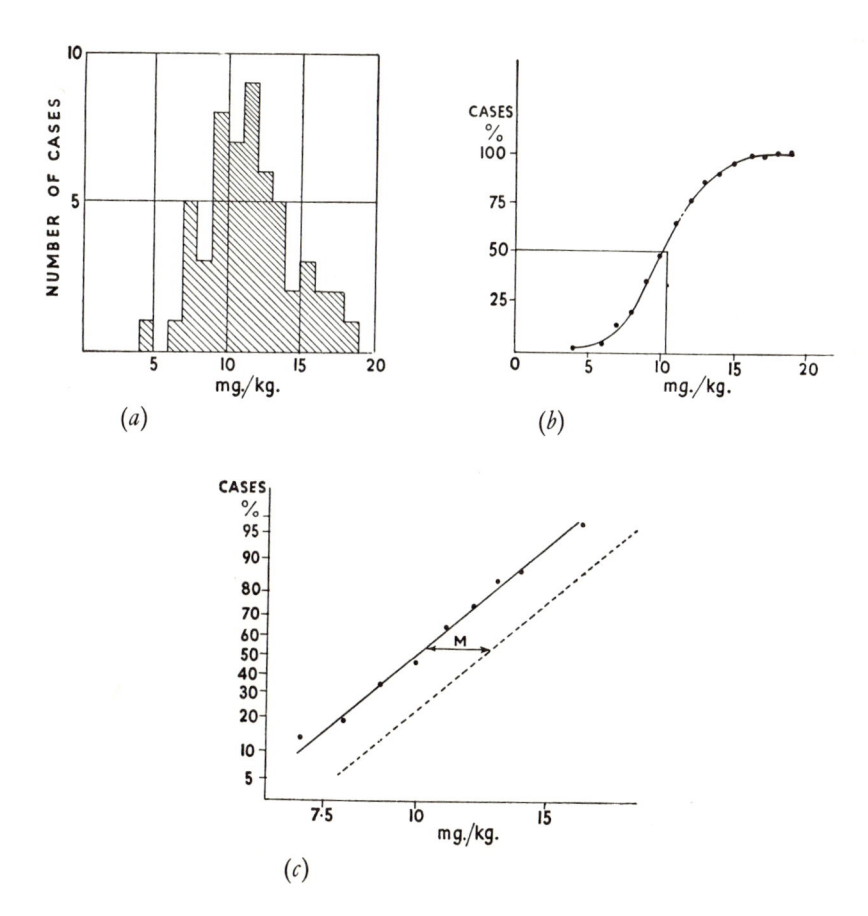

Fig. 3.10 Dosage of sodium amytal (mg per kg) needed to produce drowsiness when given by slow intravenous injection to 55 obstetric patients. (b) The same results plotted as an integrated frequency distribution. (c) The same results plotted by using a logarithmic scale for the abscissa and a probit scale for the ordinate.

Figure 3.10 shows, however, that the control of these factors does little to decrease individual variation in the response to drugs. In this case the barbiturate, sodium amytal, was slowly injected intravenously until the desired degree of drowsiness was induced. The patients were healthy women of child-bearing age and the doses were calculated in mg per kilo body weight. A comparison of Fiures 3.9 and 3.10(a) shows that the elimination of a number of possible errors has diminished but by no means abolished the scatter of results.

In cases with a wide variation in response the variation is often unevenly distributed. The *normal curve of error* or *Gaussian curve* is a symmetrical bell-shaped curve, but the curve found with drugs usually is of a skewed shape. This is shown in Figure 3.9, in which the right-hand portion of the curve shows a tail of resistant individuals. It is often found that curves of this type are converted into symmetrical distribution if the doses are plotted logarithmically. This implies that if, say, 1 per cent of the population are so susceptible that they respond to one-half the dose needed by the average individual, then 1 per cent will be so resistant that they will require twice the average dose.

Figure 3.10(a) shows that equal responses in a group of only fifty-five individuals were obtained in one case with 4 mg per kg and in another with 19 mg per kg. Figure 3.10(a) represents a frequency distribution and the diagram used to describe it is called a histogram (cf. also Fig. 3.2(a)). In Figure 3.10(b) these results are plotted in a different way as an integrated frequency distribution analogous to the digitalis data (Fig. 3.2(b)), to show the percentage of patients responding to a given dose. For example, the dose required to affect 50 per cent of the patients (ED50) is 10.5 mg per kg. Figure 3.10(c) shows yet another way of presenting the same data, using a logarithmic scale for the X axis and a probit scale for the Y axis. The symmetrical S-shaped curve of Figure 3.10(b) has now been transformed to a straight line. The significance of the probit scale is discussed in the legend to Figure 3.11. Linear transformations of this kind are frequently used for quantitative measurement of activity; for example, if another barbiturate tested in similar fashion gave results expressed by the dotted line in Figure 3.10(c), the activity ratio of the two barbiturates could be derived from the horizontal distance (M) between the two lines.

The slope of both the percentage mortality curve and the probit curve derived from it depends on the amount of scatter in the population. The greater the scatter, the flatter the slope. The amount of scatter naturally depends on the population studied. For example, a closely inbred population of animals shows less variation than an unselected mixed stock. The amount of scatter in response depends also on the drug. With some drugs such as the anaesthetics and digitalis the response is fairly uniform, whereas with other drugs there is a very wide individual variation in response.

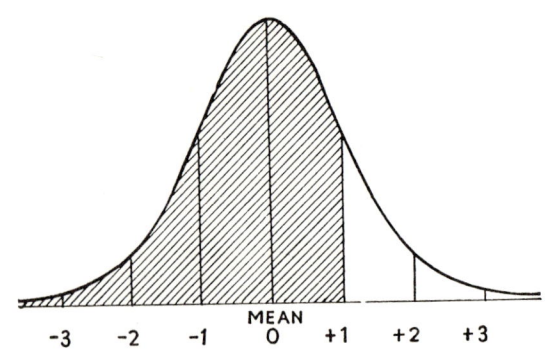

Deviation in units of standard deviation (σ).

Fig. 3.11 Explanation of probit. The figure above represents a normal or Gaussian curve. The points on the abscissa are multiples of the standard deviation called normal equivalent deviations (N.E.D.). The figure shows the relationship between a percentage scale and a N.E.D. scale. The percentage corresponding to any point on the N.E.D. axis is represented by the percentage area of the curve to the left of that point. In this example the shaded area is equal to about 84 per cent of the total area, and the N.E.D. corresponding to this percentage is +1. The probit is equal to the N.E.D. +5 and in this instance is 6. The use of the N.E.D. was introduced by Gaddum because he found that when doses are plotted on a logarithmic scale, and the percentage of animals affected on an N.E.D. scale, the points lie on approximately straight lines. The probit (probability unit) was used by Bliss in order to avoid negative numbers which occur when the N.E.D. is used.

PHARMACOGENETICS

Besides random individual variation in drug response, genetically determined differences are increasingly recognised, giving rise to the modern study of pharmacogenetics.

When the plasma concentrations resulting from the administration of a constant dose of the tuberculostatic drug isoniazid (p. 422) are measured in a large population sample, bimodal distribution curves are obtained as shown in Figure 3.12. Curves of this type suggest a genetically determined drug response. In the case of isoniazid it has been shown that human populations can be divided into slow and rapid inactivators and that the biochemical basis for high isoniazid blood levels in slow inactivators lies in the absence of an acetylating enzyme for isoniazid which is present in rapid inactivators. Slow inactivation of isoniazid is a genetic trait due to a recessive gene which occurs more frequently in certain populations (European) than in others (Japanese). The relevance of these findings is that persons who develop toxic symptoms, such as peripheral neuropathy, after treatment with isoniazid are predominantly slow acetylators.

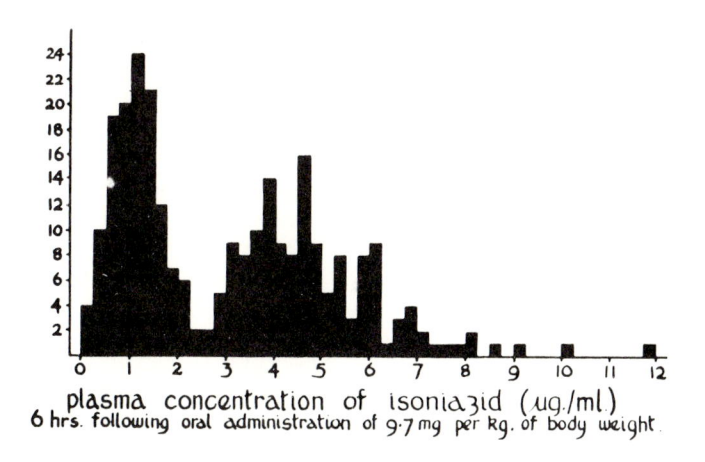

Fig. 3.12 Bimodal distribution of plasma isoniazid concentrations. 6 hours following oral administration of 9.7 mg per kg of body weight. 267 family members — 53 families. (After Price Evans, 1965, *N. Y. Acad. Sci.*)

Another drug effect depending on genetic constitution is suxamethonium apnoea (p. 306). Usually a dose of suxamethonium produces a short-lived muscular relaxation but about one subject in 3000 develops a prolonged muscular relaxation which includes paralysis of the respiratory muscles. Suxamethonium is inactivated by the enzyme serum cholinesterase and the prolonged apnoea following its administration has been shown to be due to an abnormality of serum cholinesterase by which its affinity for suxamethonium is reduced. Although the abnormality is undoubtedly genetic its precise elucidation has proved difficult because of the occurrence of several genotypes for serum cholinesterase in man with varying affinities for suxamethonium.

A genetic defect which has been estimated to affect more than a hundred million people rendering them susceptible to drug-induced haemolytic anaemia is the hereditary deficiency of glucose-6-phosphate dehydrogenase. This deficiency was discovered in connection with the haemolytic anaemia induced in some individuals by the antimalarial drug primaquine (p. 443) but it has now also been shown to induce acute haemolysis after other drugs, including sulphonamides, antimalarials and aspirin. It also increases the risk of haemolysis after ingesting fava beans.

The incidence of this trait varies according to geographical origin; it occurs particularly frequently in persons originating from Africa and the Mediterranean basin. The condition is genetically complex due to the heterogeneity of the enzyme involved. It has been suggested that the defect may carry with it certain compensating advantages, in that glucose-6-phosphate-dehydrogenase deficient individuals may show an increased resistance against falciparum malaria, which might explain the persistence of a serious genetic defect in endemic malarial regions.

THERAPEUTIC INDEX

Ehrlich recognised that a drug must be judged not only by its useful properties but also by its toxic effects. He estimated the therapeutic usefulness by measuring the minimum curative dose and comparing it with the maximum tolerated dose. In terms of Ehrlich's ideas the therapeutic index of a drug could then be defined as the ratio

$$\frac{\text{Maximum tolerated dose}}{\text{Minimum curative dose.}}$$

Unfortunately this definition fails to take into account the variability seen even in the most uniform populations, whereby a dose which is tolerated by some individuals may kill others.

A different form of therapeutic index which takes into account animal variability is expressed by the ratio

$$\frac{LD_{50}}{ED_{50}}$$

which is the ratio of the dose which kills 50 per cent of a group of animals, the median lethal dose, and the dose which produces a desired pharmacological effect in 50 per cent, the median effective dose.

This method of expressing the therapeutic index is widely used in animal experimentation because it is statistically reliable and data can be plotted on a probit scale. However, unlike Ehrlich's ratio, this ratio does not give the margin between a safe dose and a generally effective dose. Various proposals have been made to produce a more meaningful index whilst taking into account animal variability. One proposal is to employ the ratio

$$\frac{LD_1}{ED_{99}}$$

as a 'margin of safety' index giving a dose that is usually safe and a dose that is usually effective. A disadvantage of this index is that extreme probit values carry little statistical weight. Particularly serious difficulties arise when the LD and ED probit line are not parallel.

Assessment of the therapeutic value of a drug

The quantitative assessment of the therapeutic value of a drug in terms of its activity and toxicity in man is generally difficult. In principle there are two ways in which this can be attempted:

1. By quantal assays measuring in series of subjects the incidence of 'therapeutic' and toxic effects in order to establish a therapeutic ratio. Gold recorded the number of patients vomiting with increasing doses of digitoxin comparing it with the number showing inversion of the T-wave. Toxic dose determinations (vomiting) were necessarily limited to the lower ranges of the dose-response curve but it was possible to obtain a therapeutic ratio by comparing the doses producing vomiting and T-wave inversion in the same proportion of subjects.

2. By graded assays comparing the *relative* activities and toxicities of two different drugs. Seed et al compared morphine and dihydrocodeine in man measuring quantitatively by graded bioassays their relative analgesic and respiratory depressant effects. The analgesic assay was carried out by the method of Figure 3.7. Respiratory depression (the toxic effect) was measured by a rise in alveolar pCO_2. The relative analgesic and respiratory depressant activities of morphine and dihydrocodeine were not statistically different. There was thus no difference between the two drugs in terms of therapeutic ratio.

Examples of quantitative measurement of a therapeutic ratio in man are rare. This derives from the fact that the clinical consensus has been that it is not possible to summarise the multifactorial beneficial and deleterious effects of drugs employed in man in terms of a precise mathematical formula.

Since it has not been possible to apply precise and comprehensive standards of drug safety and effectiveness in man, the Food and Drug Administration of the United States has adopted a general formula, referred to as the *benefit-to-risk ratio*, in assessing new drugs. This ratio balances the therapeutic value of a drug against its inherent risks, taking into account the seriousness of the disease to be treated and the availability of less toxic (i.e. safer) and more reliable (i.e. more effective) drugs. Thus even a drug which carries a significant risk of side effects may be approved if its therapeutic value outweighs its hazards.

ASSESSMENT OF DRUG TOXICITY

Before a new drug is submitted for clinical trial it is necessary to determine its toxic effects in a number of species. The choice of species for toxicity studies will be determined by a knowledge of the pharmacological properties of the drug and its distribution, metabolism and excretion. In acute and sub-acute toxicity tests, three or more species are used, one of which should be non-rodent. Several dose levels of the drug should be studied, given by at least three different routes of administration. For long-term or chronic toxicity studies the selection of species is guided by the results obtained from acute toxicity tests and from preliminary evidence of the metabolic pattern of the drug in man. Several dose levels should be used, including those related to the proposed clinical dose. Throughout the course of these experiments detailed observations are made on the appearance, behaviour and changes in body weight; periodic haematological and urine analyses are also performed and histological examination of biopsy specimens of important organs may provide valuable information. Detailed post mortem studies should include comprehensive histological examination of a wide range of tissues including the liver, kidney, gonads and other endocrine glands, the heart, brain and the eyes. Special investigations using histochemical and electron microscopic techniques are important adjuncts for detecting changes, for example in the endoplasmic reticulum of liver cells indicative that enzyme induction has occurred.

Carcinogenic and mutagenic tests

When preliminary observations of single dose administration in human subjects have shown that the drug is worthy of initial small scale clinical trial, more extensive animal toxicity tests are initiated. These include long-term tests for carcinogenicity. The assessment of carcinogenic risk involves prolonged, detailed and exacting studies, the results of which unfortunately are not always conclusive. A lack of evidence of tumour induction is the only available criterion of non-carcinogenicity. Rats, mice and hamsters are generally regarded as the most suitable species for these tests. In special circumstances, tests with other species are sometimes used; for example, the dog is used for testing suspected bladder carcinogens of the aromatic amine group and monkeys for testing certain hormone preparations. In carcinogenicity tests it is important that the highest dose level should be within the toxic range, but should be consistent with prolonged survival of the majority of the animals; for rats and hamsters the tests should continue for at least two years.

The evaluation of a drug in respect to carcinogenic hazards should take into account the recommended clinical uses of the drug; the fact that long continued exposure to a substance is necessary before a positive response has been observed in animal carcinogenicity tests, may not preclude the clinical use of the drug on a single occasion in any one individual, nor its use where the therapeutic benefits are deemed to outweigh carcinogenic risk. To determine whether prolonged use of a drug may present a potential hazard to man by causing gene mutations or chormosome aberrations, special tests for mutagenecity are undertaken. No single test or battery of tests is likely to detect and characterise all mutagenic agents, and a variety of *in vitro* and *in vivo* non-mammalian and mammalian test systems are used; other special techniques include human cell culture tests and chromosome examinations of somatic and germ cells.

Tests for teratogenicity
These tests have become an important part of the screening programme for the development of new drugs. The adverse effects of drugs on the developing embryo when tissue differentiation occurs has necessitated the use of a variety of methods for assessing the potential risks of functional or biochemical disturbance in the embryo. This subject is further discussed on page 225.

In the development and introduction of a new drug there are four main stages: animal studies, initial observations in man, limited clinical trials and formal therapeutic trials. After the drug is marketed a system of clinical monitoring of adverse reactions is arranged, whereby voluntary reports from doctors in hospitals and general practice are sent to the company concerned with marketing the drug or to a drug monitoring registry. In addition a systematic study of selected hospitals and representative samples of general practice communities is arranged to assess the nature and incidence of adverse reactions in relation to the prescribed uses of the drug. By the use of epidemiological techniques and the collation of evidence from different countries under the auspices of the World Health Organisation it should be possible to assemble and interpret rapidly the significance of reports of adverse reactions.

ADVERSE EFFECTS OF DRUGS IN MAN

Despite all the precautions against toxic effects which result from appropriate animal studies, some toxic effects which occur in man may be of an entirely different nature from those observed in animal experiments. Some anticonvulsant drugs used in the treatment of epilepsy produce side effects which could not have been foretold by animal experiments; for example phenytoin produces hyperplasia of gums and troxidone causes photophobia. Sometimes these and other drugs may produce severe adverse effects such as megaloblastic anaemia or blood dyscrasias. A variety of skin rashes of varying degrees of severity may arise during treatment with many types of drugs. Renal damage from the prolonged use of phenacetin and other analgesics, and Parkinsonism during treatment with phenothiazine drugs are other examples of toxic hazards first revealed after the drugs had been in use for many months or even years.

It has become essential, therefore, for all who prescribe and administer drugs to have some appreciation of the various types of adverse reactions that may arise quite suddenly and unexpectedly in the course of treatment. No hard and fast rules can be laid down concerning the relation between a drug and the particular type of toxic effect associated with its use but it is important that any such serious reaction occurring in a patient should be recorded in the notes pertaining to his medical records.

Classification of unwanted effects
The unwanted effects produced by drugs in man can be conveniently classified as follows (Rosenheim).

Overdosage. These may arise from a single large dose or by cumulation after repeated doses and are usually shown as an exaggerated form of the pharmacological actions typical of the drug. Overdosage of an anticoagulant drug used for the prevention of clotting results in haemorrhage and overdosage of an adrenergic neurone blocking drug used for the treatment of hypertension results in orthostatic hypotension.

Side effects. This terms is used to describe therapeutically undesirable but unavoidable effects of drugs, such as dryness of the mouth and impairment of accommodation when atropine or related drugs are used to inhibit gastric secretion and motility in the treatment of peptic ulcer. Drowsiness is often associated with the use of methyldopa in hypertension and most antihistamine preparations are liable to give rise to this unwanted effect.

Secondary effects. These may arise indirectly as a consequence of the action of a drug, such as the occurrence of moniliasis in patients given prolonged treatment with a tetracycline; chelation with calcium is another property of such drugs and tetracycline therapy during pregnancy may result in yellow pigmentation of teeth when they erupt during normal development of the infant.

Intolerance. A lowered threshold to a normal pharmacological action of the drug, e.g. some patients may develop orthostatic hypotension after a relatively small dose of chlorpromazine.

Idiosyncrasy. This term is used to describe a qualitatively abnormal reaction to a drug. An example is the haemolytic anaemia which occurs in some patients after taking the antimalarial drug primaquine. This appears to be due to a genetic deficiency as described on page 29.

Hypersensitivity or allergic reactions. These are mediated by an antigen-antibody reaction and usually involve previous exposure and sensitisation to the drug, e.g. urticarial or asthmatic reactions caused by penicillin or aspirin. Allergic drug reactions are discussed on page 103.

THERAPEUTIC TRIALS

The object of a therapeutic trial is to determine whether a drug is of use in the treatment of disease. A trial of this kind must be carefully planned in order to eliminate the possibility that an observed effect may be due to factors unconnected with the drug. The subjects should be divided into two groups which are equivalent in all respects except for the difference in treatment. Trials should preferably be arranged in such a way that patients treated with one drug are compared with patients given another drug at the same place and at the same time.

A drug may be compared with another drug or with an inert substance but when a drug is tested in severely ill patients the administration of a placebo (dummy drug) may be unnecessary or even undesirable. In such cases it is usual to give the best available treatment to two groups of patients and to supplement in one group the drug under test. To eliminate bias, the patients are usually allotted to one of the two groups by random selection, and it is an advantage if the clinician who assesses the patient's response does not know which of the two treatments the patient has received.

The effect of the drug should be measured not only by the apparent change in the well-being and general condition of the patients but also by objective measurements depending on the type of disease, for example, changes in temperature, sedimentation rate or radiological and bacteriological evidence. If this is impossible as in trials of analgesic drugs which depend entirely on subjective changes it is particularly important that neither the patient nor the observer should know which drug has been taken.

The results of a therapeutic trial are more likely to be significant if the clinical state of the patient is sharply defined. For example the streptomycin trial described in Chapter 34 was restricted to patients with 'acute progressive bilateral pulmonary tuberculosis of presumably recent origin, bacteriologically proved, unsuitable for collapse therapy, age group 15 to 25'. This trial gave the first unequivocal evidence on a relatively small number of patients of the value of streptomycin in the treatment of pulmonary tuberculosis.

Application of statistical methods to drug trials

Statistical methods can be legitimately applied to every unbiased drug trial, i.e. one in which patients have been allocated at random to the various treatment and control groups. Statistics can be applied not only to large numbers but also to small samples, and it is particularly important in a drug trial to reduce to a minimum the number of human subjects involved. The object of the statistical analysis is to find out whether the drug under study has produced an effect which is statistically significant, i.e. whether the difference between the treatment and control group is such that it is unlikely to have arisen merely by chance. Thus the analysis usually ends with a test of statistical significance. Differences which would have arisen by chance less than 1 in 20 times are regarded by general convention as statistically *significant* and those arising less than 1 in 100 times as *highly significant*. It must be emphasised, however, that a statistically non-significant result in a drug trial does not signify that the drug is ineffective, it may simply be that insufficient subjects, or the wrong subjects, or the wrong dosage have been used. Statistical non-significance is merely a verdict of non-proven.

Amongst the many tests of statistical significance available a few are distinguished by their wide applicability to pharmacological problems involving small numbers. Information on the uses and limitations of these tests must be sought in appropriate books on statistical methods. Although they may be based on the same general principles, different tests are applicable to different situations, for example enumeration (all or none) data require different statistical treatment from measurement (graded) data. Some of the most widely used statistical tests are as follows:

The chi-square test is applicable to enumeration data and suitable for the comparison of numbers of individuals in different treatment groups. The data in Table 34.1, giving numbers of patients showing improvement after streptomycin, as compared with a control group, were assessed by a chi-square test and the difference between the two groups was found to be statistically significant.

The t-test can be applied to data resulting from the measurement of some continuous variate like weight or blood pressure. The t-test can be used in two principal ways: (1) to compare sets of two measurements in the same individual, i.e. after a drug and after a placebo, and (2) to compare the means obtained from measurements on two different groups.

The analysis of variance can be considered as an extension of the t-test applicable to more complex situations. For example the measurements recorded in Figure 3.4(b) required an analysis of variance for the assessment of their statistical significance.

Ranking tests. These are non-parametric tests applicable to scores which are not truly numerical. Although parametric tests such as the t-test are frequently applied to such data, their basically non-numerical character introduces distortions which are avoided in ranking tests. For example, two groups of school children given different diets may be compared in terms of their rank in class.

Sequential trials. In this type of experiment a continuous statistical analysis is made as the data from each subject become available. The trial is stopped when a clear-cut verdict of statistical significance or non-significance emerges. Figure 3.13 shows a chart for plotting the results of a sequential trial. For each subject who considered codeine compound tablets to be more effective, a cross was

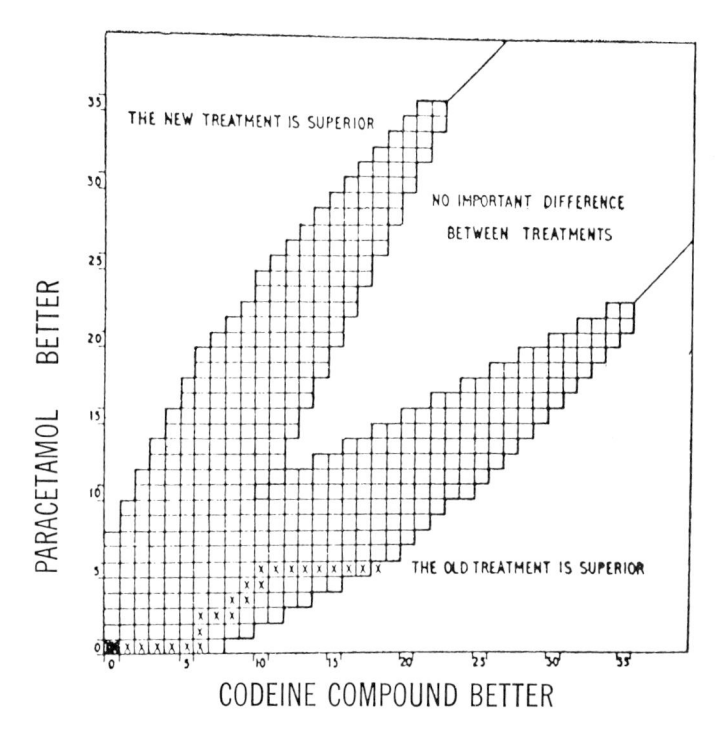

Fig. 3.13 Chart showing result of test using the method of sequential analysis. (see text) (After Newton and Tanner, 1956. *Brit. med. J.*)

placed to the right of the previous cross, and for each who preferred paracetamol tablets, a cross was placed above the previous cross. The trial ended when the boundary favouring codeine compound tablets was reached. The chief advantage of a sequential trial is the saving in the number of subjects since the number to be included in the trial need not be decided upon at the start.

FURTHER READING

Aldridge W N (ed) 1971 Mechanisms of toxicity. Macmillan, London
Armitage P 1960 Sequential medical trials. Blackwell, Oxford
Bain W A 1949 Discussion on antihistamine drugs. Proc. Roy. Soc. Med. 42: 615
Bliss C I 1952 The statistics of bioassay. Academic Press, New York
Burn J H, Finney D J, Goodwin L G 1950 Biological standardisation. Oxford University Press
Colquhoun D 1971 Lectures on biostatistics. Clarendon Press, Oxford
Finney D J 1964 Statistical method in biological assay. Griffin, London
Finney D J 1950 Biological assay. Br. Med. Bull. 7: 292
Gaddum J H 1954 Clinical pharmacology. Proc. Roy. Soc. Med. 47: 195
Gorrod J W (ed) 1973 Drug toxicity. Taylor & Francis, London
Harris E L, Fitzgerald J D (eds) 1970 The principles and practice of clinical trials. Churchill Livingstone, Edinburgh
Hill A B 1971 Principles of medical statistics. The Lancet, London
Houde R W, Wallenstein S L, Beaver W T 1965 In: de Stevens (ed) Clincal measurement of pain in analgetics. Academic Press, New York
Lader M H, Wing L 1966 Physiological measures, sedative drugs and morbid anxiety. Maudsley Mongr. Oxford University Press
Laurence D R (ed) 1959 Quantative methods in human pharmacology and therapeutics. Pergamon, Oxford
Levine R 1978 Pharmacology. Drug actions and reactions. Little Brown, Philadelphia
Loomis T A 1978 Essentials of toxicology. Henry Kempton, London
Mainland D 1963 Elementary medical statistics. Saunders, Philadelphia
Myerscough P R, Schild H O 1958 Quantitative assays of oxytocic drugs on the human postpartum uterus. Brit. J. Pharmac. 13: 207
Oldham P D 1968 Measurement in medicine. English University Press, London
Remington R D, Schork M A 1970 Statistics. Applications to biological and health sciences. Prentice Hall, London
Richards D J, Rondel R K (ed) 1972 Adverse drug reactions. Churchill Livingstone, Edinburgh
Schild H O 1942 A method of conducting a biological assay on a preparation giving repeated graded responses illustrated by the estimation of histamine. J. Physiol. 101: 115
Seed J C, Wallenstein S L, Houde R W, Bellville J W 1958 A comparison of the analgesic and respiratory effects of dihydrocodeine and morphine in man. Arch. Int. Pharmacodyn. 96: 293
Snedecor G W, Cochran W G 1967 Statistical methods. Ames, Iowa
Stewart G A, Young P A 1963 Statistics as applied to pharmacological and toxicological screening. Progr. Medic. Chem. 3: 187
Walpole A L, Spinks A (eds) 1958 The Evaluation of Drug Toxicity. Churchill, London

4. Absorption, distribution and fate of drugs

Physicochemical factors controlling absorption 34; Absorption of drugs from alimentary tract 36; Rate of absorption 36; Absorption from mouth, stomach, intestine 36; Absorption of electrolytes 36; Specific carriers 37; Salt and water absorption 37; Particle size and absorption 37; Bioavailability 38; Delayed absorption 39; Body fluid compartments 39; Blood-brain barrier 40; Penetration into fat depots 41; Binding to plasma proteins 41; Metabolism of drugs 42; Hepatic microsomal enzymes 43; Interaction of MAO inhibitors with foods and drugs 44; Drug excretion by kidney 44; Secretory mechanisms for drugs 45; Pharmacokinetics 45; Exponential elimination 46; Biological half life 47; Drug cumulation 47; Frequency of administration 48.

Drugs can be divided into two classes, placebos and substances which are intended to produce a definite pharmacological action. The use of placebos is psychotherapy and not pharmacology, and hence in this chapter it is only necessary to consider the latter class. In most cases it is necessary to produce an adequate effect for an adequate time, and therefore both the intensity and the duration of action must be considered. As a general rule, the action depends on the presence of an adequate concentration of drug in the fluids bathing the tissues and on the susceptibility of the cells to the drug. The concentration attained by the drug around the cells on which it acts depends on absorption, distribution and clearance. The physico-chemical factors which control drug absorption are important because they determine whether a drug can reach its site of action.

ABSORPTION OF DRUGS

A drug may have to penetrate a succession of cellular membranes to reach its site of action in the body. If a drug is administered orally and its site of action is on the central nervous system it must first penetrate the cells of the gastrointestinal epithelium and subsequently the blood brain barrier. Brodie has pointed out that the gastrointestinal tract, the brain, the tubules of the kidney, the eye and the placenta can be considered to be surrounded by protective membranes, which are in fact layers of cells controlling the uptake of substances into these organs. The intestine is lined by a sheath of epithelial cells so closely packed as to form a practically continuous boundary. When a substance is absorbed it must first enter the epithelial cells and be transferred across them to reach the fluid of the lamina propria and finally the blood and lymph capillaries.

Physico-chemical factors controlling absorption

Electron-microscopic studies indicate that the cell membrane is essentially a double layer of oriented lipid molecules sandwiched between two stretched polypeptide layers. The cell membrane also possesses minute pores through which hydrophilic molecules like water itself, urea, glycerol and small ions such as chloride and potassium can pass. The capillary wall and the glomeruli of the kidney contain much wider pores which allow larger molecules to pass, although they will not normally allow the passage of plasma proteins.

Drugs and nutrients may pass across membranes by processes which are passive or active. Passive transport involves processes such as diffusion which do not require metabolic energy. Active transport occurs against a chemical or electrical potential gradient and requires the expenditure of metabolic energy. The chief mechanisms of drug transfer across membranes are as follows.

Diffusion through lipid phase of cell membrane.
Non-polar substances dissolve in the cell membrane and cross it by diffusion; ions cannot penetrate in this way since they are not lipid-soluble. Penetration of non-polar substances is favoured by a high lipid/water partition coefficient and in the case of weak acids and bases by the presence of a high proportion of lipid-soluble unionised forms. An intravenous injection of thiopentone which is poorly ionised will be followed by its rapid accumulation into the brain whereas a similar injection of tubocurarine which is a fully ionised quaternary ammonium compound will not reach the brain because it cannot penetrate the blood-brain barrier.

An interesting consequence of this mechanism is that if the pH on the two sides of a membrane is different the distribution of a weak electrolyte on the two sides of the membrane will also be different. This is illustrated in Figure 4.1 which shows this phenomenon for a weak acid in the stomach. Only the unionised form is permeable and it will reach the same concentration on both sides at equilibrium, but the amount of ionised form present will depend on pH in accordance with the Henderson-Hasselbalch equation:

for an acid and
$$pK_a = pH + \log \frac{C_u}{C_i}$$

$$pK_a = pH + \log \frac{C_i}{C_u}$$

for a base where C_u is the concentration of the unionised form and C_i that of the ionised form.

In the present case the ionised form, and hence the total concentration, is much less in the acidic lumen than in the

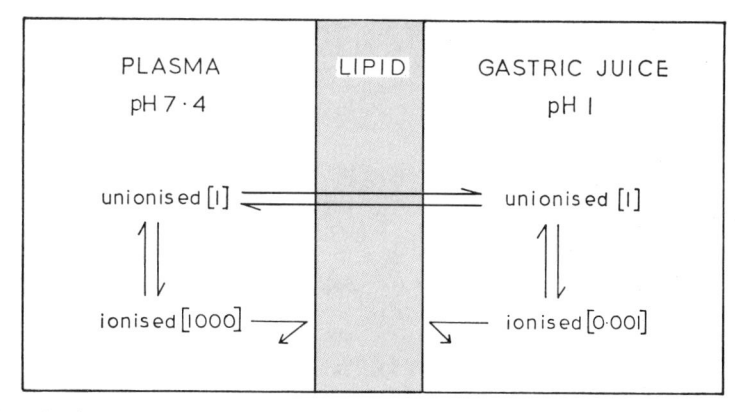

Fig. 4.1 Distribution of a weak acid between plasma and gastric juice separated by a lipid membrane permeable only to the unionised form of the drug. (Modified from Brodie, 1964, in *Absorption & Distribution of Drugs*, ed. Binns. Livingstone, Edinburgh.)

neutral blood stream. It follows that a weak acid present in the lumen is rapidly absorbed into the blood, whereas a weak base present in the blood stream is rapidly excreted into the lumen of the stomach. These relationships have been verified experimentally in man with reasonable accuracy. Thus it has been found that a weak acid such as aspirin is rapidly absorbed from the human stomach, whereas ephedrine, which is a weak base, is not absorbed.

Another factor which influences the distribution of drugs across membranes is their degree of protein binding. For example aspirin is more concentrated in blood plasma than in tissue fluids because of the greater protein content of the former. One of the reasons why few drugs distribute evenly between extracellular and intracellular fluid is the different degree of protein binding in the two media.

Filtration through pores
Hydrophilic lipid-insoluble substances can cross membranes through water-filled pores. When a hydrostatic or osmotic pressure difference exists across a membrane, water flows in bulk through the membrane pores, carrying with it any solute molecules whose dimensions are less than those of the pores. The evidence for this is that the diffusion rates for most 'hydrophilic substances depend on their molecular radius. These pores may allow the penetration of small molecules, like urea, into cells and the passage of larger molecules across the capillary wall. The water that filters across the glomerular membrane of the kidney carries with it all the solutes of plasma except large protein molecules of the size of albumin.

Facilitated diffusion
This follows the concentration gradient but does not obey simple diffusion laws. An example of facilitated diffusion is the penetration of sugars through the red cell membrane which is believed to involve a carrier mechanism.

Active transport
This is a process in which a solute moves across a membrane against an electrochemical gradient: either against a concentration gradient or, if the solute is charged, against a potential gradient, or some combination of the two. Active transport involves metabolic energy and a characteristic feature of it is that it can be blocked by metabolic inhibitors such as dinitrophenol. It can also be inhibited competitively by any other substance which utilises the same transport mechanism. Active transport often shows specificity for a particular type of chemical structure and the transport mechanism can become saturated when the concentration of the substance gets too high. Examples of active transport involving metabolic energy are the extrusion of sodium ions by nerve and muscle; the secretion of hydrogen ions by the stomach; the reabsorption of glucose and the secretion of penicillin by the tubules of the kidney.

Active transport is often envisaged in terms of a carrier mechanism. The carrier may itself be an ion with a charge opposite to that of the ion to be transferred. Alternatively a carrier may have a specific configuration capable of accepting only a limited range of molecules. Specific carriers are responsible for the absorption of glucose and of amino acids by the intestine. In the kidney at least two carrier mechanisms exist (p. 45), one for the secretion of acidic compounds including penicillin, probenecid, diodrast and phenol red and the other for basic compounds containing the quaternary ammonium group and amines. Both the acidic and the basic mechanisms are competitive so that the transport of one substance can be blocked by an excess of another substance in the same group.

Pinocytosis
This is an entirely different type of transport in which cells engulf small droplets of extracellular fluid. Pinocytosis can be observed in amoebae and in tissue culture cells and it probably also occurs in mammals. Its role is not fully

understood but it has been suggested that it might account for the uptake of protein in the gastrointestinal tract of infants or for the resorption of liquid droplets in the alveoli.

Absorption of drugs from alimentary canal

Rate of absorption

The great majority of drugs are given by mouth. If a tablet is placed under the tongue, considerable absorption occurs from the mucous membrane of the mouth, and this is a simple method of obtaining a rapid action with such drugs as nitroglycerin or isoprenaline. Some drugs, notably alcohol and aspirin, can be rapidly absorbed from the stomach, but generally absorption of a drug does not commence until it passes through the pyloric sphincter, hence the time of commencement of absorption depends on the activity of the stomach and may vary from a few minutes to more than two hours.

When a drug is swallowed with a considerable volume of water on an empty stomach, it passes rapidly through the pylorus; if the drug is irritant and swallowed with little or no fluid, it may cause closure of the pyloric sphincter and hence absorption will be irregular in onset. The absorption of drugs taken after a meal is variable. If the drug is non-irritant and taken with a large amount of fluid, the fluid may pass rapidly along the lesser curvature and into the pylorus, but if the volume of fluid is small the drug will mix with the food mass and pass more slowly through the pyloric sphincter. In general the time required for absorption of about three-quarters of a dose of drug is usually between one and three hours.

The gastric functions are deranged by many diseases and in particular by fever, hence it is unsafe to assume that the rate of absorption in a sick person will be similar to that which occurs in health. It is probable that in disease, absorption may sometimes be considerably delayed. A gross delay in absorption is often a possible reason for a drug, such as a hypnotic, failing to produce its usual effect.

Absorption from mouth

The lining of the mucous membrane of the mouth behaves as a lipoidal barrier for the passage of drugs. Their rate of absorption is determined by the proportion of unionised drug present at the pH of the mouth, which is about pH 6, and its lipid solubility.

Unionised lipid soluble compounds, including nitroglycerin, methyltestosterone and oestradiol, are absorbed through the oral mucosa. Buccal administration is especially advantageous for steroids which are acid labile or rapidly metabolised by the liver since the acidic stomach and the portal circulation are bypassed. High molecular weight compounds such as heparin and proteins such as insulin are not appreciably absorbed.

Beckett and his colleagues have developed a buccal absorption test in which the subject's mouth is rinsed for 5 min with a buffered drug solution which is then expelled and analysed. They found that absorption could be entirely accounted for by the lipid solubility of the undissociated moiety; for example at pH 9.2 over 70 per cent of a solution of amphetamine was absorbed whilst at pH 6 none was absorbed. Absorption increased linearly with the concentration of drug and there was no selectivity in the uptake of optical enantiomorphs of amphetamine suggesting diffusion rather than active transport.

Absorption from stomach

It was formerly believed that only a few exceptional substances such as alcohol are absorbed from the stomach but it is now known that drugs which are weak acids are absorbed to an appreciable extent from the stomach. Aspirin is practically undissociated at pH 1 and is therefore absorbed from the stomach. If the gastric contents are made alkaline with sodium bicarbonate, it is not absorbed. Bases are generally not absorbed from the stomach.

Absorption from intestine

Intestinal absorption may be studied *in vivo* and *in vitro*. The simplest and most reliable method is to measure the amount of drug that has disappeared at various times from the gastrointestinal tract of unanaesthetised animals. A quantity of drug is administered, the animal is killed after a specified time, and the entire gastrointestinal tract removed and assayed for remaining non-absorbed drug. Before disappearance can be equated with absorption it must of course be shown that the drug is not destroyed within the lumen of the canal.

A more controlled method of measuring disappearance of a substance from the lumen of the gut is by 'perfusion *in vivo*'. This involves perfusing the lumen of a length of gut from a drug reservoir, the blood supply being left intact, and analysing the effluent.

A frequently used *in vitro* technique is based on the use of everted sacs of small intestine. A length of rat or hamster intestine is everted so that the mucosal surface is on the outside; it is then placed in oxygenated saline-buffer containing the drug and the amount transported inside the sac (the serosal side) is measured.

Clinical methods involve the measurement of blood and urine levels of a drug after oral administration. This approach is often used to compare various doses and dosage forms of drugs, e.g. antibiotics, rather than to analyse absorption *per se*.

Intestinal absorption of electrolytes. The original suggestion made by Höber, of a lipid-pore structure of the intestinal epithelium has been largely vindicated by later work. Very small hydrophilic molecules of the size of urea or mannitol are rapidly absorbed through membrane pores; larger molecules are absorbed by diffusion through a lipid phase.

When solutions of various drugs are perfused through rat small intestine their rate of absorption is related to their degree of ionisation. Weak acids and bases are well absorbed and strong acids and bases are poorly absorbed (Fig. 4.2).

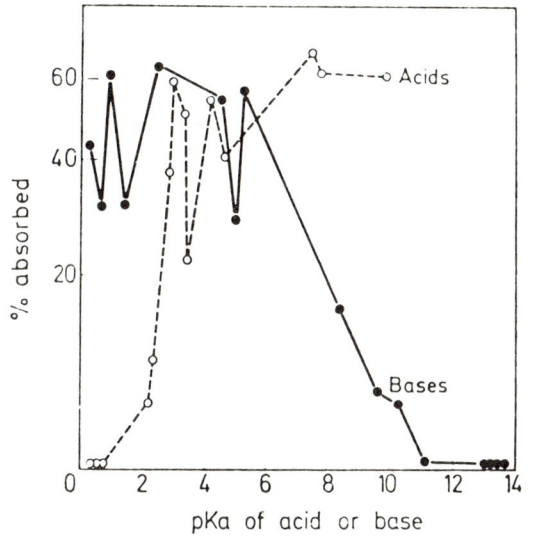

Fig. 4.2 Intestinal absorption in the rat of drugs in relation to their pK_a values. (After Schanker, Tocco, Brodie and Hogben, 1958, *J. Pharmacol.*)

Although organic ions cross the intestinal epithelium much more slowly than uncharged molecules, they can be absorbed; for example 5 to 10 per cent of an oral dose of hexamethonium is absorbed in man. The mechanism of absorption of quaternary compounds is not well understood; it has been suggested that they may be absorbed as complexes with some endogenous phosphatide.

Intestinal transport by specific carriers. Many foodstuffs, including amino acids and glucose, are taken up from the intestine by 'carriers' possessing specific attachment sites which can carry hydrophilic substances through lipoid membranes. Carrier mechanisms are usually highly specialised, for example different amino acids are believed to be carried by separate carriers. Carrier transport is characterised by stereospecificity, saturation kinetics and competition.

Some drugs which are sufficiently similar to natural substrates are transported by carrier mechanisms. For example the anticancer agent 5-fluorouracil (p. 381) is transported across the intestinal epithelium by the same carrier mechanism which transports the related natural pyrimidines uracil and thymine. It has been shown by experiments *in vitro* that active carrier transport of drugs from the mucosal to the serosal side of the intestine can take place against substantial concentration gradients.

Conceivably, carrier mechanisms will be utilised in the future for designing new drugs. For example it might be possible to couple an active drug with an amino acid, thus ensuring its rapid uptake by the intestine.

Absorption of inorganic salts and water. The mechanism of transport of sodium chloride from the intestine has been the source of much controversy. The absorption of sodium chloride from the lumen of the intestine into the blood against a considerable chemical gradient requires the expenditure of energy which may be required for the active transport of sodium or chloride or both. Different mechanisms operate in different parts of the gastrointestinal tract. Thus it is believed that in the colon Na^+ is actively absorbed and Cl^- passively absorbed, whilst in the stomach Cl^- is actively secreted and Na^+ moves passively. Complicating factors are the variable electrical potential gradients which exist across the wall of the gastrointestinal tract.

Movements of water in the intestine are largely due to osmotic gradients. It is known that a hypertonic solution placed in the lumen of the intestine becomes diluted by movement of water from blood to lumen whilst hypotonic solutions in the lumen lead to water movements in the opposite direction.

The intestinal absorption of divalent cations is slow and unreliable and the body has developed various special mechanisms for their transport. Calcium and ferrous iron are examples of divalent inorganic ions required by the body. A feature of calcium absorption is the ability of the body to increase its calcium absorptive capacity during periods of low calcium intake, provided there is an adequate supply of vitamin D (p. 363). Similarly when there is a deficiency in iron, as in pregnancy, absorption of iron from the intestine is increased. There is evidence that iron is transported by a special carrier substance, called transferrin (p. 203).

Influence of particle size on intestinal absorption

The rate of dissolution of a solid drug is an important factor determining its rate of absorption from the gastrointestinal tract. Figure 4.3 shows the effect of dissolution rate upon absorption of different preparations of aspirin.

Solution of a drug starts from the surface. Since the surface/volume ratio increases as the radius decreases, a high degree of subdivision will produce a large surface area and hence rapid solution and absorption. The relationship between surface area and rate of solution can be expressed mathematically by the Noyes-Whitney equation

$$\frac{da}{dt} = KS(C^s - C)$$

where a = amount of drug, t = time, K = a constant incorporating temperature, turbulence, pH and other factors, S = surface area of drug, C = concentration of dissolved drug and C_s = saturated concentration of drug. It is seen that the rate of solution is proportional to the surface and decreases as drug saturation is approached.

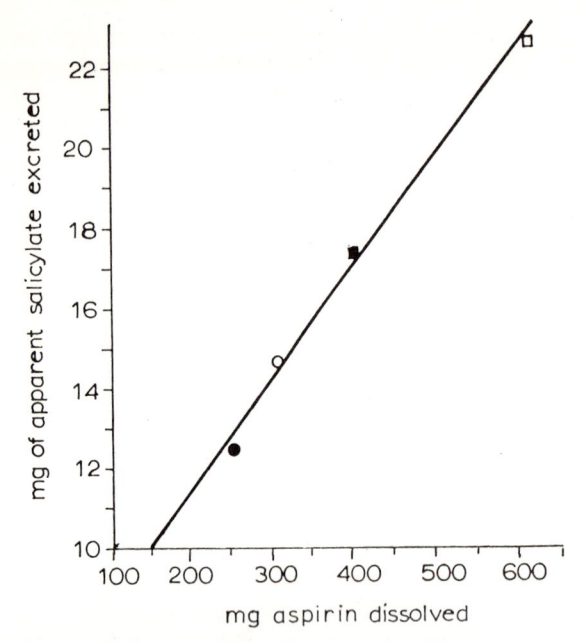

Fig. 4.3 Mean amount of salicylate excreted by 12 subjects (1 hour after the administration of 0.65 g of aspirin) against *in vitro* solution rate (mean amount of aspirin dissolved in 10 minutes) of four different formulations of aspirin. (After Levy, Gumtow and Rutowski, 1961, *Canad. Med. Ass. J.*)

In practice saturation may not be reached if the drug is absorbed as soon as it is dissolved. The above equation then simplifies to

$$\frac{da}{dt} = KSC_s$$

showing that solution rate is proportional to the saturated concentration or solubility of the drug.

The pharmaceutical formulation of a drug may have a complex effect on the rate of absorption as shown by the following example. Oral penicillin (phenoxymethylpenicillin, p. 402) may be formulated as the free acid or as the potassium salt. The potassium salt of oral penicillin is readily soluble in the acid environment of the stomach, where the penicillin acid will be liberated. The free penicillin acid is at once precipitated, giving rise to a suspension of very fine particles. Each particle becomes surrounded by a film of gastric fluid which rapidly gets saturated with penicillin, which then diffuses into the surrounding area. The dispersed weak acid becomes rapidly absorbed from the stomach producing a high peak blood level. By contrast, if the acid form of oral penicillin is ingested as such, it fails to dissolve appreciably in the acid milieu of the stomach and does not become absorbed until it reaches the intestine where the pH is more favourable for solution. The drug is then absorbed, giving rise to a lower and more protracted blood level.

Since particle size is an important factor which may influence drug action, it is now recognised that a drug formulated by one manufacturer may not be therapeutically equivalent to one prepared by another manufacturer unless compared by appropriate clinical trial. Several examples of this type of problem, usually referred to as *bioavailability* of a drug have been encountered with formulations of griseofulvin, an antifungal antibiotic; other examples include phenindione, an anticoagulant, and formulations of corticosteroids.

Bioavailability
Bioavailability means the fraction of drug reaching the site of action but since this cannot be precisely measured the usual definition of bioavailability is the percentage drug reaching the systemic circulation. By this criterion the bioavailability of an intravenous drug dose is one; that of an oral dose is less than one because of incomplete absorption and elimination by the liver through drug metabolism and excretion in the bile — the *first pass effect*.

In clinical practice bioavailability has been difficult to measure. It is sometimes defined as the time integral of plasma concentration but this can be an inadequate measure unless the plasma profile of drug is also taken into account. Thus, in a trial in which equal doses of two preparations of oral digoxin were given to normal subjects, formulation A gave high peak plasma levels and short half lives, whilst formulation B gave low peak levels and long half times, but only A produced untoward central effects such as nausea. When the two preparations were tested *in vitro*, A had a much faster dissolution rate than B. It has since become an official requirement of both BP and USP to test the rate of dissolution of digoxin.

Differences in bioavailability. These can be due to a number of factors including differences in tablet disintegration time. The bioavailability of different drugs is greatly dependent on the first pass effect. Metabolism by the liver plays a predominant part in the clearance of many lipophilic drugs; for example orally administered hexobarbitone is 99 per cent destroyed in the liver rendering its oral bioavailability extremely low. By contrast, drugs such as ephedrine or amphetamine which are hydrophilic and cleared largely by the kidneys have high oral bioavailability.

The term *bioinequivalence* refers to differences between formulations of the same drug. Bioinequivalence has been demonstrated for different preparations of digoxin, phenytoin, levodopa, aspirin and many other drugs. It has often been used as an argument for prescribing a particular drug formulation but its main relevance is when a patient is switched from one preparation to another formulation of the same drug.

Absorption from subcutaneous and intramuscular injection sites
Compared to oral administration, subcutaneously and intramuscularly injected drugs are more completely

absorbed and act faster; compared to intravenous administration they act less suddenly and are therefore less dangerous to the heart and respiration.

Two processes have to be distinguished in the absorption from subcutaneous and intramuscular injection sites: (1) diffusion of drug molecules in the extravascular tissue and (2) passage of drug molecules through the capillary wall. The first process is normally rate limiting as is shown by the powerful effect of *hyaluronidase*, an enzyme which hydrolyses hyaluronic acid, the polysaccharide which forms the groundwork of intracellular collagen. By adding hyaluronidase to the injection fluid the viscosity of the hyaluronic acid gel is reduced, diffusion rate through the interstitial groundwork is increased and drug absorption is greatly speeded up.

Absorption from a site of injection may be increased by increasing local blood flow by the application of heat or massage. Local blood flow may be a critical factor if parental injections are given to patients with a failing peripheral circulation. Thus, when a patient is given a subcutaneous morphine injection after severe trauma, the analgesic effect produced may be inadequate and further doses may be given. When his circulation is restored, however, a rapid and potentially dangerous absorption of morphine may occur.

Delayed absorption
Vasoconstrictor drugs diminish the rate of absoprtion; for example the addition of adrenaline or noradrenaline to a solution of local anaesthetic reduces the absorption of the local anaesthetic into the general circulation.

Another method of delay is to administer a drug in a relatively insoluble form. This may be achieved by converting it into a poorly soluble salt, ester, or complex which is injected either as an aqueous suspension or an oily solution. Procaine penicillin is a salt of penicillin which is only slightly water-soluble; when injected as an aqueous suspension it is slowly absorbed and exerts a prolonged action (p. 402). Esterification of the steroiid hormones, oestradiol, testosterone and deoxycortone, increases their solubility in oil and in this way slows down their rate of absorption when they are injected in an oily solution.

The physical characteristics of a preparation may influence its rate of absorption. An example of this are the insulin zinc suspensions; if insulin is allowed to react with zinc in an acetate buffer, an insoluble insulin-zinc complex results. The physical form of this complex varies according to the pH of the buffer. One form consists of a fine amorphous suspension which is relatively rapidly absorbed; another consists of a suspension of large crystals which provide a depot effect and are slowly absorbed. These two preparations can be mixed in various proportions for the treatment of diabetic patients (p. 339).

One of the most effective methods of ensuring slow and continuous absorption of certain steroid hormones is the subcutaneous implantation of cast or compressed solid pellets. The rate of absorption appears to be proportional to the surface area of the implant and for this reason a flat pellet is more efficient than a spherical one. These pellets are sometimes extruded through the skin incision and it is safer to implant several small rather than one large pellet. The tissue reaction at the site of the implant causes the formation of a fine capsule of connective tissue, through which the drug must diffuse in order to be absorbed. This capsule may cause irregular absorption or may prevent it altogether. Implants of deoxycortone acetate have been used in the treatment of Addison's disease and their effect may last for periods up to six months. Testosterone and oestradiol may also be administered in this way. An alternative method of ensuring slow absorption is the intramuscular injection of a suspension of the drug in the form of very small crystals.

DISTRIBUTION OF DRUGS IN THE BODY

Body fluid compartments

The water of the body can be considered to be distributed into compartments as shown in Figure 4.4. The total body water as a percentage of body weight varies from 50 to 70 per cent. The water content is inversely related to the amount of fat in the body: in females it averages about 52 per cent and in males it is approximately 63 per cent.

The extracellular fluid comprises the blood plasma (4.5 per cent), interstitial fluid (16 per cent) and lymph (1 to 2 per cent). The intracellular fluid (30 to 40 per cent) is the sum of the fluid contents of all cells in the body including erythrocytes. The transcellular fluid compartment (about $2\frac{1}{2}$ per cent) includes the cerebrospinal, intraocular, peritoneal, pleural and synovial fluids and digestive secretions.

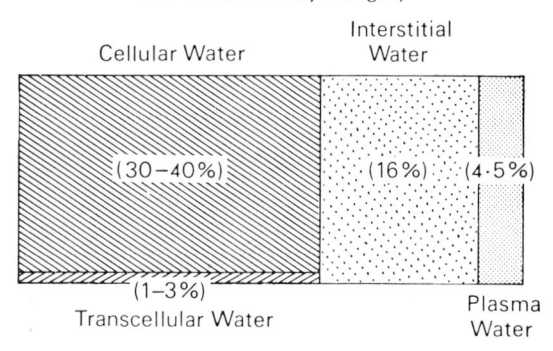

Fig. 4.4 Distribution of water in body compartments. (After Pitts, 1968, *Physiology of the Kidney and Body Fluids* Year Book, Medical Publishers.)

Distribution of drugs in fluid compartments

The following types of drug distribution can be distinguished.

Drugs distributed in the plasma compartment
They include globulins and high-molecular dextrans. Certain dyes such as Evans blue bind tightly to plasma albumin and can thus be used to estaimate the plasma volume. In another method plasma volume is measured with radioiodinated human serum albumin injected intravenously.

Drugs distributed in the extracellular fluid
Inulin, sucrose, thiosulphate, sulphate, chloride, bromide and sodium belong to this class. Unaccountably the volumes of distribution of these substances vary considerably, from about 16 per cent of body weight for inulin to 30 per cent for radiosodium. Sulphate and thiosulphate are distributed in about 22 per cent of body weight. Radioactive sulphate is frequently used to measure extracellular space.

Drugs distributed throughout the body water
Alcohol urea, sulphonamides and antipyrine are typical examples. Antripyrine is sometimes used to measure total body water but more frequently one of two isotopes of water, deuterium oxide or tritiated water are used for this purpose.

In a few cases there is an obvious relation between the distribution of drugs in the body and their site of action, for example inorganic iodine is selectively fixed by the thyroid and radioactive phosphate by bone. Frequently, however, the organs of excretion and metabolism, namely the kidneys and liver, contain higher concentrations of drugs than the organs upon which the drugs exert their action.

The rate of distribution of drugs is usually rapid if they are injected intravenously. If, for example, a dose of sodium iodide is injected intravenously, it is distributed over the greater portion of the extracellular fluid in a minute or two. In general, lipid soluble substances leave the capillaries rapidly, probably by diffusing through the capillary wall. Water soluble substances which leave the capillaries through pores also diffuse out rapidly but their rates of diffusion depend on molecular weight.

FUNCTIONS OF THE BLOOD-BRAIN BARRIER

The barrier separating blood from brain fulfils several functions. Mechanically, the cerebrospinal fluid provides a cushion which protects the brain from injury. Functionally, the blood-brain barrier maintains a tight control of the chemical milieu of the cerebrospinal fluid (CSF) and therefore of the brain, particularly in relation to the concentration in the CSF of the inorganic ions calcium, magnesium and potassium which profoundly influence neuronal excitability. The CSF also provides a path of clearance of breakdown products of cellular metabolism from the brain.

The boundary between blood plasma and the central nervous system is less permeable to a variety of water soluble substances, including dissociated acids, bases and proteins, than that between plasma and other tissue cells. This is due to the fact that, in contrast to normal capillary junctions which are separated by slits 50 to 100 A wide, the endothelial cells of brain capillaries are joined by continuous tight intercellular junctions. Drugs thus have to pass through cells rather than in-between cells to penetrate from the blood to the brain. Although anatomically the blood-brain barrier can be considered as separating the blood from the extracellular fluid of the brain, in a pharmacological sense the cerebrospinal fluid functions as an intracellular fluid. Whereas in the rest of the body charged molecules penetrate freely into the extracellular fluid but are prevented from penetrating the cell interior, in the central nervous system they exchange readily between CSF and brain tissue but are prevented from penetrating from the plasma into the CSF.

The CSF is formed by the choroid plexus of the cerebral ventricles. Its production in man is at the rate of about 0.5 ml/min and its total volume about 120 ml. The CSF is returned to the general circulation by the arachnoid granulations which act as flap valves. If the hydrostatic pressure in the subarachnoid spaces is higher than in the venous sinuses the valves open and the CSF moves in bulk into the blood stream. Drugs which penetrate the blood-brain barrier are thus removed by the bulk flow of CSF. If a compound enters the CSF slowly enough it may never achieve a high concentration because it is removed by this flow.

Figure 4.5 shows the rate of entry of three different drugs into rabbit brain. The rate depends on two factors, the degree of ionisation at pH 7.4 and the lipid/water

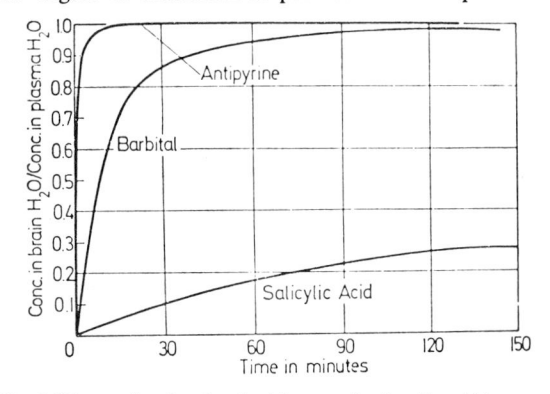

Fig. 4.5 Entry of antipyrine, barbitone and salicyclic acid into rabbit brain during a period of constant plasma concentration. (After Rall, 1971, *Handb. Exp. Pharm.*, *Vol.* 28/1.)

partition coefficient of the unionised form. The rapidly penetrating antipyrine is practically unionised at pH 7.4 and has a high lipid solubility, barbitone which is less lipid-soluble and considerably ionised, penetrates more slowly and salicylic acid which is practically completely ionised at pH 7.4 ($pK_a = 3$) penetrates most slowly.

Fully ionised quaternary compounds do not penetrate the brain significantly. When drugs are available as tertiary and quaternary forms the tertiary form has usually the greater central activity, as is the case with eserine and neostigmine; mecamylamine and hexamethonium; and atropine and methylatropine.

An important drug which is carried into the brain by active transport is the amino acid L-dopa, used in the treatment of Parkinsonism (p. 273). This substance, after oral administration, is readily taken up by the brain, where it is transformed into the physiologically active compound L-dopamine. If L-dopamine is injected as such into the blood stream it is not taken up by the brain in sufficient amounts to exert a clinical effect.

PENETRATION OF DRUGS INTO FAT DEPOTS

Fat is a major component of the body; in lean persons it accounts for about 10 per cent of body weight, in fat persons for 30 per cent or more. Since some drugs are highly fat-soluble it is obvious that the body fat plays an important part in their distribution.

Early studies with thiopentone suggested that rapid recovery from thiopentone anaesthesia was due to a shift of thiopentone into fat depots rather than a rapid breakdown of the drug as was previously believed. It is now considered, however, that whilst the lipid-solubility of thiopentone can account for its rapid penetration into the brain its redistribution in fat is too slow to explain its rapid termination of action. This is believed to be due to redistribution from the brain into a variety of tissues by way of the blood (p. 304). If, however, multiple doses of thiopentone are given, they will tend to produce a protracted release of the drug from fat depots and thus prolong anaesthesia. Other short-acting barbiturates including hexobarbitone and thialbarbitone and many hypnotic and sedative drugs such as glutethimide and diazepam are highly fat soluble.

Certain long-acting drugs owe their persistent effects to their storage in fat depots. Examples are quinestrol, a cyclopentyl ether of ethinyloestradiol and methyl-testosterone. The alpha-adrenergic blocking agent phenoxybenzamine owes its prolonged effect to two separate mechanisms: (1) a covalent, irreversible link with receptors (p. 16) and (2) storage and slow release from fat depots.

The organochlorine insecticides (p. 467) are highly lipid soluble and tend to accumulate in the body fat. Residues of these insecticides in human adipose tissue have been identified in populations throughout the world. They also occur in fish and birds.

BINDING OF DRUGS TO PLASMA PROTEINS

Many drugs are bound to plasma proteins, particularly to the albumin fraction. This binding is reversible and there is a dynamic equilibrium between the bound and unbound forms of a drug.

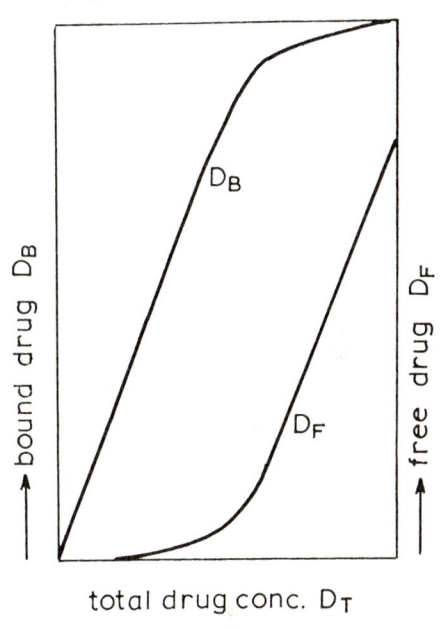

Fig. 4.6 Theoretical curves showing the concentration of free drug D_F and of plasma-bound drug D_B as a function of total drug concentration D_T. (After Keen, 1971, *Handb. Exp. Pharm.*, Vol. 28/1.)

Figure 4.6 shows the effect of protein binding on the amount of free and bound drug in plasma. As total drug in plasma is increased the concentration of free drg rises slowly at first but above the point at which the plasma proteins become saturated it rises steeply. Conversely the concentration of bound drug rises steeply at first but flattens progressively as the saturation limit of the binding sites is approached. It follows from this that the higher the total concentration of drug the greater the proportion that is free.

The binding of drugs to plasma proteins is of great significance since only the unbound or free drug is effective. On the other hand, the drug-protein complex may carry a drug to its site of action when its solubility in plasma is low as in the case of corticosteroids and vitamins A and E. Plasma protein binding slows the uptake of drugs by tissues through decreasing the concentration gradient of free drug. It also provides a continuous source of free drug to replace that removed by excretion and metabolism.

The chief protein concerned in drug transport is serum albumin, but globulins and haemoglobin can also bind drugs. Although albumin has a net negative charge at pH 7.4, it can bind both positively and negatively charged drug molecules. Drugs which bind to plasma proteins include penicillins, tetracyclines, sulphonamides, salicylates, barbiturates, phenylbutazone, digitoxin, vitamin C, histamine and others.

The degree of protein binding of drugs depends on their concentration and their affinity for plasma proteins. Some drugs are strongly bound in therapeutic concentrations, for example phenylbutazone may be up to 95 per cent bound. The degree of drug binding is also dependent on the concentration of protein in plasma. In pregnancy the concentration of plasma proteins rises and some hormones such as thyroxine become more highly bound. In hypoproteinaemic conditions binding of drugs to plasma proteins diminishes.

Competition for binding sites
The number of binding sites of albumin having a high affinity for drugs and hormones is limited. Different drugs can compete for the same sites on albumin and thus displace each other. This may have dangerous consequences. For example if a patient who is satisfactorily treated with maintenance doses of warfarin, an anticoagulant which is protein-bound, is given an analgesic such as aspirin, the salicylate may displace some of the protein-bound warfarin, and the resultant increase in free warfarin may produce a severe haemorrhage.

Interaction may also occur between drugs and normal body constitutents. Thus it has been shown that sulphonamides can compete with bilirubin for binding sites; they may thus produce jaundice and even kernicterus in new-born infants. Other potentially dangerous effects may result from the displacement by drugs of protein-bound thyroxine and of corticosteroids.

CLEARANCE OF DRUGS

Drugs are removed from the body in two ways, some are excreted unaltered but the majority are first metabolised and then excreted. The organs of excretion are the kidneys and the liver, but the liver is a relatively inefficient route for the excretion of drugs because many that are excreted in the bile are reabsorbed from the intestine. On the other hand, the liver is the most important organ concerned with the metabolism of drugs. Some substances are neither excreted nor metabolised but are fixed by tissues. Fixation of this type is obviously liable to result in cumulative poisoning. The fixation of lead in the bones is an example of this form of storage and of the resultant dangers. The liver sometimes removes substances from the blood which it cannot detoxicate. The fixation of arsenical compounds by the liver is an example of this mechanism which exposes the organ to special dangers and is one reason why so many poisons produce serious injury to the liver.

METABOLISM OF DRUGS

The biochemical changes which drugs undergo in the body may lead to pharmacological inactivation or activation. They can be classified as follows.

Inactivation
Active drugs can be inactivated by processes such as oxidation, reduction and hydrolysis. The rate of inactivation of a drug has an important influence on the duration of its effects. Thus the actions of barbiturates with rapidly oxidisable side chains are terminated mainly by metabolism into inactive compounds, whereas the actions of the long-acting barbiturates in which the side chain is slowly oxidised, are terminated largely by excretion of the unchanged drug.

Conjugation
Active drugs can also be detoxicated by conjugation reactions which are synthetic processes requiring a source of energy. This energy is provided by adenosine triphosphate (ATP) through a mechanism which involves the intermediate formation of an active nucleotide. Conjugation reactions include glucuronic acid conjugation (progesterone is reduced to pregnanediol and subsequently conjugated to form pregnanediol glucuronide); acetylation of the amino group of sulphonamides and of isoniazid; and O-methylation of catecholamines. The detoxication products are usually more water soluble and less lipid soluble than the original compounds and therefore more readily excreted by the kidney.

Conjugation reactions are generally two-stage reactions, the first being the biosynthesis of a coenzyme donor and the second a transfer reaction. For example in the case of glucuronide formation the first stage consists in the synthesis of uridine diphosphate glucuronic acid and the second in the transfer of glucuronic acid to a substrate. Other conjugation reactions require as coenzymes glutathione, coenzyme A or adenosine coenzymes.

Transformation
Drugs can be transformed into other pharmacologically active compounds. Some drugs are inactive *in vitro* but become active *in vivo*; thus prontosil, a red dye, is reduced in the body to the active antibacterial compound sulphanilamide (p. 385) and proguanil is oxidised to an active antimalarial (p. 440). Some active drugs are

rendered more active by metabolism and then detoxicated. Examples are:

	Activation	Inactivation
chloral hydrate →	trichloroethanol →	urochloralic acid
phenacetin →	p-acetamidophenol → (paracetamol)	p-acetamidophenyl glucuronide.

The pharmacological activity in these cases is dependent on two factors, the rates of activation and inactivation. Some drugs are converted to less active metabolites before complete inactivation, e.g.,

heroin → 6-acetylmorphine → morphine → morphine glucuronide.

The oxidative metabolism of methyl alcohol and of ethyl alcohol gives rise to highly toxic intermediates, as follows:

Methyl alcohol	Ethyl alcohol
CH_3OH	$CH_3.CH_2OH$
↓	↓
Formaldehyde	Acetaldehyde
HCHO	$CH_3.CHO$
↓	↓
Formic acid	Acetic acid
HCOOH	CH_3COOH
↓	↓
CO_2 and H_2O	CO_2 and H_2O

Normally the toxic acetaldehyde formed from ethyl alcohol is rapidly metabolised to acetate but if this stage of metabolism is slowed down, toxic symptoms develop (p. 488).

Drug metabolism catalysed by hepatic microsomal enzymes

Some drugs are metabolised by normal metabolic processes, that is by enzymes which have natural substrates in the body, thus the plasma cholinesterases hydrolyse procaine and suxamethonium. Many drugs are metabolised by enzymes which are located in the intracellular microsomes of liver cells and which seem to be largely concerned with the metabolism of compounds which are foreign to the body.

The endoplasmic reticulum of liver cells is a tubular lipoprotein network extending throughout the cytoplasm. It can be subdivided into rough and smooth reticulum. The rough endoplasmic reticulum is studded with ribosomes concerned with protein synthesis. The reticulum contains enzymes which metabolise foreign compounds, steroids and lipids. During disruption of liver cells the reticulum fragments form numerous small vesicles known as microsomes. Microsomal enzymes are closely associated with lipoprotein membranes and are difficult to solubilise, but lipid soluble drugs can penetrate the endoplasmic reticulum and interact with the microsomal enzymes.

Amongst the principal reactions catalysed by microsomal enzymes are oxidations requiring molecular oxygen and reduced $NADH_2$ as coenzyme. The oxidation of $NADH_2$ itself is the first step in the microsomal oxidation of many drugs and it can be inhibited competitively by other drugs interacting with the same system.

Cytochrome P450

Cytochromes are conjugated proteins having iron-porphyrin complexes as their prosthetic groups. They function as respiratory catalysts by virtue of their iron complexes oscillating between the ferrous and ferric state. Cytochrome P450 has been well characterised and is known to play a fundamental role in the oxidation in the liver of various lipophilic compounds including food additives, industrial organic compounds and an increasing number of drugs. Lipophilic compounds are metabolically rather inert but they can be attacked by certain monooxygenases which carry out hydroxylation reactions in the liver rendering them more hydrophilic so that they can be excreted by the kidney.

Cytochrome P450 acts as a coenzyme capable of binding ferrous oxygen. The cytochrome is localised intracellularly in the endoplasmic reticulum membrane and its oxygen transfer reaction can be followed spectroscopically in microsomal extracts. Cytochrome P450 is widely involved in microsomal drug oxidations; it can also oxidise carbon monoxide to carbon dioxide.

Activation of microsomal enzymes

Remmer made the interesting observation that repeated administration of a drug can stimulate the activity of microsomal enzymes. He found that after repeated administration of barbiturates to animals their hypnotic effect was greatly diminished and concluded that this was due to an accelerated metabolism of barbiturate by enzymes. These changes in enzymatic activity are due to the formation of new enzyme and they are accompanied by morphological changes of the endoplasmic reticulum which can be observed by electronmicroscopy.

In experiments with ^{14}C phenobarbitone it has been found that the first step in stimulating the microsomal system consists in the binding of the drug to the microsomes. This is followed by an increase in phospholipid content due to the formation of new endoplasmic reticular membranes and enzyme synthesis by the rough endoplasmic reticulum. When synthesis is completed the rough reticular membranes lose their ribosomes and transform to smooth membranes which are abundant in electron micrographs of drug-stimulated hepatic tissue. When treatment with phenobarbitone ceases, these changes slowly reverse and the levels of protein, enzyme and coenzyme activity return to normal.

The activation of drug metabolising enzymes involves the genetic apparatus of the cell. It has been suggested that compounds such as phenobarbitone combine with a normally occurring repressor substance, the ensuing derepression and synthesis of messenger RNA leading to new enzyme formation.

Interaction of drugs and microsomal enzymes
Stimulation of microsomal enzymes occurs particularly with substances having high lipid solubility and a slow rate of metabolism. Amongst barbiturates, phenobarbitone has these properties and is therefore an effective stimulant. Drugs such as barbitone and hexobarbitone are less effective, the former because it is relatively lipid insoluble and the latter because it is rapidly metabolised. Many non-barbiturate drugs can also stimulate the endoplasmic reticulum, including phenylbutazone, imipramine, chlorcyclizine, ether and nitrous oxide. The organochlorine insecticides produce a slow but long-lasting stimulation of drug metabolising enzymes. The stimulation of microsomal enzymes is relatively unspecific. Thus treatment by phenobarbitone will promote the inactivation of a variety of drugs and hormones including cortisol and testosterone.

Some substances inhibit microsomal enzymes and in this way prolong the effects of drugs. One of these, SKF 525, has been shown to cause a tenfold increase in the sleeping time of dogs given hexobarbitone. Substances may produce biphasic effects consisting of inhibition and stimulation. For example glutethimide, a hypnotic drug, produces an initial inhibition of phenobarbitone metabolism followed by strong stimulation.

Interaction of monoamine oxidase inhibitors with food and drugs

Monoamine oxidase is an enzyme which catalyses the oxidative deamination of monoamines (p. 76) leading to the formation of aldehyde, ammonia and hydrogen peroxide

$$RCH_2 NH_2 + O_2 + H_2O \rightarrow RCHO + NH_3 + H_2O_2.$$

The wall of the intestine and the liver are rich in monoamine oxidase and thus protect the organism against the toxic effects of amines such as tyramine and tryptamine absorbed from the gastrointestinal tract. Such amines may be formed in the intestine by bacterial decarboxylation of amino acids or they may be present as such in food. Large quantities of tyramine are contained in cheese (turos = Gr. for cheese), salted herring and yeast extract; some cheeses contain as much as 1 g/kg tyramine.

Inhibitors of monoamine oxidase (iproniazid, phenelzine, p. 260) are used in the treatment of depressive illness and hypertension, and if patients receiving these compounds eat tyramine-rich food they may exhibit symptoms due to the systemic absorption of tyramine. They include severe headaches, sudden hypertension and sometimes intracranial haemorrhage. The symptoms develop suddenly, often when the patients are at rest, and may be dangerous, but they disappear when the offending food is withdrawn.

Sudden rises in blood pressure may also occur when monoamine oxidase inhibitors are administered in conjunction with drugs such as amphetamine or imipramine which interfere with central adrenergic transmission. In this case the monoamine oxidase inhibitors probably act indirectly by interfering with the metabolism of endogenously liberated catecholamines.

EXCRETION OF DRUGS BY THE KIDNEY

Various renal mechanisms (p. 154) are involved in the elimination of drugs and their metabolites.

Glomerular filtration. Compounds of molecular weight 5000 or less pass the glomerulus freely, so that the free plasma fraction of nearly all drugs is rapidly filtered through the glomerulus.

Passive reabsorption in proximal tubules. About 80 per cent of sodium chloride and water are reabsorbed iso-osmotically in the proximal tubules. This would result in a fivefold concentration of drugs in the tubule compared to plasma, which provides the driving force for their passive reabsorption. Very small molecules such as urea are absorbed through pores whilst weak undissociated acids and bases are absorbed by 'non-ionic' diffusion.

Active secretion in proximal tubules. Both anionic and cationic secretion mechanisms operate in the proximal tubules.

Active reabsorption in proximal tubules. This mechanism is important for the reabsorption of glucose, amino acids and urate but its importance for drug reabsorption is uncertain.

Active and passive reabsorption in distal tubules. Marked changes of concentration and pH of the tubular fluid occur in this region (p. 159). Other events, such as secretion of urates (p. 292) may also occur in this region.

The concept of renal clearance discussed on page 153 is also applicable to drugs. In calculating renal clearances of drugs it is necessary to take into account their free concentration in plasma rather than total concentration. Drug clearances are often related to the inulin clearance which measures glomerular filtration rate. If the clearance ratio drug/inulin is >1 the drug must undergo net secretion, if <1 it undergoes net reabsorption.

Excretion of weak electrolytes

The excretion rates of weak electrolytes depend on urinary pH because only the undissociated acids and bases are reabsorbed in the tubules. Weak bases are excreted slowly in alkaline urine because they are largely undissociated and reabsorbed; in acid urine they are rapidly excreted because they are largely dissociated. The converse is true of weak acids, which are excreted faster in alkaline urine. Since urinary pH varies between strongly acid (pH 4.5) and weakly alkaline (pH 8.0) it follows that the excretion rates of bases are more affected by changing urinary pH than those of acids.

The following factors, amongst others, determine drug excretion by the kidneys:

1. The pK of the drug. Even small differences in pK are important. Thus, making the urine alkaline affects the excretion rate of phenobarbitone more than of barbitone because at, say, pH 7.8 phenobarbitone (pK_a 7.2) is only 17 per cent unionised and therefore largely excreted whilst barbitone (pK_a 7.8) is 50 per cent unionised and largely reabsorbed.
2. The lipid solubility of the unionised drug.
3. The rate of urine flow. A fast urine flow will tend to diminish the rate of reabsorption in the tubules particularly of poorly lipid soluble substances. Highly lipid soluble substances, however, such as pentobarbitone, equilibrate so rapidly across the tubular membrane that they are unaffected by the rate of urine flow.

An important aspect of electrolyte excretion in the kidney is that it tends to promote the excretion of drug metabolites because most drugs are rendered more polar by the microsomal enzyme mechanisms. Hence the metabolic products are better excreted than the original drugs.

Secretory mechanisms affecting drugs

Two secretory mechanisms affecting the elimination of drugs by the kidney have been clearly established: (1) the organic anion (or hippurate) transport system, (2) the organic cation mechanism. Both operate in the proximal tubules.

Table 4.1 Compounds secreted by proximal tubules

(A) Acidic compounds	(B) Basic compounds
penicillin	morphine
phenylbutazone	pempidine
salicylate	choline
acetazolamide	dopamine
ethacrynic acid	procaine
para-aminohippuric acid	quinine
phenol red	histamine
dinitrophenol	5-hydroxytryptamine
	tetramethylammonium
	neostigmine
	pyridopyridostigine
	tetraethylammonium
	hexamethonium

Early work on the anionic system concerned mainly phenol red and para-aminohippuric acid (PAH) but it is now known that many other organic acids are also excreted by this mechanism and that they compete with each other for a common carrier. The anionic mechanism can be inhibited by metabolic inhibitors such as dinitrophenol. Some compounds secreted by this process are shown in Table 4.1A; they include penicillin, salicylates and phenylbutazone.

Some of the drugs secreted by the cationic renal mechanism are shown in Table 4.1B. This process has been shown to be dependent on metabolic energy, to be saturable and competitive. The cationic transport mechanism can be clearly differentiated from the anionic by their different pH optima and different susceptibilities to metabolic inhibitors. The cationic tubular process secretes primary, secondary and tertiary amines and quaternary ammonium compounds. It can be specifically inhibited by positively charged antimonials and arsenicals.

There is some evidence that other specific secretion mechanisms operate in the kidney; for example there may exist a mechanism for secreting catechols.

PHARMACOKINETICS

It is necessary for the rational administration of drugs to study not only their pharmacological effects but also their *rates* of absorption, distribution and clearance. The branch of pharmacology dealing with these problems is called pharmacokinetics. Pharmacokinetics is a relatively new branch of pharmacology, which deals with changes in the distribution of drugs in the body, describing them as mathematical functions of time and concentration of drug.

In pharmacokinetic terminology the body is divided into 'compartments', hypothetical spaces in which drugs are assumed to be uniformly distributed. Compartments are considered to be bounded by membranes and changes in concentration of drugs are considered to involve their exchange between different compartments. 'Transport' from one compartment to another may represent real transport from one location to another or it may represent the transformation from one chemical state to another within the same location.

A simple assumption, frequently applicable, is that the rates of transport of drugs from one compartment to another are proportional to their concentrations, in which case they can be expressed by first order rate constants. This simple postulate is, however, by no means always applicable. For example the transport between two compartments may involve a saturable carrier and the transport rates then generally cease to be proportional to concentration.

It is usual to postulate a minimum number of compartments consistent with a reasonable description of events. Approximations are frequently used. Thus is a drug is injected into the blood stream, subsequently diffuses into the extracellular spaces and is finally excreted, the system strictly involves at least two body compartments, blood stream and extracellular fluid, but it is often treated as a single compartment if drug distribution between the compartments is rapid relative to drug elimination. Another frequently adopted approximation is to neglect 'deep' compartments such as fat and bone which communicate with the extracellular fluid but do not equilibrate with it rapidly.

Exponential elimination rate

In the simplest model a drug which has been injected intravenously is assumed to be instantaneously and uniformly distributed and removed at a rate proportional to its concentration. A hydraulic analogy for this single compartmental model is shown in Figure 4.7. The rate of elimination of the drug can then be described by

$$C = C_0 e^{-kt} \qquad (1)$$

where C_0 = initial concentration of drug, C = concentration at time t, and k = elimination rate constant. In logarithmic form

$$\ln C = \ln C_0 - kt \qquad (2)$$

Thus if a drug is exponentially eliminated a plot of log concentration against time should give a straight line. Figure 4.8 shows for an exponentially cleared drug the relation to be expected between dose (or initial concentration) of drug and its duration of action as measured by the time needed to reach a threshold drug concentration in the body. The duration of action of the drug varies as the logarithm of the dose. Thus if 10 units produce an action lasting one day then 100 units will produce an action lasting two days and 1000 units three days.

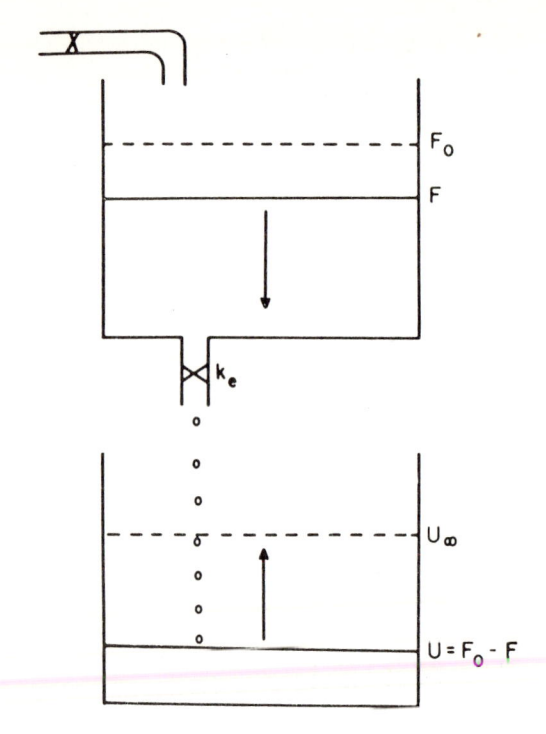

Fig. 4.7 Hydraulic analogy of the one-compartment body model. F_0 is the level for the amount corresponding to the original dosage in the body and F is the level for the amount of drug at any time. The valve setting of k determines the rate of urinary excretion. The level U in the urine compartment corresponds to the amount of drug excreted at any time. (After Garrett, in *Schering Workshop on Pharmacokinetics*, 1969, Pergamon.)

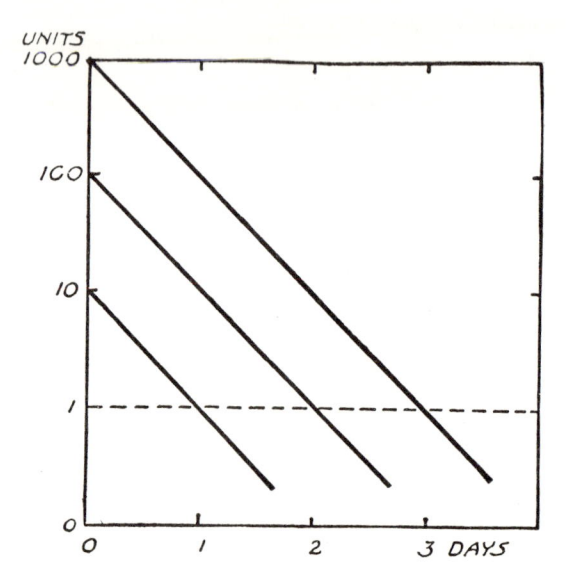

Fig. 4.8 Relation between dosage and duration of action in the case of a drug cleared exponentially. If the action lasts until the drug remaining in the body is reduced to a threshold level (e.g. 1 unit) then the duration varies as the logarithm of the dosage.

Table 4.2 Half-life of drugs in man (hours). (After Dost, 1968, *Grundlagen der Pharmakokinetik*, Thieme.)

Very short to short		Long to very long	
tubocurarine	0.2	aspirin	6
penicillin	0.5	sulphadimidine	7
vitamin B$_1$	0.35	tetracycline	9
insulin	0.7	glutethimide	10
PAS	1.0	dicoumarol	32
ampicillin	1–2	sulphadimethoxine	20–40
isoniazid	1–3	vitamin D	40
erythromycin	1.5		
cortisol	1.7		
streptomycin	2–3		
prednisolone	3.4		
ethylbiscoumacetate	2.4		
imipramine	3.5		

This relation implies that it is in practice impossible to produce a prolonged action by giving massive doses of a drug that is rapidly excreted. With nearly all active drugs there is a limit to the quantity that can safely be introduced into the body at one time, and hence massive dosage, besides being ineffective, is a dangerous method for the production of prolonged action. Two methods by which prolonged action can be obtained with a rapidly cleared drug are delayed absorption or frequent dosage; a third method is to interfere with the excretion of the drug by the kidneys (p. 154).

Many drugs are eliminated at an apparently exponential rate so that their appropriate first order rate constants and corresponding half lives of drug elimination can be computed.

The biological half-life of a drug is the time required for its concentration in the body to fall to one half. In an exponential process the half-life ($t_{1/2}$) is related to the elimination rate constant (k) by the expression

$$t_{1/2} = 0.69/k \qquad (3)$$

As shown in Table 4.2, the half-lives of elimination of different drugs vary over more than a hundredfold range and this is an important fact which must be taken into account in drug administration. For example the half-life in man of the anticoagulant ethylbiscoumacetate is 2.4 hours, whilst that of dicoumarol is 32 hours. Hence when treatment with dicoumarol is stopped it may take a week or so for the prothrombin time to return to normal, whilst when treatment with biscoumacetate is stopped the prothrombin time returns to normal within less than a day.

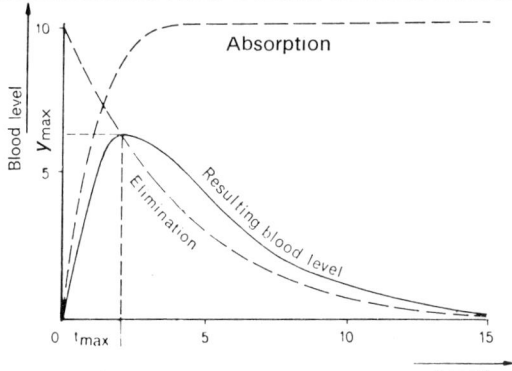

Fig. 4.9 Theoretical curve (solid curve) showing blood level of a drug during simultaneous absorption and elimination (Bateman curve). Dashed absorption curve shows theoretical blood level after the same oral dose not affected by any elimination process. Dashed elimination curve shows blood level expected after intravenous injection of same dose. t_{max} = time to maximal blood level; y_{max} = maximal blood level. (After Dost, *Grundlagen der Pharmakokinetik*, 1968, Thieme.)

More complex pharmacokinetics

When both absorption (e.g. from the gut) and elimination are taken into account a more complex model applies. This model can be expressed by the so-called Bateman function shown in Figure 4.9, which can be considered to result from the interaction of two processes, absorption and elimination (indicated by the dashed curves). The Bateman function is of considerable theoretical interest in pharmacokinetics and some of its mathematical consequences are as follows.

1. The time t_{max} after which the blood concentration becomes maximal, is concentration-independent; given a particular drug and method of administration the maximal blood level will occur at the same time whether the dose is large or small.

2. The concentration maximum, y_{max}, is proportional to the dose. Thus if the dose is doubled the maximal blood concentration is also doubled.

An even more complex pharmacokinetic relationship results if drug distribution and metabolism are also taken into account. The essential components of the scheme are then as shown below

```
                          drug in tissue
                             fluids
                               ↑↓
  drug in          drug in              intact drug
   depot    →    circulation    →      in urine etc.
 (e.g., gut)                ↓
                          drug         metabolites in
                       metabolism    →   urine etc.
```

Compartmental analysis and the use of computers

Curves of drug elimination are nowadays frequently obtained by means of radioactive tracers. They are often complex, reflecting the fact that a number of compartments may be involved. Drug elimination curves can sometimes be resolved graphically into two first order curves as in Figure 4.11 but it is often necessary to employ more elaborate mathematical tools for analysing curves into their components and fitting them to experimental data.

Mathematical expressions for dealing with compartmental analysis have been derived which consist essentially of sums of exponentials and the problems of fitting mathematical curves to experimental data by least square statistical methods have been investigated. In the early studies in this field by Teorell and others, analogue computers were mainly used but increasingly the more powerful digital computers are being used for the purpose. Although, as has been pointed out, drug elimination curves can frequently be treated successfully as simple exponential functions it is probable that more complicated, computer-derived analyses of drug distribution and elimination will be increasingly employed.

CUMULATION OF DRUGS

Cumulation results when the intake of a drug exceeds its clearance from the body. The laws governing the

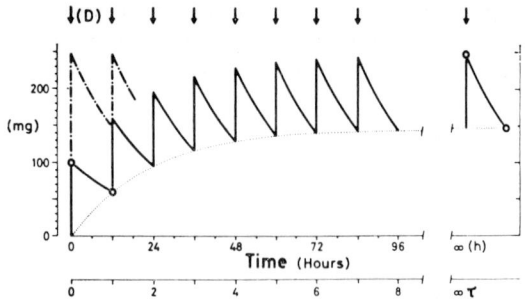

Fig. 4.10 Accumulation of a drug during the intermittent administration of the maintenance dose $D = 100$ mg. The curve describes the calculated amount of drug in the body. The drug has a half-life of $t_{1/2} = 16$ hr. Dosage interval $\tau = 12$ hr. Stippled line shows the administration of a loading dose (246 mg) such that followed by maintenance doses (100 mg), a horizontal, if fluctuating, blood level results. (After Dettli, in *Schering Workshop on Pharmacokinetics*, 1969, Pergamon.)

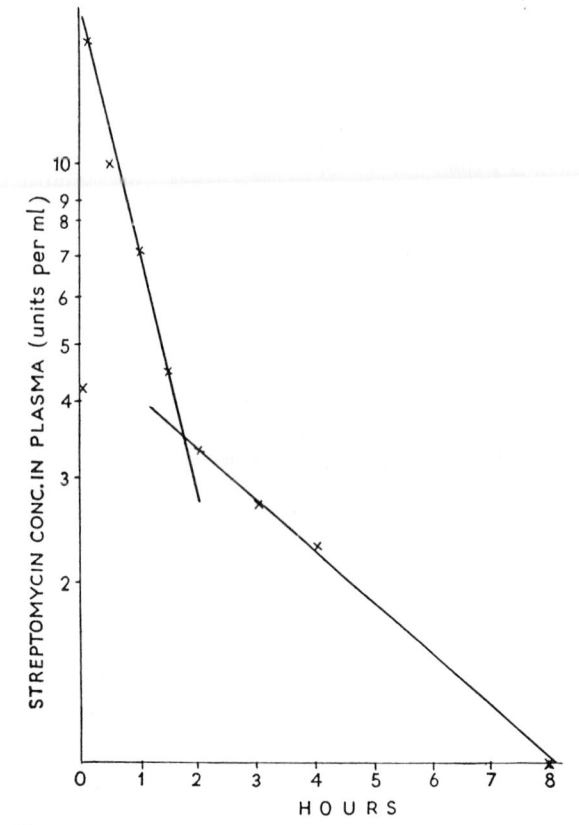

Fig. 4.11 Plasma concentration of streptomycin after intravenous administration of 100 000 units to a patient with pulmonary tuberculosis. (After Adcock and Hettig, 1946, *Arch. int. Med.*)

cumulation of drugs that are cleared in an exponential manner are relatively simple. If a drug is given at regular intervals and if a constant fraction of the drug present in the body is cleared in the interval, then it is possible to calculate the extent to which the drug will cumulate. The amount of drug in the body will rise until the amount cleared in the interval between the doses is equal to a single dose.

For example, if 1 g of drug is given four-hourly and one-fifth of the drug in the body is cleared in four hours, then the amount in the body will rise until 5 g is present. At this point the rate of clearance will equal the rate of entry and no further cumulation will occur.

Figure 4.10 shows the type of cumulation curve to be expected if equal doses of a drug are administered at regular intervals assuming exponential clearance. In the initial stages the drug level in the body builds up until a stage is reached at which drug elimination during the dose interval is equal to the dose administered. After this point the drug level will vary only within the range of dose fluctuations.

Figure 4.10 also illustrates the case where an initial 'loading' dose has been administered followed by a constant 'maintenance' dose so that the drug level in the body remained constant throughout, fluctuating only within the range of the maintenance doses. The dosages required to obtain this state of affairs can be calculated (if certain simplifying assumptions are made). For example it may be shown that if a loading dose is chosen which is twice the maintenance dose, and the dose interval is equal to the half life of the drug, a horizontal though fluctuating blood level is reached from the beginning.

As a concrete example we may consider sulphadimidine ($t_{1/2} = 7$ hours). If a loading dose is chosen which is twice the maintenance dose and a regular dose interval of seven hours is adopted an approximately horizontal blood level should be established from the start. Where such calculations have been made they have been found to be in reasonable agreement with experimental measurements of blood levels of drug.

PLASMA CONCENTRATIONS AND CLINICAL EFFECT

The plasma concentrations achieved in different patients receiving the same oral doses vary greatly, largely due to different rates of metabolism. The relationship between plasma concentration and clinical effect is less variable and has been studied in detail with several drugs. Clinical plasma concentration ranges producing therapeutic and toxic effects are shown in Table 4.3.

FREQUENCY OF ADMINISTRATION

The wide variations that have been shown to occur in the fate of drugs in the body indicate that the frequency with which drugs should be given varies greatly. Salicylates and most sulphonamide drugs are examples of drugs which are sufficiently rapidly absorbed and excreted, to make it necessary to give these drugs frequently if it is desired to maintain a steady concentration in the blood.

With digitalis on the other hand, since clearance is very slow, there is no particular advantage in giving frequent doses and its action can be maintained just as well by a single daily dose as by the traditional dosage three times a day. Insulin and thyroxine, which resemble each other in that both are hormones regulating metabolism, provide a very striking contrast as regards duration of action. Insulin produces its full action in from two to three hours after subcutaneous administration, and its action ceases after five to eight hours. A single dose of thyroxine, on the other hand, only produces its full action after several days, and its action lasts at least a fortnight. Insulin dosage has to be timed very carefully in relation to the daily carbohydrate intake, whereas in the case of thyroxine the question of importance is the total amount taken during a week.

There is usually no objection to taking even very slow-acting drugs in small divided doses three times a day, since this is popularly regarded as the normal manner for taking medicines, but it is important for the practitioner to know whether the effects produced by the drug depend on the amount taken during the previous six hours or the amount taken during the previous week.

With most drugs which have important therapeutic actions, it is necessary to produce an effective concentration in the body as quickly as possible, and to maintain this concentration for an adequate time. This is achieved by initial intensive doses followed by maintenance doses. The logical method would be to commence with a large dose, but this may be dangerous because the individual susceptibility of the patient is usually unknown. Hence it is frequently necessary to build up the body concentration of the drug gradually, thus giving the practitioner the chance of observing the reactions of the patient. If the method of intensive dosage followed by maintenance doses is used, it is of course essential to distinguish clearly between the two scales of dosage, and to be careful not to continue the intensive dosage for too long.

Intravenous injection is sometimes the only available method of administering a drug, and where a rapid and intense action is desired it is an exceptionally effective method. When a steady prolonged action is needed, however, intravenous administration is peculiarly unsuited and intramuscular or oral administration is preferable. When a drug does not irritate the gastrointestinal tract and is well absorbed, oral administration is generally best since the delay in absorption tends to diminish the fluctuations resulting from excretion of the drug in the intervals between the doses. Thus oral administration promotes a uniform concentration in the body fluids.

Table 4.3 Plasma concentrations of standard drugs.[1] (After Sjökvist *et al.* (1976) in Avery, Principles of Clinical Pharmacology.)

Drug	Therapeutic range	Side-effects
Digoxin	1–2 ng/ml	>2 ng/ml
Digitoxin[2]	10–25 ng/ml	>35 ng/ml
Quinidine[3]	2–4 µg/ml	>6 µg/ml
Procainamide	4–8 µg/ml	>8–12 µg/ml
Lignocaine	2–5 µg/ml	>9 µg/ml
Theophylline	10–20 µg/ml	>20 µg/ml
Phenylbutazone[2]	60–80 µg/ml	>80–100
Salicylate[2]	150–300 µg/ml	>300 µg/ml
Phenytoin (di-phenylhydantoin)	10–20 µg/ml	>25 µg/ml
Phenobarbitone	15–30 µg/ml	>35 µg/ml
Ethosuximide	40–80 µg/ml	>100 µg/ml
Lithium	0.5–1.5 mEq/l	>1.6 mEq/l
Nortriptyline	50–180 ng/ml	>200 ng/ml

1. Antibiotics are excluded because the bioassay methods used seem to be less reliable than chemical procedures.
2. More clinical data needed.
3. Improved chemical methodology needed.

FURTHER READING

Binns T B (ed) 1964 Absorption and distribution of drugs. Livingstone, Edinburgh
Brodie B B, Heller W M (ed) 1972 Bioavailability of drugs. Karger, Basel
Curry S H 1977 Drug disposition and pharmacokinetics. Blackwell, London
Dost W H 1968 Grundlagen der pharmakokinetik. Thieme, Stuttgart
Gaddum J H 1944 Administration of drugs. Edin. Med. J. 51: 305
Gamble J L 1950 Chemical anatomy, physiology and pathology of extracellular fluid. Harvard University Press, Cambridge, Mass
Gibaldi M 1977 Biopharmaceutics and clinical pharmacokinetics, 2nd edn. Lea and Fibiger, Philadelphia
Griffin J P, d'Arcy P F 1975 A manual of drug interaction. John Wright, Bristol
Krüger-Thiemer E 1977 Pharmacokinetics In: Kinetics of drug action, J van Rossum ed. Handb. exp. Pharm. 47
Rall D P 1971 Drug entry into brain and cerebrospinal fluid. In Handb. exp. Pharm. 28/II
Raspé G ed 1970 Schering workshop on pharmacokinetics. Pergamon, Oxford
Schanker L S 1964 Physiological transport of drugs. Adv. Drug Res. 1: 72
Weiner I M 1971 Excretion of drugs by the kidney. In Handb. exp. Pharm. 28/II
Williams R T 1959 Detoxication mechanisms. Wiley, New York

SECTION TWO

Neurohumoral transmission and local hormones

5. Cholinergic transmission

Physiology of the autonomic system 53; Theory of humoral transmission 55; Chemical organisation of peripheral nervous system 56; Drugs stimulating cholinergic receptors 57; Anticholinesterases 60; Ganglion blocking drugs 63; Neuromuscular blocking drugs 65; Presynaptic interference 68; Muscarinic receptor blocking drugs 69.

The term *auto-pharmacology* was introduced by Dale to denote the study of chemical regulators produced by the body. Modern pharmacology can indeed be considered in two main categories, namely, those substances which are produced by the body, and those which are foreign to it. In this chapter we shall discuss a particular aspect of autopharmacology, peripheral cholinergic transmission.

PHYSIOLOGY OF THE AUTONOMIC NERVOUS SYSTEM

Regulation of the activity of smooth muscle, cardiac muscle and glands is carried out by the autonomic or involuntary nervous system. The autonomic nerves do not travel directly from the central nervous system to the structures they innervate but their preganglionic medullated fibres pass out from the cranial, thoracolumbar and sacral regions and form relays in peripheral ganglia from which a second, postganglionic non-medullated fibre passes to the tissues. The activity of skeletal muscles is controlled by the somatic or cerebrospinal nervous system.

The motor nerves supplying skeletal muscle take their origin from cells in the anterior horn of the spinal cord and thence run directly to the motor end plate without forming a ganglionic synapse.

In spite of these anatomical differences the autonomic and cerebrospinal systems have certain similarities in their overall organisation. Figure 5.1 shows a comparison of the cerebrospinal and sympathetic nervous systems at the level of the thoracic outflow. Each forms a reflex arc consisting of afferent, internuncial and efferent neurones. In the somatic system the internuncial neurone is located entirely within the spinal cord whilst in the autonomic system it emerges from the spinal cord as a preganglionic fibre.

Gaskell and Langley defined the autonomic as an entirely efferent system, but many modern workers prefer to include with it those afferent nerves which convey messages from visceral stimuli and which run alongside sympathetic and parasympathetic efferent fibres.

Most smooth muscles and glands have a double autonomic nerve supply, an augmentor and an inhibitor supply, and in most cases these fibres reach the structure by different routes, and the different supplies show distinct reactions to drugs.

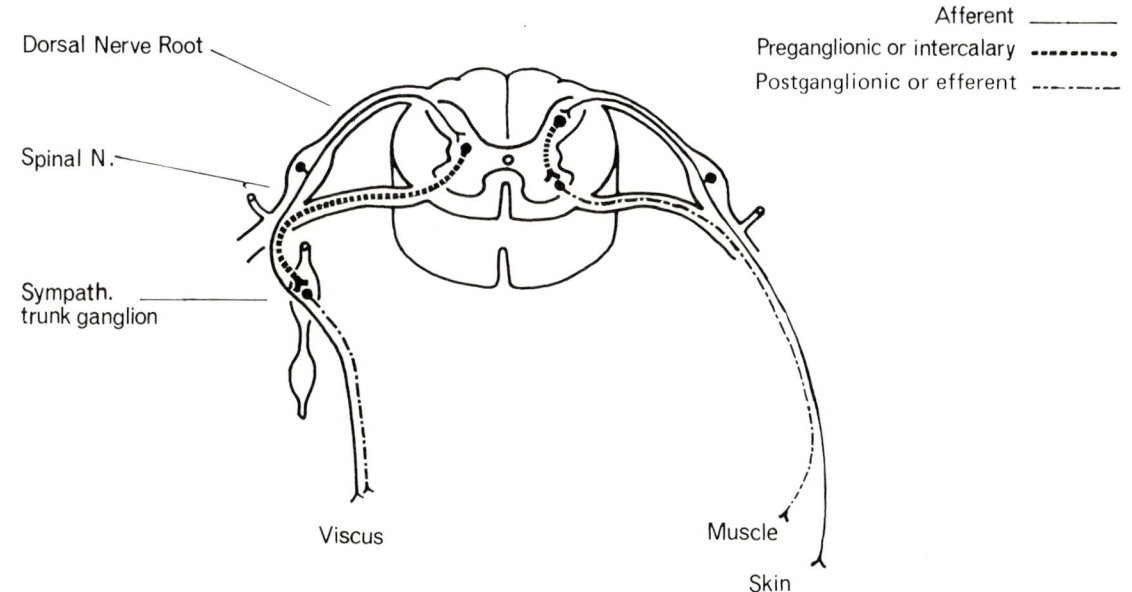

Fig. 5.1 Schematic representation of autonomic and somatic reflex arcs revealing their fundamental similarity. (After Mitchell, 1950, Anatomy of the Autonomic Nervous System, Livingstone, Edinburgh.)

The two sets of nerves supplying these tissues are the sympathetic and the parasympathetic or craniosacral autonomic. The sympathetic outflow leaves the spinal cord as minute medullated nerves (the white rami communicantes) which pass out by all the thoracic and the upper lumbar nerves. These fibres have cell stations in the ganglia of the sympathetic cord and in the cardiac, solar, and hypogastric plexuses, but in a few cases the cell stations occur scattered around the organ which the nerves supply. The postganglionic non-medullated fibres, which commence in the ganglia, follow various paths. The fibres from the sympathetic cord pass back to the spinal nerves in the grey rami communicantes, whilst those from the coeliac and mesenteric ganglia pass directly to the organs which they supply.

The parasympathetic fibres leave the central nervous system in two groups, the cranial group by the cranial nerves III, VII, IX, X and XI, and the sacral outflow by the sacral nerves II, III and IV. The cell-stations of the parasympathetic system are generally situated close to the organ which they supply. Hence, as a general rule the postganglionic fibres are shorter in the parasympathetic than in the sympathetic system. In the gastrointestinal tract the network of the myenteric plexuses constitutes the postganglionic parasympathetic fibres.

Central control of the autonomic system

The autonomic system is regulated by a series of controlling centres. Some organs such as the gut possess local nerve plexuses which can carry out fairly complex functions but control is exercised chiefly by centres in the brain and medulla. During the latter half of the last century a series of 'vital centres' were located in the medulla. The chief of these were the vagal centre, the respiratory centre, the vasomotor centre, the cough centre, and the vomiting centre. In recent years it has been proved that these medullary centres are controlled by centres in the hypothalamus.

The hypothalamus contains centres regulating the sympathetic and parasympathetic systems which regulate metabolism and the expression of the emotions. Stimulation of the sympathetic hypothalamic centres produces all the changes fitting the animal for active exertion. For example electrical stimulation of the hypothalamus in cats produces an increase in muscle blood flow. Functions controlled by the hypothalamus (hyp) include: bladder control (ant. hyp), heat loss (ant. hyp), thirst and appetite (separate regions of mid. hyp), sexual behaviour (post. hyp).

The hypothalamic region appears not only to regulate and correlate the activity of the autonomic nervous system but also to regulate the water, salt and carbohydrate metabolism. The hypothalamus regulates urine secretion, and the tonicity of the blood. The regulation of water and salt metabolism is perhaps the most important function of the hypothalamus since this involves the maintenance of the blood plasma at a normal composition, and any derangement of this composition deranges the activities of all the organs of the body.

It is now known that the cerebral cortex also has autonomic representation. Thus Penfield has shown that electrical stimulation of the human cerebral cortex during cranial operations may produce an increase in gastrointestinal activity.

Chief functions of the autonomic system

The autonomic nervous system regulates those functions which are not under conscious control. The nervous control of most of the glands and smooth muscles in the body is complex. The muscles of the small intestine, for example, receive a motor supply from the vagus and an inhibitory supply from the sympathetic, but in addition there is a local nerve plexus (Auerbach's plexus), which, when separated from all central nervous control, can execute the reflexes involved in the passage of a wave of peristalsis down the gut.

The system of control is even more complicated in the case of the gastric glands, for the secretion can be stimulated by the vagus, but the regulation of the secretion is for the most part carried out by local chemical reflexes. The entrance of food into the pyloric part of the stomach causes the secretion of a hormone, gastrin, which passes by the bloodstream and excites the secretion of the gastric glands possibly by way of the release of histamine.

Another interesting feature relates to hollow muscular organs, because a nerve, when it causes contraction of the body of such an organ, generally causes relaxation of the sphincter guarding the outlet. For example, stimulation of the sacral nerves causes contraction of the body of the bladder and relaxation of the sphincter of the bladder, while stimulation of the sympathetic produces the opposite effects.

The chief effects of stimulation of the sympathetic and parasympathetic nerves are summarised in Table 5.1. The sympathetic system is not essential to life. Animals which have been completely sympathectomised can survive and reproduce but they cannot cope with emergencies such as exposure to cold and shock. The sympathetic-adrenal system usually functions as a unit to produce a series of changes which put the body in a condition suitable for immediate violent activity (fight or flight): the heart rate and blood pressure is increased, the blood flow is redistributed towards muscles and the heart, the blood sugar rises and the bronchi and pupils dilate.

An increase in parasympathetic activity renders the body incapable of violent action. Most of the effects produced by the parasympathetic resemble the conditions which occur in sleep and during digestion. It is organised for localised discharge and controls discrete functions such as the emptying of the bladder and rectum and accommodation of the lens.

Theory of humoral transmission of the nerve impulse

The finding that such drugs as adrenaline and pilocarpine produced almost exactly the same effects as were produced by stimulation of the sympathetic and parasympathetic nerves respectively, led naturally to the theory that these drugs acted by stimulating the nerve endings of the postganglionic fibres of these systems. A complete theory of the selective action of drugs on nerve endings was worked out on this assumption. The sympathetic nerve endings were believed to be stimulated by adrenaline and to be paralysed by ergotoxine. The parasympathetic nerve

Moreover, after section and complete degeneration of the postganglionic sympathetic nerve fibres to the pupil, the dilator effect of adrenaline on the pupil could still be observed. Indeed the denervated pupil was more sensitive to adrenaline than the innervated pupil. Since degeneration of all visible nervous structures did not reduce the action of the appropriate drugs, it was necessary to postulate that the drugs acted upon nerve endings that could not be demonstrated histologically. An alternative explanation was propounded by Elliot who suggested that adrenaline might be the chemical stimulant liberated on each occasion when a sympathetic impulse arrives at the periphery. Elliott's suggestion was made in 1904 but the final proof of chemical transmission was not established until 1921 when Otto Loewi carried out his fundamental experiments on the frog heart.

Table 5.1 Effects of stimulation of sympathetic and parasympathetic nerves on the chief organs of the body in man

Organ	Sympathetic	Parasympathetic
Blood vessels	Constriction, except the blood vessels of the heart and voluntary muscles which are dilated	*Nil* (except in certain special cases e.g. the genital organs where vasodilatation occurs)
Heart	Acceleration and increased contractility of atrium and ventricle; improved A-V conduction	Slowing: diminished contractility of atrium and A-V block
Eye (iris)	Contraction of radial muscle (mydriasis)	Contraction of circular muscle (miosis)
(ciliary muscle)		Contraction
Skin (sweat secretion)	Increase	
(erection of hairs)	Increase	
Salivary glands	Slight viscid secretion	Free secretion and vasodilatation
Stomach (motility)	Inhibition	Increase
(secretions)	Inhibition	Increase
(sphincters)	Contraction or relaxation	Relaxation or contraction
Intestinal movements	Inhibition	Increase
Gall bladder	Relaxation	Contraction
Liver	Glycogenolysis	
Spleen	Contraction	
Pancreatic secretion		Increase
Bronchial muscles	Relaxation	Contraction
Bronchial secretion		Increase
Suprarenal glands	Release of adrenaline and noradrenaline	
Bladder (fundus)	Relaxation	Contraction
(sphincter)	Contraction	Relaxation
Uterus	Contraction and relaxation	

endings were believed to be stimulated by pilocarpine, acetylcholine and physostigmine and to be paralysed by atropine.

This theory explained so many facts and was such a convenient mnemonic that it was universally accepted, although there were many details for which it did not provide a satisfactory explanation. For example, acetylcholine caused contraction of certain striped muscles, pilocarpine stimulated the sweat glands, and this action was antagonised by atropine, but there was no evidence for the existence of any parasympathetic nerve endings in these structures.

Loewi's findings can be summarised as follows:

1. Stimulation of the vagus caused the appearance of a substance in the Ringer-perfusate of the frog heart capable of producing in a second heart an inhibitory effect resembling vagus stimulation. Loewi concluded that a substance had leaked out which normally transmits the effects of vagus stimulation. The substance was called 'vagus-stoff' and later identified as acetylcholine.

2. Stimulation of the sympathetic caused the appearance of a substance capable of accelerating a second heart.

Loewi concluded later, from fluorescence measurements, that this substance was adrenaline. (In the frog heart adrenaline, not noradrenaline, acts as adrenergic transmitter.)

3. Although atropine prevented the inhibitory action of the vagus on the heart it did not prevent release of 'vagus-stoff'. When the perfusate collected during vagus stimulation of an atropinised heart was transferred to a second heart it caused it to be inhibited. Atropine thus prevented the effects rather than the release of transmitter.

4. When 'vagus-stoff' was incubated with ground-up frog heart muscle it became inactivated. This effect is due to enzymatic destruction of acetylcholine by cholinesterase.

5. Physostigmine (eserine) prevented destruction of 'vagus-stoff' by heart muscle, providing evidence that the potentiation of vagus stimulation by physostigmine is due to an inhibition of cholinesterase which normally destroys the transmitter substance acetylcholine. A diagrammatic representation of Loewi's experiments on 'vagus-stoff' is shown in Figure 5.2.

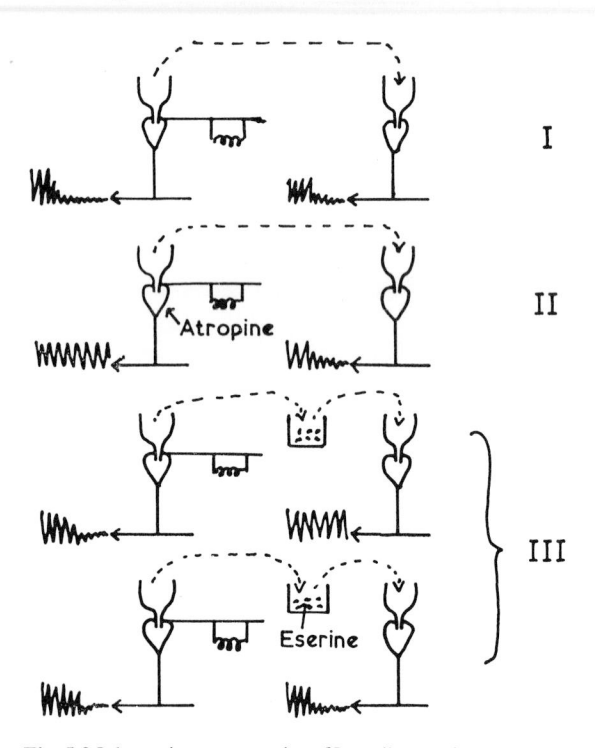

Fig. 5.2 Schematic representation of Loewi's experiments on isolated frog heart. I. Vagus stimulation causes release of transmitter substance ('vagus-stoff') capable of inhibiting second heart. II. Atropine prevents effect of transmitter on donor heart, not transmitter release. III. Transmitter destroyed by ground-up heart muscle (action of cholinesterase). Destruction of transmitter prevented by eserine.

The experiments of Loewi thus established the humoral nature of postganglionic sympathetic and parasympathetic transmission and the mode of action of atropine and eserine. According to this theory, the vagus inhibits the frog's heart, not by the transmission of an electrical stimulus from the nerve to the muscle, but by causing the liberation of acetylcholine, and this drug acts upon the muscle cells. Similarly, the sympathetic nerves act by causing the liberation around the cells, of noradrenaline. Hence the administration of noradrenaline or of acetylcholine naturally produces effects closely similar to those produced by stimulation of autonomic nerves. According to this view atropine acts on receptors on the effector cells and renders them incapable of being acted on by acetylcholine released from nerve endings. Eserine potentiates vagus stimulation not by a subliminal stimulation of nerve endings but by preventing the destruction of the released acetylcholine by an enzyme, cholinesterase.

This theory provided an explanation for findings which were formerly unexplained. Thus it had been observed by Anderson that after denervation of the pupil, pilocarpine continued to constrict it whilst eserine became ineffective. The explanation is that since eserine acts by preventing the destruction of acetylcholine it has no effect on denervated organs in which no acetylcholine is being liberated, but pilocarpine which, like acetylcholine, acts directly on receptors continues to be effective after denervation.

Chemical organisation of the peripheral nervous system

The fundamental discoveries of Loewi provoked intensive research, and the work of Dale and his co-workers has revealed a general system of humoral transmission of impulses at nerve endings which is diagrammatically represented in Figure 5.3.

Dale proposed the terms cholinergic and adrenergic to denote transmissions by acetylcholine-like and adrenaline-like substances. The motor nerves of striated muscle and the preganglionic fibres of the parasympathetic and sympathetic systems, including the preganglionic fibres which innervate the adrenal medulla, are cholinergic. The postganglionic fibres of the parasympathetic are cholinergic, whilst those of the sympathetic system are mostly adrenergic, with certain exceptions which are cholinergic such as the fibres innervating the eccrine sweat glands in man and certain sympathetic vasodilator nerves. Cholinergic nerves release acetylcholine and adrenergic nerves release noradrenaline. Some adrenergic nerves release dopamine.

More recent evidence suggests that the picture outlined in Figure 5.3 may be oversimplified. There is evidence that autonomic nerve endings may be endowed with sets of *presynaptic receptors* capable of modulating and inhibiting transmitter release. Presynaptic receptors have been

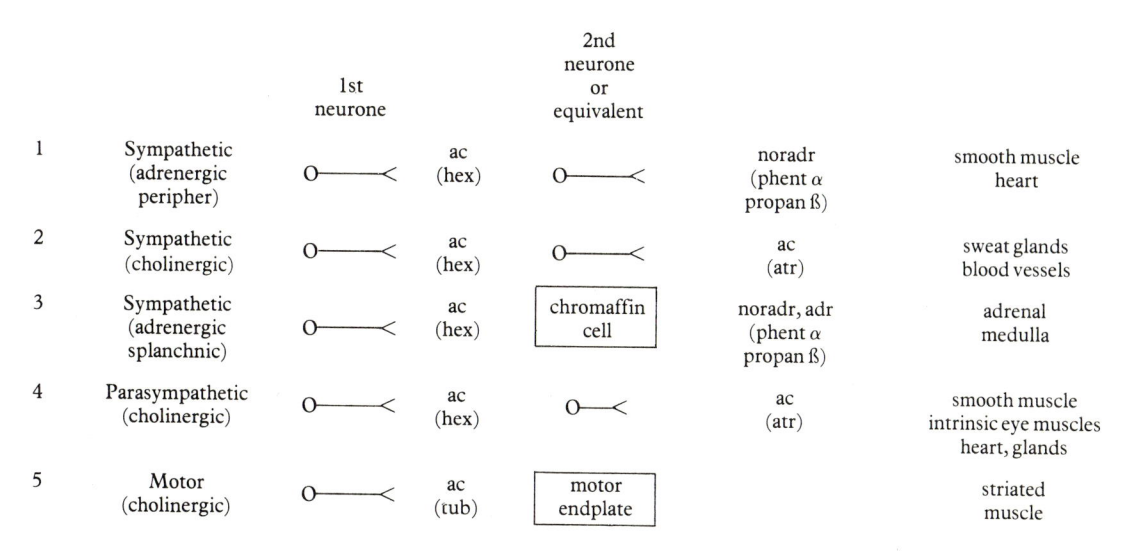

		1st neurone		2nd neurone or equivalent		
1	Sympathetic (adrenergic peripher)	O—<	ac (hex)	O—<	noradr (phent α propan ß)	smooth muscle heart
2	Sympathetic (cholinergic)	O—<	ac (hex)	O—<	ac (atr)	sweat glands blood vessels
3	Sympathetic (adrenergic splanchnic)	O—<	ac (hex)	chromaffin cell	noradr, adr (phent α propan ß)	adrenal medulla
4	Parasympathetic (cholinergic)	O—<	ac (hex)	O—<	ac (atr)	smooth muscle intrinsic eye muscles heart, glands
5	Motor (cholinergic)	O—<	ac (tub)	motor endplate		striated muscle

Fig. 5.3 Substances liberated at nerve endings and typical antagonists. 1. Typical sympathetic pathway to smooth muscle, heart muscle and glands; preganglionic cholinergic and postganglionic adrenergic fibres. 2. Sympathetic pathway to sweat glands and vasodilator fibres; preganglionic and postganglionic cholinergic fibres. 3. Sympathetic cholinergic innervation of suprarenal medulla. 4. Parasympathetic pathway to smooth muscle, heart muscle and glands; preganglionic and postganglionic cholinergic fibres. 5. Cholinergic innervation of motor end plate of striated muscle. Symbols without brackets are transmitter substances: ac acetylcholine; adr adrenaline; noradr noradrenaline. Symbols in brackets are typical antagonists: hex hexamethonium; tub tubocurarine; phent phentolamine = α-adrenoceptor blocker; propan propranolol = ß-adrenoceptor blocker.

studied particularly in relation to noradrenergic function and will be further discussed on page 82.

Sensory nerves are of many kinds, and there is evidence that some of these may be stimulated by acetylcholine. Pain sensations are believed to be due to the stimulation of sensory nerve endings by specific substances released by the injured tissues. Keele and his colleagues have shown that substances which occur in the body such as bradykinin, 5-hydroxytryptamine and histamine produce pain when they are applied to the exposed surface of the dermis after the epidermis has been removed by forming a blister.

The mode of transmission of impulses in the central nervous system has been shown to be organised in a manner which is similar in principle to that in the periphery though vastly more complicated. The pharmacology of the CNS is discussed in Chapter 17 and subsequent chapters.

Drugs affecting peripheral cholinergic mechanisms
These drugs can be classified in two main groups:
1. Drugs which imitate or augment the actions of the cholinergic transmitter substance acetylcholine. In this group are included:
   a. Substances which act on cholinergic receptors such as choline esters and pilocarpine.
   b. Substances which inhibit cholinesterase and thereby potentiate the released acetylcholine.

   In this group can also be included substances such as calcium which promote the release of transmitter from cholinergic nerve endings.
2. Drugs which interfere with cholinergic transmission. This group can be subdivided into:
   a. Antagonists which block cholinergic receptors. These can be further classified into those which act on
      (i) muscarinic receptors, e.g. atropine,
      (ii) nicotinic receptors in ganglia, e.g. hexamethonium,
      (iii) nicotinic receptors in the motor end plate, e.g. tubocurarine.
   b. Substances which inhibit the release of transmitter, e.g. hemicholinium or magnesium.

DRUGS WHICH STIMULATE CHOLINERGIC RECEPTORS

Acetylcholine
The discovery of the pharmacological action of acetylcholine arose from work on adrenal glands. Adrenal extracts were known to produce a rise of blood pressure owing to their content of adrenaline. In 1900 Reid Hunt found that after such extracts had been freed of adrenaline they produced a fall of blood pressure instead of a rise. He attributed the fall to their content of choline but at a later

stage concluded that a more potent derivative of choline must be responsible. With Taveau he tested a number of choline derivatives and discovered that the acetic acid ester, acetylcholine, was some 100 000 times more active in lowering the rabbit's blood pressure. It is now known that adrenal glands contain choline as well as acetylcholine, the latter is concentrated mainly in the adrenal medulla where it acts as the transmitter of splanchnic nerve stimulation for the release of adrenaline from medullary cells.

Although Hunt's studies suggested that acetylcholine may be a normal constituent of tissues, its physiological function was not apparent at that time and it remained for many years an interesting pharmacological curiosity.

Muscarine and nicotine actions of acetylcholine. In a study of the pharmacological actions of acetylcholine carried out in 1914 Dale distinguished two types of activity which he designated as 'muscarine' and 'nicotine' actions of acetylcholine. Muscarine actions are those which can be reproduced by the injection of muscarine, the active principle of the poisonous mushroom *Amanita muscaria*. The muscarine actions are characterised by the fact that they can be abolished by small doses of atropine.

On the whole these actions correspond to those of parasympathetic stimulation as shown in Table 5.1. There are two important exceptions to this analogy; acetylcholine produces generalised vasodilation in the body and it also causes secretion of sweat glands in man. Although these effects are not produced by parasympathetic stimulation they are classified with the muscarine actions since they are abolished by small doses of atropine. After the muscarine actions have been eliminated by atropine, larger doses of acetylcholine produce another set of effects, closely similar to those of nicotine. They include stimulation of all autonomic ganglia, of voluntary muscle and of secretion of adrenaline by the medulla of the suprarenal gland.

The muscarine and nicotine actions of acetylcholine are demonstrated in Figure 5.4 on the blood pressure of an anaesthetised cat. Small and medium doses of acetylcholine produce a transient fall in blood pressure due to arteriolar vasodilation and slowing of the heart. Atropine abolishes these muscarine actions of acetylcholine. A large dose of acetylcholine given after atropine produces nicotine actions; the rise in blood pressure is due to a stimulation of sympathetic ganglia and consequent vasoconstriction and also to a stimulation of adrenal medullary cells and a consequent release of adrenaline into the circulation.

Dale's classification was originally made on pharmacological grounds, but it has proved to correspond closely to the main physiological functions of acetylcholine in the body. The muscarine actions correspond to those of acetylcholine released at the postganglionic nerve endings of parasympathetic and cholinergic sympathetic fibres. The nicotine actions correspond to those of acetylcholine released at the ganglionic synapses of the sympathetic and parasympathetic systems, the motor endplate of voluntary muscle and the endings of the splanchnic nerves around the secretory cells of the suprarenal medulla (Fig. 5.3).

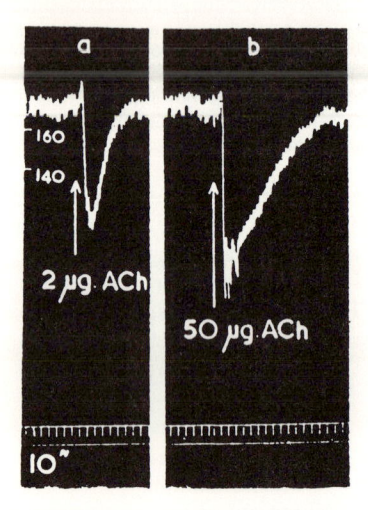

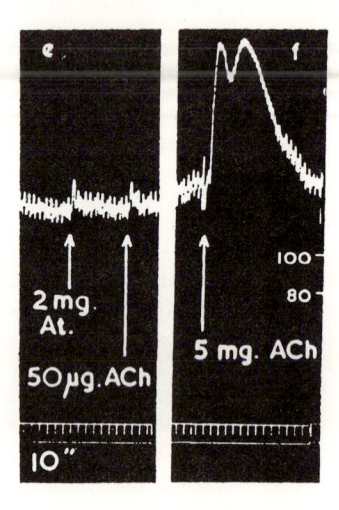

Fig. 5.4 The muscarine and nicotine actions of acetylcholine demonstrated on the blood pressure of a cat. (a) Transient fall of blood pressure due to arteriolar vasodilation by small dose of acetylcholine. (b) A greater fall of blood pressure by a larger dose of acetylcholine; this is due to slowing of the heart as well as vasodilation. (e) The muscarine actions of acetylcholine in (a) and (b) are blocked by atropine. (f) A very large dose of acetylcholine in the presence of atropine produces a rise of blood pressure due to stimulation of sympathetic ganglia and of the adrenal medulla. (Burn, 1963, *The Autonomic Nervous System*, Blackwell Scientific Publications.)

Pharmacological chemistry. Acetylcholine is an unstable ester of choline and acetic acid

$$CH_3-N^+(CH_3)_2-CH_2-CH_2OH \qquad CH_3-COOH$$

Choline   Acetic acid

$$CH_3-N^+(CH_3)_2-CH_2-CH_2-O-\underset{\underset{\displaystyle}{\|}}{C}-CH_3$$

Acetylcholine

The pharmacological properties of the acetylcholine molecule are due primarily to its strongly basic cationic head represented by the quaternary ammonium group. The positive charge is essential for the interaction of acetylcholine with a receptor site which is negatively charged. This also applies to other substances which react with the acetylcholine receptor. Figure 5.5 shows activity ratios of two substances which act on the acetylcholine receptors of the frog rectus; nicotine, a weak base, whose ionisation depends on pH, and tetramethylammonium, a strong base which is fully ionised throughout the range. It is seen that the activity ratio varies with pH in such a way as to indicate that only the ionised, positively charged, form of nicotine is active.

The activity of acetylcholine is greatly reduced by changing the configuration of the cationic head. Table 5.2 shows the effect of replacing the quaternary methyl groups of the cationic head by ethyl groups. The activity declines progressively due to a less accurate fit of the molecule on the receptor.

The carbon side chain containing the ester linkage is also important for activity. Tetramethylammonium, which represents the isolated cationic head of acetylcholine has muscarine and nicotine actions but is much weaker than acetylcholine itself.

Table 5.2 Equiactive doses of compounds in which the quaternary methyl groups of acetylcholine are successively replaced by ethyl groups (after Holton & Ing, 1949, *Brit. J. Pharmacol.*)

	Fall in blood Pressure (cat)	Contraction of Intestine (guinea pig)
$CH_3COOCH_2CH_2-\overset{+}{N}Me_3$ (acetylcholine)	1	1
$-\overset{+}{N}Me_2Et$	3	2.5
$-\overset{+}{N}MeEt_2$	400	700
$-\overset{+}{N}Et_3$	2000	1700

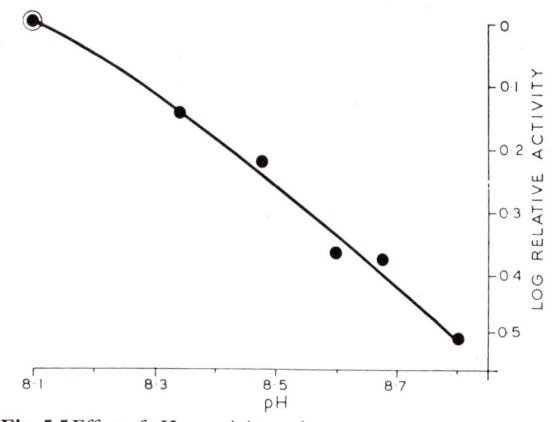

Fig. 5.5 Effect of pH on activity-ratio tetramethylammonium/nicotine. Tetramethylammonium (TMA) is a strong base which remains fully ionised independently of pH: nicotine is a weak base ($pK_a = 8$) which becomes progressively less ionised with increasing pH. The tracing shows that the activity ratios of the two drugs depend on pH in a manner to be expected if only the ionised form of the nicotine molecule had pharmacological activity. The solid line represents the theoretical activity ratios derived on this assumption. It is seen that the acetylcholine receptor functions here as a moderately efficient pH electrode. Each point represents a separate comparative assay carried out on the frog rectus abdominis preparation at a given pH. The results (log scale) are expressed relatively to the activity ratio at pH 8.1. (Data by H. O. Schild.)

Other choline esters

Other esters of choline also have acetylcholine-like activity but they are all less active than acetylcholine; however some are more useful therapeutically because they are less readily inactivated by cholinesterase. Two of the most important are acetyl-ß-methylcholine (methacholine, mecholyl) which is resistant to pseudocholinesterase though not to true cholinesterase, and carbamoylcholine (carbachol) which is resistant to both cholinesterases. Another difference is that methacholine has only muscarine actions whilst carbachol has both nicotine and muscarine actions. In consequence of their greater stability these compounds are active when given either by mouth or parenterally.

$$CH_3-\underset{\|}{\overset{O}{C}}-O-CH-CH_2-\overset{+}{N}(CH_3)_3 \cdot Cl^-$$
$$CH_3$$
Acetyl-ß-methylcholine chloride
Methacholine

$$NH_2-\underset{\|}{\overset{O}{C}}-O-CH_2-CH_2-\overset{+}{N}(CH_3)_3 \cdot Cl^-$$
Carbamoylcholine chloride
Carbachol

Methacholine is given subcutaneously in doses of 15 mg to terminate attacks of paroxysmal tachycardia. Carbachol in subcutaneous doses of ¼ to 1 mg has been found valuable for the relief of postoperative retention of urine, since the administration of the drug often obviates the necessity of passing a catheter. It also stimulates colonic movements and promotes the passage of flatus. The drug however produces certain unpleasant effects namely salivation, nausea, sweating, shivering and faintness. Overdosage can cause bronchoconstriction and alarming cardiovascular collapse due to excessive slowing of the heart. Carbachol is sometimes used by local application in eye drops to constrict the pupil and lower intraocular pressure.

Muscarine and pilocarpine
Both these substances are natural products whose actions have been known long before those of acetylcholine were discovered. Although they are not choline esters they possess a quaternary or tertiary nitrogen group which enables them to react with the muscarinic acetylcholine receptor. Muscarine is of historical interest but it is of no therapeutic importance. Its chemical structure has only recently been established.

A feature of the action of pilocarpine is that it has a particularly powerful stimulant action on sweat secretion. It is used as a miotic for the initial and maintenance treatment in primary open-angle glaucoma. After topical instillation miosis begins in 15 to 30 min and lasts 4 to 8 h. Pilocarpine also stimulates salivary secretion and bronchial secretion, and the last mentioned action is so marked that it greatly interferes with the use of pilocarpine as a diaphoretic. Pilocarpine also has typical parasympathomimetic actions on the heart and on plain muscle; it is chiefly used in therapeutics to produce constriction of the pupils.

Anticholinesterases
Small amounts of acetylcholine are continuously released at cholinergic nerve endings and probably also formed in certain non-nervous structures. For example, it has been suggested that the rhythmic movement of cilia which have no nervous supply is controlled by acetylcholine synthesised by the mucous membrane of the trachea. Substances which inhibit cholinesterase produce acetylcholine-like effects in the body because they promote the accumulation of acetylcholine.

It is known that at least two distinct cholinesterases exist in the body, called true cholinesterase and pseudocholinesterase. Both enzymes can be shown to hydrolyse not only acetylcholine but a variety of other esters. True cholinesterase hydrolyses acetylcholine faster than other choline esters, whilst pseudocholinesterase destroys butyrylcholine at a faster rate than acetylcholine. True cholinesterase, also known as acetylcholinesterase, is found in the grey matter of the central nervous system, in autonomic ganglia, motor end plates and in the red blood cells of most mammals. It is believed to be concerned with the destruction of acetylcholine released at nerve endings. Pseudocholinesterase occurs in plasma, intestinal mucosa and smooth muscle, the liver and in the white matter of the central nervous system. The term pseudocholinesterase probably comprises a series of esterases, some of which are capable of hydrolysing not only choline esters but also other pharmacologically active esters such as procaine, succinylcholine and atropine. The physiological function of pseudocholinesterase in the body is not known.

Mode of action of cholinesterase
It is generally held that only a small fraction of an enzyme protein, the active site, reacts directly with the substrate. The active site of acetylcholinesterase has been investigated by Wilson, Bergmann and Nachmansohn who have concluded, mainly on the basis of studies with inhibitors, that the active site contains two subsites as shown in Figure 5.6. One, the anionic site, is chiefly concerned with specificity; the other, the esteratic site, is concerned with the hydrolytic process. The anionic site is negatively charged and resembles the acetylcholine receptor in reacting with positively charged cations. The esteratic site contains a group G which may be an imidazole group. Figure 5.6 shows the enzyme-substrate complex which is believed to be formed before acetylcholine becomes hydrolysed.

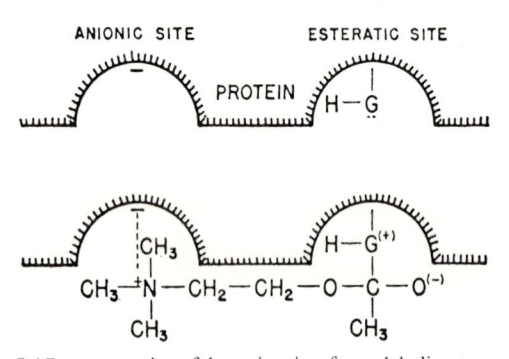

Fig. 5.6 Representation of the active site of acetylcholinesterase and the enzyme-substrate complex with acetylcholine. (After Wilson, 1960, *The Enzymes*, Vol. 4, eds. Boyes, Hardy and Myrbäck, Acad. Press, New York.)

Mode of action of anticholinesterases
The destruction of acetylcholine can be inhibited by substances which themselves combine with the active site of cholinesterase. These substances are of two kinds:

1. *Reversible inhibitors* such as physostigmine and neostigmine, the action of which is due to the formation of a reversible complex between the enzyme and the inhibitor molecule. The duration of action of compounds of this type depends on the rate of dissociation of the enzyme-inhibitor complex and the rate at which the free inhibitor is removed from the body by metabolism and excretion.

2. Irreversible inhibitors such as the organophosphorus compounds diisopropylfluorophosphonate (DFP), tetraethylpyrophosphate (TEPP), parathion and malathion, some of which are used as pesticides in agricultural and veterinary practice (p. 468). These substances inhibit not only cholinesterase but other hydrolytic enzymes, e.g. trypsin and chymotrypsin. The action of these compounds is probably due to phosphorylation of the esteratic site of the active enzyme centre of cholinesterase. Since they form a virtually irreversible complex with the enzyme, their duration of action depends on the rate at which new cholinesterase is formed. Hence their effects in the body are more prolonged than those of the reversible inhibitors.

The phosphorylated enzyme which results from the reaction of alkylphosphates with acetylcholinesterase can be regenerated by oxime and hydroxime compounds which displace the phosphate group from its attachments. The oxime-phosphonate is then split off leaving the regenerated enzyme. A compound of this kind is pyridine-2-aldoxime mesylate (*pralidoxime*, P_2S) which can be used as an antidote especially in conjunction with atropine in the treatment of poisoning by alkylphosphate anticholinesterases (p. 469).

Physostigmine (eserine) is an alkaloid which occurs in the calabar bean; it combines reversibly with cholinesterase and by thus promoting accumulation of acetylcholine in the tissues produces both muscarine and nicotine effects. It does not act on tissues whose postganglionic parasympathetic nerves have been made to degenerate. Physostigmine causes increased movement of the gut but is not used clinically for this purpose since it frequently produces nausea and vomiting. It also causes a slowing of the heart, a fall in blood pressure, and muscular twitchings. Physostigmine also has an action on the c.n.s. and may cause headache in small doses; large doses can produce bradycardia, cardiac arrest and respiratory failure. Physostigmine may be used clinically in the treatment of glaucoma, but it is less well tolerated than pilocarpine because it frequently causes hyperaemia of the conjunctiva and iris. Since physostigmine readily crosses the blood-brain barrier it is an effective antidote for central anticholinergic intoxication by drugs such as atropine or scopolamine.

Neostigmine (prostigmin). This synthetic compound (Fig. 5.7) has actions similar to those of physostigmine but it is less toxic. It is used for its muscarine effects in the prevention of paralytic ileus and also for relief of postoperative urinary retention. Its nicotine actions are made use of in the treatment of myasthenia gravis and in anaesthesia to reverse the effects of tubocurarine. Neostigmine is one of the main drugs used in the treatment of *myasthenia gravis*, a neuromuscular disorder in which the voluntary muscles are much more rapidly fatigued than normally. When neostigmine methylsulphate is injected intramuscularly in doses of 0.5 to 1.5 mg, rapid relief of signs and symptoms is produced (Fig. 5.8). When higher doses are used, or when it is injected intravenously to reverse the effects of tubocurarine, atropine (0.5 mg) is usually given to prevent its undesirable muscarinic actions. Neostigmine bromide is absorbed from the alimentary tract and can be administered by mouth in doses of 15 to 45 mg. Although treatment of myasthenia by anticholinesterases is highly effective and may be life saving, its management is difficult in view of the twin hazards of myasthenic crisis due to underdosage and 'cholinergic crisis' due to overdosage with anticholinesterase drugs. In the latter case further drug treatment may aggravate paralysis due to the production of depolarisation block (p. 66).

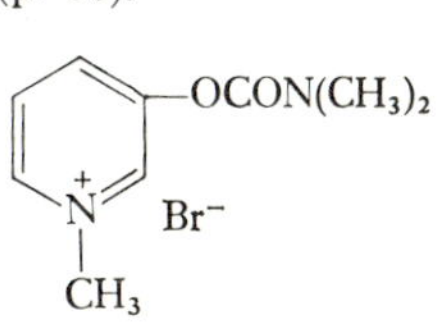

Pyridostigmine bromide
(mestinon)

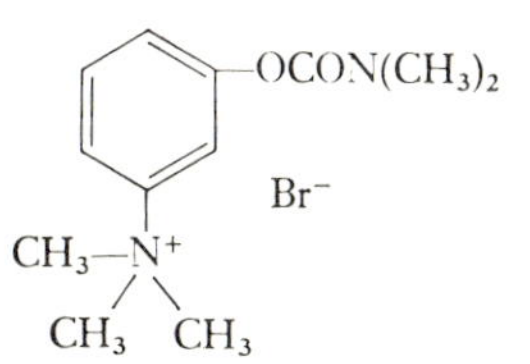

Neostigmine bromide
(prostigmine)

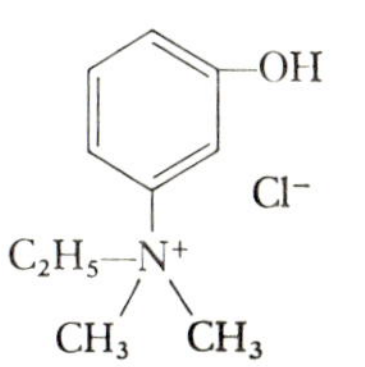

Edrophonium chloride
(tensilon)

Fig. 5.7.

Pyridostigmine bromide (mestinon) a compound related to neostigmine in structure and pharmacological actions, is now widely used in the treatment of myasthena gravis. Although it is less active than neostigmine, when administered in equiactive doses its effects are slightly more prolonged. It is given by mouth in doses of 60 to 240 mg.

Edrophonium chloride (tensilon) is a related compound which lacks the dimethyl carbamic ester group. The action of edrophonium is much shorter than that of neostigmine and it is given intravenously in doses of 2 to 10 mg as a diagnostic test, but not for the treatment, of myasthenia gravis.

Diisopropylfluorophosphonate (dyflos, DFP) interacts particularly with pseudocholinesterase in blood and tissues but in higher concentrations will also inhibit true cholinesterase; it produces muscarine and nicotine actions in animals which resemble those produced by physostigmine. In man it has been shown to increase intestinal activity and has been used in the treatment of postoperative paralytic ileus. When applied locally to the eye it produces constriction of the pupil and in patients with glaucoma this effect results in a prolonged fall in intraocular pressure. An undesirable side effect which may arise is painful spasm of the ciliary muscle.

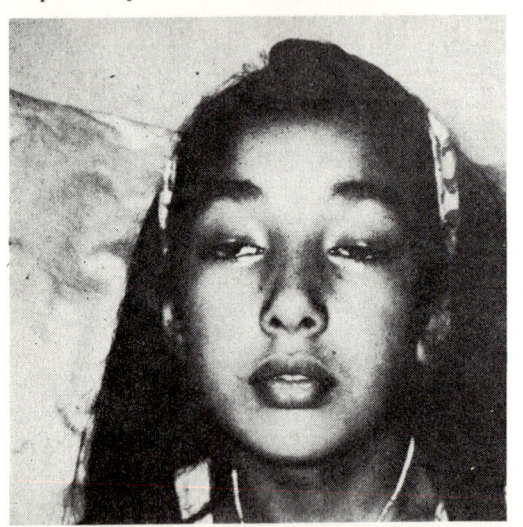

Ganglion-blocking drugs

Langley and Dickinson showed in 1889 that after painting a solution of nicotine on the superior cervical ganglion, or

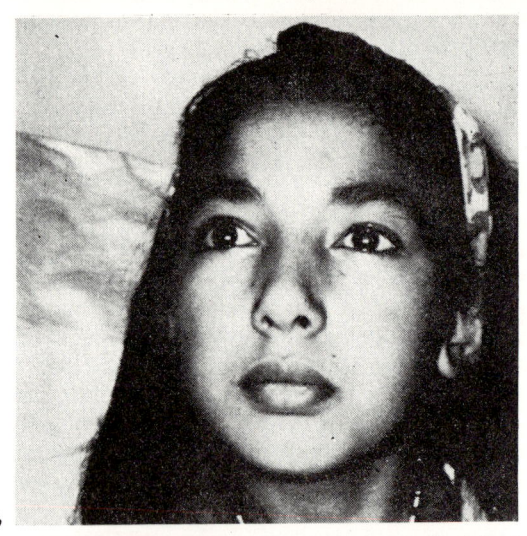

Fig. 5.8 Effect of anticholinesterase on patient with myasthenia gravis. (a) Typical bilateral ptosis and mask-like face, before injection. (b) Relief of ptosis and increased mobility of facial muscles, 10 minutes after intramuscular injection of 0.5 mg neostigmine methylsulphate.

Several compounds with powerful anticholinesterase activity are used as insecticides and poisoning by these compounds has occurred amongst agricultural workers (p. 469). These insecticides are absorbed through the skin, conjunctiva and alimentary tract or by inhalation. The onset of poisoning is insidious and is characterised by anorexia, nausea, excessive sweating and salivation. In more severe cases there is constriction of the pupils, pulmonary oedema and muscular twitching first of the eyelids and later of most voluntary muscles; death occurs from neuromuscular paralysis.

DRUGS WHICH BLOCK CHOLINERGIC RECEPTORS

The actions of acetylcholine can be antagonised by a variety of drugs which can be divided into three main groups. They will be discussed in sequence as those which antagonise:

1. ACh actions on nicotinic receptors in autonomic ganglia.
2. ACh actions on nicotinic receptors in the motor endplate.
3. ACh actions on muscarinic receptors of smooth muscle, heart muscle and glands.

There is a good deal of overlap between these three groups. For example, although tubocurarine is most active on the motor endplate, large doses also paralyse the ganglionic synapse.

after an intravenous injection of nicotine, stimulation of the preganglionic fibres produced no dilatation of the pupil or constriction of the vessels of the ear, whilst stimulation of the post-ganglionic sympathetic fibres produced these effects in the normal manner. They concluded that nicotine paralysed the transmission of the nervous impulse across the ganglion. Nicotine has thus served as a prototype of drugs producing ganglionic block, but in reality its action is extremely complex, since it produces paralysis only after an initial stage of stimulation and it acts not only on autonomic ganglia but also on striated muscle, medullary centres, sensory receptors of the skin, the chemoreceptors of the carotid sinus and the hypothalamus. Later work has led to the discovery of drugs which produce ganglionic block but do not affect other structures in the body.

Transmission at ganglionic synapses

In order to understand the action of ganglion-blocking drugs it is necessary to appreciate the manner in which the nerve impulse is transmitted in autonomic ganglia.

Transmission of the nerve impulse at the ganglionic synapse may be pictured as follows. When an impulse reaches the endings of the preganglionic fibre it causes a release of acetylcholine. Acetylcholine combines with receptors on the surface of the postganglionic fibre and alters the permeability of the surface. Ions leak out and this causes a short lasting electrical negativity, or depolarisation, of the cell membrane. When depolarisation has reached a critical magnitude it gives rise to a

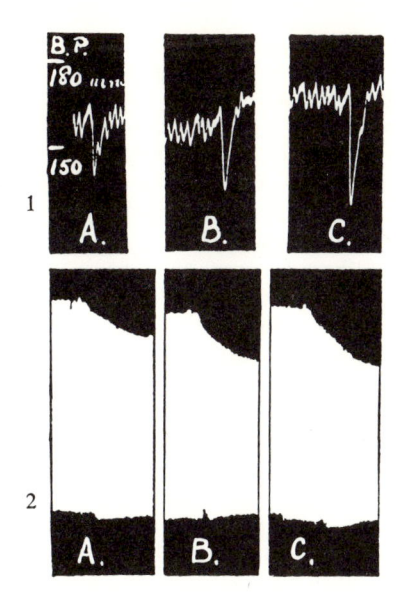

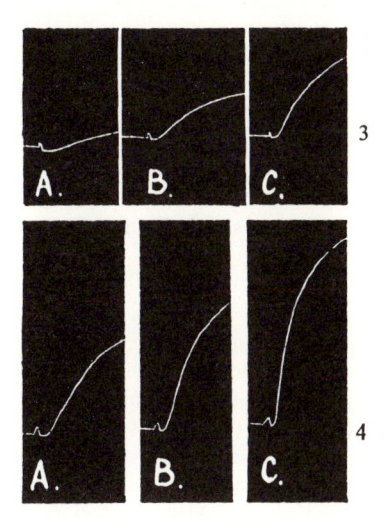

Fig. 5.9 Identification of released acetylcholine by parallel quantitative assays. The stomach of a cat was perfused with Ringer-Locke solution containing eserine. The effluent collected during vagal stimulation was compared with two doses of acetylcholine in the ratio 1:2 on the following preparations: (1) blood pressure of cat, (2) isolated frog heart, (3) isolated frog rectus abdominis, (4) isolated dorsal muscle of the leech.

In each test the effluent (B) had the same activity relative to the standard acetylcholine solutions (A and C). (After Dale & Feldberg, 1934, *J. Physiol.*)

propagated electrical impulse in the postganglionic fibre. The action of acetylcholine is evanescent since it is rapidly hydrolysed by cholinesterase.

Some of the evidence that acetylcholine acts as a humoral transmitter of the nerve impulse at the ganglionic synapse is as follows:

1. When the superior cervical ganglion of a cat is perfused with eserinised Locke's solution the perfusate collected during electrical stimulation of the preganglionic fibre contains a substance with the properties of acetylcholine. The perfusate collected in the absence of stimulation or during retrograde stimulation of the postganglionic fibre is inactive.

The identification of the released substance as acetylcholine is based on biological assay methods. Figure 5.9 illustrates the method of *parallel quantitative assays* frequently used on such occasions. In this method the perfusate is compared with a standard solution of acetylcholine by several different tests. It is considered unlikely that a substance would show the same activity relative to acetylcholine by different tests unless it was acetylcholine itself. If the released substance is acetylcholine it would be expected to have other properties including rapid destruction by cholinesterase when incubated with blood and protection against this effect by eserine; an increased response of a test preparation which has previously been treated with eserine; antagonism by atropine of its effects on smooth muscle.

2. When acetylcholine is injected into the fluid perfusing the ganglion it produces stimulation of the postganglionic neurone as shown by action potentials in the postganglionic fibre and contraction of the nictitating membrane.

3. Addition of a low concentration of eserine to the fluid perfusing a ganglion potentiates the effects of preganglionic nerve stimulation.

4. Section and degeneration of the preganglionic fibre causes a loss of acetylcholine and choline acetylase in the ganglion.

Interference with ganglionic transmission
This can happen in several ways:

1. By interference with the release of acetylcholine. This type of block may be produced experimentally by hemicholinium compounds, botulinus toxin, local anaesthetics, by an excess of magnesium or a deficiency of calcium ions, but it is of little practical importance.

2. By preventing the effect of acetylcholine. Certain drugs, e.g. tetraethylammonium and hexamethonium, prevent the depolarisation of the ganglion by acetylcholine. These drugs compete with acetylcholine for receptors and when they are present in sufficient concentration prevent the access of acetylcholine to the receptors.

3. By producing a prolonged acetylcholine-like action. When acetylcholine acts in high concentrations or for a

prolonged time on ganglia or motor endplates it eventually renders them inexcitable to the action of acetylcholine. This effect can also be produced by other substances, for example, nicotine on ganglia and decamethonium on motor endplates. This type of paralysis has been called depolarisation or desensitisation block.

All the ganglion-blocking drugs in current clinical use are competitive antagonists of acetylcholine and produce a block of transmission without previous stimulation, by the second mechanism described above. Their clinical uses are discussed on page 120.

Tetraethylammonium
The ganglion blocking action of this compound was discovered by Burn and Dale in 1915. These authors studied the effects of tetramethylammonium (TMA) and tetraethylammonium (TEA) on the cat's blood pressure. They found that whilst the former produced a rise of blood pressure due to a nicotinic stimulant effect on sympathetic ganglia, the latter produced very little effect on its own. If however TMA was administered after TEA its pressor effects were abolished. TEA also abolishes the effects of acetylcholine on ganglia and thus blocks transmission of the nerve impulse in ganglia.

$$CH_3-\overset{\overset{CH_3}{|}}{N^+}-CH_3 \qquad C_2H_5-\overset{\overset{C_2H_5}{|}}{N^+}-C_2H_5$$
$$\underset{|}{CH_3} \qquad \underset{|}{C_2H_5}$$

Tetramethylammonium (TMA)   Tetraethylammonium (TEA)

It was later shown by Acheson and Moe that intravenous injections of TEA produce a fall in blood pressure in animals and man (p. 113) due to abolition of the normal vasoconstrictor tone. The drug was introduced into clinical practice for the treatment of hypertension but its use was discontinued because of its short lasting action and its widespread effects on other structures besides autonomic ganglia. For this reason a search has been made for compounds with a more selective action on ganglia, of which hexamethonium is an example. This drug is irregularly absorbed from the alimentary tract, but some of the later drugs such as mecamylamine are well absorbed and can be taken by mouth.

Hexamethonium
The ganglion blocking action of this compound was discovered by Paton and Zaimis. They investigated a number of compounds belonging to the polymethylene bistrimethylammonium series.

$$(CH_3)_3N^+-(CH_2)_n-N^+(CH_3)_3$$

and found that the pharmacological actions of members of this series varied according to chain length. When the methylene chain linking the two quaternary groups contained 5 or 6 carbon atoms the compounds produced ganglionic block and when the chain contained 9 or 10 carbon atoms they produced neuromuscular block. Pharmacological activity varied sharply with chain length; alteration of the length by one carbon atom may change the activity by a factor of 20 as shown in Figure 5.10. The action of hexamethonium is similar to that of TEA but is stronger and longer lasting.

After a dose of hexamethonium, electrical stimulation of the preganglionic trunk of the cat's superior cervical ganglion produces no visible physiological effect although acetylcholine continues to be released as may be shown by perfusion of the ganglion; stimulation of the postganglionic trunk causes dilation of the pupil and retraction of the nictitating membrane as before. Hexamethonium prevents acetylcholine from stimulating the ganglion but does not itself stimulate or depolarise the ganglion.

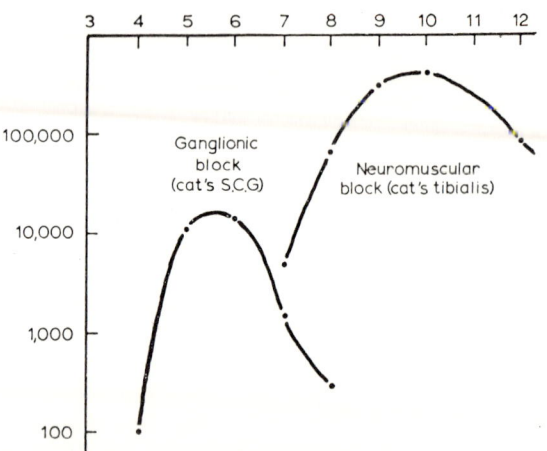

Fig. 5.10 Effect of chain length on ganglion blocking and neuromuscular activity of compounds of the bistrimethylammonium series.
Abscissa: number of carbon atoms in polymethylene chain.
Ordinate: logarithmic scale of potency, with arbitrary origins.
(After Paton and Zaimis, 1949, *Brit. J. Pharmacol.*)

The effect of hexamethonium on blood pressure is due to a release of the tonic influence which the sympathetic nerves normally exert on blood vessels. When hexamethonium is injected into an anaesthetised cat it causes a fall of blood pressure to 70 mm Hg, but when it is injected into a pithed cat, which has no sympathetic tone, it does not cause a fall in blood pressure. Hexamethonium interrupts the sympathetic pathway at the ganglionic synapse. This can be shown by experiments with noradrenaline and nicotine. Both drugs produce a rise of blood pressure when injected into a pithed cat, nicotine by stimulating the sympathetic ganglia, and noradrenaline by stimulating the plain muscle of the arterioles. After a dose of hexamethonium the vaso-constrictor effect of nicotine is abolished but that of noradrenaline is maintained or increased.

When hexamethonium is injected into a normal subject in the recumbent position it causes a rise in skin temperature and an increase of blood flow to the extremities, but there is no appreciable fall of blood pressure. When the subject stands up the arterial pressure drops abruptly; this postural hypotension is one of the main disadvantages when a ganglion-blocking drug is used clinically. Hexamethonium also causes inhibition of gastric, salivary, and sweat secretion, impairment of accommodation, and in some patients impairment of bladder and bowel function. Patients usually become tolerant to hexamethonium so that the dose has to be gradually increased.

Mecamylamine (inversine)
In contrast to hexamethonium, which is a quaternary ammonium compound, this drug is a secondary amine and hence it is much better absorbed from the gastro-intestinal tract. When tested for ganglion-blocking activity on the nictitating membrane of the cat its activity by intravenous injection is about equal to that of hexamethonium, but when administered orally to patients it is much more effective than hexamethonium owing to its more complete absorption. The side effects of mecamylamine are similar to those of the other ganglion-blocking drugs but because it is a secondary amine it penetrates the blood-brain barrier and may produce central effects such as an acute anxiety state.

Neuromuscular blocking drugs

It is necessary to distinguish between the propagation of the nerve impulse along the nerve fibre, its transmission across the neuromuscular junction, and its further propagation along the muscle membrane. The manner of propagation along the nerve fibre and along the muscle membrane is essentially similar. According to a view put forward last century by Hermann, and still generally accepted, the nerve impulse travels in steps. A stimulated portion of nerve generates electric current which in turn excites the next portion of nerve which again generates current, and so a wave of electric excitation travels right to the end of the nerve much as the process of ignition travels along the length of a fuse by local point-to-point excitation. This self-propagating electrical process changes to a chemical process at the junction of nerve and muscle. When an impulse reaches the nerve endings it causes the release of acetylcholine which diffuses to the adjacent motor endplate and depolarises it. When the endplate potential reaches a critical magnitude it excites the adjacent muscle membrane and so initiates a propagated impulse along the membrane. This eventually leads to activation of the contractile substance actomyosin by intermediate steps which involve calcium. Meanwhile the acetylcholine is destroyed by cholinesterase located in the pre- and postsynaptic membranes in close apposition to the nerve terminals. The endplate membrane repolarises quickly and once again is ready to respond to acetylcholine.

Acetylcholine in neuromuscular transmission
Information about the transmitter function of acetylcholine has come from pharmacological and electrophysiological experiments.

Dale and colleagues showed in 1936 that when a mammalian striated muscle was perfused with eserinised Locke's solution, stimulation of its motor nerve caused the appearance in the venous effluent of a substance with the properties of acetylcholine. Acetylcholine release was not inhibited by tubocurarine which abolished the contractile effect of nerve stimulation. When acetylcholine was injected into the artery perfusing a striated muscle it produced a quick contractile response which was shown to correspond to a brief asynchronous tetanus. Further evidence for the participation of acetylcholine was provided by the finding that a twitch response following nerve stimulation was converted into a tetanus in the presence of eserine.

The role of acetylcholine at the neuromuscular junction has been further elucidated by electrophysiological techniques largely through the work of Katz and his colleagues. The neuromuscular junction is composed of a presynaptic membrane which forms part of the motor nerve ending, and a postsynaptic membrane on which acetylcholine receptors are located. The two membranes are separated by a gap of 500 Å. Three essential features are involved in neuromuscular transmission and may be briefly summarised as follows:

1. Release of acetylcholine is a presynaptic event, the mechanisms of which are not fully understood. Intracellular recordings by means of microelectrodes at the motor endplate have demonstrated 'miniature endplate potentials' which are due to the effects on the postsynaptic membrane of spontaneously released packets or 'quanta' of acetylcholine. Each packet, containing several thousand molecules of acetylcholine, is able to produce a transient depolarisation of the postsynaptic membrane by about 1 millivolt (mV). The arrival of an action potential at the motor nerve endings brings about the simultaneous release of several hundreds of these packets (i.e. several million molecules of acetylcholine per impulse per endplate). In normal circumstances this is more than is required to ensure successful neuromuscular transmission; indeed it has been estimated to be about five times the threshold requirement. This large safety factor is sufficient to compensate for substantial variations in

transmitter output. A notable exception, where the safety factor is greatly reduced, occurs in the disease myasthenia gravis (p. 61).

2. Diffusion of acetylcholine across the synaptic gap from its point of release causes it to interact with acetylcholine receptors on the outer surface of the muscle membrane bringing about a local depolarisation of the postsynaptic membrane, the endplate potential (EPP). When the depolarisation reaches a threshold value, an electrical impulse is initiated which propagates along the whole muscle fibre and leads to contraction of the fibre (Figure 5.11a). The effect of acetylcholine in producing the EPP can be likened to a short-circuit across the membrane due to a transient increase in its permeability to both sodium and potassium ions. It is this change in permeability which causes the membrane to depolarise and to initiate the muscle action potential and the consequent contraction mechanisms.

3. The presence at both presynaptic and postsynaptic membranes of acetylcholinesterase provides a means of controlling the duration of action of acetylcholine, a feature which is relevant to the use of anticholinesterase drugs.

Synthesis, storage and release of acetylcholine in nerves
Acetylcholine is synthesised by the enzyme choline acetylase which is present in all cholinergic neurones and is capable of transferring acetylcoenzyme A to choline. The synthesis of acetylcholine thus requires the presence of adequate quantities of choline acetylase, free choline, coenzyme A and active acetate for the formation of acetylcoenzyme A. The formed acetylcholine is believed to accumulate within synaptic vesicles in the nerve terminal.

Both choline acetylase and acetylcholine occur throughout the axons of cholinergic nerves as well as in their endings. Choline acetylase is probably manufactured in the cell body and carried peripherally by the movement of the axoplasm. Choline is a normal constituent of the extracellular fluid which does not penetrate readily into the cell interior, yet when the acetylcholine turnover is brisk as during nerve activity, choline has to be continually replenished in the interior of the nerve. This is accomplished by a specific carrier mechanism.

The presence of calcium in the extracellular fluid is essential for transmitter release. If calcium is lowered there is a striking fall in the amount of acetylcholine released. Magnesium antagonises these effects of calcium. Since calcium is required for the process by which depolarisation brings about the release of acetylcholine, it has been suggested that depolarisation may open a gate for calcium ions, allowing them to penetrate the axon membrane. Calcium may be essential for the process which causes a transient fusion of axon and vesicular membrane leading to the release of transmitter.

Interference with neuromuscular transmission

Neuromuscular transmission can be reduced or blocked by a variety of factors acting either by presynaptic or postsynaptic interference with the acetylcholine mechanism. The most important neuromuscular blocking drugs in clinical use act postsynaptically and they will be discussed first.

Postsynaptic interference
Many compounds structurally related to acetylcholine, particularly quaternary ammonium compounds react with nicotinic acetyl-choline receptors of the postsynaptic membrane. Such substances may produce neuromuscular block by two main mechanisms.

Competitive block
One type of drug occupies the acetylcholine receptors without producing depolarisation, and prevents the build-up of a critical end plate depolarisation by acetylcholine. These drugs compete with acetylcholine for receptors according to the law of mass action and produce a parallel shift of the log-dose response curves of acetylcholine typical of competitive antagonism (p. 11). They are usually referred to as competitive neuromuscular blockers; examples are tubocurarine and gallamine.

Depolarisation block
Another type of drug reacts with acetylcholine receptors but produces depolarisation and consequent block. Examples are decamethonium and suxamethonium. Their effect resembles that of an excess of acetylcholine. Several factors probably contribute to the block: (1) The long lasting depolarisation produced by these drugs results in an inactivation of the sodium carrying mechanism required for generating a propagated impulse along the muscle fibre. This failure is probably the main cause of depolarisation block in an intact mammalian organism. (2) The receptors may become desensitised. It is known from *in vitro* experiments that when acetylcholine is applied to a motor endplate by micropipette it produces an initial depolarisation but the membrane soon becomes repolarised though acetylcholine remains present. This condition has been referred to as desensitisation of receptors towards acetylcholine. Similar transient effects have been observed with other depolarising agents and it has been suggested that the neuromuscular block produced by such agents may after an initial stage of depolarisation be due to a state of desensitisation or refractoriness of endplate receptors.

Tubocurarine
Tubocurarine is a pure alkaloid extracted from curare. It has a complex chemical structure (Fig. 5.12) and was previously believed to be a bisquaternary ammonium compound. More recent work has shown, however, that it

contains only one quaternary nitrogen group. Tubocurarine is poorly absorbed from the gastrointestinal tract and is administered intravenously. Its main effect is to cause flaccid muscular paralysis without preceding stimulation.

Eccles, Katz and Kuffler studied the action of tubocurarine on the endplate potential. When a muscle is stimulated through its motor nerve the endplate potential can normally not be recorded since it is submerged in the much larger muscle action potential. In the presence of tubocurarine, however, the endplate potential can be made visible. Tubocurarine diminishes the effect of acetylcholine on the endplate, and reduces the endplate potential to a point where it cannot excite the adjacent fibres. Stimulation of the motor nerve now produces a demonstrable local endplate potential but no propagated action potential, as shown in Figure 5.11b. Larger concentrations of tubocurarine completely abolish the endplate potential.

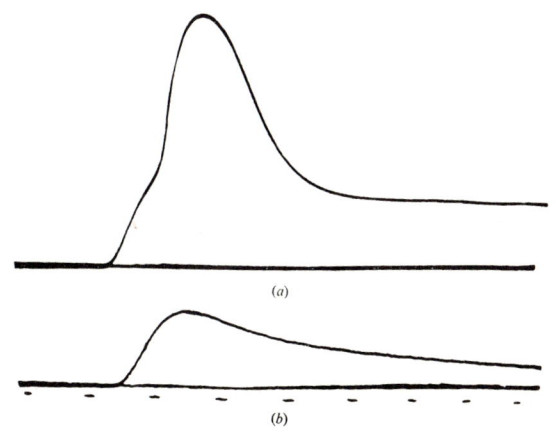

Fig. 5.11 Records obtained from a single endplate of frog muscle when a microelectrode is inserted in the muscle fibre. (a) Without tubocurarine, showing two components of the rising phase; an endplate potential from which a propagated spike arises (amplitude of maximal point 112 millivolts). (b) With tubocurarine (4×10^{-6}, showing only an endplate potential (amplitude of maximal point 9 millivolts). Time marks, m.sec. (Records kindly supplied by Professor B. Katz.)

Tubocurarine antagonises acetylcholine because it competes for the same receptors on the endplate, with which acetylcholine normally combines.

When tubocurarine chloride is injected intravenously muscular paralysis begins in the eyes and spreads to the face, neck, limbs, trunk and finally to the intercostal muscles and the diaphragm. Moderate doses of 10 to 20 mg given intravenously usually do not paralyse the respiratory muscles and have no anaesthetic or analgesic effect. The maximum effect of an intravenous injection is reached in about four minutes and begins to wear off after half an hour. Tubocurarine also has some ganglion-blocking action and hence may produce a fall of blood pressure.

The main use of tubocurarine is in anaesthesia (p. 305). It is also used to diminish the risk of injury in electro-convulsive therapy. The *dimethylether of tubocurarine* (metocurine) resembles tubocurarine in its pharmacological actions, but is two to three times more active.

The effects of tubocurarine on striated muscle are antagonised by the anticholinesterases, physostigmine and neostigmine, which cause an increased accumulation of acetylcholine at the endplate.

Gallamine triethiodide (flaxedil)
This is a synthetic compound introduced by Bovet and his colleagues in 1947. It contains three quaternary nitrogen groups (Fig. 5.12). Its mode of action is similar to that of tubocurarine and it is antagonised by anticholinesterases. Gallamine differs from tubocurarine in having an appreciable atropine-like action on the heart, but no ganglion-blocking effect. When administered intravenously to patients it may produce tachycardia and a rise of blood pressure.

Fig. 5.12.

Decamethonium
This compound was first studied in 1948. It is a member of the bis-trimethylpoly-methylene series to which hexamethonium also belongs Figure 5.10 shows that in this homologous series the compound with a chain length

of 10 carbon atoms has maximum neuromuscular-blocking activity and very little ganglion-blocking activity. Although decamethonium produces neuromuscular block and a flaccid paralysis in the cat and in man, its actions differ in several respects from those of tubocurarine. The neuromuscular block is usually preceded by spontaneous fasciculations and by a potentiation of the maximal twitch elicited by stimulation of the motor nerve. The block is not reversed by neostigmine and other anticholinesterases but, if anything, is potentiated. In denervated mammalian muscle decamethonium causes a typical contracture; it also produces spastic opisthotonus in the chick (Fig. 5.13) and a contracture of the isolated frog rectus.

Decamethonium is now mainly of theoretical interest. It was the first depolarising neuromuscular drug used but has become obsolete because of its prolonged action.

Suxamethonium (succinylcholine)
This compound which can be regarded as two molecules of acetylcholine joined together (Fig. 5.12) produces neuromuscular block by depolarisation. Its action is therefore fundamentally similar to that of decamethonium but since it is rapidly hydrolysed by cholinesterase its action is of shorter duration. This compound has largely replaced decamethonium and its clinical uses in anaesthesia are discussed on page 306. Abnormal sensitivity to suxamethonium is discussed on page 29.

Differences between competitive and depolarising block
These have been analysed particularly in the cat.

A characteristic effect of depolarising drugs is the production of initial muscular fasciculations before block. Competitive blockers produce no such stimulation. The depolarising drugs also produce a twich response when injected intra-arterially into cat muscle and a prolonged contracture in chronically denervated muscle. The latter effect can be explained by a spread of acetylcholine receptors over the whole muscle membrane after denervation.

An increase in acetylcholine concentration near the receptors tends to antagonise competitive block and aggravate depolarisation block. Thus anticholinesterases antagonise tubocurarine and potentiate decamethonium. In some cases depolarising blockers may reverse a competitive block and conversely tubocurarine may partly reverse a depolarisation block.

These distinctions are not always clear-cut; it is sometimes found that a depolarising block turns into a block which is reversible by anticholinesterases, thus becoming apparently competitive. This has been called dual block.

Evaluation of drugs producing neuromuscular block
The activity of these compounds can be determined by one of the following methods:

1. The production of neuromuscular block in the mammalian nerve muscle preparation.
2. The paralysing effect produced by the injection of graded doses into mice holding on to a rotating cylinder.
3. Slow intravenous injection into rabbits until the head drops forward and cannot be raised spontaneously.
4. Reduction of hand-grip strength and of respiratory minute volume in man after small intravenous doses.

The toxicity can be assessed by comparing the LD50 under artificial respiration with the LD50 under normal respiration.

A rapid method of obtaining information about the mode of action of these compounds is to administer them intravenously in the chick. In this species tubocurarine and allied drugs produce a flaccid paralysis whilst drugs such as decamethonium cause a spastic paralysis (Fig. 5.13).

Presynaptic interference
Acetylcholine synthesis, storage or release may be affected. Certain substances related to choline (*hemicholiniums* and *triethylcholine*) prevent the synthesis of acetylcholine so that the stores of acetylcholine in nerve endings become depleted and nerve stimulation becomes ineffective. The action of these drugs is antagonised by choline, presumably because they compete with choline for a carrier mechanism which transports it to the sites of acetylcholine synthesis.

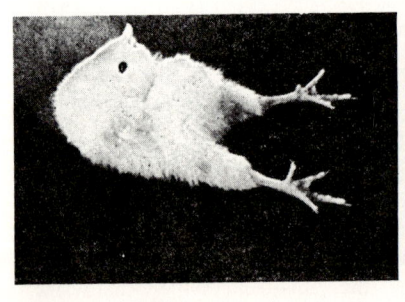

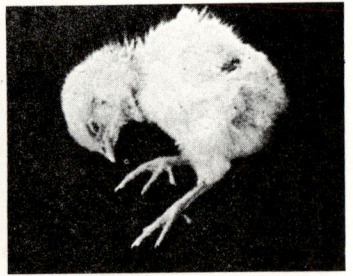

Fig. 5.13 A comparison of the effects of an intravenous injection of decamethonium iodide (left) and tubocurarine chloride (right). (After Buttle and Zaimis, 1949, *J. Pharm. Pharmacol.*)

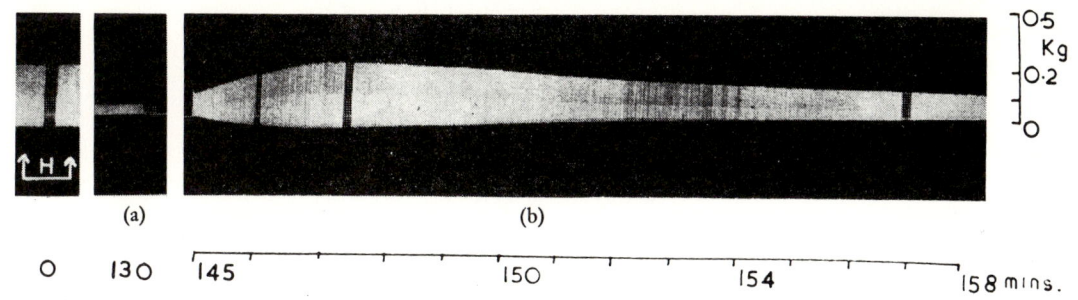

Fig. 5.14 The effect of hemicholinium and subsequent rest on the responses of the cat tibialis anterior muscle to nervous stimulation. Intravenous injection of hemicholinium (H) produced a slowly developing neuromuscular block (a); stimulation was stopped for 15 minutes and when re-applied (b) the muscle response showed transient recovery. (By courtesy of Dr. Harold Wilson.)

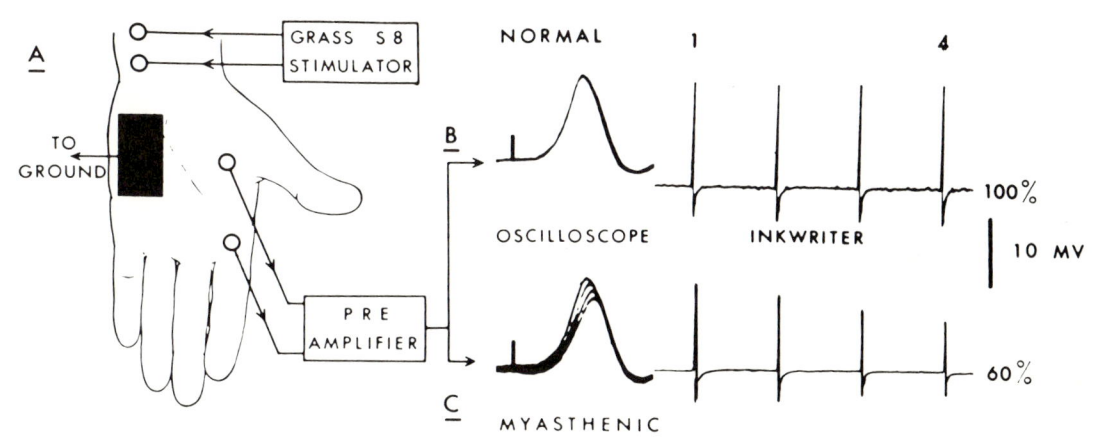

Fig. 5.15 Diagram of an electromyographic method used to study neuromuscular function in myasthenic patients. The ulnar nerve is stimulated four times at quarter-second intervals and the resultant muscle action potentials are amplified and displayed on an oscilloscope and on an ink-writer. The records were obtained from a normal subject (B) and from a myasthenic patient (C). The four equal responses in B indicate that all the muscle fibres respond to every stimulus, whereas in the myasthenic patient (C) where the transmitter output is already only about one-fifth of that of normal subjects, there is a progressive decrease in the number of muscle fibres responding to each successive stimulus. This neuromuscular failure can be measured by expressing the amplitude of the fourth response as a percentage of the first. Neuromuscular transmission measured in this way was 100 per cent in the normal subject but only 60 per cent in the myasthenic patient. (After Roberts & Wilson (1969) In 'Myasthenia Gravis', Heinemann Med. Books, London.)

Since the pharmacological effects of these drugs become apparent only when the transmitter stores have been depleted, their action is slow to develop; the most active cholinergic junctions are affected first. When injected into the cat these compounds produce a neuromuscular block which is aggravated by stimulation and relieved by rest (Fig. 5.14). It has been suggested that these drugs could be used to block excessive neuromuscular activity in tetanus, but so far they have not been employed clinically.

Acetylcholine release can be inhibited by magnesium, local anaesthetic drugs and botulinus toxin.

Myasthenia gravis is a neuromuscular disorder in which the voluntary muscles are much more readily fatigued than normally; the distinct features of this disease are a characteristic weakness of the ocular, facial, pharyngeal, limb and respiratory muscles. Although the aetiology of this disease is obscure there is considerable evidence in support of the view that in myasthenic patients the safety factor for neuromuscular transmission is reduced (Fig. 5.15). The site of the physiological defect in myasthenia, whether pre- or post-synaptic has been the subject of controversy but the most widely held view was that it is presynaptic due to reduced acetylcholine release. More recent evidence, however, is in favour of a postsynaptic acetylcholine receptor defect, due to an autosensitisation process. The post-synaptic defect in myasthenia gravis appears to result from a combination of a decrease in acetylcholine receptors associated with structural changes at the endplate and impaired function in the remaining receptors due to fixation of an acetylcholine receptor antibody.

Muscarinic receptor blocking drugs
Atropine
This alkaloid, racemic or ($\pm$)-hyoscyamine, is an ester of tropic acid and the tertiary amino-alcohol tropine.

(I) Atropine (±-Hyoscyamine)

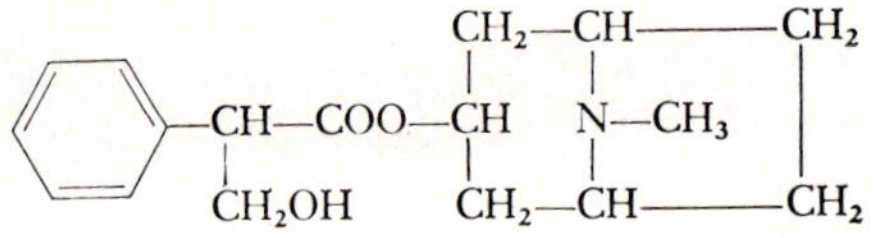

Tropic acid residue   Tropine residue

(II) Hyoscine (Scopolamine)

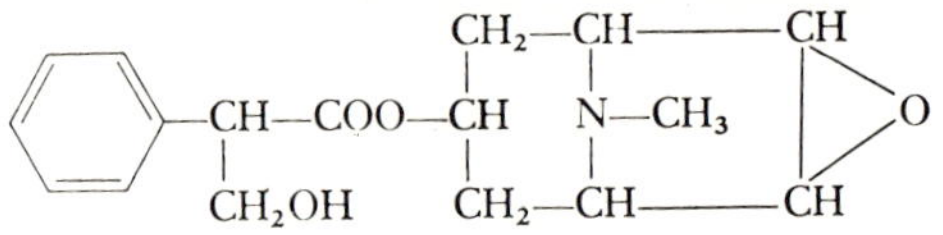

(III) Homatropine

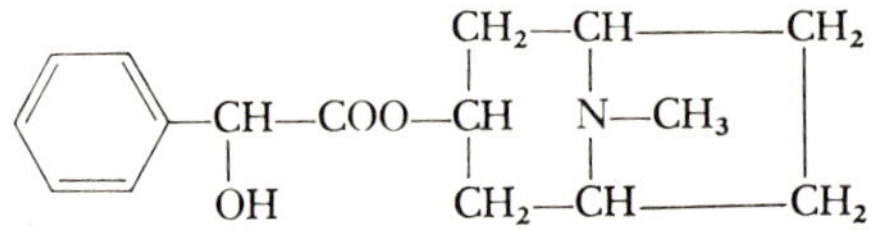

(IV) Lachesine chloride

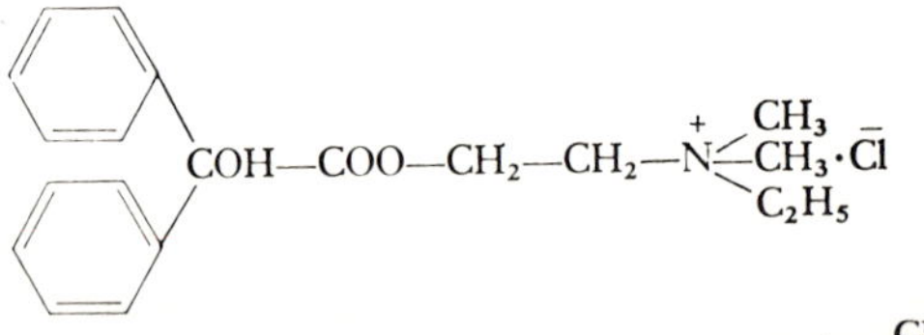

(V) Propantheline bromide

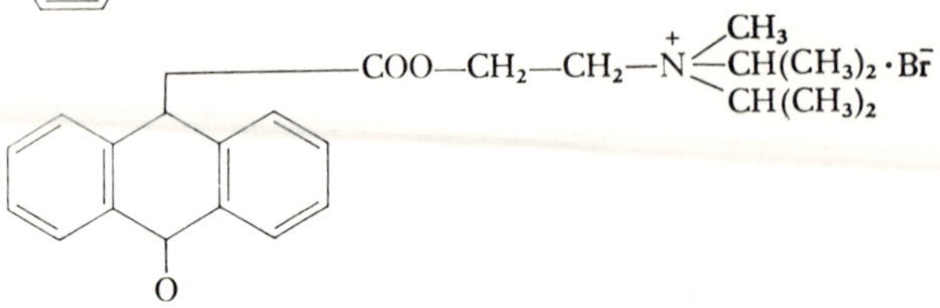

Fig. 5.16 Atropine-like drugs.

Solanaceous plants contain mainly L-hyoscyamine which is converted to the racemic compound during the process of extraction. The peripheral actions of atropine are mainly due to its content of L-hyoscyamine which is twenty times more active than the dextrorotatory isomer. Scopolamine [L-hyoscine], another alkaloid occuring in solanaceous plants, is an ester of tropic acid and scopine (Fig. 5.16).

Actions of atropine

Atropine has peripheral and central actions. The closely related drug hyoscine also has both peripheral and central actions.

Peipheral actions. Atropine is a competitive antagonist of the muscarine actions of acetylcholine as discussed on page 12. Atropine also antagonises most of the effects of stimulation of parasympathetic and cholinergic sympathetic nerves. It does not prevent the release of acetylcholine but antagonises the effects of acetylcholine at the effector level after it has been released from post-ganglionic nerve endings.

Atropine and related anticholinergic drugs have the following peripheral effects in man. They cause an increase in heart rate; decreased production of saliva, sweat and bronchial, lachrymal, nasal, gastric and intestinal secretions. They reduce vagal gastrin release and cause decreased intestinal motility and inhibition of micturition. The ocular effects (p. 88) include dilatation of the pupil, paralysis of ocular accommodation, photophobia and tendency to increased intraocular pressure.

A small subcutaneous dose of atropine (0.5 mg) produces drying of the mouth and a dual effect on the pulse rate: an initial slowing due to central stimulation followed in about twenty minutes by an acceleration due to the drug antagonising the action of acetylcholine on the pacemaker of the heart. A larger dose (1 mg) produces acceleration of the pulse and dilatation of the pupil; it also inhibits spasmodic contractions of the gut, ureter and bladder. Atropine has a particularly powerful effect in reducing secretions. Atropine also reduces gastric secretion and motility, but to produce this effect the dose must be sufficient to cause a dry mouth. Atropine relaxes bronchial spasm, but the sympathomimetic amines are of greater value in the treatment of asthma.

One peculiarity of the action of atropine is that it only produces its full peripheral action after a delay of five to ten minutes, even when given intravenously, and when given subcutaneously the full action only appears after twenty to thirty minutes.

Central actions. Atropine produces both stimulant and depressant actions on the central nervous system. In contrast, hyoscine is entirely depressant. The actions of both these drugs on Parkinsonism and on travel sickness are discussed on pages 274 and 193.

Uses in anaesthesia. Atropine and other anticholinergic drugs are given before anaesthesia to reduce excessive salivary and airways secretions caused by some inhalation anaesthetics and suxamethonium. These drugs are also given to protect against bradycardia and even cardiac arrest induced by suxamethonium, cyclopropane and manipulations involving vagal stimulation. Atropine is more effective than scopolamine in preventing reflex bradycardia but scopolamine is a more powerful antisialagogue than atropine. Scopolamine has strong central sedative and calming effects and sometimes causes dizziness and delayed awakening. Both atropine and scopolamine readily cross the blood brain barrier and even in therapeutic doses may cause confusion especially in the elderly. In toxic doses these drugs cause hallucinations and coma.

Atropine poisoning. The central actions of atropine are characteristically seen in atropine poisoning. In the early stages of poisoning there is increased talkativeness and confusion followed by a state of mania and hallucinations. Other symptoms of atropine poisoning are dryness of the mouth, and throat, dilatation of the pupil, rapid pulse, dry warm skin, flushing of the face and sometimes a scarlatiniform rash.

Atropine substitutes

The anticholinergic actions of compounds related to atropine are qualitatively similar but they differ quantitatively in their specific activities. In particular, the quaternary compounds are fully ionised in the pH range of body fluids and possess reduced lipid solubility. They thus penetrate cellular barriers less well passing with difficulty the blood-brain barrier or into the eye. When administered by parenteral and oral routes they have reduced central and ocular effects while exhibiting strong peripheral effects.

The first clinically effective atropine substitute, *homatropine*, was introduced in 1883 and is still widely used in ophthalmology (p. 88). *Homatropine* (Fig. 5.16) is an ester of mandelic acid and tropine, and it has been found that as a general rule substances with atropine-like activity are esters of an aromatic acid and a tertiary or quaternary amino alcohol. One of the most interesting results of the study of the relation between chemical constitution and pharmacological action in this series has been the realisation that there is a close relationship between compounds with acetylcholine-like and atropine-like actions. Acetylcholine itself is an ester of the quaternary amino-alcohol choline, and a short chain organic acid. If the length of the acid chain is increased, acetylcholine-like activity decreases and eventually compounds can be produced that antagonise acetylcholine and have atropine-like properties. Ing has shown that the benzilic ester of choline and the related compound *lachesine* (IV) have strong peripheral atropine-like actions.

A number of synthetic anticholinergic compounds have been developed in addition to the natural alkaloids atropine, hyoscine (scopolamine) and hyoscamine. The anticholinergic drugs have been used clinically for three main purposes, their effects on the eye, their antisecretory and antispasmodic actions in the gastrointestinal and urinary tract and on the bronchi, and their actions on the extrapyramidal motor system. These actions will be further discussed on pages 190, 181 and 274 respectively.

Quaternary compounds such as *atropine methonitrate* (eumydrin), and *hyoscine methobromide* (pamine) produce peripheral effects similar to those of the parent compounds but have less action on the central nervous system. A number of synthetic quaternary ammonium compounds such as *propantheline* (probanthine) (V) and *dicyclomine* (merbentyl) have also been shown to antagonise the muscarine actions of acetylcholine.

PREPARATIONS
Drugs mimicking acetylcholine
Bethanechol chl (Carbamylmethylcholine, Urecholine) 5–30 mg p.o.
Carbachol (Carbamoylcholine) 1–4 mg p.o., 250–500 μg sc
Methacholine chlor (Acetyl-ß-methylcholine) 10–25 mg sc
Pilocarpine hyd, miotic 1–5% (Ch. 7)

Anticholinesterases
Ambenonium chl (Mytelase) 5–25 mg 3–4x die
Distigmine brom (Ubretid) p.o. 5 mg, i.m. 500 μg dl (intest atony, urin retent)
Edrophonium chl (Tensilon) 2 mg i.v. (diagn myasthen)
Neostigmine brom (Prostigmin) 15–375 mg dl p.o.
Physostigmine salic (Eserine) 0.25–1% (eye instil)
Pyridostigmine brom (Mestinon) 60–240 mg p.o., 1–5 mg i.m. sc

Irreversible antichol
Demecarium (Ch. 7)
Dyflos (Diflupyl) 0.1% conj
Ecothiopate (Ch. 7)

Ganglion blocking drugs
See Ch. 9

Neuromuscular blocking drugs
See Ch. 22

Muscarinic receptor blocking drugs
Atropine Methonitrate (Eumydrine) 200–600 μg (infant pylorospasm)
Atropine sulph 0.25–2 mg p.o. *or* sc i.m. i.v.
Dicyclomine hyd (Merbentyl) 30–60 mg dl
Glycopyrronium brom (Robinul) 1–2 mg 3x die
Hyoscine Butylbromide (Buscopan) 20 mg i.m. i.v.
Hyoscine Methobromide (Pamine) 2.5–5 mg 3xdl ½ h before meal
Mepenzolate brom (Cantil) 25–50 mg 4x die
Pipenzolate brom (Piptal) 5–10 mg 3–4x die
Poldine Methylsulphate (Nacton) 10–30 mg dl
Propantheline brom (Probanthine) up to 45 mg dl

FURTHER READING

Burn J H 1975 The autonomic nervous system for students of physiology and pharmacology

Cheymol J (ed) 1972 Neuromuscular blocking and stimulating agents. Int. Enc. Pharm. Ther. Section 14. Vols I & II

Feldberg W, Gaddum J H 1934 The chemical transmitter at synapses in a sympathetic ganglion. J. Physiol. 87: 305

Katz B 1966 Nerve, muscle and synapse. McGraw-Hill, New York

Koelle G B (ed) 1963 Cholinesterases and anticholinesterase agents. Hand. exp. Pharmak. suppl. 15. Springer, Berlin

Lehmann H, Liddell J 1959 The cholinesterases. In: Evans, Gray (eds) Modern trends in anaesthesia, Vol 2. Butterworths, London

Loewi O 1921 Ueber humorale Übertragbarkeit der Herznervenwirkung. Pfluegers Arch. ges Physiol. 189: 239

Loewi O, Navratil E 1924 Der Angriffspunkt des Atropins. Ibid. 206: 123

Mitchell G A C 1953 Anatomy of the autonomic nervous system. Livingstone, Edinburgh

Triggle D J, Triggle C R 1976 Chemical pharmacology of the synapse.

Zaimis E 1964 General physiology and pharmacology of neuromuscular transmission. In: Disorders of voluntary muscle. Churchill, London

Zaimis E (ed) 1976 Neuromuscular junction. Handb. exp. Pharm. 42

6. Adrenergic mechanisms

Catecholamine content of tissues 73; Assay of catecholamines 73; Formation of adrenergic transmitters 74; Storage and release 75; Inactivation and fate 76; Adrenoceptors 78; Actions of adrenaline, noradrenaline, isoprenaline and dopamine 79; Presynaptic noradrenaline receptors 82; Adrenergic receptor blockers 82; Adrenergic neurone blockers 82; False transmitters 84.

Substances which mimic the effects of sympathetic stimulation have been called sympathomimetic amines by Barger and Dale, who stated that these substances imitate the actions of adrenaline 'with varying intensity and varying precision'. In this chapter we shall discuss mainly those sympathomimetic amines, called catecholamines, which are derivatives of dihydroxyphenylethylamine (dopamine) (Fig. 6.3). The catecholamines of chief pharmacological interest are adrenaline, noradrenaline, dopamine and isoprenaline. The first three occur as normal constituents of the body; isoprenaline has not been identified as a body constituent but there is some evidence that a closely related compound may occur naturally in the body.

Elliott suggested in 1904 that the similarity between the effects of adrenaline and of stimulation of sympathetic nerves might be due to the liberation of adrenaline at the nerve endings. In 1906 Barger and Dale investigated a large number of sympathomimetic amines and concluded that the primary amine, noradrenaline, produced effects which correspond even more closely to the stimulation of sympathetic nerves than did the effects of adrenaline. The significance of this finding was not fully appreciated, since at that time only adrenaline was known to occur in the body. In 1946 v. Euler showed that sympathetic nerves contained mainly noradrenaline whilst Holtz showed that the adrenal gland contained noradrenaline as well as adrenaline; it is now known that postganglionic sympathetic nerve endings release mainly noradrenaline and dopamine whereas the suprarenal medulla releases a mixture of adrenaline and noradrenaline.

Catecholamine content of tissues

Catecholamines are stored in the body in (a) special chromaffin cells, (b) postganglionic sympathetic neurones, (c) adrenergic neurones in the central nervous system.

The largest accumulation of chromaffin cells occurs in the adrenal medulla where adrenaline and noradrenaline are stored in separate cells. Peripheral tissues contain mainly noradrenaline which can be accounted for by their sympathetic postganglionic innervation. Small amounts of adrenaline in the periphery are probably due to scattered chromaffin cells. Dopamine is found in the periphery and the existence of dopaminergic nerves has been proved.

Adrenergic neurones also exist in the central nervous system and the brain contains appreciable amounts of noradrenaline and dopamine which are stored in distinct regions. It has been established that there are regions in the brain in which dopamine rather than noradrenaline is the transmitter. The main concentrations of noradrenaline occur in the hypothalamus (Fig. 6.1). Dopamine is contained especially in the *corpus striatum* which forms part of the extrapyramidal nervous system. This part of the brain is damaged in Parkinsonism and in patients with this disease the dopamine content of the brain is diminished.

The functions of catecholamines in the central nervous system are incompletely understood. There is evidence that dopamine, noradrenaline and 5-hydroxytryptamine are important central transmitters and are also concerned with the release of hypothalamic-pituitary peptides which control anterior pituitary functions (p. 322).

Measurement of catecholamines

The catecholamine content of tissues may be measured by biological or chemical assay methods.

Biological assay. Tissue extracts are usually subjected to paper chromatography to separate the different catecholamines. The papers are then eluted and the eluates assayed against standard solutions of noradrenaline and adrenaline by suitable biological tests such as a rise of the rat's blood pressure or a relaxation of the isolated rat uterus. It is also possible to estimate the adrenaline and noradrenaline content of an extract by a differential method in which the extract is assayed on two different test preparations.

Chemical assay. Adrenaline is stable in acid solution but in neutral or alkaline solution it becomes oxidised to pharmacologically inactive compounds which are coloured or fluorescent. The chemical structure of these degradation products is shown in Figure 6.2. Adrenochrome has a red colour which can be used for the colorimetric determination of adrenaline. A much more sensitive method is based on measuring the green fluorescence of adrenolutin which can be detected in concentrations as low as 10^{-8}. By the use of spectrofluorimetric methods it is possible to measure differentially the concentrations of adrenaline, noradrenaline and dopamine in various parts of the brain.

Another development is the histochemical location of catecholamines by fluorescence. In this way it has been shown that certain neurones in the brain contain predominantly noradrenaline, others dopamine and yet

▲ : 1.0 μg./g.
○ : >0.3 <0.4 μg./g.
X : >0.4 <1.0 μg./g.
— : >0.2 <0.3 μg./g. fresh tissue

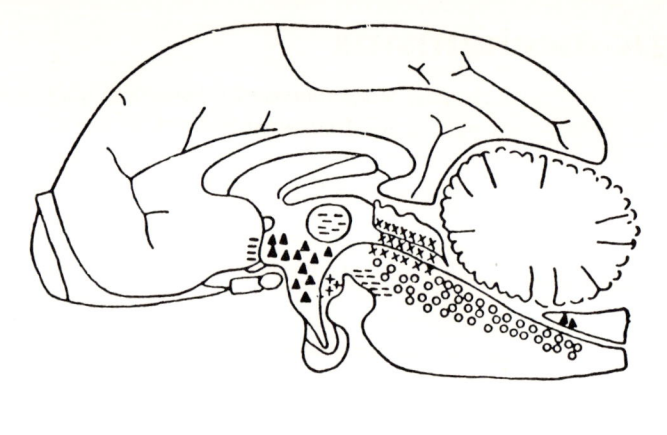

Fig. 6.1 The distribution of noradrenaline in the dog's brain. (After Vogt, M., 1954, *J. Physiol.* 123: 451).

others 5-hydroxytryptamine. Postganglionic peripheral sympathetic neurones also exhibit this green fluorescence.

Formation of adrenergic transmitters

It is important to understand the mechanism of formation of catecholamines since any interference with the metabolic pathways involved may lead to physiological disturbances due to either accumulation of a precursor or lack of a normal product.

The primary source of adrenaline in the body is the aminoacid L-tyrosine, and the most probable pathway of formation of adrenaline, proposed by Blaschko over forty years ago, is shown in Figure 6.3. Alternate routes probably exist but they are of minor importance. The four enzymes responsible for the formation of adrenaline in the body are (1) tyrosine hydroxylase, (2) dopa decarboxylase, (3) dopamine-beta-hydroxylase and (4) N-methyl transferase.

Tyrosine hydroxylase catalyses the conversion of L-tyrosine to L-dopa. It is a specific enzyme present in small amounts in catecholamine-synthesising cells. The reaction catalysed by it is the slowest, and therefore rate-limiting step, in catecholamine synthesis.

Dopa decarboxylase converts L-dopa to dopamine. This is a relatively unspecific enzyme found in a variety of tissues which promotes the decarboxylation of the laevo forms of dopa, 5-hydroxytryptophan (p. 93) and histidine (p. 94). Its coenzyme is pyridoxal phosphate.

Dopamine-beta-hydroxylase catalyses the beta hydroxylation of dopamine converting it to noradrenaline. It is a copper-containing enzyme which can be inactivated by chelating agents which remove copper. Its coenzyme is ascorbic acid.

Phenylethanolamine-N-methyl transferase occurs in adrenal medullary cells. It methylates noradrenaline converting it to adrenaline; it can also convert adrenaline further to its N-dimethyl derivative. The adrenal medulla contains adrenaline and noradrenaline and small amounts of the N-dimethyl derivative which has actions resembling isoprenaline.

Adrenaline → Adrenaline quinone

Adrenochrome (red) → Adrenolutin (green fluorescence)

Fig. 6.2 Oxidation products of adrenaline.

ADRENERGIC MECHANISMS 75

and amphetamine which deplete catecholamine stores by displacement, reserpine which inhibits amine storage and imipramine which inhibits the normal recapture of released noradrenaline.

Storage and release of catecholamines

Histochemical studies have shown that virtually all the noradrenaline in peripheral tissues is located in adrenergic nerves where it occurs in the cell bodies, in nerve axons and in greatest concentration in nerve endings. The sympathetic nerves can be made to degenerate by surgical denervation, immunosympathectomy or 'chemical denervation' by the compound, 6-hydroxydopamine. Under these conditions all noradrenaline disappears from the tissues.

Noradrenaline containing nerve endings show characteristic swellings which are believed to represent areas of synaptic contact with effector cells. Electronmicroscopic studies have revealed that these swellings contain large numbers of dense-core vesicles in which noradrenaline is stored. Adrenal medullary cells contain similar but rather larger vesicles which store either adrenaline or noradrenaline. Since the concentration of catecholamines in these vesicles exceeds the osmolarity of tissue fluid they must be bound in an osmotically inactive form, probably bound mainly to ATP which occurs in the storage vesicles in a molar ratio (catecholamine/ATP) of 4:1. The storage vesicles also contain a soluble protein, chromogranin, which may also be involved in the binding of catecholamines. The materials of which storage vesicles are composed are believed to be synthesised in the nerve cell and transported down adrenergic axons. If a ligature is

Fig. 6.3 The intermediate stages in the formation of adrenaline. (After Blaschko, 1957, *Br. med. Bull.*)

Regulation of catecholamine turnover

It is valuable to know which step in a biosynthetic pathway is normally rate-limiting, because the synthesis can be controlled most effectively at this point. The rate-limiting step in catecholamine synthesis appears to be the oxidation of tyrosine by tyrosine hydroxylase and it is interesting that this enzyme is inhibited by the end product of the biosynthetic reaction, noradrenaline. It thus seems that a high concentration of noradrenaline in cells can inhibit its own biosynthesis.

Although normally the levels of catecholamines in the adrenal medulla and in adrenergic neurones remain remarkably constant this is only achieved by a dynamic balance between rates of synthesis and utilisation. It is possible by means of radioactive tracers to measure the turnover rate of these amines, i.e. the rate at which tissue stores are being used and replaced by newly synthesised materials. Such studies have revealed that the rate of turnover of catecholamines varies when their rate of utilisation changes, e.g. during exposure to cold or stress. The synthesis of catecholamines is also stimulated by drugs which increase their rate of release such as tyramine

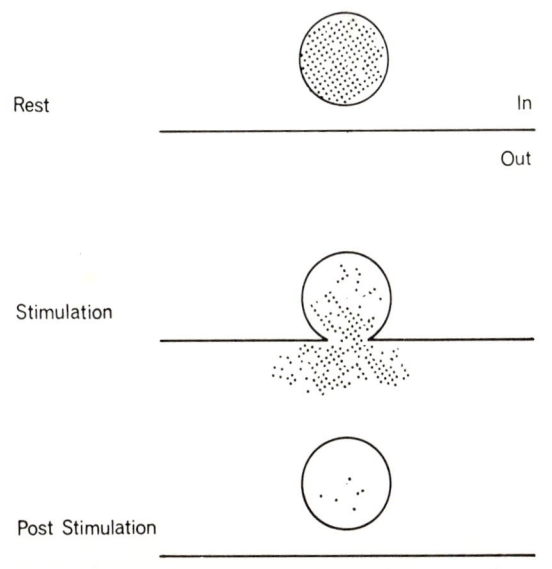

Fig. 6.4 The exocytosis hypothesis of catecholamine secretion. (After Iversen and Callingham, 1971, in *Fundamentals of Biochemical Pharmacology*, Pergamon, London.)

tied around an adrenergic nerve a rapid accumulation of catecholamine can be shown to occur by fluorescence at the proximal site of the ligature.

Douglas and Rubin have studied the mechanism of catecholamine release in the adrenal gland. Acetylcholine, the physiological transmitter at the synapse of the adrenal medullary cell produces a depolarisation of the cell accompanied by catecholamine release. An essential link between membrane depolarisation and catecholamine release is the entry of calcium into the cell. There is evidence that the contents of storage vesicles are discharged directly into the extracellular fluid by a process of exocytosis (Fig. 6.4). This is supported by the fact that catecholamines and ATP are released in the same proportions into the extracellular fluid in which they occur inside the storage vesicles.

INACTIVATION AND FATE OF ADRENERGIC TRANSMITTERS

The naturally occurring catecholamines adrenaline and noradrenaline are inactivated in the body in two ways, by enzymic degradation and by tissue uptake.

Enzymic degradation

Catecholamines are substrates for the enzyme *monoamine oxidase* (MAO) which is found in many mammalian tissues. This enzyme oxidatively deaminates monoamines which have an amine group attached to a terminal carbon atom and it thus destroys adrenaline, noradrenaline and 5-hydroxytryptamine. Ephedrine and amphetamine in which the amine group is not attached to a terminal carbon atom combine with monoamine oxidase but are not destroyed by it. They can thus act as competitive inhibitors to prevent the destruction of adrenaline and noradrenaline by amine oxidase.

A second route of enzymic inactivation of catecholamines is by way of the enzyme *catechol-O-methyl-transferase* (COMT) discovered by Axelrod. This enzyme transfers a methyl group to the 3-hydroxy group of catechols. It acts on catechol derivatives including dopa, dopamine, noradrenaline, adrenaline and isoprenaline, but not on monophenols.

The main routes of metabolism of adrenaline and noradrenaline and the reactions catalysed by the two enzymes are shown in Figure 6.5.

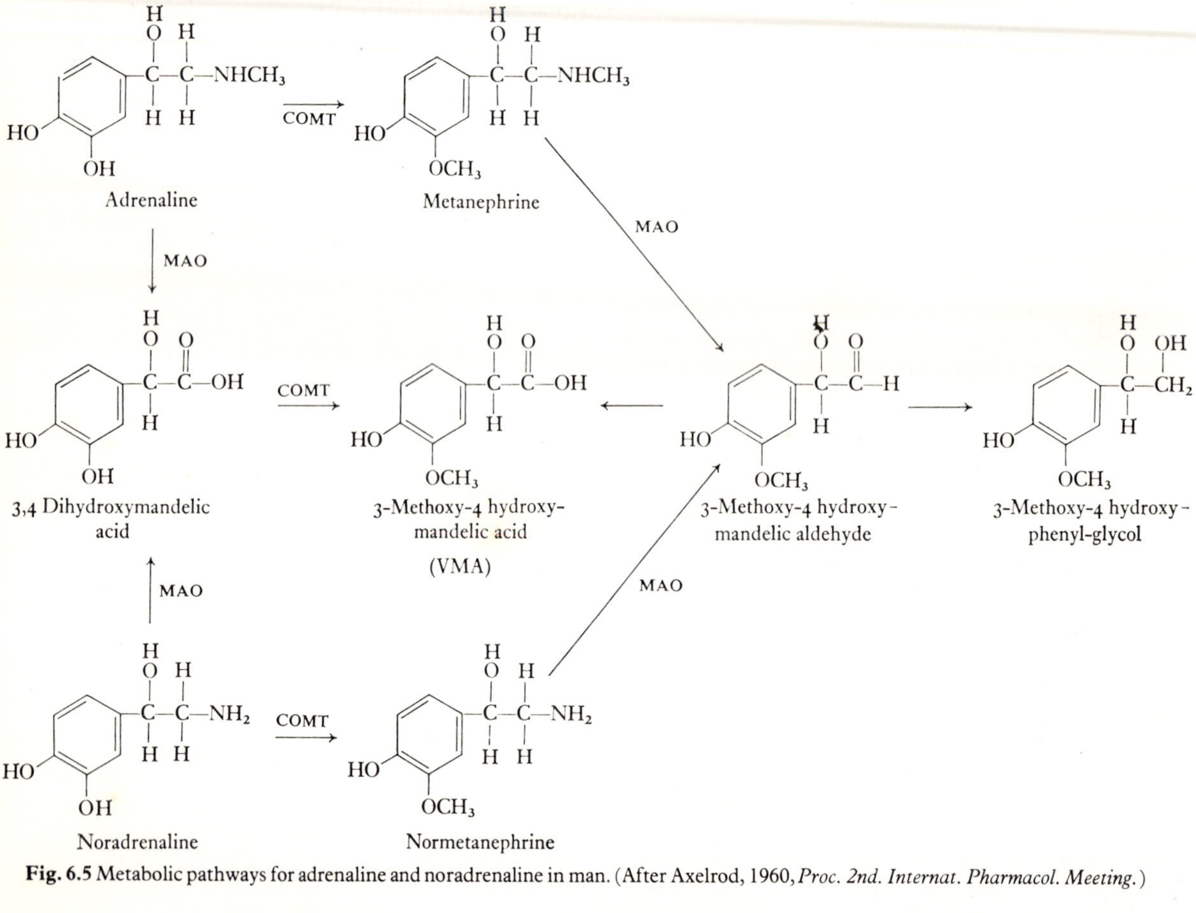

Fig. 6.5 Metabolic pathways for adrenaline and noradrenaline in man. (After Axelrod, 1960, *Proc. 2nd. Internat. Pharmacol. Meeting.*)

The two enzyme systems have different functions. Catechol-*O*-methyltransferase is concerned mainly with the rapid destruction of released catecholamines, particularly of adrenaline released from the adrenal medulla and of injected catecholamines.

Amine oxidase, on the other hand, exerts its effect on endogenous catecholamines near their site of release. Thus an inhibitor of amine oxidase such as iproniazid (marsilid) can produce an increase of the catecholamine content of the brain and the heart.

Tissue uptake

Burn and Tainter showed in 1932 that a perfused preparation which had lost its response to tyramine would regain this response after an infusion of adrenaline. They concluded that the infusion of adrenaline had replenished uptake sites and that tyramine acted indirectly by releasing adrenaline from these sites. The concept of uptake sites has been confirmed by experiments with radioactive tracers.

If an isolated heart is perfused with low concentrations of labelled noradrenaline this is rapidly taken up into the tissue where it may reach concentrations many times greater than in the external solution. This uptake is due to an active, sodium dependent, process whereby noradrenaline is transported through the axonal membrane of adrenergic nerve endings. If the nerve is allowed to degenerate the uptake of noradrenaline is abolished.

This uptake process (uptake$_1$, Iversen) can be competitively inhibited by sympathomimetic amines such as tyramine and amphetamine. It is believed that the sympathomimetic effects of these drugs are largely indirect and are due to the displacement of noradrenaline from uptake sites. Certain drugs which bear no obvious structural similarity to noradrenaline are highly effective uptake inhibitors. Some of the most potent are the tricyclic antidepressants desmethylimipramine, imipramine and amitriptyline (p. 258). Cocaine is also a strong inhibitor of noradrenaline uptake and this probably explains its effect in potentiating both sympathetic stimulation and the action of adrenaline (p. 309).

The physiological function of the neuronal uptake mechanism is to terminate the action of the transmitter after its release from nerve endings. The enzymes MAO and COMT do not appear to play a major part in this process. Two further uptake mechanisms for noradrenaline are important. Following its transport by the axonal membrane 'pump', noradrenaline is taken up by adrenergic storage vesicles in such a way that it can be released again by nerve impulses. The overall effect is thus to economise on the synthesis of the transmitter. Accumulation by storage vesicles is strongly inhibited by reserpine.

Another uptake mechanism for catecholamines is extraneuronal and has been termed uptake$_2$. This is a low-affinity, high-capacity system which has different structural requirements from uptake$_1$. For example injected isoprenaline is rapidly taken up by this system. Amines accumulated by this system are readily inactivated enzymatically.

Diminished uptake of catecholamines could explain certain supersensitivity reactions. It has long been known that post-ganglionic denervation followed by degeneration of nerve endings renders effector organs such as the pupil supersensitive to injected adrenaline. This could be due to a lack of uptake by nerves and hence a higher concentration of catecholamines around receptors.

Urinary excretion of catecholamines

When adrenaline or noradrenaline are administered to man they are excreted in the urine largely in the form of metabolites, such as 3-methoxy-4-hydroxymandelic acid (vanilmandelic acid, VMA) (Fig. 6.5). Patients with tumours of the suprarenal medulla (phaeochromocytoma) excrete very large amounts of this substance as shown in Figure 6.6. Normally little adrenaline and noradrenaline is excreted unchanged in the urine but appreciable amounts may appear after exercise and under conditions of stress. Patients with phaeochromocytoma excrete relatively large quantities of free noradrenaline as may be demonstrated by a biological assay of the urine for example on the blood pressure of a cat or by spectrofluorimetric assay.

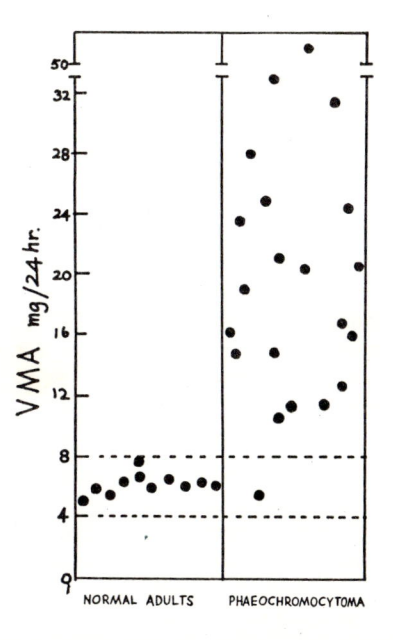

Fig. 6.6 Daily excretion of 3-methoxy-4 hydroxymandelic acid (VMA) in normal subjects and patients with phaeochromocytoma. (After Sandler and Ruthven, 1960, in *Adrenergic Mechanisms*, J. & A. Churchill, London.)

Adrenergic receptors (adrenoceptors)

A great deal of study has been devoted to the interaction of catecholamines with their receptors and the classification of catecholamine receptors. Attempts have also been made to isolate catecholamine receptors. Of special interest is the evidence that the interaction of catecholamines with receptors, particularly beta receptors, appears to be closely related to the intracellular formation of cyclic AMP.

The idea that adrenaline reacts with receptors is due to Langley (1906) who was impressed by the fact that sympathetically innervated structures retain their response to adrenaline even after denervation and complete degeneration of nerve endings. He therefore postulated a 'receptive substance' interposed between nerve and muscle on which adrenaline acts. The further concept of two kinds of adrenaline receptors arose from Dale's work on ergot. He showed that ergot abolished the stimulant but not the inhibitory actions of adrenaline on smooth muscle; when they coexisted, ergot would 'unmask' the inhibitory actions. Thus whereas adrenaline normally caused a rise of blood pressure and a contraction of the pregnant cat uterus, adrenaline given after ergotoxine caused a fall of blood pressure and relaxation of the uterus. These results can be explained by assuming that the two types of effect are due to the action of adrenaline on two different kinds of receptors, only one of which is blocked by ergot. A number of compounds were subsequently found to block the constrictor effects of adrenaline on smooth muscle but not its relaxant effects nor its stimulant action on the heart. These compounds are referred to as alpha adrenergic blockers.

In 1948 Ahlquist carried out an important study in which he investigated the order of potency of a series of sympathomimetic amines in different pharmacological test objects. He concluded that the order of potency for contraction of smooth muscle of blood vessels, nictitating membrane, uterus, ureter and radial muscle of the iris was, in descending order, adrenaline, noradrenaline and isoprenaline whilst the order for relaxation of blood vessels and uterus and stimulation of the heart was isoprenaline, adrenaline and noradrenaline. He concluded that there were two types of receptors responsible for the two types of effects which he called alpha and beta receptors. (Later work showed that relaxation of intestinal muscle by catecholamines is a mixed alpha and beta effect.)

Some ten years later it was discovered that dichloroisoprenaline (DCI) antagonised selectively those effects of catecholamines which Ahlquist had classified as beta effects thus greatly strengthening the argument for two types of adrenoceptors. DCI had no practical applications since it had agonist as well as antagonist activity but soon afterwards, Black and his colleagues introduced the beta blockers pronethalol and propranolol which became valuable clinical tools since they lacked agonist activity.

Classification of adrenergic blocking drugs

Receptor theory, discussed in Chapter 2, was originally conceived on the basis of rigid criteria involving the assumption of a unique fit between receptor, agonist and antagonist. These criteria appeared to be applicable to muscarinic acetylcholine receptors and their interaction with acetylcholine and atropine. Early evidence had suggested that atropine would exhibit a constant well defined affinity for receptors in a variety of tissues and species and it was assumed in consequence that a well defined muscarinic receptor structure could be postulated for interaction with muscarinic antagonists. This assumption has recently been borne out by careful measurements carried out at Mill Hill, London by means of radioactive receptor labelling.

By contrast, pharmacological receptor studies in the field of adrenergic receptors have indicated a much greater variability. Two types of variability have been particularly encountered: (1) variability depending on the chemical structure of various adrenergic blocking agents, particularly beta adrenergic antagonists, and (2) variability depending on differences in receptor structure in different tissues. With regard to chemical selectivity of adrenoceptors it was pointed out on page 14 (Fig. 2.5) that certain beta adrenergic blocking drugs, e.g. propranolol, appear to produce unspecific blocking effects (equal affinity for receptors in rabbit atrium and aorta) whilst others, e.g. practolol, exhibit pronounced differences in their receptor affinity in the two tissues. With regard to tissue selectivity recent work carried out by the author and colleagues has shown that although adrenoceptors in guinea pig heart and trachea exhibit a common affinity for propranolol, adrenergic receptors in guinea pig fat cells have a significantly lower affinity for propranolol.

In conclusion, it has now become necessary to postulate the existence of subclasses of beta adrenoceptors and their blocking agents, presumably caused by a less precise fit between drug and receptor.

A number of investigations have been carried out in this field, employing the standard approaches commonly used to elaborate new drugs capable of interacting with particular drug receptors.

Two types of procedures have been thus used to characterise adrenoceptors; measurement of (a) the relative potencies of agonists in different test systems and (b) the effect of antagonists preferably by determining affinity constants or pA_2 values (p. 11). Furchgott carried out a series of critical experiments from which he concluded that alpha receptors in different test systems were relatively homogenous. On the other hand there is much evidence that beta receptors are not homogenous. Lands and his colleagues have suggested a sub-classification of beta receptors based on correlating the effectiveness of agonist catecholamines in eliciting various kinds of beta adrenergic responses. They concluded that the beta responses fell into two groups. One group of responses including cardiac stimulation was considered to be mediated by $ß_1$ receptors; the other, including relaxation of the smooth muscle of blood vessels and bronchi by ß$_2$ receptors. The subclassification of beta receptors remains controversial but it is clear that beta receptors in smooth muscle and in the heart differ. This is apparent from both agonist and antagonist studies. Comparisons of the beta receptor agonists isoprenaline and salbutamol (p. 179) have shown that the latter drug is relatively more active on bronchial muscle than on the heart. On the other hand certain beta receptor antagonists e.g. practolol (p. 116) have greater affinity for beta receptors in the heart than in bronchial muscle.

Specific *dopamine* receptors (van Rossum) antagonisable by haloperidol have been postulated both in the central nervous system and peripherally.

Structural requirements for drugs which act on alpha and beta receptors
Figure 6.7 shows the log dose-response curves obtained with a homologous series of noradrenaline derivatives with increasing length of the side chain attached to the terminal amino group. The test represents a typical alpha effect, contraction of the rat *vas deferens*. The activity decreases progressively as the number of carbon substituents increases. At first the curves are shifted to the right but reach the same maximum; next the slopes and the maxima of the curves decline because the activation of each receptor produces a smaller effect, i.e. the 'intrinsic activity' or 'efficacy' declines. Finally the compounds turn into antagonists because they have "affinity' for the receptors but lack 'efficacy'.

The structural requirements for beta effects are different. In this case increasing substitution on the amino group, as in isoprenaline itself, may actually enhance activity. The catechol groups are of great importance for beta effects; the substitution of the OH groups by Cl as in dichloroisoprenaline produces a compound which antagonises beta effects.

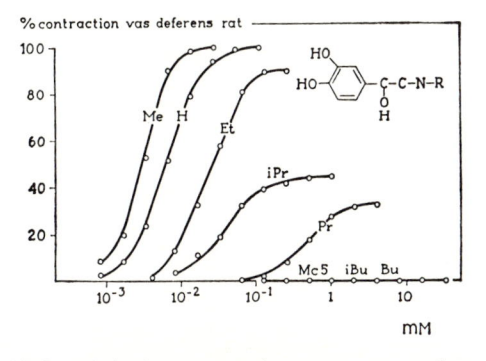

Fig. 6.7 Cumulative log concentration-response curves for a series of homologous noradrenaline derivatives. Note the gradual change from active to inactive compounds as a result of the gradual alkylation. (After Ariens, 1960, in *Adrenergic Mechanisms*, J. & A. Churchill, London.)

Catecholamines and cyclic AMP
Many effects of catecholamines such as the inotropic effect on the heart and increased release of free fatty acids are accompanied by a rapid rise of the cellular concentration of cyclic AMP (adenosine-3' 5'-phosphate) (Fig. 6.8).

Cyclic AMP (p. 319) is a cyclic nucleotide formed from ATP in the presence of magnesium ions. The enzyme responsible for synthesising cyclic AMP, called adenyl cyclase, is activated by catecholamines, particularly by adrenaline and isoprenaline and those having strong beta actions whose effects are blocked by beta adrenergic antagonists.

Adenyl cyclase is situated in the cell membrane and it has been suggested that the pharmacological effects of catecholamines on the heart and smooth muscle as well as their metabolic effects may be due to stimulation of adenyl cyclase through an action on beta receptors. There is indeed a good correlation between a rise in cyclic AMP and various pharmacological effects of catecholamines although it is a controversial matter whether there is a causal relationship between the two phenomena.

Fig. 6.8 Structure of cyclic AMP.

ACTIONS OF CATECHOLAMINES

In this section the pharmacological actions of adrenaline, noradrenaline, dopamine and isoprenaline are duscussed. Special aspects of the clinical uses of these drugs are dealt with in other appropriate chapters.

Circulation

Adrenaline
A medium dose of adrenaline injected into an anaesthetised cat produces a rapid rise of blood pressure and a reflex inhibition of the heart rate. The rise of blood pressure is due to a constriction of the blood vessels of the skin, mucous membranes and viscera. Splenic vessels are strongly constricted. Other parts of the circulation are less affected; there is slight vasoconstriction in the lung and

kidneys and no appreciable effect on brain vessels. The vasoconstrictor action is exerted on α-adrenergic receptors situated on the blood vessels themselves, adrenaline retains its pressor effect after destruction of the vasomotor centre in the medulla oblongata and after the administration of ganglion-blocking and adrenergic neurone-blocking drugs.

Adrenaline also has vasodilator effects due to an action on ß-receptors notably on the coronary vessels. Blood flow through skeletal muscle vessels is increased as has been shown by experiments in the human forearm. The vasodilator effect occurs particularly with slow intravenous infusions and it can be demonstrated most clearly after block of alpha receptors by phenoxybenzamine. Adrenaline also produces an increase in hepatic blood flow.

Adrenaline may affect resistance and capacity vessels differentially. Resistance is determined mainly by arterioles which control blood flow; capacity is determined largely by veins. In the intact animal a constriction of veins causes an increase in venous return and contributes to the increase in cardiac output produced by adrenaline.

The effect of adrenaline depends on the dose and on the state of the circulation. When the blood pressure is high a small dose may produce a fall whereas the same dose given to a spinal cat in which the blood pressure is low causes a rise. Vasoconstriction produced by adrenaline may be followed by vasodilatation; thus, when applied to a swollen mucous membrane adrenaline produces first a decongestion followed later by increased swelling. Clear evidence for a vasodilator component of adrenaline is provided by the fall in blood pressure which occurs when adrenaline is administered after an alpha adrenergic blocking drug.

If adrenaline is administered by slow intravenous infusion in man it produces an increase in pulse pressure due to a rise in the systolic and a fall in the diastolic blood pressure; the mean blood pressure remains approximately constant (Fig. 6.9). These changes are due to an increase in cardiac output accompanied by a decrease in total peripheral resistance. The decrease in peripheral resistance is due to the fact that when given in low concentrations by intravenous infusion, the vasodilator action of adrenaline on muscular arterioles overshadows its

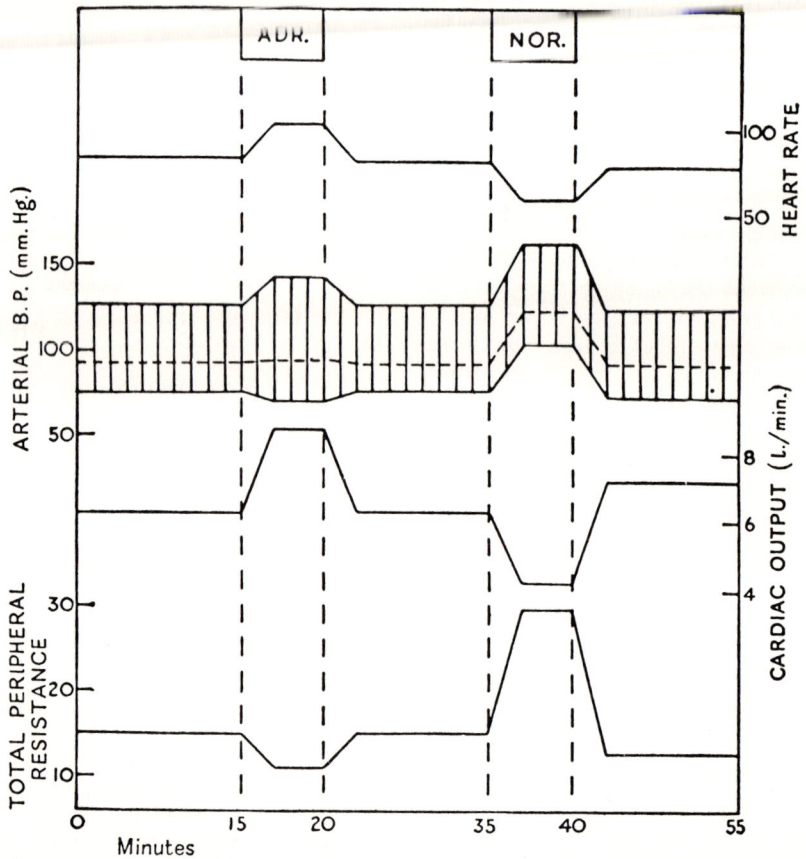

Fig. 6.9 Diagrammatic representation of the effects in man of intravenous infusions of adrenaline and of noradrenaline on the heart rate, arterial blood pressure, cardiac output and total peripheral resistance. (After Barcroft and Swan, 1953, *Sympathetic Control of Human Blood Vessels*, Edw. Arnold, London.)

vasoconstrictor action elsewhere. There is tachycardia and the subject experiences palpitations, tremor and a feeling of anxiety. Hyperthyroid and hypertensive subjects often show an exaggerated response to adrenaline.

If a more concentrated (1:1000) solution of adrenaline is rapidly injected intravenously in man it produces a sudden rise of systolic and diastolic pressure which can lead to cerebral haemorrhage. Marked ventricular arrhythmias and even ventricular fibrillation may occur, especially when the heart is already affected by disease or drugs.

Noradrenaline
Noradrenaline which in large doses acts mainly on alpha receptors has slightly more blood pressure-raising activity than adrenaline when tested in spinal cats but it lacks most of the vasodilator action of adrenaline; it does not dilate muscle vessels although it dilates coronary vessels. Alpha adrenergic blocking drugs reduce the pressor effect of noradrenaline but do not change it to a depressor effect.

Noradrenaline when administered by slow intravenous infusion in man produces a rise in both systolic and diastolic blood pressure due to a generalised vasoconstriction, a reflex slowing of the pulse rate and if anything a decrease in cardiac output (Fig. 6.9). The slowing of the heart can be abolished by atropine.

Isoprenaline
Isoprenaline, which acts on beta receptors produces a general vasodilatation and a fall of blood pressure. When given by slow intravenous infusion in man it causes a fall in peripheral resistance. The cardiac output and pulse pressure are increased, the systolic pressure may rise slightly but the diastolic pressure falls. There is a severe tachycardia which is alarming to the patient.

Heart
The catecholamines have powerful effects on impulse formation, conduction and contractility of the heart which can be demonstrated in isolated as well as intact preparations. As explained on page 132 intracellular recordings reveal that each conducted cardiac impulse is preceded by a slow local depolarisation in the region of the S-A node, called the pacemaker potential. The most characteristic effect of catecholamines is to increase the slope of the pacemaker potential so that the firing threshold is reached faster, the beat intervals become shorter and the heart rate increases.

Adrenaline, noradrenaline and isoprenaline all increase the rate of the pacemaker in the isolated heart but isoprenaline is most active; noradrenaline and adrenaline are about equiactive. The catecholamines can produce similar effects in the Purkinje fibres of the conducting system and may activate them to such an extent that their rate of firing becomes faster than that of the sinus, and ectopic foci result.

In intact animals ectopic foci occur particularly after intravenous injections of adrenaline since the reflex slowing of the sinus rate favours the development of ectopic pacemakers. Although isoprenaline is intrinsically more effective than adrenaline in producing ectopic beats it does not have this effect in the intact animal. Isoprenaline does not raise the blood pressure and hence it fails to produce a reflex slowing of the heart; it causes an increase in the rate of firing of the S-A node, which reduces the likelihood of ectopic beat formation in the conducting system.

The action of catecholamines on the pacemaker is due to an increase in sodium permeability during the slow depolarisation phase. Adrenaline causes a marked increase in conduction velocity especially in a damaged heart with low conduction velocity. It favours transmission in the atrioventricular node and may relieve heart block. It increases the slow Ca carrying inward current of the cardiac action potential (p. 132).

The catecholamines increase the strength of contraction of the heart partly by increasing the rate at which the contractile elements are activated in both auricle and ventricle.

Smooth muscle
Adrenaline produces relaxation of the bronchioles, inhibition of movements of the stomach and intestine, and relaxation of the fundus of the bladder. It causes contraction of the ileocolic sphincter and of the sphincter of the bladder. Adrenaline also contracts the pregnant uterus of many species, but inhibits the uterus in parturient women. When administered systemically it dilates the pupils by contracting the radial muscle of the iris.

Noradrenaline has less powerful effects on smooth muscle than adrenaline. It is less active in relaxing bronchial and intestinal muscle and is also less active in stimulating the radial muscle of the iris and the nictitating membrane.

Isoprenaline is three to ten times as active as adrenaline in producing bronchodilatation. It also causes relaxation of the intestine and the uterus. It is chiefly used in the treatment of asthma (p. 178).

Skeletal muscle
Orbeli found that when frog striated muscle was stimulated through its motor nerve the onset of fatigue could be prevented by simultaneous stimulation of its sympathetic nerves. In mammalian muscle, adrenaline and noradrenaline augment the response to motor nerve stimulation by an action on the neuromuscular junction. It is uncertain whether this effect is presynaptic, or postsynaptic, or both.

Central effects

The administration of adrenaline in man produces feelings of anxiety, tremor and other signs of central stimulation. When adrenaline is administered intravenously to cats it produces stimulation of the reticular activating system and consequent cortical arousal.

Interesting effects on behaviour can be observed when drugs are introduced directly into the hypothalamus of rats. After administration of adrenaline or noradrenaline the animals eat voraciously whereas after carbachol or acetylcholine they want to drink.

All three catecholamines stimulate respiration when given by intravenous infusion in man. The effect of noradrenaline and adrenaline on respiration gradually subsides due to the fall in alveolar pCO_2 but the more powerful stimulant effect of isoprenaline persists throughout the infusion period. The catecholamines stimulate depth rather than rate of respiration.

Sweating and piloerection

Both these phenomena are under the control of sympathetic nerves but the former is controlled by cholinergic nerves and the latter by adrenergic nerves. However after intradermal injection in man not only parasympathomimetic drugs but also adrenaline and noradrenaline produce sweating.

The apocrine glands in the human axilla are probably not innervated and they respond to adrenaline. Sweat glands of the horse are apocrine glands which have no innervation and are probably controlled by circulating adrenaline.

Metabolic effects

When adrenaline or isoprenaline are administered by intravenous infusion they produce a marked increase in oxygen consumption; noradrenaline has no such effect. Adrenaline increases blood sugar and lactate and decreases liver and muscle glycogen. It can thus relieve insulin hypoglycaemia provided that the store of glycogen is adequate. It also augments lipolysis, causing an increase in free fatty acids.

Dopamine

Dopamine is an important neurotransmitter in its own right in the central nervous system as discussed in Chapter 17. It also acts on peripheral blood vessels partly by a stimulant action on α- and ß-adrenoceptors and partly by an action on specific dopamine receptors identifiable by semi-specific dopamine antagonists such as haloperidol and pimozide. Large doses of dopamine in man, produce vasoconstriction by stimulating α-adrenoceptors, but smaller intravenous doses cause vasodilatation by an action on specific dopamine receptors in renal, coeliac and mesenteric arteries. When dopamine was administered experimentally by intravenous injection to patients with oliguric shock it caused an increase of inulin clearance and sodium excretion, presumably due to its renal vasodilator action.

DRUGS WHICH MODIFY ADRENERGIC ACTIVITY

Adrenergic receptor blocking drugs

Presynaptic noradrenaline receptors

The idea of presynaptic receptors arose from experiments by Brown and Gillespie who showed that the α-adrenergic blocking drug phenoxybenzamine augmented stimulation-induced transmitter release from noradrenergic nerve endings. This effect has been explained by postulating the existence of presynaptic α-receptors on noradrenergic nerve endings; their stimulation by α-adrenergic agonists producing a negative feedback inhibition of transmitter release, while α-adrenergic antagonists augment release. There is evidence that presynaptic and postsynaptic α receptors are not identical. Clonidine (p. 117) has a marked presynaptic α-stimulant action and also some post-synaptic activity. By virtue of its post-synaptic α-activity it produces vasoconstriction but by virtue of its strong presynaptic α-activity it causes reduced transmitter release of the cardiac sympathetic and slowing of the heart. Its overall hypotensive effect is probably due largely to central adrenergic presynaptic inhibition.

Other more complex presynaptic mechanisms have also been postulated. It has been suggested that the stimulation of presynaptic ß-adrenoceptors produces positive feedback, increasing stimulation-evoked noradrenaline outflow, whilst ß-blockers have the opposite effect decreasing noradrenaline outflow.

The existence of presynaptic noradrenaline receptors has only recently been recognised. Earlier work on the effects of noradrenaline was concerned entirely with postsynaptic receptors and largely with the vascular effects of noradrenaline and related catecholamines acting on alpha-adrenoceptors and the effects of blocking drugs upon their actions.

Postsynaptic alpha-adrenoceptor blocking drugs

For reasons which are not fully understood the alpha-blocking drugs are more effective in antagonising circulating catecholamines than the effects of noradrenaline released by adrenergic nerve stimulation. In man they do not effectively lower the blood pressure in hypertension but they produce a sudden fall in blood pressure when administered intravenously to patients with phaeochromocytoma in whom the blood level of noradrenaline is increased. This rapid fall in blood pressure provided a diagnostic test for phaeochromocytoma (Fig. 6.10) but measurement of urinary catecholamines and their metabolites is now the established diagnostic method of choice (Fig. 6.6).

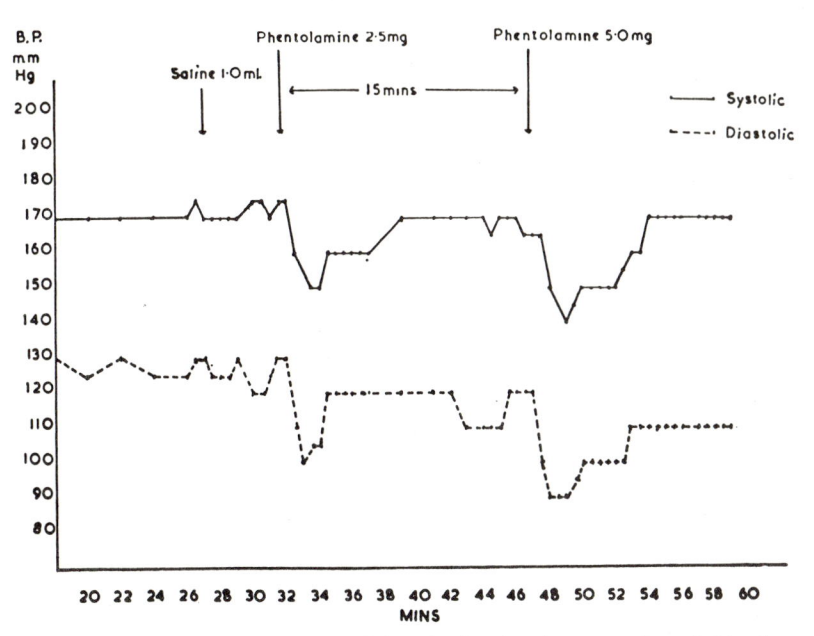

Fig. 6.10 Effects produced by normal saline and by two doses of phentolamine given intravenously on the blood pressure of a patient with phaeochromocytoma. (After Wilson, 1962, *Scot. med. J.* 7: 438.)

The alpha blockers are sometimes effective in the treatment of certain types of peripheral vascular disease, e.g. Raynaud's disease. Patients with this condition suffer from vascular spasm of the fingers due to increased sympathetic activity and the alpha-blocking drugs can produce a vasodilatation and an increase in skin temperature.

There are several groups of alpha-blocking drugs:

Phentolamine (rogitine) and *tolazoline (priscol)* produce vasodilatation which is due to a strong antagonism of the adrenergic transmitter and in the case of tolazoline also partly to a direct relaxation of the plain muscle of the arterioles.

Derivatives of chlorethylamine. These compounds are related to nitrogen mustard. Dibenamine was introduced in 1947 by Nickerson and Goodman; *phenoxybenzamine (dibenzyline)* is a less toxic derivative which can be taken by mouth. These drugs are antagonists of the alpha effects of catecholamines; their actions are slowly produced and are very prolonged. This delayed onset of action is due to the slow formation in the body of reactive intermediate compounds which combine irreversibly with the alpha receptors (p. 16). Phenoxybenzamine is given by mouth for the treatment of Raynaud's disease. The local irritant effects of this drug may produce nausea and vomiting; other untoward effects such as swelling of the nasal mucosa, tachycardia and postural hypotension are due to its antagonism of normal sympathetic tone.

Ergot alkaloids are contained in ergot, a fungus which grows on rye. Their complicated chemical structure based on lysergic acid (Fig. 221) enables them to interact with a variety of receptors including α-adrenoceptors and 5-HT receptors.

Dihydroergotamine and other dihydrogenated ergot alkaloids have α-adrenoceptor blocking activity. Other ergot alkaloids are discussed on pages 127 and 274.

Beta-adrenoceptor blocking drugs
These are structurally related to isoprenaline as shown in Figure 9.5 The first effective ß-blocker, *dichloroisoprenaline* had both agonist and antagonist activity but the subsequent drugs *pronethalol* followed by *propranolol* are competitive antagonists of isoprenaline without agonist activity.

The ß-blocking drugs decrease heart rate and the velocity of heart muscle contraction and they reduce blood pressure in patients with hypertension. Their important uses in hypertension (p. 115), cardiac arrhythmias (p. 147) and angina of effort (p. 123) are discussed elsewhere, as well as the properties of different and more selective ß-blockers.

Adrenergic neurone blocking drugs

Adrenergic neurone blocking drugs prevent the release of noradrenaline from postganglionic sympathetic nerve endings and in this way produce a fall of blood pressure in hypertensive patients. They do not prevent the release of catecholamines from the adrenal medulla nor do they antagonise the effects of catecholamines at receptor level. Most of the effective adrenergic neurone blocking drugs are guanidine derivatives including *guanethidine* and *bethanidine*; the use of these drugs in the treatment of hypertension is discussed on page 118.

Table 6.1 Differentiation of sympathetic blocking drugs

	Responses of nictitating membrane to		
	Preganglionic stimulation	Postganglionic stimulation	Noradrenaline injection
Ganglion block (e.g. hexamethonium, mecamylamine)	abolished	normal	normal or potentiated
Adrenergic neurone block (e.g. guanethidine, bethanidine)	abolished	abolished	normal or potentiated
α-Receptor block (e.g. phentolamine, phenoxybenzamine)	abolished	abolished	abolished

Assessment of adrenergic neurone block
Adrenergic neurone blocking drugs are relatively ineffective in lowering the blood pressure in acute experiments on anaesthetised animals although they do so in hypertensive animals. These drugs are usually assessed by their effects in blocking sympathetic neurones, e.g. by relaxation of the nicitating membrane in unanaesthetised cats and failure of the nictitating membrane to respond to sympathetic stimulation in anaesthetised cats.

It is possible to distinguish between different types of adrenergic blocking drugs by their effects on the adrenergically mediated retraction of the nictitating membrane of the anaesthetised cat as shown in Table 6.1.

It is interesting to compare the effects of reserpine and adrenergic neurone blocking drugs. Reserpine produces sympathetic blockade by a profound depletion of tissue catecholamines. Guanethidine also produces depletion of tissue catecholamines but the blocking effect precedes depletion: other drugs with similar adrenergic neurone blocking effects, e.g. bethanidine and debrisoquine, produce little or no depletion of catecholamine stores. Present evidence suggests that the action of adrenergic neurone blockers cannot be explained by their depletion of catecholamine stores; it seems to involve some mechanism which is not fully understood, whereby the release of transmitter following a nerve impulse in adrenergic nerves is impeded.

False transmitters
Noradrenaline is the catecholamine which is synthesised, stored and released by adrenergic nerves under normal conditions, but since the enzymatic mechanisms involved are not entirely specific for noradrenaline, other substances structurally related to it can also be stored and released by adrenergic nerves. Such substances are called *false transmitters*.

Alpha-methyldopa was the first substance shown to act in this way. This amino acid was found to lower the level of noradrenaline in tissues and it was originally thought that its effect was due to inhibition of the enzyme dopa decarboxylase concerned in noradrenaline synthesis. This explanation was abandoned after it was found that other more powerful inhibitors of dopa decarboxylase failed to lower noradrenaline levels. An alternative explanation was that α-methyldopa is converted in the body to α-methylnoradrenaline (Fig. 6.11), and that the methylated amine replaced noradrenaline in neuronal storage sites.

This alternative explanation is now generally accepted. As amines with an α-methyl group are not destroyed by amine oxidase, α-methylnoradrenaline persists longer in the storage sites than noradrenaline. Adrenergic nerve stimulation causes the release of α-methylnoradrenaline and in cases where both the methylated compound and noradrenaline are present in the storage sites the amounts of the two amines released correspond to those present in the storage sites confirming the hypothesis of release by exocytosis.

Since α-methylnoradrenaline is less active as an agonist than noradrenaline (though not completely inactive) replacement by the false transmitter produces an overall decrease in sympathetic activity which is beneficial in hypertension.

Interactions with catecholamines in the central nervous system, which are believed to contribute to the actions of drugs such as *reserpine, monoamine oxidase inhibitors, imipramine, amphetamine* and *clonidine* are discussed in other sections.

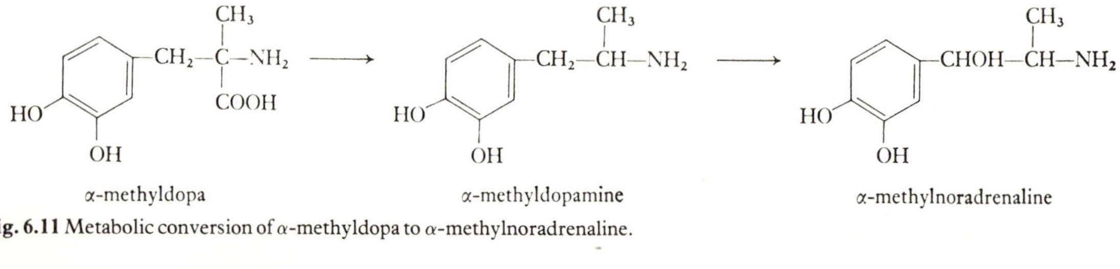

Fig. 6.11 Metabolic conversion of α-methyldopa to α-methylnoradrenaline.

PREPARATIONS

Adrenoceptor stimulants (also Ch. 9, Ch. 12)
Adrenaline (Epinephrine) 200–500 μg s.c. i.m.
Isoprenaline hyd (Isoproterenol) 5–20 mg subling, 80–400 μg aeros, 200 μg s.c. i.m. inj
Noradrenaline ac tart (Levarterenol) 2–20 μg/min i.v. inf

Dopamine hyd 2–5 μg/kg/min

Alpha-adrenergic blocking drugs
Dihydroergotoxine mesylate up to 4.5 mg p.o. dl
Phenoxybenzamine hyd (Dibenyline) 10–20 mg init p.o.
Phentolamine mes (Rogitine) 5–10 mg i.v.
Thymoxamine hyd 40 mg 4x die
Tolazoline hyd (Priscol) 25–50 mg 4–6x die init

Adrenergic neurone block
False transmitter   } See Ch. 9
Beta block

FURTHER READING

Blaschko H, Muscholl E 1972 Catecholamines. Handb. exp. Pharmac. 23
Euler U S 1956 Noradrenaline. Thomas, Springfield
Iversen L L 1967 The uptake and storage of noradrenaline in sympathetic nerves. Cambridge University Press, Cambridge
Iversen L L (ed) 1973 Catecholamines. Br. med. Bull. 29: 91
Kopin I J 1964 Storage and metabolism of catecholamines: The role of monoamine oxidase. Pharmacol. Rev. 16: 179
Moran C N (ed) 1967 New adrenergic blocking drugs: their pharmacological, biochemical and clinical actions. Ann. N.Y. Acad. Sci. 739: 541
Sandler M, Ruthven C R J 1969 The biosynthesis and metabolism of the catecholamines. Progr. Med. Chem. 6: 200
Schümann H J, Kronenberg G (ed) 1970 New aspects of storage and release mechanisms of catecholamines. Springer, Berlin
Starke K 1977 Regulation of noradrenaline release by presynaptic receptor systems. Rev. Physiol. Biochem. Pharmac. 77: 2
Trendelenburg V 1963 Supersensitivity and subsensitivity to sympathomimetic amines. Pharmac. Rev. 15: 225
Usdin E, Snyder S H (eds) 1974 Frontiers in catecholamine research. Pergamon, New York
Vane J R et al (ed) 1960 Adrenergic Mechanisms. Churchill, London

7. Autonomic control of the intrinsic muscles of the eye

Nervous control of pupil 86; Mechanism of accommodation 86; Drainage of intraocular fluid 87; Drugs affecting cholinergic mechanisms 87; Drugs affecting adrenergic mechanisms 88.

The internal muscles of the mammalian eye are all controlled by the autonomic nervous system, hence this organ provides a convenient subject on which to study the functions of the autonomic nervous system, and the manner in which these are modified by drugs.

The eye, moreover, presents the special advantage that drugs applied either to the conjunctiva or injected under the conjunctiva pass directly through lymph channels into the eyeball and hence local effects can be studied apart from those produced by central actions.

THE NERVOUS CONTROL OF THE PUPIL

The system of double nervous control which is typical of all smooth muscle and glands can be studied particularly easily in the pupil. The pupil is supplied with constrictor fibres from the parasympathetic and with dilator fibres from the sympathetic. The course of these two sets of fibres is shown in Figure 7.1.

This complicated system of nerve supply can be affected by drugs in many ways. The oculomotor centre in the brain is kept in constant check by impulses passing from the higher centres, and if these higher centres are inhibited, constriction of the pupil occurs. Such an inhibition of the higher centres occurs in sleep, and also in surgical anaesthesia. The central, Edinger-Westphal, nucleus of the oculomotor nerve is stimulated by morphine, and hence morphine produces a pin-point pupil.

Normally the sphincter is the dominant muscle but fear, excitement, and most other strong emotions produce dilatation of the pupil. This effect appears to be due chiefly to the excitement increasing the cortical inhibition of the oculomotor centre. Asphyxia appears to stimulate some centre which controls the sympathetic nerves of the eye and in marked asphyxia this action is reinforced by stimulation of the nerves supplying the suprarenal glands; this causes the secretion of excess of adrenaline, which acts directly upon the pupil, producing dilatation.

These reactions explain the pupillary changes seen in anaesthesia. During the excitement stage the cerebral stimulation causes dilatation of the pupil, an effect similar to that seen in alcoholic intoxication; in the stage of surgical anaesthesia the pupil is constricted; and in the toxic stage of medullary depression the imperfect respiration causes anoxaemia, which produces dilatation of the pupil. Any form of anaesthesia which is associated with asphyxia, such as the administration of nitrous oxide without oxygen, also causes dilatation of the pupil.

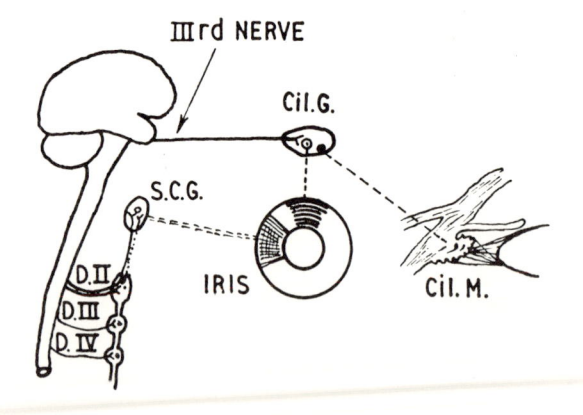

Fig. 7.1 The nerve supply of the iris. The parasympathetic supply passes by the IIIrd nerve to the ciliary ganglion (Cil.G): the medullated fibres end here, and non-medullated fibres pass to the circular muscle of the iris and to the ciliary muscle (Cil.M.). The sympathetic supply passes by the upper dorsal nerves to the sympathetic cord and to the inferior and superior cervical ganglion (S.C.G.). The postganglionic fibres originating from the S.C.G. innervate the radial muscle of the iris. (In the cat they also innervate the nicitating membrane or third lid.)

Mechanism of accommodation

Accommodation consists in an increase in the curvature of the lens which is brought about as follows.

The lens is attached to the ciliary body by a series of strands called suspensory ligaments which form the zonule (Fig. 7.2). When the eye is unaccommodated, i.e. set for distant vision, these strands exert tension on the lens and keep it in a flattened state. If the tension in the zonule is relieved the lens changes configuration and adopts its natural more spherical shape; the eye is then accommodated for near vision.

The ciliary body contains smooth muscle which is cholinergic and innervated by the third nerve. When this muscle contracts it moves the ciliary body inwards and forward and by decreasing the tension in the zonule increases the curvature of the lens.

Stimulation of the third nerve or application to the conjunctiva of a drug with an acetylcholine-like action such as pilocarpine, carbachol or an anti-cholinesterase such as eserine produces accommodation for near vision. By contrast drugs which block muscarinic receptors such as atropine and hyoscine, and those which block parasympathetic ganglia, e.g. hexamethonium and mecamylamine, paralyse accommodation. Sympathomimetic drugs such as ephedrine and phenylephrine which produce dilatation of the pupil do not paralyse accommodation, though they may limit its range.

Drainage of intraocular fluid
The aqueous humour is contained in the anterior and posterior chambers (Fig. 7.2). It is secreted from the epithelium covering the ciliary body, passes over the lens through the pupil into the anterior chamber and drains away through the angle of the anterior chamber, or filtration angle, into a plexus known as the canal of Schlemm. The relation of the aqueous humour to blood plasma resembles that of the cerebrospinal fluid to plasma. Aqueous humour has a much lower concentration of protein than plasma and although its mineral composition is generally similar it is sufficiently different to be regarded as a secretion product rather than as a simple ultrafiltrate of blood.

Intraocular pressure
Intraocular pressure can be defined as that pressure required to prevent fluid from passing out of a needle inserted into the anterior chamber (Davson). The normal intraocular pressure is 15 to 20 mmHg; this is sufficient to promote drainage of the aqueous and maintain the curvature of the corneal surface. Drainage is rendered more difficult by a dilatation of the pupil (mydriasis) which leads to a folding up of the iris and its withdrawal into the angle of the anterior chamber. Mydriatic drugs may thus produce an increase in the intraocular pressure especially in patients predisposed to glaucoma. Conversely, a constriction of the pupil (miosis) tends to open up the access to the canal of Schlemm and miotic drugs can thus be used to lower a dangerously increased intraocular pressure.

The intraocular pressure may also be influenced by drugs which affect the blood vessels. Thus, application of adrenaline to the conjunctiva produces vasoconstriction and may lower intraocular pressure, whilst histamine which produces capillary vasodilatation raises the intraocular pressure.

Acetazolamide (Diamox) has been found to lower the intraocular pressure in glaucoma after systemic administration. Acetazolamide inhibits the enzyme carbonic anhydrase (p. 164) which is concerned in the secretion of aqueous humour. It thus acts on the formation rather than on the drainage of intraocular fluid.

Dichlorphenamide (Daranide) has similar actions.

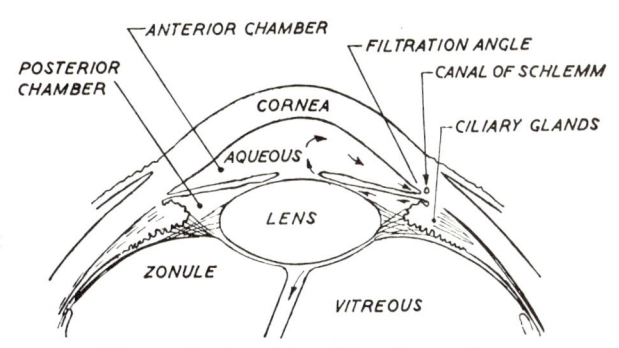

Fig. 7.2 Diagram showing origin and fate of aqueous humour.

ACTION OF DRUGS ON THE EYE

Drugs affecting cholinergic and adrenergic mechanisms are discussed in the preceding two chapters; the actions of these drugs on the eye will be considered below.

Cholinergic mechanisms

Anticholinesterases
  Eserine. If a 1 per cent solution of eserine (physostigmine) (p. 61) is instilled in the conjunctival sac the pupil constricts after a few minutes. The ciliary muscle contracts and a spasm of accommodation ensues in which the lens cannot change its shape and its far point and near point become identical. Objects appear enlarged (macropia) because owing to the lack of accommodation effort they are perceived to be further away.

Twitching of the eyelids may occur. The actions of eserine on the pupil and on accommodation can be antagonised by atropine and related drugs.

Eserine reduces the intraocular tension in both normal subjects and in patients with glaucoma. The spasmodic contraction of the intraocular muscles provoked by the first application of the drug frequently causes pain but this disappears after the contraction has been established. Eserine frequently causes hyperaemia of the conjunctiva and iris and is not well tolerated if applied for prolonged periods.

Eserine may be used to prevent the formation of adhesions in iritis by constricting the pupil.

Dyflos (diisopropylfluorophosphonate), an irreversible inhibitor of cholinesterase (p. 61), has a more prolonged action than eserine and only a single drop of a 0.1 per cent solution is required daily. *Ecothiopate* (phospholine iodide) and *Demecarium* (tosmilen) are related anticholinesterases with a prolonged action. These powerful long-acting miotics are used in the treatment of glaucoma when short-acting miotics are inadequate but they sometimes give rise to cataract.

Systemic effects such as acute abdominal spasm and bronchospasm may occur as a result of continued local application of this group of compounds. Other side effects include severe frontal headache due to spasm of accommodation, twitching of the eyelids and suffused conjunctival vessels.

Parasympathomimetic agents

Pilocarpine. In contrast to eserine, pilocarpine constricts the pupil even after degeneration of the postganglionic parasympathetic nerve endings. Pilocarpine produces similar effects to eserine on the pupil, accommodation and intraocular pressure.

Pilocarpine is an important clinically used miotic for the treatment of glaucoma. Pilocarpine penetrates the eye well and after local instillation to the conjunctiva produces a reduction of intraocular pressure which is maximal in two to four hours. Pilocarpine is generally better tolerated than other miotics. *Ocusert pilocarpine* is a new drug delivery system with a centrally located reservoir of pilocarpine. When it is placed under the upper or lower eyelid pilocarpine diffuses out across two polymer layers which serve as rate controlling membranes. The ocusert is claimed to require replacement only once a week and to provide better longterm control of intraocular pressure than pilocarpine eyedrops.

Carbachol may be used in chronic glaucoma when resistance to pilocarpine has developed or when a stronger, longer-acting drug is required. Carbachol may cause more spasm of accommodation and headache than pilocarpine.

Anticholinergic agents

Atropine. If a 1 per cent solution of atropine (p. 69) is applied to the conjunctiva it produces effects which are the opposite of those produced by pilocarpine or eserine. Within fifteen minutes the pupil dilates and the nearpoint recedes until accommodation is completely paralysed. The paralysis of accommodation (cycloplegia) may last two to three days and the mydriasis eight to ten days. The dilated pupil allows light to enter freely so that photophobia results; at the same time objects appear reduced in size (micropia) for reasons opposite to those explained in relation to eserine macropia.

Atropine is used extensively in ophthalmology. By eliminating accommodation it permits an exact determination of refraction. Atropine dilates the pupil and facilitates examination of the fundus of the eye. Repeated application causes complete immobilisation of the ciliary muscle and iris and hence will ensure rest in the inflamed eye.

The main disadvantage of atropine is its effect on intraocular pressure. This action is of no importance in a normal eye but if the intraocular pressure is already unduly high, atropine may cause a rapid further rise and induce an attack of acute glaucoma. This effect, once started, cannot be stopped and may destroy the function of the eye.

Homatropine produces the same effects as atropine, but its action lasts a shorter time and passes off in about twenty-four hours. Homatropine hydrobromide (2 per cent) therefore is a much more convenient drug than atropine for examination of the eye, but atropine is better if it is desired to immobilise the intrinsic muscles of the eye in the treatment of iritis. A 1 per cent solution of *lachesine* chloride produces effects in the eye which are similar to, but of shorter duration, than those of atropine. Atropine sometimes produces conjunctival irritation and in these patients lachesine may be used in place of atropine.

Cyclopentolate acts more quickly than atropine and produces mydriasis within half an hour after application of a 0.5 per cent solution.

Tropicamide 0.5% produces a mydriasis of short duration with minimal effect on accommodation.

Adrenergic mechanisms

Adrenaline and noradrenaline

The human orbit contains several varieties of smooth muscle which are sympathetically innervated; these include the radial iris muscle, the superior palpebral muscle which raises the upper eye lid and the vasoconstrictor muscles of the conjunctiva. Electrical stimulation of the sympathetic chain produces dilatation of the pupil by the action of released noradrenaline on the radial muscle. When adrenaline is injected intravenously in a cat it produces a transient mydriasis and retraction of the nictitating membrane or third lid. These effects of injected adrenaline are greatly increased if the postganglionic sympathetic nerve supply has been cut and allowed to degenerate.

Local application of a solution of adrenaline (1 per cent) to the conjunctiva produces vasoconstriction but usually no dilation of the pupil. However, when adrenaline is instilled in eyes with primary open-angle glaucoma it induces a prolonged fall in intraocular pressure, conjunctival vasoconstriction and slight mydriasis. The mechanism of the fall in intraocular pressure is not clearly understood. It has been suggested that it may involve both a facilitation of outflow and a decrease in production of aqueous humor.

Adrenaline is often used in conjunction with a miotic such as pilocarpine to reduce further the intraocular pressure in glaucoma.

Phenylephrine

This sympathomimetic amine is more stable than adrenaline and when applied locally (3 to 10 per cent) is absorbed from the conjunctiva. It can thus produce dilatation of the pupil for fundal inspection without the disadvantage of paralysis of accommodation as with the atropine-like drugs. It also produces a constriction of the conjunctival blood vessels; when the drug is absorbed by the nasolachrymal duct it may result in an uncomfortable vasoconstriction in the nose. Phenylephrine is often used to supplement anticholinergic drugs to achieve maximal mydriasis.

PREPARATIONS

Eye-drops

Miotics
Acetylcholine chloride (Miochol) powder
Carbachol 3 per cent
Demecarium Brom (Tosmilen) 0.25, 0.5 per cent
Ecothiopate (Phospholine Iodide) 0.03–0.25 per cent
Neostigmine (Prostigmin) Methylsulph 3 per cent
Physostigmine Salic 0.25 per cent
Pilocarpine Nitr 1–4 per cent
Pilocarpine ocuserts

Other drugs reducing i.o. pressure
Adrenaline 0.5, 1 per cent
Phenylephrine 10 per cent

Mydriatics and cycloplegics
Atropine Sulph 0.5, 1 per cent
Atropine Sulph Eye ointment (opulets)
Cyclopentolate Hyd 0.1–1 per cent
Homatropine Hydrobromide 1, 2 per cent
Hyoscine Hydrobromide 0.2 per cent
Tropicamide (Mydriacil) 0.5, 1 per cent

Notes

Minims are single dose containers
Ocuserts are elliptical sustained release units for placing under the eyelids, they release pilocarpine at the rate of 20 or 40 $\mu g/h$
Opulets (atropine) are single use capsules
Neutral adrenaline does not cause pupillary change but reduces i.o. pressure
Phenylephrine is a mydriatic but reduces i.o. pressure

FURTHER READING

Davson H 1963 The physiology of the eye. Churchill, London
Havener W H 1966 Ocular pharmacology. Mosby, St Louis
Leopold I H 1962 The eye as a pharmacological laboratory. Clin. Pharmacol. & Therap. 3: 561
Potts A M 1965 The effect of drugs upon the eye. In: Physiol. Pharmacol IIB: 329

8. Local hormones and allergy

True hormones and local hormones 90; Kallikrein-Kinin system 90; Prostaglandins 91; SRS-A 92; 5-Hydroxytryptamine 93; Melatonin 94; Histamine 94; H_1 and H_2 histamine receptors 96; H_1-antihistamines 97; Allergy 98; Antigens and Antibodies 98; Types of hypersensitivity reactions 99; Anaphylaxis 100; Mechanism of anaphylactic histamine release 102; Hypersensitivity to drugs 103.

TRUE HORMONES AND LOCAL HORMONES

When Bayliss and Starling introduced the word hormone they intended it to apply to an active principle formed in one organ and carried by the bloodstream to others in which it produced its specific effect. Dale pointed out that in addition to the true hormones there existed substances in the body of an equally intense physiological activity whose normal action was restricted to the site of their liberation. He called such substances locally acting chemical stimulants; others have called them *local hormones* or *tissue hormones* or simply pharmacologically active substances in tissues. Acetylcholine and noradrenaline were formerly included in this group but since their neurotransmitter function has been clearly established they are usually excluded. A heterogenous group of pharmacologically active substances in tissues whose functions have not as yet been well defined will be described in this chapter. Some of these substances, e.g. 5-HT are likely to be neurotransmitters whilst others, e.g. prostaglandins appear to be involved in a variety of normal and pathological functions including reproductive functions and platelet aggregation. The role of some of these substances, especially histamine, in allergy and anaphylaxis will also be discussed.

THE KALLIKREIN-KININ SYSTEM

The body makes use of an elaborate set of defence mechanisms in which proteolytic enzymes play an important role. These defences include blood clotting, fibrinolysis, the immunological serum complement system and the kallikrein-kinin system; their overall effect is to produce haemostasis, removal of blood clots, activation of antibody reactions and vasodilation following tissue damage. It is in the latter type of activity that kinin formation is particularly involved. A related proteolytic system of great importance, the renin-angiotensin system is discussed on page 111.

During the 1930s, workers in Germany described kallikrein, a substance in human urine, which produced a fall of blood pressure when injected intravenously in dogs. Kallikrein is inactive in isolated preparations but Werle showed that it is capable of liberating by enzymic action an active substance from serum proteins called *kallidin*. Independently, Rocha e Silva and his colleagues showed that certain snake venoms incubated with plasma proteins give rise to a pharmacologically active product which they called *bradykinin*. Kallidin, bradykinin and related peptides are now referred to collectively as *kinins*.

An outline scheme of the kallikrein system is shown in Figure 8.1. Kallikreinogen is an inactive precursor of kallikrein which can be activated in various ways. A physiological activator is Hageman factor (clotting factor XII, p. 210) which is also needed for blood clotting and fibrinolysis. Patients with the Hageman trait, in whom this factor is missing, show disturbances in blood clotting as well as in kinin formation.

Kallikreins are kininogenase enzymes which rapidly produce kinins from kininogen. The blood pressure fall in the dog after kallikrein injection is due to the rapid formation of kinin in the blood stream. Several forms of kallikrein are recognised including plasma kallikrein and glandular kallikrein which occurs in pancreas, salivary gland and urine. Kallikrein can be assayed directly by intravenous injection in dogs and indirectly by incubating it with the appropriate serum fraction and measuring the amount of kinin formed by biological assay on an isolated smooth muscle preparation. Other substances with kininogen activity are trypsin and certain snake venoms. The action of kallikrein is inhibited by DFP.

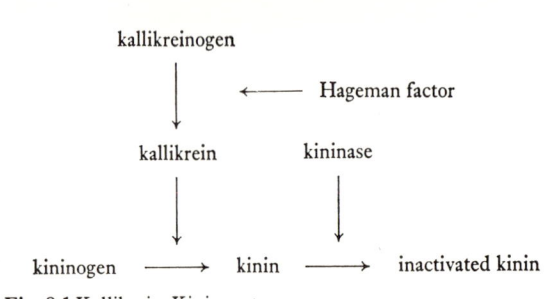

```
kallikreinogen
      |
      |  ←—— Hageman factor
      ↓
  kallikrein         kininase
      |                 |
      ↓                 ↓
 kininogen ——→ kinin ——→ inactivated kinin
```

Fig. 8.1 Kallikrein-Kinin system.

Kininogen is an α-2-globulin of plasma. The type of kallikrein determines which kinin will be released from kininogen; plasma kallikrein liberates bradykinin and glandular kallikrein liberates kallidin.

Several kinins have been chemically identified and synthesised. Amongst the most important are the nonapeptide *bradykinin* and the decapeptide lysbradykinin or *kallidin* (Fig. 8.2). Plasma can convert kallidin into bradykinin. Plasma and serum also contain kininases which destroy kinins.

Arg-Pro-Pro-Gly-Phe-Ser-Pro-Phe-Arg
Bradykinin

Lys-Arg-Pro-Pro-Gly-Phe-Ser-Pro-Phe-Arg
Kallidin

Fig. 8.2

Actions and possible roles of kinins
Kinins are pharmacologically highly active. Bradykinin stimulates isolated smooth muscle preparations including rat uterus, guinea pig ileum, rabbit and cat duodenum; other smooth muscle structures including rat duodenum and colon are relaxed. No specific antagonist against kinins has been developed so far.

Bradykinin is one of the most powerful vasodilator substances known. It lowers the blood pressure in all animals tested. In the intact animal it increases cardiac output and produces coronary vasodilatation. An interesting property of kinins is the production of intense pain when injected intraarterially or applied to an exposed blister base (p. 286). Although nerve endings eventually become desensitised to this effect the formation of bradykinin is likely to be an important factor in the pain associated with tissue injury. Kinins have systemic and local effects on the circulation. They cause a release of adrenaline from the adrenal medulla. They are likely to play an important part in inflammation; whenever tissues are damaged the kinin forming system is readily activated. Kinins may cause vasodilatation during activity in submaxillary and other glands. They probably play a role in allergic reactions. Kinins produce bronchoconstriction.

Related polypeptides
Substance P (Euler and Gaddum) is a polypeptide with actions similar to, but distinguishable from bradykinin. Chemically it is an endecapeptide. It occurs in extracts of intestine and brain.

Several new pharmacologically active peptides have been discovered by Erspamer and his colleagues in lower vertebrates or invertebrates. They include *eledoisin* from the salivary gland of *Eledone*, *physalaemin* from the skin of *Physalaemus* and *caerulein* from the skin of *Hyla caerulea*. The latter has pharmacological actions resembling gastrin. Each of these substances has been chemically characterised. A further group of peptides represented by *bombesin*, *alytesin* and *ranatensin* have been isolated by these workers from the skin of amphibian species. These bombesin-like peptides have a stimulant action on several types of smooth muscle, notably those of the intestinal and urinary tracts and uterus.

PROSTAGLANDINS

In contrast to most other pharmacologically active tissue products, prostaglandins are acidic in nature and soluble in fat solvents. The occurrence of depressor and smooth muscle stimulating activity in human seminal fluid was discovered independently by Goldblatt and v. Euler in 1933-34. The activity was due to lipid soluble acidic material which was named prostaglandin (PG). It was later found that many different tissues contained prostaglandin.

The isolation and chemical characterisation of prostaglandins was carried out by Bergström and colleagues in Sweden using modern methods of gas-liquid chromatography, mass spectrometry and X-ray crystallography. Chemically they can all be considered derivatives of 'prostanoic acid', a 20-carbon fatty acid containing a five-membered ring with two adjacent sidechains. The structure of two prostaglandins, PGE_1 and PGE_2 is shown in Figure 8.3. The subscripts 1 and 2 stand respectively for one and two double bonds in the chain. Different members of the series are distinguished by the presence of double bonds, hydroxyl or carbonyl groups. Those derived from natural sources are designated by the letters E, Fα, A and B.

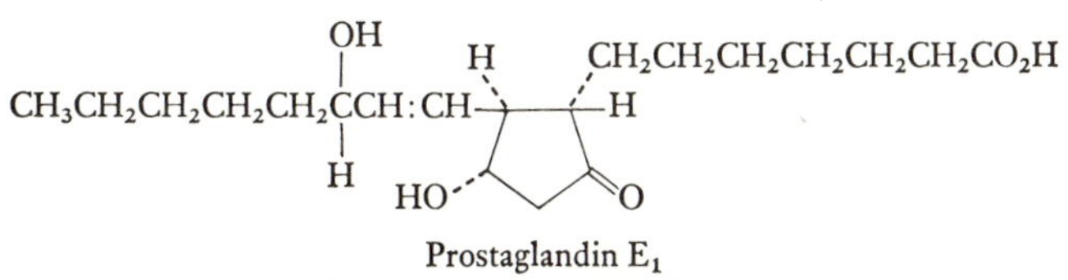

Prostaglandin E_1

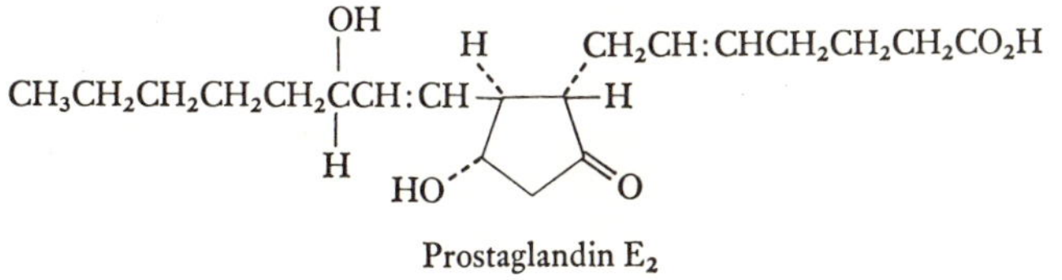

Prostaglandin E_2

Fig. 8.3

Metabolism

Prostaglandin synthetase is a multiple enzyme complex which catalyses the conversion of precursor arachidonic acid and other long chain unsaturated fatty acids into prostaglandins. The synthetase enzyme is usually obtained from bovine seminal vesicles but it also occurs in the microsomal fraction of other tissues. Prostaglandin synthetase is inhibited by aspirin and other nonsteroidal anti-inflammatory drugs such as indomethacin and flufenamic acid and this antienzyme effect has been proposed as the mechanism of action of the aspirin-like drugs (p. 286).

Other synthetic pathways. Several unstable intermediates with short half-lives are produced during prostaglandin biosynthesis. The first intermediates recognised were cyclic enderoperoxides called PGG_2 and PGH_2. They were shown to transform into thromboxanes A_2 and B_2. Thromboxanes are particularly active as platelet aggregators. More recently an alternative pathway of enderoperoxide metabolism has been demonstrated leading to the formation of *prostacyclin*. This pathway is believed to be promoted by contact with the blood vessel wall. Prostacyclin inhibits platelet aggregation, in contrast to thromboxane which promotes aggregation, suggesting that both pro- and anti-aggregation factors are being produced through arachidonic acid metabolism.

Degradation. An important degrading enzyme is 15-OH-prostglandin dehydrogenase. It is believed that prostaglandins are not stored in the body except in special locations such as seminal vesicle. They are normally synthesised as required, followed by rapid degradation.

Pharmacological actions. Although structurally related, different prostaglandins vary greatly in their pharmacological activities. Furthermore, each particular prostaglandin produces a variety of effects in different organ systems and this very variety of actions greatly restricts their clinical uses. Attempts are now being made to produce new synthetic prostaglandin-like compounds with more restricted ranges of pharmacological actions. So far prostaglandins have been used clinically only in limited fields such as myometrial stimulation. Potentially the prostaglandin group is of considerable clinical interest and we discuss below some of their main actions.

Female reproductive tract. Prostaglandins have a predominantly stimulant effect on uterine smooth muscle and since sperm is a concentrated source of prostaglandins it has been suggested that they may have a function in the transport of sperm by activating uterine movements. Prostaglandins are absorbed from the vagina and may thus affect the female genital tract both by their local action and after systemic absorption. PGE_1 and $PGF_2\alpha$ are powerful stimulants of the pregnant myometrium and have been used to produce uterine contractions at term and during pregnancy for inducing abortion (p. 222).

As has been mentioned, the aspirin-like anti-inflammatory drugs inhibit prostaglandin synthesis. They also inhibit uterine movements in experimental animals and this has suggested that prostaglandins may be concerned with uterine motility.

$PGF_{2\alpha}$ has been shown to produce regression of the corpus luteum and interruption of pregnancy in various species including rabbit, sheep and rhesus monkey. The mechanism of the luteolytic effect is uncertain, it might possibly be due to a primary vascular action of prostaglandin.

Platelet aggregation. Aspirin inhibits the second stage of platelet aggregation during which the *platelet release reaction* (p. 209) occurs. It has been shown that the inhibitory effect of aspirin is due to the transient formation in the body of prostaglandin precursors which are powerful inhibitors of platelet aggregation. Some of these precursors (thromboxanes) have been chemically identified.

Smooth muscle. Prostaglandins act on smooth muscle but their actions are often limited by their side effects, e.g. PGE_1 produces bronchodilatation in asthmatics but it also irritates the respiratory passages.

Central nervous system. Prostaglandins have powerful effects on the central nervous system. PGE_1 injected into the cerebral ventricles of unanaesthetised cats produces stupor and catatonia beginning 20 to 30 min after injection and lasting several hours. The microionophoretic application of PGE_1 and $PGF_2\alpha$ to neurones in the brain stem produces firing in a proportion of these neurones.

Prostaglandins administered into the cerebral ventricles of various species raise body temperature and since pyrogen-induced fever in cats produces an increase in prostaglandin-like material in the cerebrospinal fluid it has been suggested that prostaglandins may play a part in temperature regulation.

SRS-A

The term *slow reacting substance* (SRS) was used by Feldberg and Kellaway to describe an unknown smooth muscle stimulating principle which appeared together with histamine in the perfusate of guinea pig lung after injection of cobra venom. SRS-A is the name given by Brocklehurst to a smooth muscle stimulating substance which appears with histamine in the perfusate of the isolated guinea pig lung following an anaphylactic reaction.

SRS-A is acidic in nature but its exact chemical constitution has not been established. It produces a slow contraction of the guinea pig ileum and of human bronchial muscle. The presence of SRS-A in a perfusate can be detected by means of a biological assay after the effects of any histamine present have been eliminated by an antihistamine drug.

5-HYDROXYTRYPTAMINE

5-hydroxytryptamine (serotonin, 5-HT) has been the subject of much research during recent years. This substance was discovered by Erspamer in 1940 in the salivary glands of the octopus and called by him enteramine. Rapport in 1948 independently isolated the substance from serum and identified it as 5-hydroxytryptamine.

5-HT occurs in cells of the enterochromaffin (argentaffin) system which is present in all vertebrate species; it occurs in the gastrointestinal tract, the central nervous system, blood platelets and mast cells. Two other indolalkylamines have been shown to be normal constituents of the mammalian organism: tryptamine in the brain and urine and melatonin in the pineal gland.

Formation

The formation of 5-HT from L-tryptophan is shown in Figure 8.4. The limiting step in the biosynthesis of 5-HT is the hydroxylation of L-tryptophan in the 5-position by the enzyme tryptophan-5-hydroxylase. The subsequent decarboxylation step is carried out by an enzyme which is closely related to dopa decarboxylase. 5-HT is destroyed by amine oxidase.

Actions

5-HT stimulates many types of smooth muscle. Its stimulant effect on the isolated rat uterus and on the rat stomach strip is made use of for its bioassay. It can also be measured by fluorimetric methods which are increasingly used.

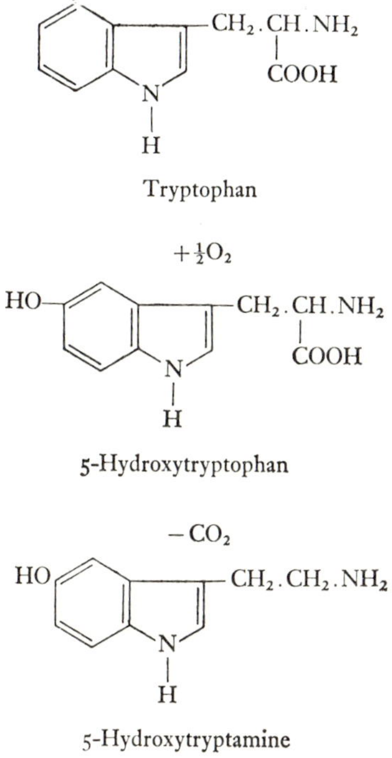

Tryptophan

5-Hydroxytryptophan

5-Hydroxytryptamine

Fig. 8.4

The action of 5-HT on the circulation is complex. It usually produces a fall of blood pressure and in some species such as the rat it causes a powerful capillary dilatation. It also affects nervous tissue. When 5-HT is applied to a blister base it causes pain and when perfused through the superior cervical ganglion it causes stimulation of the post-ganglionic fibres. When injected into the cerebral ventricles it causes drowsiness.

Experiments with antagonists show that 5-HT acts on two types of receptors.

D-receptors are present in the isolated uterus and probably also in the central nervous system and are blocked by phenoxybenzamine (p. 16). They are also blocked by the hallucinogenic drug lysergic acid diethylamide (LSD, p. 265) and its derivative brom-LSD (BOL). Another anti-5-HT compound acting on D-receptors is methysergide (p. 128).

M-receptors are blocked by morphine. When 5-HT acts on isolated guinea pig ileum it is believed to act on M-receptors situated on postganglionic cholinergic nerve endings which then release acetylcholine. Hence the effect of 5-HT in this preparation is blocked by atropine. The effect on M-receptors of the endogenous morphine-like polypeptide enkephalin is discussed on page 241.

Possible functions

Various functions have been assigned to 5-HT but none has been unequivocally established.

Functions in the CNS. Changes in the 5-HT content of the brain tend to be correlated with altered behaviour suggesting that 5-HT may act as a central neurotransmitter. Thus reserpine which causes central depression also depletes the brain of 5-HT. Procedures which increase the 5-HT content of experimental animals such as administration of 5-hydroxytryptophan together with an amine oxidase inhibitor to prevent the destruction of 5-HT, produce hyperpyrexia and excitement.

Further evidence that 5-HT may be a neuro-humoral transmitter is based on the evidence that 5-HT is contained in certain neurones together with the enzymes for its synthesis and inactivation, that it produces neuronal stimulation when applied by microiontophoresis and that it can be released by nerve stimulation. Its presence in the brain (p. 236) can be demonstrated by histochemical fluorescence methods.

Particularly high concentrations of 5-HT occur in the raphe system of the medulla and midbrain. This system has an important function in sleep and Jouvet has shown in cats that surgical lesions or elimination of its 5-HT content by p-chlorophenylalanine, which inactivates tryptophan-5-hydroxylase, leads to permanent insomnia, an effect which can be alleviated by administering 5-hydroxytryptophan. This evidence suggests that sleep may be dependent on 5-HT neurones.

A possible involvement of 5-HT in human depressive illness is discussed on page 259.

5-HT also plays a part in central temperature regulation; it has been found that intrathecal administration of 5-HT in cats raised body temperature whilst noradrenaline lowered it.

Peristaltic function. The intestine contains large amounts of 5-HT in the enterochromaffin cells of the mucosa. 5-HT stimulates intestinal smooth muscle and it has been suggested that it may be implicated in the peristaltic reflex.

Vascular functions. 5-HT increases capillary permeability and causes oedema of the paws of rats when injected subcutaneously. This reaction is used in assessing anti-inflammatory agents. 5-HT probably participates in the anaphylactic reaction of mice and rats but not of man.

Clinical implications

Lembeck discovered that carcinoid tumours (malignant argentaffinoma) had a high 5-HT content, and that patients with carcinoid excreted 5-HT and its degradation product, hydroxyindoleacetic acid, in urine. These patients have attacks of intestinal colic, bronchoconstriction and flushing attributable to 5-HT, although the flushing may be partly due to kinin formation. It has been suggested that 5-HT may be involved in pregnancy toxaemia and in migraine; patients with migraine excrete increased amounts of 5-HT in urine following an attack.

It is possible that 5-HT metabolism is involved in some forms of mental deficiency. For example in phenylketonuria there is a failure to oxidise phenylalanine to tyrosine and also a deficiency of 5-HT in blood suggesting that oxidation of both phenylalanine and tryptophan may be impaired.

Melatonin

Melatonin, an important indole derivative synthesised in the body, is found in the pineal gland. Melatonin is N-acetyl-5-methoxytryptamine (Fig. 8.5). In mammals the pineal gland is the only organ containing the enzyme which catalyses the last step in melatonin synthesis. Melatonin is released into the circulation and produces various, mostly inhibitory, effects; among others it depresses ovarian growth and the secretion of thyroid hormone. The synthesis of melatonin in the pineal gland varies diurnally; exposure to light depresses melatonin formation and darkness has the opposite effect. Axelrod has suggested that rhythmic fluctuations in the secretion of melatonin may provide the body with a 'biological clock' which synchronises rhythms in other organs.

Many indole derivatives have pharmacological effects. *Psilocybin* (p. 489) a naturally occurring derivative of 4-hydroxytryptamine, is an antagonist of 5-HT. It has hallucinogenic effects in man similar to LSD which is also

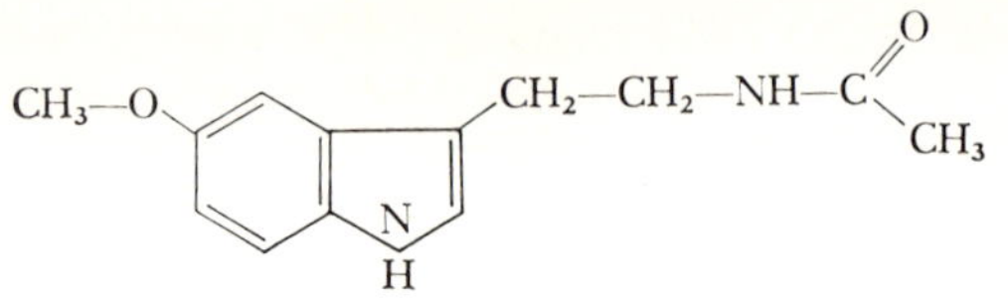

Fig. 8.5 Melatonin.

a 4-substituted indole derivative. *Methysergide*, a synthetic compound used in the prophylactic treatment of patients with migraine (p. 128) is related to LSD and is also an antagonist of 5-HT.

HISTAMINE

Although histamine was synthesised in 1907, it was not until the 1920's that it was recognised as a naturally occurring body constituent. It is contained largely in metachromatically staining mast cells and the related blood basophils. Mast cells can be considered as unicellular endocrine organs capable of secreting heparin, hyaluronic acid, histamine and in some species, 5-hydroxytryptamine. Mast cell histamine is held within granules combined with the acid mucopolysaccharide heparin (p. 212). The pathological tissue of urticaria pigmentosa is extremely rich in both mast cells and histamine.

Histamine is also found in other tissues, particularly in the gastric mucosa. Histochemical fluorescence has shown that gastric mucosal histamine is contained in a special type of enterochromaffin-like cell.

The chemical structure of histamine is shown in Figure 8.6.

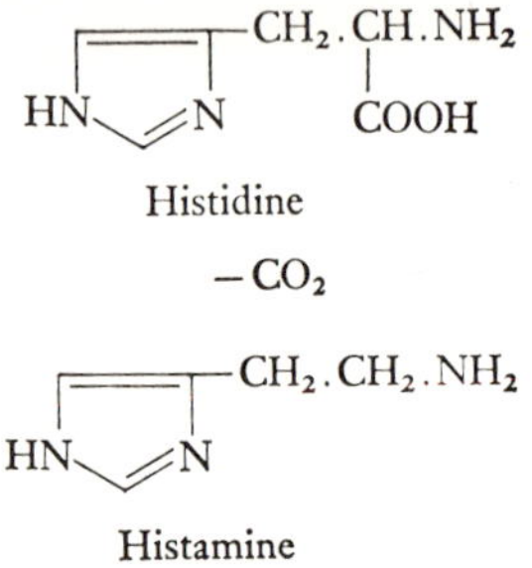

Fig. 8.6

It is stable in acid and this property is made use of in extracting it from tissues. It can be assayed biologically by its effects in contracting the isolated guinea pig ileum or uterus or in lowering the cat's blood pressure. Histamine can also be assayed chemically by fluorimetric methods.

Formation and destruction

Mammalian histamine is formed by the intracellular decarboxylation of histidine (Fig. 8.6). This reaction is catalysed by the enzyme histidine decarboxylase which requires pyridoxal phosphate as coenzyme. Histidine decarboxylase is specifically inhibited by α-methylhistidine. The histamine forming capacity (HFC) of tissues has been extensively studied. Schayer and his colleagues consider newly formed or 'induced' histamine to be a regulator of the microcirculation in various forms of stress. Kahlson and colleagues have studied 'nascent' histamine in rapidly growing tissues. They found urinary histamine to be greatly increased in pregnant rats and showed that this was due to an increased HFC in the foetal liver. An increase in HFC also occurs during wound healing and when sensitised human leucocytes are treated with a specific antigen.

Histamine is inactivated by two enzymes in the body, histaminase and the methylating enzyme imidazole-N-methyltransferase. Histaminase is inhibited by aminoguanidine and other carbonyl reagents. Histaminase is widely distributed in the body, high concentrations occur in the human placenta which is the origin of the increased blood histaminase level found in human pregnancy. High concentrations of the methylating enzyme occur in the CNS.

Pharmacological actions

The chief actions of histamine are contraction of most smooth muscle, dilatation and increased permeability of capillaries, and stimulation of secretions particularly of the oxyntic glands of the stomach. It also causes secretion of adrenaline from the supra-renal glands. The action on the circulation is complex and varies according to the species of animal. In mammals it causes constriction of the larger blood vessels and dilatation of the capillaries, but the smaller arterioles are constricted in some species, for example the rabbit, and dilated in others, such as the cat, dog and man. Hence histamine produces a rise of blood pressure in the former and a fall of blood pressure in the latter. It contracts the smooth muscle of the gut, the uterus of most species and the bronchioles. Different species vary greatly, both regarding the effects produced by histamine and their sensitivity to the drug. The guinea-pig is killed by an intravenous injection of 0.8 mg/kg., whilst 1000 times this dose is needed to kill a mouse.

The predominant effect in the guinea-pig is bronchoconstriction which causes death from asphyxia. In the cat a large dose of histamine produces extreme capillary dilatation, haemoconcentration and a reduction of the circulating blood volume; in the dog, hepatic vasoconstriction and engorgement of the liver with a consequent pooling of blood in the splanchnic area. In man the skin, mucous membranes and bronchioles are highly susceptible to the action of histamine. It is an interesting fact that the tissues which are most reactive to histamine in various species are those in which the most intensive anaphylactic and allergic responses occur.

Actions in man

Man is relatively insensitive to the hypotensive effects of histamine; when injected subcutaneously or intravenously the usual effects are flushing of the skin and a rise in skin temperature. If histamine is slowly infused intravenously it produces a cutaneous vasodilation of the face and neck which gradually extends over the rest of the body; there is a marked increase in blood flow through the limbs with a rise in heart rate and cardiac output, but no significant change in blood pressure. When a single dose of histamine is injected intravenously it produces a sharp fall in blood pressure and a rise in cerebrospinal fluid pressure which is followed by an intense but short-lasting headache when these pressure changes subside. When histamine is given by mouth it produces no pharmacological effects presumably because it is acetylated in the intestinal tract.

The most definite effect produced by histamine injections is stimulation of the secretion of gastric juice. The subcutaneous injection of 1 mg histamine acid phosphate can be used as a clinical test for gastric function (p. 187); a larger injection of histamine (5 mg) can be tolerated if an H_1-antihistamine is previously administered. There is evidence that histamine plays a physiological role in gastric secretion. It is present in the gastric mucosa of all species studied and its concentration is maximal in the areas where the parietal cells are most concentrated, although it is not contained in the parietal cells themselves. After a meal and after the injection of the acid secretory hormone gastrin (p. 185) the HFC of the gastric mucosa increases and it has been suggested that this causes the histamine containing cells to form new histamine, which then diffuses towards the parietal cells causing them to secrete acid.

The action of histamine on capillaries can be easily demonstrated on the human skin. If a scratch is made through a drop of histamine solution a local redness is produced which is followed by a wheal surrounded by a flare. This is a reaction similar to that which occurs when the skin is slightly injured by drawing a blunt pencil firmly across it. This combination of effects was called by Lewis the triple reaction, which he attributed to the release of 'H-substance'.

Histamine causes a dilatation of skin capillaries and an increase in their permeability to plasma proteins; this results in an exudation of plasma under the epidermis and the formation of a wheal. The surrounding flare is believed to be due to a local axon reflex through the sensory fibres which enter the posterior roots of the spinal cord. The evidence of an axon reflex being involved is that the histamine flare is unchanged immediately after section of sensory nerves to the skin but is abolished after these nerves have degenerated.

Histamine causes itching especially when it is introduced into the most superficial layers of the skin. When histamine is applied to a blister base it causes itching

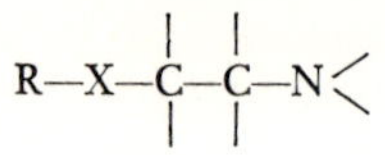

(I)

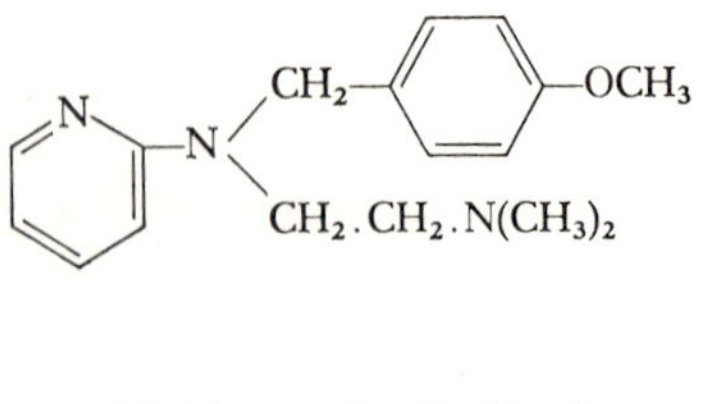

(II) Mepyramine (Anthisan)

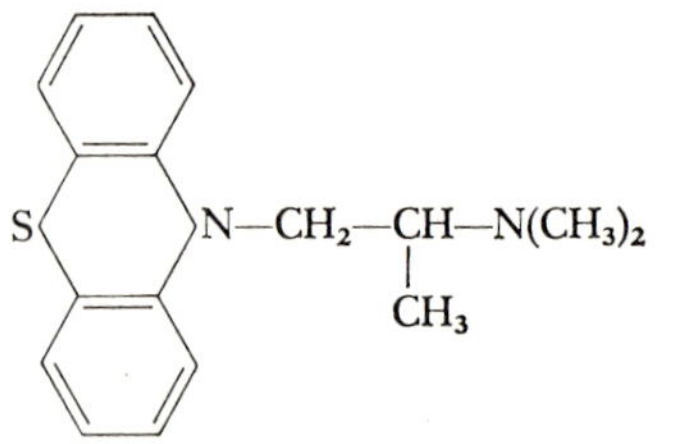

(III) Promethazine (Phenergan)

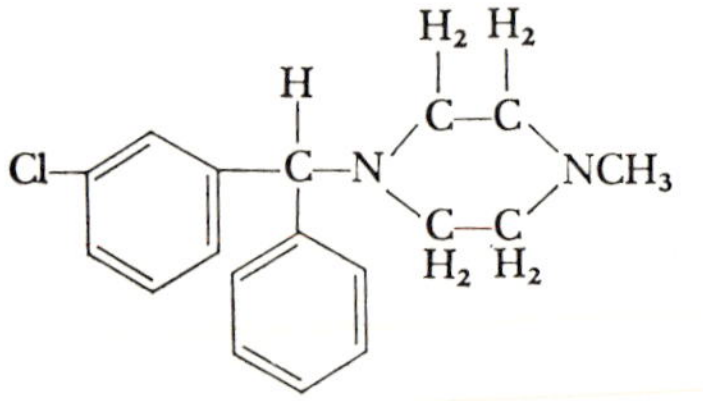

(IV) Chlorcyclizine (Histantin)

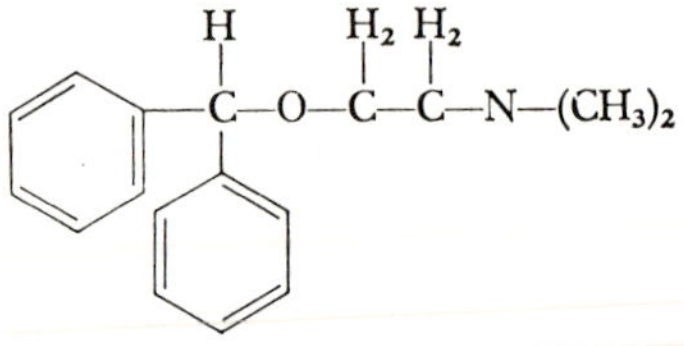

(V) Diphenhydramine (Benadryl)

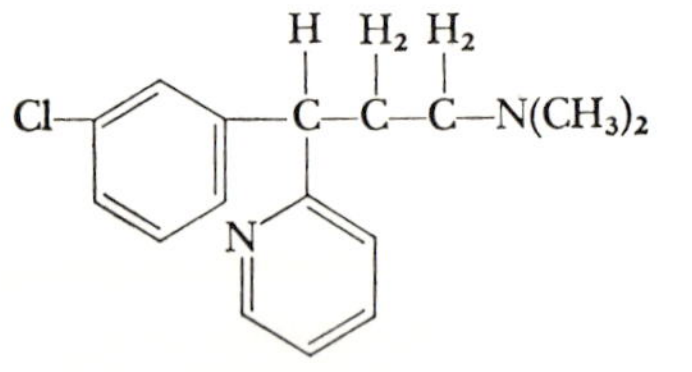

(VI) Chlorpheniramine (Piriton)

Fig. 8.7 Chemical structures of H_1 histamine antagonists.

in low concentrations and pain in higher concentrations. The pain produced by histamine is potentiated by acetylcholine, and the intense burning pain of a nettle sting can be explained by the fact that nettles contain high concentrations of both histamine and acetylcholine.

Possible transmitter functions. High concentrations of histamine are found in postganglionic sympathetic nerves, but in contrast to noradrenaline their histamine content does not diminish after nerve section. The explanation may be that histamine occurs in the mast cells of the connective tissue sheath rather than the sympathetic neurone itself and may have no direct transmitter function. Histamine also occurs in certain parts of the central nervous system, particularly the hypothalamus (Adam), in this case not in mast cells but in synaptosomes, suggesting a possible transmitter function for histamine in the central nervous system. A possible involvement of histamine in normal gastric acid secretion is discussed on page 187.

Histamine receptors

It is possible to distinguish, by means of specific antagonists, two types of histamine receptors (p. 13):

H_1 receptors. These are blocked by typical H_1-antihistamines such as mepyramine. They are found in human and guinea pig bronchial muscle and in the guinea pig ileum, isolated preparations of which have a common affinity for mepyramine (Table 2.2). Antagonism by H_1 antagonists is competitive and specific.

H_2 receptors. Another group of antagonists, block various actions of histamine unaffected by H_1 antagonists such as stimulation of acid gastric secretion. Other effects of histamine antagonised by H_2 but not H_1 antagonists are the paradoxical relaxation of isolated rat uterus and stimulation of the isolated heart. Quantitative investigations with H_2 antagonists have shown that the receptors mediating these various effects of histamine have common affinities for the same H_2 antagonist, suggesting a

common H_2 receptor. It is interesting that H_2 antagonists also block the secretory effects of the gastrin analogue pentagastrin (p. 186) which supports the notion that the gastric secretory hormone, gastrin, may produce its effect by way of histamine. H_1 and H_2 receptors can also be distinguished by their differential response to agonists; for example H_2 receptors are selectively stimulated by 4-methylhistamine and H_1 receptors by 2-methylhistamine.

Pharmacological chemistry. Histamine exists as an equilibrium mixture of several different tautomeric species. At the pH of extracellular fluid, 7.4, the predominant species is the histamine monocation. This tautomeric species stimulates both H_1 and H_2 receptors. There are, however, profound chemical differences between *antagonists* affecting the two receptors. The H_1 antihistamines (Fig. 8.7) have in common a side chain with a charged side chain endgroup, generally ammonium, whilst the ring structure is not critical. By contrast the H_2 antagonists (Fig. 13.7) contain an essentila imidazole group and an uncharged side chain. H_1 antagonists are lipophilic and capable of penetrating the blood-brain barrier and producing central effects, whereas H_2 antagonists are hydrophilic and do not readily penetrate the CNS.

A simultaneous occurrence of H_1 and H_2 receptors has been demonstrated in several tissues. For example the depressor action of a small dose of histamine in the cat is abolished by an H_1 receptor antagonist such as mepyramine but in order to abolish the depressor effect of a large histamine dose an H_2 receptor antagonist must also be added. In guinea pig bronchial muscle a small dose of histamine produces bronchoconstriction by an action on H_1 receptors, but larger doses of histamine given after mepyramine produce bronchodilatation by an action on H_2 receptors.

Clinical effects of H_1 antagonists are discussed below and structures of H_2 antagonists acting on gastric acid secretion on page 187.

H_1-Antihistamines

The first antihistamines were discovered by a systematic approach of a group of French workers in the late 1930s trying to find synthetic substances which antagonised histamine in isolated preparations. Some powerful specific antihistamines including mepyramine were discovered during these early investigations. It was subsequently shown that the antihistamines were competitive receptor antagonists capable of antagonising the contractile effects of histamine in isolated intestinal and bronchial smooth muscle. Later on it was established that the mepyramine-sensitive histamine effects were exerted on a common H_1 receptor and that further series of histamine effects including those on acid gastric secretion were exerted on a common H_2 receptor as discussed. The H_1 receptor antagonists are usually referred to simply as antihistamines or conventional antihistamines. The chemical structures of some characteristic H_1-antihistamines are shown in Figure 8.7.

Assessment of antihistamine activity

The antihistamines vary in the intensity and duration of their actions and a number of methods have been used to assess their activity.

1. Determination of the intravenous toxic dose of histamine in guinea pigs after subcutaneous injection of antagonist. Halpern has shown that promethazine can protect guinea-pigs against the immediate effects of 1000 lethal doses of histamine although the animals may eventually die from perforated gastric ulcers.
2. Protection against bronchospasm induced in guinea-pigs by histamine aerosols.
3. Antagonism of histamine contraction of isolated guinea-pig intestine; determination of pA_2 value.
4. Reduction of wheal response in man to intradermal histamine after oral administration of the antagonist (Fig. 8.8).

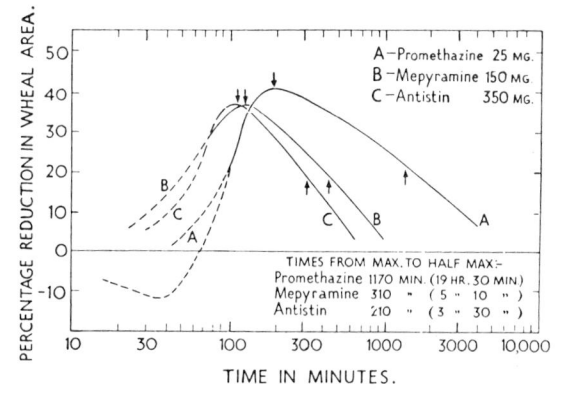

Fig. 8.8 The effect on normal subjects of oral administration of antihistamine drugs on the response to intradermal injections of histamine. The onset and duration of action of approximately equally effective doses of antihistamine drugs is represented by the percentage reduction in wheal area. The time of onset of maximum action of the drugs is indicated by ↓ and of half maximum action by ↑. The full action of promethazine begins in three hours and reaches half action in nineteen and a half hours; with mepyramine the action begins in two hours but reaches half maximum action in about five hours. (After Bain, 1949, *Proc. Roy. Soc. Med.*)

In assessing the activity of these drugs not only the magnitude of the effect but also its duration must be taken into account. As shown in Figure 8.8 the action of promethazine is long-lasting and for this reason the frequency of administration required is less than for other drugs with a shorter duration of action.

Other pharmacological actions

Other effects of H_1-antihistamines are exerted on central histamine receptors; both H_1- and H_2-histamine receptors have been found in the brain. The H_1-antihistamines penetrate the blood-brain barrier more readily than the H_2-antihistamines and they depress various functions of the central nervous system; they produce drowsiness, reduce the rigidity and tremors of Parkinsonism, and are very effective in counteracting motion sickness. The extent to which these effects are produced by different compounds varies; for example, drowsiness is produced by diphenhydramine (benadryl) but less so by phenindamine (thephorin). The H_1-antihistamines also produce central stimulation, they may activate the EEG and in toxic doses may cause convulsions.

Therapeutic uses of H_1-antihistamines

Antihistamine drugs are absorbed from the alimentary tract and are usually given by mouth; they can also be administered intravenously, for example in the treatment of anaphylactic shock. Local administration in ointments or aqueous solution is undesirable since it may produce skin sensitisation.

These drugs have been used against every type of allergic condition; they suppress allergic reactions of the skin and mucous membranes, but do not remove the cause of the reaction, hence the symptoms may reappear when the drug is stopped. They are relatively successful in the treatment of acute urticaria, allergic pruritus, allergic rhinitis and hay fever. In chronic diseases, however, although itching and sneezing may be relieved, the general condition of the skin and mucous membranes remains unaltered.

The use of antihistamine drugs to relieve nausea and vomiting in pregnancy, travel sickness and irradiation sickness is discussed on page 193. The antihistamines are frequently used for their hypnotic and sedative actions. They are effective hypnotics (p. 247) which do not cause respiratory depression and are particularly useful in children and old people. They are also used for pre- and post-operative sedation to relieve apprehension and fear.

Toxic effects

Side reactions of the H_1-antihistamine drugs have been reported by most observers, but only in a few cases were the symptoms so severe as to warrant discontinuing the drug. The commonest complaint is drowsiness and dryness of the mouth; headache, dizziness and tinnitus also occur, most frequently in ambulant patients. It is a curious fact that the local administration of antihistamine drugs for the relief of skin allergies may in some cases produce hypersensitivity of the skin to these drugs.

ALLERGY

Allergy, a word coined by v. Pirquet in 1906, means altered reactivity. The term allergy is currently used to denote a condition of hypersensitivity in man attributable to some underlying antigen-antibody reaction. The study of allergy forms part of the larger study of immunology and only certain aspects of special pharmacological interest will be discussed here.

Antigens

An antigen is a substance which can elicit a specific immunological response. As a rule organisms do not respond immunologically to their own body constituents, so that antigens are normally foreign to the body. Nevertheless the body may become sensitised towards its own tissues, e.g. its own thyroid or testis. Such autosensitisation reactions may be due to pathological alterations of body proteins which render them 'foreign' to the immunologically competent cells. Alternatively autosensitisation may be due to the leakage of normally sequestered body constituents, such as the lens proteins, into the general circulation.

Antigens are large-molecular compounds, either proteins or polysaccharides. When small molecules such as aspirin become antigenic they probably first react chemically with body proteins which in this way are rendered 'foreign' to the body.

Antibodies

Antibodies are formed in the body in response to the introduction of an antigen. They are manufactured in the spleen, lymph node cells and bone marrow by special cells rich in ribonucleic acid, called plasma cells. The antibodies are subsequently shed and occur in the γ-globulin fraction of the blood plasma.

The γ-globulins are a heterogeneous group of proteins which can be separated by ultra-centrifugation, electrophoresis and chromatography into different components. One sub-group, called reaginic antibodies, is of special interest for the study of allergy since it has the capacity of attaching itself to human tissues and sensitising them. Other γ-globulins are capable of neutralising antigen but incapable of attachment to tissues.

Considerable progress has been made in the elucidation of the chemical structure of antibodies. They are known to be made up of polypeptide subunits held together by disulphide bridges as shown in Figure 8.9. The most important property of antibodies is their specificity. This is manifested in two ways:

1. Antibodies interact specifically with antigen. The combining sites of antibodies are highly selective and can discriminate between closely related antigens. The combining sites for the antigens are located on the Fab and Fd portions on the antibody model shown. Antibodies are bivalent, i.e. they have two sites capable of combining with antigen, whilst antigens are multivalent. In this way lattices are built up which can precipitate as was proposed by Marrack.

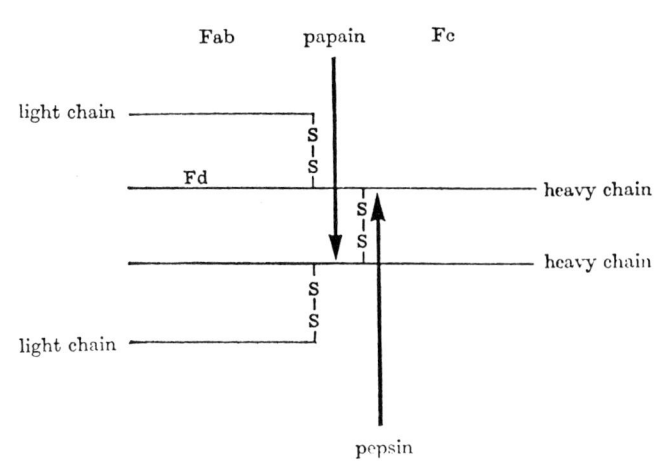

Fig. 8.9 Diagrammatic four-chain structure of an immunoglobulin molecule showing the probable sites of cleavage by papain and pepsin. The number of inter-heavy chain disulphide bridges has not been established with certainty. (Cohen, *Proc. Roy. Soc.* B, 1967.)

2. Certain antibodies attach themselves to tissues and produce anaphylactic sensitisation. Here again, specificity is apparent. For example, the antibodies of the horse cannot attach themselves to guinea-pig tissues. The combining sites with tissues are located on the Fc portion.

Types of hypersensitivity reactions

Allergic reactions are often subdivided according to their time course into immediate and delayed hypersensitivity reactions. Another, more fundamental, subdivision is into reactions mediated by serum antibodies and those mediated by sensitised cells. Coombs and Gell have introduced a useful classification of hypersensitivity reactions as follows.

Type 1. Anaphylactic-type. The antigen reacts with a specific class of antibody bound to mast cells or circulating basophils. This reaction leads to the release of pharmacologically active transmitters.

Type 2. Cytotoxic type. Antibodies bind to antigen present on the cell surface causing cell disruption. Type 2 reactions require complement.

Type 3. Hypersensitivity reactions mediated by antigen-antibody complexes in serum, e.g. serum-sickness.

Type 4. Cell-mediated hypersensitivity of the delayed type.

Reactions due to cell-fixed antibodies

The prototype is the anaphylactic reaction which depends on the binding of circulating antibody to tissues, a process called sensitisation. When cell-bound antibody subsequently comes in contact with a specific antigen a violent reaction, the anaphylactic reaction, ensues. Anaphylactic reactions are mediated largely, though not necessarily exclusively, by the release of pharmacologically active substances.

Anaphylactic sensitisation may be active or passive. In active sensitisation the antigen is administered to an animal which produces antibodies; they are subsequently bound by tissue cells which thus become sensitised. In passive sensitisation the antigen is administered to subject A which produces circulating antibodies; the serum of A is transferred to subject B whose tissues bind the antibody and become sensitised.

Reactions due to circulating antibodies

Serum sickness is a condition due to the formation in the circulation of soluble antigen-antibody complexes. These complexes can produce effects which resemble anaphylaxis. Serum sickness may occur a week or so after the injection of a large amount of an antigenic protein such as horse serum; it arises at a time when antibodies begin to appear in the blood whilst antigen still circulates. The chief symptoms of human serum sickness are cutaneous eruptions, fever and painful joints. The rashes usually cause intense itching.

The Arthus reaction is an acute inflammatory reaction which occurs when antigen is injected into the skin of an animal whose blood contains large amounts of circulating antibody. The reaction occurs inside the blood vessels. Although the Arthus reaction as such is not relevant to human pathology it can be regarded as a model reaction of pathological events which occur in human disease, e.g. in certain types of glomerulonephritis.

Hypersensitivity reactions mediated by sensitised cells

These are also referred to as delayed reactions and their prototype is the *tuberculin reaction*. When the skin of a patient or a guinea pig with tuberculosis is injected with tuberculin (a protein derived from the tubercle bacillus) there is no immediate effect but after about four hours redness and induration develop around the site of injection which reach a maximum in 24 to 48 hours.

Landsteiner and Chase have shown that tuberculin hypersensitivity and other types of delayed hypersensitivity cannot be transferred to non-sensitised animals by serum antibodies of sensitised animals but they can be transferred by intact lymphocytes of sensitised animals. Although delayed hypersensitivity is presumably caused by antibodies carried in the cellular elements of blood, it would seem that these antibodies are so closely bound up with the lymphocytic blood cells, that they cannot be separated from them. The lymphocytes participating in specific immune responses can be subdivided into two classes, the thymus-dependent *T lymphocytes* which are responsible for delayed hypersensitivity reactions and the bone-marrow-derived *B lymphocytes* which are the precursors of antibody secreting cells. T cells and B cells have been shown to interact. Co-operation between T and B cells has been demonstrated in the production of antibody (the 'helper' effect). T lymphocytes can also act as 'killer' cells by lysing sensitised target cells *in vitro*.

Many allergic skin reactions due to food, drugs and chemicals are of the delayed type. For example contact with primula or poison ivy, or in some individuals, contact with the leaves of tomato or even potato may produce sensitisation which leads to a characteristic delayed reaction and dermatitis on further contact. Similarly, skin contact with drugs such as penicillin, sulphonamides and procaine or with metals such as nickel or mercury may lead to a delayed type of hypersensitivity and to contact dermatitis. Hypersensitivity to drugs is further discussed below.

Anaphylaxis

This condition was discovered by Portier and Richet in 1898, who found that when a dog injected with sea anemone poison was given a second dose after an interval of several days, the second dose produced more severe toxic effects than the first dose. They called this condition anaphylaxis because they believed that the first injection of this toxic protein had rendered the animal unprotected ($αναφυλαξις$ — unprotectedness) towards the second injection. Arthus, however, showed in 1903 that similar effects could be produced with non-toxic proteins. In this case the first dose produced no symptoms at all, while the second dose produced a severe toxic reaction.

The anaphylactic reaction can be demonstrated most clearly in the guinea-pig. If a small dose of protein (antigen) is injected the animal shows no obvious reaction. But if the same dose is reinjected after an interval of three to four weeks, the guinea-pig dies within a few seconds from asphyxia, due to bronchoconstriction.

A corresponding phenomenon can be demonstrated in isolated tissues. If the isolated lung of a normal guinea-pig is perfused with Ringer's solution and egg albumen is added to the perfusion fluid, no reaction occurs, but if a similar experiment is performed with the lungs of a guinea-pig which three weeks previously has had a sensitising dose of the same protein, intense bronchoconstriction is produced.

If the isolated uterus of a normal guinea-pig is suspended in Ringer's solution and egg albumen is added to the solution no reaction occurs, but if this experiment is performed on the uterus of an animal which has previously been sensitised to egg albumen a maximal contraction of the uterus occurs (Dale-Schultz reaction). Dale found that the sensitised uterus would only react once to the specific antigen and that afterwards it became desensitised to the antigen.

Anaphylactic reactions in man
Systemic anaphylactic reactions in man are rare but they may occur from the intravenous injection of a protein to which the patient is sensitised. They can arise from the accidental injection of an antigen during skin testing or from the sting of a bee or a wasp. Amongst drugs, penicillin is particularly liable to produce severe anaphylactic reactions; they are due partly to degradation products of penicillin which react with body proteins and form antigens (p. 406).

Anaphylactic reactions in man usually begin with itching and flushing of the skin, followed by severe dyspnoea due to laryngospasm and bronchospasm, and a profound fall of blood pressure. They can be fatal, but rapid relief is often obtained by the administration of adrenaline and an intravenous antihistamine drug.

Clinical allergy
Examples of allergic reactions which occur clinically are asthmatic attacks produced by the inhalation of dust or feathers by sensitised patients, hay fever due to contact of pollen with the mucous membranes of the nose and conjunctiva and urticaria from ingestion of certain foods such as strawberries or shellfish.

The antibodies responsible for human allergic disease are called reagins. The readiness with which reagins are formed in different individuals varies and in this sense allergy may be said to have a genetic basis.

Reaginic antibodies
Ishizaka has shown that human reaginic antibodies belong to a separate immunoglobulin class called IgE. They can be distinguished from other antibodies by their heat lability and susceptibility to sulph-hydryl reagents. Human IgE antibodies can sensitise human and primate tissues but probably not the tissues of guinea pigs and other rodents.

Reaginic antibodies are believed to be responsible for allergic conditions in man such as allergic bronchial

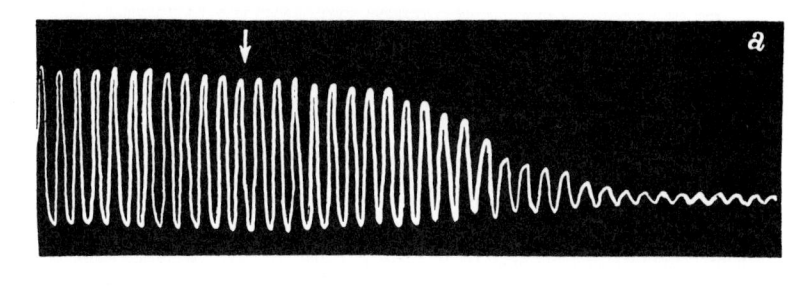

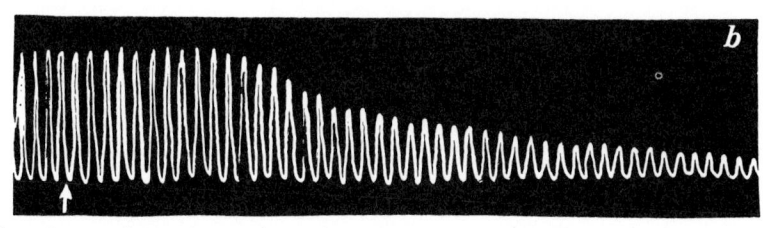

Fig. 8.10 Release of a bronchoconstrictor substance from guinea-pig lungs during anaphylactic shock. Record of excursions of artificially ventilated guinea-pig lung perfused with Tyrode solution. (a) Guinea-pig sensitised to egg-albumen; at the arrow egg albumen was added to the perfusion fluid and the resulting bronchoconstriction produced a marked decrease in excursions. (b) Normal guinea-pig; at the arrow the perfusion fluid emerging from the sensitised lung was perfused through the lungs of a non-sensitised guinea-pig and caused similar effects. (After Bartosch, Feldberg and Nagel, 1932, *Arch. f. Physiol.*)

asthma, hay fever and allergic urticaria; their detection and measurement is therefore of great importance. They can be detected by biological reactions, usually involving histamine release or by chemical measurements.

Biological reactions. Tests include (a) passive sensitisation of human or monkey tissues with reaginic human serum followed by addition of specific antigen, e.g. pollen, leading to histamine release. One of the best methods is passive sensitisation of chopped human lung obtained at operation. (b) Application of antigen to actively sensitised leucocytes of allergic patients and measurement of histamine release (Lichtenstein and Osler). (c) Intracutaneous injection of serum of a sensitised patient into a non-sensitised individual, followed 24 hours later by antigen to produce a wheal and flare reaction (Prausnitz-Kuestner).

Chemical methods include tests for the detection of (a) total IgE (radioimmunosorbent test, RIST) and (b) antigen-specific IgE (radioallergosorbent test, RAST).

Desensitisation
This term is currently applied to two rather different processes.

1. The failure of a sensitised preparation to respond to a second dose of antigen. This form of desensitisation may be due to exhaustion of antibody or of an essential enzyme system activated by the antigen-antibody reaction.

2. Clinical hyposensitisation. This consists of a course of graded injections of antigen, e.g. of a suspension of pollen into a hypersensitive patient in order to render him less sensitive. In this case desensitisation is believed to be due to the formation of *blocking antibodies*. In contrast to reagins the blocking antibodies do not attach themselves to the skin but they can combine preferentially with the antigen and thus prevent its reaction with reagin attached to the skin.

Mechanism of the anaphylactic reaction
The events which lead to an anaphylactic reaction are as follows. As a consequence of the injection of an antigen into an animal specific antibodies are formed which circulate in the blood. Some of the circulating antibodies, the anaphylactic antibodies, become bound to tissue cells, particularly to mast cells and basophils; this process is called sensitisation. A second dose of antigen injected some weeks later into a sensitised animal will react with the tissue-bound antibody and elicit an anaphylactic reaction.

The dominant symptom in the anaphylactic reaction varies according to species. In the guinea pig it is bronchospasm which causes an asthma-like condition capable of killing the animal from asphyxia. The chief effect in the rabbit is a constriction of the pulmonary vessels which produces a failure of the right side of the heart. In the dog the chief effect is on the vessels of the splanchnic area and the liver; these organs are greatly engorged and the obstruction of the portal circulation causes a rapid fall of blood pressure and death from circulatory failure.

The specificity of anaphylaxis is remarkable. When an animal is sensitised to a protein it reacts to that protein and

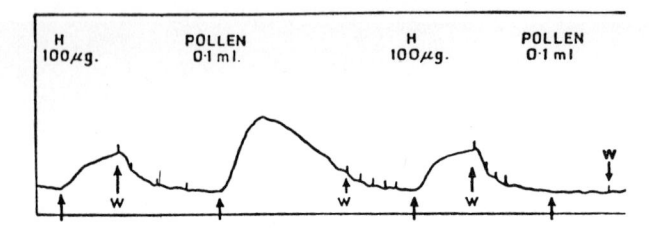

Fig. 8.11 Contractions of bronchial muscle taken from a patient with pollen asthma during an operation for bronchiectasis and suspended in Ringer's solution. The first dose of pollen extract caused a contraction but the second dose of pollen extract was ineffective. In spite of this desensitisation to pollen extract the muscle continued to respond to histamine. The desensitised muscle has not lost its responsiveness to histamine but fails to release histamine when antigen is added. (After Schild, Hawkins, Mongar and Herxheimer, 1951 *Lancet.*)

to that protein alone. Traces of protein, moreover, are sufficient both to establish sensitivity and to provoke an anaphylactic reaction. A guinea pig can be sensitised by 0.0001 ml of serum and asthma can be provoked in sensitive human subjects by the inhalation of traces of a specific protein in the form of dust.

Evidence that the anaphylactic reaction in different species varied in a manner similar to their reactions to histamine led to the hypothesis that the bronchoconstriction and other symptoms of anaphylaxis might be due to the release of endogenous histamine. In 1932 Feldberg, Dragstedt and others showed that histamine is indeed released in anaphylaxis in quantities sufficient to account for the observed effects. It was shown that when the lung of a guinea pig which had previously been sensitised to ovalbumen, was perfused with Ringer's solution, the injection of a dose of ovalbumen into the perfusate caused the appearance of a pharmacologically active principle in the venous effluent which had all the properties of histamine. It produced bronchoconstriction if injected into a second lung (Fig. 8.10) and a contraction of the isolated guinea pig uterus and ileum. Other smooth muscle stimulants are also released in anaphylaxis. SRS-A (p. 92) is released in the anaphylactic reaction of the guinea pig and man and is probably a major factor in human allergic disease. 5-HT appears to be the main factor in rodent anaphylaxis but its release in human allergy has not been clearly demonstrated. A participation of prostaglandins in the anaphylactic reaction of the guinea pig has been demonstrated but the mechanism of their release is not clear; they may be released as a secondary consequence of the powerful bronchoconstriction occurring during the anaphylactic reaction. In the presence of blood, bradykinin may also be formed.

Various organic bases such as tubocurarine, morphine and the synthetic compound 48/80 release histamine if applied to unsensitised tissues. They produce effects which resemble those of histamine, for example if morphine is injected intradermally it produces a characteristic triple response.

Such substances may act by a simple ion exchange mechanism displacing histamine from its binding with heparin. Some histamine releasers act in a more complex fashion, inducing reactions which are akin to the anaphylactic reaction and can be used as model systems for its investigation.

Mechanism of anaphylactic histamine release and its inhibition

Tissue histamine is contained in mast cells. When an antigen-antibody reaction takes place on a sensitised mast cell, an extrusion of mast cell granules and a release of histamine occurs. Anaphylactic histamine release is dependent on extracellular calcium; calcium probably constitutes the effective stimulus for initiating histamine release. Mast cell histamine release is inhibited by raised intracellular levels of cyclic AMP and this may be the mechanism by which ß-adrenergic catecholamines inhibit anaphylactic histamine release. Anaphylactic histamine release is specifically inhibited by disodium cromoglycate which is an effective therapeutic agent in the prevention of allergic bronchial asthma (p. 181). It has been shown that cromoglycate prevents the uptake of labelled calcium by the mast cell membrane and this may be the basis of its clinical effect.

Actions of H_1 antihistamines in allergy

The H_1 antihistamines counteract the effects of allergic histamine release in the skin and mucous membranes, but they are remarkably ineffective in the clinically important allergic condition of bronchial asthma.

An experimental demonstration of the interactions of a specific antigen, histamine and an H_1 antihistamine, mepyramine, in isolated sensitised human bronchial muscle is shown in Figure 8.11-13. It shows the responses *in vitro* of isolated bronchial rings from a patient with pollen asthma who had part of his lung removed because of bronchiectasies. The results of this investigation can be summarised as follows:

1. Sensitised human bronchial muscle contracts in response to antigen and is subsequently desensitised. It also responds to histamine but the histamine response is maintained after desensitisation to the antigen (both effects are typical of isolated organ anaphylaxis) (Fig. 8.11)
2. Interaction of antigen with sensitised human lung causes histamine release (Fig. 8.12)
3. There is a marked, over 1000-fold, difference between the concentrations of the H_1-antihistamine, mepyramine, required to antagonise external histamine and those required to antagonise (presumably) internally released histamine (Fig. 8.13)

The reasons for this discrepancy are not fully understood, but at least two factors are probably involved. Firstly, histamine is released from mast cells situated in close proximity to the bronchial smooth muscle cells. During the anaphylactic reaction the latter thus become exposed to very high concentrations of histamine which cannot be readily antagonised by a competitive antihistamine drug. Secondly, it is known that other bronchoconstrictor substances such as SRS-A are also released and take part in the total reaction. It is significant in this context that physiological antagonists such as catecholamines and substances which interfere with the release mechanism such as cromoglycate and catecholamines are much more effective in asthma than the classical antihistamines.

Clinically the antihistamines are more effective in allergic conditions involving capillaries such as hay-fever and urticaria. This may be due to the fact that in these conditions the mast cells are further removed from the site of action of histamine, resulting in a longer diffusion path and hence lower concentration of histamine at the active site.

Hypersensitivity to drugs

The reaction of individuals to drugs varies very greatly, and a dose which may be suitable for one person may produce toxic effects in a more sensitive person. The term 'hypersensitivity' should be reserved, however, for those cases in which a normal or subnormal dose of a drug produces a violent reaction, which is wholly unlike the normal response to the drug. This reaction, may take the form of a skin rash, a rise in temperature, or swelling and increased secretion of mucous membranes. For instance, in some individuals a dose of aspirin or penicillin produces asthma, associated with intensive urticarial eruptions. It is believed that about one person in 10 000 is sensitive to aspirin. Sensitisation to sulphonamides, thiouracil compounds, barbiturates and many other drugs is also known to occur.

It is probable that hypersensitivity reactions produced by low molecular chemical substances depend on these substances or their degradation products first reacting with tissue proteins and thus becoming antigenic. Landsteiner investigated this problem systematically. He showed that a highly specific sensitisation of guinea-pigs could be produced by the administration of proteins conjugated with drugs. The treated animals showed the usual lethal anaphylactic response to the protein-drug complex when this was injected intravenously; in many cases this also occurred when only the drug was injected.

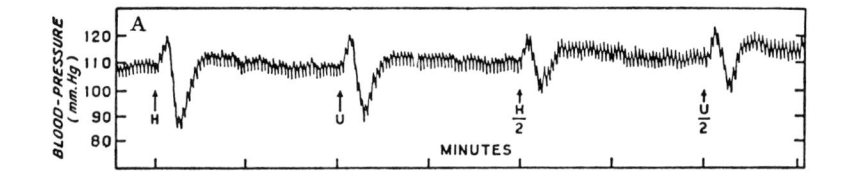

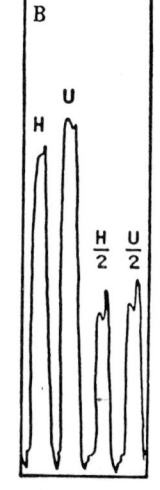

Fig. 8.12 Histamine release from isolated human sensitised lung tissue. When pollen extract is added to the bath in which a piece of sensitised lung tissue is suspended, histamine is released and diffuses into the surrounding fluid. The figure illustrates two methods of assaying the released substance (U) against histamine (H). A. Record of cat arterial blood pressure. B. Contractions of isolated guinea-pig ileum. (After Schild, Hawkins, Mongar and Herxheimer, 1951, *Lancet*.)

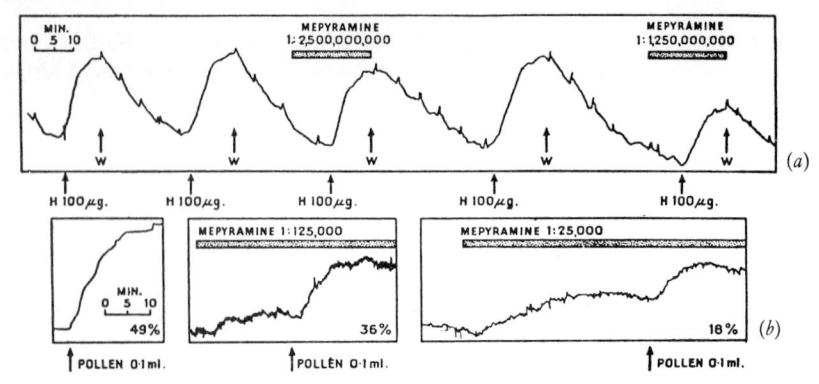

Fig. 8.13 Contractions of isolated sensitised human bronchial muscle. Low concentrations of mepyramine are sufficient to antagonise the contractions produced by histamine added to the bath. High concentrations of the antihistamine are required to antagonise the contractions produced by the addition of the specific antigen to the bath.

Another allied problem is the skin sensitisation that occurs in certain individuals after prolonged exposure to certain chemical compounds. This trouble occurs not uncommonly in industrial workers. Dinitrochlorobenzene and paraphenylenediamine are examples of drugs which cause such effects. Skin sensitivity of the contact dermatitis type can be produced experimentally in animals. If a small quantity of dinitrochlorobenzene is applied locally to the skin of a guinea pig, the whole skin of the animal becomes hypersensitive to this compound within about a week. Thus if further application of the compound is made to any other area of the skin, a characteristic skin reaction develops which resembles contact dermatitis in man. The reaction develops slowly and is maximal twenty-four to forty-eight hours after application, after which it gradually subsides. Skin reactions to chemicals are in most cases of the delayed hypersensitivity type.

The laboratory detection of drug allergy is frequently difficult. A useful test for drug allergy is the lymphocyte transformation test in which the suspected drug is applied to a culture of the patient's lymphocytes. This causes a stimulation of the genetic apparatus of the lymphocyte manifested by cell division and increased incorporation of labelled thymidine.

Formation of a complete antigen by a drug

Drugs of molecular weight under 1000 must first bind to a macromolecule, usually a protein, in order to become capable of inducing antibody synthesis. For this purpose a strong, generally covalent, bond between drug and macromolecule must be formed. Drugs such as sulphonamides and barbiturates which do not bind covalently to proteins presumably become allergenic by first forming a protein-reactive degradation product. Antibodies against drug-protein complexes are highly specific. Once formed it is often possible to elicit an immediate allergic reaction with the responsible drug (hapten) or degradation product alone. By contrast, eliciting of a delayed hypersensitivity reaction is believed to require the prior formation of a hapten-protein conjugate.

In penicillin allergy the penicilloyl group called the *major determinant* is in most cases responsible for antibody formation but some of the most dangerous penicillin allergies are due to other degradation products called *minor determinants*. A difficulty in detecting penicillin allergy by immunological tests is that the reactions of immediate type are probably due to reaginic antibodies whilst the antibodies detected by serum tests are often not reaginic. Benzylpenicilloyl-specific serum antibodies are very frequent. Thus Levine in New York found that 97% of unselected hospital patients had such antibodies. Some of these patients had never received penicillin, suggesting that their antibodies were due to the widespread presence of penicillin in the environment.

PREPARATIONS

Histamine and analogues
Histamine Acid Phosphate Injection s.c. 0.5–1 mg; 5 mg after the administration of an antihistamine
Betahistine Hyd H_1-histamine analogue
Ametazole Hyd (Betazole), H_2-histamine analogue

Histamine-H_1 antagonists
Brompheniramine Maleate (Dimotane) 4–8 mg
Chlorpheniramine Maleate (Piriton) 10–40 mg daily
Clemastine Fumarate (Tavegil) 1 mg night and morning
Dimethindene Maleate (Fenostil) 2.5 mg night and morning
Dimethothiazine Mesylate (Banystyl) Tablets 20 mg; also antiserotonin action
Diphenhydramine Hyd 50–200 mg daily
Diphenylpyraline Hyd 5–20 mg daily
Mebhydrolin (Fabahistin) 50–100 mg 3 times daily
Mepyramine Maleate (Anthisan) 300–600 mg daily
Phenindamine Tartrate (Thephorin) 25–50 mg 1–3 times daily
Promethazine Hyd (Phenergan) 20–50 mg daily
Triprolidine Hyd (Actidil) 5–7.5 mg daily

Histamine-H_2 antagonist
Cimetidine (Tagamet). See Ch. 13

Antiemetics and antinauseants
Dimenhydrinate etc. See Ch. 13

FURTHER READING

Austen K F, Becker E L (eds) 1968 Biochemistry of the acute allergic reactions. Blackwell, Oxford

Berti F, Samuelsson B, Velo G P (ed) 1977 Prostaglandins and thromboxanes. Plenum, New York

Black J W et al 1972 Definition and antagonisms of histamine H_2-receptors. Nature, 236: 385

Erspamer V (ed) 1966 5-Hydroxytryptamine and related indolealkylamines. Handb. exp. Pharmac. Vol. 19

Erdös G (ed) 1970 Bradykinin, kallidin and kallikrein. Handb. exp. Pharmacol. Vol. 25

Gell P G H, Coombs R R A (eds) 1968 Clinical aspects of immunology. Blackwell, Oxford

Horton E W 1972 Prostaglandins. Heinemann, London

Humphrey J H, White R G 1970 Immunology for students of medicine. Blackwell, Oxford

Karim S M M (ed) 1976 Prostaglandins. Chemical and biochemical aspects. MTP Press, Lancaster, England

Mongar, J L, Schild H O 1962 Cellular mechanisms in anaphylaxis. Physiol. Rev. 42: 226

Rocha e Silva M 1966 Histamine; chemistry, metabolism, physiological and pharmacological actions. Handb. exp. Pharm. 18: 1, 2)

Roitt I M 1977 Essential immunology. Blackwell, Oxford

Schachter M (ed) 1960 Polypeptides which affects smooth muscles and blood vessels. Pergamon, Oxford

Schild H O 1962 The mechanisms of contact sensitisation. J. Pharm. Pharmacol. 14: 1

Schild H O, Hawkins D F, Mongar J L, Herxheimer H 1951 Reactions of isolated human lung and bronchial tissue to a specific antigen. Histamine release and muscular contraction. Lancet 2: 376

Turk J L 1978 Immunology in clinical medicine. Heinemann, London

SECTION THREE

Pharmacology of organ systems

9. The circulation

The peripheral circulation 109; Experimental hypertension 111; Drugs which reduce blood pressure 112; Diuretics 113; Vasodilators 114; Beta blockers 115; Interference with catecholamine metabolism 117; Central antihypertensives 117; Adrenergic neurone block 118; Ganglion block 120; Hypertensive emergencies 121; Coronary vasodilators and antianginals 121; Central vasoconstrictors 124; Sympathomimetics 124; Angiotensin 127; Ergotamine 127; Shock 129.

THE PERIPHERAL CIRCULATION

The most essential task of the circulation is the supply of an adequate quantity of oxygen to the tissues. The oxygen requirements of individual tissues vary continuously and the body must therefore be able to adjust their blood supply rapidly. The blood flow through a tissue depends on two factors, head of pressure and resistance, but since homoeostatic mechanisms tend to keep the blood pressure constant the flow depends mainly on the vascular resistance. The vessels controlling resistance are the arterioles and precapillary sphincters.

Zweifach, who studied the blood flow through capillaries of the skin, considers that true capillaries arise from intermediate structures, called *metarterioles*, which connect arterioles and venules (Fig. 9.1). The flow of blood through the capillaries is controlled by rings of smooth muscle at their origin called *precapillary sphincters* which perform rhythmic contractions so that in a resting organ only a fraction of capillaries is open at any time. When an organ functions, i.e. a muscle contracts or a gland secretes, new capillaries open up and the blood flow increases greatly.

Arterio-venous anastomoses (Fig. 9.1) occur especially in the skin, forming low resistance pathways through which a large amount of blood can flow as when a rapid loss of heat from the body is required.

The basic principles of the exchange of fluid between capillaries and the extracapillary tissue spaces were established by Starling in 1896. This exchange is governed by two factors, the difference in hydrostatic pressure between capillary lumen and interstitial fluid and their difference in colloid osmotic pressure. At the arterial end of the capillary the hydrostatic pressure (about 32 mmHg) is higher than the colloid osmotic pressure of plasma proteins (about 25 mmHg), hence fluid leaves the capillaries. At the venous end of the hydrostatic pressure is only about 15 mmHg, hence fluid is drawn back into the capillaries. This delicate balance is upset under a variety of conditions, e.g. when (1) capillary venous pressure is elevated, as in congestive heart failure, (2) colloid osmotic pressure is lowered, as in certain forms of nephritis, (3) capillaries become permeable to plasma proteins through the action of drugs such as histamine.

The *postcapillary venules* and *veins* are the main capacitance vessels of the circulation containing about two thirds of the total blood volume. Both resistance and capacitance vessels are under sympathetic control and can be constricted by alpha-sympathomimetic drugs.

THE ARTERIAL BLOOD PRESSURE

This depends on the output of the heart and the resistance offered by the blood vessels as expressed by the equation:

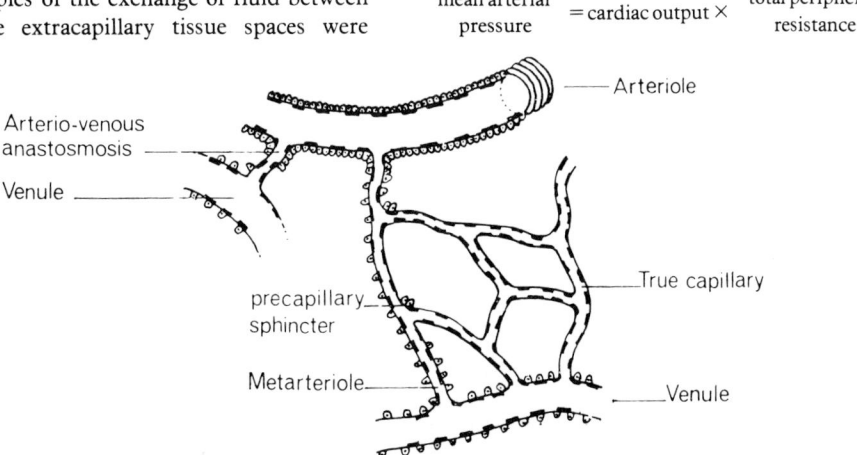

$$\text{mean arterial pressure} = \text{cardiac output} \times \text{total peripheral resistance}$$

Fig. 9.1 Diagram of the microcirculation based on Zweifach's analysis. (After Kelman, 1971, *Applied Cardiovascular Physiology*, Butterworth's.)

The waveform of the blood pressure is asymmetrical, its mean lying closer to the diastolic than to the systolic point. A persistent rise in diastolic pressure can be regarded as important evidence of an increased peripheral resistance. The pulse pressure, given by the difference between systolic and diastolic pressures, depends on stroke volume and arterial distensibility. In arteriosclerosis, when the arterial wall becomes less distensible, the pulse pressure is increased.

The systolic blood pressure in a healthy young adult during complete rest is usually between 110 and 120 mm and the diastolic pressure between 60 and 70 mmHg. The blood pressure at rest may be taken as a measure of the lowest pressure that will ensure a sufficient supply of blood to the brain, and therefore, in a healthy individual, the lower the blood pressure during rest the more efficient is the circulation. The average diastolic pressure increases with age and is usually about 100 mmHg in a man of 65 years. It has become apparent with the extensive use of antihypertensive drugs that even a mild degree of uncorrected hypertension carries an unfavourable prognosis. Thus it has been shown, in studies in the United States, that treatment with antihypertensive drugs in a group of men with diastolic pressures between 90 and 114 mmHg produced a significant reduction in morbidity and mortality compared with untreated controls.

THE ACTION OF DRUGS ON THE CIRCULATION

Drugs can affect the circulation by altering the output of the heart, by altering the peripheral resistance, or by altering the volume or viscosity of blood in circulation. These variables, however, are interdependent. For instance, the output of the normal heart can only be increased if the venous return is increased and this is usually brought about by a change in the circulating blood volume due to mobilisation of the blood depots. In this way cardiac output is increased during exercise, body heating, and after adrenaline. Drugs which dilate arterioles, decrease the peripheral resistance and cause an increase in cardiac output by facilitating venous return. This is true of the nitrites and most anaesthetics. These same drugs in larger doses increase the capacity of the peripheral bed and in this way cause a decrease in the circulating blood volume with a corresponding decrease in cardiac output.

Drugs which alter the blood pressure usually alter the distribution of blood in the body. Most drugs which produce vasoconstriction decrease the blood flow through the skin and viscera thus automatically increasing the blood flow through the brain and muscle.

Changes in blood flow are difficult to interpret since they may be caused either by a direct action on the vessels, by reflex adjustments in vasomotor tone following changes in blood pressure, or by a change in pressure-head.

The arterioles of the skin, muscles and viscera have a vasoconstrictor and in some special cases a vasodilator nerve supply and also possess intrinsic tone independent of nerve supply. For instance, after sympathectomy in animals the blood pressure falls initially but later recovers completely and in man sympathectomy is also followed eventually by a recovery of vascular tone, although the recovery is usually more marked in the upper limbs than in the lower limbs. Although vasodilator fibres emerge from the central nervous system by the posterior nerve roots, by special nerves such as the chorda tympani and the nervus erigens and by sympathetic cholinergic pathways, it is doubtful whether they have any functional significance in the maintenance of blood pressure. The arterioles are kept in a state of partial contraction by their vasoconstrictor nerve supply and therefore the production of vasodilatation by drugs generally involves a reduction of the sympathetic vasoconstrictor activity.

Measurement of blood flow and blood pressure

The blood flow through the arm may be measured by means of plethysmographs which temporarily obstruct venous return. Blood flow through the arm is mainly muscle flow and that through the hand, skin flow. Other methods of determining blood flow include the measurement of changes in temperature and light absorption and the use of radioactive labelling. An ingenious method of measuring blood flow through the brain based on the Fick principle has been used by Kety and Schmidt. In this method nitrous oxide is inhaled and the cerebral blood flow is estimated by determining the concentration of the gas in serial samples of arterial blood and blood from the internal jugular vein.

The measurement of blood flow in man and the effect of drugs upon it is becoming increasingly complex and highly specialised. Thus several different types of catheter flowmeter have been developed which can be introduced into a large vessel such as the aorta or pulmonary artery to measure their blood flow. These flow probes are of three main types (1) electromagnetic, (2) thin metal film probes, in which an electric current passed through the film raises its temperature whilst the flow of blood over its surface tends to lower it, the rate of heat loss being measured, (3) Doppler flowmeters, which depend on the fact that if a beam of ultrasound is directed into a flowing column of blood the reflected echo depends on the velocity of the flow.

Whilst arterial blood pressure is still normally measured by sphygmomanometer the continuous assessment of blood pressure, by an automatically controlled sphygmomanometer is difficult. It is frequently preferable to use for this purpose an electromanometer connected to an indwelling arterial cannula. Blood pressure transducers convert pressure changes into electrical signals by affecting capacitance, resistance or inductance. The transducer must not distort the pressure wave, the connections to it should be short and the natural frequency of the system as high as possible.

Another measurement requiring specialised skills is the measurement of central venous pressure which can be more informative in the functional assessment of the cardiovascular system than measurement of the arterial pressure. The central venous pressure provides information about the functional state of the heart and the circulating blood volume. It is measured by a suitable pressure transducer connected to a catheter with its tip close to the right atrium.

HYPERTENSION AND ANTIHYPERTENSIVE DRUGS

Hypertension may accompany many disorders including renal disease, disease of the adrenal glands and toxaemia of pregnancy. In most patients with high blood pressure, however, no primary disorder is evident and the condition is then referred to as essential hypertension. Malignant hypertension is a progressive form of hypertension associated with papilloedema of the optic fundi in which the diastolic pressure is 140 mm or more.

Experimental hypertension

The cause of essential hypertension is not known but it is possible to produce in animals, by various experimental procedures, conditions which have some resemblance to human hypertensive disease and which may help to elucidate its mechanism. These experimental conditions may also be used to test antihypertensive drugs. The following are some of the main types of experimental hypertension.

Hypertension following renal artery constriction
In 1898 Tigerstedt and Bergman observed that saline extracts of kidney produced a rise of blood pressure when injected intravenously. They partially purified the active substance and called it 'renin'. Goldblatt showed in 1934 that constriction of the renal arteries of dogs produces persistent high blood pressure. The rise of blood pressure is due to a substance liberated by the kidney; it also occurs when an ischaemic kidney is grafted into a normal animal or when blood from an ischaemic kidney is transfused into a normal animal.

Later work has shown that renin is a protein of the kidney which is itself inactive but interacts with a component of the alpha-globulin fraction of plasma to produce the active compound angiotensin as shown by Braun-Menendez and his colleagues and by Page and Helmer.

Renin has the properties of an enzyme. Purified solutions of renin do not produce vasoconstriction in organs perfused with Ringer's solution but cause a slow and prolonged rise of blood pressure when injected into the blood stream. Angiotensin is a low molecular polypeptide which, in contrast to renin, produces vasoconstriction in isolated organs and contraction of isolated smooth muscle. The pharmacological properties of angiotensin are discussed on page 127.

Renin is secreted by the renal *juxtaglomerular (J-G) cells* located in the wall of the afferent glomerular arteriole. Renin secretion is stimulated by low intrarenal perfusion pressure which is mechanically transmitted as the degree of stretch against the vessel wall. The J-G cells are richly innervated by sympathetic nerves. Beta-adrenoceptor stimulation by isoprenaline increases renin secretion, whilst beta-adrenoceptor blockers such as propranolol inhibit renin secretion and tend to lower renin plasma levels.

The role of the renin-angiotensin system in human hypertension has been the subject of much study. There is no doubt that in patients in whom the renal blood flow has been pathologically restricted a hypertension closely similar to that in the 'Goldblatt kidney' develops which can be cured by removal of the afflicted kidney.

Attempts have been made to measure the renin content of plasma in essential hypertension. This can be done by incubating purified plasma with a suitable globulin substrate and measuring the amount of angiotensin formed by its effect in raising the blood pressure of an anaesthetised rat. Alternatively a radioimmunoassay of angiotensin I may be used. Such measurements have shown that the renin content of plasma varies greatly but is usually elevated in malignant hypertension.

It has been suggested that the production of renin by the kidney may be important particularly in the early stages of hypertension. In the later stages, disturbances in adrenal cortical function, involving salt retention may supervene.

Hypertension due to corticosteroids
It is possible to produce hypertension in rats by administration of a high salt diet combined with corticosteroids. In man the condition of primary aldosteronism (Conn's syndrome) is attended by hypertension which can be relieved by aldosterone antagonists such as spironolactone (p. 163). There is evidence of a close relationship between the renin-angiotensin system and aldosterone secretion. It has been shown in animals and man that angiotensin stimulates the release of aldosterone from the adrenal cortex. Aldosterone promotes salt retention by the kidney which is an important factor in hypertension.

Figure 9.2 shows the effect of a low salt diet on plasma renin levels in two normal subjects. It is seen that a low salt diet increases the plasma renin level. This can be regarded as part of a compensatory mechanism in which renin produces angiotensin, angiotensin promotes aldosterone secretion, which in turn corrects the salt deficiency by increasing sodium reabsorption in the renal tubules. In malignant hypertension however, this compensatory mechanism seems to be deranged.

Although in essential hypertension aldosterone secretion may be normal, it is usually markedly increased in malignant hypertension.

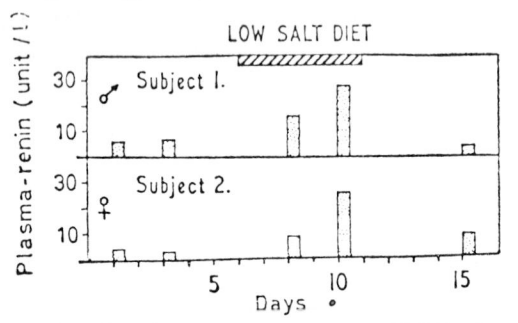

Fig. 9.2 The effect of salt depletion on the plasma renin levels in normal subjects. (After Brown et. al., *Aldosterone*, Blackwell, 1964.)

Hypertension due to neurological and psychological factors
Hypertension can be produced in animals by section of the afferent nerves from the carotid sinus and aortic arch. Persistent hypertension can also be produced in rats of suitable genetic constitution by repeated exposure to strong sensory stimuli such as a strong air blast. This is of interest in view of the undoubted importance of genetic factors in human hypertension.

General measures for the reduction of blood pressure in hypertension

Prior to the introduction of the modern antihypertensive drugs it was disputed whether hypertension should be treated at all. It was argued that hypertension was only a symptom and that a reduction of the blood pressure might be harmful since it could interfere with regulatory processes. This viewpoint has now been shown to be wrong as it has been demonstrated, in controlled trails, that untreated hypertensive patients have more frequent cerebral and other cardiovascular accidents than patients whose blood pressure has been lowered by drugs.

Although hypertension may exist without exhibiting symptoms, it is more usual that, after an elevated blood pressure has persisted for some time, clinical manifestations arise. They include headache, dizziness, nose bleeding, breathlessness on exertion and at a later stage retinal changes, encephalopathy, heart failure and stroke. Since the danger to life arises from the secondary effects of the high blood pressure on the brain, heart and kidneys, it is desirable to lower the blood pressure and maintain it at a reduced level.

A blood pressure reduction of sufficient intensity and duration will usually relieve the reversible secondary manifestations and the extent of relief does not depend on the method employed to lower the blood pressure but on how effectively and consistently it has been reduced.

Restricted sodium intake. A severe restriction in sodium intake reduces the blood pressure in hypertension. Drastic dietetic methods are undoubtedly effective but irksome to patients and now rarely employed. However, some salt restriction is desirable since it has been shown that the antihypertensive effect of oral diuretics is reduced by a high salt diet.

Sympathectomy. This is sometimes effective, especially in malignant hypertension, but the lowered blood pressure following sympathectomy is seldom maintained.

Rest and sedation. The degree of contraction of the arterioles, venules and veins is under the control of the vasomotor centre which in turn is influenced by higher centres and also by the cardiovascular baroreceptor nerves. The arterial resistance depends mainly on the degree of arteriolar constriction whilst the capacity of the circulation depends largely on the degree of constriction of the venules. Both are important factors in determining the blood pressure.

It is thus clear that all drugs which depress the vasomotor centre must have an important effect on the blood pressure. Thus, barbiturates, anaesthetics, alcohol, chlorpromazine, morphine and other central depressants will produce a fall in blood pressure when given in large amounts, although their widespread actions make then unsuitable as hypotensive drugs.

Rest and sedation have an important influence on blood pressure in hypertension. Figure 9.3 shows the results obtained in a hypertensive patient by administration of a barbiturate. It is seen that a centrally acting barbiturate produced as profound a fall of blood pressure as a ganglion blocking drug. Rest in bed in hospital often produces a marked lowering of blood pressure and this factor must be taken into account when hypotensive drugs are assessed in hospital patients. Sedative drugs are widely used in the treatment of hypertension but they produce little effect in subjects with a persistently elevated diastolic blood pressure and they cannot replace the more effective specific hypotensive drugs.

Drugs which reduce blood pressure

Drugs which reduce the blood pressure after an acute injection in normotensive anaesthetised animals are not necessarily effective in the treatment of human hypertension; conversely many drugs which produce a fall of blood pressure in patients with hypertension produce little or no hypotensive effect in acute animal experiments.

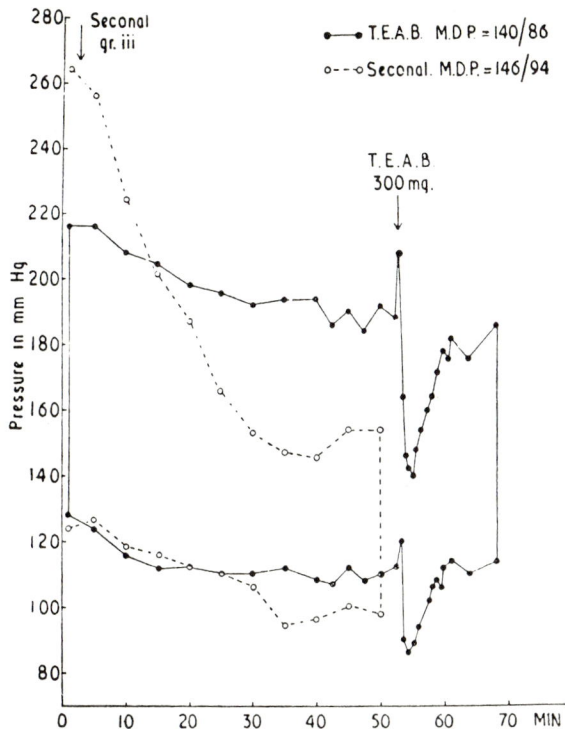

Fig. 9.3 The effect on the blood pressure of a patient with hypertension, of a centrally acting barbiturate compared with that of tetraethyl ammonium bromide, one of the first ganglion blocking drugs. (After Frew and Rosenheim, *Clin. Sci.*, 1949.)

Indeed some antihypertensive drugs, e.g. clonidine or adrenergic neurone blockers may produce an initial rise of blood pressure after their intravenous administration in experimental animals. Nevertheless, in view of their long-range antihypertensive effects in patients (and as a rule also in animals rendered hypertensive) they can be classed as hypotensive drugs.

Theoretically, a drug which lowers blood pressure in hypertension could act by a variety of mechanisms, including the following:

1. Reduction of cardiac output
2. 'Unspecific' peripheral vasodilatation
3. Reduction of circulating blood volume
4. Block of α-adrenoceptors
5. Adrenergic neurone block
6. Interference with catecholamine biosynthesis and metabolism
7. Ganglion block
8. Depression of vasomotor centre in the medulla
9. Action on higher central blood pressure regulating mechanisms
10. Reflex vasomotor depression
11. Inhibition of renin release.

These various mechanisms have all been explored in the search for an effective and relatively non-toxic antihypertensive drug. Some of the earlier drugs such as the gangion blockers were clinically effective but too disabling for routine use as suggested by the then current caricature of the 'hexamethonium man', staggering, half-blind, constipated and impotent. The gangion blockers were followed by a remarkable succession of newer antihypertensive drugs, with new modes of action, having the general objective of rendering long-term antihypertensive treatment bearable to the patient. The present consensus is that mechanisms (1), (2), (3), (5), (6) and (9) provide the most acceptable basis for clinically useful antihypertensive drug action.

Some of the properties required of an antihypertensive drug are as follows. It should:

1. produce a blood pressure reduction of sufficient degree and duration in all types of hypertension including malignant hypertension;
2. give rise to a normally functioning cardiovascular system in which homoeostatic reflexes are maintained; it should not induce orthostatic hypotension or excessive reflex tachycardia during effort; it should be effective in the recumbent position and during sleep;
3. be free of side effects unconnected with its hypotensive action; for example, it should not produce parasympathetic block, diarrhoea or nausea; it should not interfere with sexual function and should not cause sedation and drowsines; it should not produce central stimulation, excitation or giddiness;
4. be adequately absorbed from the gastrointestinal tract;
5. not give rise to tolerance;
6. allow of combination with other drugs.

Few if any anti-hypertensive drugs presently in use possess all these properties.

It is possible that drugs will in future become available which are truly antihypertensive rather than merely hypotensive. Such drugs would affect the fundamental causes of hypertension and the use of sodium-eliminating diuretics as adjuncts in hypotensive therapy is a move in this direction.

Much research has gone into the investigation of the mechanism of action of antihypertensive drugs. In some cases their mode and site of action has been reasonably well established; in others it has remained doubtful or unknown.

The main types of antihypertensive drugs will now be discussed.

Diuretics
A *thiazide* (p. 160) or related diuretic drug usually serves as the basis of antihypertensive treatment either in conjunction with other antihypertensive drugs or as the sole treatment in cases of mild hypertension. The precise mechanism of the blood pressure lowering action of diuretics is uncertain. Diuretics reduce plasma and extracellular fluid volume and total exchangeable sodium,

they tend to diminish blood volume and decrease blood pressure and cardiac output. After prolonged treatment with diuretics, however, plasma volume and cardiac output return partially to normal whilst at the same time peripheral resistance decreases. The present view is that reduction of plasma volume and total extracellular fluid by diuretics is the main factor in their antihypertensive effect. Another contributing factor may be a change in reactivity of the blood vessel wall possibly connected with tissue sodium depletion. It can be shown that thiazides reduce the vasoconstrictor response to noradrenaline in hypertensives.

Clinically the thiazides are well tolerated: they lower both supine and standing blood pressure and maintain their antihypertensive effect during prolonged administration. Thiazides increase the urinary excretion of potassium and the resulting hypokalaemia may be associated with a mild hypochloraemic alkalosis. A good way to prevent the hypokalaemia is to increase dietary potassium intake and decrease dietary sodium chloride. Potassium supplements may be given if the serum potassium level falls below 3 to 3.5 meq/l but supplements are generally not required except in special cases of vomiting and diarrhoea or in digitalis intoxication which is aggravated by low serum potassium. In some patients thiazides may produce a mild hyperglycaemia or an increase in blood uric acid. Some patients exhibit skin rashes and other allergic reactions with thiazides.

Certain drugs related to thiazides e.g. chlorthalidone produce similar effects in hypertension.

Other diuretics. In clinical use normalisation of blood pressure with thiazides alone can be achieved only in mildly hypertensive subjects. On the other hand, all oral diuretics including the thiazides, chlorthalidone, ethacrynic acid, frusemide and aldosterone antagonists potentiate the effects of other antihypertensive drugs and enable them to be used at lower doses and with less side effects. There is, however, no correlation between their diuretic and antihypertensive properties and for most purposes the thiazide group is as effective as the more potent and specific diuretics as adjunct to antihypertensive therapy.

The *loop diuretics* (p. 161) *frusemide* and *ethacrynic acid* are chemically distinct but similar in their pharmacological actions. Both have a more rapid onset of action and a greater diuretic effect than the thiazides. They are usually reserved for hypertensive patients with impaired renal function or when a rapid effect is required to control fluid overload. They have little advantage over thiazides in patients with uncomplicated hypertension.

Potassium sparing diuretics may be used in conjunction with thiazides for the treatment of hypertension. *Spironolactone* is a competitive inhibitor of aldosterone. In essential hypertension it acts as an inhibitor of aldosterone-mediated exchange of Na and K in the distal tubule replenishing thiazide-induced potassium loss. It has some antihypertensive activity of its own and enhances the antihypertensive action of thiazides, but there is some danger that it may produce hyperkalaemia.

Triamterene may be given together with a thiazide to decrease potassium loss. Contrary to spironolactone it has no hormonal activity and is not an effective antihypertensive when used alone. *Amiloride* is a potassium sparing diuretic with similar actions to triamterene.

Vasodilators
Orally active vasodilator drugs are increasingly used in the treatment of hypertension usually in conjunction with a diuretic and a beta blocker. The vasodilator drugs provide the most direct means of reducing total peripheral resistance and thus lowering blood pressure, but have potential disadvantages if used alone. These include 1. a reflex increase in heart rate leading to an increase in cardiac output; 2. an increase in plasma renin activity; 3. sodium and water retention and expansion of extracellular fluid and plasma volume.

Hydrallazine (Apresoline) (Fig. 9.4) is a derivative of phthalazine. When injected intravenously in animals it produces a fall in blood pressure which is slow in onset, takes several minutes to reach a maximum and is long lasting. Even large doses of this drug do not reduce the blood pressure below a level of about 80 mmHg. The mechanism of the hypotensive action of hydrallazine is believed to be partly a direct action on blood vessels and partly central.

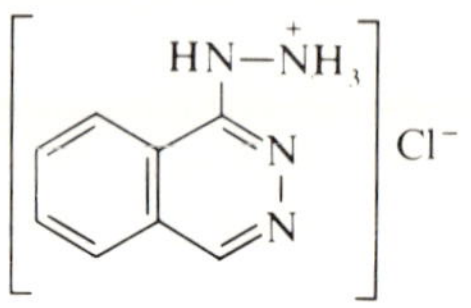

Hydrellezine
Hydrochloride

Fig. 9.4 Hydrallazine hydrocloride.

Hydrallazine has been found to increase the cardiac output and renal blood flow in man. Absorption of hydrallazine after oral administration is irregular. It is usually given by mouth in gradually increasing doses. Hydrallazine is now seldom administered alone since the use of large doses may lead to a lupus erythematosus-like syndrome. It also has a cardiac stimulant action and should therefore be avoided in patients with angina.

Several new antihypertensive drugs have been recently introduced which are believed to act mainly on peripheral blood vessels as vasodilators. They produce a fall in blood pressure in hypertensive patients and are frequently given in conjunction with a ß-adrenoceptor blocking drug to prevent a reflex rise in heart rate. They include *guancydin* and *minoxidil*. Other antihypertensive drugs are claimed to be α-blockers. They include *prazosin* and *indoramin*.

Prazosin is a new vasodilator antihypertensive agent which acts partly by α-adrenergic block. It may also reduce central sympathetic outflow. It dilates both arterioles and veins and in hypertensive patients lower diastolic blood pressure and reduces left-ventricular pressure allowing the heart to function more efficiently. The dose of prazosin must be increased gradually since the first dose has caused collapse and unconsciousness in a proportion of patients.

Beta blockers
Propranolol is the prototype ß-adrenoceptor blocking drug. It is a competitive antagonist of isoprenaline with an identical sidechain (Fig. 9.5) which allows it to interact with ß-receptors and thereby block the effects of adrenergic stimulation mediated through these receptors. Propranolol is an unselective ß-blocker with equal affinity for ß-receptors in heart and smooth muscle (p. 14).

When propranolol is used in man it acts as ß-receptor antagonist in at least four places: (1) block of cardiac chronotropic and inotropic ß-receptors resulting in a decrease in heart rate and myocardial contractility; (2) block of vascular vasodilator ß-receptors leaving α-receptor-mediated vasoconstriction unopposed; (3) block of central ß-adrenergic receptors; (4) block of renal ß-receptors thus inhibiting renin release. When propranolol is given to a hypertensive subject it first causes a fall in pulse rate and cardiac output accompanied by peripheral vasoconstriction with little or no change in blood pressure. The vasoconstriction is due to compensatory sympathetic reflexes and unopposed α-adrenergic activity on blood vessels. If the oral administration of propranolol is continued for several weeks the haemodynamic picture changes and blood pressure begins to fall progressively. At this stage the cardiac effects of propranolol persists but the initial vasoconstriction subsides so that the total effect is a diminished systemic blood pressure.

There is no generally accepted explanation of the haemodynamic readjustment and the blood pressure fall after propranolol in spite of the undoubted clinical antihypertensive effectiveness of this and other beta blockers. Several mechanisms have been postulated:

1. Some form of 'autoregulation' or 'resetting' of blood pressure bringing it gradually back to normal with continued administration of ß-blocker.
2. A possible central effect: propranolol has been shown to produce a fall of blood pressure in animals when injected into the fourth cerebral ventricle.
3. An effect through the renin-angiotensin system. Propranolol lowers the renin level of plasma and is clinically more effective in high-renin than in low-renin hypertension.

Clinical use. Propranolol has become one of the most extensively used drugs for the treatment of moderately severe hypertension, especially when combined with a diuretic. One of its advantages is that cardiovascular reflexes are maintained and hence it is not liable to cause orthostatic hypotension. It does not interfere with sympathetic α-adrenergic neurotransmission and does not cause diarrhoea or impairment of sexual function. Contrary to guanethidine, propranolol does not counteract the effects of tricyclic antidepressants.

Clinically the side-effects of propranolol are usually relatively minor ones such as fatigue, cold extremities, unpleasant central stimulant effects, vivid dreams and dizziness. A potential disadvantage in some patients is that propranolol inhibits sympathetic bronchodilation by blocking ß$_2$-receptors as well as the cardiac ß$_1$ receptors. It normally causes a slight increase in airways resistance but in predisposed patients it may bring about an attack of asthma. A fundamental disadvantage of propranolol, related to its antisympathetic activity in the heart, is that it may occasionally precipitate failure in a heart dependent on catecholamine stimulation. If propranolol is used alone it tends to cause sodium retention and oedema which may be prevented by the concurrent use of a diuretic.

Other ß-blockers. The chemical structures of various ß-adrenoceptor antagonists are compared with isoprenaline in Figure 9.5 which shows that compounds which interact with ß-receptors, either to stimulate or to block, have obvious structural similarities. The side chain which determines interaction with the receptor is identical or similar in the agonist, isoprenaline, and in the various antagonists. Whether the effect of a compound will be predominantly activation or blockade depends on the nature of the aromatic ring. For stimulating activity two hydroxyl groups in 3-, 4- position of the aromatic ring are optimal. Their replacement with chlorine atoms, as in dichlorisoprenaline, results in a marked reduction of stimulant activity and the emergence of receptor blocking properties. A fused aromatic ring and the insertion of an oxygen bridge between ring and side chain, as in propranolol, results in a powerful competitive antagonist.

A large number of newer ß-blockers have been introduced differing in potency, selectivity, stimulant activity and membrane stabilising action.

Potency. Beta blockers are competitive antagonists and their receptor affinities can be precisely measured. It is of some interest to establish pA$_2$ values for beta blockers, but in clinical practice this is relatively irrelevant since dosage is established by trial and error. Certain beta blockers are unselective in having similar affinities for ß-receptors in heart and smooth muscle. Amongst these unselective ß-blockers *pindolol* has somewhat greater receptor affinity than *oxprenolol* and *propranolol*.

Selectivity. An undesirable property of ß-blockers is that they may increase airways resistance in patients with

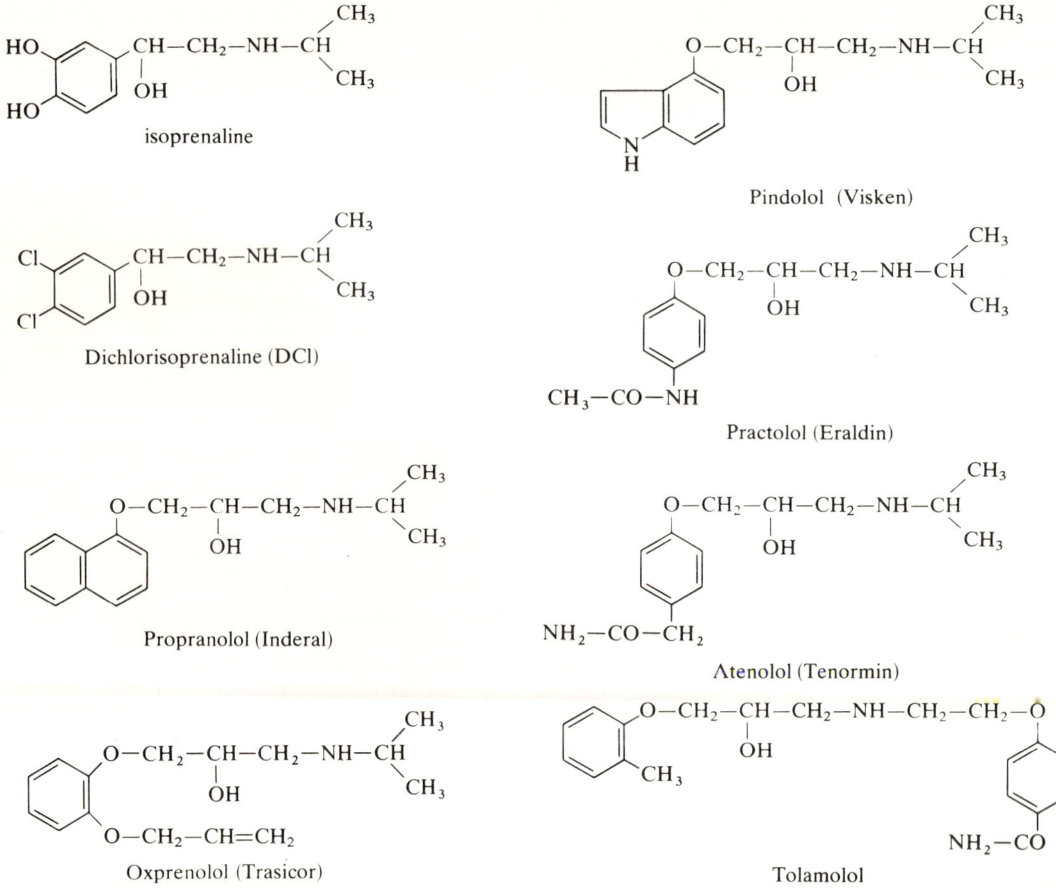

Fig. 9.5 Chemical structures of isoprenaline and beta-adrenoceptor blocking agents.

obstructive lung disease by blocking tonic sympathetic drive to ß-adrenoceptors dilating bronchial smooth muscle. The search for 'cardioselective' ß-blockers is based on the notion that ß-receptors might not be homogenous and that some drugs might be able to distinguish between subclasses of ß-receptors (ß₁ receptors in the heart and ß₂ receptors in smooth muscle).

The first compound described with greater blocking potency on ß₁ receptors than on ß₂ receptors was *practolol* (pA₂ atria: 6-7; pA₂ trachea: 4-5). In clinical use practolol did not produce brochoconstriction. Unfortunately it is apt to produce allergic reactions of the eyes and skin and in rare cases a sclerosing peritonitis which have greatly restricted its use. Other beta blockers for which there is evidence of cardioselectivity are: *atenolol, acebutolol, tolamolol* and *metoprol*.

Beta-adrenoceptor stimulant activity. Many beta blockers are partial agonists, i.e. they stimulate the ß-receptor in addition to preventing access of catecholamines to the receptor. *Propranolol* and *sotalol* lack this stimulant activity but *oxprenolol, pindolol* and *alprenolol* and *practolol* all have some agonist activity. The clinical relevance of partial agonist activity is not clear. Whilst marked sympathomimetic activity is undesirable, particularly in the treatment of angina pectoris, drugs with a moderate degree of sympathomimetic activity might be expected to lack the undesirable negative chronotropic and inotropic effects of propranolol.

Membrane stabilising activity. L-propranolol has a strong quinidine-like action but this is unlikely to be relevant to its ß-blocking activity since D-propranolol which lacks ß-blocking activity has a similar quinidine-like action. There is evidence that the antiarrhythmic activity of propranolol is due to its ß-blocking activity rather than to its membrane stabilising activity.

Labetalol blocks both α- and ß-receptors. The acute effects of labetalol in man resemble the result of giving a mixture of an α- and a ß-blocker in that it causes a rapid fall in blood pressure due to a fall in peripheral vascular resistance but no compensatory tachycardia or rise in cardiac output. Labetalol effectively lowers blood pressure in hypertension. After an oral dose the blood pressure falls in 2 to 4 hours unlike the effect of a ß-blocker alone which takes a day or more to develop. Intravenous labetalol causes an immediate fall in blood pressure in patients with severe hypertension which is dose-related.

Unlike propranolol, labetalol causes postural hypotension due to its α-blocking action. This is a common reason for patients to stop taking the drug. For this reason a pure ß-blocker is a preferable first choice for the long-term treatment of hypertension.

Interference with catecholamine metabolism
Methyldopa (Aldomet). Alpha-methyldopa inhibits the enzyme dopa-decarboxylase which catalyses an essential step in the formation of noradrenaline (Fig. 6.3) and of 5-hydroxytryptamine. Since methyldopa has been shown to deplete tissues of their noradrenaline content, its decarboxylase-inhibiting effect seemed to provide a satisfactory explanation of its hypotensive action. Further experiments, however, have thrown doubt on this explanation and it is now believed that the hypotensive action of methyldopa is due to the formation of alpha-methylnoradrenaline which displaces noradrenaline in adrenergic nerve endings. Animal experiments have confirmed this by showing that when the sympathetic nerves to the heart are stimulated after treatment of the animal with methyldopa, both noradrenaline and methylnoradrenaline are released.

When methyldopa is administered to a hypertensive subject it produces a progressive decrease in blood pressure and reduction in heart rate. The reduction in pressure is greater in the erect than in the supine position but the cardiovascular reflexes are reasonably well maintained.

Methyldopa is usually administered orally but it can be given intravenously in emergencies. The dose is 0.5 to 3.0 gm daily, generally combined with a diuretic. The blood pressure fall is almost as great in the lying as in the standing position and postural and exertional hypotension are much less of a problem than with adrenergic neurone blockers or pargyline. Retention of salt and water may occur but this can be prevented by the simultaneous administration of a thiazide diuretic. The main side effect of methyldopa is drowsiness which usually decreases after prolonged use but is rarely quite absent. Headaches, dizziness, weakness and nightmares may occur especially in the early stages of administration. Some patients develop diarrhoea or impotence.

Potentially serious complications are various manifestations of hypersensitivity including jaundice, pyrexia, rashes and rarely haemolytic anaemia. Liver function tests often show abnormalities during early treatment with methyldopa; fever may suggest hepatitis. After prolonged treatment with large doses a positive Coombs test may develop, often without evidence of haemolytic anaemia. Great caution must be exerted when manifestations of hypersensitivity occur.

Nevertheless the present consensus is that methyldopa is a very useful drug, especially for the treatment of nonmalignant hypertension. It has no adverse effects on the foetus and is frequently employed for the control of hypertension in pregnancy. Tolerance occurs but this is rarely progressive. The effects of methyldopa are antagonised by small doses of amphetamine-like drugs.

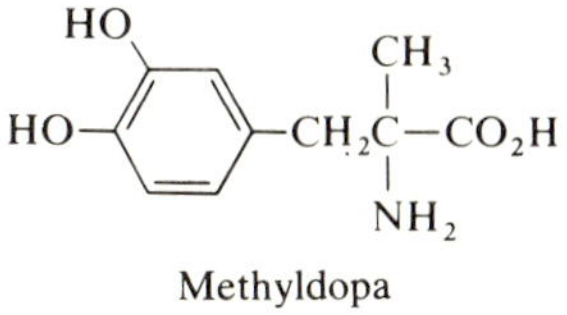

Methyldopa

Fig. 9.6 Methyldopa.

Central antihypertensive action
Indian workers (Bhargava and colleagues) have shown that when noradrenaline is injected into the cerebral ventricles of anaesthetised dogs it produces bradycardia and a fall of blood pressure, suggesting the existence of central sympathetic centres which regulate blood pressure. At present one of the important antihypertensive drugs, clonidine, is considered by most workers to act centrally.

Clonidine (Catapres) is an imidazoline derivative synthesised in 1962. Its chemical structure is shown in Figure 9.7.

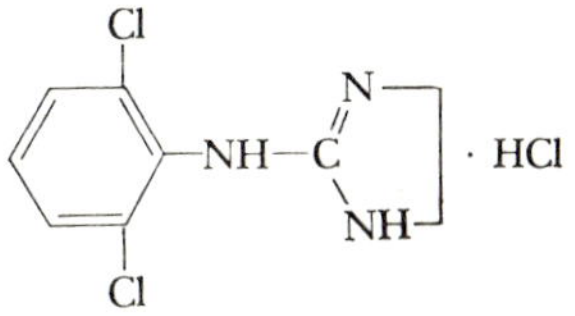

Fig. 9.7 Clonidine hydrochloride.

When injected into the cerebral ventricles or vertebral artery of a cat, clonidine produces a decrease of blood pressure and heart rate accompanied by a reduction in the electrical discharges in sympathetic nerves. It has been shown that part of its effects on the heart and blood vessels are due to a reduction of sympathetic impulses at the level of the central nervous system. Recent work suggests that clonidine also has peripheral action preventing stimulation of the heart by sympathetic nerves. The action is believed to be due to a presynaptic inhibitory effect of clonidine whereby release of the transmitter substance, noradrenaline, is reduced. The regulation of noradrenaline release by presynaptic receptor systems is discussed on page 82.

In man, oral or intramuscular clonidine produces a fall of blood pressure due to the combined effects of a reduced cardiac output and a decrease in peripheral resistance; it also causes marked bradycardia. Intravenous injection of clonidine produces an initial rise in blood pressure followed by a prolonged fall. Renal blood flow is maintained. If clonidine is administered alone it may cause a retention of sodium and chloride but if it is combined with a thiazide diuretic this is prevented, and the hypotensive effect of clonidine augmented. Clonidine does not cause appreciable orthostatic hypotension.

For the treatment of hypertension, clonidine is administered orally starting with doses of 0.2 to 0.3 mg per day, which are gradually increased until the blood pressure readings are satisfactory. It is usually administered in combination with an oral diuretic. In patients with hypertension, clonidine is approximately as effective in controlling blood pressure as methyldopa. In patients treated with clonidine the blood pressure on standing is only slightly lower than when lying and there is no fall of blood pressure after exercise as with adrenergic neurone blockers. In contrast to the latter, male patients on clonidine do not experience failure of ejaculation or impotence. Clonidine may cause constipation but its main side effects are sedation, which may be marked, and dryness of the mouth. Clonidine produces no long-term tolerance; it should not be withdrawn suddenly in hypertensive patients, as this may cause a rapid rise of blood pressure attended by an increase in the urinary output of catecholamines. The rebound blood pressure rise may be prevented by the α-blocking drug phentolamine.

Small doses of clonidine have been found of value in the prophylactic treatment of migraine (p. 129).

Adrenergic neurone-blocking drugs
The mode of action of adrenergic neurone-blocking drugs has already been discussed (p. 83). Briefly, these drugs act within the sympathetic nerve terminal to prevent the release of transmitter whilst in small doses they do not impair conduction of impulses along sympathetic nerves nor prevent the combination of transmitter with receptors. They can also release noradrenaline from stores in nerve endings and inhibit the capacity of re-uptake of noradrenaline by nerves. They inhibit the release by amphetamine and similar drugs of noradrenaline stored in nerve endings.

The adrenergic neurone blockers can be used in the treatment of moderate and severe hypertension. They are as effective as the ganglion blockers but lack the serious disadvantages of parasympathetic block produced by the latter. They are, however, not indicated as drugs of first choice in the elderly due to their tendency to produce postural and exertional hypotension.

Bretylium. Bretylium is a derivative of xylocholine, the first adrenergic neurone blocker to be discovered. It is a quaternary ammonium compound which lowers the blood pressure by selectively depressing adrenergic nerve function. It prevents transmitter release from sympathetic nerve endings but not from the adrenal medulla. At the same time it causes the responses to circulating catecholamines to be increased.

From the clinical point of view bretylium has proved disappointing as an antihypertensive. Its main drawback is a rapid development of tolerance, believed to be due to increasing hypersensitivity to the action of catecholamines. The use of bretylium for the control of arrhythmias is discussed on page 147.

Guanethidine. This derivative of guanidine (Fig. 9.8) is well, though incompletely absorbed from the gastrointestinal tract. It is a valuable antihypertensive drug with a prolonged action useful for the treatment of severe hypertension in patients who do not respond to other drugs.

When guanethidine is injected intravenously into an anaesthetised cat its first effects are sympathomimetic; it produces a rise of blood pressure, acceleration of the heart and retraction of the nictitating membrane. Somewhat later the signs of adrenergic neurone blockade become apparent: the blood pressure decreases, particularly if the animal is tilted, the nictitating membrane relaxes and it now fails to respond to stimulation of its adrenergic nerves. The initial sympathomimetic effect can be explained by a release of noradrenaline from adrenergic nerve endings; the subsequent block is due to a failure of the mechanism whereby post-ganglionic nerve impulses release adrenergic transmitter. This interference constitutes the basic action of guanethidine and occurs even in the absence of transmitter depletion.

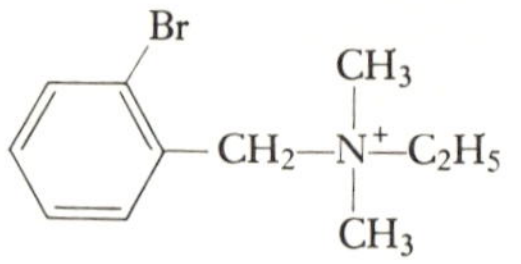

Bretylium

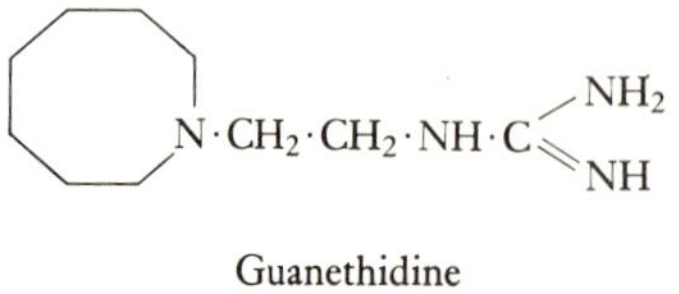

Guanethidine

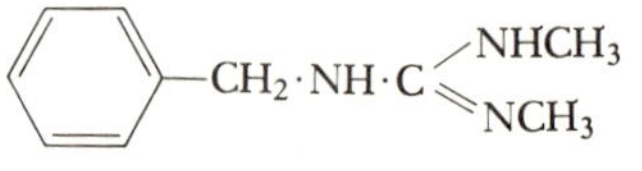

Bethanidine

Fig. 9.8 Adrenergic neurone-blocking drugs.

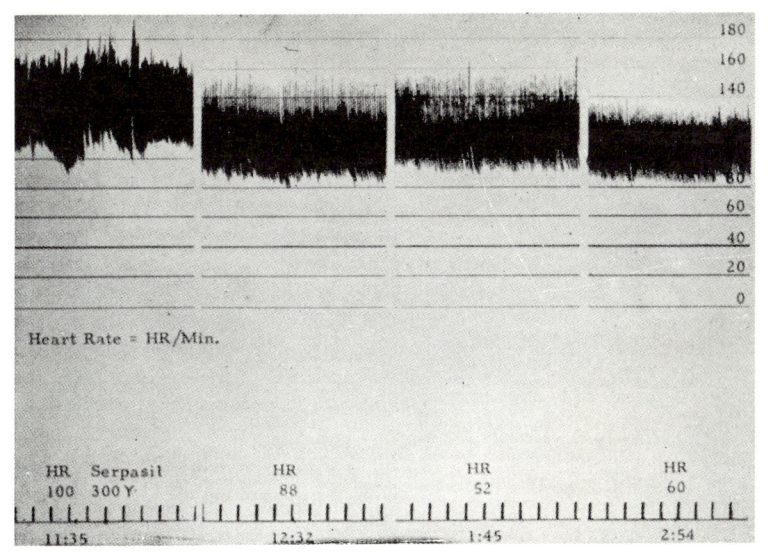

Fig. 9.9 Gradual fall in blood pressure after the intravenous injection of 0.3 mg per kg of reserpine in an unanaesthetised dog. (After Plummer et al, 1954, *Ann. N.Y. Acad. Sci.*)

When administered orally in man, guanethidine produces a progressive fall in systolic and diastolic blood pressure. Since there is a pronounced postural variation, the blood pressure of patients receiving guanethidine should be recorded both lying down and standing up. The excretion of guanethidine is very slow and a single dose may continue to exert an effect for several days. It therefore need only be administered once daily, usually in the morning. Even so, patients may experience postural hypotension on getting up next morning. This is probably because hypertensive patients experience a fall of blood volume during the night which enhances the effect of sympathetic blockade. The initial dose of guanethidine is 10 to 20 mg, which is increased by 10 mg daily until satisfactory blood pressure control is achieved.

The most common untoward effects are postural and exertional hypotension and diarrhoea. The former is treated by lying the patient flat, the latter by reducing the dose of guanethidine or combining it with a small dose of a ganglion blocker such as mecamylamine or pempidine. Some degree of bradycardia is usual with guanethidine. Sexual function is frequently affected and there may be muscular weakness or parotid pain. Transient neurological changes sometimes occur in arteriosclerotic subjects. The concurrent administration of an oral diuretic greatly enhances the effect of guanethidine and prevents salt and water retention.

After prolonged use, there is usually some tolerance to adrenergic neurone blocking drugs, but with guanethidine this is not important.

Bethanidine. This compound (Fig. 9.8) is a derivative of guanidine with a fundamentally similar action to guanethidine but its effect is more rapid and shorter and it does not produce diarrhoea. Bethanidine is administered orally in doses of 20 to 200 mg daily together with an oral diuretic. It is a clinically useful antihypertensive drug with a short duration of action and lacking central side effects.

Debrisoquine is another adrenergic neurone blocking drug resembling bethanidine in its short duration of action and relative absence of side effects such as diarrhoea.

Imipramine and other tricyclic antidepressants interfere with the antihypertensive action of adrenergic neurone blockers by inhibiting their active uptake into sympathetic nerve endings.

Other antihypertensive drugs
Reserpine. Reserpine is a hypotensive and tranquillising drug which is further discussed on page 256. It produces a depletion of catecholamines *in vivo* and *in vitro*, i.e. from intact sympathetic nerves and also from isolated suspensions of catecholamine containing nerve granules. It thus reduces the effects of adrenergic nerve stimulation. It also diminishes the effects of drugs such as ephedrine and tyramine which act by releasing noradrenaline from nerve endings. On the other hand reserpine potentiates the action of adrenaline and noradrenaline. Reserpine causes a depletion of 5-HT from the brain and other tissues.

When a dose of reserpine is administered intravenously to an unanaesthetised dog it produces a slowing of the heart rate and a gradual fall of blood pressure which reaches its maximum only after several hours (Fig. 9.9). A similar delayed fall in blood pressure is observed when this drug is given parenterally to a hypertensive patient. Central vasomotor reflexes such as the rise in blood pressure which occurs after occlusion of the carotid sinus are also inhibited.

Reserpine is absorbed from the gastro-intestinal tract and oral administration of this drug to hypertensive patients in doses of 0.5 to 1 mg daily results in a gradual fall in blood pressure after about ten days. Reserpine has a sedative effect and this sometimes may be desirable in anxious hypertensive patients, but it also produces drowsiness, nightmares and sometimes profound mental depression. Another side effect of reserpine is an increase in gastrointestinal tone and motility; it also frequently causes stuffiness of the nose.

Reserpine is now used mainly in cases of mild hypertension, usually orally and in combination with a thiazide diuretic.

Ganglion blocking drugs
The mode of action of the ganglion blocking drugs is discussed on page 63. These drugs were the first potent antihypertensive drugs introduced into clinical medicine, but they have now been largely superseded by other drugs which are as effective but have less disturbing side actions. A particular advantage of the ganglion blocking drugs is their rapid onset of action which makes them suitable for the control of hypertensive emergencies.

Hexamethonium. This quaternary ammonium compound is now mainly used by intravenous injection. It is given by slow infusion until the blood pressure begins to fall.

Mecamylamine and pempidine. These drugs are amines which are well absorbed from the alimentary tract and may produce satisfactory control of blood pressure but they are seldom now used clinically because of their undesirable side effects. By their parasympathetic blocking effects they may cause blurring of vision, retention of urine and constipation which may lead to paralytic ileus. Small doses of pempidine are sometimes used in conjunction with guanethidine when this produces uncontrollable diarrhoea.

Trimethaphan is a rapidly acting ganglionic blocking drug given intravenously (p. 121).

Pargyline
Pargyline is an inhibitor of monoamine oxidase, the enzyme which is responsible for the metabolism of catecholamines and 5-hydroxytryptamine in tissues and regulates the level of noradrenaline stored in sympathetic nerve endings.

The administration of pargyline and other amine oxidase inhibitors to hypertensive patients leads in the course of two or three weeks to a progressive fall of blood pressure which occurs particularly in the upright position.

Pargyline is used as an antihypertensive drug but has important disadvantages. It is liable to give rise to severe orthostatic hypotension. It also produces central nervous effects leading to euphoria or depression and it is incompatible with various drugs such as sympathomimetic amines, morphine and general anaesthetics, and also with certain types of food. Thus some cheeses contain tyramine which is dependent on momoamine oxidase for its inactivation. When monoamine oxidase is inhibited by pargyline the ingestion of this type of cheese may produce a severe hypertensive crisis (p. 44).

Reflex hypotension
Veratrum alkaloids. The action of the veratrum alkaloids on the circulation was investigated by Bezold and Hirt in 1867 and they suggested that the fall of blood pressure produced by these drugs was due to a vagal reflex initiated by the stimulation of sensory receptors in the heart. Later work has shown that these drugs stimulate sensory receptors in a number of areas including the coronary vessels, the lungs and the carotid body and in this way produce a reflex bradycardia and fall of blood pressure.

The veratrum alkaloids can be divided into two groups according to their pharmacological actions.

1. Tertiary amine esters such as protoveratrine A and B produce a fall of blood pressure by reflex stimulation of the sensory receptors mentioned above. In larger doses these drugs stimulate or sensitise all excitable tissue, for example, they cause repetitive firing of isolated nerve and skeletal muscle fibres.
2. Secondary amines such as veratramine slow the heart rate by a direct action on the sino-auricular node.

Alkavervir is a purified mixture of alkaloids from green hellebore (*Veratrum viride*). When this preparation is injected intramuscularly in hypertensive patients it produces a decrease in systolic and diastolic blood pressure and a fall in heart rate. The main drawback of the veratrum alkaloids is that in doses which produce a fall in blood pressure they usually cause unpleasant side effects, particularly salivation, nausea and vomiting. They are therefore seldom used alone in the control of hypertension but they are sometimes combined with other drugs.

Adrenergic alpha-receptor blocking drugs
These drugs (p. 82) block the receptors in blood vessels on which the adrenergic transmitter acts and they would therefore be expected to reduce the blood pressure. They do in fact lower the blood pressure, especially after an intravenous injection but for reasons not fully understood they have proved disappointing in the long term treatment of hypertension. Their main field of use is for the treatment of peripheral vascular disease, and to reduce the blood pressure in phaeochromocytoma (p. 83).

Although the classical α-blockers have not been clinically effective in the treatment of essential hypertension, it is possible that some of the recently introduced drugs may owe their activity to α-blockade. Two of the newer antihypertensives, *prazosin* and *indoramin* have strong α-blocking activity and the new antihypertensive *labetalol* has both ß- and α-blocking activity.

Dopamine receptor stimulation. Dopamine causes vasodilatation by stimulating specific dopamine receptors in the mesenteric and renal arterial bed. Attempts have been made to develop dopamine receptor stimulants with antihypertensive activity. A drawback is that dopamine receptor stimulants frequently have a central emetic action. This work is still in the experimental stage.

Drugs used in hypertensive emergencies
An acute marked rise of blood pressure is a medical emergency requiring rapid treatment to avoid severe cardiovascular complications. The vasodilator drugs diazoxide and sodium nitroprusside are most widely used in such cases.

Sodium nitroprusside (nipride) $Na_2Fe(CN)_5NO,2H_2O$ is a powerful vasodilator which relaxes both resistance and capacitance vessels. The heart rate is usually reflexly increased. It acts directly on blood vessels and the dramatic decrease in peripheral resistance lowers the blood pressure and thereby the afterload on the heart, causing myocardial function to improve.

Nitroprusside is given by slow intravenous infusion and acts within a few seconds. It is best administered in an intensive care unit. It is also used for controlled hypotension during general anaesthesia. Nitroprusside is converted in the body to cyanide which is metabolised in the liver to thiocyanate.

Diazoxide is chemically closely related to thiazides but it produces sodium retention rather than diuresis. It is, however, a potent hypotensive when injected intravenously. The peripheral vasodilator effect of diazoxide which is exerted largely on precapillary resistance vessels, supports indirectly the view that the thiazides also have a direct hypotensive effect. Diazoxide is used by intravenous injection in acute hypertensive emergencies, including eclamptic fits in pregnancy, when it produces an immediate fall of blood pressure which lasts for 4 to 12 hours.

Alternatively the blood pressure can be reduced within minutes by intravenous administration of a short-acting ganglion blocking drug such as *trimethaphan* (arfonad). *Hydrallazine* given intravenously may also reduce the blood pressure rapidly.

Combined drug administration in hypertension
The judicious use of antihypertensive drugs involves careful supervision and adjustment of dosage; it has been found that combinations of two or more drugs substantially diminish the undesirable side effects of the more potent drugs. Although various combined preparations are available it is generally advisable to prescribe individual drugs separately because this permits easy adjustment of dosage which is not possible when using tablets containing fixed proportions of the constituent drugs.

In the standard treatment of chronic hypertension, drug combinations are almost invariably used. The most usual combination is an oral diuretic plus one other drug, though in very mild hypertension a diuretic alone may be sufficient. An effective drug combination in moderately severe hypertension is the use of a thiazide diuretic with a beta blocker and perhaps a vasodilator. Beta blockers have now become almost standard therapy in hypertension. Vasodilators may be indicated since a high peripheral resistance is the major haemodynamic disturbance in essential hypertension. The vasodilatation produces a reflex increase in heart rate and cardiac output which can be prevented by beta blockade. Beta blockers also prevent increases in plasma renin activity. Diuretics, besides having an antihypertensive effect of their own, counteract sodium and water retention and the concomitant expansion of extracellular fluid and plasma volume.

Alternative forms of antihypertensive medication are the use of a diuretic together with methyldopa or with clonidine. Both these drugs may cause some degree of drowsiness. In severer forms of hypertension an adrenergic neurone blocker such as guanethidine or bethanidine may be indicated. Although the latter drugs tend to produce orthostatic hypotension and are therefore not ideally suited for elderly or arteriosclerotic patients they have the advantage of absence of drowsiness and lack of interference with mental alertness.

CORONARY VASODILATOR AND ANTIANGINAL DRUGS

Effect of oxygen lack on the heart

The central nervous system is injured by oxygen lack more rapidly than any other tissue but with this exception the heart is more susceptible to oxygen lack than any other important organ in the body. The oxygen supply of the heart depends upon the blood flow through the coronary arteries and this in turn depends on the pressure in the aorta and resistance in the coronary circuit. The maximum amount of blood flowing through the coronary arteries in experimental animals may rise to as much as 20 per cent of the total output of the left ventricle. The heart's activity from minute to minute depends on the efficiency of the coronary circulation because cardiac muscle cannot enter into oxygen debt. In this regard it differs entirely from voluntary muscle which can enter into extensive oxygen debt and thus can maintain activity for some time in the absence of any oxygen supply. For instance a sprinter can run the 100 yards without breathing. During this sprint a large amount of energy has been obtained by the conversion of glycogen into lactic acid. This is an anaerobic process which requires oxygen after the exercise, and recovery is effected by a comparatively slow process of oxygenation that takes from half an hour to an hour. The heart however has very little power of running into oxygen debt, for any accumulation of lactic acid immediately depresses its activity. Hence its activity is dependent from minute to minute upon an adequate supply of oxygen. For this reason any interference with the coronary circulation at once injures the heart.

This is a very important general principle that controls the performance of the heart, for as soon as a heart begins to fail a vicious circle is established because the feebler the heart beat the poorer is the coronary circulation and the worse the oxygen supply to the heart.

Coronary insufficiency can be defined as an imbalance between the available oxygen supply and the oxygen requirements of the myocardium. If the oxygen supply of the heart falls short of its requirements precordial pain (angina) results.

The coronary reserve of patients with angina differs from that of normal subjects. In these, exercise can increase the blood flow through the coronaries several-fold but in anginal patients the ability to increase blood flow in exercise is limited because of atherosclerotic changes in the blood vessels. Exercise will then tend to produce pain and a characteristic reduction of the S-T segment of the electrocardiogram due to anoxia of the heart muscle.

Effect of coronary dilators in angina

The beneficial effect of amyl nitrite in angina pectoris was discovered by Lauder Brunton in 1867 who describes his discovery as follows:

'Many years ago when I was a resident physician I had a case of angina pectoris under my care. I used to go all hours of the day and night and take tracings of the man's pulse. I found during an attack the pulse became very hard indeed and the oscillations became very small. It therefore occurred to me that if one were to dilate the coronaries the man's pain ought to subside. I knew that nitrite of amyl had the effect and tried it with the result that no sooner had the flushing of the face occurred and the vessels began to dilate than the pain disappeared.'

The effect of nitrites in relieving the pain of angina can be explained in two ways, either by increased oxygen supply to the heart muscle due to coronary vasodilatation or by decreased oxygen requirements of the heart.

There has been some controversy as to which is the most important factor. It can be shown that nitrites are effective coronary vasodilators not only in isolated preparations but also in normal human subjects when their coronary blood flow is measured by cardiac catherisation using a nitrous oxide or a thermistor method. In anginal patients, however, experiments have shown little or no increase in coronary blood flow with sublingual nitroglycerin. This suggests that the relief of pain might be a consequence of circulatory readjustments whereby the oxygen requirement of the heart is reduced. The oxygen consumption of the heart depends on two principal factors, ventricular 'preload' (dependent on ventricular end-diastolic fibre length) and ventricular 'afterload' (ventricular wall tension during systole). Nitroglycerin affects both parameters. It causes a reduction in ventricular preload by venous dilatation and peripheral pooling of blood. It also decreases afterload by peripheral vasodilatation. These changes are accompanied by an improvement in anginal pain.

The nitrites dilate blood vessels by a direct action on their smooth muscles. Other drugs, e.g. thyroxine primarily increase oxygen consumption and produce coronary vasodilatation as a secondary effect. The administration of thyroxine in man frequently gives rise to precordial pain. This is an example of a coronary vasodilator which cannot be used clinically since it increases the oxygen consumption of the heart more than its oxygen supply. Another example is adrenaline which is a coronary vasodilator but is useless in angina pectoris and may even precipitate attacks of precordial pain.

Actions of nitrites

Both nitrites and organic nitrates are employed as coronary vasodilators, but the group is collectively referred to as nitrites. The nitrites chiefly used in therapeutics are amyl nitrite and octyl nitrite, but sodium nitrite is also effective. The inorganic nitrates are inactive but organic nitrates such as glyceryl trinitrate (nitroglycerin) and penta-erythritol tetranitrate act like nitrites and are widely used.

The fundamental action of all these drugs is a direct relaxant effect on smooth muscle. Their most conspicuous effect is on blood vessels.

The nitrites produce vasodilatation most readily in the vessels of the skin, and their action is most marked in the blush area. The action of amyl nitrite on the blush area is very intense, and the drug may cause a rise in surface temperature of 3°C in this region. The nitrites cause a quickening of the pulse which may be preceded by a slowing of the pulse. The quickening is a reflex effect due to the fall in blood pressure, the slowing is due to stimulation of the vagal centre in the medulla.

The nitrites increase coronary blood flow. They also dilate the cranial vessels and may produce a brief but intense headache. Large doses of nitrites produce methaemoglobinaemia.

Amyl nitrite

This is a volatile and inflammable liquid with an ether-like smell which is available in small crushable glass capsules. The capsule is crushed in a handkerchief and the vapour is inhaled. Amyl nitrite acts quickly since it is rapidly absorbed into the blood stream; it is also rapidly excreted. A dose of 0.2 ml takes about two minutes to produce its maximum fall of blood pressure, and its action lasts about 10 minutes. Amyl nitrite is used when a very rapid action is required but its side effects are more unpleasant than those of other nitrites. Apart from its undesirable pungent smell it may also produce marked flushing, headache and an increase in intraocular pressure. Like all nitrites it may produce methemoglobinaemia on repeated use.

Octyl nitrite is a liquid which is less volatile than amyl nitrite and has a slightly more prolonged action.

Glyceryl trinitrate, nitrogylcerin
This is probably the most widely used drug in angina. It is an odourless liquid which explodes on concussion. It is compounded with mannitol in small tablets containing 0.5 mg nitroglycerin. The tablets when sucked are absorbed from the buccal mucous membrane; they act in a few minutes and their action lasts for about 20 minutes.

In the treatment of an anginal attack or when the patient feels that an attack is impending a tablet containing 0.5 mg nitroglycerin is placed under the tongue. It is important that the tablet should be placed under the tongue and not swallowed, because absorption from the buccal mucous membrane is rapid, whereas there is little or no absorption in the stomach, and hence, if the drug is swallowed, it does not act until after it has passed into the intestine.

Pentaerythritol tetranitrate is available as tablets which are swallowed. Their onset of action is slow and they produce a vasodilator effect which lasts for several hours. Because of the slow onset of action they are of no value in the treatment of acute attacks and their preventive use frequently proves disappointing.

Sorbide nitrate (isosorbide dinitrate) is another long-acting organic nitrate which has been used by sublingual application in conjunction with propranolol.

Perhexiline maleate is absorbed from the gastrointestinal tract. It is used in the prophylaxis of angina of effort.

Nifedipine is a new drug which is pharmacologically related to verapamil (p. 146) in antagonising the postexcitation influx of calcium ions into cardiac and vascular smooth muscle cells. It lacks the antiarrhythmic properties of verapamil but is a more powerful calcium ion antagonist which dilates coronary arteries and arterioles. It lowers the blood pressure and improves maximal exercise capacity and chest pain on exercise. Unwanted effects include flushing and dizziness.

Prenylamine is used prophylactically in angina of effort.

Tolerance
Frequent administration of nitrites leads to tolerance, for example, an industrial worker who is exposed to nitroglycerin may develop severe headaches which disappear after repeated exposure. The tolerance disappears if he ceases to be exposed to nitrite for a few days, and in order to avoid loss of tolerance he may carry the compound in his clothing whilst away from work.

Tolerance also develops during medical use of nitrites and limits their clinical use.

Other coronary vasodilators
In addition to the nitrites certain other drugs which dilate blood vessels by a direct action can be classes as coronary dilators.

Xanthine derivatives (p. 165)
Theophylline, caffeine and theobromine are derivatives of xanthine which relax smooth muscle and produce vasodilatation Theophylline and other xanthine derivatives are inhibitors of phosphodiesterase the enzyme which promotes the destruction of cyclic AMP. Its various pharmacological actions may thus be due to an increased level of intracellular cyclic AMP. Their action is complicated by the fact that they also have a central vasoconstrictor effect which counteracts the peripheral vasodilatation. The peripheral effect is strongest with theophylline and the central effect with caffeine.

Theophylline also has a relaxant effect on bronchial muscle, a stimulant effect on the heart and a diuretic action. Clinically this drug is usually employed in its water soluble form as theophylline ethylenediamine or aminophylline. Aminophylline dilates coronary vessels and has been used for the prevention of anginal attacks but its clinical efficacy in angina is not established.

Papaverine
Papaverine is one of the naturally occurring alkaloids of opium. It has no analgesic activity, but is a powerful relaxant of smooth muscle.

Intravenous injections of 30 to 100 mg papaverine hydrochloride are used in the treatment of pulmonary arterial embolism. The object of the treatment is to relieve arterial spasm, permit the passage of the embolus beyond a major arterial bifurcation and to open up a collateral circulation.

Papaverine has no value in angina.

Dipyridamole
This is a powerful coronary vasodilator injected intravenously, but has no convincing clinical value in angina.

Sodium nitroprusside (sodium nitroferricyanide) (p. 121)
This is converted in the body to cyanide which is metabolised in the liver to thiocyanate. It is toxic unless infused slowly and may be used as a short-lasting vasodilator of systemic or coronary vessels. Its powerful vasodilator action is sometimes made use of in ventricular infarction or severe angina pectoris.

Propranolol (p. 115)
Stimulation of the heart by either circulating adrenaline released from the adrenals or noradrenaline released from sympathetic nerve endings may give rise to wasteful oxygen consumption by the heart with consequent relative

hypoxia and anginal pain. Propranolol can indirectly lower the oxygen requirements of the heart by blocking the beta receptors on which these catecholamines act. There is evidence that the administration of propranolol significantly increases the exercise tolerance of patients with angina of effort.

The starting dose of propranolol in angina is 10 mg four times daily which may be increased as necessary up to 200 mg daily until the patient responds satisfactorily or undesirable side effects appear. Objective evidence of response is provided by a reduction of the resting heart rate to about 60 beats per minute. Side effects include occasionally nausea and dizziness but the most serious drawback is that propranolol may precipitate heart failure either by causing an incipient failure to become manifest or by making an established failure worse. This can sometimes be prevented by the concurrent administration of digitalis. Propranolol may cause excessive bradycardia which may be relieved by the intravenous administration of 1 mg atropine. Propranolol may also cause bronchoconstriction and precipitate an asthmatic attack by blocking beta receptors which dilate bronchial muscle.

When used for the prevention of anginal attacks propranolol is best administered before meals. Its beneficial effect can be increased by the concomitant administration of nitrites given after meals. The two drugs act synergistically since the nitrite, contrary to the beta blocker, causes coronary dilatation whilst the beta blocker prevents the increase in heart rate which usually follows the administration of nitrites.

Other ß-blockers
Certain newer ß-blockers used for the relief of angina differ from propranolol in certain aspects of their pharmacological action.

1. Cardioselectivity. A high affinity for ß-receptors in the heart relative to bronchial muscle (p. 116) is a potential advantage in patients with a history of asthma and bronchitis. Cardioselective ß-blockers include *practolol*, *atenolol* and *tolamolol*. The use of practolol has now been restricted because of a characteristic oculocutaneous hypersensitivity syndrome produced by this drug, but there is no evidence, so far, of a similar reaction with other ß-blockers.

2. Beta-adrenoceptor stimulant activity. Certain ß-adrenoceptor antagonists are partial agonists, i.e. they stimulate the receptor themselves in addition to preventing access of catecholamines to the receptor. They include *pindolol* whilst propranolol lacks stimulant activity. The stimulant property might be a clinical advantage in counteracting excessive bradycardia and hypotension but a possible clinical disadvantage in the treatment of angina pectoris.

VASOCONSTRICTOR DRUGS
Centrally acting vasoconstrictor drugs
The presence of a vasoconstrictor centre in the medulla is indicated by the following experiments. Firstly, if animals are decerebrated by transection through the mesencephalon the blood pressure and vascular reflexes remain normal, but after section through the lower part of the medulla, the blood pressure falls to a low level and the normal vascular reflexes are abolished. Secondly, stimulation of a well defined area on the floor of the 4th ventricle by means of unipolar electrodes or by the application of acetylcholine causes vasoconstriction, acceleration of the heart, liberation of adrenaline from the suprarenal glands and other typical sympathomimetic effects. Other centres regulating vasomotor tone are situated in the hypothalamus and in the spinal cord. Drugs may act on the vasomotor centre either directly or reflexly. Heymans has shown that the vasoconstriction produced by lobeline and nicotine is reflex and due to stimulation of the chemoreceptors of the carotid sinus.

Most drugs which stimulate the central nervous system stimulate the vasomotor centre in the medulla and thus cause a rise of blood pressure in the normal animal. The action of these drugs is best shown in decerebrate unanaesthetised animals since all anaesthetics lower the sensitivity of the vasomotor centre. *Picrotoxin, leptazol* and *nikethamide* are examples of drugs which produce a rise of blood pressure through stimulation of the vasomotor centre. In man a rise of blood pressure only occurs if convulsive doses are used or if the blood pressure is abnormally low to start with. If convulsions are produced by means of leptazol the systolic pressure may rise by as much as 100 mmHg. This, however, is partly due to mechanical factors since the blood pressure rises much less if the convulsions are prevented by a neuromuscular blocking drug. In failure of the peripheral circulation nikethamide and other central stimulants produce a transient rise of blood pressure; they are used for this reason in acute circulatory collapse.

Carbon dioxide stimulates the vasomotor centre but dilates blood vessels by a peripheral action. When inhaled in a concentration of 5 per cent the central effect predominates and a rise of blood pressure occurs. The blood flow in a normal hand is reduced during inhalation of CO_2 but in a sympathectomised hand it is increased. The cerebral blood flow is increased up to 75 per cent by the inhalation of 5 to 7 per cent CO_2.

Peripheral vasoconstrictors
Sympathomimetic drugs
A number of compounds containing the basic skeleton of phenylethylamine and phenylisopropylamine have actions which resemble those of sympathetic nerve stimulation. These substances have been called by Barger and Dale sympathomimetic amines.

Table 9.1 Structure and actions of sympathomimetic amines

	4	3				Vasoconstrictor (α)	Bronchodilation (β)	CNS excitation
Phenylethylamine	H	H	H	H	H	(+)		
Dopamine	OH	OH	H	H	H	(+)		
Noradrenaline	OH	OH	OH	H	H	+		
Adrenaline	OH	OH	OH	H	CH$_3$	+	+	(+)
Isoprenaline	OH	OH	OH	H	CH(CH$_3$)$_2$		+	
Phenylephrine	H	OH	OH	H	CH$_3$	+		
Metaraminol	H	OH	OH	CH$_3$	H	+		
Amphetamine	H	H	H	CH$_3$	H	+		+
Methamphetamine	H	H	H	CH$_3$	CH$_3$	+		+
Mephentermine	H	H	H	CH(CH$_3$)$_2$	CH$_3$	+		
Ephedrine	H	H	OH	CH$_3$	CH$_3$	+	+	+
Methoxamine	OCH$_3$*	OCH$_3$§	OH	CH$_3$	H	+		
Salbutamol	OH	CH$_2$OH	OH	H	C(CH$_3$)$_3$		+	

* 2—position in ring
§ 5—position in ring

It is known that at least three sympathomimetic amines occur in the body and in addition some 200 have been synthesised. They differ from each other in regard to activity and duration of action, affinity for alpha or beta receptors, and stimulant effects on the central nervous system. Stability is conferred by (1) the absence of OH groups in the ring which prevents autoxidation by molecular oxygen and destruction by catechol-O-methyltransferase and (2) the presence of an extra methyl group in the side chain, as in ephedrine, which protects against the action of amine oxidase. The chemical structure of some of the sympathomimetic amines is shown in Table 9.1.

Dopamine is the immediate precursor of noradrenaline (Fig. 6.3). It acts on both alpha and beta adrenergic receptors and there is evidence that it also acts on a specific dopamine receptor. Evidence for the existence of specific vascular dopamine receptors is based on the antagonism of dopamine action by the specific dopamine antagonists haloperidol or pimozide. In man, dopamine decreases peripheral resistance by producing vasodilatation in renal and mesenteric arteries through an action on dopamine receptors. Dopamine also has an inotropic effect on the heart through dopamine receptor stimulation.

Specific dopamine receptors in the CNS are discussed in Chapter 17. Injected dopamine does not penetrate the CNS but it may produce vomiting by acting on medullary centres lying outside the blood-brain barrier.

Adrenaline. In clinical practice adrenaline is used more for its local effects on blood vessels than for its general action on the circulation. It is a powerful local haemostatic. For example, a plug of cotton wool soaked in adrenaline solution is an effective method of arresting epistaxis. Adrenaline is also used with local anaesthetics to produce local vasoconstriction. In such cases a solution of 1 in 100 000 or even less is sufficient to produce the desired effect. The total amount of adrenaline used with local anaesthetics should not exceed 1 mg and even this dose may be unsafe especially in hyperthyroid patients.

Subcutaneous injection of adrenaline produces a beneficial effect in anaphylactic shock and related conditions. It is also of value in the relief of urticaria occurring as an allergic reaction in a sensitive patient.

The accidental intravenous injection of an antigen in an allergic patient sometimes produces acute generalised oedema with swelling of the mucous membranes of the respiratory tract; in these circumstances an immediate intramuscular injection of a large dose of adrenaline solution (1 to 2 ml of 1 in 1000) may be life saving.

Adrenaline is of no value in combating traumatic shock. In this condition the arterioles are reflexly constricted as a compensatory mechanism and the heart is accelerated. Further stimulation of the heart is undesirable and further vasoconstriction might increase capillary stasis and plasma loss.

Noradrenaline. Slow intravenous infusions of noradrenaline are used in spinal anaesthesia and during operations for sympathectomy or phaeochromocytoma in which the supply of endogenous noradrenaline is suddenly reduced. However, there is the danger that when the noradrenaline infusion is stopped the blood pressure may fall precipitously. Another danger of noradrenaline infusion is that local tissue necrosis may result from extravasation of the solution.

Phenylephrine. This drug differs from adrenaline in lacking a hydroxyl group in the 4 position on the ring. It is entirely vasoconstrictor with strong alpha receptor stimulant activity and little effect on beta receptors. It has no effect on the central nervous system.

Phenylephrine may be used to restore the blood pressure in general anaesthesia and has the advantage of not inducing cardiac irregularities. It raises the blood pressure by peripheral vasoconstriction and this may bring about a reflex bradycardia which can be made use of in the treatment of sinus tachycardia.

Phenylephrine is widely used as local vasoconstrictor and decongestant of mucous membranes of the nose and larynx. It is also used as a vasoconstrictor in conjunction with local anaesthetics. When applied to the conjunctiva it causes dilatation of the pupil without cycloplegia.

Metaraminol (Aramine). Like phenylephrine, metaraminol is a 3-hydroxyphenyl derivative. It has a prolonged vasoconstrictor action and is used mainly for the treatment of hypotension; it increases both systolic and diastolic arterial pressure. Metaraminol has some stimulant effect on the heart but this is normally overshadowed by reflex bradycardia due to the pressure rise.

Metaraminol may be given by intravenous infusion or intramuscular injection. When doses of 2 to 10 mg are injected intramuscularly, the pressor effect reaches a peak in about half an hour and lasts for about one hour. The injection may be repeated.

Amphetamine. Amphetamine differs from the sympathomimetic amines so far discussed in lacking OH groups on the benzene ring. Its important central effects are discussed on page 262. The vasoconstrictor effect of amphetamine is partly due to a release of noradrenaline from storage sites in sympathetic nerve endings. This also applies to ephedrine. In a spinal cat the effects of both drugs are abolished by pretreatment with reserpine which depletes noradrenaline, but are restored after an infusion of noradrenaline.

Amphetamine can be administered orally. If a sufficient dose is administered in man it may cause a rise of blood pressure which lasts several hours. When administered locally by a spray to mucous membranes, it causes vasoconstriction and decongestion. Amphetamine may produce urine retention by contracting the sphincter of the bladder.

Methamphetamine has powerful central effects (p. 126) and is one of the amphetamine preparations most commonly abused in Britain. It has pressor effects which are due largely to an increase in cardiac output. It has been used to raise the blood pressure in spinal anaesthesia and in hypotension due to ganglionic block.

Mephentermine is a long acting vasoconstrictor which increases blood pressure in man largely by increasing the cardiac output.

Ephedrine. Ephedrine is the oldest known sympathomimetic drug. It occurs naturally in the shrub *Ephedra sinica* and was used in Chinese medicine for thousands of years under the name Ma-huang. Ephedrine produces its effects largely indirectly by releasing noradrenaline and this is probably the explanation of its rapid reduction of effect (tachyphylaxis) when it is administered repeatedly in rapid succession.

Ephedrine produces both the alpha and beta effects of catecholamines but differs from them in (a) its efficacy after oral administration, (b) its weaker but much longer duration of action due to resistance to amine oxidase and O-methyltransferase, (c) its central stimulant activity. In man ephedrine produces peripheral vasoconstriction and raises the blood pressure. Its most important therapeutic application is for the prevention of asthmatic attacks as discussed on page 180.

Methoxamine (Vasoxine). This sympathomimetic drug acts only on alpha receptors and produces no stimulation of the heart. It has no central effects. It has a relatively prolonged action producing a rise in both systolic and diastolic blood pressure and a reflex bradycardia. It can be used to counteract a fall of blood pressure in general anaesthesia.

Salbutamol is a bronchodilator which is discussed on page 179.

Vasoconstrictor drugs for local application

Sympathomimetic drugs are often inhaled or applied locally to produce shrinkage of mucous membranes of the nose and larynx. For this purpose a rapid and prolonged action is desirable with few after-effects such as irritation and vasodilatation, and preferably absence of cortical stimulation. Unfortunately these drugs lose their vasoconstrictor effect if used over long periods and produce an increasing amount of after-congestion. Their prolonged use is often associated with a vasomotor rhinitis which ceases when medication is stopped.

Propylhexedrine (Benzedrex) is a volatile sympathomimetic base which when inhaled produces vasoconstriction of the nasal mucous membranes. It has relatively little central stimulant effect and for this reason has largely replaced amphetamine inhalers (benzedrine) which were used by addicts as a source of the drug.

Naphazoline (Privine) and Xylometazole (Otrivine) These synthetic compounds are derivatives of imidazoline and some of their actions resemble those of adrenaline. In animals they produce vasoconstriction, a rise of blood pressure, dilatation of the pupil, retraction of the nictitating membrane and relaxation of the intestine. They are used in concentrations of 0.05 to 0.1 per cent to produce local vasoconstriction of the nasal mucosa. When used frequently naphazoline, because of its more prolonged action, may produce considerable after-congestion.

The use of vasoconstrictor drugs in conjunction with local anaesthetisc is discussed on page 313.

Angiotensin amide (Hypertensin)

Angiotensins are polypeptides which are formed by the action of the enzyme renin on angiotensinogen, an α_2-globulin present in plasma. Angiotensin I is a pharmacologically weakly active decapeptide which is degraded by *converting enzyme* to the active octapeptide angiotensin II. The amino acid composition of angiotensins varies slightly in different species; the composition of angiotensin II of horse and probably also man is shown in Figure 9.10.

H-Asp-Arg-Val-Tyr-Ileu-His-Pro-Phe-OH

Fig. 9.10 The composition of angiotensin II (horse).

Angiotensin amide is a synthetic derivative containing 5-valyl angiotensin II and is the form used clinically. Its actions are closely similar to natural angiotensin II. A number of synthetic analogues of angiotensin II have been prepared some of which have the same order of activity as the naturally occurring product. Potent antagonists of angiotensin II which probably act by competitive antagonism have recently been synthesised. Thus, the compound in which the phenylalanine (Phe) moiety of the molecule is changed to isoleucine (Ileu) is a powerful antagonist of the blood pressure effects of angiotensin II.

Besides its effect on blood pressure, angiotensin II has a number of interesting pharmacological and physiological actions. Thus it contracts the smooth muscle of the isolated uterus and guinea pig ileum. It also causes a release of aldosterone and produces a release of catecholamines from the adrenal medulla.

Effects on blood vessels. Angiotensin amide constricts blood vessels, especially the precapillary arterioles and acts particularly on the blood vessels of the skin and splanchnic areas. The blood flow in these regions is therefore reduced but it is relatively well maintained in skeletal muscle and coronary vessels. Angiotensin is a powerful pressor drug which is about forty times as active as noradrenaline. It does not seem to have any direct effect on the heart.

The pressor effect of angiotensin during prolonged infusion is better sustained than that of noradrenaline and, unlike the latter, extravasation of the solution does not produce local tissue necrosis. Since angiotensin produces constriction of the renal and hepatic circulation, prolonged infusions may be harmful.

In the treatment of severe hypotension, angiotensin amide is administered as an intravenous infusion in concentrations of 1 mg/litre in 0.9 per cent sodium chloride, at a rate of 1 to 10 μg per minute.

Teprotide is a synthetic nonapeptide which inhibits the enzyme responsible for converting angiotensin I to the active angiotensin II. It can temporarily reduce the blood pressure in patients with hypertension.

Vasopressin

The pressor hormone of the posterior pituitary (p. 329), when injected into anaesthetised animals produces a rise of blood pressure which lasts for about thirty minutes and is due to splanchnic vasoconstriction. In the unanaesthetised animal the rise is often preceded by a fall in blood pressure which is due to a transient failure of the heart caused by coronary vasoconstriction. Vasopressin acts on the arterioles, capillaries and venules. When injected subcutaneously in man it produces intense pallor, especially of the face, which is due to contraction of the capillaries and subpapillary venous plexuses of the skin. It also causes a slight rise in blood pressure and a decrease in pulse pressure.

Ergotamine

This is one of the alkaloids of ergot; it is a peptide alkaloid derived from lysergic acid (Fig. 15.5) and its structure is shown in Figure 9.11. Like other ergot alkaloids ergotamine has a variety of pharmacological actions including α-adrenergic stimulant and blocking activity, stimulation of the uterus and vasoconstriction. Its almost specific activity in the treatment of migraine is believed to be due to its vasoconstrictor action.

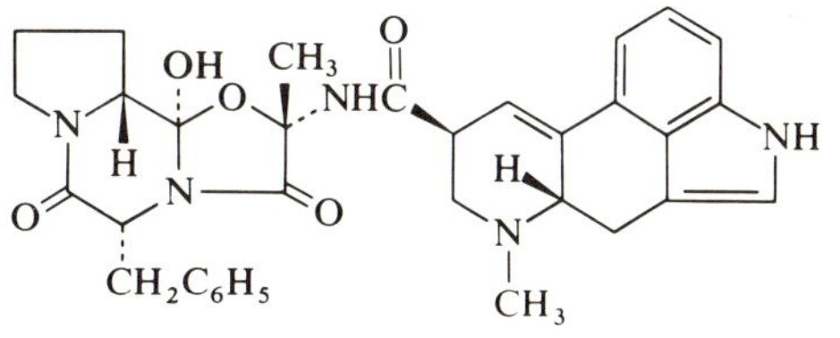

Fig. 9.11 Ergotamine.

Migraine. Migraine headaches are intermittent with intervals of freedom from headache between attacks. A typical attack is characterised by a preliminary aura probably due to constriction of intracranial vessels followed by an intense, generally hemicranial headache due to dilatation and oedema of extracranial vessels in the external carotid bed. The action of ergotamine in patients with migraine was studied by Graham and Wolff who showed that this drug reduced the pulsations of the temporal artery in man and that the intensity of headache would diminish in proportion to the decrease in pulsations (Fig. 9.12) and attributed the beneficial effects to vasoconstriction.

The vasoconstrictor effect of ergotamine is due to interaction with two types of receptor 1. α-adrenergic receptors on which ergotamine acts as a partial agonist of low efficacy and high affinity 2. stimulation of 5-HT receptors which are highly sensitive to ergotamine. Experimental evidence of the likely involvement of 5HT in migraine was provided by the demonstration that migraine attacks begin with a sudden fall in serum 5-HT levels.

128   APPLIED PHARMACOLOGY

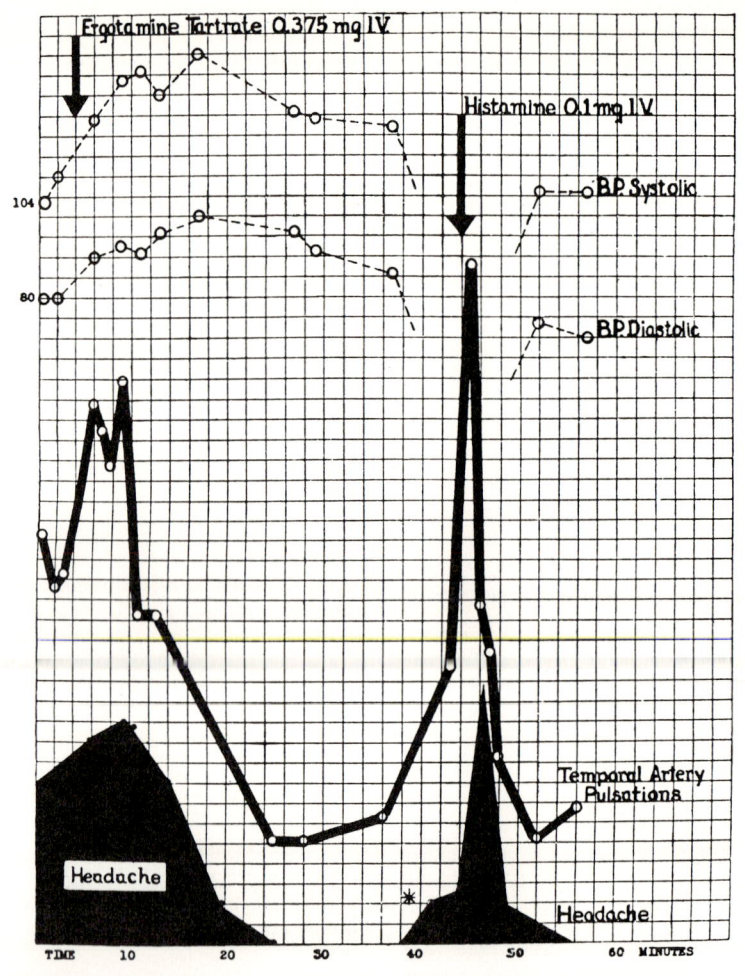

Fig. 9.12 The effect of ergotamine and of histamine on the amplitude of pulsations of the temporal artery of a patient with migraine. The figure shows that there is a close relation between the intensity of the headache and the photographically recorded amplitude of pulsations. Ergotamine decreased the intensity of headache and the amplitude of pulsations whilst histamine produced the opposite effect. (After Graham and Wolff, *Arch. Neurol. and Psychiat*, 1938.)

Ergotamine tartrate relieves attacks of migraine in most people. The earlier the drug is given during the attack the better the results, and patients usually continue to respond to the drug, however frequently it is used. Other types of headache are not relieved, on the contrary, ergotamine produces headache and vertigo in some patients and sometimes nausea and vomiting. Ergotamine may be administered by subcutaneous injection or orally. The subcutaneous dose is 0.25 to 0.75 mg; when given by mouth it is often combined with caffeine in tablets containing 1 mg ergotamine tartrate and 100 mg caffeine. Three of these tablets may be taken at the beginning of the attack and if necessary one every half hour; the total dose should not exceed six tablets. The beneficial effect of caffeine in migraine may be due to a reduction of cerebral blood flow. Overdoses of ergotamine may cause severe limb ischaemia.

Drugs in migraine prophylaxis
Migraine is a severely disabling condition, for which a reliable prophylactic agent would be of great value. The antipyretic analgesics such as aspirin and paracetamol are relatively ineffective in this condition. In addition to ergotamine which is effective in the migraine attack, two other drugs have been claimed to be effective in the prophylaxis of migraine.

Methysergide (deseril) is a lysergic acid derivative closely related to LSD (p. 265). It has strong anti-5HT activity. It has been found effective in the prophylactic treatment of migraine and other types of vascular headache, reducing the frequency and intensity of attacks. It is of no value in treating an acute attack of migraine.

Side effects are usually mild and transient, consisting of gastrointestinal and central symptoms, but severe side effects in some cases have necessitated limitation of the use of the drug. The most serious complication is the occurrence of retroperitoneal fibrosis which may lead to obstruction of the urinary tract. The drug is used under careful supervision in the management of patients with intractable migraine in which it is sometimes highly successful.

Clonidine (catapres; dixarit) is an antihypertensive discussed on page 117. When given prophylactically in small doses (0.025 to 0.5 mg twice daily) it has been found to lessen the frequency and severity of migraine headaches. It is effective when given to women for a few days before menstruation. It may cause dryness of the mouth and drowsiness.

CIRCULATORY COLLAPSE (SHOCK)

Shock is a life-threatening circulatory condition in which there is a serious reduction of cardiac output with inadequate perfusion of vital organs. Impaired renal function is shown by oliguria or anuria, impaired cerebral function by confusion or coma, impaired hepatic function by progressive metabolic acidosis due to the accumulation of lactic acid.

Shock can occur either because the function of the heart itself is impaired (cardiogenic shock) or because the cardiac return is reduced (hypovolaemic shock or peripheral circulatory failure). The first condition may occur for example in myocardial infarction, the second may be the result of blood loss, plasma loss as in extensive burns or after accidents, or loss of extracellular fluids as in severe gastrointestinal infections. Shock may also occur as a consequence of poisoning.

The two types of circulatory failure can be distinguished by measuring the central venous pressure. When cardiac function is impaired the central venous pressure is always raised whilst with inadequate venous return it is not normally raised and frequently reduced.

Treatment of shock

The initial treatment of hypovolaemic shock consists of laying the patient flat to increase arterial perfusion of the brain. Arterial oxygen saturation may be improved by oxygen therapy.

Transfusion
This is the most important step in the treatment of shock when the central venous pressure is low. Plasma or plasma substitutes are given initially, followed by blood transfusion and administration of electrolyte solutions. Patients in shock often have acidosis which may be corrected by administration of sodium bicarbonate.

Drugs
Drugs have an auxiliary function in the treatment of shock. The drugs mainly employed are:

1. Morphine and other opioid analgesics. They are required in traumatic shock; otherwise only in the presence of pain. They are best given intravenously to avoid absorption delay and in small doses to obviate further circulatory depression.
2. Circulatory drugs. Extreme constriction of peripheral vessels is harmful in shock and for that reason noradrenaline infusion is now seldom used, but a milder long lasting vasoconstrictor such as metaraminol is occasionally indicated. A different approach, advocated for patients in severe shock, is to give an α-adrenergic blocking agent such as phenoxybenzamine to counteract harmful adrenergically mediated peripheral vasoconstriction.
3. Inotropic agents to improve contractility of the heart. Central venous pressure may rise during transfusion indicating impaired cardiac function. In such cases a catcholamine may be given of which isoprenaline is the most useful since it increases cardiac contractility by virtue of its ß-stimulant action without increasing peripheral resistance. Another useful short-term cardiac inotropic agent is glucagon.

Dextrans are polysaccharides of variable molecular weight consisting of predominantly straight chain polymers of glucose in which the linkages between the glucose units are almost entirely of the α-1,6 type. They are produced by bacterial fermentation of sucrose. Dextrans of low molecular weight (50 000 or less) are rapidly excreted in the urine whilst those of higher molecular weight remain in the circulation and are slowly metabolised after storage in reticulo-endothelial tissue.

Dextran 40 injection is used primarily for assisting capillary blood flow and preventing intravascular aggregation of blood cells, whilst Dextran 70, 110 or 150 injections are used mainly to maintain or restore the blood volume. Transfusion of a 6 per cent dextran solution in 5 per cent dextrose should be regarded as an emergency measure and repeated administration should be avoided because dextrans have antigenic properties.

Polyvinlypyrrolidone (PVP) is a synthetic polymer which has been used as a plasma substitute. When administered intravenously it may cause an increase in sedimentation rate and rouleaux formation and toxic effects in infants.

Other colloids which have been used as plasma substitutes are gelatin, pectin, methyl cellulose and modified human globin.

PREPARATIONS

Antihypertensives

Beta-adrenergic blocking agents
Acebutolol (Sectral) s ß$_1$ angina 200 mg twice daily
Atenolol (Tenormin) s ß$_1$ angina 200 mg twice daily
Labetalol (Trandate) α hypert 300–600 mg daily
Metoprol (Lopressor) ß$_1$ hypert 200–400 mg daily, angina 100–200 mg daily
Nadolol 60–160 mg daily
Oxprenolol (Trasicor) s hypert 160 mg daily init., angina 120–240 mg daily
Pindolol (Visken) s hypert 15–45 mg daily, angina 7.5–15 mg daily
Practolol (Eraldin) ß$_1$ s angina 200–600 mg daily. Serious skin, eye reactions
Propranolol (Inderal) hypert, angina 10–40 mg 3 or 4 times daily
Sotalol (Betacardone) hypert, angina 240–600 mg daily
Timolol (Blocadren) 15–45 mg daily
key   s = intrinsic sympathomimetic activity
        ß$_1$ = some degree of cardioselectivity
        α = α and ß blocking activity

Ganglion blockers
Mecamylamine Hyd (Inversine) 2.5–25 mg daily
Trimetaphan Camsylate (Arfonad) 0.05–1 g over 2 h by slow i.v. infusion

Adrenergic neurone blockers
Bethanidine Sulph (Esbatal) 10 mg thrice daily init
Debrisoquine Sulph (Declinax) 10 mg twice daily init
Guanethidine Monosulph (Ismelin) 10–20 mg daily init
Guanoclor Sulph (Vatensol) 10 mg daily init
Guanoxan Sulph (Envacar) 10–20 mg daily init

Central vasodilators
Clonidine Hyd (Catapres) 0.15–0.3 mg daily init
Deserpidine (Harmonyl) 0.25 mg daily init
Hydrallazine Hyd 50 mg daily init
Reserpine (Serpasil) 0.1–0.5 mg daily

Catecholamine metabolism interference
Methyldopa Hyd (Aldomet) 0.5–3 g daily
Pargyline Hyd (Eutonyl) 10–25 mg daily init

Reflex antihypertensive
Alkavervir (Veriloid) 9–15 mg daily

Miscellaneous antihypertensives
Diazoxide inj (Eudemine) 300 mg i.v.
Prazosin Hyd (Hypovase) 2 mg thrice daily init
Sodium Nitroprusside Injection (Nipride) 0.5–8 μg/kg/min

Coronary vasodilators and antianginal drugs
Aminophylline Injection 250–500 mg slow i.v.
Amyl Nitrite Vitrellae (crushable glass capsules) 0.2 ml
Dipyridamole (Persantin) 50 mg 3 × daily
Glyceryl Trinitrate Tablets 0.5–1 mg
Nifedipine (Adalat) 10 mg 3 × daily
Octyl Nitrite Vitrellae
Pentaerythritol Tetranitrate 10–30 mg
Perhexiline Maleate 100 mg 2 × daily
Prenylamine Lactate 60 mg 3 × daily
Sorbide Nitrate 5–20 mg subling 2–3 × daily
Verapamil see Ch. 10
Beta blockers see above

Systemic vasoconstrictors
Adrenaline Injection 0.1% s.c. 0.2–0.5 ml
Angiotensin Amide (Hypertensin) 5–20 μg i.v. infus
Desmopressin 1–4 μg i.v. or i.m.
Ephedrine Hyd 15–60 mg
Metaraminol Tartrate (Aramine) 2–10 mg i.m. or s.c.
Methoxamine Hyd (Vasoxine) 5–20 mg i.m. 5–10 mg i.v.
Noradrenaline Injection (Levophed) 4–20 μg/min
Oxedrine Tartrate (Sympatol) 50–100 mg s.c., i.m., i.v.
Vasopressin Injection 0.1–1 ml (2–20 U) s.c., i.m.

Local vasoconstrictors
Adrenaline Solution 0.1 per cent
Naphazoline Nitrate (Privine) 0.05–0.1 per cent
Oxymetazoline Hyd (Otrivine) 0.05 per cent
Phenylephrine Hyd (Narex) 5 mg s.c. or i.m. 0.5 mg i.v.
Propylhexedrine (Benzedrex) 250 mg per inhaler

Antimigraine drugs
Clonidine Hyd (Dixarit) 50–75 mg morning and evening
Dihydroergotamine Mesylate Injection 1–2 mg i.m., s.c.
Ergotamine Tartrate (Femergin) Injection 0.25–0.5 mg
Pizotifen Malate 0'5 mg 3 × daily for migraine prophylaxis
Methysergide (Deseril) migraine prophylaxis; danger retroperitoneal fibrosis

Plasma substitutes
Dextran 40 Inj av mol wt 40 000
Dextran 70 Inj av mol wt 70 000
Dextran 110 Inj av mol wt 110 000
Gelatin (Gelofusine) av mol wt 30 000

FURTHER READING

Barcroft H, Swan H J C 1952 Sympathetic control of human blood vessels. Arnold, London
Davies S D, Reid J H (ed) 1975 Central action of drugs in blood pressure regulation. Pitman Medical, London
Genest C C, Koiw E, Kuchel O (ed) 1977 Hypertension. McGraw Hill, New York
Gross F (ed) 1966 Antihypertensive therapy. Springer, Berlin
Gross F (ed) 1979 Antihypertensive agents. Handb. exp. Pharm. 39
McMahon G F 1978 Management of essential hypertension. Futura Publishing, New York
Onesti G, Kim K E, Moyer J H (ed) 1973 Hypertension, mechanism and management. Grune Stratton, New York
Page I H, Bumpus F M (ed) 1974 Angiotensin. Handb. exp. Pharm. 31
Peart W S 1965 The renin angiotensin system. Pharm. Rev 71: 143
Winbury M M 1964 Experimental approaches to the development of antianginal drugs. Adv. Pharmac. 3: 1

10. The heart

Cardiac action potential 131; Calcium current 132; Cardiac output 133; Disordered rhythms 134; Cardiac glycosides 135 Effects on contractility and output 136; Actions on vagus and conduction 137; Mode of action of cardiac glycosides 140; Digitalis receptor 140; Radioimmunoassay 141; Pharmacokinetics of digoxin and digitoxin 141; Digitalis in congestive heart failure 143; Clinical uses 143; Toxic actions 143; Antiarrhymthmic agents 144; Quinidine 144; Procainamide 145; Lignocaine 145; Phenytoin 146; Verapamil 146; Beta blockers 147; Cardioversion 147; Clinical uses of antiarrhythmics 147; Aminophylline 149; Isoprenaline 149.

The heart is the most important muscle in the body and possesses certain remarkable characteristics. In the first place it has a unique capacity for continuous exertion, since it functions throughout life without ever resting. The heart of a man of seventy years has made more than 2500 million contractions without ever having had repose for a full second.

The efficiency of the heart as a pump is a matter of the greatest importance, both in health and in disease. In health it is the chief factor limiting the capacity for any muscular exertion that lasts more than a few seconds, whilst in many diseases the fate of the patient is largely determined by the condition of the heart. Another outstanding characteristic of the healthy heart is that it has great powers of reserve, for its performance during bodily rest represents only a fraction of its full capacity, and it can rapidly increase its output manyfold.

The heart is a complex pump of remarkable efficiency and in order to understand the treatment of heart disease it is necessary to study carefully the laws regulating the normal working of this machine.

Transmission of the wave of excitation in the heart

The normal contraction of the heart depends on a wave of excitation which starts in the sino-auricular node and passes over the auricles and ventricles. The muscular contraction is accompanied by a wave of change in electric potential, and this latter can be assessed in the intact animal by the electrocardiograph. By this means it is possible to measure very accurately the time relations of the passage of a wave of excitation. A typical human electrocardiogram is shown in Figure 10.4.

The wave of excitation spreads from the sino-auricular node all over both auricles at a rate of about a metre a second. The auriculo-ventricular node, the bundle of His and the Purkinje system, into which the bundle of His divides, together form a specialised path of conduction between the auricles and ventricles. This arrangement is shown as a diagram in Figure 10.1. Section of the bundle of His, either experimentally or by disease, produces a complete block between the auricles and ventricles.

In the human heart the interval between the commencement of the auricular and ventricular contractions is about 0.15 seconds. The wave of excitation is checked at the A-V node and thereafter travels through the bundle and the ventricular muscle. The delay between the contractions of the auricles and of the ventricles provides time for the auricles to drive the blood into and distend the ventricles.

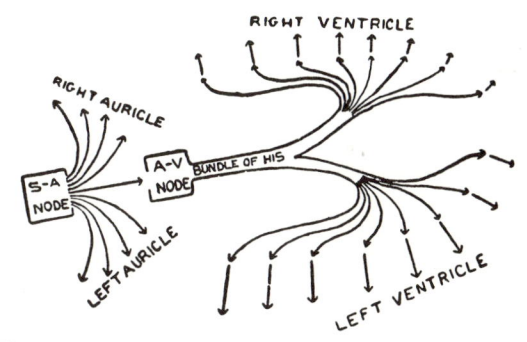

Fig. 10.1 The course of the wave of excitation in the heart.

The cardiac action potential

When the membrane potential of cells constituting the sino-auricular node is measured by intracellular electrodes it exhibits rhythmical changes illustrated in Figure 10.2. A. During diastole a slow depolarisation, the pacemaker potential, develops which carries the membrane potential from −80 to about −60 mV; the pacemaker potential gives rise to a propagated action potential, indicated by the rapid upstroke of the curve, which is followed by a slow phase of repolarisation. Pacemakers also exist elsewhere in the heart, for example in the Purkinje system. Normally these latent pacemakers do not generate impulses because their rhythm is too slow and the action potential from the sinus excites them before they reach threshold. Under abnormal conditions, however, latent pacemakers may become dominant.

The rhythmical changes of electrical potential at the pacemaker site can be explained in terms of changes in membrane conductance to ions. According to the ionic theory when the depolarisation reaches a critical threshold value, a sudden increase in sodium permeability (g_{Na}) occurs which initiates a complex sequence of events, the action potential. The increase in g_{Na} can be interpreted as the activation of a sodium carrier system. A large sodium

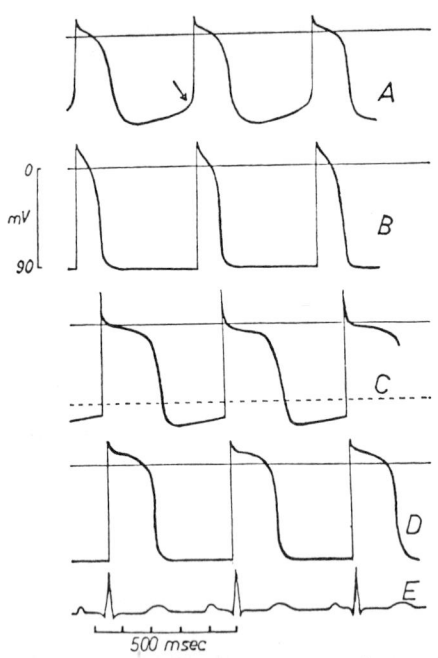

Fig. 10.2 The membrane potential in the course of two cardiac cycles of a fibre of the sinoatrial node (A), of the atrium (B), of the Purkinje system (C), and of the ventricular myocardium (D) of a dog heart drawn on the same time axis as the electrocardiogram (E). Note diastolic depolarisation in (A) and (C), the different shape and duration of the action potentials of different cardiac tissues and the atrioventricular delay indicated by the delay in the upstroke between (B) and (C). The beginning of the propagated action potential is indicated by the arrow (↘). (After Trautwein, *Pharmacol. Rev.* 1963.)

conductance is maintained for only about one millisecond, after which the sodium carrier becomes progressively inactivated. When the sodium carrier is not available the heart is inexcitable and is in its absolute refractory period. During the following relative refractory period the sodium carrier becomes progressively reactivated.

The calcium current

The theory of Hodgkin and Huxley gave a quantitative account of the action potential of squid nerve explaining it in terms of specific ionic channels and voltage-dependent gating mechanisms. Attempts by Noble and others to apply similar considerations to heart muscle required wide ranging modifications of the original theory to account for the differences between the action potentials in cardiac muscle and in nerve. The cardiac action potential lasts much longer than the nerve action potential and has a different shape, the repolarisation process in heart muscle being extremely slow compared to the depolarisation process. A distinguishing feature of the cardiac action potential (Reuter, 1967) is that in addition to the sodium current present in nerve, a calcium current contributes to depolarisation in the heart. A recent reconstruction of the likely sequence of ionic events in a cardiac Purkinje fibre is shown in Figure 10.3, the top diagram indicating the membrane potential, the lower diagram the sequence of ionic conductance changes. Inward conductance is split into two components, a rapid transient strong sodium current and a slow weaker calcium current which remains activated throughout the voltage plateau and helps to maintain it. An outside potassium current underlies the repolarisation process. The resultant changes in ion concentrations are eventually restored through energy requiring metabolic processes.

Inward calcium current is believed to play a critical role in the contractile events of cardiac muscle. Since calcium is responsible for activating the contractile proteins of heart muscle (Ebashi and Endo) it is possible that calcium ions entering the heart during each beat directly activate the contractile process. Alternatively, since the quantity of calcium entering with each action potential is small, a regenerative release of calcium from the sarcoplasmic reticulum with each calcium current inflow may take place. It is widely accepted that calcium current provides a link between electrical and mechanical excitation in heart muscle. In support of this view is the finding that adrenaline whilst increasing the force of contraction of heart muscle also increase calcium current inflow.

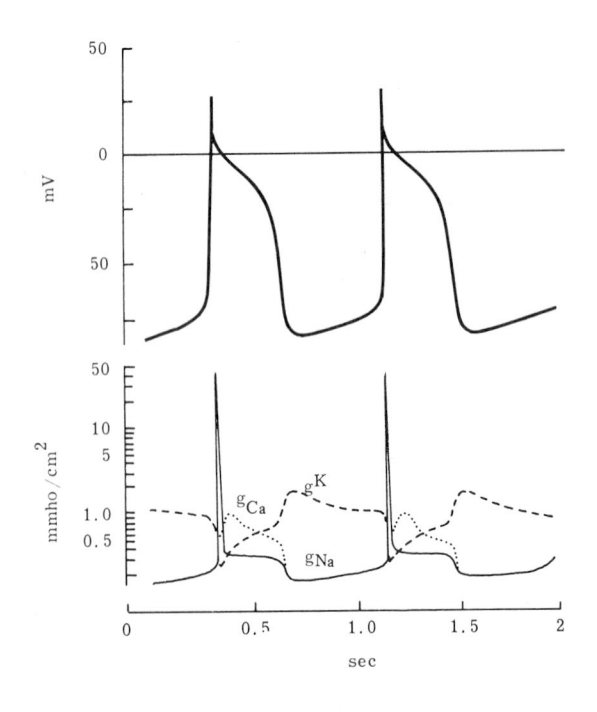

Fig. 10.3 Origin of pacemaker potential. Hypothetical conductance changes underlying recorded potential charges. (After Noble, 1975, in Nayler, *Contraction and Relaxation in the Myocardium*, Academic Press, London.)

Properties of heart muscle

The activity of the heart is conditioned by certain characteristics of heart muscle. In the first place heart muscle gives an all or none response. This means that any stimulus, which is adequate to excite this muscle at all, causes a contraction which is the maximum that the muscle is capable of performing in the condition in which it finds itself at the moment of excitation. Another fundamental property of heart muscle is that contraction is followed by an absolute refractory period during which the heart muscle is incapable of excitation. This is followed by a relative refractory period during which the heart muscle can respond to stimulation, but the stimulus must be stronger than normal.

The contractile power of the heart muscle recovers more slowly than does its excitability, and the duration of the refractory period following a contraction depends on the duration of the period of rest before the contraction, hence by gradually increasing the frequency of stimulation the heart can be worked up to a rapid feeble beat.

In common with all other forms of muscle, the force of contraction of the heart muscle varies as the initial length of the muscle fibres. Hence within certain limits, the greater the distension of any chamber of the heart, the more powerful is its contraction. This was termed by Starling, the law of the heart.

The work done by the heart is regulated by the pressure which regulates the initial filling. The greater the initial filling the more forcible is the contraction, and the greater is the pressure against which it can expel its contents. Any increase in the venous inflow into the heart will therefore increase the work done by the heart. The practical importance of this 'law of the heart' is that it forms an automatic adjustment which ensures that the work done by the heart varies in proportion to the quantity of blood supplied to it by the venous inflow.

The heart is a pump, but its supply of energy depends on the oxygen contained in the blood which it pumps. Hence the activity of the heart depends on the efficiency of the coronary circulation. The coronary circulation is discussed in Chapter 9.

Reflex mechanisms controlling the heart's activity

The pacemaker of the heart has a natural rhythm that can be estimated either by measuring the frequency of the excised heart, or that of a heart in which both the vagus and sympathetic have been cut. The sympathetic apparently exercises no constant action on the heart, but causes rapid acceleration of the heart in excitement. The vagus, however, exercises control of the heart, and the pulse rate observed in a patient is not the frequency of the uncontrolled pacemaker, but the frequency of the pacemaker under a considerable amount of vagal control. The degree of vagal control can be estimated by giving a dose of atropine to abolish the action of the vagus.

It has long been known that a rise of blood pressure stimulates the vagus and causes slowing of the pulse. At one time it was believed that this effect was produced either by stimulation of the sensory nerve endings of the vagus in the aorta or by a direct effect on the vagus centre. Heymans proved that the blood pressure was regulated chiefly by the carotid sinuses. These are situated at the bifurcation of the common carotids. A rise of blood pressure at this point stimulates the cardio-inhibitory centre and causes bradycardia and a fall of blood pressure. A fall of blood pressure at this point inhibits the vagal centre, stimulates the cardio-accelerator centre and the vasomotor centre, and also causes increased adrenaline secretion, which augments these latter effects. In man digital pressure upon the carotid sinus usually causes a sharp fall of blood pressure of about 30 mmHg.

Cardiac output

The heart, blood vessels, lungs and blood can be regarded as a single functional system which supplies oxygen to the tissues and removes carbon dioxide. The circulation has, of course, numerous other functions, but the supply of oxygen is by far the most urgent. The importance of an uninterrupted supply of oxygen to the tissues is indicated by the fact that arrest of the circulation to the brain produces unconsciousness in about five seconds.

The functions of the circulation are concerned with external and internal respiration. The external respiration, i.e. the exchange of gases in the lungs, is discussed in Chapter 12. As regards the internal respiration, the supply of oxygen to the tissues depends upon two factors, namely: (1) the amount of oxygen that the tissues can take from a unit volume of blood and (2) the amount of oxygen supplied by the blood. This depends amongst other factors on the cardiac output, which equals the stroke volume of the heart multiplied by the frequency. The demand of the tissues for oxygen varies very greatly from minute to minute, and these changes are compensated for by variation of all three of the factors mentioned, namely, oxygen utilisation, pulse rate and stroke volume.

Cardiac output may be measured by application of the Fick principle which states that

$$\text{cardiac output} = \frac{\text{oxygen consumption}}{\text{arterio-venous oxygen difference}}$$

The main technical difficulty in applying Fick's principle is to obtain representative samples of mixed venous blood. An important technique has been the use of direct catheterisation of the right auricle by means of a catheter introduced through the basilic vein (Forssmann, 1929). Representative samples of mixed venous blood may be obtained by this method which also provides reliable measurements of right auricular pressure.

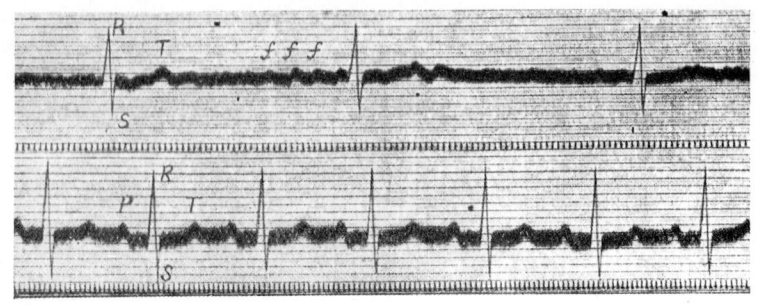

Fig. 10.4 Electro-cardiograms. Lower record from normal subject; upper record from case of auricular fibrillation. (Sir Thomas Lewis.)

More recently, measurement of cardiac output by techniques based on the Fick principle is being displaced by indicator dilution techniques which do not require samples of mixed venous blood or the measurement of the body's oxygen consumption. With this type of technique a dye is rapidly injected into the venous side of the circulation, preferably directly into the right atrium. The resulting dye concentration-time profile is then assessed in the arterial blood. Cardiac output can be calculated from the quantity of dye injected and the area of the curve of dye concentration against time.

Disordered rhythms of the heart

These are of particular pharmacological interest because they are more amenable to treatment by drugs than most other types of cardiac disorder. Cardiac arrhythmias may involve changes in one or more of the following functions: automaticity, conduction velocity and refractory period. Each of these is related in a characteristic way to the cardiac action potential. Thus in considering the potential records shown in Figure 10.2, the slope of the pacemaker potential determines the degree of automaticity; for example the S-A node (A) has a characteristic pacemaker potential and exhibits automaticity whilst the auricle (B) possesses neither. The rate of rise of the action potential determines the conduction rate and the duration of the action potential determines the length of the refractory period. Since the shape of the action potential of heart muscle depends ultimately on its ionic permeability, particularly to sodium, calcium and potassium, it follows that cardiac arrhythmias must involve changes in ionic permeabilities which are amenable to influence by drugs.

An important type of disordered rhythm is auricular (atrial) fibrillation. This frequently appears in old-standing cases of mitral disease, and ultimately develops in about 80 per cent of cases of mitral disease. Records of the arterial pulse of the apex beat of the ventricle in this condition show that the ventricle is contracting rapidly, irregularly and inefficiently. A considerable proportion of the ventricular contractions are so inefficient that they produce no radial pulse.

The characteristic feature of the arterial pulse in auricular fibrillation is its absolute irregularity; no two succeeding waves are of the same strength, and the interval between every two beats is different. Records of the venous pulse show no record of auricular contraction. These observations are confirmed by records of the electrical variation of the heart. Figure 10.4 shows records from a normal adult and from a patient with auricular fibrillation. The lower record shows the following characteristics of a normal electrocardiogram: a P wave due to the spread of activity over the atrial muscle, a PR interval during which the atrial cells are completely depolarised whilst the conducting tissue is not yet depolarised, a QRS complex involving successive depolarisation of the interventricular septum, right ventricle and apex, and a T wave representing ventricular repolarisation. The upper (abnormal) record shows absence of the P wave. Moreover, the R waves occur at irregular intervals.

Auricular fibrillation may involve one or both of the following pathological processes (1) a disturbance of impulse formation when an ectopic focus in the auricle discharges at a very rapid rate and (2) a disturbance of impulse conduction leading to re-entry of the stimulus in the same circuit.

Sir Thomas Lewis suggested that in auricular fibrillation small waves of contraction are coursing in a circus movement around the auricle about 450 times a minute. These waves are marked 'f' in the upper record of Figure 10.4.

Under normal conditions the wave of excitation passes over the auricle in about 0.035 second, and is succeeded by a refractory period. The whole auricle is still in a refraction condition at the time when the wave of excitation has completed its course. In auricular fibrillation the wave of excitation proceeds more slowly than normal; hence, by the time that the wave of excitation has traversed the auricle a part of the auricle has recovered its excitability, and in terms of the circus movement theory waves of excitation can re-enter and continue to travel round and round the auricle in a circle. The result of this activity of the auricle is that a shower of impulses pours down upon the auriculoventricular node.

The rate of excitation is greater than that to which the node of the ventricle can respond, but the ventricle contracts at a rate far greater than its maximum efficient rate. In consequence, the ventricle exhausts itself with a rapid inefficient beat.

A difficulty raised by the circus theory is that it postulates a discrete excitation circuit which has been difficult to locate. An alternative, suggested by a computer model, is that there is no stable circuit but that variable re-entry circuits occur. The present view is that both ectopic focus theories and circuit theories are plausible and that both mechanisms may apply in individual cases.

Antiarrhythmic drugs may influence auricular fibrillation in several ways. They may depress the spontaneous diastolic depolarisation of ectopic pacemakers, thus diminishing automaticity, or they may lengthen the refractory period of the auricle so that a re-entering stimulus meets a refractory cell and the circus movement is arrested. Another theoretical possibility is that a drug may increase overall conduction velocity so that the ectopic circus movement is more likely to meet a refractory cell and become extinguished. In clinical practice it is seldom possible to determine which basic mechanism is deranged and the use of antiarrhythmic drugs is governed less by theoretical considerations than by a process of trial and error.

Auricular flutter is another form of disordered rhythm of the heart. In this case the auricle contracts about 300 times per minute, and the ventricle is stimulated to a rapid and inefficient beat.

ACTION OF DRUGS ON THE HEART

Although many drugs affect the heart, only a few are of value in the treatment of heart disease. Of these the most important are: cardiac glycosides used in the treatment of congestive heart failure, generally in conjunction with diuretic drugs; quinidine, procainamide, lignocaine, phenytoin, propranolol, bretylium, verapamil and others for the control of certain disorders of rhythm, and the nitrites and beta blockers used for the treatment of angina of effort. Aminophylline and adrenaline are cardiac stimulants which are used in the emergency treatment of heart failure; isoprenaline is a cardiac stimulant which may be used in heart block to improve conduction.

Cardiac glycosides

Digitalis is the most important drug used in cardiac therapeutics but the history of the drug is interesting in showing the variety of beliefs concerning a drug that can be deduced from clinical observation, when this is uncontrolled by any scientific observations. Digitalis was originally used as a remedy for tuberculosis, and also as an emetic, but in 1775 Withering showed that it had a powerful diuretic action and also an action on the heart. It was used as a diuretic, but Pereira stated that it acted as a cardiac depressant and recommended it 'to reduce the force and velocity of the circulation'. After about 1860 it was considered a cardiac tonic, and was believed to raise blood pressure. During the first half of the nineteenth century digitalis was also used for treatment of numerous diseases of the central nervous system, including epilepsy, general paralysis of the insane and delirium tremens.

The action of digitalis in auricular fibrillation of the heart was elucidated by Mackenzie, but it is only more recently that digitalis glycosides have been generally acknowledged to be the supreme remedy for congestive heart failure, whatever its cause.

Chemistry of cardiac glycosides
The chief active principles of the leaves of *Digitalis purpurea* are three glycosides, namely, digitoxin, gitoxin and gitaloxin. Gitalin, which was previously considered to be a pure glycoside contained in the leaves of *Digitalis purpurea* is now known to be a mixture of glycosides. Another pure glycoside, digoxin, has been isolated from the leaves of *Digitalis lanata*, a plant indigenous to the Balkans. Digitoxin and digoxin are both crystalline substances. They are chemically closely related differing only by the hydroxyl group of digoxin at C12 (Fig. 10.5), but the additional hydroxyl group alters the physico-chemical properties of the compound rendering digoxin more polar and water-soluble. The composition of

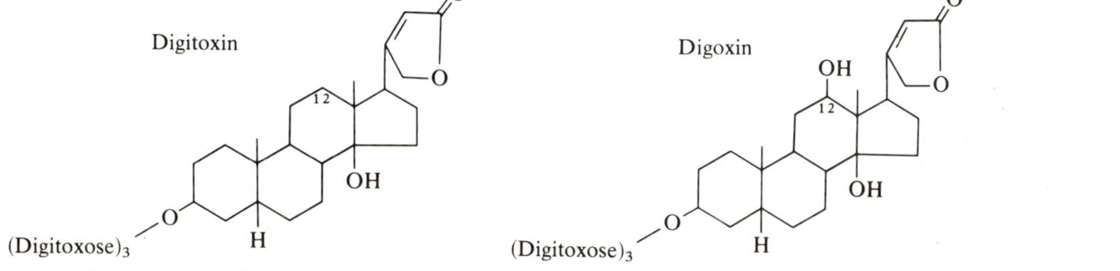

Fig. 10.5 Structural chemical formula of digitoxin and digoxin.

commercial digitoxin varies slightly, but digoxin is a well-defined substance of constant composition. Nativelle's digitaline, which was isolated in 1869, is probably identical with digitoxin. Stoll has shown that these glycosides are degradation products, for example, the parent substance of digoxin is a glucoside of acetyldigoxin called lanatoside C.

The digitalis glycosides are easily broken down, e.g. digitoxin breaks down to form one molecule of digitoxigenin and three molecules of a sugar, digitoxose. Digitoxose is a 2-desoxy-monosaccharide. Three molecules of digitoxose are attached in series to a molecule of the aglycone digitoxigenin.

The seeds of *Strophanthus gratus* contain the glycoside g-strophanthin or ouabain. G-strophanthin is a well defined crystalline substance but other strophanthins such as the glycosides derived from *Strophanthus kombe* are ill-defined mixtures of uncertain composition. The strophanthins are readily soluble in water. Their absorption from the gastro-intestinal tract is uncertain and they are used only for intravenous injection.

All the cardiac glycosides have a common chemical structure, being combinations of sugars with aglycones or genins. The genins are chemically related to the steroid hormones but differ from them in possessing a 5- or 6-membered lactone ring (Fig. 10.5) which is essential for their cardiac action. Hydrogenation of the unsaturated double bond in the lactone ring greatly reduces cardiac activity.

Experiments on the isolated heart have shown that the aglycones produce pharmacological actions similar to those produced by the glycosides, but there is a striking difference as regards the firmness of their combination with the cardiac tissue. The glycosides are fixed firmly whereas the aglycones can easily be washed out. Hence in the intact animal the aglycones produce only a transient action. The aglycones, furthermore, are even less water soluble than the glycosides and are poorly absorbed from the gastro-intestinal tract.

Effects on contractility and output of the heart
Boehm showed in 1872 that digitalis increased the output of an isolated frog's heart which was pumping serum from a low venous into a high arterial reservoir. He computed the work of the heart as the product of the cardiac output and the difference in height of the two reservoirs and concluded that digitalis in therapeutic doses increased the work of the heart through a direct action on the contractility of heart muscle.

We shall discuss the evidence for a direct muscular action of digitalis in some detail since these studies are a good example of pharmacological analysis and of the difficulties which are involved in applying the results of animal experiments to man.

Experiments on animals. To be relevant these should be designed to show in an unequivocal way the effect of digitalis on the force of contraction of heart muscle, and at the same time they should, as far as possible, approximate to the conditions obtaining in man; two aims which are usually incompatible.

One of the simplest ways of assessing the effects of a drug on the force of contraction of heart muscle is by the use of the isolated papillary muscle of the cat. In this preparation the fine papillary muscle attached to the tricuspid valve is suspended in Locke's solution. The muscle is stimulated electrically at a regular rate and its contractions recorded isometrically. Figure 10.6 shows a gradual failure of the muscle during the control period and a gradual recovery of the force of contraction after

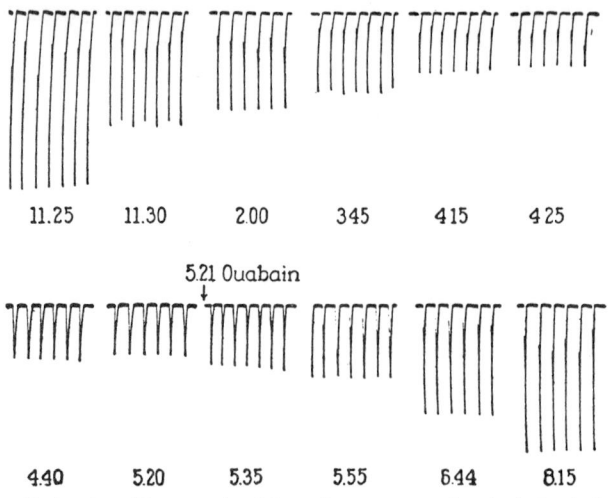

Fig. 10.6 Isometric contractions of isolated papillary muscle of the cat in response to electrical stimulation. The period shows the gradual failure of the muscle during the control period (11.25-5.20) and gradual recovery of tension after the addition of strophanthin to the bath. (After Gold, 1946, *J. Amer. med. Ass.*)

strophanthin has been added to the bath. Concentrations as small as 1:40 to 1:70 million of strophanthin produce this effect. These concentrations are of the same magnitude as those likely to occur in the tissues of patients who have received a therapeutic intravenous dose of this drug.

A general way of assessing the contractility of heart muscle is by means of its force-velocity relationship. Sonnenblick has shown that cardiac glycosides alter the force-velocity relation of isolated cat papillary muscle during isometric contraction increasing velocity for a given load as well as the maximum velocity of shortening (Fig. 10.7). Basically similar effects are produced in the intact human heart.

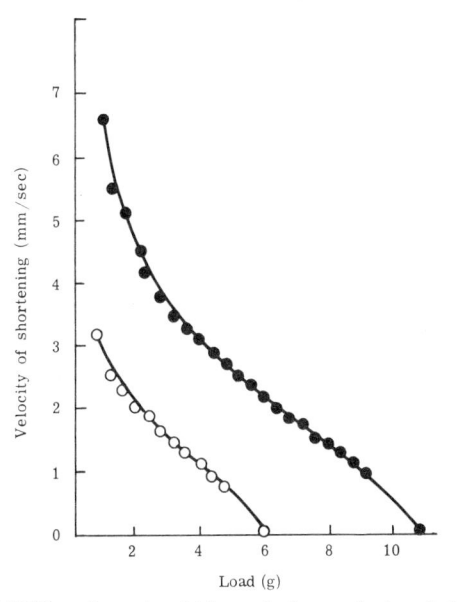

Fig. 10.7 Effect of strophanthidin on the force-velocity relation of the cat papillary muscle. (Adapted from Sonnenblick *et al.*, after Smith & Haber, 1973, *New Engl. J. Med.*) A control curve is O—O—O; after addition of strophanthidin the curve is shifted upward and to the right ●—●—●, increasing the maximum velocity of shortening as well as the maximum isometric force developed.

It is much more difficult to measure alterations in the contractility of the heart in the whole animal since the results are often obscured by simultaneous changes in venous return, heart rate and arterial pressure, all of which affect diastolic volume and hence the force of contraction. These factors can be eliminated in the mammalian heart-lung preparation in which the peripheral circulation is excluded. If in this preparation the heart is fatigued or depressed by drugs, the right auricular pressure rises, the ventricles dilate and the cardiac output falls. After digitalis the right auricular pressure falls, the ventricles become smaller and the cardiac output is restored.

Effects on oxygen consumption
The main factors determining oxygen consumption of heart muscle are ventricular wall tension and contraction velocity, both of which are increased by cardiac glycosides. Hence digitalis increases oxygen consumption in a normal heart. In a failing heart the situation is more complicated since two opposing factors affect oxygen consumption after digitalis administration, an increase due to the greater contraction velocity and a decrease due to the smaller size of the heart and decreased wall tension. Experimentally it has been found that in a failing heart digitalis may not increase and even decrease oxygen consumption. In such cases the mechanical efficiency of the heart expressed as the ratio:

$$\frac{\text{external work}}{\text{oxygen consumption}}$$

is increased by digitalis.

Evidence in man. The changes produced by digitalis in the failing heart-lung preparation are similar to those produced in patients with heart failure when the heart is dilated and incapable of expelling its contents adequately.

Digitalis has been found to increase cardiac output in heart failure, not only in cases of auricular fibrillation, but also in patients with normal rhythm. Radiological studies have shown that after digitalis the diastolic shadow is decreased (Fig. 10.16) and the excursions of the ventricles are increased. This means that although the heart has become smaller in size it expels its contents more fully. If the heart is dilated digitalis increases the cardiac output, but if the heart is of normal size digitalis may not increase the cardiac output by may even decrease it.

The beneficial effect of digitalis in heart failure is due mainly to its action in improving the contractility of the heart muscle, but the subsequent changes in arterial and venous pressure also contribute to this effect. In heart failure the ventricular beat is rapid and often irregular, the venous pressure is raised, and the systolic pressure is frequently low. Improvement of any of these abnormal conditions may, in itself, improve the function of the heart. For example, an increase of the systolic pressure improves the oxygen supply of the heart by increasing the coronary blood flow; a slower and more regular beat increases the diastolic filling and prolongs the periods of rest between beats. A lowering of an excessive right auricular pressure by means of venesection may also improve the cardiac output.

Actions of digitalis on the vagus and on conduction
Traube showed in 1851 that digitalis slowed the heart in dogs and that slowing was abolished by cutting the vagi. The vagal action of digitalis has been variously attributed to a sensitisation of the heart towards vagus stimulation, to a direct stimulation of the vagus centre in the medulla and to reflexes arising either from the carotid sinus and the

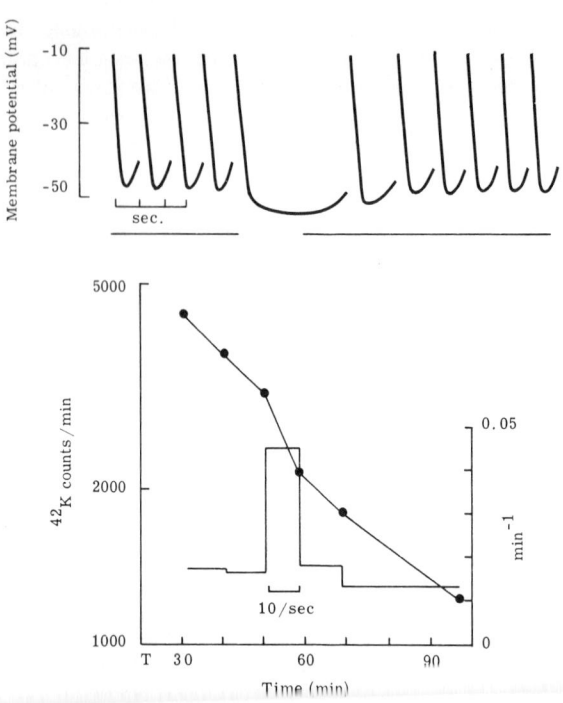

Fig. 10.8 Mechanism of action of acetylcholine on pacemaker activity in cardiac muscle. *Top*: Hyperpolarization of frog sinus membrane during vagal stimulation (Hutter and Trautwein, 1956). *Bottom*: Increase of K^{42} efflux produced by vagal stimulation in frog sinus venosus. The points show the radioactivity in the tissue on a logarithmic scale (left ordinate). The bars show fraction of K^{42} in tissue lost per minute. During the period labelled 10 sec, the left vagus nerve was stimulated at 10 sec. (From Hutter, 1961, *Br. Med. Bull.*)

aortic arch, or from an improvement in the contractility of the heart itself. Heymans found that in dogs, digitalis sensitised the carotid sinus mechanism and that slowing was abolished after denervation of the carotid sinus and aortic arch.

The effects of vagus stimulation are mediated by the release of acetylcholine from vagal nerve endings. Acetylcholine acts on muscarinic receptors in the heart muscle which can be blocked by atropine. The basic action of acetylcholine on cardiac pacemaker activity consists in a selective increase of the potassium permeability of the cell membrane causing hyperpolarisation and inhibition (Fig. 10.8)

Both the S-A node and the A-V node are under vagal control. Stimulation of the right vagus slows impulse formation in the S-A node and stimulation of the left vagus impairs conduction in the A-V node and may even produce heart block. Digitalis produces the following actions by stimulation of the vagus:

1. A slower rate of impulse formation in the S-A node. When the heart rate is controlled by the S-A node, this effect of digitalis results in a slowing of the heart rate. This effect of digitalis can be demonstrated in experimental animals, but it is relatively unimportant in the clinical use of digitalis.

2. Impaired conduction of the A-V node. The impairment of A-V conduction by digitalis is shown both by a prolongation of P-R interval and by the development of heart block (Fig. 10. 9).

In human auricular fibrillation about 400 impulses per minute may reach the A-V node. These impulses do not all reach the ventricle so that a certain degree of heart block is already present. If a patient with auricular fibrillation and heart failure is put to rest in bed the degree of heart block increases and the ventricular rate falls. This is due to increased vagal tone consequent upon an improved circulation. If digitalis is given to the patient, the degree of heart block is greatly increased and the ventricular rate is correspondingly slowed. Initially the heart block is mainly due to vagal stimulation because when an intravenous dose of atropine is administered at this stage the heart rate increases to the original level or above it.

The action of digitalis on A-V conduction is, however, complex and is produced partly by vagal stimulation and partly by a direct effect of digitalis on the conducting tissue. In patients who are fully digitalised the direct effect of digitalis becomes predominant and its vagal effect small so that atropine then produces only a small increase in the heart rate. This direct effect can be attributed to a prolongation of the effective refractory period of the A-V

Fig. 10.9 Action of digitalis on auriculoventricular conduction. I. and II. Patient had received digitalis for ten days. **I.** Prolonged P–R interval (0.33 second). **II.** Occasional auriculo-ventricular block. **III.** Digitalis stopped for ten days. Normal conduction, P–R interval (0.2 second). (Lead 2. Right arm, left leg. Time 30 per second.) (Figures supplied by Professor Murray Lyon.)

node and of the conducting tissue. The effective refractory period is the shortest interval between two stimuli each of which produces a conducted and effective response.

3. Shortening of the refractory period of auricular muscle.

Stimulation of the vagus shortens the refractory period of auricular muscle and favours the establishment of auricular fibrillation. Auricular fibrillation can be produced experimentally in animals by the local application of acetylcholine to the surface of the auricle. Acetyl-ß-methylcholine (methacholine) when injected into a patient with auricular flutter may convert the flutter to fibrillation (Fig. 10.10). Digitalis through its vagal action produces similar effects, for in patients with auricular flutter it may convert the flutter to fibrillation and in patients with auricular fibrillation it increases the rate at which the auricles fibrillate.

Other actions of digitalis
Digitalis increases the excitability of heart muscle and induces the formation of abnormal foci of excitation in cardiac muscle; in this way digitalis, when present in high concentration, may give rise to a variety of cardiac arrhythmias. A characteristic effect of digitalis is to cause a reduction or inversion of the T wave of the electrocardiogram. Digitalis has a direct effect on blood vessels, producing vasoconstriction. Clinically this effect is not important; on the contrary, digitalis may increase peripheral blood flow in patients with heart failure by improving the circulation and diminishing reflex sympathetic activity.

Nausea and vomiting frequently occur during the therapeutic use of digitalis and may be due to several different causes. Firstly, the digitalis glycosides are irritant, and if given by mouth act as local emetics. Secondly, these drugs stimulate the vomiting centre in man and in animals. For example, vomiting can be readily induced in pigeons by intravenous injection of a cardiac glycoside. Finally, these drugs can produce vomiting by a reflex action arising from the heart. Sensory impulses from the heart can produce vomiting, as is shown by its occurrence as a result of over-exertion; and it is believed that nausea and vomiting may arise as a secondary effect

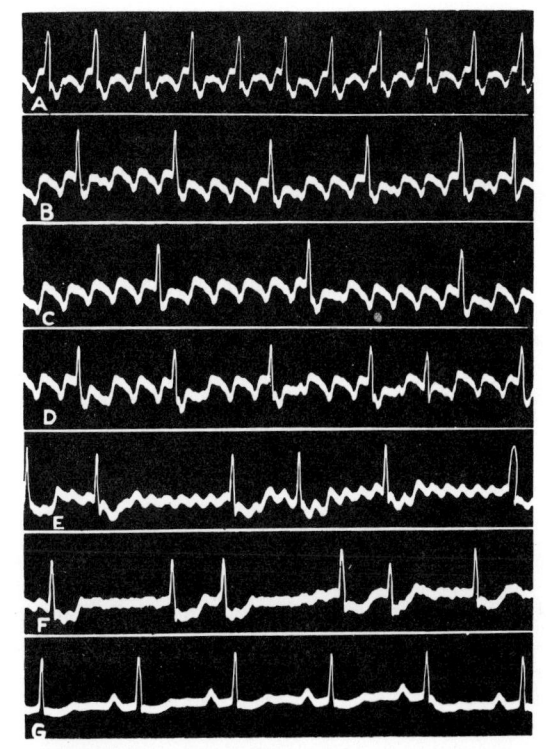

Fig. 10.10 Effect of mecholyl in a patient with thyrotoxicosis and auricular flutter.
A. Control. Auricular flutter with 2:1 rhythm.
B. Five min. after a subcutaneous injection of 50 mg. acetyl ß-methylcholine-chloride; 4:1 block.
C. 6:1 block.
D. Beginning fragmentation of flutter waves.
E. Coarse auricular fibrillation.
F. Fine auricular fibrillation.
G. Resumption of normal rhythm 1½ hours after injection of the drug. (After Nahum and Hoff, 1935, *J. Am. med. Ass.*)

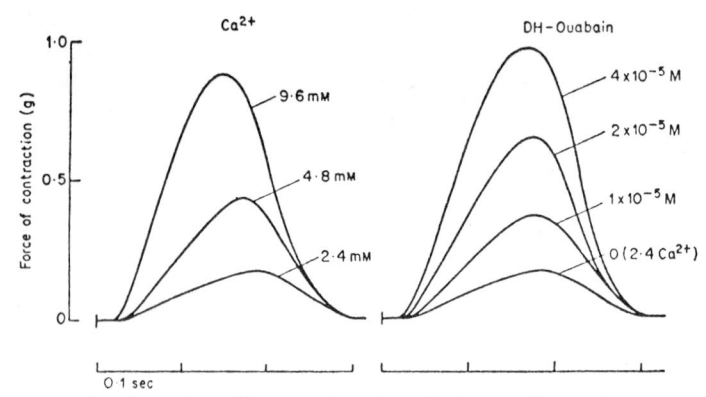

Fig. 10.11 Isometric tension curves of a guinea-pig papillary muscle under the influence of increasing concentrations of Ca^{2+} (left) and dihydro-ouabain (right). 35°C. Resting tension 0.4 g, stimulating frequency 1/sec. (After Reiter, 1970. In Cuthbert, ed., Calcium and Cellular Functions. Macmillan, London.)

due to the increased activity of the heart following digitalis therapy.

Mode of action of cardiac glycosides

The most important effect of cardiac glycosides is that they improve the ability of heart muscle to exert tension. It has been shown both experimentally and clinically that these glycosides increase not only the maximal tension exerted by heart muscle but also the steepness (dp/dt) of its isometric contraction curve reflecting an increase in the velocity of shortening of the contractile proteins (Fig. 10.11). It is of interest that the inotropic effect of a cardiac glycoside can be closely mimicked by increasing the concentration of external calcium as is also shown in Figure 10.11.

Present evidence suggests that two basic mechanisms are concerned in the effect of cardiac glycosides on heart muscle (1) interference with the movements of sodium and potassium across the cell membrane, (2) increased concentration of free intracellular calcium.

1. Movements of sodium and potassium across the cell membrane were initially studied in red blood cells. When red corpuscles are suspended in Ringer solution in the cold they lose potassium and gain sodium by passive diffusion but if they are subsequently rewarmed they take up potassium and expel sodium by an active process. This active transport process is readily inhibited by cardiac glycosides as was shown by Schatzmann in 1953. Active membrane transport is associated with splitting of ATP and involves a sodium-potassium activated adenosinetriphosphatase, which can be inhibited by cardiac glycosides. Cardiac glycosides and potassium compete for this enzyme and this may explain the antagonistic effect of high serum potassium towards certain toxic effects of digitalis. Conversely, a low serum potassium, such as occurs with rapid diuresis, favours the occurrence of digitalis-induced ectopic beats.

2. There is much evidence that calcium forms an essential link between the electrical events in the membrane and the contractile element. It has been suggested that the glycosides increase the force of contraction by increasing the concentration of free intracellular calcium. The precise mechanism by which this is brought about is not known. According to one theory digitalis glycosides affect intracellular calcium distribution so that during inflow of the cardiac calcium current (p. 132) an increased amount of free calcium becomes available to activate the contractile machinery. Another theory concentrates on transmembrane calcium exchanges and the existence of two different carrier mechanisms for the extrusion of sodium ions by the cardiac cell membrane. The first of these, sodium-potassium ATPase, extrudes sodium in exchange for potassium; when this mechanism is inhibited by digitalis, sodium will tend to accumulate in the cell. The second carrier exchanges sodium for calcium, so that in consequence of a higher internal sodium, more calcium will enter the cell. The cardiac glycosides are thus assumed to promote calcium entry indirectly by increasing the intracellular concentration of sodium by a mechanism involving inhibition of Na,K-ATPase.

Digitalis receptor

Repke has proposed that the Na,K-ATPase of the myocardial cell membrane represents the molecular point of attack or 'receptor' for cardiac glycosides. Several arguments can be advanced for this hypothesis. (1) Cardiac glycosides, particularly polar glycosides such as ouabain bind specifically to membrane receptors resembling Na,K-ATPase. (2) Potassium has a marked effect on the rate and equilibrium constants of the glycoside-receptor complex. A high potassium concentration inhibits glycoside binding in agreement with the beneficial effects of raised serum potassium in digitalis intoxication. (3) There is a connection between Na, K-ATPase inhibition

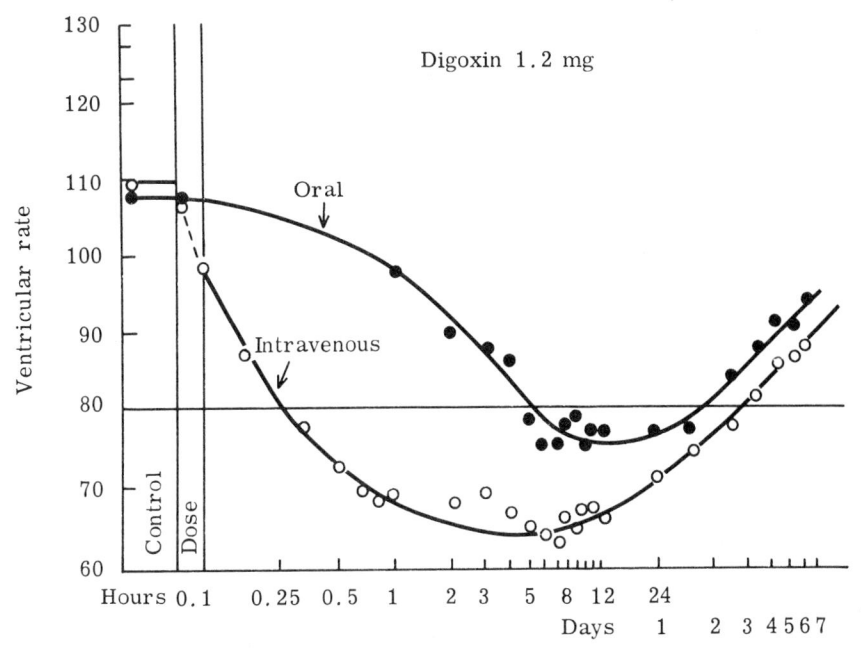

Fig. 10.12 Curve of the ventricular rate response in patients with atrial fibrillation after a single dose of digoxin. (After Gold et al., 1953, J. Pharmac. exp. Ther.)

and free intracellular calcium level and hence the inotropic effect of digitalis. The ATPase-receptor hypothesis has proved highly stimulating, though controversial. Some authors consider Na,K-ATPase inhibition to be the mechanism of the toxic, rather than the inotropic, effect of cardiac glycosides.

Onset and duration of action
The onset of the action of cardiac glycosides is slow. This is due to both pharmacokinetic delay and a slow interaction with receptors. Figure 10.12 shows the time course of the action of digoxin after oral and intravenous application measured by its effect on heart rate in auricular fibrillation. The oral delay is largely pharmacokinetic. The intravenous delay is remarkably long, probably partly due to a slow interaction with receptors.

Radioimmunoassay of digoxin
Methods by which minute quantities of cardiac glycosides can be measured in plasma and tissues are now widely employed. In a typical radioimmunoassay an aliquot of digoxin-containing serum is mixed with a known quantity of tritiated digoxin and the mixture incubated with anti-digoxin antibody. From the quantity of tritiated digoxin bound by antibody the concentration in the original serum can be calculated since both samples of digoxin compete for the same antibody sites. In another method digoxin is measured by its inhibition of red corpuscle ATPase using Rb[86] as marker.

There is good correlation between daily digoxin doses and plasma levels (Fig. 10.13) and some correlation between plasma levels and toxic effects although it has been shown that concentrations of digoxin in heart muscle may be up to 100 times greater than in plasma.

Pharmacokinetics of digitoxin and digoxin
The two main clinically used glycosides, although closely similar in chemical structure and pharmacological action, differ in their pharmacokinetic properties due to the non-polar lipid soluble character of digitoxin and the polar water-soluble character of digoxin.

Digitoxin is completely absorbed from the gut and is equally effective given orally or parenterally. Due to its lipid solubility it undergoes extensive enterohepatic recirculation. It is reabsorbed in the kidney tubules, hardly any of it being excreted. Digitoxin is metabolised in the liver; stimulation of microsomal liver enzymes, e.g. by a barbiturate, tends to lower its steady state blood concentration. It is 97 per cent bound to plasma proteins and has a long biological halflife (about eight days).

Digoxin, although reasonably well absorbed from the intestine, is not so completely and reliably absorbed as digitoxin and differences in the bioavailability of different brands of digoxin tablets have been detected. (The subject of bioavailability is discussed on p. 38). Digoxin is only about 20 per cent bound to plasma proteins and has a shorter half life than digotoxin. Due to its polar nature digoxin is excreted by the kidneys and is found in the urine either as unchanged digoxin or a closely related compound. If kidney function is impaired, digoxin may accumulate in the body and produce symptoms of digitalis intoxication. Figure 10.14 shows a pharmacokinetic

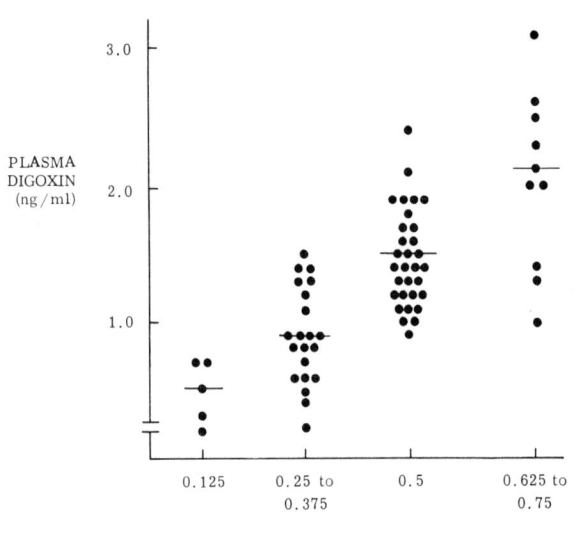

Fig. 10.13 Plasma digoxin concentrations, by radioimmunoasser, plotted against oral dose of digoxin in 68 patients. All had normal or near-normal renal function. The horizontal bars represent mean values. (After Chamberlain et al., Br. med. J.)

analysis of digoxin blood levels after oral administration. Digoxin plasma levels can be described by two exponential processes characterised by two half-times. Line B represents the dominant slow process ($t_{1/2} = 31$ h) reflecting slow elimination of digoxin by the kidney. Line C represents an initial fast process $t_{1/2} = 1$ h) representing distribution and tissue binding.

Principles of administration of digitalis

The general principle is to produce as rapidly as convenient an effective concentration of drug in the body (loading dose) and maintain the effect by smaller doses sufficient to balance the rate of elimination (maintenance doses). A theoretical example illustrating the principle of the maintenance dose is given in Figure 10.15 showing (a)

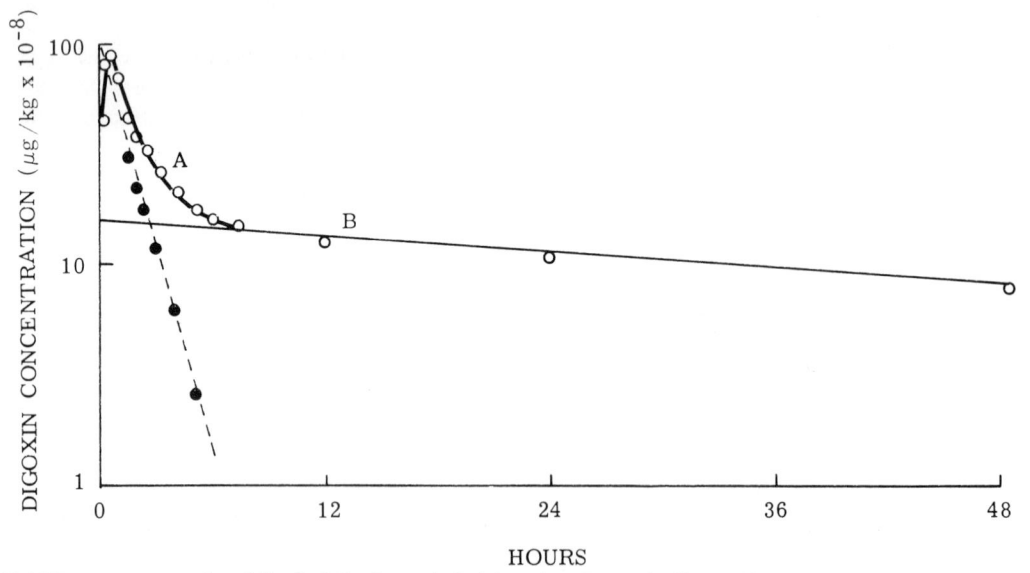

Fig. 10.14 Serum concentration of digoxin following oral administration. Composite figure. Line B is the best straight line that can be drawn back to zero time. It represents the dominant T of digoxin of 31 h associated with metabolism and excretion of the glycoside. The steep straight line, derived by substracting line B from the descending limb of curve A, represent distribution and binding of digoxin to the tissue. (After Doherty, Perkins and Mitchell. Arch Int Med 1961.)

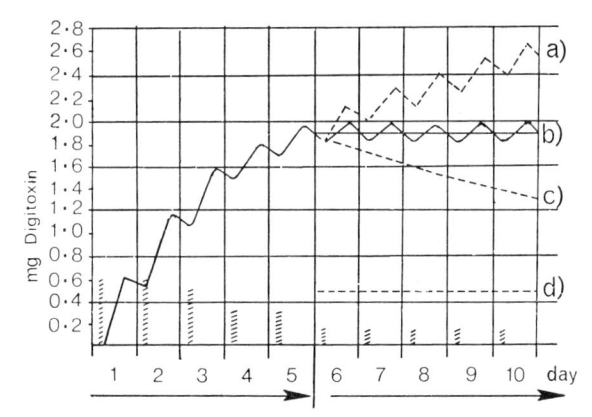

Fig. 10.15 Hypothetical curve (b) showing concentration of digitoxin in the body after administering the following oral doses: Day 1 and 2, 0.6 mg; day 3, 0.5 mg; day 4 and 5, 0.3 mg; subsequent days average: 0.136 mg which represents the daily maintenance dose for this patient. If patient had continued taking 0.3 mg digitoxin after reaching the maintenance level, curve (a) would result, leading to toxic cumulation. If patient had discontinued taking digitoxin after reaching maintenance level, curve (c) would result, leading to decompensation (d). (After Baumgarten. Die Herzwirksamen Glycoside. Georg Thieme. Leipzig. 1963.)

the build-up of an excessive concentration, leading to toxic cumulation, if the daily dose is too large; (b) the build-up of a steady maintenance level if doses are optimally adjusted; (c) the progressive decline of drug concentration leading to decompensation, if drug administration is stopped when the maintenance level has been reached.

Digitalis in the treatment of congestive heart failure

The cardiac glycosides are useful in the treatment of congestive heart failure because of a remarkable combination of properties possessed by no other group of drugs. The sympathomimetic drugs strengthen the heart but at the same time they accelerate the rate, facilitate A-V conduction and cause vasoconstriction. The digitalis glycosides, by contrast, strengthen the heart without producing appreciable vasoconstriction and at the same time they slow the heart rate and regularise the ventricle in auricular fibrillation by depressing A-V conduction. Their action is persistent, an effective concentration can be maintained in the tissues for many months, and no tolerance is acquired.

In most cases of heart failure the cardiac output is low, blood flow through the capillaries is slowed down and the oxygen content of the venous blood is decreased owing to more complete abstraction of oxygen by the tissues. Since the oxygen carried by the blood is almost fully utilised and the damaged heart cannot increase its output effectively, the circulation lacks reserve powers and the tissues suffer from oxygen deficiency at the slightest exertion. In these cases of 'low output heart failure' digitalis produces the greatest benefit.

In heart failure the kidney functions are impaired because the circulation is impaired. Digitalis relieves oedema and improves urinary secretion because it relieves venous congestion; it has no direct action on the kidney and does not produce diuresis in normal subjects. Cardiac dropsy is, however, relieved more rapidly if diuretic drugs are administered together with digitalis.

Clinical use of digitalis

In congestive heart failure the aim of treatment is to increase the cardiac output, reduce the work of the heart and relieve oedema. In the past the standard way of treatment was the use of digitalis combined with low sodium diet and rest, adding a diuretic if necessary. More recently the idea that a cardiac glycoside should be given to all patients with congestive heart failure has been questioned. Some clinicians prefer diuretics for initial and maintenance treatment of patients with mild congestive failure, adding digitalis where necessary.

Digitalis is most effective when congestive failure is associated with hypertension or coronary disease. It is the drug of choice in heart failure with auricular fibrillation. Under these conditions digitalis has a dual action: (1) By its action on A-V conduction it damps down the stream of impulses reaching the ventricle and in consequence the beat of the ventricle becomes slower, more regular and more forceful. Digitalis does not stop auricular fibrillation, indeed the fibrillating rate may be increased after digitalis. By its inotropic action it improves the action of the heart. Figure 10.16 shows the beneficial effects of oral digitalis in a patient with heart failure and auricular fibrillation. In both auricular fibrillation and flutter digitalis may convert the arrhythmia to normal sinus rhythm. In patients with severe heart failure and a very rapid ventricular pulse DC cardioversion (p. 147) is now sometimes used to manage supraventricular arrhythmias.

Digitalis is of limited usefulness in certain types of high output failure. Opinion is divided on the benefits and dangers of digitalis in acute myocardial infarction.

Toxic actions of digitalis

No useful effect is produced unless an adequate dose of digitalis is given, but an overdose produces dangerous toxic effects, especially when potassium depletion arises from concurrent use of a thiazide diuretic. The most common cause of digitalis intoxication is intracellular potassium depletion which is not necessarily reflected in the serum potassium level. There are striking variations in individual tolerance to digitalis. Age is an important factor, infants and children tolerating relatively larger doses than adults while old people are increasingly susceptible to intoxication. Anorexia, headache, nausea and vomiting are the first signs of mild intoxication. As a general rule it is undesirable to reduce the apex rate below sixty. Frequent extra-systoles and auricular tachycardia with incomplete

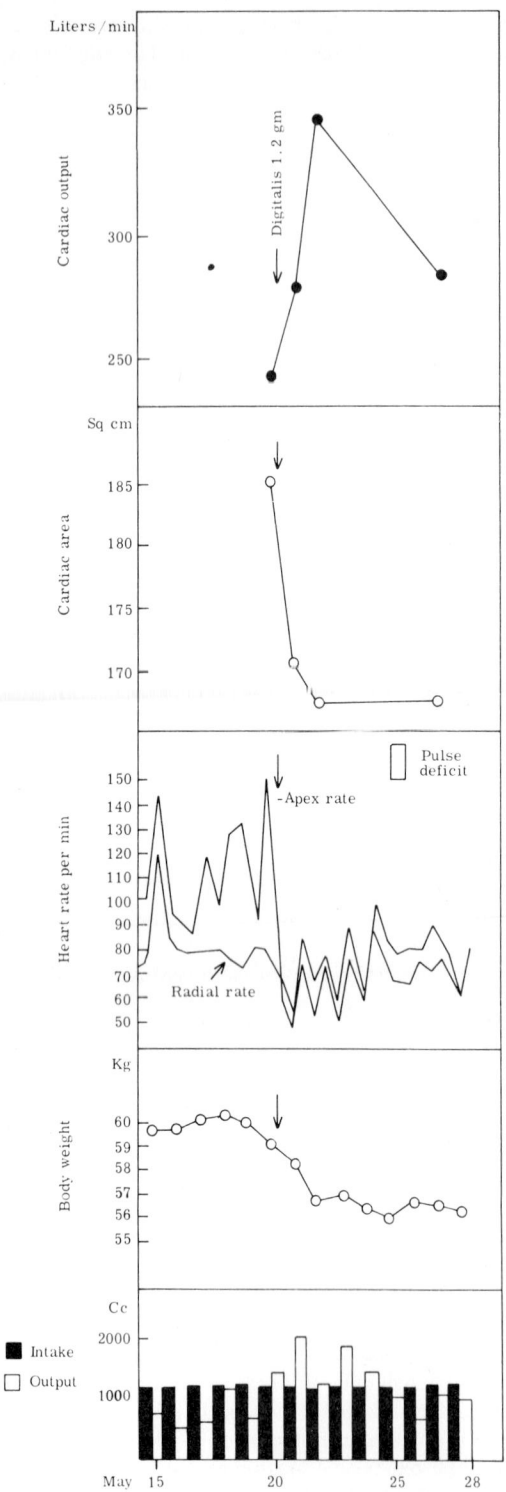

Fig. 10.16 Effect of a single oral dose of digitalis in a patient with heart failure due to auricular fibrillation. Note increase in cardiac output occurring with a decrease in the size of the heart. (After Stewart and Cohn, 1932, *J. Clin. Invest.*)

heart block are serious signs of intoxication. Particularly dangerous is the occurence of multiple ventricular extrasystoles in the form of coupled or irregularly spaced beats. These may lead to ventricular tachycardia, and eventually to fatal ventricular fibrillation.

In the majority of cases of digitalis intoxication the only treatment necessary is to stop the drug, withhold diuretics and if necessary administer potassium, usually by mouth. When the patient is seriously ill, for example with auricular tachycardia, A-V block, or ventricular tachycardia, potassium chloride may be slowly infused intravenously under continuous electrocardiographic control. If kidney function is impaired intravenous potassium may be too dangerous. In such cases 250 mg phenytoin (p. 146) given slowly intravenously may control the arrhythmia. Calcium potentiates the effects of digitalis on the heart and there is some evidence that the administration of a calcium chelating agent such as disodium edetate (p. 474) may reduce the toxic effects of digitalis by lowering free serum calcium.

ANTIARRHYTHMIC AGENTS

Antiarrhythmic drugs interfere with the ionic mechanisms responsible for the cardiac action potential. As explained, the sequence of events leading to the action potential is intiated by an inward movement of Na^+. This is followed by an inward displacement of Ca^{++} beginning during the rising phase and maintained throughout the plateau phase of the action potential. Many of the known antiarrhythmic drugs including quinidine, procainamide and lignocaine act at the level of the cell membrane to reduce the inward Na current. The antiarrhythmic activity of some other drugs, such as verapamil, probably depends on their ability to reduce the inward current carried by Ca^{++}. An important group of antiarrhythmic drugs interfere with the sympathetic control of the heart by blocking the effect (propranolol) or inhibiting the release (bretylium) of the adrenergic transmitter noradrenaline. The clinically important action of digitalis glycosides in controlling the ventricular response in auricular fibrillation has already been discussed.

Quinidine

Quinidine is the dextrorotatory isomer of quinine. Wenckebach (1917) noted that when patients with malaria who had auricular fibrillation were given large doses of quinine, the fibrillation in some cases ceased. Quinidine was found more effective in producing this effect than was quinine.

The effect of quinidine on the cardiac action potential has been investigated by intracellular recording. Quinidine slows the rate of rise of the action potential and causes the tail of the repolarisation phase to be prolonged (Fig. 10.17), increasing the effective refractory period. It also increases the threshold of electrical excitability and

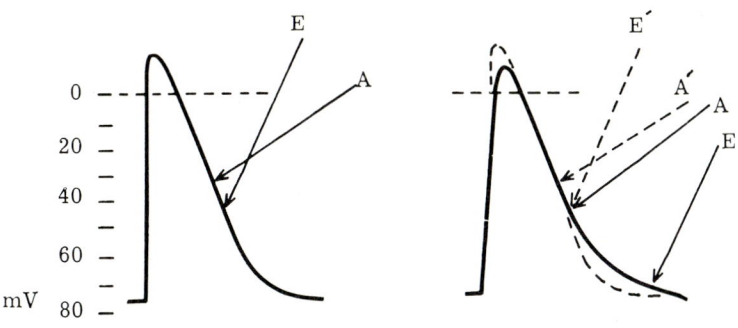

Fig. 10.17 Effect of quinidine (9 mg/kg) on cardiac intracellular potentials: left control; right after quinidine. A—absolute refractory period. E—effective refractory period. There is no change in resting potential after quinidine but the rate of rise of the action potential is slowed and the tail of repolarization prolonged. (After Vaughan Williams, 1975. In Nayler, *Contraction and Relaxation in the Myocardium*. Academic Press, London.)

slows the rate at which an excitatory stimulus is propagated.

These various actions of quinidine can be explained by an effect on the cell membrane to reduce the rate of entry of sodium. Quinidine and the pharmacologically related drug procainamide also depress the contractility of the heart. They depress automaticity, particularly in ectopic sites.

Actions of quinidine

In the normal heart the main action is a decrease in heart rate which is not abolished by atropine and which is due to a prolongation of the refractory period of the S-A node. In auricular fibrillation, quinidine produces one of two effects. It may either completely abolish fibrillation and restore normal rhythm, or it may slow the rate of fibrillation, sometimes converting it to flutter without restoring normal rhythm. Presumably in the first case the action of quinidine on the refractory period and excitability predominates and in the second case the action on conduction predominates. Interpreted in terms of the circus movement theory, the circus movement persists because the time taken for an impulse to complete a circuit remains longer than the refractory period of the muscle.

It is undesirable to slow the rate of fibrillation or flutter without restoring normal rhythm since as the number of impulses reaching the A-V node decreases, A-V conduction improves and the ventricular rate tends to rise. This may result in a dangerous tachycardia. Auricular rates around 200 are particularly dangerous, since the ventricle may then follow each auricular stimulus. The best way of preventing this is by premedication with digitalis which depresses A-V conduction more effectively than quinidine.

Figure 10.18 shows the difference between the mode of action of digitalis and quinidine. The patient received an amount of digitalis that slowed the ventricular rate to a dangerous extent and resulted in appearance of idioventricular impulses. Quinidine, however, caused the appearance of a normal rhythm.

Clinical uses of quinidine. In the past quinidine was used to convert auricular fibrillation and flutter to a normal sinus rhythm. This use has now declined because of the ready availability of DC-countershock treatment. Quinidine is however still used to maintain a normal sinus rhythm after conversion in these patients. The chief limitation of quinidine is its toxicity and in some patients with severe heart failure serious cardiovascular reactions including asystole may occur after administration of small doses of quinidine.

Procainamide (Pronestyl) (Fig. 10.19)
This compound is the amide corresponding to the ester procaine. Procaine has considerable quinidine-like activity, but its clinical usefulness is limited on account of its rapid hydrolysis by procainesterase. Procainamide is much more stable than procaine; it can be administered orally or by intravenous injection. When taken by mouth it is absorbed from the gastro-intestinal tract and most of it is excreted unchanged in the urine. The electrophysiological properties and antiarrhythmic actions of procainamide are similar to those of quinidine and the two drugs may be used interchangeably for prophylaxis and maintenance treatment. Because its half-life is relatively short oral procainamide must be given every 3-4 hours.

The chief toxic effect of procainamide is a fall of blood pressure which is due in part to a depression of heart muscle. It may also produce disturbances of intraventricular conduction and even cardiac arrest necessitating the use of an electrical pacemaker or of isoprenaline. If used for longterm treatment it may cause neutropenia and a symptom resembling disseminated lupus erythematosus.

Lignocaine (Lidocaine)
This local anaesthetic drug (p. 311) has effects on cardiac arrhythmias which differ in some respects from those of quinidine and procainamide. Although it resembles these drugs in depressing automaticity in the ventricles it differs from them in not affecting conduction velocity and failing to increase the refractory period.

146 APPLIED PHARMACOLOGY

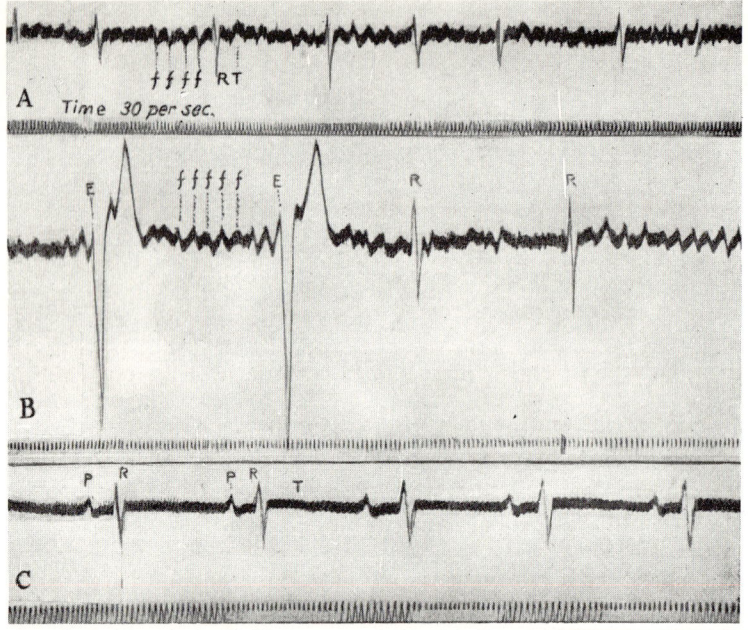

Fig. 10.18 e.c.g. records of a patient with auricular fibrillation, treated with digitalis and quinidine. **A.** Before treatment. Auricular fibrillation. Rates — auricle, 411 per minute; ventricle, 74 per minute. **B.** Effect of full digitalisation. Fibrillation rate in auricle slightly increased to 460 per minute. Ventricle slowed to 41 per minute, and idioventricular impulses (E) occurred. Digitalis stopped and quinidine given. **C.** Effect of quinidine. Normal rhythm. Rates — auricle and ventricle, 65 per minute. (Figures supplied by Professor Murray Lyon.)

Lignocaine is given by intravenous injection for the rapid control of ventricular arrythmias particularly those occurring during heart surgery and in myocardial infarction. Certain ventricular arrhythmias following myocardial infarction seem to presage ventricular fibrillation. On the detection of this, lignocaine may be given by slow intravenous injection. It is used mainly when a rapidly acting agent is required for short periods; it is of no use for the long-term treatment of auricular or ventricular arrythmias.

Lignocaine has become one of the most widely used drugs in coronary care units. It is also often employed to treat digitalis-induced ventricular arrythmias. It may produce toxic effects on the central nervous system including drowsiness, disorientation, twitching and convulsions.

Fig. 10.19 Procaine HCl and Procainamide HCl.

Phenytoin (Epanutin)
This antiepileptic drug (p. 270), which is structurally related to barbiturates, has been shown to have antiarrhythmic properties. Like quinidine and procainamide, it reduces the automaticity of ectopic pacemakers but unlike these it shortens the refractory period and enhances the conductivity of cardiac muscle.

Phenytoin is clinically effective in reversing ventricular arrhythmias, particularly when they are caused by digitalis, but has no place in the treatment of auricular fibrillation. Phenytoin can be administered orally. Its toxic effects (p. 270) include ataxia, visual disturbances and vertigo. Large initial doses may be required to achieve an effective plasma level.

Verapamil
Verapamil (Cordilox) has been shown to reduce experimentally the slow inward calcium current during the cardiac action potential. It exerts pronounced effects on cardiac rhythms including a slowing of the sinus rate and a prolongation of the P-R interval. Clinically it has been found to have antiarrhythmic properties and has been employed in the treatment of atrial flutter and other supraventricular ectopic rhythms especially those believed to involve re-entry mechanisms. There is also some evidence that verapamil reduces anginal attacks, increasing exercise tolerance. Verapamil is a dangerous drug which may cause sinus arrest, A-V block and negative inotropic effects and should be used under expert supervision.

Newer antiarrhythmic drugs

Efforts have been made to develop antiarrhythmic drugs for use in cardiac infarction with which therapeutic plasma concentrations can be achieved rapidly followed by maintenance oral administration. *Mexiletine,* which may be administered parenterally or orally has been found to control ventricular arrhythmias with dose-dependent side effects. *Ajmaline* an alkaloid obtained from Rauwolfia serpentina is effective in ventricular arrythmias and has been shown to block selectively conduction in the His-Purkinje system.

A quinidine-like drug which may be used in auricular fibrillation to maintain the beneficial effect of cardioversion is *disopyramide*. A quinidine-like drug which is well absorbed by mouth is *aprindine*.

Great progress has been made recently in methods of human intracardiac electrography by which the effects of new drugs on the different components of the specialised conducting tissue can be investigated.

Adrenergic beta-receptor blockade

Stimulation of adrenergic beta receptors either by noradrenaline released from sympathetic nerves or by circulating adrenaline increases automaticity of ectopic pacemakers by increasing the rate of diastolic depolarisation of the cardiac action potential. Conversely, drugs which reduce the activity of adrenergic receptors reduce automaticity and improve certain types of arrythmias. Two classes of adrenergic blocking drugs have been used in this context: beta adrenergic blockers such as propranolol; and adrenergic neurone blockers such as bretylium.

Propranolol (Inderal) (p. 115). The antiarrhythmic effect of propranolol can be attributed to two separate mechanisms: (1) its beta blocking effect and (2) an independent quinidine-like effect. There has been some controversy about the relative importance of these two factors but most observers agree that when small doses are used the beta blocking effect is predominant. Large doses of propranolol produce a negative inotropic effect on the heart due to the lack of sympathetic drive.

Propranolol may be given intravenously but more usually it is administered orally. It is effective in the prophylaxis and treatment of sinus tachycardias, particularly paroxysmal and exercise-induced tachycardias. It does not convert auricular fibrillation to sinus rhythm. It is generally effective in controlling excessive heart rates in hyperthyroidism (p. 334). Propranolol can be administered in conjunction with digitalis, whose vagal effect it potentiates by antagonising sympathetic stimulation. Digitalis can counteract the negative inotropic effect of propranolol whilst the latter can abolish ectopic rhythms produced by digitalis.

The main drawback of propranolol treatment is its negative inotropic action which may lead to heart failure.

Certain newer beta blockers (p. 115) may be substituted for it possessing 'intrinsic' sympathomimetic (partial agonist) activity. These compound stimulate heart muscle and may therefore be less likely to precipitate heart failure. Certain cardioselective beta blockers (p. 116) have the advantage that they are less liable to cause bronchoconstriction in asthmatic patients.

Bretylium. This adrenergic neurone blocking drug was one of the first of its class used in the treatment of hypertension (p. 118) but its use for this purpose has been abandoned because of the rapid occurrence of tachyphylaxis. Bretylium has been shown to possess antiarrhythmic properties in experimental animals, being effective in terminating ventricular fibrillation. It has been used clinically in the treatment of otherwise intractable ventricular arrhythmias.

Cardioversion

The use of electroshock treatment to convert auricular fibrillation to normal sinus rhythm is a relatively new technique employed in certain severe cardiac arrhythmias. Brief high voltage DC pulses are applied to anaesthetised patients through external electrodes fixed to the chest. The current pulses depolarise the heart muscle and in this way abolish abnormal recirculating wave patterns, allowing a normal sinus rhythm to become reestablished. If the electrical pulses are applied at a certain vulnerable point of the cardiac cycle, just before the apex of the T wave, they may precipitate ventricular fibrillation. For this reason the defibrillator is fitted with a device which turns off the current immediately after the R-wave of the electrocardiogram.

Cardioversion has been claimed to be initially successful in abolishing auricular fibrillation in 90 per cent of cases but its effect is often transient. In order to maintain the improvement, drug treatment may be combined with cardioversion. Patients with decompensated auricular fibrillation are usually digitalised prior to cardioversion, but it is advisable to stop giving digitalis 24 hours before attempting cardioversion since this seems to increase the susceptibility of the heart towards digitalis-induced arrhythmias.

Clinical uses of antiarrhythmic agents

Cardiac arrhythmias are caused by disturbances of impulse formation, or conduction, or both. The antiarrhythmic drugs depress spontaneous diastolic depolarisation thus reducing the automaticity of ectopic foci and they affect conduction by altering conduction velocity and the duration of the refractory period.

Sinus tachycardia such as occurs in thyrotoxicosis seldom requires symptomatic drug treatment, but propranolol may be useful to treat palpitations. *Sinus bradycardia* which may occur in acute myocardial infarction can sometimes be controlled by cautious doses of atropine or by temporary pacing.

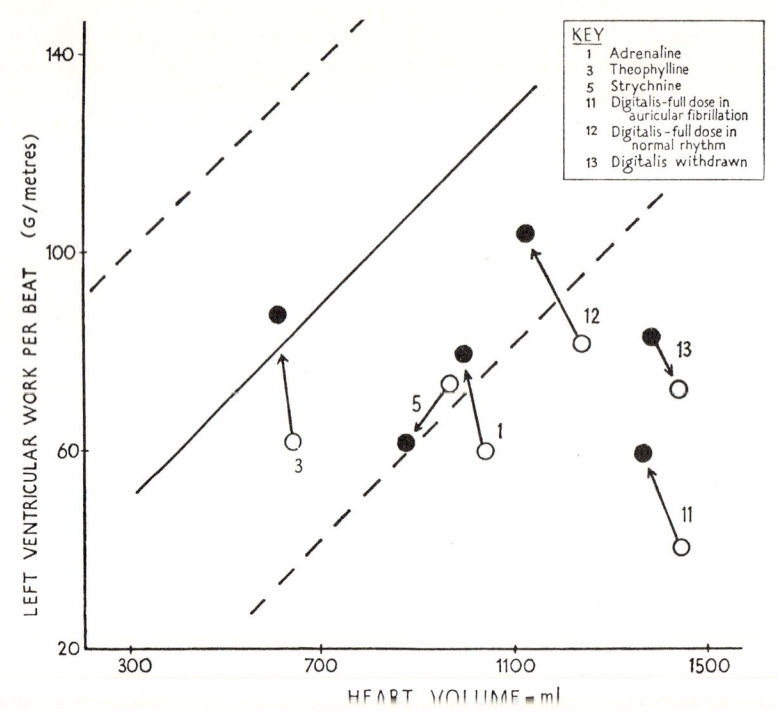

Fig. 10.20 These figures illustrate the effects of drugs on patients suffering from cardiac disease. The true cardiac stimulants increase left ventricular work without an increase in the size of the heart. Strychnine neither stimulates nor depresses the heart since the size of the ventricle is decreased in proportion to its work. (From Starr et al, 1937, *J. Clin. Invest.*)

Paroxysmal auricular tachycardia can sometimes be stopped by vagal pressure. Otherwise an anticholinesterase drug such as neostigmine or edrophonium (p. 61) may be employed to increase vagal tone. In *auricular fibrillation* or *flutter* digitalis is the drug of choice with the ultimate hope of restoring normal sinus rhythm. In some cases DC cardioversion may be necessary. In some cases propranolol may be combined with digitalis allowing a reduction of the dose of the glycoside. Frequently arrhythmias develop during cardioversion and lignocaine is used to treat ventricular arrhythmias occurring in these cases. Following cardioversion procainamide or quinidine may be given for a longer period in order to maintain normal sinus rhythm.

Ventricular tachyarrhythmias are dangerous especially in patients with coronary artery disease. Lignocaine is the drug of choice for the rapid control of ventricular premature systoles because it does not depress A-V conduction. If the condition progresses to paroxysmal ventricular tachycardia one of the following drugs may be used: lignocaine, procainamide, propranolol, quinidine, diphenylhydantoin. The latter is however, mainly used in the treatment of digitalis-induced arrhythmias. If the paroxysmal tachycardia endangers life, DC cardioversion may be attempted to convert the arrhythmia.

Ventricular flutter and *fibrillation* may be treated by immediate DC cardioversion; when the action of the heart has been restored antiarrhythmic drugs are used to prevent recurrence. Lignocaine may be infused for 2-3 days followed by oral procainamide, quinidine, propranolol or phenytoin.

CARDIAC STIMULANTS

Cardiac stimulants are drugs which increase the force of contraction of heart muscle. Their action can be assessed on the isolated heart, on the heart-lung preparation, and on the intact circulation. Starr and his co-workers have used diagrams as shown in Figure 10.20 to illustrate the effect of a drug in producing cardiac stimulation or depression in intact man. In these diagrams the work of the heart, as estimated from the cardiac output and the peripheral resistance, is plotted against the volume of the heart determined from X-ray pictures. The dotted lines indicate the probable range of normal values obtained from several hundred determinations. Applying Starling's concept, a heart is said to be stimulated when the work per beat of the heart for a given diastolic size is increased, and is said to be depressed when the reverse occurs. Accordingly when a drug stimulates the heart the position in the diagram shifts upward or to the left; when it depresses, it moves downward or to the right. Movement along a diagonal line implies neither stimulation nor depression. Amongst many drugs tested in this way it was found that adrenaline, digitalis and theophylline were true stimulants when administered in therapeutic doses. This is shown in Figure 10.20, which also shows that strychnine is not a cardiac stimulant.

Aminophylline (theophylline ethylenediamine)
This may be given intravenously, or by mouth. It is irritating to the gastro-intestinal tract and when given intravenously must be injected slowly since it produces powerful stimulation of the heart, which may be fatal. It is most effective when given by intravenous injection in acute attacks of cardiac dyspnoea, where it produces an abrupt fall in venous and intrathecal pressure, reduction of pulmonary oedema and improvement in respiration. The fall in venous pressure results from peripheral vasodilatation of capillaries and venules, and improved cardiac output due to coronary vasodilatation and direct stimulation of heart muscle. Compared with digoxin the action of aminophylline is more rapid but less persistent and it tends to accelerate rather than slow the heart by stimulating the pacemaker. Caffeine has a similar but weaker action on the heart.

Adrenaline
Adrenaline is a true cardiac stimulant, but its action is very transient. In acute poisoning by cardiac depressants it stimulates the heart temporarily, raises the blood pressure and thus restores coronary circulation. It may be of value to start a heart beat in cases of sudden emergency such as drowning. Intravenous injections are dangerous and may produce acute cardiac dilatation, pulmonary oedema and ventricular fibrillation.

Isoprenaline
Isoprenaline may be used to stimulate cardiac automaticity in partial or complete heart block by its effects on beta adrenergic receptors in the heart. It has the advantage over adrenaline that it does not raise the systemic blood pressure and can be administered sublingually; it can also be given by mouth as a sustained release preparation which is effective for about eight hours. A disadvantage of isoprenaline in cardiogenic shock is its failure to increase coronary perfusion pressure.

Isoprenaline may benefit patients by either overcoming a conduction block or by accelerating an ectopic ventricular pacemaker even though the conduction block persists. In cases of cardiac arrest it is seldom possible, without an electrocardiogram, to distinguish between ventricular asystole and ventricular fibrillation. Isoprenaline is most likely to be effective in the former case; ventricular fibrillation can generally only be effectively treated by an electrical defibrillator.

Dopamine
Dopamine (p. 82), the third cardioactive endogenous catecholamine, has so far been used only experimentally in man. In a direct comparison between dopamine and isoprenaline in patients after coronary bypass surgery both drugs increased cardiac output in a dose-dependent fashion, but isoprenaline achieved this partly at least by an increased heart rate, whereas dopamine did not affect the heart rate increasing cardiac output entirely by increased stroke volume. *Dobutamine* is a synthetic sympathomimetic amine with a dopamine-like action. It produces an inotropic effect with little or no increase in heart rate and has been used with some success in patients with severe congestive heart failure.

PREPARATIONS

Cardiac glycosides
Deslanoside (Cedinalid) 0.8–1.2 mg i.v. initially
Digitoxin 1–1.5 mg rapid digitalisation; 50–200 μg (microgram) daily maintenance
Digoxin 1–1.5 mg rapid digitalisation; 250–750 μg daily maintenance
Lanatoside C 1–1.5 mg po daily
Medigoxin (Lanitop inj); 300 μg medigoxin = 500 μg digoxin

Antiarrhythmic drugs
Aprindine Hyd 200 mg init; 100–150 mg daily aftw
Beta blockers see Ch. 9
Bretylium Tosylate 5 mg/kg i.m.
Disopyramide (Rythmodan) 300 mg, then 150 mg six hourly
Lignocaine Hyd (Lidocaine, Xylocaine) 50–100 mg by slow i.v. inj
Mexiletine Hyd 100–250 mg by slow i.v. inj
Phenytoin Sodium 5 mg/kg by slow i.v. inj
Procainamide Hyd (Pronestyl) 250 mg — 1 g per os; durules 500 mg slow release
Quinidine Sulph prophyl 200 mg 3–4 x daily; treatment 200–400 mg 2–4 hourly
Verapamil Hyd (Cordilox) 40–80 mg

Cardiac stimulants
Adrenaline Injection (1:1000) 0.2–0.5 sc
Aminophylline Ch. 12
Dobutamine Hyd
Isoprenaline 0.5–10 μg/min infusion

FURTHER READING

Baumgarten G 1963 Die herzwirksamen glycoside. Thieme, Leipzig
Braunwald E, Ross J, Sonnenblick E H 1967 Mechanisms of contraction of the normal and failing heart. Churchill, London
Castellanos A, Lemberg L 1969 Electrophysiology of pacing and cardioversion. Butterworth, London
Chung K 1969 Digitalis intoxication. Excerpta Medica, Amsterdam
Dreifus L S, Likoff W (ed) 1973 Cardiac arrhythmias. Grune and Stratton, New York
Fisch C, Surawicz B (ed) 1969 Digitalis. Grune and Stratton, New York
Glynn J M 1964 The action of cardiac glycosides on ion movements. Pharmac. Rev. 16: 381
Gold H 1948 Digitalis. J. Am. med. Ass. 136: 1027
Hamer J (ed) 1979 Drugs for heart disease. Chapman Hall, London

Julian D G 1978 Cardiology. In: Progress in clinical medicine. Churchill Livingstone, Edinburgh

Krikler D M, Goodwin J F (ed) 1975 Cardiac arrhythmias. Saunders, London

Mason D T, Spann J F, Zelis R 1970 The clinical pharmacological and therapeutic applications of the antiarrhythmic drugs. Pharmac. Therap. 11: 460

Nayler Winifred G (ed) Contraction and relaxation in the myocardium. Academic Press, London

Rushmer R F 1976 Cardiovascular dynamics. Saunders, Philadelphia

Starling E H 1918 The law of the heart (Linacre Lecture, 1915). Longmans Green, London

Stock J P P, Williams D O 1974 Diagnosis and treatment of cardiac arrhythmias. Butterworth, London

Stoll A 1959 Cardiovascular glycosides. J. Pharmac. 7: 849

Trautwein W 1963 Generation and conduction of impulses in the heart as affected by drugs. Pharmac. Rev. 15: 277

Watanabe Y, Dreifus L S Cardiac arrhythmias. Electrophysiological basis for clinical interpretation. Grune and Stratton, New York

11. The kidneys

Functions of the kidney 151; Urinary clearance 153; Excretion of drugs 154; Hormonal control 155; Reabsorption of sodium bicarbonate 157; Diuretic drugs 158; Reabsorption and excretion of sodium, potassium and water 158; Thiazide diuretics 160; Mercurials 161; Frusemide 162; Ethacrynic acid 162; Spironolactone 163; Triamterene 163; Forced alkaline diuresis 164; Choice of diuretic 165; Drugs in radioscopy 166.

FUNCTIONS OF THE KIDNEY

The kidneys are the chief organs that excrete nonvolatile substances from the body, whilst the lungs excrete all volatile substances. The only channels, other than the kidneys, through which non-volatile substances are excreted are the liver and intestine which excrete a limited number of substances, such as bile pigments, heavy metals and morphine. The glands of the bronchial tract and the stomach, and the salivary glands, in addition to excreting chlorides also excrete iodides and bromides, whilst the skin can excrete large quantities of water and sodium chloride as sweat. With these chief exceptions, the body is dependent upon the kidneys for the removal of all end products of metabolism and of all substances absorbed from the alimentary canal that cannot be metabolised and are not needed by the body.

The normal kidney is impermeable to large molecular substances and hence does not normally excrete blood proteins or substances such as dextran when these are introduced into the blood stream.

The chief functions of the kidneys are as follows:

1. The maintenance of the osmotic pressure of the blood at a constant level. This is effected chiefly by the excretion of varying quantities of water.

2. The maintenance of the alkaline reserve of the blood by the excretion of any non-volatile acids formed in metabolism and by the formation of ammonia to neutralise excess acid.

3. The excretion of the whole of the waste products of nitrogenous metabolism, and in particular the excretion of urea and uric acid.

4. The excretion of the inorganic constituents of the food which are not required by the body, and of those organic constituents that are not needed and cannot be metabolised.

The kidneys, therefore, may be considered as the organs chiefly responsible for keeping constant from day to day the composition of the body as a whole and of the blood in particular.

Work done by the kidneys

The kidneys must not be regarded as filters, but as chemical works. They perform a large amount of work in altering the concentrations of solutions, although this is not so obvious as is the work of an organ such as the heart, which produces movement.

The kidneys in the production of this work consume about as much oxygen per gram weight as does the heart. The average oxygen consumption of the whole body of a dog at rest is 0.01 ml per gram per minute, and that of the dog's heart is 0.05 ml per gram per minute, whilst the oxygen consumption of the kidney of the rabbit during normal activity is 0.05 ml per gram per minute. Barcroft and Brodie calculated that during diuresis the dog's kidneys used 11 per cent of the total oxygen consumed in the body. This large oxygen consumption is rendered possible by an abundant blood supply. The blood flow through the human kidneys is about 1.3 litres per minute. The output of the heart during bodily rest is about 5 litres per minute, and therefore about one-quarter of the cardiac output passes through the kidneys.

These figures are of fundamental importance, because they emphasise the fact that the kidney, like the heart, is entirely dependent upon an abundant oxygen supply for the maintenance of its normal functions.

STRUCTURE OF THE KIDNEY

The renal unit, which is shown in Figure 11.1, consists of a glomerulus connected to a tubule some 2 or 3 cm long, which leads to a collecting tubule. Each tubule consists of a proximal segment of irregular epithelial cells which immediately joins the glomerulus and has the largest diameter; an intermediate thin segment, consisting of flat cells, and a distal segment with regular columnar epithelial cells (Fig. 11.2). Each human kidney contains about a million of these units. Hence the total length of tubules in the two kidneys is about 60 kilometres, whilst the total surface of the glomerular membranes is more than 2 square metres. These figures are only approximations, but they indicate the remarkable complexity of the mechanism that is packed within the kidneys.

Mechanism of kidney function

The functions of the kidney are very complex and the mechanisms involved are only partially understood. The activities of the kidney can most easily be understood if it be remembered that besides being an organ of excretion it also is an organ of retention. Its task is to clear the body of unwanted substances without losing any substances of value to the body.

152   APPLIED PHARMACOLOGY

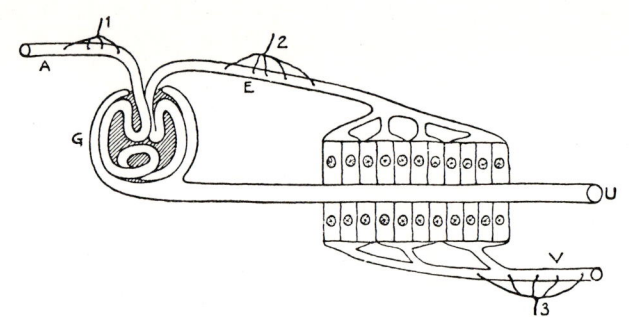

Fig. 11.1 Diagram of renal unit. A—Vas afferens of glomerulus. E—Vas efferens passing from glomerulus to tubule. G—Glomerulus. U—Tubule passing toward ureter. V—Venule. The possible sites at which the sympathetic vasoconstrictors may exert their action are marked 1, 2 and 3. (After Verney, 1928.)

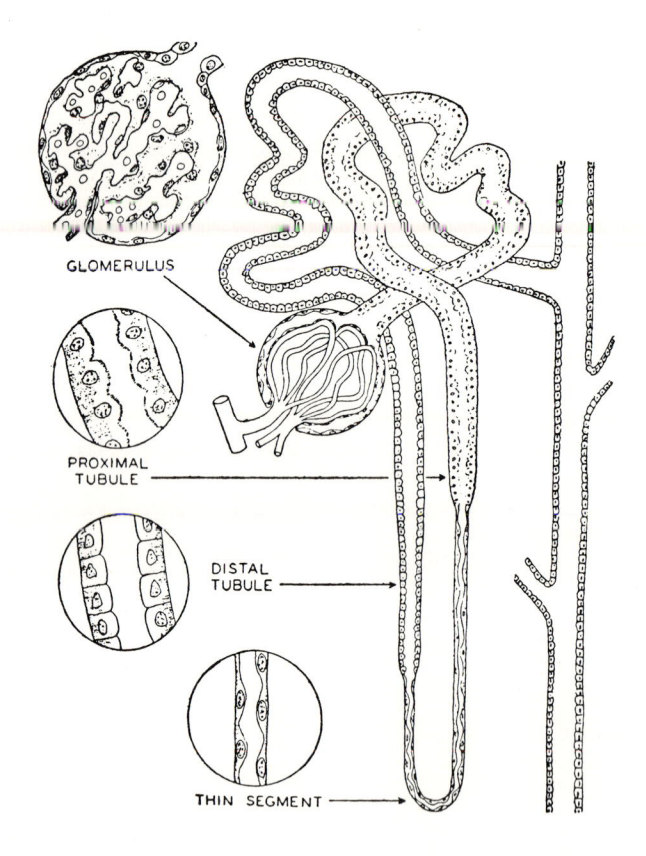

Fig. 11.2 Diagrammatic representation of a human nephron. (After Homer Smith, 1937. *The Physiology of the Kidney*.)

The basic mechanism of excretion is the filtration by the glomerulus of a colloid-free ultrafiltrate and the elaboration of this filtrate by the tubules. The most striking feature of this elaboration is the reabsorption of about 99 per cent of the water and sodium chloride, and the whole of the glucose in the filtrate.

According to current theories the glomeruli of the human kidneys filter 130 ml/min of fluid, which is about one-sixth of the volume of the plasma passing through them. The tubules reabsorb 129 ml/min of this fluid. The normal daily activity of the kidneys is indicated by figures in Table 11.1.

Table 11.1

	Quantities in 24 hours		
	Filtered by glomeruli	Reabsorbed by tubules	Excreted in urine
Water (litres)	185	183.5	1.5
Sodium chloride (g)	1200	1185	15
Sodium bicarbonate (g)	400	400	—
Glucose (g)	185	185	—
Urea (g)	44	14	30
Creatinine (g)	1.7	0	1.7

These figures, even though they are not exact, indicate the scale of the activity of the kidneys.

The power of the kidneys to excrete foreign substances is shown by the following examples. When phenol red passes through the kidney about half of the dye is removed and excreted. In this case a fraction of the dye remains in the plasma, but some iodised contrast agents are almost completely removed after a single passage through the kidney.

Renal tubular function

Cushny put forward the hypothesis that the plasma constituents could be divided into nonthreshold and threshold substances. According to this hypothesis the whole of the nonthreshold substances are excreted, but the tubules reabsorb the threshold substances in such a manner that the reabsorbed fluid contains them in the same concentration as they occur in normal plasma; hence only the excess of the threshold substances are excreted.

Cushny's hypothesis had the great merit of emphasising the fact that renal excretion is so arranged that its effect is to maintain constant the composition of the *milieu intérieur*, but it provided an oversimplified picture of the activities of the kidney. It is now known that the tubules can reabsorb the different constituents of urine independently of each other. For example, glucose, phosphate and sulphate are reabsorbed from the proximal convoluted tubules by interrelated active processes. Normally these constituents are removed completely from the tubular urine but there is a limiting rate for the active reabsorption of each. Approximately 80 per cent of the sodium chloride and water content of the glomerular filtrate is also reabsorbed from the proximal tubule.

The ultimate composition of the urine is determined in Henle's loop and the distal tubule from which further absorption of water and sodium occurs. The reabsorption of sodium ions in the distal tubule is mainly controlled by aldosterone and involves a coupled exchange of sodium from the urine for hydrogen or potassium ions from the tubular cells. Water reabsorption occurs in Henle's loop and the distal tubule and is facilitated by the antidiuretic hormone (ADH), in the absence of which reabsorption is reduced and the urine flow greatly increased.

The tubules can also secrete certain substances, for example penicillin, para-aminohippurate, many quaternary ammonium compounds and the iodine-containing contrast agents such as diodone (diodrast). The speed of excretion of these substances can only be explained on the assumption that they are secreted by the tubules.

If the principle of tubular secretion is accepted as a possibility, the excretion of any substance in urine can be explained either by filtration plus reabsorption, or by tubular secretion, or by a combination of these processes. If, however, the rate at which a substance is filtered through the glomeruli is known, then the rate of excretion in excess of this must be due to the action of tubular secretion. The yardstick which gives a measure of the glomerular filtration rate is provided by the inulin clearance.

The urinary clearance

The urinary clearance of a substance is a measure of its rate of removal from the plasma by the kidneys and may be defined as the volume of plasma virtually cleared of the substance in 1 minute. Clearance is expressed as ml per minute and is computed by dividing the quantity of substance excreted in the urine in 1 minute by the quantity contained in 1 ml of plasma.

The urinary clearance of a substance depends on its method of excretion. Shannon and Homer Smith showed that inulin, a polysaccharide with a molecular weight of about 6000 is filtered through the glomeruli but is neither reabsorbed nor secreted by the tubules of a normal human kidney. Hence its clearance is a measure of the rate of formation of the glomerular filtrate. In man the inulin clearance by the two kidneys is approximately 130 ml per minute.

The clearance of most other constituents of plasma is less than the inulin clearance because they are partly reabsorbed and returned to the bloodstream. For example, the clearance of urea in man is only about two-thirds of the inulin clearance and the clearance of sodium and chloride is usually only a small fraction of the inulin clearance. The normal clearance of glucose is zero because it is completely reabsorbed by the tubules unless its concentration in the plasma is abnormally high.

The clearance of those constituents of plasma, however, which are excreted by the tubules is usually higher than the inulin clearance. For example, the clearance of diodone (diodrast) is about 800 ml per minute. It appears that this substance is completely removed from the plasma in a single passage through the kidney, hence the volume of plasma cleared of diodrast in 1 minute corresponds to the total flow of plasma through the kidneys during that period. A plasma flow of 800 ml corresponds to a flow of approximately 1.3 litres of blood through the kidneys each minute. Figure 11.3 is a diagrammatic representation of the way in which the kidney is believed to excrete these substances.

The amazing flexibility of the kidneys' activities is perhaps best illustrated by their power to excrete water. They can excrete water at a rate of 750 ml per hour, which is equal to the maximum rate at which water can be absorbed from the gut. On the other hand, in a desert climate the urinary secretion may fall to 15 ml an hour and the kidneys manage to get rid of the waste products in this small volume.

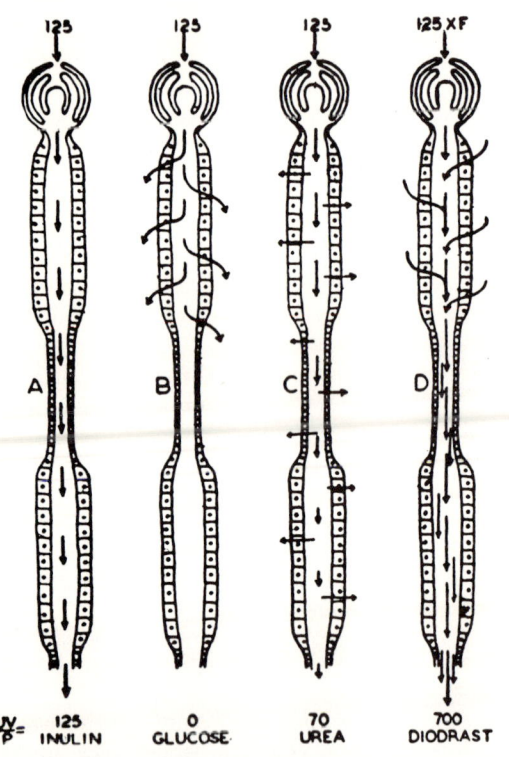

Fig. 11.3 Scheme to illustrate the excretion of (A) inulin, which is excreted solely by filtration with no tubular reabsorption; (B) glucose, which is filtered, but at normal plasma level and rate of filtration is completely reabsorbed by the tubule; (C) urea, which is filtered, but in part escapes from the tubular urine by diffusion; (D) diodrast, which is excreted both by filtration and tubular excretion. UV/P is the clearance in each instance, i.e. the virtual volume of blood cleared per minute. (U and P are the concentrations per unit volume of urine and plasma, and V is urine flow per minute.) The inulin clearance is taken as equal to the rate of filtration of plasma. F is the fraction of diodrast filterable from the plasma; 1−F being the fraction bound to plasma proteins. (After Homer Smith, 1943. *Lectures on the Kidney*.)

These variations in urine volume are not so surprising when the volume of the glomerular filtrate (7.8 litres per hour) is considered. The normal urine volume is 0.8 per cent of the glomerular filtrate, whilst the volumes in extreme diuresis and in dehydration are respectively 10.2 and 0.2 per cent.

In order to effect these concentrations the kidney tubules must work against very large osmotic pressures.

The osmotic pressure of the blood is about seven atmospheres, or 100 pounds to the square inch, which corresponds to a depression of freezing point $\Delta = -0.56°C$. The kidney can, however, secrete urine at concentrations ranging from $\Delta = -0.08°C$ to $\Delta = -3.2°C$. In the latter case the concentration must be effected against a pressure of about 28 atmospheres.

Excretion of drugs by the kidney

Since drugs are abnormal constituents of the body they might be expected to be filtered through the glomeruli and not be reabsorbed in the tubules. Careful search has been made for substances which show this behaviour, and they are extremely rare. Sulphathiazole is believed to fulfil these conditions and its clearance is therefore similar to that of inulin, but the great majority of drugs are extensively reabsorbed by the tubules.

Penicillin is actively secreted by the tubules and its clearance may approach that of diodone. The secretion of penicillin by the tubules may be inhibited by probenecid which also inhibits tubular secretion of sodium para-aminohippurate. It is believed that this substance interferes with specific enzymes involved in the secretion of penicillin and *p*-aminohippurate by the tubules. Another remarkable action of probenecid is that it increases the urinary clearance of uric acid by inhibiting the reabsorption of uric acid by the tubules (p. 292). For this reason probenecid is used for the treatment of chronic gout. It would seem that the enzymes involved in the reabsorption of uric acid by the tubules are closely related to those concerned with the secretion of penicillin and *p*-aminohippurate (p. 45).

A number of quaternary ammonium compounds, for example tetraethylammonium, N-methylnicotinamide and neostigmine are also actively secreted by the tubules. The mechanism of renal transport of these substances is different from that involved in the secretion of penicillin; they are not inhibited by probenecid, but are effectively blocked by a variety of quaternary ammonium compounds.

When weak bases are excreted in the urine their rate of excretion may vary according to the pH of the urine. Figure 11.4 shows the excretion of pethidine and its degradation product norpethidine by the kidneys after an intramuscular injection of 100 mg of pethidine. It shows that these amines are excreted much more rapidly in acid than in alkaline urine.

The mechanisms of excretion of drugs by the kidneys and the effect of pH upon their rate of excretion are discussed in more detail on page 44.

Nephrotoxic effects of drugs

During excretion drugs may damage the kidney particularly when they are taken for a long time. Phenacetin, one of the antipyretic analgesic drugs has been

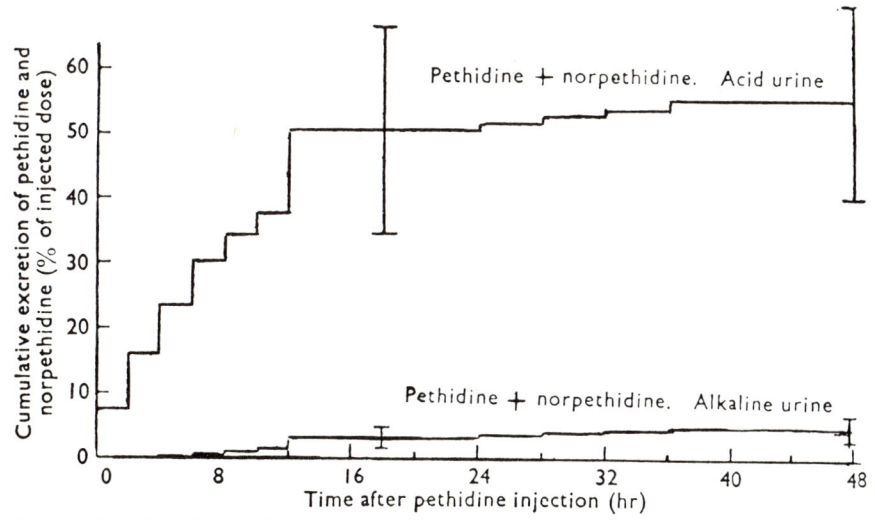

Fig. 11.4 Cumulative excretion of pethidine and norpethidine in highly acid urine and in alkaline urine during 48 hr period after injection of 100 mg of pethidine hydrochloride. Each line gives the means of results from six normal subjects. The vertical lines give the standard deviations. (After Milne, 1963, Brit. J. Pharmacol.)

shown to produce interstitial nephritis and renal papillary necrosis when used continuously and in large amounts (p. 291). The mechanism of this action is not understood.

There is some evidence that other drugs including some widely used antipyretic analgesics can damage the kidney.

HORMONAL CONTROL

There is good evidence that the rate of urine excretion is influenced by hormones secreted both by the posterior pituitary gland and by the adrenal cortex. If the nerve tract from the hypothalamus to the posterior pituitary gland be severed, a condition akin to diabetes insipidus develops. Under these conditions, injection of vasopressin in very small amounts produces a remarkable diminution in urine volume. A similar but less spectacular effect can be produced in the normal subject when water diuresis is produced by drinking one or two pints of water. In this case administration of vasopressin inhibits the diuresis.

Verney and his co-workers have shown that when small amounts of hypertonic solutions of sodium chloride or dextrose are injected into the carotid artery of the dog, they cause a temporary inhibition of water diuresis (Fig. 11.5) which is abolished by removal of the posterior pituitary gland. It appears that these effects are due to the stimulation of specific osmo-receptors which control the secretion of antidiuretic hormone which acts directly on the kidney, promoting the reabsorption of water. The effect of the antidiuretic hormone is thus to counterbalance the original increase in osmotic pressure of the blood.

If the whole pituitary gland is removed, the state of diabetes insipidus is not induced because the lack of posterior pituitary hormone is balanced by lack of adrenal cortical secretion due to the absence of stimulation from the anterior pituitary (adrenocorticotrophin). A large rate of urine flow cannot be attained in the absence of the adrenal glands and even partial destruction, as in Addison's disease, renders the subject easily liable to water intoxication.

Adrenal cortical insufficiency
Adrenal cortical insufficiency results in a profound disturbance of renal function. There is a failure to retain sodium, a reduction of plasma volume and a consequent lowering of the glomerular filtration rate: at the same time there is a retention of nitrogen and potassium. These disturbances are due to a deficiency of the naturally occurring mineralocorticoid hormone aldosterone and they can be corrected by the administration of deoxycortone acetate (DOCA) or fludrocortisone (fluorohydrocortisone) (p. 345).

Another feature of adrenal cortical insufficiency is a delay in excreting a water load. When normal subjects are given water to drink they excrete most of it within two hours, but in patients with Addison's disease this reponse is delayed. The ability to excrete water rapidly is restored by the administration of cortisone, hydrocortisone or cortrophin (ACTH) but not by aldosterone.

Diabetes insipidus
This is characterised by thirst, weakness and loss of weight and by the daily excretion of large volumes of urine of low

156 APPLIED PHARMACOLOGY

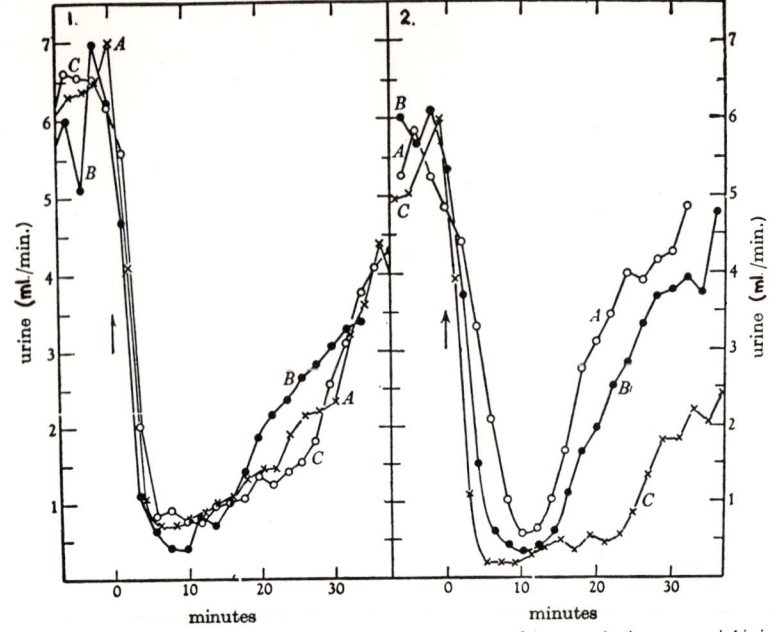

Fig. 11.5 The anti-diuretic effects of hypertonic solutions of sodium chloride and of dextrose by intra-arterial injection. The observations were carried out in the unanaesthetised dog and the test dose of water was given approximately 45 minutes before zero. 1 shows the effects on urine flow of three solutions each calculated to produce about the same increase in osmotic pressure; A and C = sodium chloride; B = dextrose. The anti-diuretic responses are very similar and are compared in 2 with the responses produced by intravenous injections of posterior pituitary extract. A = 1 milliunit (mU), B = 2 mU, and C = 3 mU. The injections of sodium chloride and of dextrose produced a release of anti-diuretic hormone equivalent to 2.5 mU. (After Verney, 1947.)

specific gravity. The urine does not contain sugar. In the treatment of this disease vasopressin (p. 329) is given by subcutaneous injection; vasopressin tannate in oil (pitressin tannate) is designed to delay and prolong the absorption of the antidiuretic factor. Another form of administration is a nasal snuff of vasopressin which is absorbed from the nasal mucous membrane.

Figure 11.6 shows the satisfactory effects of such treatment in a case of diabetes insipidus.

A synthetic analogue of vasopressin with stronger antidiuretic activity has recently been introduced. This analogue, *1-desamino-8-D-arginine vasopressin (DDAVP, desmopressin)*, is a highly selective antidiuretic agent with little vasopressor and oxytocic activity. It has a prolonged action, a single intranasal dose producing antidiuresis lasting 20 hours.

THE pH OF URINE

The kidneys assist the respiratory centre in maintaining the neutrality and the alkaline reserve or buffer power of the blood and excrete daily an amount of acid corresponding to 20 to 50 ml of normal acid. The quantity of acid is insignificant when compared to the quantities of acid excreted by the lungs as carbon dioxide, since these

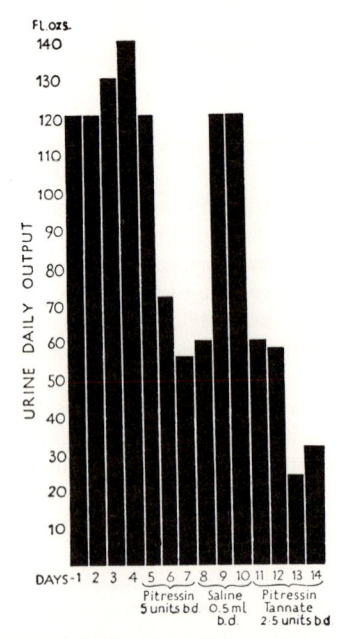

Fig. 11.6 The effect of posterior pituitary extract on the daily output of urine in a patient with diabetes insipidus. The figure shows the effects of subcutaneous injections of vasopressin (pitressin), compared with half the dose of pitressin tannate in oil. A control observation was made with normal saline.

excrete about 1500 G of CO_2 daily, but the acid secreted by the kidneys is non-volatile acid that cannot be excreted by the lungs, and if it were retained in the body it would rapidly exhaust the alkaline reserve of the blood.

The reaction of the urine ranges from pH 4.8 to 8 but normally the urine is considerably more acid than the blood. There are three mechanisms by which the kidneys maintain the alkali reserve of the blood and regulate the pH of the urine (Fig. 11.7). Each of these mechanisms depends fundamentally on an exchange of hydrogen ions formed in the tubular cell with sodium ions present in the tubular urine.

Reabsorption of sodium bicarbonate
The mechanism of reabsorption of bicarbonate-bound base has been investigated by Pitts and his colleagues and is illustrated in Figure 11.7a. An essential link in this process is the formation of carbonic acid from carbon dioxide within the tubular cell through the catalytic action of carbonic anhydrase. The carbonic acid subsequently dissociates to yield hydrogen ions which are exchanged for bicarbonate-bound sodium from the tubular urine. The sodium bicarbonate thus formed within the tubular cell is returned to the blood whilst the unstable carbonic acid formed in the tubular urine is broken down to water and carbon dioxide which then diffuses back across the tubule into the blood. The net result of this process is the conservation of sodium bicarbonate which under normal conditions is completely reabsorbed from the tubular urine. However, when the amount of sodium bicarbonate in the urine is excessive, it is not completely reabsorbed and the urine becomes alkaline.

Phosphate buffer system
The pH of the urine is mainly controlled by phosphate buffers. The glomerular filtrate which has a pH of about 7.4 contains mainly dibasic phosphate which is transformed into the acid mono basic form as the urine flows along the renal tubules. This transformation also depends on the exchange of hydrogen ions for sodium ions and thus on the carbonic anhydrase system (Fig. 11.7b). Since the rate of formation of carbonic acid by carbonic anhydrase depends on the tension of carbon dioxide in the blood a delicate mechanism is provided for the preservation of the carbon dioxide-bicarbonate ratio which determines the pH of the blood.

Formation of ammonia
A third mechanism for the conservation of sodium and elimination of excess chloride consists in substituting ammonium ions for sodium ions during the excretion of neutral salts. As shown in Figure 11.7c the interaction of hydrogen ions formed in the tubular cell with chloride ions in tubular urine would result in the formation of hydrochloric acid. The kidney however cannot excrete free hydrochloric acid since it is unable to tolerate a urinary pH below about 4.5. It protects itself against a more acid pH by forming ammonia from amino acids. The ammonia reacts with the hydrochloric acid, and the ammonium chloride thus produced is excreted in the urine.

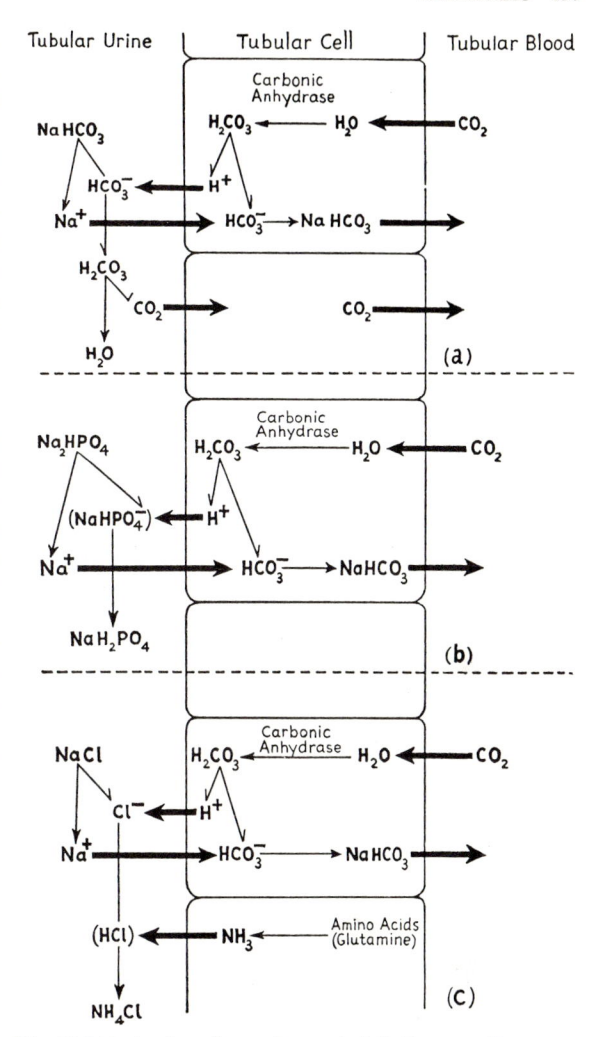

Fig. 11.7 Mechanisms for renal control of alkali reserve. See text. (After Pitts, 1953, *Harvey Lectures*.)

Change of pH of urine
The urine can be rendered alkaline by administering sodium or potassium citrate, or any other harmless salt that is oxidised in the body to form bicarbonates. The quantity required to render the urine alkaline is about 10 g a day. The administration of acid sodium phosphate in doses of 6 g per day turns an alkaline urine acid, although this dosage does not produce any certain increase in the acidity of most normal urines. Ammonium chloride has a more powerful effect and in doses of 5 g a day will reduce the reaction of the urine to about pH 5.3 (orange colour with methyl red).

The drug is capable of producing greater acidity if continued, but at the same time is liable to produce renal irritation and haematuria, hence the administration of ammonium chloride must be reduced when the urinary pH falls to 5.3. By the use of a ketogenic diet it is possible to alter the urinary pH to slightly below 5 without producing renal irritation.

The pH of the urine can therefore be controlled, and by the administration of suitable drugs can be changed from acid to alkaline, or *vice versa*, in 1 or 2 days. The extreme range of reaction that can be produced is from pH 5 to 8.5 or possibly 9.

DIURETIC DRUGS

All substances that increase urine flow may be classed as diuretics, and in this sense water itself is the foremost diuretic agent. Since, however, the main purpose of using diuretics is to promote the excretion of water, it is customary to restrict the use of the term diuretic to those substances which induce a net loss of water from the body. From a therapeutic point of view diuretics can be defined as compounds which remove excess extracellular water in disease; it is however customary to exclude substances such as digitalis which have no diuretic action in the normal kidney but promote urine flow in heart failure by improving the circulation.

Drugs may influence the excretion of water by the kidney in two ways, by increasing glomerular filtration or by diminishing reabsorption of water in the tubules. The latter appears to be the chief mechanism by which most diuretics act, but it is often difficult to assess the relative importance of the glomerular and tubular factors. For example, theophylline may produce a 15 per cent increase in filtration rate and this corresponds to an extra litre of water filtered by the glomeruli in one hour. There is also evidence that theophylline depresses tubular reabsorption, and it cannot be estimated how much of the increased urine output is due to the increase in glomerular filtrate and how much is due to specific inhibition of tubular reabsorption. It must be concluded, therefore, that theophylline is both a glomerular and tubular diuretic.

Evaluation of diuretics

The evaluation of diuretic drugs, as with all drugs used clinically, must take into account their toxicity as well as their pharmacological activity. Since treatment with diuretics may continue for long periods, it is necessary to test such drugs not only for their acute toxicity but also for the occurrence of renal and other types of tissue damage after chronic administration. The activity of diuretics can be assessed experimentally in rats. The animals are given a dose of water by stomach tube equivalent to 5 per cent of their body weight and the time taken to reach a maximum rate of water excretion is determined. This method can be used for the quantitative comparison of diuretic activity by administering to groups of rats two different drugs each at two or more dose levels.

Diuretic drugs can also be assayed in man; a simple method is to record the loss in body weight produced in patients with cardiac oedema. This method can be used as a quantitative assay by comparing the effects of two diuretics at more than one dose level.

The full clinical evaluation of a diuretic involves also the assessment of other factors such as tolerance after repeated use and the occurrence of toxic effects which may become evident only after prolonged administration.

Efficacy and potency of diuretics. It is necessary to distinguish between the efficacy of diuretics and their relative activities or potencies which is simply the ratio of doses producing the same effect. Gold and his colleagues measured the activity of diuretics in terms of the weight loss obtained in oedematous patients, but since the effect of diuretics depends on their dose, the term *efficacy* in relation to diuretics has come to mean the maximal effect which may be obtained by increasing dosage. In this sense efficacy can be measured in experimental animals, in normal man and in patients.

Efficacy of a diuretic varies according to the parameter by which it is assessed, whether the effect is measured by excretion of sodium, excretion of water or weight loss. It also depends on the duration of the urine collection periods; thus short collection periods will enhance the apparent efficacy of short acting drugs and long collection periods that of long acting drugs. Relative efficacy is thus difficult to assess and the main importance of the concept derives from the fact that certain diuretics have outstanding efficacy when measured by various criteria. Thus all the thiazide derivatives produce approximately the same ceiling effects but frusemide has a much greater ceiling effect whether this is measured under experimental or clinical conditions. Before discussing individual diuretics it is necessary to consider the ways in which sodium excretion is regulated by the kidney.

Reabsorption and excretion of sodium, potassium and water

The process of reabsorption of sodium by the tubules, which affects 99 per cent of sodium filtered through the glomeruli, can be divided into several phases. About 80 to 85 per cent of sodium is reabsorbed in the proximal tubules along with chloride, bicarbonate and water. This process is iso-osmotic; both the fluid which is reabsorbed and that remaining in the tubular lumen have the same osmotic pressure as the plasma. During the next stage the urinary filtrate enters the loop of Henle situated in the renal medulla. Whilst traversing Henle's loop the urine undergoes a remarkable series of concentration and dilution changes shown in Figure 11.8.

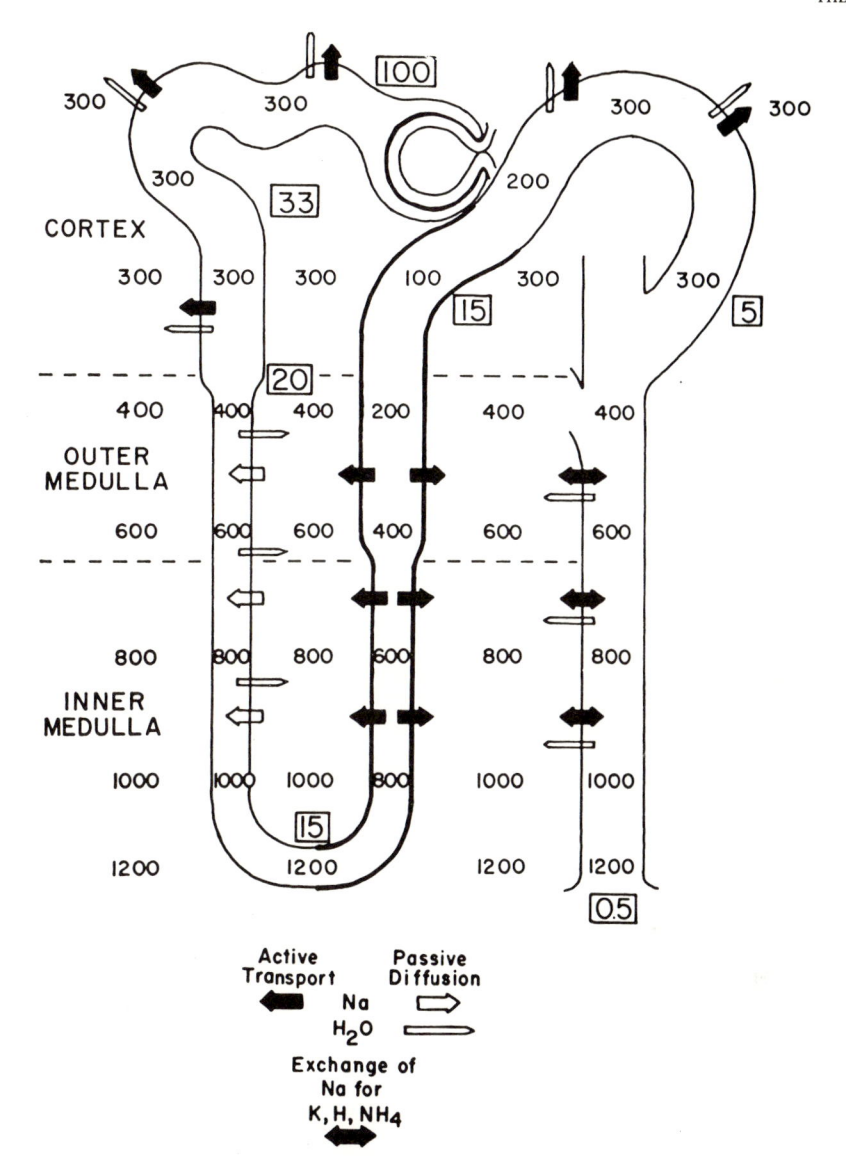

Fig. 11.8 Exchanges of water and ions in the nephron. Concentrations of tubular urine and peritubular fluid in mosmol/l; large, boxed numerals: estimated per cent of glomerular filtrate remaining within the tubule at each level. (After Pitts, 1968, *Physiology of the Kidney and Body Fluids.* Year Book Med. Publ., Chicago.)

The concentration changes in Henle's loop are believed to be due to a countercurrent multiplication effect by virtue of which the filtrate at the bottom of the hairpin pool becomes greatly concentrated, changing from its iso-osmotic level of 300 to 1200 mosmol/l whilst water is abstracted from the filtrate into the hypertonic surroundings. The urine becomes again diluted in the ascending loop of Henle by sodium chloride extrusion which results in the appearance of a hypotonic urine in the distal tubule. (There is now some doubt whether the actively reabsorbed ionic species at this site is the sodium ion (Fig. 11.8) or, as suggested by more recent work, the chloride ion.) In the distal nephron, consisting of the distal convoluted tubule and collecting duct, the filtrate undergoes further profound transformation which determines largely the ultimate composition of the urine. At this stage more sodium and water are reabsorbed. Sodium reabsorption is an active process which depends on aldosterone. Water reabsorption is a passive process depending on osmotic forces and the presence of the antidiuretic hormone (ADH).

During dehydration when the concentration of circulating ADH is high, the cells of the distal nephron are readily permeable to water, whilst during water diuresis when the ADH titer is low the epithelium of the distal tubules and collecting ducts is impermeable to water (Fig. 25.4).

Yet another process resulting in net sodium reabsorption is the exchange of sodium for hydrogen discussed earlier. The final regulation of pH by this process occurs in the distal nephron, although some exchange of hydrogen for sodium is believed to occur all along the nephron. Figure 11.8 shows an outline scheme of water and sodium reabsorption, based on Pitts, 1968.

The average renal clearance of potassium represents about 20 per cent of glomerular filtration. Two separate steps are involved. The proximal tubules reabsorb almost all the potassium filtered through the glomeruli, whilst in the distal tubule net secretion of potassium into the urine takes place.

Classification of diuretics
The main effect of diuretics is to increase sodium excretion by action on the tubules and they should ideally be classified according to the precise tubular site on which their saluretic effect is exerted. Unfortunately this cannot be done with any degree of confidence since in many cases localisation study of the site of action of diuretics has yielded contradictory results or suggested that diuretics act concurrently at different sites. We shall be mentioning the outcome of some of these localisation studies, which are based largely on clearance and micropuncture techniques, without entering into the frequently intricate argument by which the conclusions were arrived at. Diuretics which have clinical relevance will be mainly discussed, but others, including some now of only theoretical interest will also be briefly referred to.

Clinical use of diuretics
The clinical use of diuretics has greatly increased since the introduction of the thiazides and the recognition of their value and that of potassium sparing diuretics in the treatment of hypertension. The newer group of powerful 'loop' diuretics are also widely used clinically. By contrast other diuretic drugs such as the mercurials which previously formed the mainstay of therapy have lost clinical importance. Osmotic diuretics, e.g. mannitol, are occasionally used to produce diuresis in acute renal oliguric failure. Certain substances, e.g. acetazolamide, cause diuresis but they are clinically used for a different purpose, such as glaucoma treatment.

Benzothiadiazine diuretics (thiazides)
Chlorothiazide and related thiadiazine derivatives are powerful diuretics which are effective when given by mouth. Their introduction has been the most important advance in diuretic therapy since the discovery of the organic mercurials.

Chemical structure
The discovery of chlorothiazide arose from the observation that sulphonamides inhibit the activity of carbonic anhydrase. The synthesis of a series of benzene disulphonamide derivatives with high diuretic activity culminated in the production of a number of benzothiadiazine dioxides with the general structure

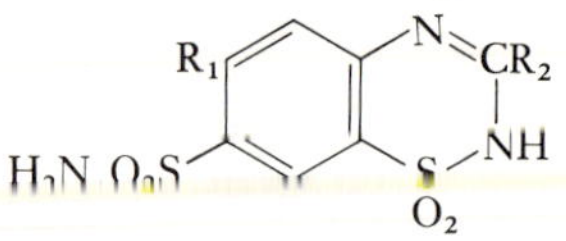

The introduction of a halogen group at R_1 enhanced diuretic activity as in chlorothiazide and its dihydro derivative. Hydrochlorothiazide is about twenty times more active than the parent compound. Substitution of the chlorine atom in hydrochlorothiazide by a trifluoromethyl group produces a compound hydroflumethiazide which is also about twenty times more active than chlorothiazide. Compounds with even greater diuretic activity have been produced by substitution in the R_2 position as in bendrofluazide.

Diuretic action of thiazides
Thiazides are readily absorbed from the gastro-intestinal tract and produce a moderately intense diuretic action. Thiazides increase the urinary excretion of sodium and water by inhibiting sodium reabsorption in the cortical portion of the ascending limb of Henle's loop and in the

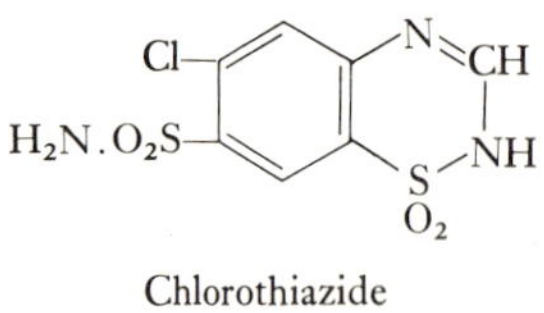

Chlorothiazide

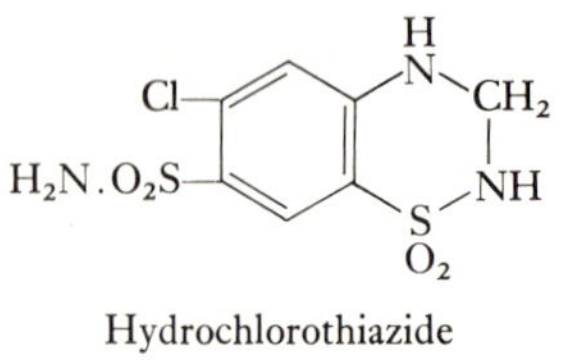

Hydrochlorothiazide

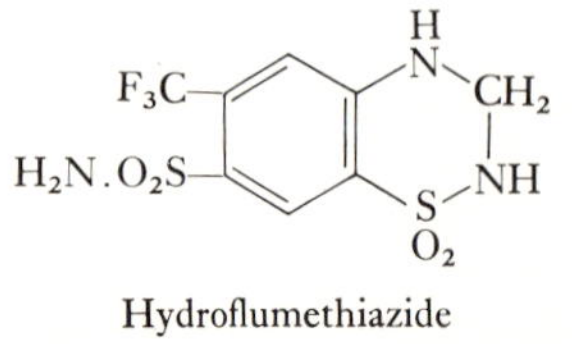

Hydroflumethiazide

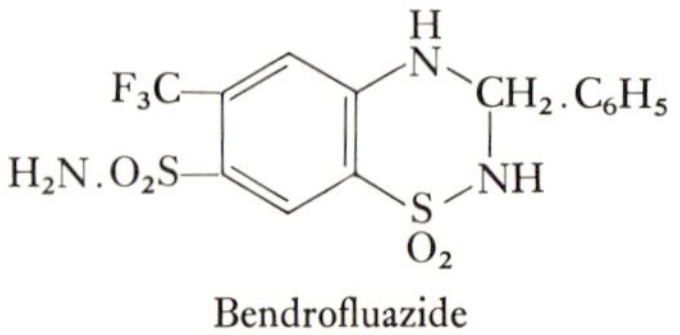

Bendrofluazide

first part of the distal tubule. By increasing the rate of delivery of tubular fluid to the distal exchange sites they cause a loss of potassium and hydrogen ions into the urine. In patients receiving prolonged thiazide treatment the serum potassium level often falls and the hypokalamia may be associated with hypochloraemic alkalosis.

A thiazide diuretic generally forms the basis of antihypertensive therapy (p. 113). The thiazide initially lowers blood pressure by reducing plasma volume. The hypotensive effect is better maintained by giving the thiazide together with a ß-blocking or vasodilator drug.

Undesirable effects of thiazides. When thiazides are administered over long periods they stay clinically remarkably effective. They produce relatively few side effects, the most frequent of which are due to potassium depletion. Potassium deficiency may give rise to lassitude and muscle weakness but the deficiency is difficult to assess objectively since nearly all body potassium is intracellular and a whole body counter for potassium is seldom available. For clinical purposes a normal plasma potassium can provide an indirect indication that the intracellular potassium concentration is adequate.

The effects of potassium deficiency can be avoided by providing a diet containing meat, fruit and vegetables. When thiazide treatment is intensive or prolonged it is often necessary to provide a supplement 20 to 40 mEq potassium. It has been found that in patients receiving a thiazide a high sodium diet aggravates urinary potassium loss. Potassium depletion increases the sensitivity of the heart to digitalis. It is therefore necessary to reduce the maintenance dose of digitalis when patients are given a thiazide diuretic in conjunction with digitalis. Prolonged treatment with thiazide diuretics may cause uric acid retention and precipitate an attack of gout in predisposed patients. It may also produce hyperglycaemia. Hypersensitivity to thiazide diuretics, manifested by skin rashes or thrombocytopenic purpura, sometimes occurs.

Chlorthalidone (Hygroton)
The effect of chlorthalidone is similar to that of the thiazide diuretics but it is more prolonged so that when chlorthalidone is used for maintenance therapy it need be administered only every second day; in doses of 100 mg three times weekly, it seldom causes serious potassium depletion. Chlorthalidone is often administered together with antihypertensive drugs.

Clorexolone (Nefrolan)
This is another long-action diuretic.

Loop diuretics
This term has been widely employed in the recent American literature to denote diuretics with an action primarily on the medullary portion of the thick ascending limb of Henle's loop. Both sodium and chloride are transported out of the ascending limb at this site accumulating hypertonically in the medullary interstitium. There has been much controversy whether, in this physiochemical process, sodium is actively reabsorbed followed passively by chloride, or whether, on the contrary, chloride transport is the active process, but it is now widely accepted that at this site in the ascending limb of Henle's loop chloride is transported actively and sodium passively.

It appears that the events in Henle's loop are of fundamental importance in relation to the capacity of the kidney to elaborate a concentrated or a diluted urine. Under the influence of certain diuretics the kidney becomes 'isosthenuric', i.e. tending to excrete urine isotonic with plasma. Diuretics which produce this type of effect are believed to exert an important part of their action on the active chloride transport mechanism in the ascending part of Henle's loop.

The term loop diuretic is usually applied to some of the newer diuretics such as frusemide and ethacrynic acid which probably act in this way. It is interesting that some of the oldest diuretics, the mercurials, may also act in this manner.

Mercurial diuretics
Organic mercury compounds have held in the past an important position amongst diuretic drugs; their main disadvantage is that their usual method of administration is by intramuscular injection.

Mercury has long been known to produce diuresis; for example, calomel combined with digitalis has been used since the eighteenth century to produce diuresis in oedema. Although organic mercurials are generally less potent as diuretics than an equivalent amount of an ionised inorganic mercury salt, they are much more useful since they are less toxic and produce a more prolonged action.

Mersalyl (Salyrgan) is one of the most satisfactory organic mercurial diuretics. It has the following chemical structure:

$$\text{C}_6\text{H}_4 \begin{cases} \text{OCH}_2-\text{CO}_2\text{Na} \\ \text{CO}-\text{NH}-\text{CH}_2-\text{CH}(\text{OCH}_3)-\text{CH}_2-\text{HgOH} \end{cases}$$

Mersalyl sodium

It contains about 40 per cent of mercury in nonionisable form and is freely soluble in water. It is administered intramuscularly in 10 per cent solution, and the usual dose is 0.5–2 ml.

The toxicity of organic mercurials may be reduced by forming a complex with theophylline and if preparations containing equal amounts of mercury are tested in cats, it can be shown that mersalyl with theophylline is only half as toxic as mersalyl alone.

Mode of action of mercurial diuretics

Experiments by Govaerts with transplanted kidneys proved that the mercurial diuretics act directly on the kidney.

Mercury reacts with the sulphydryl groups of proteins and it has been suggested that the mercurial diuretics produce their effects by a reversible inhibition of sulphydryl enzyme systems. Another theory is that they act on a sodium-potassium dependent ATPase concerned in sodium reabsorption.

Clinical effects

Although the mercurials have now been relegated to a place of secondary importance they are still used in the treatment of oedema and ascites in cardiac failure.

The mercurial diuretics produce diuresis in normal individuals and in patients with oedema. In the latter a single dose may bring about the excretion of 5 litres or more of urine in a day. The predominant effect of mercurials on chloride excretion may cause a hypochloraemic alkalosis in which mercurials lose their diuretic activity. Ammonium chloride (p. 157) can prevent the development of this refractory state and restore sensitivity if refractoriness due to metabolic alkalosis has developed.

Frusemide (Lasix)

Frusemide was discovered in the course of attempts to replace the heterocyclic part of the benzothiadiazine molecule. First investigations suggested an action similar to thiazide diuretics with a higher ceiling effect. Later studies showed important differences from the thiazides and it is now believed that the main action of frusemide is to inhibit the active chloride reabsorption mechanism in the ascending loop of Henle.

Actions. The main difference between thiazides and frusemide in animal experiments is the greater ceiling effect or efficacy of the latter in relation to sodium excretion. In contrast to thiazides, frusemide does not depress glomerular filtration rate and this may help to explain its greater ceiling effect.

Frusemide is well absorbed when given orally, and produces a rapid action. It is strongly bound to plasma proteins. Frusemide is classed as a 'high ceiling' diuretic since its peak diuretic effect is greater than that of thiazides. Excretion of calcium and magnesium are increased by about the same percentage as sodium and there is a marked increase in potassium excretion due to its increased secretion by the distal tubule. A characteristic effect of large doses of all the high ceiling diuretics is that they may cause a metabolic alkalosis due to excessive chloride loss accompanied by an increase in the concentration of bicarbonate in the extracellular fluid.

Clinical uses

Frusemide has a broad dose-response curve and therapy may be started with small doses, increasing dosage gradually if required. When administered orally it acts within an hour and given parenterally the diuretic effect is almost immediate. It can be given intravenously in the emergency treatment of pulmonary or cerebral oedema or to bring about a forced diuresis in severe barbiturate poisoning. Given by mouth it is often effective in patients with refractory oedema who have failed to respond to thiazides; it is particularly useful in patients with impaired kidney function and a low glomerular filtration rate.

Although it can lower blood pressure it has no particular advantage as an antihypertensive drug, when its short powerful effect may lead to annoying urinary frequency. In elderly men with prostatic obstruction the rapid diuresis caused by frusemide may cause acute urinary retention.

Frusemide is a powerful drug with relatively few serious side effects; its main disadvantage is the fluid and electrolyte imbalance it produces. A large dose may produce weakness, dizziness, nausea and vertigo. Prolonged administration may produce hypovolaemia with severe prostration, potassium deficiency and hypochloraemic alkalosis. It is important to remember the need for chloride as well as potassium supplement in these cases. Frusemide produces hyperuricaemia and may precipitate an attack of gout in susceptible individuals.

Bumetanide

This is a potent new diuretic producing effects similar to frusemide at about one-fortieth the dosage. Like frusemide it causes a rapid natriuresis associated with increased urinary output of potassium. Bumetadine is well tolerated, but if administered for long periods it produces hyperuricaemia like other saluretics. Although similar in its total effect to frusemide its long-term merits have not yet been fully evaluated.

Frusemide

Ethacrynic acid

Ethacrynic acid (Edecrin)

Ethacrynic acid was discovered by Beyer and his colleagues as a result of a search for a non-mercurial SH-blocker. The outcome was the discovery of an entirely new type of powerful diuretic, although interestingly there is now some doubt whether its diuretic effect can be explained by its relatively weak SH-blocking action.

Ethacrynic acid affects the ability of the kidney to elaborate either a concentrated or diluted urine by interfering with the active transport of chloride in the ascending loop of Henle. Under the influence of ethacrynic acid the kidney tends to excrete urine isotonic with plasma, a condition also found in some kidney diseases.

Actions
Ethacrynic acid is rapidly absorbed and rapidly cleared from the blood. Its excretion by the kidney is by filtration and secretion through the proximal tubular transport system for acids.

It differs from thiazides in having a greater ceiling response and in causing much greater chloride excretion, which may lead to a condition of hypochloraemic alkalosis. Its effect on potassium excretion is similar to that of thiazides.

Clinical effects and toxicity
Due to the great diuretic efficacy of ethacrynic acid it frequently causes disturbances which can be attributed to a rapid reduction of the circulating blood volume such as dizziness, vertigo, headache and orthostatic hypotension. Overdosage may produce a dangerous reduction of plasma sodium and particularly chloride and hypochloraemic alkalosis. Severe potassium depletion may also occur. For these reasons it is generally considered to be a drug for use mainly in hospital where daily electrolyte estimations can be made.

The main indication for ethacrynic acid is in patients who are refractory to thiazides. It is very effective in acute conditions such as pulmonary oedema with left ventricular failure. It may also be used in barbiturate poisoning to induce a strong diuretic effect. It is often necessary to give salt and water with it to compensate for the low blood volume, and to administer potassium supplements. In hypochloraemic alkalosis, chloride must be administered.

Ethacrynic acid may produce gastrointestinal symptoms such as anorexia, nausea and vomiting and sometimes diarrhoea. A serious, but fortunately rare, complication of high ceiling diuretics is inner ear deafness which has been observed after ethacrynic acid and, in a transient form, after frusemide. It is usually administered with food in a starting dose of 50 mg daily which is increased until the desired effect is obtained.

Potassium-sparing diuretics
Excessive potassium loss is an unwanted effect of most oral diuretics in common use. Potassium excretion is brought about by the secretion of potassium by the distal tubules and it seems likely that the increased flow through the distal tubules during diuresis by itself stimulates potassium secretion. Aldosterone is an important factor increasing the secretion of potassium in exchange of sodium by the distal tubules.

Oral potassium supplements cause heart burn and abdominal discomfort and patients frequently neglect taking them. The potassium-sparing diuretics are more reliable than potassium supplements in raising the serum potassium level during diuretic therapy. Since only a small fraction of urinary sodium is normally reabsorbed at the distal exchange sites, the potassium-sparing agents are weak diuretics when used alone. Their main use is in conjunction with thiazides or loop diuretics.

Spironolactone
Whilst the proximal nephron reabsorbs a constant fraction of sodium filtered through the glomerulus, the distal nephron reabsorbs a smaller but highly variable fraction. The mechanism by which sodium is absorbed and potassium and hydrogen excreted in the distal tubule is controlled by aldosterone, excess of which causes retention of salt and water in the body whilst promoting the excretion of potassium and hydrogen ions.

Spironolactone is structurally related to aldosterone and acts as its receptor antagonist. In some cases of oedema there is an excessive secretion of aldosterone; in such cases spironolactone increases excretion of sodium and chloride in the urine accompanied by diuresis, reduces the excretion of potassium and hydrogen ions and decreases the titratable acidity of the urine.

Clinical uses. Spironolactone is a mild diuretic which is especially valuable where there is excessive secretion of aldosterone and when potassium depletion must be avoided. It is used in patients with oedema due to hepatic cirrhosis in which potassium loss is dangerous and in the nephrotic syndrome. In heart failure it may be administered concurrently with a thiazide diuretic.

The action of spironolactone is slow in onset and it may take several days until a full effect is produced. A danger of spironolactone treatment is that it may cause hyperkalaemia especially in patients with impaired renal function.

Triamterene (Dytac)
This drug produces effects which are similar to those of spironolactone. It was formerly believed that triamterene acted as an aldosterone antagonist but subsequent work by Herken and colleagues on adrenalectomised animals showed that triamterene was active in the absence of aldosterone and it is now considered to produce its diuretic effect by direct action on the distal tubule. It differs from spironolactone in its speed of action, producing diuresis within 2–4 hours of oral ingestion.

Like spironolactone, triamterene promotes potassium retention and it is therefore usefully combined with potassium eliminating diuretics such as the thiazides.

When administered on alternate days with a thiazide, electrolyte disturbances are unlikely to occur.

Spironolactone

Triamterene

Amiloride resembles triamterene in its mode and site of action and likewise has a mild natriuretic and potassium-sparing effect.

Osmotic diuretics

Reabsorption of sodium and consequently water from the proximal tubules is prevented if a non-absorbable anion is present. In this way potassium nitrate and parenteral sodium sulphate act as diuretics. A related action is that of the osmotic diuretics urea, sucrose and mannitol which promote water excretion by not being reabsorbed in the proximal tubules.

Urea and potassium nitrate were previously widely used as oral diuretics but they are now rarely employed. They are relatively ineffective compared to the newer diuretics, must be given in large amounts and produce nausea and headache. Intravenous *mannitol* is sometimes administered in the treatment of drug poisoning in order to force diuresis but care must be taken not to overload the circulation. Intravenous mannitol may also reduce intraocular or cerebral pressure by withdrawing fluid into the circulation.

Forced alkaline diuresis

Forced alkaline diuresis can be employed to increase the rate at which some acidic drugs, particularly salicylates and phenobarbitone are eliminated from the body in cases of poisoning. It is a dangerous technique which requires strict control and is best carried out in an intensive care unit. It is usual to combine an alkaline intravenous infusion (500 ml/h of 1.2% sodium bicarbonate) with a diuretic (20 mg/h frusemide or 20 g/h mannitol) and give 1 litre 5% dextrose plus 20 mg frusemide whilst monitoring central venous pressure and urine volume. The chief dangers are hypokalaemia and hyponatraemia and overloading the circulation to a degree which may cause either pulmonary oedema or cerebral oedema with convulsions.

Obsolete diuretics

Some diuretics which have become obsolete have clinical applications in other fields.

Acetazolamide (Diamox)

Acetazolamide

This drug inhibits carbonic anhydrase in the renal tubule causing reduced tubular reabsorption and increased excretion of bicarbonate which carries with it sodium, potassium and water. As a consequence diuresis, alkalinization of urine and mild metabolic acidosis occur. Since the diuresis depends on bicarbonate excretion, refractoriness to the diuretic effect rapidly develops as the blood bicarbonate falls. For this reason acetazolamide is now seldom employed as a diuretic.

Acetazolamide and other carbonic anhydrase inhibitors reduce aqueous production thus lowering intra-ocular pressure. These drugs are of great value in the long-term treatment of primary open-angle glaucoma and other forms of chronic glaucoma. They are also used for the treatment of acute glaucoma in conjunction with miotics and osmotic agents.

Acetazolamide has been used in epilepsy especially in children in combination with other drugs.

Xanthines

The chief xanthine derivatives are as follows: (1) caffeine (tri-methyl xanthine), which occurs in coffee and tea. (2) theobromine (di-methyl xanthine) which occurs in cocoa. (3) theophylline (di-methyl xanthine, isomeric with theobromine). These substances are often conjugated with other compounds to improve their solubility; for example theophylline ethylene diamine (aminophylline) and theobromine sodium salicylate (diuretin).

Of the three xanthine derivatives theophylline has the strongest, and caffeine the weakest diuretic action. Caffeine has a strong excitant action on the central nervous system, and theophylline is a cardiac stimulant; it is also liable to produce vomiting.

The mode of action of these drugs in producing diuresis in experimental animals has long been a matter of dispute. According to one view, the diuresis is due to the drugs dilating the afferent arterioles of the glomerulus to a greater extent than the efferent arterioles, thereby increasing the effective filtration pressure and hence

Caffeine

Theobromine

Theophylline

glomerular filtration rate. Another view is that they exert an effect on the renal tubule cells, reducing their reabsorptive capacity. The present view is that either or both mechanisms may operate. The xanthine diuretics are now mainly of pharmacological interest; clinically their use as diuretics has become absolute.

Choice of diuretic

The production of diuresis in a healthy individual is a very simple matter, but it is very difficult to produce benefit by means of drugs when the kidneys are so injured by disease that they are unable to perform their normal functions.

An important use of diuretics, however, is where the impairment of kidney function is secondary to circulatory failure. Although in these cases the essential treatment is improvement of the circulation by rest and digitalis, it is usually necessary to reduce the extracellular fluid by limiting the intake of salt and increasing its excretion by the administration of diuretics. There is some evidence that the salt retention is due to an increased secretion of aldosterone by the adrenal cortex.

For the treatment of moderate oedema one of the orally administered *thiazide diuretics* is usually the drug of first choice. From the therapeutic point of view there is little to choose between the various members of this group, the effective dose of which ranges from 1 g of chlorothiazide to 10 mg or less of bendrofluazide. *Chlorthalidone*, because of its smooth action, may be a useful alternative to the thiazides for prolonged therapy. The risk of potassium depletion is likely to arise during prolonged administration and supervision of the patient with periodic biochemical monitoring is required. Concurrent treatment with digitalis may require occasional adjustment of the maintenance dose of digitalis.

The thiazide diuretics are widely used in the treatment of hypertension (p. 113). They are often combined with other antihypertensive drugs, the dose and toxicity of which can thus be reduced. In moderate doses the thiazides may be given for long periods without causing harm, if potassium depletion is avoided. Prolonged administration of thiazides may cause an elevation of blood sugar and the insulin requirements of diabetic patients may be increased. These diuretic drugs also raise the blood uric acid level and may precipitate an attack of gout in a predisposed patient.

The introduction of high-ceiling diuretic compounds such as *frusemide* and *ethacrynic acid* has provided powerful means for the treatment of resistant cases of fluid retention. An initial oral dose is usually sufficient to produce a rapid diuresis; repeated administration requires careful adjustment of dosage to avoid excessive loss of fluid and electrolytes. In patients with severe heart failure frusemide may be given orally, or in urgent cases by intravenous injection. In resistant cases ethacrynic acid may be given. These drugs have also been given intravenously in the treatment of acute pulmonary oedema.

Spironolactone or *triamterene* are sometimes useful in the the treatment of oedema associated with hepatic cirrhosis and nephrosis. When administered alone they seldom produce a significant diuresis but when given orally in conjunction with a thiazide or other diuretic they often cause a sodium chloride diuresis without excessive loss of potassium.

In disease of the kidneys the chief treatment is to relieve their work as far as possible by rest and diet. A kidney severely injured by disease cannot be forced to do more work by means of drugs. Therefore diuretics are useless in the treatment of acute nephritis or advanced sclerosis of the kidneys. The administration of cortisone or ACTH to patients with nephrotic oedema sometimes induces a diuresis. This method of treatment, however, involves special risks. Instead of producing diuresis these drugs may cause an increased retention of fluid and a flare-up of infections to which nephrotic patients are already particularly prone.

In anuria which sometimes follows operations on the urinary tract, the kidneys can sometimes be forced to start excreting by means of diuretics and may then continue to do so. In anuria of this type administration of a solution of 6 per cent *sodium sulphate* or 5-20 per cent *mannitol* as an intravenous drip can be an effective method of forcing the urine flow to start. Other measures include the use of renal dialysis in the form of the 'artificial kidney'. While the anuric kidneys are given time to recover, the blood is circulated through long coils of collodion tubes surrounded by a saline solution into which the plasma ultrafiltrate diffuses. Or a saline solution may be passed constantly through the peritoneal cavity; the ultrafiltrate diffuses into it from the blood plasma in the peritoneal capillaries. Surgical treatment by kidney transplant is an encouraging prospect.

DRUGS USED IN RADIOSCOPY OF THE KIDNEY AND OTHER ORGANS

X-ray photographs can be taken of most of the cavities in the body by introducing into them suspensions or solutions of substances opaque to X-rays. The higher the atomic weight of an element the greater is its power to arrest X-rays. The problem is to find suspensions or solutions of inert substances containing atoms of high atomic weight. The two elements chiefly used are barium (at. wt. 137) and iodine (at. wt. 127). Suspensions of barium sulphate are used as test meals for the study of intestinal function. Iodised oils can be introduced into many cavities of the body, e.g. subdural space, uterus and Fallopian tubes. The method is of particular value for the photography of the bronchi.

To render the pelvis of the kidney and the ureter opaque to X-rays, methods of retrograde pyelography or of intravenous pyelography are used. Certain complex organic compounds of iodine have been synthesised which are excreted rapidly by the kidneys and can be used to render the ureters opaque to X-rays. Lichtenberg discovered uroselectan (iopax) which contained 43 per cent of iodine.

Diodone (diodrast, iodopyracet), sodium diatrizoate (hypaque) and methiodal (skidan) all contain iodine and are used as contrast agents for the investigation of renal function. In certain individuals these compounds produce an allergic reaction when injected intravenously and a solution of adrenaline (1 in 1000) should be at hand when these drugs are used.

PREPARATIONS

Thiazides and related diuretics
Bendrofluazide (Aprinox) 2.5-20 mg daily
Bumetanide (Burinex) 1mg in the morning
Chlorothiazide (Saluric) 0.5-2 g daily
Chlorthalidone (Hygroton) 50-200 mg daily
Clopamide (Brinaldix) 20-60 mg daily
Clorexolone (Nefrolan) 10-25 mg daily, long acting
Cyclopenthiazide (Navidrex) 250 µg-1 mg daily
Ethacrynic acid (Edecrin) 50 mg after breakfast
Frusemide (Lasix) 40-120 mg daily or on alternate days
Hydrochlorothiazide (Hydrosaluric) 25-100 mg 1-3x daily
Hydroflumethiazide (Hydrenox) 25-100 mg daily
Mefruside (Baycaron) 25-50 mg daily
Methyclothiazide (Enduron) 2.5-10 mg daily
Metozalone 5-10 mg daily
Polythiazide (Nephril) 0.5-4 mg daily, long duration
Quinethazone 50-100 mg daily

Potassium sparing diuretics
Amiloride (Midamor) 5-20 mg daily
Spironolactone 100-200 mg daily
Triamterene (Dytac) 150-250 mg daily

Other diuretics
Acetazolamide 250 mg-1g daily
Dichlorphenamide (Daranide) 50-200 mg daily
Mannitol 300 mg/kg i.v. as single dose
Mersalyl Injection 0.5-2 ml

FURTHER READING

Lant A F, Wilson G M 1966 The evaluation of diuretics in man. Int. Enc. Pharm. Therap. 6: 473
Pitts R F 1959 The physiological basis of diuretic therapy. Thomas, Springfield
Smith H W 1956 Principles of renal physiology. Oxford University Press, London
Verney E B 1947 Antidiuretic hormone and factors which determine its release. Croonian Lecture. Proc R. Soc. B. 135: 25
Vogel H G, Ullrich K J (eds.) 1978 New aspects of renal function. Excerpta Med, Amsterdam
de Wardener W E 1973 The kidney. Churchill Livingstone, Edinburgh

12. Respiration and bronchi

Mechanism of normal respiration 167; Respiratory failure 168; Oxygen administration 168; Carbon monoxide poisoning 170; Cyanide poisoning 170; Respiratory stimulants 171; Respiratory and cough depressants 173; Bronchial asthma 176; Sympathomimetics 177; Disodium cromoglycate 181; Aminophyline 182; Corticosteroids 182.

MECHANISM OF NORMAL RESPIRATION

The chief functions of respiration are the supply of oxygen to the body and the removal of carbon dioxide. The evaporation of water in the respiratory passages also assists in regulating the temperature of the body. This function is of great importance in animals that have few sweat glands, such as the dog, but is less important in man.

Any failure of respiration produces the double effect of depriving the body of oxygen and of allowing carbon dioxide to accumulate. These two effects occur simultaneously, and both combine to produce the symptoms of asphyxia. Lack of oxygen and excess of carbon dioxide produce quite distinct effects. The sensations in asphyxia are due almost entirely to the excess of carbon dioxide, while most of the injurious effects produced on the tissues by asphyxia are due to the lack of oxygen.

The interchange of gases between the tissues and air occurs in two stages: (1) in the lungs between the blood and the alveolar air (external respiration); and (2) in the tissues between the blood in the capillaries and the tissues (internal respiration).

The interchange of respiratory gases

The interchange of gases between the blood and the alveolar air depends upon the following factors. (a) The difference in the tensions of the gases of the blood and the gases of the alveolar air. (b) The rate of blood flow through the lungs. (c) The area over which the exchange is taking place. (d) The resistance offered by the alveolar walls to the diffusion of gases.

The tension of gases in the alveolar air depends upon the composition of the air inspired, and upon the ventilation of the lungs; the latter depends upon the rate of respiration and the volume of each respiration.

In health the lungs are provided with considerable reserve powers which are reflected in the wide variations produced in the rate and depth of breathing. Thus the normal resting subject breathes about 6 litres of air per minute, whilst a trained athlete, exerting maximal effort inspires up to 190 litres per minute. The limiting factor for oxygen uptake is the minute volume of the circulation and the efficiency of the lungs depends on the large surface area of the alveoli, which is about 70 sq m.

The volume of air breathed is regulated by the respiratory centre, a term which is conveniently used to describe a functionally integrated group of nerve cells located in the pons and upper two-thirds of the medulla. The respiratory centre is very sensitive to any change in the pH of the blood; since the pH of the blood in the absence of metabolic disturbance depends on the tension of carbon dioxide in the blood, the slightest change in CO_2 tension immediately affects the respiratory centre. This centre is stimulated by any rise in the CO_2 tension, and the consequent increase in the volume of respiration results in the excretion of the excess of CO_2 and the reduction of the tension to normal. The volume of respiration can thus be adjusted to maintain the CO_2 tension in the blood and in the alveolar air at the normal level.

The respiratory movements are partly under voluntary control and they are also affected by a number of reflexes. Respiration is thus accelerated by painful or emotional stimuli and by stimulation of nerves supplying the pharynx or nasopharynx. Respiratory movements are also partly controlled by the baroreceptors of the carotid sinus; they are inhibited and stimulated respectively by a rise or fall in the blood pressure in the sinus. Lack of oxygen or excess of carbon dioxide stimulates respiration through an action on the chemoreceptors of the carotid body.

The rate of blood-flow through the lungs is rapid but much less so than the rate at which oxygen is taken up by haemoglobin and at which carbon dioxide diffuses into the alveolar air. In many lung diseases, however, parts of the lung are not adequately ventilated by the inspired air and other parts may be poorly perfused with blood, so that the blood leaving the lungs may have a reduced oxygen and raised carbon dioxide content.

The blood in its passage through the lungs becomes almost completely saturated with oxygen at the pressue of oxygen existing in the alveolar air; this degree of saturation represents about 95 per cent of the saturation produced by pure oxygen at atmospheric pressure.

Since the arterial blood is nearly completely saturated with oxygen when ordinary atmospheric air is breathed, the breathing of pure oxygen does not increase the volume of oxygen in the blood more than 3 to 4 per cent, but the breathing of pure oxygen raises the amount of oxygen in solution and hence the oxygen tension in the arterial blood and thus may improve the respiration of the tissues.

The tension of carbon dioxide in the alveolar air differs

in different individuals, but remains extraordinarily constant in any particular individual. An adequate rate of exchange of carbon dioxide between the tissues and blood and between blood and alveolar air is maintained by the enzyme carbonic anhydrase which is contained in the red blood cells. This accelerates the rate at which carbonic acid is decomposed into or formed from carbon dioxide and water.

Influence of carbon dioxide and of oxygen on the respiratory centre

The respiratory centre is governed by the carbon dioxide tension of the blood. Increase in the CO_2 tension produces the marked subjective symptoms associated with asphyxiation. Any decrease in the carbon dioxide tension causes apnoea. Apnoea lasting for some minutes can be easily produced by means of forced respiration, for this in a few minutes can reduce the alveolar CO_2 tension to about one-half the normal.

The respiratory centre is not stimulated directly by oxygen lack, but a diminished partial pressure of oxygen in the arterial blood stimulates respiration reflexly by stimulating the chemoreceptors of the carotid and aortic bodies. In a normal adult the breathing of pure oxygen decreases pulmonary ventilation only very slightly (by about 10 per cent). This is probably due to the inactivation of the minimal chemoreceptor drive which is present at normal oxygen levels. The situation is different in respiratory failure when chemoreceptor drive becomes dominant as discussed below, and in newborn and particularly premature babies when the administration of oxygen reduces breathing.

Provided the body can dispose of excess carbon dioxide, lack of oxygen produces no distressing subjective symptoms; it may cause sleepiness and lassitude or it may cause a sense of contentment and well-being that persists until unconsciousness occurs. The reason why exposure to carbon monoxide is so dangerous is that the oxygen content of the blood can be reduced to a dangerously low level without the occurrence of any feeling of distress.

Respiratory failure

The lungs of a man at rest transfer over 300 litres of oxygen in 24 hours from air to the blood and eliminate it in the form of carbon dioxide. The arterial oxygen tension in a normal healthy man is about 90 mmHg and that of carbon dioxide about 40 mmHg. It is usually considered that an arterial oxygen tension below 60 mmHg and arterial carbon dioxide above 49 mmHg is indicative of respiratory failure. This may arise from (a) inadequate ventilation of the lung, (b) insufficient perfusion of the lung with blood and (c) a deficient gas exchange between alveolar air and blood.

A common clinical cause of respiratory failure is severe chronic bronchitis. The basic treatment of respiratory failure is the provision of oxygen. The minimum arterial oxygen level compatible with life is about 20 mmHg and the object of treatment of respiratory failure is to raise the arterial oxygen tension to at least 50 mmHg. This may be accomplished in two ways, either by administering oxygen to a spontaneously breathing patient or by providing artificial ventilation.

Oxygen administration

Patients with mild or moderately severe respiratory failure may be able to eliminate carbon dioxide adequately but fail to oxygenate the blood sufficiently unless oxygen is added to the inspired air. High concentrations of oxygen should not be used because in patients with inadequate oxygenation and retention of carbon dioxide, the respiratory centre is no longer responsive to changes in CO_2 tension and is primarily under the influence of chemoreceptors whose lack of oxygen provides the 'ventilatory drive'. When high concentrations of oxygen are administered the oxygen lack is suddenly removed and the respiratory centre may fail to drive the respiratory muscles. This is referred to as oxygen apnoea.

Even in the absence of complete apnoea, the administration of oxygen leads to diminished ventilation and a further rise in pCO_2 in these patients causing progressive impairment of consciousness. A compromise can sometimes be achieved between the desired increase in arterial pO_2 and the rise in pCO_2, based on the fact that in severe hypoxaemia oxygen dissocation of haemoglobin lies in the steep part of the curve where a small increase in arterial pO_2 causes a large increase in oxygen saturation so that even a small admixture of oxygen to air becomes clinically effective.

When oxygen is administered it is initially given in low concentrations (24 per cent) and the patient's progress is followed by serial pCO_2 measurements. The concentration of oxygen in the inspired air is gradually increased providing the pCO_2 does not rise and the patient shows no signs of hypopnoea. The concentration of oxygen may be increased every hour or so until it reaches 35 per cent. The most satisfactory way of administering these measured concentrations of oxygen is by a standard mask which works on a high air-flow venturi principle. If it is desired merely to raise inspired oxygen concentration, a simple and effective method is to administer oxygen by nasal catheter. It is important to remember that a considerable quantity must be given if any effect is to be produced. Total ventilation is normally 5–8 litres per minute but a fevered subject breathes at least 10 litres of air a minute and this volume contains 2 litres of oxygen. An extra litre of oxygen a minute is the smallest quantity that will produce any effect, and an extra 2 litres are usually required to produce any benefit; the amount usually administered is 4 to 6 litres per minute.

Oxygen therapy is of most value when anoxaemia is due to the failure of oxygen to pass from the alveolar air into the haemoglobin of the blood, and the blood leaves the lungs only partially saturated with oxygen. Hence any increase in the oxygen tension in the alveolar air will tend to increase both the quantity and the tension of the oxygen in the blood leaving the lungs. The blood leaving the lungs in the anaemic type of anoxaemia is nearly completely saturated, and therefore any increase in the oxygen tension in the alveolar air cannot produce any great increase in the quantity of oxygen entering the blood, although it can increase the amount of oxygen dissolved in the blood.

Artificial ventilation
Some mechanical ventilators operate by producing a subatmospheric pressure outside the lungs but more usually they work by positive pressure ventilation. Their application requires endotracheal intubation or tracheostomy. The former can be performed quickly and easily but it is time-limited since it cannot be applied for longer than about eight days (except in very small children) due to the laryngeal damage it causes. Once switched on, the patient usually synchronises with the ventilator, provided that the minute volume is adequate, but sometimes fails to do so in which case a sedative drug such as diazepam may be required.

Artificial ventilation is needed in conditions such as poisoning, poliomyelitis and laryngeal obstruction in which the lungs are not primarily affected, but with the advent of respiratory units it is also being increasingly employed as a temporary measure in cases of severe respiratory failure to prevent the occurrence of progressive anoxaemia. Examples of pulmonary conditions in which intubation and artificial ventilation has been used are exacerbations of chronic lung disease, pulmonary oedema and, in rare cases, severe bronchial asthma.

Artificial respiration may be needed for indefinite periods in respiratory paralysis due to poliomyelitis. Drinker's respirator (iron-lung) is a rigid airtight box in which the patient is enclosed with his head emerging. Respiration is effected by rhythmical suction from an air pump. The patient can be fed whilst under treatment, and life can thus be maintained for long periods.

A very effective method of giving artificial respiration for long periods is by intermittent positive pressure ventilation (IPPV) in which air or oxygen are administered either through a tracheostomy tube or by a tube inserted into the trachea through the mouth. An advantage of this method is that any accumulation of mucus or fluid in the trachea or bronchi can be readily removed by insertion of a catheter. A disadvantage is that secondary infection of the lungs is liable to occur if patients are ventilated by a tracheostomy tube for more than a few days.

Emergency respiratory resuscitation
This is required in the first aid treatment of such conditions as drowning, electrocution, carbon monoxide poisoning, in emergencies in medical practice such as respiratory arrest during anaesthesia or in asphyxia neonatorum.

The most important consideration in the choice of method of resuscitation is the speed with which it can be brought into effective use, for the chances of a successful result depend on how soon after respiration has ceased the resuscitation begins. The chances of survival decline rapidly if respiration has stopped for two minutes; Drinker estimated that the chances of resuscitating an individual with primary respiratory failure (with the circulation still active) are 97 per cent if the respiration has stopped for 1 minute; 75 per cent if stopped for 2 minutes and 25 per cent if stopped for 5 minutes.

Mouth to mouth breathing is a rapid and effective method of artificial respiration. Schafer's prone-posture method has the special merit that it can be carried out with unskilled assistance and the chance of injury to the liver, which is always engorged in asphyxia, is reduced to a minimum.

Eve's rocking method is one of the best methods for the ventilation of the lungs in an apnoeic subject. It depends on the principle of employing the diaphragm as a piston in the thorax. The patient is tied on a stretcher, ladder or door, which is placed on a trestle or convenient structure to act as a fulcrum, and is rocked through an angle of 45 degrees, up and down at a rate of about ten times a minute. In the head-down position, the abdominal viscera slide against the diaphragm and produce expiration. In the head-up position, inspiration is produced by the abdominal organs falling downwards and pulling the diaphragm down. It has been shown that in this way the excursion of the diaphragm is about 5 cm. The tidal air volume produced in apnoeic anaesthetised dogs by Eve's method is about 50 per cent greater than that produced by a modified Schafer method of resuscitation.

Oxygen poisoning
The effects of breathing 100 per cent oxygen for prolonged periods have been observed in many species of animals. The animals develop congestion and oedema of the lungs which in many instances is fatal. Observations of this type have also been made on normal healthy men. Comroe and his colleagues, using close-fitting masks, have shown that when 100 per cent oxygen was inhaled continuously for 24 hours at atmospheric pressure, 82 per cent of the subjects complained of substernal distress, cough, sore throat and nasal congestion. When 75 per cent oxygen was inhaled only 55 per cent of the men were affected and no symptoms occurred when 50 per cent oxygen was used. There is probably little chance of oxygen poisoning occurring under the usual clinical conditions, since the

administration of oxygen by catheter or oxygen tent, rarely produces concentrations higher than 50 per cent. The lung damage by oxygen inhalation is characterized by an irritant reaction of the respiratory tract with capillary congestion, thickening of alveolar membranes, oedema, atelectasis and alveolar haemorrhage.

A peculiar form of oxygen poisoning is *retrolental fibroplasia* seen in premature infants exposed to excessive concentrations of oxygen. The condition is characterised by the obliteration of the developing blood vessels in the immature retina and frequently leads to blindness. The changes are produced by high arterial pO_2 levels (100 mmHg and above) but do not seem to occur with lower pO_2 levels. The condition develops relatively rapidly and has been recorded in a baby whose arterial pO_2 remained at about 150 mmHg for 3-4 hours. It is essential therefore to keep the arterial pO_2 in these babies well below 100 mmHg.

CARBON MONOXIDE POISONING

Carbon monoxide combines with haemoglobin to form carboxyhaemoglobin, which is 200 to 300 times as stable a compound as oxyhaemoglobin. A concentration of about five parts of CO in 10 000 is sufficient to transform half the haemoglobin in the blood into a compound which is useless as a carrier of oxygen, and this may cause unconsciousness. Any higher degree of haemoglobin unsaturation is dangerous to life, and high concentrations of CO may cause death in a few seconds.

Carbon monoxide is a colourless, odourless gas, which may be present in some types of household gas (up to 20 per cent) and in the exhaust gases of motor cars (up to 7 per cent); moreover, it is formed by combustion of any fuel unless the oxygenation is extremely good. The inhalation of coal gas was a frequent mode of suicide, poisoning by exhaust gases in garages is common, and other forms of accidental poisoning by carbon monoxide are not uncommon. The gas is a peculiarly dangerous form of poison, because the anoxaemia it produces does not cause respiratory distress. The first effect is stupor and usually the subject continues at whatever task he is employed until he becomes unconscious. Exposure for some hours to a concentration of a few parts of CO per 10 000 of air produces dizziness and headache, whilst a few parts per 1000 produces unconsciousness in about half an hour.

Although the skin is classically described as cherry red in colour, due to the carboxyhaemoglobin in the blood, it is more usually pale and slightly cyanosed. The diagnosis can be confirmed with certainty by spectroscopic examination of the blood. The specific action of carbon monoxide poisoning is the deprivation of the tissues of oxygen, and it has no other direct toxic actions of importance. Prolonged anoxaemia produces various secondary toxic actions on the brain, for example, oedema of the brain which causes intense headache. More severe intoxication can cause permanent injury to the brain, and may result in loss of memory or even insanity. Fortunately these effects are rare and the great majority of cases which recover show no permanent after-effects.

Treatment of carbon monoxide poisoning
Speedy treatment is very important, because the effects depend not only on the amount of CO inhaled, but also on the duration of the asphyxia that it produces. The essential treatment is the thorough ventilation of the lungs with the highest concentration of oxygen available. Carboxyhaemoglobin can be dissociated, and the rate at which it can be dissociated is proportional to the oxygen tension in the blood.

The patient must be removed from the gas source and 100 per cent oxygen administered by a close-fitting mask. Mechanical ventilation through a cuffed endotracheal tube should be used if there is respiratory inadequacy. Any circulatory deficiency and gross degrees of metabolic acidosis should be corrected. An early assessment of the neurological state and treatment of any cerebral oedema are important.

CYANIDE POISONING

In cyanide poisoning the oxygen-carrying capacity of blood is unimpaired, but the tissues are incapable of utilising the oxygen provided. The toxic effect of cyanide is to inhibit the oxidation of reduced cytochrome whereby cellular respiration is suppressed. Cyanide produces this effect by reacting reversibly with the trivalent iron of cytochrome oxidase in mitochondria which is essential for cellular respiration.

Hydrocyanic acid and its salts are extensively used in industry and for fumigation, but the majority of deaths from cyanide poisoning are due to suicide. The diagnosis of cyanide poisoning is, in the first instance, frequently based on circumstantial evidence since the victim is usually found near the source of the cyanide. Respiration is at first rapid but quickly becomes slow and laboured, vomiting and convulsions are followed by coma and death. The odour of bitter almonds in the breath is a characteristic sign but is not present in all cases. The venous blood is bright red since the uptake of oxygen by the tissues is diminished and cyanosis does not occur until the final stages of respiratory failure. The diangosis may be confirmed by spectroscopic examination of the blood.

Treatment of cyanide poisoning
Cyanide poisoning is rapidly fatal, large doses produce death within a few minutes.

With smaller doses the toxic effects are more protracted and it may be possible to tide the victim over with artificial respiration and amyl nitrite inhalation until the specific antidote, cobalt edetate, can be administered.

The traditional treatment of cyanide poisoning has been to produce immediate methaemoglobinaemia by administering amyl nitrite by inhalation and sodium nitrite by injection. Methaemoglobin combines with cyanide to form non-toxic cyanmethaemoglobin. Sodium thiosulphate is then given to convert into cyanate (SCN) any cyanide which is dissociated from cyanmethaemoglobin.

More recently cobalt edetate has been employed for the treatment of cyanide poisoning. Cobalt forms stable complexes with cyanides and the complexes are thought to reduce the potential toxicity of cobalt.

RESPIRATORY STIMULANTS

There is a great clinical demand for drugs which will produce a powerful stimulant action on the centres which regulate respiration and circulation. Drugs of this type are required in the treatment of emergencies such as respiratory failure during anaesthesia, in asphyxia neonatorum and in poisoning by various drugs.

The respiratory stimulants may be classified as follows:

1. Those which act on the respiratory centre, carotid sinus, or both, e.g. carbon dioxide and the analeptic drugs leptazol, nikethamide, doxapram and picrotoxin. The sympathomimetic amines ephedrine, amphetamine and methylamphetamine also act on the respiratory centre and have the additional advantage that they improve its blood supply when the blood pressure is depressed.

2. Those which act reflexly by a general afferent stimulation, e.g. inhalation of ammonia vapour (dilute solution of ammonia, B.P.C.). The respiratory centre can be excited reflexly by any method of stimulating sensory nerves. The flicking of an apnoeic baby with a wet towel is an example of this form of therapy.

Carbon dioxide (Fig. 12.1)

Carbon dioxide is the most powerful of respiratory stimulants. Pure air contains about 0.03 per cent of CO_2, and in a badly ventilated room the air may contain up to 0.3 per cent of CO_2. The additon of 1 per cent CO_2 to the inspired air increases the volume of air breathed per minute about 25 per cent, 4 per cent CO_2 increases it 100 per cent, and 7 per cent CO_2 increases it over 500 per cent.

The respiratory stimulation by 4 per cent carbon dioxide is not unpleasant and may not even be noticed by the subject but concentrations of 7 per cent or more cause dyspnoea, dizziness, headache and faintness. High concentrations of CO_2 produce unconsciousness, muscular rigidity and tremors and finally generalised convulsions. Mixtures of 30 per cent carbon dioxide in oxygen have been used in psychiatric treatment; these mixtures are administered for periods of two minutes by which time they produce unconsciousness and convulsions.

A definite therapeutic indication of carbon dioxide is that it must be added to the oxygen used in certain types of pump oxygenators to avoid reducing the carbon dioxide tension of the blood.

Oxygen with carbon dioxide

Intermittent inhalation of oxygen with 5 to 7 per cent carbon dioxide was widely used in the past to stimulate respiration. For example, it was used postoperatively to prevent the condition of atelactasis or massive collapse of the lungs due to a combination of shallow breathing and accumulation of mucus. The bronchi become plugged with mucus and portions of the lungs collapse and, if the condition is not relieved, the collapsed lung is invaded by bacteria and pneumonia results. Carbon dioxide inhalation also stimulates coughing which is the natural defence against atelactasis.

It is now recognised, however, that carbon dioxide inhalation may produce harmful effects and its postoperative use has been largely abandoned. The reason is that under conditions of impaired breathing carbon dioxide is already retained and its addition to the inspired air aggravates the symptoms of hypercapnia. The sensitivity of the respiratory centre to CO_2 may then be reduced or even abolished so that it cannot be stimulated to activity by an increase in the pCO_2.

Clinical evidence of hypercapnia

Depression of the central nervous system is the most important sign of hypercapnia. With an increasing carbon dioxide tension there is a progressive impairment of consciousness. At twice the normal CO_2 tension (80 mmHg) drowsiness and confusion are frequent and the ability to concentrate is impaired. At 120 mmHg, coma is almost invariable. The coma is accompanied by depression of all the reflexes. The intracranial pressure is increased and may occasionally be so high as to produce papilloedema. Other clinical features include severe headache, tremors and peripheral vasodilatation.

ANALEPTIC DRUGS

The term *analeptic* is derived from the Greek word — to restore or repair — and was originally applied to drugs which restored body functions after depression by disease or poisons. Later the term was applied more particularly to drugs which stimulate the central nervous system. In the present discussion the term is applied to drugs which stimulate the central nervous system, particularly the centres controlling respiration and blood pressure, and which are used to antagonise depression by an overdose of general anaesthetics or hypnotics.

Mechanism of action

Recent studies involving the application of drugs by multibarrelled microelectrodes to mammalian brain and spinal cord suggest that central stimulant drugs such as strychnine and picrotoxin interfere with inhibitory pathways in the c.n.s. Strychnine is believed to lower the threshold of spinal cord synapses by antagonising glycine presumed to be the inhibitory transmitter acting at spinal interneurones. Picrotoxin, another powerful central stimulant, may block inhibitory pathways mediated by GABA. It has been shown that picrotoxin can ree-stablish electrical conduction in cat cuneate nucleus after its block by GABA.

Qualitatively similar but stronger GABA-antagonistic effects are produced by the alkaloid bicucculine (Curtis).

These postulated mechanisms are not definitely proven as the functions of inhibitory c.n.s. transmitters are not fully established. The analysis of drug interactions after their application by microelectrodes in the c.n.s. is difficult since their concentrations at the site of action cannot be quantitatively measured. Nevertheless, it is now widely assumed that the action of analeptics can be explained by their interference with ubiquitous inhibitory pathways in the central nervous system.

The analeptic drugs are used for two main purposes, (1) to produce stimulation of failing respiration and peripheral circulation; (2) to antagonise the cerebral depressant effect of poisoning by hypnotic drugs. The use of analeptic drugs for the treatment of poisoning is, however, being increasingly questioned.

Picrotoxin

Picrotoxin is a white crystalline substance, sparingly soluble in water, which is prepared from the fishberry, *Cocculus indicus*. It is a powerful analeptic but its disadvantage is that the dose required for stimulation of respiration is very close to that which produces convulsions. The action of picrotoxin is transient and the drug disappears rapidly from the blood. It has been used in the treatment of barbiturate poisoning by intravenous injections repeated at half-hourly intervals, but is now replaced by more satisfactory methods such as endotracheal intubation and positive pressure ventilation.

Leptazol (cardiazol)

This compound (pentamethylene tetrazole) is a cortical and medullary stimulant which has been used to counteract the depressant effects of overdosage with alcohol, opiates, and hypnotics.

Strychnine

This is an alkaloid obtained from the seeds of *Nux vomica*. It has a bitter taste and in small doses acts as a simple bitter and stimulates the secretion of gastric juice. It also increases the movements of the human stomach as shown by intragastric balloon experiments.

The chief action of strychnine on the central nervous system is on the spinal cord which is first affected; increasing doses stimulate all parts of the brain since strychnine has a marked facilitative action on central synapses. In small doses strychnine produces exaggerated reflex responses whereby the motor component of the reflex is augmented and the inhibitory component diminished. The work of Eccles and his colleagues has provided evidence that strychnine interferes with the action of an inhibitory transmitter in the spinal cord. It may compete with the inhibitory transmitter for receptor sites on the postsynaptic membrane.

The sensations of touch, smell and hearing are rendered more acute by strychnine, an effect which is attributed to the action of the drug on the sensory functions of the brain. The sense of vision is particularly affected; not only is the visual acuity increased but the field of vision is enlarged. This is believed to be due to an action on the retina, an effect which can be demonstrated by local application of the drug to the conjunctiva of one eye.

Strychnine poisoning

Large doses of strychnine produce tonic or spinal convulsions. The convulsions occur in response to sensory stimuli and consist of a simultaneous contraction of most of the muscles of the trunk and limbs; the flexors and extensors contract simultaneously but since the extensors are the more powerful, the trunk and limbs are extended rigidly. The convulsions last for about a minute and then all the muscles relax. A few convulsions (2-6) suffice to kill a mammal, the usual cause of death being asphyxia.

The treatment of strychnine poisoning must be quickly applied since patients seldom survive more than five or six convulsions. The convulsions may be controlled in the first instance by a volatile anaesthetic until it is possible to administer intravenously thiopentone sodium or pentobarbitone sodium. In animals it has been shown that the interneurone blocking drug mephenesin specifically antagonises strychnine convulsions but its clinical use for this purpose is limited because of its toxicity when administered intravenously.

CLINICALLY USED RESPIRATORY STIMULANTS

These drugs have limited application as central respiratory stimulants. They act on medullary centres or reflexly on chemoreceptors of the carotid body to increase pulmonary ventilation and may be used to stimulate breathing in anaesthesia and poisoning, in respiratory disease or in the treatment of respiratory distress in the newborn.

Nikethamide
A powerful, if short-acting, respiratory stimulant when given intravenously. Its injection is followed by coughing and occasionally vomiting. Signs of arousal are usually apparent whilst the rate and depth of respiration increases. It may be given repeatedly by intermittent injections.

Doxapram
A useful respiratory stimulant acting particularly on chemoreceptors. In view of its short-lived action it may be administered by continuous intravenous infusion. It has been found beneficial in patients receiving oxygen therapy who show a progressive increase in pCO_2.

Ethamivan
A respiratory stimulant with analeptic activity employed in the newborn.

Aminophylline
Stimulates the respiratory centre and is used in the treatment of Cheyne-Stokes breathing.

SYMPATHOMIMETIC AMINES

Certain sympathomimetic amines have useful awakening and respiratory stimulant properties. The relative potency of several amines in shortening anaesthesia in animals is shown in Table 12.1 below.

A characteristic feature of the action of these amines is that only shallow anaesthesia can be influenced and deep anaesthesia cannot be reversed by increased doses of these drugs. The awakening effect occurs within 5 to 15 minutes and lasts for 2 to 3 hours; even with large doses muscular twitching is not produced.

Action of morphine on the respiratory centre
Morphine and heroin have a powerful depressant action on the respiratory centre. Small doses of morphine in animals reduce both the frequency and volume of respiration and increase the tension of CO_2 in the blood. This is also true for other analgesics and it has been shown that pethidine and methadone when tested on rabbits have a respiratory depressant action in proportion to their analgesic activity.

The effect of morphine on the respiration of normal subjects resembles that of reducing the concentration of CO_2 in the alveolar air. Linhard found that in a normal subject the administration of 6 per cent CO_2 produced a sixfold increase in the volume of air breathed, but after 15 mg morphine had been given the same concentration of CO_2 only caused a fourfold increase in the volume of air breathed. This method of assessing respiratory depressant action has been used in testing other analgesics in normal human volunteers. It can be seen from Figure 12.2 that in approximately equipotent analgesic doses morphine, methadone and pethidine cause similar degrees of respiratory depression. It has been found, however, that in contrast to morphine and methadone, pethidine in doses which produce analgesia during labour, does not depress the respiration of the new-born infant. The respiratory depression produced by morphine, methadone and pethidine can be antagonised by nalorphine.

The depression of the respiratory centre by anaesthetics is a serious complication of anaesthesia. The cough reflex is paralysed at the end of the second stage of anaesthesia, and in the third stage of anaesthesia the sensitivity of the respiratory centre to carbon dioxide is reduced.

The cough reflex
Coughing is a very effective method of clearing the larger bronchi for it produces a violent blast of air through these. The velocity of air in the bronchial tree may be increased

Table 12.1 The relative potencies of some sympathomimetic compounds in shortening anaesthesia. (After Jacobsen, 1939, Acta med. Scand.)

Substance	Potency
ß-Phenylisopropylamine sulphate (amphetamine sulphate)	1
N-Methylamphetamine hydrochloride	1–2
N-Propylamphetamine hydrochloride	½–1
N-Isopropylamphetamine hydrochloride	⅛–¼
Ephedrine hydrochloride	1/20–1/10
ß-Phenylethylamine hydrochloride	0

RESPIRATORY AND COUGH DEPRESSANT DRUGS

Drugs which depress the medullary centres affect the respiration in two ways: they depress the respiratory centre and make it less sensitive to the stimulus of carbon dioxide, and they also depress the cough centre. The first of these actions is harmful, but the second effect is often desired in therapeutics.

nearly 10-fold during violent breathing, but in the act of coughing it is increased 20-fold.

Coughing is therefore a protective reflex action which removes irritants from the larger bronchi and upper air passages. The movements associated with the act of coughing are believed to be co-ordinated by a 'cough centre' which is situated close to the vagal centre and to the vomiting centre. The cough reflex is like the vomiting reflex in that it does not occur in full anaesthesia, but can

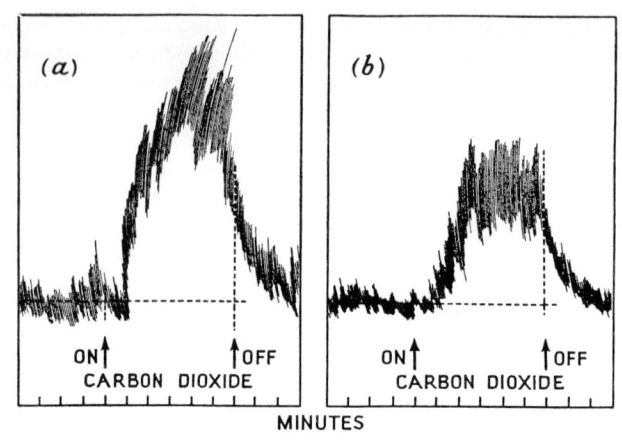

Fig. 12.1 Typical records obtained with Gaddum's respiration recorder in a normal man: (a) initial response to breathing 5 per cent carbon dioxide in oxygen; (b) response half an hour after intramuscular injection of methadone 10 mg. (After Prescott, Ransom, Thorp and Wilson, 1949, *Lancet*.)

occur in the unconscious subject. During consciousness the reflex can be inhibited by conscious effort, but there is a limit to this power of inhibition. Coughing is excited by various sensory stimuli, but stimulation of the sensory endings of the vagus or glossopharyngeal is the most powerful stimulus. The vagus supplies sensory fibres to the larynx and bronchi, and, in addition, the abdominal vagus supplies sensory fibres to the stomach and many other abdominal organs.

The strongest cough reflex is excited by stimulation of the larynx and trachea. Stimulation of the pharynx and large bronchi produces less effect and the sensitivity decreases rapidly as the bronchi become smaller. Stimulation of the sensory endings of the abdominal vagus also induces coughing. A well-marked example of this is the coughing that accompanies emesis. The vagus also carries the secretory fibres to the bronchial mucous glands, and stimulation of any of the sensory branches of the vagus tends to increase the secretion of these glands.

Action of drugs on cough

Coughing is usually a useful reflex which removes undesirable material from the respiratory passages, and therefore care must be taken in interfering with it. Drugs may modify cough by (a) depression of the cough centre, (b) local action on the pharynx and larynx or (c) by decreasing the viscosity of bronchial secretion.

The chief conditions that can be alleviated by medical treatment are as follows:

1. Hyperirritability of the throat and bronchi. This leads to a frequent, dry, hacking cough, which does not remove any phlegm, but is distressing to the patient. Pleural inflammation can also produce a similar effect and the distress is usually increased by the cough causing pain.

2. Excessive cough due to undue tenacity of the mucus. This form of cough is treated by increasing the bronchial secretion, and thus rendering it more fluid.

3. Excessive bronchial secretion causing accumulation of fluid or mucus in the bronchi. When severe bronchitis is produced, either by bacterial infection or by irritant gases, the bronchial secretion may be so great as to threaten to drown the patient. Milder bronchitis may cause some of the bronchi to be plugged with mucus, and if the respiratory movements and the cough reflex are depressed this may result in massive collapse of a portion of the lung.

Assessment of drugs acting on cough centre

There are several methods of producing cough experimentally in animals and in man which can be used to assess the effect of drugs on the cough centre.

1. The introduction into the trachea of an irritant chemical such as sulphur dioxide or ammonia. A method has been used in man to elicit a minimal cough response by

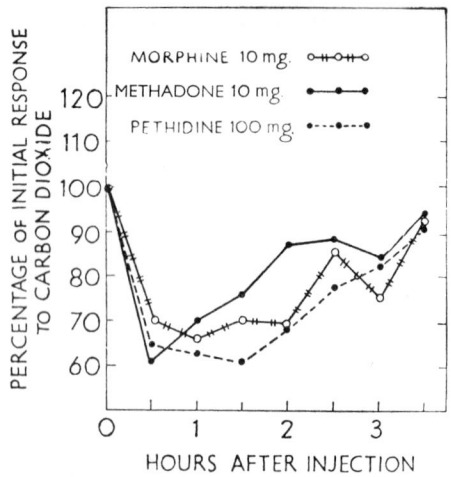

Fig. 12.2 Depression of respiratory stimulation by 5 per cent carbon dioxide in normal man. Approximately equivalent analgesic doses of morphine, methadone and pethidine produce the same degree of respiratory depression. (After Prescott, Ransom, Thorp and Wilson, 1949, *Lancet*.)

the sudden introduction of small amounts of ammonia into the inspired air. In experiments of this kind methadone was found to be about fifteen times more active than codeine; when the concentration of ammonia inhaled was increased, methadone was still effective whereas even large doses of codeine were ineffective.

2. Electrical stimulation of the central end of the cut superior laryngeal nerve of the cat; this causes a brief respiratory gasp which resembles a cough. Table 12.2 shows that methadone is more active and codeine and pethidine are less active than morphine in suppressing experimentally induced cough.

3. Administration of an aerosol containing antigen to a sensitised guinea pig (Herxheimer's micro-shock method). Minute amounts of the aerosol produce a dry cough and later a condition resembling an asthmatic attack. The procedure can be used to assay drugs which suppress cough and also to study drugs which are effective in bronchial asthma.

Table 12.2 Intravenous dose of morphine and related drugs required for suppression of cough produced by electrical stimulation of the superior laryngeal nerve in cats. (After Green and Ward, 1955, *Brit. J. Pharmacol.*)

Drug	Dose mk/kg	Relative activity
Morphine sulphate	0.4	100
Codeine (base)	4.0	10
Pethidine hydrochloride	1.0	40
Methadone hydrochloride	0.05	800

Action of drugs on the cough centre
A troublesome and useless cough usually requires the use of some depressant of the cough centre, in addition to local treatment. The opium alkaloids (p. 280) and related compounds are effective suppressants of cough. These drugs are often prepared as a syrup or linctus which has a soothing effect on the inflamed upper respiratory tract.

Morphine has a marked action in reducing the sensitivity of the cough centre and is very useful in stopping useless cough; even small doses (6 mg) usually produce marked relief. Its action in depressing the sensitivity of the respiratory centre to CO_2 and its liability to produce addiction are serious disadvantages.

Methadone depresses the cough reflex in doses as small as 2 mg and in these doses produces little or no respiratory depression.

Heroin (diamorphine) has three or four times as strong an action on the cough centre as morphine but it is even more dangerous than morphine as regards addiction.

Codeine effectively suppresses cough of a mild type in doses of 15–30 mg. Although it is much less active than morphine or methadone, codeine has the advantage that it is not liable to produce drug dependence.

In acute pleurisy, where there is considerable pain, which is aggravated by coughing, it is usually necessary to use morphine rather than codeine, because the latter has such a feeble action in alleviating pain.

Pholcodeine is more active than codeine as a cough suppressant but less active than morphine.

Dextromethorphan (romilar), another cough suppressant, is related chemically to levorphanol but like pholcodeine it has no analgesic or addictive properties. It is used in doses of 10 to 20 mg.

Local action of drugs on cough
Undue irritability of the pharynx and larynx is a common cause of persistent and useless cough, which is frequently worst at night, and may cause troublesome insomnia. The simplest method of treatment is to give lozenges containing some demulcent such as liquorice. Sprays are more effective, and may consist of liquid paraffin to which some volatile oil or menthol has been added. There is, however, some danger in using oily sprays, since the drops may enter the trachea; prolonged use may cause lipoidal pneumonia. Sprays containing ephedrine relieve cough because they diminish congestion of the throat and counteract mild bronchospasm. Inhalation of a volatile substance is a method of producing an action further down on the larynx and trachea. The inhalation of the vapour from a teaspoonful of compound tincture of benzoin in a pint of boiling water is an oldfashioned but effective remedy.

Irritant cough of the type that disturbs sleep at night appears to be frequently associated with bronchial spasm. Ephedrine hydrochloride (30 mg) frequently produces relief in such cases but may prevent sleep unless combined with a sedative. Alternatively antihistamine drugs may be used.

Expectorants
A number of drugs, which are used to relieve cough, act by irritating the sensory endings of the vagus in the stomach and thereby cause an increased secretion of the bronchial mucous glands. This relieves the persistent cough, which is due to the presence of sticky mucus in the upper air passages.

The secretion of the bronchial mucous membrane can be increased and made more fluid by the administration of *potassium iodide*. This drug increases various secretions, as is evident by the excessive lachyrymal and nasal secretion which occurs in iodism. Slow-acting emetic drugs such as *ipecacuanha, ammonium carbonate* and *squill* are used in sub-emetic doses; although their delayed action renders them unsuitable as emetics, it makes them useful as expectorants.

Mode of action of expectorants. Gordonoff studied the action of expectorants by injecting lipiodol into the bronchi of rabbits and following its fate by serial radiographs. He showed that saponins, ethereal oils, potassium iodide and ipecacuanha had a secretolytic action and increased the rate at which lipiodol in the lungs was dispersed. He concluded that expectorants act by diluting thick viscid secretions through increased activity of bronchial glands, the resultant fluid being partially reabsorbed whilst some of the unabsorbable material is rendered absorbable by the digestive action of the parenchyma of the lungs. The remaining particles are expelled from the alveoli into the bronchioles and bronchi by the kinetic energy of expired air, and further elimination is brought about by coughing or by the ciliary movement of the bronchial epithelium.

Basch and his colleagues collected, by postural drainage or by bronchoscopic suction, the sputum of patients with bronchiectases and found that drugs such as potassium iodide, ammonium chloride, ipecacuanha and senega consistently decreased the viscosity of secretions.

Inhalation of CO_2 and of steam produced an even greater liquefaction of sputum, while oxygen had the opposite effect in that it increased the viscosity of sputum. They concluded that these expectorants reduce the amount of sputum within the bronchial tree by stimulating reabsorption and rendering the remainder more liquid, so that it is coughed up more easily.

PHARMACOLOGY OF BRONCHIAL ASTHMA

Functions of the bronchi

The alveoli of the lungs are very delicate thin-walled cells about 0.25 mm in diameter, and their total area is about 70 square metres. The whole minute volume of the circulation passes through this great capillary area and the thinness of the walls permits very rapid equilibrium being established between the gases in the blood and the alveolar air.

The bronchial tree consists of branching tubes, lined with ciliated epithelium and furnished with secretory cells, the walls of which can be contracted by the bronchial muscles. The trachea and bronchi are lined with ciliated epithelium down to, but excluding a short length of, the terminal bronchioles.

Under normal conditions the mucous glands secrete a small amount of mucus which is carried up the bronchi and trachea by the ciliated epithelium, passes into the pharynx and is swallowed. Any irritation greatly increases the secretion of mucus. The vagus carries the secretory fibres of the bronchial glands and these fibres are cholinergic. Hence parasympathomimetic drugs, and notably pilocarpine, greatly increase the secretion of mucus. The activity of the glands can also be excited by a variety of reflexes. Any increase in mucous secretion tends to encourage coughing, which is chiefly effective in clearing the large bronchi.

Bronchial musculature

These muscles constitute about half the total weight of the lungs. They are arranged as a network over the bronchi. At each inspiration the bronchi become longer and wider and at each expiration they become shorter and narrower. Contraction of the bronchial muscles narrows the lumen of all the parts of the bronchial tree, but it is most effective in constricting the terminal bronchioles.

The chief normal activities of the bronchial muscles which are established with certainty are that they are contracted by the vagus and dilated by the sympathetic. Hence they contract during sleep and dilate during excitement or violent exercise.

As regards the pharmacology of the bronchial muscles, they are contracted by parasympathomimetic drugs and by a variety of other drugs, for example morphine. Histamine has a very strong bronchoconstrictor action, and in the guinea-pig histamine produces so powerful a constriction of the bronchi that the animal dies of asphyxia. Recent work has shown that the bronchoconstrictor effect of drugs such as histamine applied by aerosol is partly reflex. Peripheral stimulation sets up a reflex which stimulates vagal efferents causing further stimulation. This complex effect underlines the importance of central mechanisms in allergic bronchoconstriction. Other substances which produce bronchoconstriction are prostaglandins, bradykinin and SRS-A.

Dilatation of the bronchial muscles can be produced by sympathomimetic drugs, by atropine-like drugs and by drugs which relax most types of plain muscle — papaverine, nitrites and xanthine derivatives. The most important derangement of function of the bronchial muscles is the condition of bronchial asthma in which there is a tendency to transient attacks of dyspnoea by bronchial obstruction.

Bronchial asthma

Bronchial asthma is a complex disease in which allergic, psychological and bronchitic elements are inextricably bound up. All these factors must receive attention in the treatment of asthmatic patients, but here we are only concerned with palliative drug treatment to alleviate the acute attack. For relevant immunology see Chapter 8.

The symptoms of bronchial asthma are due to a combination of spasm of the plain muscle of bronchioles, oedema and swelling of mucous membranes and obstruction by secretions. Inspection with the bronchoscope has shown that during asthmatic attacks the mucous membrane of the trachea and bronchi is oedematous and swollen and the lumen is filled with thick tenacious secretions. If these secretions are aspirated the patient is partly relieved but further relief is obtained by an injection of adrenaline. Within a few minutes of the injection a quantity of thick secretions appears in the trachea. This is due to adrenaline relieving the intense

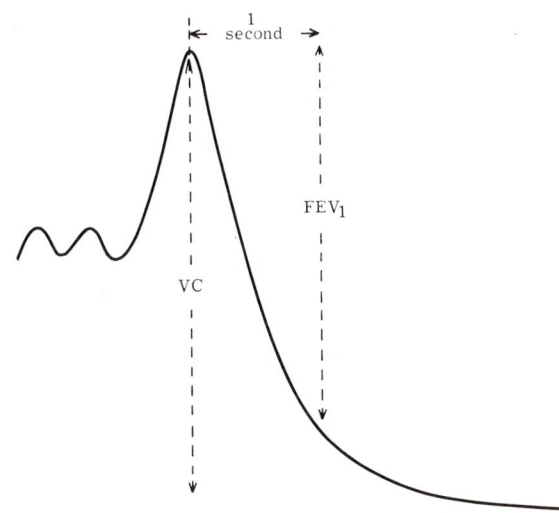

Fig. 12.3 Fast spirogram recording normal respiration, maximal inspiration and forced expiration. FEV_1 = forced expired volume in 1 second. VC = vital capacity. (After Sykes, McNicol and Campbell, 1976. In *Respiratory Failure*, Blackwell, Oxford.)

constriction of the small bronchioles and the urticaria-like swelling of their mucous membrane both of which help to retain secretions within the bronchiolar lumen. An asthmatic attack usually terminates with a bout of coughing and in children the administration of an emetic helps to expectorate the secretions.

Palliative treatment of asthma. The pharmacological actions required in the treatment of bronchial asthma are: relaxation of bronchial muscle, decrease of oedema and swelling, sedation, expectoration and improved oxygen supply. No known drug possess all these actions but the sympathomimetic catecholamines relax bronchial muscle and also appear to exert a characteristic anti-allergic effect manifested by inhibition of release of chemical mediators of allergic reactions such as histamine. They are the most effective drugs in the treatment of the acute asthmatic attack.

Assessment of severity of bronchial asthma
In order to assess airways function fully, it is necessary to measure the two parameters of airways resistance and lung compliance. Methods for measuring these parameters in man have been worked out by Comroe and his colleagues but the procedures are complex, involving the use of body plethysmographs and oesophageal balloons. It is possible, however, to obtain a clinical assessment of airways obstruction in bronchial asthma and the effects of bronchodilator drugs upon it by applying relatively simple measurements.

One of the most useful is the measurement of forced expiratory volume which is the volume of air expelled from the lungs over a given period when the subject makes a maximum expiratory effort from a position of full inspiration. If the time interval adopted is one second, the measure is called FEV_1 (Fig. 12.3). When the expiratory effort is continued to the limit of expiration the expired volume is referred to as the forced vital capacity (FVC). Other measures used for assessing bronchial function are the maximum ventilatory capacity and the expiratory peak flow rate. In order to assess lung function various static lung volumes and capacities may be evaluated. They are shown in Figure 12.4. Most of the lung volumes can be evaluated by spirometry except for the residual volume which must be determined by other means, usually by the helium dilution method. An increase in residual volume and in functional residual capacity is characteristic of the overinflation of the lungs seen in chronic bronchial asthma even between attacks. The FEV_1 is often expressed as a percentage of the forced vital capacity (FVC); this relation, referred to as forced expiratory ratio, is about 75 per cent in a normal lung.

In bronchial asthma airways resistance is increased markedly. In moderate asthma, when there may be a threefold increase in airways resistance, the FEV_1 is reduced to about half of the predicted normal and in severe asthma the FEV_1 may be 10–20 per cent of predicted. Vital capacity is usually reduced in asthma. An important indicator to be watched in asthma is the arterial oxygen tension. Some decrease of arterial pO_2 is seen regularly, even in quite mild cases, but if the bronchial obstruction impairs breathing so severely that arterial oxygen tension falls to 70 mmHg or below, urgent therapeutic measures must be taken. By contrast arterial pCO_2 does not usually rise in asthma except in the severest cases indicating that the patient is in a precarious state.

The effect of bronchodilator drugs in patients with asthma can be assessed by performing tests before and after the administration of a bronchodilator drug e.g. isoprenaline given by aerosol (Fig. 12.5). Alternatively histamine or an acetyl-choline-like drug may be administered and the reduction of its effect by administering a long lasting bronchodilator drug such as ephedrine may be measured (Fig. 12.8).

Sympathomimetic drugs

Adrenaline (Epinephrine)
Adrenaline was isolated from the suprarenal gland in 1901 almost simultaneously by Takamine, who named it adrenalin, and by von Fürth, who named it suprarenin. Its effectiveness in allergic conditions, particularly in spasmodic asthma, was soon recognised. Its action includes constriction of mucosal blood vessels and diminution of oedema by virtue of its α-adrenoceptor stimulant activity but more particularly it is a powerful bronchodilator agent by virtue of its strong ß-adrenoceptor stimulant activity. The receptors involved in the bronchodilator effects of adrenaline are generally classified within the β_2 subclass concerned with tracheal and other smooth muscle relaxation (p. 15). The activation

Lung Volumes and Capacities

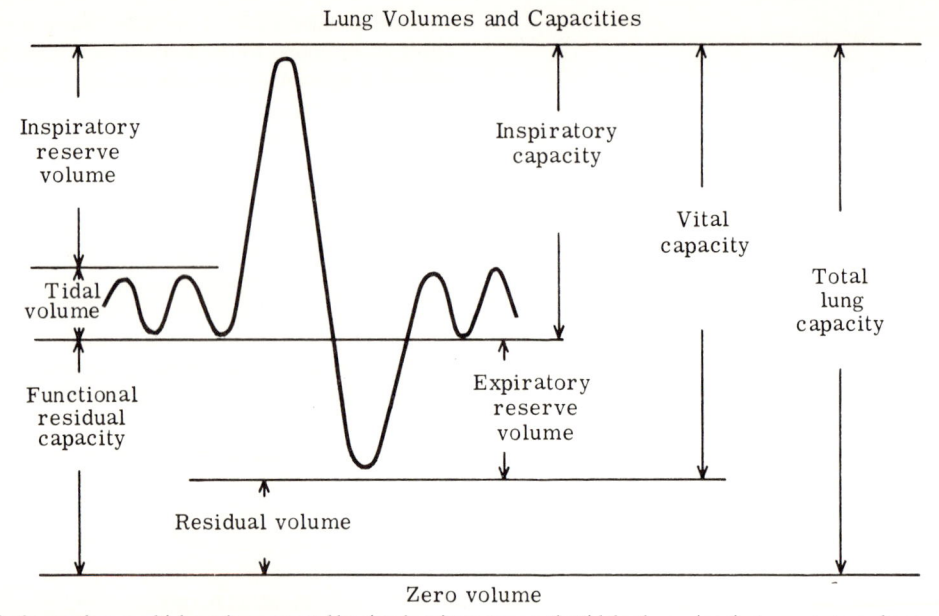

Fig. 12.4 The lung volumes which can be measured by simple spirometry are the tidal volume, inspiratory reserve volume, expiratory reserve volume, inspiratory capacity and vital capacity. The residual volume cannot be measured by observation of a simple spirometer trace and it is therefore impossible to measure the functional residual capacity or the total lung capacity without further elaboration of methods.

of ß-adrenergic receptors induces an increased formation of intracellular cyclic AMP and this effect is believed to be connected with the muscular relaxation although the mechanism by which the two phenomena are linked is not understood.

A further mechanism by which ß-adrenergic catecholamines can affect bronchial asthma is their anti-anphylactic activity by virtue of which they tend to prevent the release of mediators of allergic bronchoconstriction such as histamine from tissues mast cells.

A subcutaneous injection of 0.3–1.0 ml of a 1:1000 solution of adrenaline hydrochloride may be given in a severe asthmatic attack and usually produces relief in a few minutes. If no relief is obtained within about 5 minutes the injection may be repeated but some patients fail to respond even to repeated injections and in these cases another drug such as intravenous aminophylline must be tried. Adrenaline may also be administered by aerosol spray although it has now been largely replaced by isoprenaline and other drugs for this purpose. When adrenaline is given by spray a 1:100 solution is used, which must on no account be confused with the 1:1000 solution used for injection.

Adrenaline produces relief by relaxing the bronchioles and this relief causes a fall in the pulse rate and blood pressure, although in a normal person adrenaline might produce the reverse effect on these functions. The disadvantages attending the use of adrenaline are that it cannot be given by mouth, its action only last for a short time, and in certain individuals it causes tremors, palpitations, rise of blood pressure and increased pulse frequency.

Isoprenaline (Isoproterenol)
This is a synthetic sympathomimetic drug (p. 81) with predominantly beta-adrenergic effects including a powerful bronchodilatation which is stronger, weight for weight, than that of adrenaline. Its effect on an asthmatic patient is shown in Figure 12.5. The spirometer tracing shows that during the asthmatic attack the patient is almost incapable of inspiration or expiration and the lungs are in an almost completely inflated condition. The situation corresponds to that of an extreme case of emphysema in which the residual air is markedly increased and the vital capacity decreased. Within five minutes of inhaling a spray of isoprenaline the thorax becomes deflated, breathing returns to normal and the vital capacity increases from 1300 ml to 2900 ml.

Isoprenaline is usually administered by inhalation as an aerosol. It may also be administered by sublingual tablet since owing to its vasodilator properties it is readily absorbed from the mucous membrane of the mouth. In children it can be given rectally. Parenteral administration is seldom used since it produces marked tachycardia which is aggravated by the fall in blood pressure due to the drug.

When administered by inhalation, isoprenaline is usually given by a pressurised aerosol. When the inhaler is squeezed a single squirt of the spray is produced, delivering either 0.08 or 0.4 mg of isoprenaline. There is evidence that a phase of increased mortality attributed to

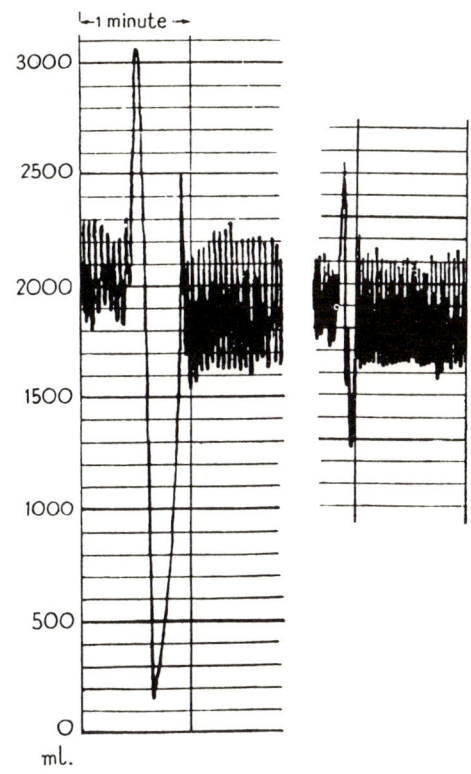

Fig. 12.5 Spirometer tracing of a patient in an asthmatic attack. The tracing on the right was taken during an acute attack. The tracing on the left was taken immediately afterwards when 3 per cent isoprenaline was inhaled for two minutes. (After Herxheimer, 1949, *Thorax*.) (Basilinis are different.)

asthma during recent years was connected with the excessive use of pressurised aerosols of concentrated isoprenaline. The sequence of events might be that a patient who fails to obtain relief from asthma, doses himself repeatedly with isoprenaline which becomes increasingly less effective in causing bronchodilatation due to receptor desensitisation. At the same time more isoprenaline gets taken up into the circulation causing stimulation of the heart and possibly a fatal ventricular fibrillation. It has been shown in anaesthetised dogs that isoprenaline may cause cardiac arrest especially under conditions of hypoxia.

Metabolism of isoprenaline. Isoprenaline is metabolised by catechol-O-methyltransferase (p. 76) to a methoxy-derivative which is a moderately potent beta blocker and its formation may thus account for some of the tolerance which develops to inhaled isoprenaline. It is believed, however, that marked tolerance is mainly due to receptor desensitisation. Isoprenaline is taken up by cells through uptake-2 mechanism for catecholamines (p. 77) which may account for its rapid absorption when inhaled. When given orally isoprenaline is transformed to an inactive ethereal sulphate.

Protokylol is a derivative of isoprenaline which is well absorbed from the gastrointestinal tract, when given orally. After oral administration bronchodilatation appears within 30 to 90 minutes and persists for 4 hours. Its cardiovascular effects are similar to isoprenaline.

Salbutamol (Ventolin)

Although isoprenaline produces a rapid and powerful bronchodilatation its inhalation is often accompanied by palpitation and tachycardia; it also has the disadvantage of short duration of action. There have been many attempts to improve on isoprenaline and one of the resulting compounds is salbutamol (Fig. 12.7). This is more stable than isoprenaline because it is not destroyed by catechol-O-methyltransferase and it can therefore be administered also by mouth. Its most important pharmacological property is that whilst having activity of the same order as isoprenaline on beta-2-receptors of bronchial muscle it has much less activity on beta-1 receptors in the heart (Fig. 12.6).

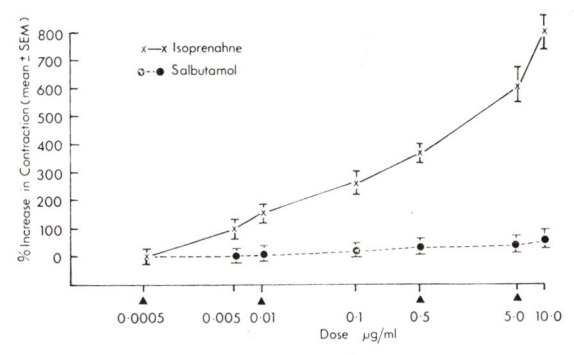

Fig. 12.6 Effect of isoprenaline and salbutamol on tension developed during isometric contraction by human heart muscle stimulated to contract at a regular rate. (After Nayler, *Postgrad. Med. J.*, 1971.)

The lack of cardiac stimulation by salbutamol has important physiological consequences. Even moderate attacks of asthma are associated with hypoxaemia which may be dangerous when arterial oxygen is reduced to the level where the steep part of the haemoglobin-oxygen dissociation curve is reached. Isoprenaline, even when it relieves airways obstruction, may aggravate the anoxaemia by increasing the oxygen consumption of the heart. By contrast salbutamol, which lacks cardiostimulatory effects, tends to improve or at least not aggravate, arterial hypoxaemia thus avoiding the attendant dangers to the heart and circulation.

Salbutamol may be administered by inhalation or orally. When given by pressurised aerosol it produces its effect somewhat more slowly than isoprenaline but bronchodilatation lasts much longer. Doses producing bronchodilatation cause little or no cardiac stimulation (Fig. 12.6). After a dose of 0.2 mg by inhalation (=two

180   APPLIED PHARMACOLOGY

puffs of 'Ventolin' inhaler) effective bronchodilatation persists for 3 hours or more. Salbutamol may also be administered orally in doses of 5-10 mg. Although effective in a proportion of patients, oral administration of salbutamol may produce objectionable limb tremor as a side effect.

Isoetharine is an isoprenaline derivative with an ethyl group on the alpha carbon. It is absorbed by mouth and has considerable ß$_2$ stimulating bronchodilator activity.

Orciprenaline (Alupent)
This compound is a derivative of resorcinol (Fig. 12.7). It is more stable than isoprenaline and may be administered by aerosol or orally. It produces greater tachycardia than salbutamol. *Terbutaline* is a derivative of orciprenaline which appears to be more active on bronchial muscle and less active on the heart than the parent compound.

Ephedrine (p. 126)
Figure 12.8 shows the effect of ephedrine in experimental asthma. Patients with chronic asthma are more sensitive to histamine than normal subjects and usually respond to an intravenous injection of histamine with an asthma-like attack and a decrease in vital capacity. These attacks may be prevented by isoprenaline or by ephedrine, but whilst isoprenaline acts almost at once, ephedrine, even when injected intramuscularly, has a latent period of action and the peak of its action occurs only after about two hours.

Ephedrine has a much weaker bronchodilator action than isoprenaline and its beneficial effects in asthma are partly due to decongestion of mucous membranes. Owing to its prolonged effect ephedrine hydrochloride is of

$HOCH_2$
HO—⬡—$CHOH.CH_2.NH.C(CH_3)_3$

Salbutamol

HO—⬡—$CHOH.CH_2.NH.CH(CH_3)_2$
   HO

Orciprenaline

HO
HO—⬡—$CHOH.CH_2.NH.CH(CH_3)_2$

Isoprenaline

Fig. 12.7 Structural formulae of bronchodilator drugs.

special value in the prevention of asthmatic attacks and it can be most useful in those asthmatic patients whose chronic asthma rarely causes acute attacks but a continuing hyperinflation of the lungs. It can be taken by mouth and, therefore, the patient can administer it to himself at need. It begins to produce relief in three quarters of an hour, if taken by mouth, and in 10 minutes, if given intramuscularly. The action persists for 4 to 6 hours. The drug may produce a rise of from 10 to 40 mmHg in the systolic blood pressure. Ephedrine has a stimulant action on the central nervous system and its regular use may

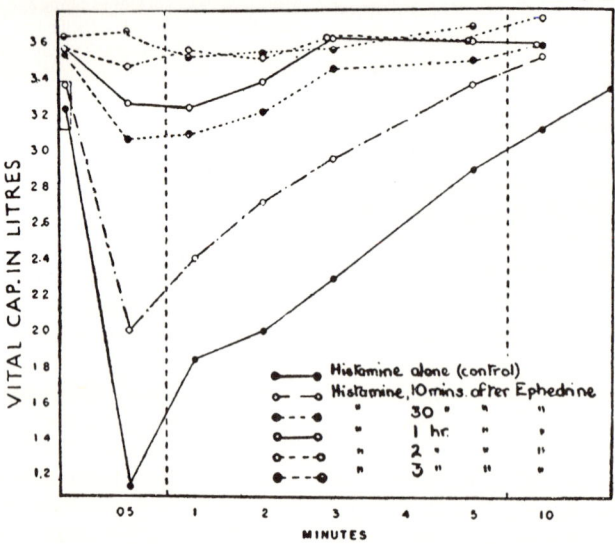

Fig. 12.8 This figure shows the decrease in vital capacity produced by intravenous injections of histamine (0.04 mg) in an asthmatic subject and the action of ephedrine (30 mg i.m.) in antagonising the effects of histamine. Injections of histamine at 1 and 2 hours after ephedrine had practically no effect on vital capacity. (After Curry, *J. Clin. Investig.*, 1946.)

produce insomnia, it is therefore often combined at night with a hypnotic or it may be taken in the morning an hour before getting up. It may cause retention of urine in elderly subjects.

The pharmacological action of ephedrine is partly indirect due to the release of noradrenaline from nerve endings, hence if it is administered repeatedly in rapid succession either in animal experiments or in man its effects diminish (tachyphylaxis). Clinically it is found that if ephedrine is administered three times daily for several weeks tolerance develops, but sensitivity can be re-established by omitting its administration for a few days.

Atropine

Since the motor nerves of the bronchi are cholinergic, atropine would appear the obvious remedy for asthma, but in actual fact it is not nearly as effective as the sympathomimetic drugs. Atropine produces excessive dryness and has an anti-expectorant action. The sputum becomes much more tenacious and adherent to the walls of the bronchi, an effect which is generally undesirable. Stramonium leaves contain atropine and scopolamine and are a frequent ingredient of asthma remedies. They are commonly incorporated in combustion powders which also contain potassium nitrate to assist combustion. The smoke inhaled is irritant, however, and temporary relief may be followed by a further attack of asthma. Atropine or its quaternary derivative atropine methyl nitrate is sometimes added to improve the effectiveness of aerosol preparations of adrenaline or isoprenaline.

Antihistamine drugs

The intensive brochoconstriction which kills guinea pigs in anaphylactic shock is due largely to histamine released from the lungs. Histamine is also liberated from the lungs of patients with allergic asthma when they are brought into contact with the specific antigen to which the patient is sensitive (Fig. 8.13). In isolated preparations antihistamine drugs prevent bronchoconstriction due to added histamine but very high concentrations are required to antagonise the anaphylactic bronchoconstriction. The relative failure of antihistamines in bronchial asthma is probably due to two factors: (1) the high local concentration of released histamine; (2) the release of other bronchoconstrictor substances which are not antagonised by antihistamines.

The clinical use of H_1-antihistamines in allergic asthma has given disappointing results. Some authors have concluded that mepyramine was no more effective in bronchial asthma than were dummy tablets, either of which apparently benefited one-third of the patients, whilst in the remainder the frequency and duration of attacks were unaltered. Other, however, concluded that *slight* asthmatic attacks may be suppressed by mepyramine or promethazine given at night, and that the action extended into the early morning and abolished the frequent 'early morning wheeze'. These drugs produce drowsiness and should therefore be given at night; when used in combination with ephedrine they counteract the wakefulness produced by the latter. There is no good evidence that the H_2-antihistamines antagonise the bronchoconstrictor effects of histamine or of allergic bronchonstriction in man.

Disodium cromoglycate (Intal, Cromolyn sodium)

This drug (Fig. 12.9) relieves bronchial asthma by interfering with the cellular mechanism which causes the release of histamine (and presumably other bronchoconstrictor substances) during the allergic reaction. As previously discussed (p. 102), it is possible to interfere with allergic histamine release. Disodium cromoglycate produces this desirable action in relatively low concentrations without showing undue toxicity. The mode of action of cromoglycate is unknown. It has been shown to inhibit histamine release from tissue mast cells. It may interfere with an early step in the allergic histamine release reaction involving calcium entry into the cell.

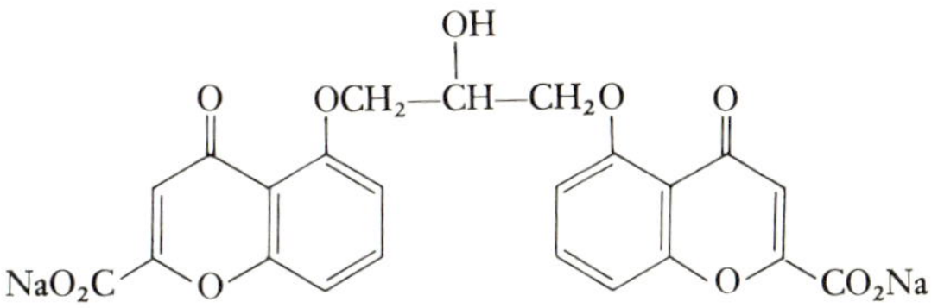

Fig. 12.9 Chemical structure of disodium cromoglycate.

Clinical action. Disodium cromoglycate is administered by inhalation of a powder through a 'spinhaler' usually in combination with isoprenaline. But there is evidence that it is also effective in the absence of isoprenaline and that it is an effective prophylactic antiasthmatic agent. Cromoglycate is ineffective in the treatment of acute attacks of asthma, including status asthmaticus. It appears to be more effective as a prophylactic drug in patients hypersensitive to a specific allergen ('extrinsic asthma') than in patients with 'intrinsic asthma'.

The effectiveness of cromoglycate has been demonstrated in clinical trials by several different criteria: patient preference, evaluation of symptoms by patients and doctors, diminished use of other anti-asthma drugs, spirometric lung function tests. Cromoglycate inhibits the development of exercise-induced asthma.

Response to the prophylactic effect of cromoglycate is very variable and has to be established by trial and error. Some patients respond in a few days, others in a few weeks, others don't seem to respond. If there is no response within a month treatment should be discontinued. In patients responding to cromoglycate, concomitant bronchodilator and cortocosteroid treatment may be cautiously reduced but corticosteroids should never be abruptly stopped in asthmatic patients.

Cromoglycate may also be administered by nasal insufflation (rynacrom) in patients with allergic rhinitis. Controlled trials have shown a significant improvement of symptoms of patients using this form of treatment during the pollen season.

Aminophylline
Aminophylline is theophylline ethylenediamine and is water soluble. The chemical structure of theophylline is shown on page 165.

Aminophylline relaxes all smooth muscle and its relaxant effect on bronchial muscle can be demonstrated on isolated human bronchi suspended in Ringer's solution or on the bronchi of anaesthetised guinea pigs. Aminophylline also increases the force of contraction of the heart, dilates coronary vessels, promotes diuresis and produces central stimulation. It is one of the most effective drugs in severe asthma and is often effective in patients who are refractory to catecholamines. Aminophylline is useful not only in allergic bronchial asthma but also in 'cardiac asthma' since it helps to reduce pulmonary oedema by strengthening the left heart and producing diuresis. Aminophylline may also improve Cheyne-Stokes breathing apparently by a central action.

Aminophylline is usually administered intravenously in doses of 250 to 500 mg in 10 ml. The injection should be administered slowly over a period of 5 to 10 minutes and may be repeated after 15 to 30 minutes. Rapid injections may produce severe toxic effects including cardiac arrest. Aminophylline is also effective orally but it often produces nausea and vomiting when administered by the oral route. Another route of administration is by rectal instillation of aminophylline; this is well absorbed and non-irritating. Intramuscular administration is highly irritating and painful.

Diprophylline is a neutral theophylline derivative which can be used intramuscularly without producing local pain.

Choline theophyllinate (choledyl). Because of the high incidence of gastric intolerance to aminophylline several related preparations have been introduced for oral use in bronchial asthma. Choline theophyllinate is one of these; it is as effective as aminophylline and reported to produce less gastric irritation.

Oxygen and helium. The administration of oxygen to asthmatic patients is beneficial when there is cyanosis. The use of a mixture of 80 per cent helium and 20 per cent oxygen has been advocated in cases of severe asthma refractory to adrenaline. Helium owing to its lower density has only about two fifths of the flow resistance of nitrogen or oxygen and this diminishes the respiratory effort required from the patient. The disadvantage of helium is that it has to be administered in a closed circuit or in a tent.

Depressants of the central nervous system are widely used in asthma to lessen nervous tension and to promote sleep at night. Barbiturates or antihistamine drugs with sedative properties such as promethazine are useful in preventing attacks of asthma especially at night.

Corticosteroids
The administration of corticotrophin or cortisol or one of the synthetic cortisol substitutes such as prednisolone or prednisone may be necessary in the management of patients with recurrent or chronic asthma and is sometimes a life saving method of relieving patients with status asthmaticus. The corticosteroids are discussed on page 346.

For the control of chronic asthma various regimes of intermittent short courses or continuous treatment with *prednisolone* have been devised to minimise the risk of adverse effects. For intermittent treatment daily doses of 15-20 mg for 3 consecutive days each week have been advocated, whilst for continuous treatment daily doses of 7.5-10 mg, gradually decreased to 2.5-5 mg have been used. Complete withdrawal of the drugs, however, is usually followed by recurrence of the attacks. Long-acting preparations of cortioctrophin such as *corticotrophin gel* and *tetracosactrin zinc phosphate* are alternative methods of treatment; they are given by intramuscular injection two or three times weekly. Regular supervision of all patients requiring corticosteroid therapy is essential for prompt detection of adverse effects.

Attempts have been made to find corticosteroids which can be inhaled as an aerosol and would thus suppress asthma without causing appreciable systemic side effects. A recent preparation which is effective when administered by aerosol is *beclomethasone diproprionate*, which is given in a daily dosage of 0.3-0.4 mg (two inhalations taken 3 or 4 times during the day). In contrast to catecholamine inhalation this treatment is valueless for acute attacks but may be used to suppress bronchial asthma on a long term basis. This form of treatment is as yet not fully evaluated. Its main drawback so far has been the occurrence of localised infections with *Candida albicans* in the mouth and throat.

Effects of corticosteroid treatment. The effects of corticosteroids are not manifested at once; after oral administration they may take 3-4 days to show activity. Their first effect is an improvement in dyspnoea. The patient becomes again responsive to bronchodilators, to which he seemed to have become resistant; at the same time the massive hypersecretion of viscous bronchial mucus becomes less, respiration becomes more efficient and arterial pO_2 improves. After an initial period of treatment with corticosteroids it must be decided whether the patient requires a maintenance dose. Sometimes a small maintenance dose of 5-7.5 mg prednisone is sufficient but it may be difficult to wean the patient completely from corticosteroids. For this reason the decision to use corticosteroids in bronchial asthma has been called a grave one (Herxheimer, 1975). It is generally agreed, however, that they are by far the most effective drugs for the treatment of severe asthma.

The fundamental danger, when corticosteroids are used for some time, is a partial atrophy of the adrenal cortex. This may be difficult to establish from simple measurements of plasma cortisol levels which can vary even under normal conditions from 20 µg per 100 ml in the morning to 5 µg or less in the evening. A particularly dangerous and insidious consequence of a low plasma cortisol level is osteoporosis of the spine.

Status asthmaticus

This term is used to describe a very severe and sustained attack of asthma, when the patient has usually failed to respond to treatment with sympathomimetic drugs, further treatment with which may lead to cardiac arrest. A patient in status asthmaticus should be regarded as a medical emergency to be admitted promptly to an intensive care unit. Immediate treatment is required with oxygen at a flow rate of 4 litres per minute and a slow intravenous injection of 250 mg of aminophylline.

On admission to hospital endotracheal intubation enables prompt aspiration of tenacious sputum and bronchial secretions and the control of respiratory failure by intermittent positive pressure ventilation (IPPV). It is important to maintain an adequate fluid balance, for a patient who has had severe dyspnoea for more than a day or two is unable to eat and drink normally. Corticosteroid therapy is essential; hydrocortisone sodium succinate (500–1000 mg) intravenously initially, followed by oral prednisolone.

Sedation by intravenous injection of diazepam or intramuscular injection of sodium phenobarbitone may be necessary. Morphine should not be used in the treatment of status asthmaticus because although it may relieve the intense anxiety of the patient, it abolishes the cough reflex, depresses the respiratory centre and may accentuate the bronchospasm.

PREPARATIONS

Cyanide antidotes
Amyl nitrite vitrellae 0.2 ml
Cobalt edetate injection 300 mg
Sodium nitrite injection 3%

Respiratory stimulants
Doxapram hyd 0.5–1 mg/kg i.v.
Ethamivan 100–250 mg i.v.
Nikethamide inj. 0.5–2 g i.v.

Cough depressants
Codeine phosph 10–60 mg
Dextromethorphan 15–30 mg po up to 4x daily
Isoaminile citr 40 mg 3–5x daily
Methadone linctus 2 mg every 4 h
Pholcodine linctus 5–15 mg
Simple linctus citric acid 125 mg

Drugs for bronchial dilatation, liquefaction, allergy
Acetylcysteine spray (mucolytic)
Adrenaline 200–500 µg s.c. or i.m.
Beclomethasone diproprionate aerosol 100 µg 3–4x die (corticosteroid)
Corticotrophin inj s.c. or i.v.
Ephedrine 15–60 mg po, s.c., i.m.
Fenoterol brom 200–400 µg 3x die ($ß_2$ sympathom)
Hydrocortisone sod succ 100–300 mg i.v.
Ipatropium 20 mg metred aerosol (anticholinerg)
Isoetharine hyd 10–20 mg 3x die ($ß_2$ sympathom)
Isoprenaline sulph (Aleudrine) 1% aerosol
Methoxyphenamine hyd (Orthoxine) 50–100 mg po every 3–4 h (ß sympathom)
Orciprenaline sulph (Alupent) 20 mg po 4x die (ß sympathom)
Potassium iodide 250–500 mg
Pseudoephedrine hyd 30–60 mg po 2–4x die
Rimiterol hyd aerosol 200 µg 1–3 metred doses ($ß_2$ sympathom)
Salbutamol sulph (Ventolin) aerosol 100 µg every 4 h ($ß_2$ sympathom)
Sodium Cromoglycate (Intal) insuffl 20 mg 4x die (anti-allerg)
Terbutaline sulph po or aerosol 250 µg ($ß_2$ sympathom)
Tetracosactrin inj (corticotroph)

FURTHER READING

AMA Drug Evaluations 3rd edn 1977 Cromolyn sodium (Intal)
Assem E S K, Schild H O 1965 Inhibition by sympathomimetic amines of histamine release by antigen in passively senitized human lung. Nature 224: 1028
Austen K F, Becker E L (ed) 1968 Biochemistry of the Acute Allergic Reaction. Blackwell, Oxford
Bouhuys A (ed) 1970 Airways dynamics. Physiology and pharmacology. Charles Thomas, Springfield
Boyd E M 1954 Expectorants and respiratory tract fluids, Pharmacol. Rev. 6: 521
Bucher K 1965 Antitussive drugs. Physiological Pharmacology, 2: 175
Comroe J H, Forster R E, Dubois A B, Briscoe A W, Carlsen Elisabeth 1962 The lung. Year Book Med. Publ. Chicago
Fletcher C M (ed) 1971 Symposium on salbutamol. Postgrad. Med. J. Suppl. 47
Herxheimer H 1975 A guide to bronchial asthma. Academic Press, London
Sykes M K, McNicol M W, Campbell E J M 1976 Respiratory failure. Blackwell, Oxford
Widdicombe J G 1963 Regulation of tracheobronchial smooth muscle. Physiol. Rev. 43: 1

13. The alimentary canal

Chief functions of the alimentary canal 184; Salivary secretion 184; Secretion of gastric juice 184; Effects of drugs on gastric secretion 185; Parasympathomimetics 185; Gastrin 185; Pentagastrin 186; Histamine 187; H_2 receptor antagonists 187; Achlorhydria 188; Urogastrone 189; Atropine-like drugs 190; Carbenoxolone 190; Antacids 190; Vomiting 191; Emetics 192; Apomorphine 192; Hyoscine 193; H_1 antihistamines in sea-sickness 193; Chlorpromazine 193; Secretin 194; Cholecystokinin-pancreozymin 194; Pharmacology of bile 194; Gallstones 195; Chenodeoxycholic acid 196; Lipid-lowering agents 196; Purgatives 197; Drugs acting on intestinal muscle 200; Diphenoxylate 200; Mebeverine 200; Opiates 200.

CHIEF FUNCTIONS OF THE ALIMENTARY CANAL

The gastro-intestinal system can be divided, according to its functions, into three portions.

The upper portion comprises the mouth, the stomach, and the upper portion of the duodenum. In the mouth the food is triturated and moistened, and digestion is commenced by the saliva, while unsuitable material is rejected by the aid of taste and smell. The functions of the stomach are more complicated than those of any portion of the alimentary canal, for it receives substances of a most varied nature, and at irregular intervals, and it has to reduce these masses to a more or less uniform consistency, and forward the product to the duodenum at a fairly uniform rate.

The pylorus and upper portion of the duodenum together form a complex reflex mechanism, whose main function is to protect the small intestine from receiving unsuitable material. Hopelessly unsuitable material is rejected by vomiting, but the reflexes which cause closure of the pyloric sphincter ensure that the food is only forwarded after it has reached a suitable stage of division and of digestion, and also ensure that concentrated solutions are suitably diluted before they enter the small intestine. The functions of the pyloric sphincter are well indicated by its name (πυλουρος = a gate-keeper or warden).

The middle portion of the alimentary canal extends from the middle of the duodenum to the ileocolic sphincter, and its functions are relatively simple, namely, to complete digestion and to absorb over 90 per cent of the substances which it receives.

The lower portion of the gut consists of colon, and the rectum. The residues entering it are reduced to a semi-solid consistency, are stored in this form, and are periodically evacuated. The mechanisms which regulate the periodical evacuation of the colon and rectum are dependent upon a rational diet and a reasonable amount of exercise.

Salivary secretion

The salivary glands have a double nerve supply: sympathetic fibres, stimulation of which causes vasoconstriction, and a scanty flow of viscid saliva. They also receive a parasympathetic supply, stimulation of which causes a copious flow of saliva, accompanied by vasodilatation. Vasodilation in the salivary glands following parasympathetic stimulation is believed to be due to the action of true vasodilator cholinergic fibres and possibly also to the release of kallikrein from the gland causing the formation of bradykinin.

The salivary secretion is excited by (*a*) the psychic reflex excited by the sight or smell of food and (*b*) the chemical stimulation of the taste endings in the mouth.

All substances with a strong taste when introduced into the mouth excite a flow of saliva; this effect is produced particularly by substances with a bitter taste, for example quinine and strychnine. Any cause of nausea or vomiting will also excite a flow of saliva. The parasympathomimetic drugs, e.g. physostigmine and pilocarpine, produce a copious flow of saliva. The effect is inhibited by atropine.

Many drugs are excreted in the saliva, for instance, iodides, salicylates, and mercury.

Secretion of gastric juice

The two main physiological mediators of acid gastric secretion are the parasympathetic mediator acetylcholine and the antral hormone gastrin. Gastric secretion is conveniently divided into three phases based on the location of afferents initiating the secretory response, referred to as the cephalic, gastric and intestinal phase.

Cephalic phase

Afferent impulses initiated by the taste and smell of food, or the mere thought of an appetising meal, are relayed through the vagal nucleus and vagal efferent fibres to the stomach. The entire cephalic phase can be blocked by vagotomy. The cephalic phase can be studied by the procedure of sham feeding. A dog is prepared with oesophageal and gastric fistulas. Secretion is collected from the gastric fistula and its volume and acid content measured. Vagal stimulation may also be brought about by insulin hypoglycaemia or by the administration of the glucose analogue 2-deoxyglucose both of which cause acid gastric secretion.

The vagus has a dual action on gastric secretion. It stimulates the parietal cells directly and it also acts on antral gastrin cells (g-cells) to stimulate gastrin release which in turn causes the parietal cells to elaborate hydrochloric acid.

Gastric phase
The stimulus for the gastric phase of acid secretion is partly a nervous cholinergic mechanism through distention of the stomach and partly a chemical mechanism operating through food degradation products such as amino acids and peptides which release gastrin. It can be shown in man, by radio-immunoassay, that gastrin is released when the antral mucosa is exposed to protein digestion products. Intragastric acidification inhibits gastrin release. In the anaesthetised cat, electrical stimulation of the vagus causes a release of immunoreactive gastrin accounting for the known connection between vagal activity and gastrin release. Recent work has shown that in various mammalian species, including man, gastrin is present within the abdominal vagus nerve, whilst it is not demonstrable in cervical and thoracic portions of the vagus.

Intestinal phase
The proximal duodenum in man is rich in gastrin. Intestinal gastrin has been shown to contribute to the serum gastrin response to a meal.

EFFECTS OF DRUGS ON GASTRIC SECRETION

Appetite, when it is deficient, can be stimulated by the excitation of the taste endings in the mouth, and drugs which will produce this effect are frequently prescribed in medicine. The substances used chiefly to stimulate the gustatory nerves in the mouth are the bitters, examples of which are gentian, quassia, quinine and nux vomica or strychnine. Many so-called tonics owe their action to the bitters which they contain.

Carlson found that bitters had no effect on gastric secretion in normal men or dogs when introduced directly into the stomach, but that when introduced into the mouth they inhibited hunger contractions.

Parasympathomimetic drugs
These drugs cause an increased flow of gastric juice.

Carbachol is the most powerful since it acts both on the secretory cells by virtue of its muscarine action and on the ganglion cells of the intramural plexuses by virtue of its nicotine action.

Bethanechol (carbamylmethylcholine) is a parasympathomimetic agent with muscarinic actions. It is not inactivated by cholinesterase so that its actions are prolonged. Because of its lack of nicotinic actions it may be preferred to carbachol for the treatment of gastric retention following vagotomy. It is given by mouth or subcutaneously.

Neostigmine stimulates gastric secretion by inhibiting the destruction of endogenous acetylcholine. These drugs also produce a powerful stimulation of stomach movements (Fig. 13.1) and because of this are rarely used therapeutically to increase gastric secretion.

Gastrin
Edkins showed that extracts of mucosa from the antral region of the stomach stimulated gastric acid secretion in anaesthetised cats. Gregory and Tracy in 1964 described

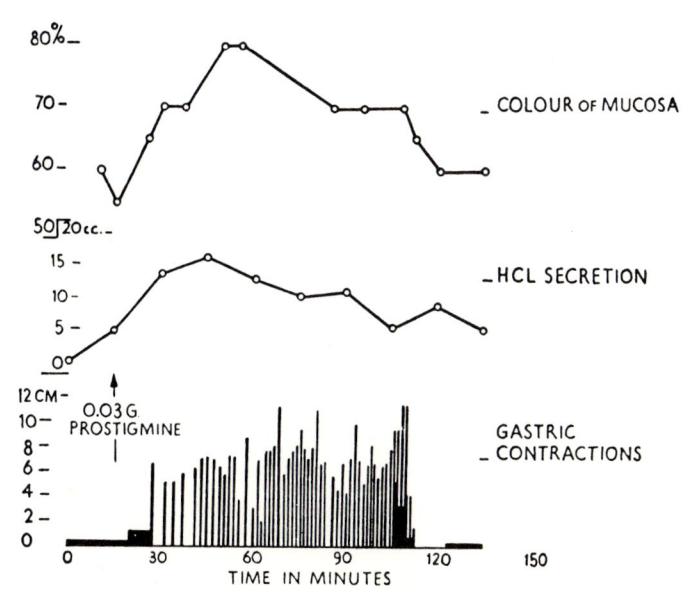

Fig. 13.1 The effect of neostigmine on gastric function. Within 20 min, 30 mg neostigmine bromide produced violent contractions of the stomach and a marked increase in gastric secretion. (After Wolf and Wolff, 1947, *Human Gastric Function*.)

the isolation from hog antral mucosa of two closely similar polypeptide hormones gastrin I and gastrin II. Each has a molecular weight of about 2000 and is a powerful stimulant of acid gastric secretion when injected subcutaneously into conscious dogs. The structure of the two gastrins is known and they have been chemically synthesised. As shown in Figure 13.3 both polypeptides are many times more active than histamine as gastric secretory stimulants in the dog. These polypeptides have also been shown to stimulate gastric secretion in man. Human antral mucosal gastrin is chemically closely related to, but not identical with, hog gastrin.

```
  1       2       3       4       5      6-10      11
Pyro  —  Gly  —  Pro  —  Trp  —  Leu  — (Glu)5 —  Ala  —

 12      13      14      15      16      17
Tyr  —  Gly  —  Trp  —  Met  —  Asp  —  Phe  —  NH₂
 |
 R
              Minimal fragment for activity
```

Gastrin I, R = H
Gastrin II, R = SO₃H

Fig. 13.2 Structure of human little gastrin (G17). Pyro = Pyropryoglutamyl.

Chemical structure of gastrins

All biologically active forms of gastrin found in human serum and tissues are single chain polypeptides. With the advent of radio-immunoassay it has become apparent that most peptide hormones are heterogeneous. Gastrin, secretin and cholecystokinin have all been shown to exist in more than one active form. In the case of gastrin several additional forms have been isolated and sequenced.

The major biologically active forms of gastrin found in serum and tissues are 'big gastrin' (G-34 I and II) and the heptadecapeptide 'little gastrin' (G-17 I and II) (Fig. 13.2). I and II refer to the absence or presence of sulphate on the tyrosine side chain of the polypeptides which does not appear to affect their biological activity. Very recently 'minigastrin' has been found to contain 14 amino acids (G-14). Another form of gastrin identified by radio-immunoassay with larger apparent molecular weight than G-34 has been referred to as 'big-big gastrin'.

Antibodies used routinely for gastrin radio-immunoassay (RIA) are specific for the carboxyterminal biologically active portion of the gastrin molecule; the antibodies do not distinguish between the various gastrin components. More accurate measurement of individual components would require fractionation of serum on gel filtration columns. The components vary in their biological properties. G-17 is highly active and is cleared from the circulation more rapidly than G-34; their half lives in man are approximately 6 and 40 min. The difference in clearance rates probably accounts for the observation that G-34 is normally the most abundant form of gastrin in the circulation.

Only four amino acids of gastrin at the carboxyl end of the molecule are necessary for its biological activity (Fig. 13.2) and they are included in the synthetic pentapeptide *pentagastrin* (pentavlon). Pentagastrin acts on the human stomach to stimulate the secretion of acid and pepsin. When pentagastrin is infused intravenously it produces maximal acid secretion in about half the subjects in a dose of 0.6 μg per kg per hour.

The gastric acid response to pentagastrin may be used clinically for several purposes: (1) to detect whether the stomach can respond to a secretory stimulant; (2) to detect excessive secretion as in some cases of duodenal ulcer; (3) to test for the completeness of vagotomy since the pentagastrin response due to the mutual potentiation of gastrin and vagus stimulation is reduced after complete vagotomy.

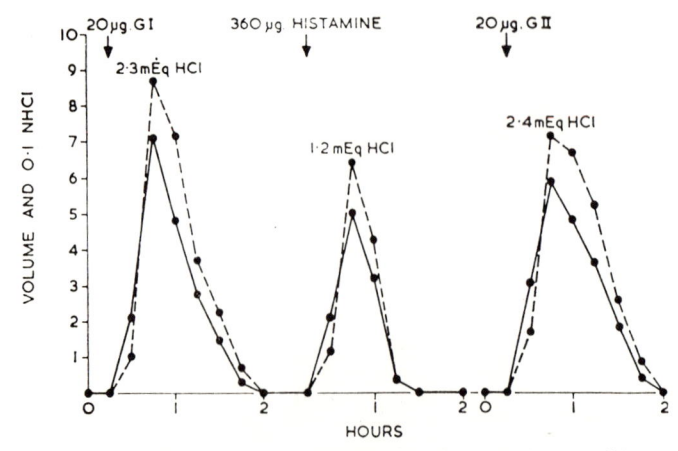

Fig. 13.3 Responses (on different occasions) of a conscious dog provided with a denervated pouch of the gastric fundus to the subcutaneous injection (at arrows) of: (left) 20 μg gastrin I (GI) (centre) 360 μg histamine base, and (right) 20 μg gastrin II (GII). The total acid outputs (mEq HCl) for each response are shown. - - - - - - - acid ——— volume, (From Gregory and Tracy, 1964, *Gut*.)

THE ALIMENTARY CANAL

Pepsin secretion

The final gastric juice contains a proteolytic enzyme, pepsin, which is secreted as a precursor, pepsinogen. Pepsinogen is converted to pepsin by acidification. At a pH of less than 3.5 pepsin is a powerful proteolytic enzyme, capable of splitting primary peptide linkages in proteins. The strongest stimulant of pepsinogen secretion is acetylcholine. Vagal activation during both cephalic and gastric phases causes pepsinogen secretion. This mechanism is blocked by atropine.

Histamine

When injected subcutaneously in dogs histamine (p. 94) causes a marked increase in gastric secretion. Wolf and Wolff have shown that 5 to 10 minutes after the subcutaneous injection of 0.5 mg histamine in man, the bloodflow in the stomach increased and the gastric mucosa became deep red. This was associated with an increase in acid production. Twenty-five minutes after the injection there were strong contractions of the stomach wall. The peak of the response in gastric secretion to histamine was reached in 45 minutes and the effects subsided in about 90 minutes (Fig. 13.4). Histamine as well as pentagastrin can be used diagnostically, to determine whether the stomach is capable of secreting acid; the dose employed is usually 1.0 mg histamine acid phosphate subcutaneously. In the 'augmented' histamine test a larger dose (3 mg histamine acid phosphate) is given, preceded by 100 mg mepyramine maleate. The H_1-antihistamine drug prevents headache and other systemic effects of histamine without interfering with its gastric secretory action.

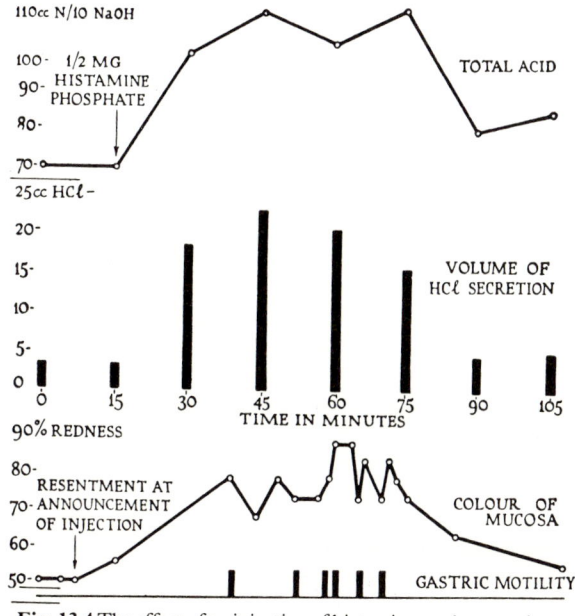

Fig. 13.4 The effect of an injection of histamine on the secretion, motility and colour of mucosa of the human stomach. (After Wolf and Wolff, 1947, *Human Gastric Function*.)

Betazole (histalog) is pyrazolethylamine and is an isomer of histamine. It is a relatively specific stimulant of H_2 receptors and as such is effective in stimulating acid gastric secretion without producing important histamine-like side effects. When administered in a dose of 50 mg as a diagnostic agent it produces a stimulation of acid secretion which is slower in onset but more prolonged than that of histamine. It produces less flushing and headache than a dose of histamine equiactive on gastric secretion.

Possible involvement of histamine in normal gastric secretion

Three substances occurring naturally in the body are capable of stimulating gastric acid secretion, acetylcholine, gastrin and histamine. Whilst the role of the first two is reasonably well understood, the role of histamine in gastric secretion has always been controversial. McIntosh proposed in 1938 that gastric mucosal histamine might be the common mediator for other stimulants of acid secretion. Although the theory of histamine as a final common path has been difficult to substantiate experimentally it is supported by circumstantial evidence and it could account for the remarkable clinical activity of histamine H_2 antagonists in antagonising not only gastric secretion induced by histamine and pentagastrin but also certain effects of cholinergic stimulation, e.g. cholinergic reflex stimulation of acid secretion in duodenal ulcer patients. The usual explanation given is that exogenous gastrin or pentagastrin acts by a histamine link and that cholinergic stimulation may act by way of a release of endogenous gastrin.

Histamine H_2 receptor antagonists

The pharmacological basis of H_2 antagonism is discussed on page 14. This group of drugs was developed through a rational application of receptor theory after it became established that histamine produced its actions by way of two sets of receptors: a mepyramine-sensitive H_1 receptor and a second type of receptor named H_2 receptor responsible for the stimulation of acid gastric secretion and certain other effects of histamine on heart and uterus. More recently it has been demonstrated that H_2 receptors (as well as H_1 receptors) also occur in the brain and that striatal H_2 receptors, capable of stimulating cAMP production, can be activated by histamine and blocked by antidepressant drugs such as amitriptyline and imipramine. The action of a typical H_2 antagonist on gastric secretion is shown in Figure 13.5. It illustrates the inhibitory effect of a dose of cimetidine on histamine-stimulated gastric secretion in the Heidenhain pouch dog.

Clinical uses of H_2 antagonists

H_2 antagonists which have been used in man include the compounds burimamide, metiamide and cimetidine. These histamine H_2-receptor antagonists are, like

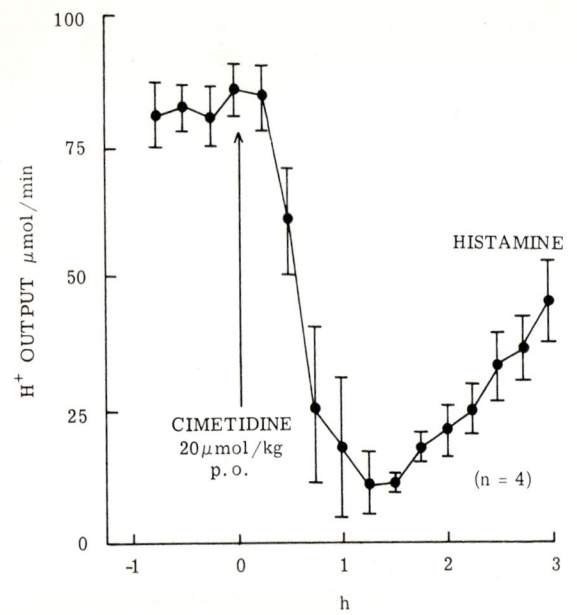

Fig. 13.5 The inhibitory effect of a single oral dose of cimetidine on maximal histamine-stimulated gastric secretion in the Heidenhain pouch dog. (After Parsons. Cimetidine. Excerpta Medica Amsterdam 1977.)

histamine, imidazole derivatives but they differ chemically from histamine in two important respects: their sidechains are longer and they are uncharged at physiological pH in contrast to the charged histamine monocation (Fig. 13.7). Like histamine itself, these compounds are derivative of imidazole, but they lack any histamine-like stimulant activity. Burimamide and metiamide both contain a structural thiourea group in their side chain and it was considered that this might be related to the finding of agranulocytosis in some animals during chronic toxicity tests with metiamide. Agranulocytosis after metiamide has also been reported in man. In cimetidine, the thiourea group has been replaced by the 'bioisosteric' cyanoguanidine group. So far no cases of agranulocytosis have been reported after cimetidine, although cases of transient leucopenia have occurred. Cimetidine and metiamide are both specific H_2-histamine antagonists giving closely similar pA_2 values and the former drug is now exclusively employed clinically.

Human studies of H_2 receptor blockade have shown that effective pharmacological control of gastric acid secretion has now become practicable. Although gastric acid output can be neutralised by antacids or inhibited by anticholinergics, adequate dosage with either type of agent is severely limited in clinical practice. Cimetidine has been shown to reduce basal acid output in man and to improve healing in doudenal and gastric ulcer patients. Figure 13.6 shows the results obtained with cimetidine treatment of duodenal ulcer in a multicentre double-blind trial.

Randomly selected patients were given cimetidine 2 g daily or 1 g daily or placebo for 28 days. Antacid tablets for the relief of pain were allowed as required. Duodenal ulceration was proved at endoscopy on entering the study. Endoscopic ulcer healing was defined as complete disappearance of all ulcers and erosions. Differences in ulcer healing between cimetidine and controls were statistically highly significant.

Fig. 13.6 Healing of duodenal ulcers in patients treated with 1g and 2g cimetidine daily compared to placebo. (After Bardhan et al in Cimetidine. Excerpta Medica Amsterdam 1977.)

The *Zollinger-Ellison* syndrome is caused by a gastrin secreting tumour (gastrinoma) which usually originates from the pancreas. These patients have a high basal acid secretion and frequent duodenal ulcers. Although the treatment of choice is total gastrectomy a full clinical remission of symptoms may be achieved with an H_2 antagonist such as cimetidine.

Hypochlorhydria and achlorhydria

Achlorhydria or absence of hydrochloric acid occurs in a considerable number of apparently normal persons without producing any clinical symptoms. It also accompanies many organic diseases and is a feature of

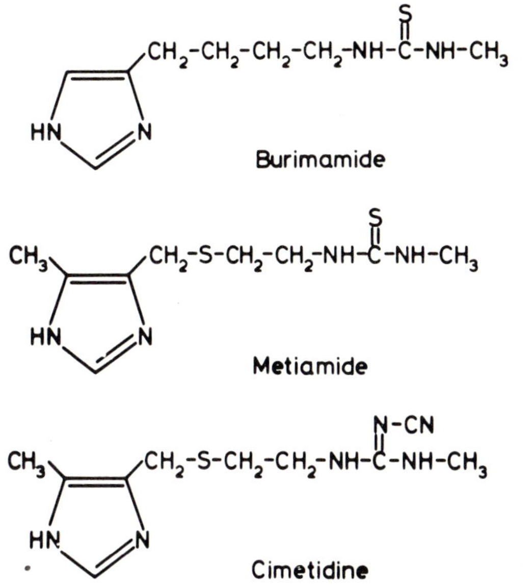

Fig. 13.7 Structures of H$_2$-receptor antagonists

gastric carcinoma and also of pernicious anaemia. The latter is distinguished by absence of gastric secretion in response to an injection of histamine.

The daily amount of acid normally secreted is so large that it is not possible to administer this quantity to a patient who is deficient in acid production. Although it has formerly been the custom to encourage replacement therapy with diluted hydrochloric acid, to do so adequately would require the administration of a pint of tenth-normal hydrochloric acid with each meal. This is hardly practicable and to overcome this difficulty acid protein preparations, for example, glutamic acid hydrochloride, have been given in capsules, from which the acid is liberated in the stomach. This form of therapy, however, does not provide the enzymes which are essential constituents of gastric juice.

INHIBITION OF GASTRIC SECRETION

The secretion of gastric juice can be inhibited in various ways.

Stimulation of any sensory nerve inhibits the psychic secretion of gastric juice. Emotional influences such as fear, anxiety, self reproach and resentment decrease the vascularity of the gastric mucosa and diminish gastric secretion and motility. Active hostility may produce the opposite effect.

Vagotomy relieves the pain of peptic ulcer, decreases the volume and the acidity of gastric secretion and reduces the motility of the stomach. Gastric acid secretion is inhibited by prostaglandin E$_1$.

Anything which produces irritation of the fundus, such as concentrated alcohol, at first stimulates gastric secretion but produces, as an after effect a prolonged inhibition of the secretion of gastric juice. Hydrochloric acid in concentrations over 0.2 per cent when it enters the pylorus inhibits the secretion of gastric juice. Inhibition can also be produced by ice-cold water and by the entrance of fats and oils into the pylorus.

The inhibitory effect of fat has been considered to be due to the liberation of 'enterogastrone' from the intestinal mucosa. *Urogastrone*, a polypeptide similar to but not identical with enterogastrone, has been isolated from human urine and chemically identified. It has been shown to inhibit the response to gastric secretion produced by the injection of histamine, gastrin or insulin in animals and man. The therapeutic value of urogastrone is at present under investigation.

CONTROL OF HYPERCHLORHYDRIA BY DRUGS

Besides the recently introduced H$_2$ antagonists discussed above, a number of well-tried agents have long been employed clinically with the aim of alleviating the symptoms of gastric hypersecretion and peptic ulceration. Particularly important are drugs inhibiting vagal secretory activity and the antacids. A drug with a different mode of action which has been used clinically in gastric ulcer is *carbenoxolone* sodium.

Drugs which inhibit secretory stimulation by the vagus

Vagal secretory activity may be inhibited by drugs which act (*a*) on the central nervous system, (*b*) on the ganglion cells of the intramural plexuses, or (*c*) on the effector cells.

Many patients with peptic ulcer, especially of the duodenum, suffer from anxiety and insomnia and sedative drugs such as chlordiazepoxide and diazepam are of value in their treatment.

Ganglion-blocking drugs such as mecamylamine and pempidine can abolish the fasting secretion of free acid and inhibit gastric motility. These drugs are rarely used as inhibitors of gastric secretion but are sometimes used to diminish the excessive motility produced by adrenergic neurone blocking drugs such as guanethidine.

Atropine reduces the secretory and motor activity of the stomach. In the dog it completely abolishes gastric secretion induced by parasympathomimetic drugs, but secretion provoked by histamine is not completely antagonised even by large doses of atropine. In man atropine produces a moderate reduction of gastric juice in response to a test meal, but increasing the dose above 1 mg does not enhance this inhibitory effect. Wolf and Wolff found that atropine inhibits the secretion of mucus as much or more than the acid secretion so that the concentration of acid in the stomach remains the same or becomes slightly higher. These authors attribute the beneficial effects of atropine to the reduction of motor activity of the stomach. Atropine also strongly inhibits pepsin secretion. The effective dose of tincture of belladonna is about 0.5 ml, equivalent to 0.15 mg atropine, given every 4 hours, an amount which usually produces dryness of the mouth. Atropine is being increasingly replaced by synthetic drugs. A tertiary amine with atropine-like activity frequently used in antidyspepsia mixtures is *oxyphenylcyclimine* (Daricon).

A large number of quaternary ammonium compounds with atropine-like activity such as *oxyphenonium* (Antrenyl), *propantheline* (Probanthin) and *poldine methylsulphate* (Nacton) have been introduced for the treatment of hyperchlorhydria and peptic ulcer. These compounds generally also possess some ganglion-blocking activity which enhances their effect. Studies of their effects on gastric secretion in man have shown that they reduce fasting secretion to about the same extent as therapeutic doses of atropine. These atropine substitutes are sometimes effective in reducing the pain and distress of patients with peptic ulcer. This effect is probably due more to inhibition of gastric motility than to reduction in gastric acidity.

Drugs affecting gastric mucus

Many conditions which lead to inflammation of the gastric epithelium and ultimately to ulceration are associated with an impaired rate of synthesis of gastric mucus as measured by the rates of incorporation of radio-actively labelled sugars. Various drugs inhibit mucus production including corticosteroids and non-steroidal anti-inflammatory drugs such as aspirin, indomethacin and phenylbutazone. They all cause gastro-intestinal inflammation, erosions and gastric ulcers. These drugs inhibit prostaglandin synthetase thereby impairing the microcirculation of the gastric epithelium.

Carbenoxolone sodium, a licorice derivative with anti-inflammatory activity, has effects on gastric mucus production which are in some ways the opposite of those produced by the ulcerogenic drugs. Carbenoxolone has been shown to accelerate healing in human gastric ulcers, though not in duodenal ulcers. It has been observed that patients taking carbenoxolone have an abnormally thick layer of mucus on their gastric mucosa.

The chief side effects of carbenoxolone sodium are salt and water retention and hypokalaemia.

ANTACIDS

These substances are important because they produce marked relief of gastric pain associated with hyperchlorhydria. The manner in which they produce this effect is not clear, for measurements of the acid content of the gastric juice during the treatment of hyperchlorhydria with frequent large quantities of these drugs, indicate that the free acid is not abolished. It has been suggested that the aim should be not complete neutralisation to pH 7.0 but rather to inhibit peptic activity which practically ceases at pH 5.

The following properties are desirable in an antacid. It should be (1) insoluble, neutral in aqueous suspension but capable of neutralising acid; (2) rapidly effective and maintain its effect for several hours; (3) non-irritant to the stomach and intestine and not cause diarrhoea or constipation, it should not produce acid-rebound or excessive eructation; (4) not liable to disturb the acid-base balance and cause alkalosis or make the urine alkaline with the danger of precipitating calculi in the urinary tract.

An assessment of the neutralising power of various alkalis is given in Table 13.1 which shows the amounts required to bring to pH 3.5 a solution of hydrochloric acid equivalent to the average daily secretion of acid in the gastric juice.

Table 13.1

Milk	1.5 litres
Magnesium oxide	3 g
Aluminium hydroxide gel	5 g
Calcium carbonate	8 g
Magnesium trisilicate	12 g
Sodium bicarbonate	12 g

Antacids differ in the rate at which they neutralise acid and in the degree of alkalinity which they can produce.

Sodium bicarbonate

This has a rapid action and raises the pH to about 7.4. It liberates carbon dioxide which evokes the eructation of gas, thereby giving a sense of relief and of satisfaction. This evolution of carbon dioxide causes a stimulation of gastrin and a secondary rise in acid secretion. The sodium chloride formed is absorbed in the intestine and the total fixed base in the body is increased. Frequent doses of sodium bicarbonate thus produce alkalosis, which may be insidious in onset. The predominant effects are mental changes which may vary from increased irritability to drowsiness and coma; headache, nausea, vomiting and tetany may also occur. Because of its tendency to produce systemic alkalosis, sodium bicarbonate should not be used for the long-term treatment of peptic ulcer. It must not be given to patients on a sodium-restricted diet.

Magnesium oxide

An insoluble powder which forms magnesium chloride in the presence of hydrochloric acid. The action of magnesium oxide in neutralising the hydrochloric acid of the stomach is more delayed than that of sodium bicarbonate, but it is more prolonged since being insoluble it provides a reservoir of antacid in the stomach. In the presence of excess magnesium oxide the pH of the gastric contents becomes slightly alkaline due to the formation of a small amount of magnesium hydroxide. Some of the magnesium chloride formed in the stomach is excreted unchanged by the intestine and acts as a mild saline purgative. Most of the magnesium chloride, however, is changed to magnesium carbonate in the intestine and excreted as such. Since no appreciable amounts of chloride are lost from the body when magnesium oxide is administered, this substance, in contrast to sodium bicarbonate, does not produce systemic alkalosis.

Milk of magnesia is a suspension of magnesium hydroxide which is frequently used as an antacid and a mild laxative in children.

Magnesium trisilicate

An insoluble powder which interacts slowly with the gastric juice with the formation of magnesium chloride and colloidal silica. About 75 per cent of the available magnesium is neutralised during the first hour and the remaining magnesium is neutralised slowly during the following three hours so that it has a slow continuous antacid effect. In addition it has adsorptive properties. When magnesium trisilicate is present in excess it produces a pH of 6.5 to 7 so that even large doses do not give an alkaline reaction. The usual dose is 0.6 to 1.8 g four times daily.

Aluminium hydroxide gel

This is a 4 per cent suspension of aluminium hydroxide which is used as a gastric antacid since it neutralises hydrochloric acid forming aluminium chloride and water. Aluminium hydroxide gradually raises the pH of the gastric contents to about 4 and maintains this value for several hours. In the alkaline milieu of the intestine aluminium chloride reacts to form insoluble aluminium compounds releasing chloride which is reabsorbed. Since no chloride is lost from the body and no aluminium hydroxide is absorbed there is no danger of alkalosis. Prolonged use may lead to constipation. The usual dose is two teaspoonfuls four or six times daily; administration by continuous intragastric drip has also been used.

Colloidal aluminium hydroxide combines with phosphates in the gastro-intestinal tract and may produce a phosphorus deficiency. The increased excretion of phosphate in the faeces results in a decrease in the excretion of phosphate in the urine and this may be utilised by administering aluminium compounds, particularly the basic aluminium carbonate orally, for the prevention and treatment of phosphatic renal calculi.

Calcium carbonate

Calcium carbonate has a constipating effect which may be modified by suitable admixture with magnesium oxide. Calcium carbonate is an effective antacid but has the disadvantage that calcium may be partly absorbed increasing the level of serum calcium. This may cause systemic effects such as headache and nausea and in rare cases renal damage.

Bismuth oxycarbonate

This has a very feeble antacid action. This insoluble salt of bismuth has been widely used in the belief that after oral administration it coated and protected the inflamed gastric mucosa. Radiological evidence, however, suggests that it is not possible to achieve a uniform coating of the mucous membrane in this way.

VOMITING

Vomiting is a protective function which serves to remove from the stomach unsuitable materials that have been swallowed. The faculty of vomiting is possessed by most mammals except rodents; the frequency with which it occurs varies greatly in different species. It is a normal physiological occurrence in cats and dogs but only occurs occasionally in man. It can be induced much more readily in children than in adults.

The act of vomiting is accomplished by a complex series of movements which are controlled by a centre situated in the medulla. When vomiting occurs, the pyloric portion of the stomach contracts tightly, the cardiac portion relaxes, and the cardiac sphincter opens. The contents of the stomach are then expelled by a simultaneous contraction of the diaphragm and the muscles of the abdominal wall. The fundus of the stomach plays a passive part in the emptying of the stomach. Vomiting is usually preceded by the sensation of nausea, and is accompanied and followed by a profuse secretion of saliva, profuse bronchial secretion, coughing, pallor of the face, sweating, fall of blood pressure, rapid pulse and irregular respiration. The vasomotor disturbance may cause vertigo or even fainting. Vomiting is associated with antiperistaltic movements of the bowel, and after repeated vomiting the ejected fluid usually contains bile. Persistent vomiting finally results in faecal matter from the lower bowel appearing in the stomach contents.

Vomiting centre

Wang and Borison have shown that the central mechanism concerned with vomiting consists of two closely related and functionally separate units in the medulla oblongata; an emetic centre situated in the region of the fasciculus solitarius and the underlying lateral reticular formation, and a chemoreceptor trigger zone on the surface of the medulla close to the vagal nuclei. The emetic centre is excited by visceral afferent nerves such as those arising from the gastrointestinal tract. The chemoreceptor trigger zone appears to be the site of action of drugs with a central emetic action such as apomorphine, morphine and cardiac glycosides. If the trigger zone is destroyed animals are unable to vomit in response to apomorphine, but they vomit in response to drugs which irritate the stomach such as copper sulphate. When the emetic centre is destroyed both types of drug are ineffective. Wang and Chinn made the interesting observation that the trigger zone is also concerned in the mediation of motion sickness since they were unable to induce motion sickness in dogs in whom this area was destroyed.

The chief ways whereby emesis may be produced are as follows:

1. Various unpleasant sensations including repulsive sights or smells and acute pain.
2. Stimulation of the vagal sensory nerve endings in the pharynx, e.g. by tickling the throat.
3. Stimulation of the sensory nerve ending in the stomach and duodenum, e.g. by local emetics.
4. Stimulation of the vomiting centre by drugs — central emetics.
5. Disturbance of the labyrinth as in travel sickness.
6. Various stimuli to the sensory nerves of the heart and viscera.

Drugs which produce vomiting

The chief methods of inducing vomiting by drugs are by (1) local emetics and (2) central emetics.

Local emetics

Emetics may be assumed to exert a local or peripheral action if they excite vomiting more readily when given by mouth than when given hypodermically. Local emetics irritate sensory nerve endings in the stomach, but this irritation produces no conscious sensation beyond a general feeling of nausea.

Local emetics do not produce their effect until they enter the pyloric half of the stomach and therefore, in order to produce vomiting rapidly, the emetic should be given with a considerable volume of fluid to ensure it reaching the pyloric part of the stomach as rapidly as possible. In the treatment of poisoning either a central emetic, such as apomorphine, or lavage of the stomach is usually preferred to local emetics. The chief disadvantage of the latter is that they often fail to act in cases of poisoning where there is depression of the central nervous system. Since they are irritant substances they produce injury to the stomach if they fail to produce emesis and are retained.

Local emetics, when given in sub-emetic doses, are useful expectorants and this is their chief use in modern medicine.

Most irritant substances act as emetics when given by the mouth, and common emetics suitable for use in emergencies are mustard and water, and warm hypertonic solutions of salt.

Salts of heavy metals such as copper sulphate and zinc sulphate, when given in a 1 per cent solution, produce vomiting in a few minutes; their rapid action prevents their damaging the stomach mucosa. These metallic salts are absorbed very slowly and therefore there is little danger of their producing poisoning. They do not produce purgation or prolonged nausea as an after-effect, and in small doses they produce an astringent action on the bowel.

Ipecacuanha. The emetic action of ipecacuanha is due to the presence in it of two alkaloids, emetine and cephaeline. These alkaloids irritate all mucous membranes, causing lachrymation and conjunctivitis, and increased secretion from the nose and bronchi. Ipecacuanha, on account of its delayed action, is not suitable for the treatment of poisoning, but in sub-emetic doses it is used extensively as an expectorant.

Central emetics

Drugs, such as picrotoxin and nikethamide which have a general excitant action of the central nervous system, stimulate the vomiting centre, together with all other centres. Morphine is remarkable in that it depresses the respiratory and cough centres but stimulates the vagal and vomiting centres. It regularly produces vomiting in dogs, usually does so in children and frequently produces nausea in adults.

Apomorphine. This drug is produced by the partial breakdown of morphine, and has a very remarkable selective action upon the vomiting centre. The subcutaneous injection of apomorphine (6 mg) in man produces vomiting within a minute, and the effect lasts for a few minutes. Larger doses produce vomiting which continues for an hour or more and may result in collapse. When apomorphine is given by mouth about twice the hypodermic dose is required to produce vomiting, and the effect is not produced for half an hour.

The specific action of apomorphine on the vomiting centre is proved by the observation that as little as 1 μg of apomorphine is sufficient to induce vomiting in dogs when applied directly to the medulla. Therapeutic doses of apomorphine produce a hypnotic action, but toxic doses produce general cerebral excitation and convulsions.

Dopaminergic activity of apomorphine. Apomorphine is structurally related to dopamine and is a powerful stimulant of dopamine receptors (p. 239). When injected subcutaneously in rats apomorphine produces typical 'stereotyped' movements characteristic of central dopamine receptor stimulation. These effects can be antagonised by dopamine receptor blocking agents such as haloperidol or chlorpromazine. The emetic effect of apomorphine is believed to be due to the stimulation of dopamine receptors in the medullary chemoreceptor trigger zone.

Due to its dopamine receptor stimulating activity,

apomorphine is capable of controlling the symptoms of Parkinsonism but it is seldom used for this purpose due to its strong emetic action. Apomorphine has been shown to be clinically effective in patients with Parkinsonism whose tremor was unresponsive to levodopa treatment. Excessive vomiting produced by apomorphine may be counteracted by chlorpromazine.

Prevention of vomiting and travel sickness

Travel sickness may afflict any susceptible person who travels by land, sea or air. The way in which motion produces sickness is not fully understood. It is probable that alternating acceleration in a vertical plane is the chief factor in the motion of the sea and that the periodicity of this alternating acceleration is important. It has been found that sickness rates are highest in medium craft such as destroyers. In small craft and rowing boats the periodicity is too rapid to have the maximum effect, and in large liners it is too slow.

Motion sickness is most readily produced when the head is held upright and least readily when it is horizontal; the position of the rest of the body is not important. With the onset of nausea the stomach becomes dilated and inert and normal peristalsis ceases. The presence of food in the stomach tends to stimulate the atonic stomach and diminish nausea. To this end sailors recommend the nibbling of dry biscuits or bread at frequent intervals. Drugs given by mouth when the sickness has begun may not be absorbed and administration should therefore begin before the onset of nausea.

The most varied assortment of drugs has been used in preventing and treating travel sickness, some such as amphetamine, ephedrine or caffeine have been chosen because they are known to stimulate the brain, others such as barbiturates because they produce depression of the central nervous system. These drugs have no effect in controlling motion sickness produced experimentally by vertical acceleration, centrifugal motion or by the swing test. However, the anticholinergic and the H_1-antihistamine drugs have a protective effect under these conditions.

Hyoscine

The belladonna alkaloids, atropine, hyoscyamine and hyoscine (p. 70) have a specific effect in motion sickness. It has been shown experimentally on soliders travelling by air and sea that hyoscine hydrobromide when given about an hour before encountering rough weather in a dose of 0.6 mg protects about half, and in twice this dose protects nearly three-quarters of susceptible subjects. The effect lasts for 4 to 6 hours. The only side effect noted was dryness of the mouth. Atropine sulphate 1.0 mg and laevohyoscyamine hydrobromide 1.0 mg are of the same order of efficacy as 0.6 mg hyoscine. For protection against sea-sickness of long duration it is necessary to give large doses of hyoscine (0.75 mg 3 times daily). This usually produces side effects such as persistent drowsiness, giddiness and blurring of vision which are so distressing that patients may refuse to continue the treatment. Hyoscine is therefore not a good drug to use for the prevention of sea-sickness in long voyages.

H_1-antihistamine drugs

The protective effect of the antihistamine compound diphenhydramine (benadryl) (p. 96) against sea-sickness was discovered soon after its introduction for the treatment of allergic conditions. A number of other antihistamine drugs have since been found to prevent travel sickness. Several large-scale investigations have been carried out on soldiers and airmen during transatlantic sea voyages in which placebos as well as various drugs were used. Each subject was required to record the occurrence of vomiting and side effects. The most effective and least disturbing drugs were the antihistamine compounds meclozine (ancolan), cyclizine (marzine) and promethazine (phenergan) when given by mouth three times daily in doses of 50 mg, 50 mg and 25 mg respectively. These three drugs gave equal protection, but promethazine produced rather more drowsiness than the other two.

Chlorpromazine (p. 252)

This drug has a marked antiemetic effect which is due to an action on the central nervous system. Wang has shown that when 0.2 mg of chlorpromazine is placed on the floor of the fourth ventricle of a dog, the intravenous dose of apomorphine required to produce vomiting is increased several times. When a small dose of chlorpromazine is administered parenterally to dogs it prevents the emetic effect of apomorphine without altering the emetic response to oral copper sulphate. This suggests that chlorpromazine prevents vomiting by an action on the chemoreceptor trigger zone.

Chlorpromazine prevents vomiting arising during pregnancy, in uraemia and from X-ray and nitrogen mustard therapy. It is usually administered by mouth or intramuscularly. The main side effect of chlorpromazine is drowsiness, but this can be counteracted by the administration of amphetamine; other side effects are discussed in Chapter 18. The distressing condition of intractable hiccough can usually be abruptly terminated by an intravenous dose of 50 mg of chlorpromazine. Alternatively perphenazine may be used which is highly effective in preventing postoperative vomiting and hiccough.

Pregnancy-vomiting can also be prevented by the antihistamine drugs and in the management of this condition the antihistamine drugs and chlorpromazine are about equally effective. Chlorpromazine is much less effective than the antihistamine drugs in preventing travel sickness.

Metoclopropamide prevents postoperative nausea and vomiting probably by blocking central dopamine receptors. By dopamine receptor block it may produce dyskinesia and extrapyramidal reactions. Clinically metoclopramide increases the resting tone of the gastro-oesophageal sphincter and thus promotes gastric emptying.

Cinnarizine (Stugeron)
This drug has the properties and uses of an H_1-antihistamine but it is mainly used for the symptomatic treatment of nausea and vertigo due to labyrinthine disturbances (Meniere's disease) and for the prevention and treatment of motion sickness. It acts in about 30 minutes and produces little or no drowsiness.

Clinical use of antiemetic drugs. Many women suffer nausea and vomiting in early pregnancy. This was formerly treated with antihistamines but it is now considered undesirable to give any drug during the first three months of pregnancy because of the risk of causing fetal abnormalities. Nevertheless a pregnant woman may be so nauseated as to make the use of an antiemetic justifiable.

Nausea frequently occurs during preanaesthetic medication with drugs such as pethidine or the opiates, but it is considered undesirable to use antiemetic drugs routinely for preoperative use because of their central depressant effects. Antiemetic drugs are frequently used in the postoperative period when either an antihistamine or a phenothiazine may be administered. Antiemetic drugs are also given when nausea is due to cytotoxic drugs.

DUODENAL HORMONES

The food mass, which is stored in the fundus of the stomach, is passed into the duodenum in driblets. The entrance of food into the duodenum causes the secretion of both bile and pancreatic juice. Bayliss and Starling showed that the entrance of acid into the duodenum caused the liberation of the hormone **secretin** from the duodenal mucosa, and that this hormone passed into the blood stream and excited the secretion of bile and of pancreatic juice.

The chemical structure of secretin has been elucidated. It is a polypeptide containing 27 amino acids which is chemically related to glucagon. When secretin is injected intravenously it causes pancreatic secretion which, although it contains some enzymes, represents chiefly the aqueous alkaline component. Secretin also stimulates secretion of the aqueous component of bile.

Certain other intestinal peptides structurally related to secretin include, besides glucagon, *vasoactive intestinal peptide (VIP)* and *gastric inhibitory peptide (GIP)* both formed of 9 amino acids. It is not known whether they have a normal hormonal function, but pancreatic cholera or watery diarrhoea, a frequently lethal disease, has been attributed to the release of VIP by a pancreatic islet cell tumour.

Cholecystokinin-pancreozymin is a hormone from the duodenal mucosa. It consists of 33 amino acids with a carboxyterminal end identical to gastrin. It stimulates the digestive secretions of the pancreas increasing the secretion of amylase, lipase and trypsin. It also causes a contraction of the gallbladder and is used for testing gallbladder function.

PHARMACOLOGY OF BILE

Formation and excretion of bile
The bile excreted by the liver is a dilute solution which contains about 0.4 per cent of organic solids. The presence of bile in the gut is required only during the digestion of food, and this dilute bile is stored in the gall bladder where about nine-tenths of its water content is absorbed and mucin is added. The concentrated bile is evacuated periodically into the small intestine. Evacuation is brought about by relaxation of the sphincter of Oddi at the termination of the common bile duct and by contraction of the gall bladder. The wall of the gall bladder contains plain muscle, and it can contract and produce a pressure of about 30 cm of water.

Pharmacology of bile flow
A true cholagogue is a substance which increases the amount of bile secreted by the liver; but since the bile is normally concentrated tenfold in the gall bladder it is almost impossible to judge whether a drug increases the amount of bile entering the gall bladder.

The entrance into the duodenum of olive oil, partially digested egg yolk, or cream is a particularly effective stimulus for the production of contractions of the gall bladder. A variety of other stimuli are effective, and immediate contractions of the gall bladder can be induced by the introduction into the duodenum, by a duodenal tube, of hypertonic solutions of magnesium sulphate. Numerous drugs are reputed to increase the flow of bile but the evidence rests mainly on the fact that they hasten the passage of the intestinal contents and somewhat check putrefactive processes, hence more bile pigment appears in the faeces.

The ability of the gall bladder mucosa to absorb and concentrate substances excreted by the liver may be impaired by inflammatory disease or calculus formation, the diagnosis of which may be confirmed by radiological examination. Iodine-containing compounds which are opaque to X-rays can be used to outline the gall bladder and the extra-hepatic ducts.

Iopanoic acid (Telepaque) is a water-insoluble contrast medium which is rapidly absorbed from the intestinal tract.

$$\text{Iopanoic acid}$$

(structure: benzene ring with three I substituents, NH$_2$, and CH$_2$.CH(COOH).CH$_2$.CH$_3$ side chain)

After oral administration it reaches its maximum concentration in the gall bladder in about 12 hours during which it produces a dense shadow in the chlolecystogram; thereafter it is eliminated by the intestine and also partly in the urine. The patient is usually instructed to take 6 tablets of iopanoic acid (3 g) after a light meal in the evening. The following morning, after X-ray examination, a high-fat meal is given and 2 or 3 hours later, further films are taken to determine the ability of the gall bladder to contract.

Iopanoic acid is relatively free from side effects though nausea, vomiting or diarrhoea may sometimes occur. It should not be administered to patients with acute nephritis or where absorption from the intestinal tract is impaired.

Iodipamide methylglucamine (Biligrafin) is a water-soluble preparation which can be injected intravenously for radiography of the biliary tract. It is rapidly excreted in the bile and this enables the hepatic and common bile ducts to be visualised by X-ray examination within 20 minutes after intravenous injection of 20 ml of a 30 per cent solution.

It is usual to inject a test dose of 1 ml to detect any sensitivity reactions.

Biliary spasm

The pain produced by the passage of gall stones down the bile duct (biliary colic) often demands immediate relief. Morphine relieves the pain owing to its central depressant action, but its local effect is unfavourable since it actually raises the pressure in the bile duct by constricting the sphincter of Oddi. Pethidine also constricts the sphincter of Oddi and raises the pressure in the common bile duct although it relaxes other plain muscle, e.g. that of the ureter. Atropine is commonly used for its antispasmodic action in combination with morphine.

The nitrites produce a striking fall of intrabiliary pressure and if biliary colic is due to spasm a tablet of glyceryl trinitrate taken sublingually or the inhalation of amyl nitrite will often relieve the attack (Fig. 13.8).

Cholelithiasis

Cholelithiasis is a common disease frequently requiring surgical intervention. Attempts have also been made to deal with cholelithiasis by pharmacological means to effect a reduction or disappearance of gallstones.

Organic constituents of bile

The major organic constituents of bile, constituting about 50 per cent of organic components of human bile, are the bile acids: cholic acid, chenodeoxycholic acid, deoxycholic acid and lithocholic acid. These acids differ from each other primarily in the number of hydroxyl groups and their position. The second most abundant group of organic compounds in bile are the phospholipids, the major ones being the lecithins. A third organic component, cholesterol, is present in small amounts contributing about 4 per cent of the total solids of bile. Bile cholesterol may be

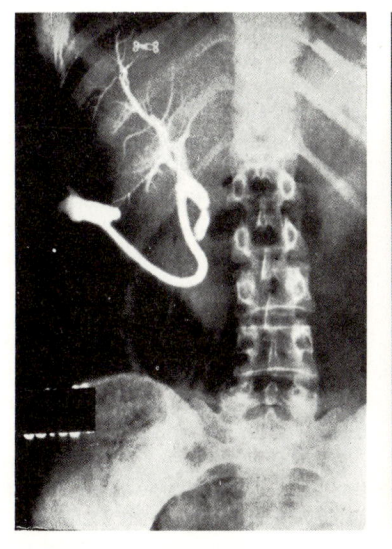

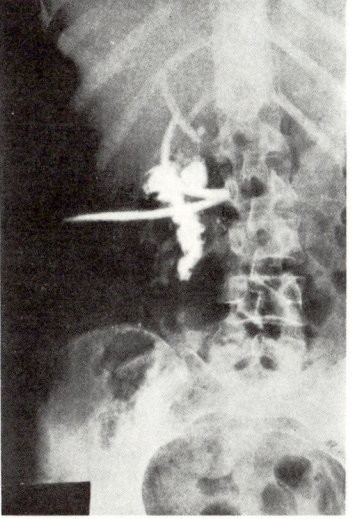

Fig. 13.8a Spasm of the lower end of the common bile duct produced by an injection of 10 mg morphine sulphate. Note filling of the hepatic ducts with the radio-opaque substance.
b Relief of spasm following the inhalation of amyl nitrite. (After Butsch, McGowan and Walters, 1936, *Surg. Gym. and Obst.*)

excreted when it helps to regulate the body stores of cholesterol. A fourth major group of organic compounds are the bile pigments, including bilirubin, constituting about 2 per cent of total organic solids.

Once secreted, bile acids undergo an interesting cycle. First they are stored in the gallbladder until digestion of a meal. They are then discharged into the small intestine where they take part in the digestion and absorption of lipids. In the terminal ileum they are largely reabsorbed and travel via the portal blood to the liver where they are taken up by hepatocytes and resecreted. The whole cycle is called the *enterohepatic circulation*.

The formation of gallstones
In many individuals the quantity of bile produced by the liver may be normal; however, the bile is qualitatively abnormal. To be stable, bile must contain certain proportions of bile acids, phospholipids and cholesterol. If there is a relative excess of cholesterol it may precipitate to form gallstones.

There have been many claims that drugs will dissolve gallstones but in general they have not withstood the test of time. Recently, however, experience has been accumulating that a prolonged oral administration of *chenodeoxycholic* acid may be effective in bringing about a dissolution of cholesterol gallstones in man. Other bile acids were apparently ineffective. Several human experiments with chenodeoxycholic acid have been reported. Several have been successful but in all cases the proportion of successes has been variable. The doses of chenodeoxy cholic acid given were usually 1 g daily for 6 months or more. As an example, in one trial 3 out of 12 patients had their stones dissolved, 3 showed a reduced size and the remainder no change.

Changes in bile chemistry have been reported after using chenodeoxycholic acid: there is a significant increase in the cholesterol solubilising capacity of the bile. This treatment is still in the experimental stage and its toxicity in man is not fully explored. Histological changes in the liver, including mild fatty changes, have been reported.

LIPID LOWERING AGENTS

Hyperlipidaemia is a common feature of atherosclerosis, the complications of which lead to ischaemic heart disease, myocardial infarction and stroke. Since the high lipid content of plasma is believed to be the main cause of atheromatous lesions of blood vessels attempts have been made to develop drugs which reduce the concentration of plasma lipids.

Hyperlipidaemia reflects changes in lipoprotein concentration of plasma: cholesterol, phospholipids and free fatty acids are insoluble in water and they circulate in the plasma as lipoproteins. A number of lipoprotein abnormalities have been described and the World Health Organization has proposed an international classification of these disorders into five main groups. The most important atherogenic factors are the cholesterol and triglyceride levels which can serve as useful therapeutic guidelines.

An essential part of treatment of hyperlipidaemia is dietary restriction of saturated fats but several drugs have been introduced which are capable of lowering blood lipids by various mechanisms.

Cholestyramine
Cholestyramine is the insoluble chloride salt of a basic anion exchange resin. It binds bile acids in the intestine preventing their reabsorption. This has two consequences, it decreases the absorption of exogenous cholesterol and it increases the metabolism of endogenous cholesterol into bile acids in the liver. The plasma cholesterol concentrations are thus lowered.

Cholestyramine combined with dietary control has been shown to lower plasma lipoproteins in type II hyperlipoproteinaemia. The drug is effective in relieving pruritis in biliary obstruction. Since cholestyramine is not absorbed its toxicity is low but it may cause bloating, nausea and constipation.

Clofibrate (Atromid — S)
Clofibrate reduces elevated plasma concentrations of triglycerides and to a lesser extent of cholesterol. It particularly reduces elevated concentrations of very low density lipoproteins. It is most effective in type III hyperlipoproteinaemia.

Clofibrate has been used in the long-term treatment and prophylaxis of patients with coronary heart disease but there is no definitive evidence that it reduces total mortality. There is some evidence of undesirable effects by clofibrate, for example an increased incidence of cholelithiasis. It should generally be reserved for patients with clofibrate-responsive hyperlipidaemia in whom there is a serious risk of ischaemic heart disease.

Several other drugs have been used in the treatment of hyperlipidaemia.

Dextrothyroxine (p. 331) is a thyroxine analogue with a high ratio of hyperlipidaemic to metabolic activity. It is effective in type II hyperlipoproteinaemia but it may cause metabolic stimulation and signs of hyperthyroidism.

Niacin (nicotinic acid) is a vitamin discussed on page 368. It produces flushing in most subjects. It has antilipidaemic activity but may produce untoward effects such as impairment of glucose tolerance. There is no definite evidence that it reduces mortality in ischaemic heart disease.

Several steroid preparations have been used for their action in reducing hyperlipoproteinaemia. They include the progestational agent *norethindrone* and the anabolic steroid *oxandrolone*.

ACTION OF DRUGS ON INTESTINAL MOVEMENTS

Drugs can affect the movements of the gut in two ways: (1) by reflexly altering the peristaltic activity and (2) by stimulating or depressing the neuromuscular mechanism of the gut. The former group are collectively referred to as purgatives and are discussed below. The latter group comprises the parasympathomimetic and sympathomimetic drugs and their antagonists as well as the opium alkaloids and other drugs affecting the neuromuscular apparatus.

Purgatives
The passage of food through the intestine may be accelerated by increasing the volume of non-absorbable residue, or altering its consistency, or by irritating the mucosa of the gut and reflexly increasing peristalsis.

Bulk laxatives
This group of substances derived from plants are polysaccharide polymers which are not broken down by the normal digestive processes of the human upper gastro-intestinal tract. They are believed to act by virtue of their ability to retain water in the gut lumen and so promote peristalsis. Their *in vitro* water-holding capacity is reflected in their *in vivo* ability to increase stool bulk.

Methylcellulose (celevac, cologel), certain plant gums, e.g. *sterculia* (Normacol), *agar* (Agarol) and *bran* have this type of action. They are widely used because of the 'natural' way they increase faecal bulk.

Other laxatives producing their action by virtue of their physical properties include the following:

Dioctyl sodium sulphosuccinate is a surface active compound which acts in the gastro-intestinal tract in a manner similar to a detergent. It loosens faecal material and produces softer stools.

Liquid paraffin consists of a mixture of the higher paraffins of the methane series. It is non-irritant and non-absorbable, and acts chiefly by softening the faecal mass. A comparatively small quantity of liquid paraffin is necessary for this purpose.

There are several disadvantages associated with the use of liquid paraffin. The chief practical objection is that the oil may leak through the anal sphincter and soil underclothing. Emulsions of liquid paraffin and agar-agar are more viscous and less liable to produce this effect. Numerous proprietary emulsions are available but many contain phenolphthalein and continuous use of the latter drug is deleterious.

Liquid paraffin may interfere with the normal digestion and absorption of food. Patients who use the drug continuously often have indigestion. A serious objection is that liquid paraffin dissolves α- and β-carotenes, which are the chief precursors of vitamin A, and prevents their absorption so that they are excreted in the faeces. This is particularly important where the diet contains little preformed vitamin A. Some liquid paraffin may be absorbed and form paraffinomas in the mesenteric lymph ducts.

Saline purgatives
The chief effect of saline purgatives is to hasten the passage of the gut contents through the small intestine and to cause an abnormally large volume to enter the colon. The distension produced by this fluid causes purgation about an hour after it has entered the colon.

A considerable number of non-toxic slowly diffusible salts act as saline purgatives. All soluble salts of magnesium and certain salts of sodium, particularly the sulphate, phosphate and tartrate, act in this manner.

Magnesium sulphate (Epsom Salts) is a typical saline purgative. It has a bitter taste and may be given with orange juice. This salt does not irritate the gut and is absorbed very slowly. The osmotic pressure of the salt in solution in the intestine retains sufficient fluid within the gut to maintain a solution of the salt isotonic with the body fluids. A 6.5 per cent solution of magnesium sulphate is isotonic and therefore 8 g of this salt retain in the gut about 120 ml of water, which would about double the volume of the faeces.

The entrance of hypertonic salt solutions into the duodenum causes closure of the pylorus, and may produce vomiting. It a hypertonic solution reaches the intestine it withdraws fluid from the intestinal wall and the volume of solution is therefore only slowly increased. Hence an amount of saline purgative dissolved in sufficient water to produce an isotonic or hypotonic solution causes more rapid purgation than the same amount dissolved in a hypertonic solution. Saline purgatives should be given on an empty stomach, for under these conditions the solution passes directly through the stomach into the duodenum, and the large bulk of fluid in the small intestine causes increased peristalsis. A saline purgative given on a full stomach will only pass in driblets into the intestine, and produces much less action.

Magnesium salts when injected intravenously do not produce purgation but depression of the central nervous system, neuromuscular block and relaxation of smooth muscle. The amount of magnesium absorbed from the gastrointestinal tract is usually too small to produce these effects, but a few cases have been reported in the literature in which, after the administration of magnesium sulphate to small children, sufficient was absorbed to produce unconsciousness. These central effects of magnesium can be reversed by the intravenous injection of calcium salts.

Magnesium citrate and *magnesium hydroxide*, act as mild laxatives by virtue of their magnesium content. The latter is also an antacid.

Sodium sulphate (Glauber's Salt) is not absorbed in the intestine and is as effective as magnesium sulphate as a saline purgative. Whilst its taste is probably more unpleasant than that of magnesium sulphate it also lacks the potential toxicity of the magnesium ion.

Irritant purgatives

Many drugs increase peristalsis by irritating the mucosa of the gut, presumably because they set up a local reflex which originates in the mucosa and is transmitted by the intramural plexuses to the intestinal plain muscle. A purgative of this type should possess the following properties:

1. It must not irritate the stomach or cause vomiting.
2. It must produce only a mild stimulation of the gut, for otherwise it will cause griping, and if it is strongly irritant and there is obstruction of the intestine, it will produce severe inflammation.
3. It must not produce systemic effects in the event of some of it being absorbed.

The following are the more important irritant purgatives.

Vegetable laxatives. The organic acids contained in such fruits as figs and prunes act as mild laxatives. They are assisted in this action by the additional bulk provided by the non-absorbable residue.

Castor oil. This vegetable oil is obtained from the seeds of *Ricinus comunis*. It is non-irritant and can be safely applied to the eye after injury to the conjuctiva. It has no action on the stomach, but in the small intestine it is hydrolysed by lipase with the liberation of ricinoleic acid which is irritant to the gut mucosa. It probably irritates both the small and large intestine and produces a soft stool in three to six hours. There is no danger in giving large doses of castor oil since its action is self-limiting as the purgation eliminates the unhydrolysed oil. Castor oil depends for its hydrolysis on the presence of bile and pancreatic juice and has no purgative action in patients with obstructive jaundice.

One of the main uses of castor oil is to prepare patients for X-ray examination of the kidneys or the intestines.

Anthracene purgatives are so called because they owe their activity to certain active principles which are derivatives of anthracene. Most of the drugs contain emodin (tri-hydroxy-methyl-anthraquinone) and several contain chrysophanic acid (di-hydroxy-methyl-anthraquinone). In such drugs as aloes, senna, cascara sagrada and rhubarb, the active principles are combined with sugars to form glycosides which must by hydrolysed before the emodin is free to act.

Some of the emodin is excreted by the kidneys. The administration of rhubarb by mouth colours the urine yellow due to the presence of chrysophanic acid; this colour changes to a purple-red when the urine is made alkaline. Emodin is also excreted in the milk.

Mode of action of anthracene purgatives. These drugs exert their effects on the colon. It was thought at one time that the glycosides are absorbed from the small intestine, converted to emodin in the liver and subsequently excreted in the large intestine where they exert their action. More recent work has shown that the glycosides are inactive when introduced into the human colon. It is now believed that the anthracene laxatives pass unchanged into the colon where bacteria hydrolyse the glycoside bond to produce free derivatives which then stimulate directly the myenteric plexus and produce defaecation.

Cascara sagrada is the mildest of these purgatives when given in ordinary doses.

Rhubarb contains a considerable quantity of tannin, which acts as an astringent and is liable to produce constipation as an after-effect. For this reason rhubarb is often prescribed with a saline purgative such as a magnesium salt (Gregory's powder).

Senna is a mild purgative which is widely used as an infusion of senna pods or senna leaves. A single dose usually produces an evacuation of the bowel within eight hours which is accompanied by griping. Senokot is a biologically standardised dry extract of senna. The biological standardisation is based on the measurement of the number of wet faeces produced after administration of the preparation to mice.

Aloes stimulates the uterus as well as the large intestine. This can be shown by injecting into a cat aloin, a water soluble mixture of active principles from aloes and recording the contractions of the uterus. Preparations containing aloes should not be used in pregnancy.

Danthron is an anthraquinone purgative given at bedtime.

The anthracene purgatives are specially suitable for administration at night to produce purgation next morning. All these drugs are liable to cause spasmodic contraction of the intestine, and senna in particular is liable to cause griping. This may be prevented by the administration of belladonna or some volatile oil, e.g. oil of peppermint or oil of clove.

Phenolphthalein is tasteless and resembles the anthracene purgatives in its general mode of action. Part of the drug is absorbed and is excreted in the bile, and hence this drug will produce purgative effects for three or four days. Owing to its mode of excretion, phenolphthalein has a cumulative action if taken regularly; for this reason its addition to paraffin and agar-agar emulsions is undersirable.

The chief toxic effects produced by phenolphthalein are skin rashes and occasionally renal irritation. A large overdose can produce severe intoxication, and hence it is unwise to supply this drug for use in children in the form of chocolate tablets and sweetmeats.

Bisacodyl (Dulcolax) is another compound with similar actions; it can be given by mouth, but is usually administered as a suppository to produce a stimulant action on the rectal mucosa which results in peristaltic action and defaecation in 15–30 minutes.

Oxyphenisatin belongs to the same group of purgatives.

Lactulose is a synthetic disaccharide which is not hydrolysed in the human small intestine. It is practically unabsorbed from the gastro-intestinal tract but in the colon it is broken down by bacterial action into acetic and lactic acids which stimulate bowel movements. It is used for the treatment of chronic constipation and has been shown to relieve the central nervous symptoms of patients with portal-systemic encephalopathy presumably by exerting a local osmotic effect in the colon.

Certain powerful purgatives such as mercurial compounds, croton oil and colocynth produce rapid purgation but they are unsafe and should not be used.

Therapeutic use of purgatives

The chief causes of constipation are:
 1. Failure of sufficient food residue to reach the colon.
 2. Inactivity or spasmodic contraction of the colon.
 3. Dyschezia, that is, failure of the entry of the faeces into the rectum to produce the defaecation reflex.

The rational treatment of the first type of constipation is to increase the quantity of water and cellulose taken in the diet. This is the virtue of the adage 'an apple a day keeps the doctor away'. Chronic constipation due to inactivity of the colon should also be treated by increasing the non-absorbable residue of the diet, i.e. by vegetables and fruit. When drugs are required the inert substances should be used in the first instance. When stronger measures are necessary the most suitable drugs are the anthracene purgatives for they can be taken in small doses without producing tolerance. A further advantage is that they do not affect the small intestine and hence do not interfere with the absorption of food.

When spasm of the colon is the cause of the constipation small doses of belladonna may suffice to relax the spasm. The success attributed to the anthracene purgatives in these cases is often due to atropine or volatile oils which are incorporated in such preparations. The mercurial and drastic purgatives should be avoided for reasons already stated.

In dyschezia the colon is normal and the constipation is due to insensitivity of the rectum. This is usually brought about by the hurry and bustle of modern life and repeated failure to answer the call to defaecate. Haemorrhoids or irritation of the anus may also delay the response. Purgatives are of little use. The bowel must be cleared by an enema of soft soap (5 per cent) or by the insertion into the rectum of a mild irritant, for example, a suppository containing 1 to 3 g of glycerine or of 10 mg of bisacodyl. These substances produce contractions of the large intestine with evacuation of its contents. Thereafter the patient is encouraged to establish more regular bowel habits.

The failure to obtain the usual daily evacuation of the bowel produces in many people of regular habits an immediate sense of discomfort, but on the other hand some perfectly healthy people defaecate only once a week. The headache associated with mild constipation is probably produced reflexly by an unusual tension in the rectum or colon. Alvarez showed that the mental haziness, malaise and headache which is so often attributed to the absorption of toxins from the colon can be produced by stuffing the rectum with cotton wool.

Occasional constipation may be produced by a sudden change of diet, a decrease in the amount of fluid taken daily, or an increase in the amount of fluid lost, e.g. by sweating. Castor oil is well suited for such cases; it is not violent and does not usually produce griping. Alternatively an anthracene purgative may be taken at night or a saline purgative in the morning.

Abuse of purgatives

Purgatives are very widely used. A recent British study showed that 29 per cent of a general practice population took purgatives. In a rural Bantu population in South Africa 20 per cent of a selected group took purgatives and a further 20 per cent used enemas. Purgative consumption increases with age. In the British group over 50 per cent of patients aged 60 or more took them more than once a week.

Much folklore, custom and cultural mystique surround the workings of the bowels. This tends to make purgation a ritual rather than a therapeutic procedure supported by the belief that an irregular or infrequent bowel habit is a source of ill health.

Drugs which act on intestinal smooth muscle

Stimulation of activity

A powerful stimulation of the smooth muscle of the gastrointestinal tract is sometimes required in postoperative atony.

The treatment of postoperative atony is often a difficult matter. Relief may sometimes be obtained by enemas. At other times it may be necessary to use stronger drugs which stimulate the smooth muscle directly.

Neostigmine (Prostigmin) is an anticholinesterase whose actions are discussed on page 61. It has both muscarinic and nicotinic actions and is used as an anticurare agent and in the treatment of myasthenia gravis.

Its muscarine effects are manifested by a powerful stimulant action on the intestine and the bladder. It can be administered in the early postoperative period when parenteral medication for intestinal atony is necessary. Excessive abdominal cramps can be alleviated by giving atropine.

Stimulation of gastointestinal activity can be brought about by upsetting the normal balance of parasympathetic and sympathetic innervation of the intestine. Thus the adrenergic neurone blocking drug guanethidine frequently causes diarrhoea.

Inhibition of activity
Many patients suffer from abnormal intestinal motility (the irritable colon syndrome) and any drug which effectively reduces the motor activity of the intestine is of practical interest.

Inhibition of gastrointestinal activity may be brought about by drugs which stimulate adrenergic receptors and more importantly by drugs which block the parasympathetic system either by blocking the muscarinic receptors of the intestinal smooth muscle or by blocking the nicotinic receptors of the ganglia of Auerbach's plexus or both. Anticholinergic drugs used for the purpose of diminishing motor activity in the gastrointestinal tract are usually referred to as *'antispasmodic' drugs*. The anticholinergic drugs comprise atropine and its tertiary and quaternary derivatives but side effects due to generalised parasympathetic blockade limit their usefulness.

Atropine. Anxiety and fear in sensitive persons may produce increased peristalsis and result in bouts of diarrhoea. Atropine, or one of the related drugs such as propantheline, may be used to diminish the activity of the gut in conjunction with a sedative drug. Lienteric diarrhoea, associated with achlorhydria may respond to treatment with dilute hydrochloric acid (BP) taken with fruit juice at meal times.

Another class of 'antispasmodic' compounds do not act specifically on cholinergic receptors but interfere with the neuromuscular apparatus of Auerbach's plexus.

Diphenoxylate is a derivative of pethidine which reduces intestinal motility and has been shown to abolish the mucosal peristaltic reflex. The proprietary preparation Lomotil contains diphenoxylate and a small dose of atropine. Lomotil has become a commonly employed non-specific antidiarrhoeal agent which has displaced opium tincture (paregoric) because its liability to cause addiction is very small. Adverse effects which include skin rashes, nausea and abdominal distension have been reported. Although prolonged use of diphenoxylate may give rise to dependence, the risk is negligible with short-term administration. *Loperamide* (Imodium) inhibits peristalsis by an action on the enteric plexus. It is given orally for the control of diarrhoea. *Mebeverine* (colofac) is a synthetic compound which has relaxant effect on colonic smooth muscle and has been found to relieve the symptoms of the irritable colon syndrome. It is relatively free of central effects and has no atropine-like action. In general the assessment of 'antispasmodic' drugs in the treatment of functional disorders of the intestine is difficult because the results of treatment are usually judged by subjective evaluation and the conditions are characterised by spontaneous remissions and relapses.

Morphine and opiates (p. 279)
The mechanism of action of morphine on the alimentary tract is complex and furthermore varies in different species. In the guinea pig the peristaltic reflex produced by filling isolated segments of the intestine is completely abolished by small doses of morphine. This reflex is mediated by Auerbach's plexus and its aboliton by morphine is believed to be due to a reduction of the release of acetylcholine from the nerve endings of the plexus. In the dog, morphine produces initially an increase in the propulsive activity of the ileum, followed by a secondary, rapidly developing decrease in propulsive activity. Although morphine may initially produce defaecation and increased intestinal movement due to stimulation of the vagus centre, the main effect is to delay the passage of the intestinal contents through the alimentary canal. The latter effect is exerted locally due to an action of morphine on the myenteric plexus.

In man, morphine increases the tone and rhythmic contractions of the intestine but diminishes propulsive activity. Its overall effect is constipating. The pyloric, ileocolic and anal sphincters are contracted and the tone of the large intestine is markedly increased. Morphine also reduces awareness of the normal stimuli for defaecation and patients with diarrhoea who are treated with morphine or opium may notice the call for defaecation only after the intestinal contents have left the body.

Morphine increases the tone of the intestine, but papaverine diminishes it. Opium, which contains papaverine as well as morphine, may be slightly more effective than morphine in reducing the motor activity of the gut, but the difference is very small.

Codeine phosphate which is much less active than morphine is often effective in mild diarrhoea and in doses of up to 180 mg daily has the advantage of fewer undesirable effects, for example, in producing drug dependence and respiratory depression.

PREPARATIONS

Histamine H_2 antagonist
Cimetidine 200 mg 3x die + 400 mg nocte

Antacids
Aluminium hydroxide gel (appr 4% Al_2O_3) 5–30 ml
Magnesium carbonate, heavy and light, 250–500 mg

Magnesium oxide, heavy and light, 250–500 mg
Magnesium trisilicate 0.5–2 g
Sodium bicarbonate 1–5 g

Laxatives
Bulk
Bran (Fybranta) with calc phosph, 6–12 tabs
Methylcellulose (Celevac) 500 mg, 3–6 tabs night and morning
Sterculia (Normacol)
Physical prop
Dioctyl sodium sulphosuccinate 50–100 mg
Liquid paraffin 10–30 ml
Saline
Magnesium oxide, heavy and light, 2–5 g as laxative
Magnesium hydroxide mixture (cream or magnesia) 25–50 ml
Sodium sulphate 1–8 g
Sodium phosphate. Phosphates enema
Irritant
Bisacodyl (Dulcolax) 5–15 mg
Cascara 1–2 tabs
Castor oil 5–20 ml
Danthron 25–50 mg
Lactulose (Duphalac) 10–20 g
Oxyphenisatin ac 5–20 mg
Phenolphthalein 50–300 mg
Senna (Senokot) 0.5–2 g

Antispasmodics
Muscarinic receptor blocking drugs, Ch. 5
Diphenoxylate (Lomotil) 5–40 mg daily
Loperamide hyd 4–16 mg daily
Mebeverine hyd (Colofac) 100 mg 3–4 daily

Emetics
Apomorphine hyd 2–8 mg s.c. or i.m.
Copper sulph 250 mg po
Ipecacuanha paediatric emetic draught 10 ml

Antiemetics
Chlorpromazine tab 25–50 mg
Cyclizine tab 25–50 mg
Dimenhydrinate tab 25–50 mg
Hyoscine tab 300–600 μg
Meclozine tab 25–50 mg
Perphenazine tab 4–8 mg

Gallstone dissolving
Chenodeoxycholic acid (Chendol) 10–15 mg/kg

Lipid lowering
Cholestyramine 10–16 g daily
Dextrothyroxine 4–8 mg daily
Clofibrate (Atromid-S) 20–30 mg/kg daily

FURTHER READING

Avery Jones F, Gunner J W P, Lennard Jones J E 1968 Clinical gastroenterology. Blackwell, Oxford
Bianchi L, Gerok W, Sickinger K (ed) 1977 Liver and bile. MTP Press, London
Bouchier I A D Gallstones. Modern trends in gastroenterology 5. Butterworths, London
Cunnings J H 1976 The use and abuse of laxatives. In: Recent advances in gastroenterology 3. Churchill Livingstone, Edinburgh
Davenport H W 1977 Physiology of the digestive tract. Year Book Medical Publishers, Chicago
Gregory R A 1962 Secretory mechanisms of the gastrointestinal tract. Arnold, London
Heaton K W 1972 Bile salts in health and disease. Churchill Livingstone, Edinburgh
Jacobson E D 1977 Gastric secretion. In: Gastrointestinal physiology. Mosby, St Louis
Johnson L R Gastrointestinal hormones. In: Gastrointestinal physiology. Mosby, St Louis
Jorpes J E, Mutt V (ed) 1973 Secretin, cholecystokinin, pancreozymin and gastrin. Handb. exp. Pharmac: 34
Misiewicz J J 1976 Clinical pharmacology and therapeutic potential of H_2 receptor antagonists. In: Topics in gastroenterology 4. Blackwell, Oxford
Parsons M E 1975 Antagonists of the histamine H_2 receptors. In: Topics in gastroenterology 3. Blackwell, Oxford
Walsh J H, Roth B E 1976 Hormone-secreting tumours of the gastrointestinal tract. In: Recent advances in gastroenterology 3. Churchill Livingstone, Edinburgh
Wastell C, Lance P (ed) 1978 Cimetidine. Westminster Hospital Symposium. Churchill Livingstone, Edinburgh

14. The haemopoietic system

Types of anaemia 202; Iron turnover 202; Therapeutic uses of iron 204; Macrocytic anaemias 205; The cobalamins 206; Folic acid 207; Drug-induced blood dyscrasias 208; Platelet aggregation 209; Blood coagulation 210; Fibrinolysis 211; Heparin 212; Oral anticoagulants 212; Control of local haemorrhage 215.

The haemopoietic system
The blood and the bone marrow are the chief components of the haemopoietic system, but in addition, the spleen and liver are important accessory organs. The spleen is a blood store and also acts as graveyard for the red blood corpuscles; the liver manufactures many of the chief constituents of the plasma and is concerned with the breakdown of the haemoglobin liberated by the destruction of red blood corpuscles. In addition the kidney contains a factor called *erythropoietin* which stimulates red cell synthesis.

Red blood corpuscles are formed and developed in the bone marrow and have an average life of about 120 days. They require constant renewal and the bone marrow is therefore one of the few tissues in the body in which active growth continues throughout life. It has been estimated that a normal man replaces the red cells of about 50 ml of blood daily and only uses about a quarter of the capacity of his bone marrow. The oxygen-carrying power of blood depends on the haemoglobin content of the red blood corpuscles. One gram haemoglobin contains about 3.3 mg or iron and its production depends on the supply of iron. In order to maintain the normal amount of haemoglobin in circulation therefore, the body must have an adequate supply of iron and must also make new red blood cells to carry the haemoglobin. Anaemia is a condition which may arise from failure either to make sufficient red corpuscles or to synthesise an adequate quantity of haemoglobin.

Types of anaemia
Severe haemorrhage is the simplest method by which anaemia can be produced, but a healthy person on an iron rich diet has remarkable powers of regenerating red blood corpuscles, and the haemoglobin content of the blood after a severe haemorrhage may be restored to normal within a month. Chronic anaemia is due either to some dietary deficiency or to disease or disorder of some organ concerned in the manufacture of the factors essential for the formation of red blood corpuscles. In many cases it is a simple matter to rectify chronic anaemia provided the type of anaemia and its cause are known. Reliable diagnosis is essential and requires determination of the red and white cell count, the haemoglobin content and examination of a stained blood film. In special cases other diagnostic methods such as sternal marrow puncture may be necessary. The symptoms of anaemia are mainly due to anoxia and are usually more severe if the anaemia develops rapidly. The following is a convenient classification of anaemias:

1. Deficiency of factors essential for normal blood formation
   (a) Deficiency of iron:
Chronic nutritional hypochromic anaemia including the hypochromic anaemias of pregnancy, infancy and childhood.
Post-haemorrhagic anaemia, acute and chronic.
   (b) Deficiency of the antipernicious anaemia factor.
Addisonian pernicious anaemia.
Pernicious anaemia of pregnancy.
Tropical macrocytic anaemia.
Macrocytic anaemia of sprue, idiopathic steatorrhoea and of liver disease.
   (c) Deficiency of vitamin C and of thyroxine.
Anaemias of scurvy and of myxoedema.

2. Depression of the bone marrow
Aplastic or hypoplastic conditions of the bone marrow may affect the formation and development of the red cells, leucocytes or platelets. Complete aplastic anaemia is a condition where the bone marrow at autopsy is entirely yellow and the formation of all these blood cells is deficient. Aplastic anaemia affecting only red cells or only platelets is rare, but agranulocytosis, a condition in which leucocytes and other cells of the myeloid series are absent occurs relatively frequently as a result of the administration of certain drugs, exposure to radio-active substances or to severe infection.

3. Excessive destruction of red blood cells
Haemolytic anaemia due to formation of defective red corpuscles or to poisons or infection.

Iron turnover
The body of a 70 kg man contains about 4 g of iron, 65 per cent of which circulates in the blood as haemoglobin. About one-half of the remainder is stored in the liver, spleen and bone marrow, chiefly as ferritin and haemosiderin, from which fresh haemoglobin can be made; the rest, which is not available for haemoglobin systhesis, is present in other tissues in the form of cytochrome, myohaemoglobin, etc. The haemoglobin content of normal blood is 15.5 g per 100 ml.

Approximately 8 g of haemoglobin, which is equivalent to 26 mg of iron, is liberated daily by the breaking-down of red cells. Nearly all of this iron is used for resynthesis of haemoglobin and only about 1 mg daily is lost in the bile and urine. The loss of iron is greater in women during menstruation, pregnancy and lactation but normally does not exceed 4 mg daily. The extra demands each day for growth and for storage of iron in children and adolescents seldom amount to more than 1 mg. The requirements of iron for the normal person are extremely small and are amply provided if the daily diet for a man contains 5 mg and for a woman or growing child 15 mg of iron. The average diet provides between 15 and 20 mg iron daily, and good supplies of iron are present in green vegetables, peas, beans, oatmeal, eggs, liver, chocolate and dried fruits; on the other hand, fish, chicken, milk and white bread are relatively poor sources.

Iron transport and storage
Transferrin is a globular protein in plasma concerned with iron transport. Each transferrin molecule contains two binding sites capable of combining with ferric iron, Fe^{+++}, and carrying it by the blood stream to sites of action such as bone marrow or placenta. Iron is fixed only on locations where it is required, thus reticulocytes have a considerable iron uptake whilst none is taken up by mature cells. Tracer experiments have shown that transferrin combines with receptors on the reticulocyte surface. Iron is subsequently carried into the cell interior whilst being reduced from the trivalent to the divalent form required for the synthesis of haemoglobin.

Apoferritin and *ferritin* are concerned with iron storage. Apoferritin is a large protein formed by duodenal cells which reacts with ferric iron to form the storage protein ferritin containing a ferric hydrophosphate micelle surrounded by a protein shell. The iron content of ferritin is variable; when fully saturated each molecule contains 5000 atoms of iron. Ferritin is found in liver, bone marrow, spleen, kidney, brain and placenta besides the intestinal mucosa. *Haemosiderin*, another storage form of iron is an aggregate of ferritin molecules.

Iron absorption
The ferritin content of the duodenal mucosa is believed to play an important part in controlling iron absorption; it has been shown experimentally that iron absorption is much less when the mucosal ferritin content is high than when it is low. Since the ferritin stores in the duodenal mucosa are in dynamic equilibrium with stores elsewhere it follows that the amount of iron absorbed depends on the state of the iron reserves in the body. Thus normal dogs made rapidly anaemic by bleeding do not immediately absorb more iron than normal dogs, but only do so after some of the iron reserves have been used up in forming new red cells.

In man, if extra iron is given by mouth to a normal subject, he does not absorb it but excretes practically all of it in the faeces. A healthy male absorbs only enough iron to replace the small daily loss but in states of iron deficiency food iron absorption may increase to around 50 per cent of that ingested, or 7.5 mg daily from a diet containing 15 mg. The demands of the foetus also increase the absorption of iron, and pregnant women, whether or not they are anaemic, absorb between 2 and 10 times more than normal women.

Iron salts must be ionised to be absorbed and several factors may influence the iron available for this purpose. Iron salts are scarcely dissociated at a pH above 5.0 and iron deficiency is common in patients with achlorhydria. In the normal subject therefore the conditions for iron absorption are optimal in the upper part of the small intestine. Absorption of iron may be inhibited by an excess of phosphorus in the diet, since iron forms insoluble or undissociated compounds with inorganic and organic phosphates such as phytic acid.

Ferrous salts are more readily absorbed than ferric salts. It has been shown by means of radioactive iron salts that normal subjects utilise between 1.5 and 10 times more ferrous than ferric salt (Fig. 14.1). Ascorbic acid, which is a powerful reducing agent, can be incorporated in preparations of ferrous salts to prevent their oxidation and thus promote their absorption.

Causes of iron deficiency
The chief causes of iron deficiency are:

Inadequate dietary intake. The normal dietary intake of iron is inadequate for women who have borne several children in quick succession. Since the iron content of milk is low, iron intake may also be inadequate in babies who are maintained too long on a milk diet or in premature babies who have insufficient body stores of iron. Iron deficiency also occurs in elderly persons who eat little meat, which is the main source of iron in a normal diet.

Malabsorption. Inadequate absorption of iron from the small intestine occurs when the food is hurried through the upper part of the intestine, as in patients with partial gastrectomy. Iron is also poorly absorbed in patients with coeliac disease and idiopathic steatorrhoea.

Loss of blood. This occurs in women who have excessive menstrual bleeding or in patients with chronic blood loss from the alimentary tract. One hundred millilitres of blood contains about 50 mg of iron; the loss of a pint of blood by haemorrhage involves a loss of 300 mg iron, which can be replaced from the iron reserves of the body. If these reserves are adequate, they are capable of replacing an iron loss from haemorrhage involving as much as one-third of the blood volume. If, however, by repeated haemorrhage, the haemoglobin level is reduced to below 50 per cent of its normal value, the iron reserves will be exhausted and the

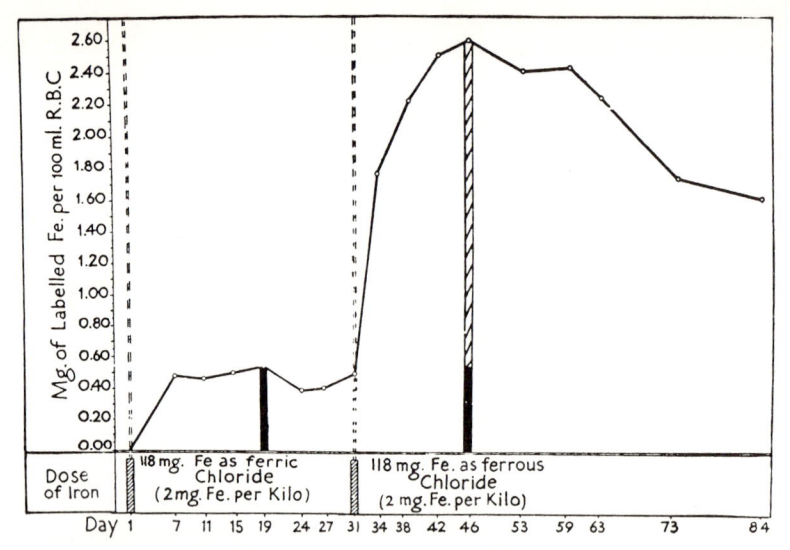

Fig. 14.1 The absorption of two preparations of radioactive iron by a subject with hypochromic anaemia. The amount of iron absorbed was measured as the amount of radioactive iron which appeared as haemoglobin in the peripheral blood. A dose of 2 mg/kg of ferric chloride was given by mouth and only 6.2 per cent of the total dose was utilised. On the other hand, when a similar dose of ferrous chloride was given 26 per cent of the total dose was utilised. (After Moore, C.V. et al., 1944. *J. Clin. Invest.*)

iron available from a normal diet will then only produce a rise of 2 per cent of haemoglobin per week.

Chronic haemorrhage may cause a constant drain from the iron reserves, for a loss of only 10 ml of blood daily involves a fivefold increase in the normal amount of iron lost. This may easily be beyond the capacity of a normal diet. If the bleeding is into the alimentary tract, for example from a peptic ulcer, the loss may be partially offset by the reabsorption of some of the haemoglobin iron.

Therapeutic uses of iron

Iron salts are frequently prescribed as 'tonics' to persons suffering from general ill health; this use of iron is irrational unless there is evidence of iron deficiency. Iron deficiency anaemia, from whatever cause, can usually be adequately treated by the administration of suitable iron salts. Many of the preparations of iron that are used are quite ineffective because the amount of iron they contain is minute or the amount absorbed is completely inadequate. Organic iron preparations such as haemoglobin or red bone marrow extract are pleasant to take but are almost useless for the treatment of anaemia because of their low content of iron. Reduced iron is effective but requires to be given in large doses.

The main principle of iron therapy is the use of ferrous salts in adequate doses. A number of preparations of ferrous iron salts are available for oral administration; they are probably equally effective in raising the haemoglobin level, provided they are administered in doses which contain equal amounts of elemental iron.

Oral administration
Most cases of iron deficiency anaemias can be treated successfully by mouth. It must be appreciated, however, that no more than 20 per cent of an administered dose of iron is absorbed so that adequate doses must be given.

Soluble ferrous salts when kept in solution oxidise to the ferric state, unless the solution contains a reducing agent such as ascorbic acid or glucose. Moreover, the oral administration of iron salts in solution presents certain difficulties, for they have an unpleasant taste, stain the teeth black, they are nearly all astringent and are liable to irritate the stomach and produce constipation and colic. Orally administered iron is absorbed best when taken before meals, but is tolerated better when taken with or immediately after meals.

Ferrous sulphate. This compound contains 30 per cent of elemental iron, therefore a tablet of 200 mg contains 60 mg of iron. It is usually available in sugar-coated tablets. These tablets are often attractively coloured but are dangerous to children who may swallow them in mistake for sweets. They cause severe gastric haemorrhage in infants, sometimes with fatal results. If a tablet of ferrous sulphate is administered 3 times daily to a patient with iron-deficiency anaemia the haemoglobin level begins to rise after 7 to 10 days and thereafter rises at the rate of about 1 to 2 per cent daily.

In slow release preparations the iron salt is incorporated in a special matrix from which it is released slowly. These preparations are taken before breakfast; they are relatively non-irritant since most of the iron is released after passing the stomach. They are more expensive than ordinary ferrous iron preparations but may be tried if the latter are not well tolerated.

Ferrous gluconate contains only 12 per cent of iron and is usually available in tablets of 300 mg containing 35 mg of iron. Compared with ferrous sulphate in doses containing the same amounts of iron it is equally effective in raising the haemoglobin level and is also as likely to produce gastrointestinal disturbances. As shown in Figure 14.2 ferrous sulphate, gluconate, and succinate are about equally effective in raising the haemoglobin level of patients with hypochromic anaemia but an equivalent dose of a ferric compound is ineffective.

Ferrous fumarate contains 65 mg of iron in each 200 mg tablet and is an alternative preparation of iron which can be used if a patient is unable to tolerate ferrous sulphate. The chelated compounds *ferrocholinate, ferrous glycine sulphate complex* (ferrous aminoacetosulphate) are also effective when administered in doses containing adequate amounts of elemental iron.

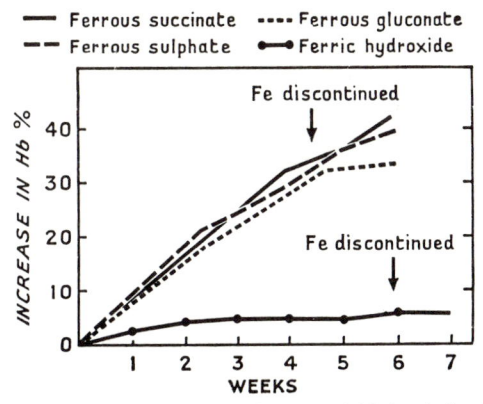

Fig. 14.2 The average weekly rise in haemoglobin level of patients with hypochromic anaemia treated with different iron salts. Each patient received the equivalent of 210 mg of iron daily in three divided doses of 70 mg taken as tablets after meals. (After O'Sullivan, Higgins and Wilkinson, 1955, *Lancet*.)

Ferric ammonium citrate. In contrast to the preparations so far mentioned this substance contains ferric iron which must be reduced to the ferrous state before absorption. It is hygroscopic and must be administered in solution. It is usually well tolerated but must be given in large doses.

Gastrointestinal irritation may occur after the administration of iron but this can usually be minimised if the preparation is taken after food. Iron therapy should be continued for several weeks after the haemoglobin level has returned to normal in order to replenish the body stores of iron.

Parenteral administration
This method of administration is used in patients unable to tolerate or absorb iron when given by mouth or who have severe iron deficiency during late pregnancy. Early intramuscular preparations were unsuccessful because they were either too irritant or insufficient iron was absorbed from the site of injection. Intravenous preparations produced both local and systemic toxic reactions such as pyrexia, flushing of the skin, palpitaions, precordial pain and locally induration and thrombophlebitis. Intravenous iron is now seldom used but preparations of iron complexed with dextran or sorbitol have become available which are less irritant and can be given by deep intramuscular injection.

Iron dextran injection (Imferon) *and iron sorbitol injection* (Jectofer) can be injected intramuscularly. A 2 ml ampoule of these preparations contains 100 mg of iron which is the amount required for a rise of haemoglobin of about 4 per cent. The amount of iron required to correct the anaemia may be roughly calculated. Indications for parenteral iron preperations are limited to special situations in which a serious iron loss cannot be readily corrected or oral iron may produce severe damage, e.g. in ulcerative colitis.

Toxic effects after intramuscular injection of iron dextran are limited mainly to pain and brown staining of the skin but systemic allergic reactions including fever, lymphadenopathy and arthralgia have been reported. In some cases severe allergic reactions, some of them fatal, have occurred especially after intravenous injections.

Since even parenteral preparations of iron raise the haemoglobin level only after a latent period, the quickest way of increasing the haemoglobin level is to give one or more blood transfusions.

Acute iron poisoning
An increasing number of cases of acute iron poisoning have occurred as the result of young children swallowing attractively coloured tablets of iron in mistake for sweets. This example serves to emphasise the importance of instructing patients to ensure that medicines are kept well out of reach of young children.

The ingestion of excessive doses of iron salts in this way gives rise to severe gastric irritation and haemorrhage and profound circulatory collapse.

Desferrioxamine mesylate (Desferal) (p. 474) is a powerful chelating agent which readily binds with iron to form a non-irritant complex. It can be administered intragastrically after gastric lavage, and intra-muscularly. In severe poisoning desferrioxamine mesylate can be given by slow intravenous infusion. Desferrioxamine is used to prevent iron accumulation by increasing iron excretion in patients with thalassaemia.

MACROCYTIC ANAEMIAS

The formation of red blood corpuscles in the bone-marrow may be interrupted at various stages before the normal red cell is fully mature and this results in the release into the peripheral circulation of macrocytic cells which have a larger diameter than normal erythrocytes. The commonest cause of disturbance in the bone marrow is associated with a deficiency of vitamin B_{12} which is necessary for normal blood formation. Deficiency of this factor results in pernicious anaemia.

Pernicious anaemia

In this disease there is a marked fall in the total red cell count, and to a lesser extent in the haemoglobin level; this is associated with achlorhydria and often complicated by the occurrence of subacute combined degeneration of the spinal cord.

In 1926 Minot and Murphy tried the effect of feeding large quantities of raw liver to patients with pernicious anaemia and found that this produced a rapid and remarkable relief in the symptoms of the disease. A similar effect was later shown by Castle and Locke (1928) as a result of feeding patients with meat that had undergone partial digestion in a normal stomach, or by feeding with raw or dried pig's stomach. These results led to the conclusion that the effective substance was elaborated in the stomach during digestion of proteins. Castle and his associates later suggested that in the normal gastric juice of human subjects there was a substance (intrinsic factor) which acted on a constituent of the diet (extrinsic factor) to produce a specific factor necessary for the normal maturation of red cells. This specific or antianaemic factor was probably stored in the liver. Patients with pernicious anaemia were believed to be lacking in intrinsic factor.

These views have been modified as a result of the isolation of vitamin B_{12} (cyanocobalamin) and its identification as the anti-pernicious anaemia factor. It is now believed that the extrinsic factor of Castle is vitamin B_{12} and that the intrinsic factor is a protein present in the gastric juice which aids the absorption of vitamin B_{12}. In patients with pernicious anaemia there is a deficiency of intrinsic factor and the absorption of vitamin B_{12} from the gastrointestinal tract is greatly reduced. Studies with radioactive vitamin B_{12} have shown that whereas a healthy person absorbs about 70 per cent of an oral dose of vitamin B_{12}, a patient with pernicious anaemia absorbs 10 per cent or less. Hence these patients require much larger amounts of vitamin B_{12} in their diet and the responses originally observed by Minot and Murphy to oral liver treatment were due to the very large amounts of vitamin B_{12} present in the liver.

Intrinsic factor

Human intrinsic factor (IF) has been isolated from gastric juice and shown to be a glycoprotein of molecular weight approximately 50 000 capable of combining on a molar basis with vitamin B_{12}. The IF-B_{12} complex is transported from the stomach to the ileum where it interacts with a specific receptor in the presence of calcium ions prior to being absorbed by mucosal cells and taken up into the blood stream. A minimal amount of vitamin B_{12} can be absorbed in the absence of IF but in its presence absorption is increased many times. Lack of IF causes megaloblastic anaemia whether in cases of pernicious anaemia or after gastrectomy.

It is believed that immunological factors play an important role in pernicious anaemia. A blocking antibody, capable of interfering with the formation of the IF-B_{12} complex has been detected in the serum of pernicious anaemia patients.

The cobalamins

In 1948 vitamin B_{12}, a red crystalline substance, was isolated from liver extracts by Lester Smith and by Rickes and his colleagues. The complete structural formula of cyanocobalamin was determined by Todd and Hodgkin in 1955. The molecule is very complex and is built round an atom of cobalt. Although vitamin B_{12} is the only cobalt containing compound so far found in nature its general structure resembles that of the natural porphyrin derivatives such as haem and chlorophyll. The yield of this vitamin from liver is extremely small and for this reason other sources of the vitamin have been sought. Vitamin B_{12} can be isolated from the culture broth of *Streptomyces griseus*, the mould used for the production of streptomycin. Compounds with vitamin B_{12} activity have also been found in the waste-liquors resulting from the production of other antibiotics.

Two forms of vitamin B_{12}, cyanocobalamin and hydroxocobalamin, are used in therapy. Both are clinically highly effective in the treatment of pernicious anaemia.

When either cyanocobalamin or hydroxocobalamin is injected subcutaneously it produces considerable remission of symptoms and a haematological response comparable with that produced by an extract of liver. The effective dose by mouth is about 100 times that required by injection. If the vitamin is given by mouth with normal gastric juice there is adequate absorption and a remission of symptoms is obtained (Fig. 14.3).

Hydroxocobalamin is as effective as cyanobalamin in producing a haematological response. It is bound more strongly to plasma proteins and has a more prolonged action; it is now the preparation of choice since less frequent injections are necessary.

Cobalamins in the treatment of pernicious anaemia

Hydroxocobalamin provides a complete substitution therapy for pernicious anaemia. The bone marrow reverts from the megaloblastic to the normoblastic type of erythropoiesis, the blood count becomes normal, subacute combined degeneration of the cord is arrested and peripheral neuritis and glossitis are cured. The gastric atrophy and achlorhydria however persist. The treatment of pernicious anaemia is divisible into two phases: intensive treatment until the blood picture is restored to

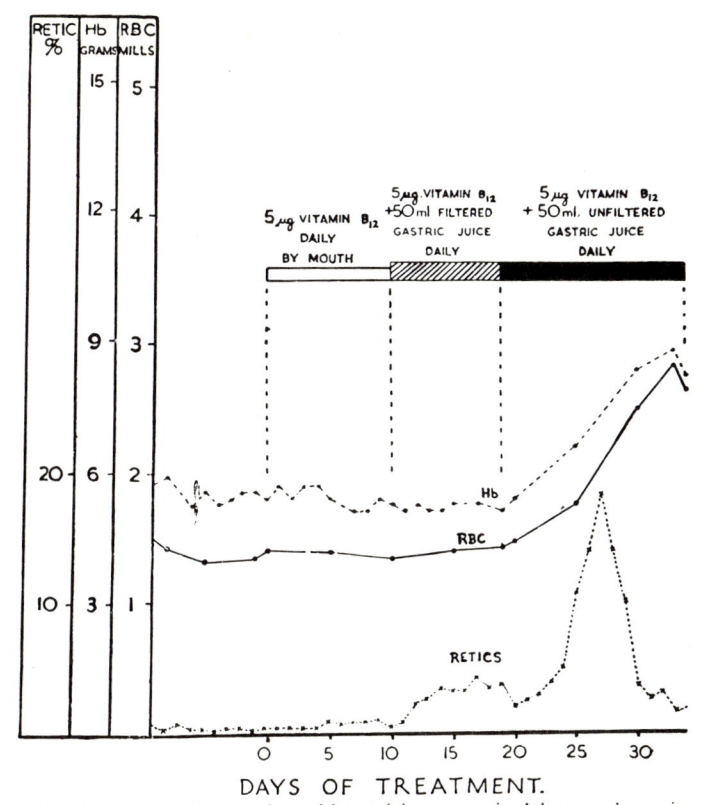

Fig. 14.3 The effect of vitamin B_{12} given by mouth to a patient with pernicious anaemia. Adequate absorption occurred when vitamin B_{12} was given with normal gastric juice but did not occur when the gastric juice had previously been passed through a Seitz filter, which removed the intrinsic factor. The figure also shows that the patient was unable to provide enough intrinsic factor in his stomach to ensure absorption of the vitamin. (After Ungley, C.C., 1950. Br. med. J.)

normal, followed by maintenance treatment. Since an adequate regeneration of red cells does not immediately take place after injection of a cobalamin there is a delay of 4 or 5 days before any marked clinical improvement can occur; the blood count should increase by about 1 million red cells within 10 days. It may be necessary if the patient is severely ill, to begin treatment with a blood transfusion, in addition to the administration of a cobalamin.

Treatment may be commenced with intramuscular injections of 1000 µg of a cobalamin once or twice weekly, gradually increasing the interval between doses to two or three weeks. The dose and the frequency of administration must be increased if necessary till the blood picture is restored to normal. Maintenance treatment has to be continued for life and it is preferable to give injections as infrequently as possible. Injection of 1000 µg hydroxocobalamin every two months is enough for maintenance. Oral preparations of vitamin B_{12} should not be used since they require the presence of the intrinsic factor for absorption. There is now no justification for using liver preparations.

When the rapid production of red cells makes heavy demands on the iron depots, a course of iron therapy for two or three months may be necessary during the phase of intensive treatment with liver extract.

Cobalamines have also been found to produce symptomatic improvement in diabetic neuropathy, trigeminal neuralgia and other types of peripheral neuropathy.

Folic acid (pteroylglutamic acid) (p. 369)
This substance is present in the liver and can also be extracted from green leaves. In the body, folic acid is converted into a derivative known as folinic acid or citrovorum factor which is the physiologically active form. In pernicious anaemia, folic acid was shown by Spies and his coworkers to produce an initial clinical improvement comparable with that obtained with liver extract; after daily administration of 10 to 20 mg folic acid by mouth a reticulocyte response was observed within 5 to 10 days. Treatment with folic acid, however, does not arrest the development of subacute combined degeneration of the spinal cord and may indeed precipitate its onset. Furthermore, although the initial increase in red cells produced by this drug is satisfactory, continuous treatment fails to maintain a satisfactory blood count.

Although folic acid is unsatisfactory in the treatment of pernicious anaemia it improves other types of macrocytic anaemias such as the megaloblastic anaemia of pregnancy, idiopathic steatorrhoea and tropical sprue. These anaemias are characterised by absence of neurological manifestations, good response to folic acid and poor response to cyanocobalamin.

Because of the frequency of megaloblastic anaemia in pregnancy a case has been made out for the prophylactic administration of folate during pregnancy. As iron is also required, a single preparation containing 0.3 mg of folic acid and 100 mg of iron may be used once daily. The risk of adverse effects by folates is small, although folate must never be substituted for cobalamin therapy in true pernicious anaemia.

DRUG-INDUCED BLOOD DYSCRASIAS

The red blood corpuscles, leucocytes and probably the blood platelets are formed in the bone marrow, whilst lymphocytes are produced from the lymph glands. Marrow poisons produce a variety of effects on the blood. Mild interference with red blood corpuscle formation causes punctate basophilia, whilst severe intoxication produces aplastic anaemia. Inhibition of platelet formation causes thrombocytopenic purpura. Interference with white blood corpuscle formation causes leucopenia and finally agranulocytosis.

The mechanism by which drug induced blood dyscrasias are produced is poorly understood. Cytotoxic drugs used in cancer chemotherapy or as immunosuppressants produce a dose-dependent leukopenia which probably reflects interference with the DNA apparatus of the cell. Many other drugs which are not obviously cytotoxic, nevertheless occasionally cause anaemia, thrombocytopenia and agranulocytosis. This type of effect is usually unrelated to dose but it seldom occurs unless the drug responsible has been given for some time. Occasionally a blood dyscrasia occurs immediately after starting a second course of drug suggesting an allergic reaction. Antibodies are seldom found, but they have been detected with some drug reactions, e.g. antibodies to blood platelets in thrombocytopenic purpura after the use of quinine or quinidine. Besides allergy, genetic and metabolic factors are involved in haematological drug reactions. Unfortunately we have no information why certain individuals suddenly develop a specific susceptibility of their bone marrow to a particular drug.

Aplastic anaemia and agranulocytosis. Benzene is the simplest example of a non-selective bone marrow poison since it reduces the formation of red and white blood corpuscles and of blood platelets. These effects can be regularly produced in experimental animals, and they occur relatively frequently in industrial poisoning; X-rays, radium and the nitrogen mustards can produce similar effects.

Chloramphenicol depresses all elements of the bone marrow so that anaemia, thrombocytopenia and agranulocytosis occur. Similar effects are produced by organic gold compounds and by phenylbutazone. Anticonvulsant drugs such as hydantoinates and, to a lesser extent, phenobarbitone may cause a megaloblastic anaemia which can be successfully treated with folic acid.

The production of agranulocytosis by amidopyrine and thiouracil compounds is a more selective effect, since it is not accompanied by anaemia. Agranulocytosis may be signalled by ulceration of the mouth and pharynx or by a systemic infection. These reactions probably have an allergic basis. Many other drugs including the sulphonamides, phenothiazines and tridione produce agranulocytosis occasionally.

Thrombocytopenic purpura. With severe thrombocytopenia, purpura usually precedes epistaxis, bleeding from the gums and alimentary tract and in some cases cerebral haemorrhage. Allergic thrombocytopenic purpura is occasionally produced by quinine, quinidine, acetazolamide, organic arsenicals and sulphonamides. Thrombocytopenic purpura may also be caused by the cytotoxic drugs, nitrogen mustards, tretamine, busulphan and urethane which depress the functions of the bone marrow.

Methaemoglobinaemia and haemolytic anaemia. Aniline, phenylhydrazine and their derivatives, such as acetanilide, cause the conversion of haemoglobin to methaemoglobin, and this is followed by the breakdown of corpuscles. The methaemoglobinaemia results in a characteristic cyanosis.

Nitrites and chlorates also produce methaemoglobin, but the latter drug is the more harmful because it also causes haemolysis of red blood cells. The sulphonamide drugs as a group produce sulphaemoglobin and methaemoglobin and in this way cause cyanosis.

Treatment of blood dyscrasias
The most important therapeutic measure in all drug-induced blood dyscrasia is the immediate withdrawal of the offending drug. Bacterial infection is particularly liable to occur in patients with agranulocytosis, due to lack of leucocytes in the circulating blood. An antibiotic such as penicillin or a tetracycline should be used to prevent bacterial infection. Agranulocytosis is frequently fatal and there is no convincing evidence that any specific treatment is effective against it. In order to stimulate the blood-forming tissues large doses of testosterone or anabolic steroids are sometimes given. If a hypersensitivity reaction seems likely corticosteroids such as prednisolone may be prescribed.

PHARMACOLOGY OF THROMBOSIS

The high morbidity and mortality from thromboembolic vascular disease has prompted a wide-ranging search for drugs which might be of value in the prevention and treatment of thrombosis. In order to understand the action of such drugs it is necessary to consider briefly the factors involved in clot formation.

It is now believed that both platelets and fibrin play a part in the formation of intravascular thrombi. Thrombosis is probably initiated by platelet adhesion and aggregation and completed by the formation of fibrin through the coagulation mechanism. Thrombus formation can be reversed by the action of the proteolytic enzyme *plasmin* which causes the breakdown of fibrin. It follows that clot formation can in principle be influenced at various stages including (1) platelet aggregation (2) blood coagulation, or fibrin formation and (3) fibrinolysis.

Platelet aggregation

Intravascular thrombi are made up of a head consisting of aggregated platelets, white cells and fibrin and a tail consisting mainly of fibrin with enmeshed red blood cells. Human arterial thrombi are usually rich in platelet aggregates and can be expected to be responsive to inhibitors of platelet function. Platelets have the property of adhering to subendothelial tissue, particularly collagen, whenever a breach occurs in the continuity of the vascular epithelium as is the case in atherosclerosis. Once platelets adhere to the injured vessel wall aggregation of other platelets, to form a platelet plug, rapidly occurs.

The biochemical mechanisms involved in platelet aggregation are complex and involve amongst others adenosine diphosphate (ADP) and the prostaglandin system. A variety of chemical stimuli may initiate aggregation of blood platelets many of which are intrinsic; thus ADP and adrenaline can both produce platelet aggregation by a direct action (first phase aggregation). If suitable concentrations of these substances are employed a second phase of aggregation follows, brought about by the release of ADP and other factors from the platelets themselves called the platelet release reaction. The platelet release reaction is activated by thrombin and collagen. Collagen which is present in blood vessels and perivascular tissue stimulates only second phase aggregation mediated by the platelet release reaction.

More recently it has been shown that platelets synthesise and release prostaglandins during aggregation and that oral ingestion of aspirin (known to inhibit aggregation) could block platelet synthesis of prostaglandins. Naturally occurring stable prostaglandins do not directly induce platelet aggregation, but in 1973 Willis reported that a labile material transiently appearing during biosynthesis of PGE_2 from arachidonate, could produce aggregation, thus providing a probable mechanism for the inhibitory effects of aspirin-like drugs. A number of prostaglandin intermediates have been synthesised, particularly by Swedish workers, and characterised as enderoperoxides or related thromboxanes. It has been shown that patients with a congenital bleeding disorder known as 'storage pool disease' lack responsiveness of their platelets to enderoperoxide.

Drugs inhibiting platelet aggregation
Such drugs are of potential interest for the prevention of thrombosis, though none have so far been clearly demonstrated to be clinically useful.

Adenosine is a specific antagonist of ADP-induced platelet aggregation, presumably by competition for the same receptors site.

Aspirin often causes gastrointestinal bleeding and has been shown to prolong bleeding time and to inhibit second phase platelet aggregation. The probable mechanism of this effect, by inhibition of the formation of a platelet aggregating enderoperoxide, has been discussed above. When a single dose of aspirin is administered its effect on bleeding time lasts several days corresponding to the life span of the platelet which may indicate irreversible platelet damage by aspirin.

There is clinical evidence that aspirin administration may decrease the incidence of postoperative thrombotic or embolic complications but the fairly widespread use of aspirin for the prevention of coronary or cerebral thrombosis lacks statistical support and large scale, controlled studies of the prophylactic use of aspirin are lacking.

Other non-steroidal anti-inflammatory analgesics such as indomethacin, sulphinpyrazone and meclofenamic acid share with aspirin the ability to block prostaglandin synthetase and all have been shown to inhibit second phase platelet aggregation.

Sulphinpyrazone administered over a period of several weeks prolonged platelet survival time and reduced human platelet turnover.

Prostaglandin E_1 (PGE_1) is a powerful inhibitor of ADP-induced platelet aggregation. It also inhibits the platelet release reaction in various species, including man. Although highly active *in vitro*, PGE_1 is rapidly broken down in the lung and has no clinical application. A great deal of research is being carried out in the prostaglandin field to find a stable compound with minimal systemic side effects capable of preventing platelet aggregation in vivo (see also p. 92).

Dipyridamole, a drug originally introduced as a coronary dilator, is claimed to have antiplatelet and antithrombotic activity in man. It fails to antagonise ADP-induced aggregation but has some effect in collagen-induced second phase aggregation. Dipyridamole has been shown to have limited usefulness in cardiac surgery in reducing

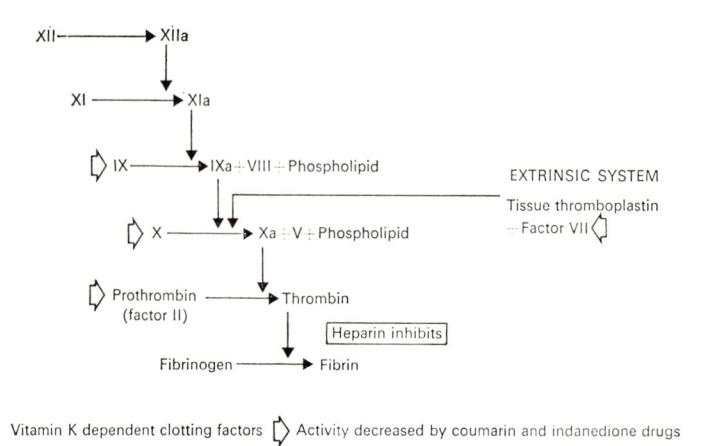

Fig. 14.4 A blood coagulation scheme. (After Ogston and Douglas, *Drugs*, vol. 1, 1971.)

the incidence of thromboembolic episodes in patients with artificial heart valves.

Blood coagulation

This involves a series of reactions which result in a fibrin clot. Although intravascular thrombosis is probably initiated by platelet aggregation, the formation of fibrin is important in holding together the aggregates of platelets and, in the case of venous thrombi, in providing the framework of the tail. In the later stages of clotting, thrombin interacts with fibrinogen to form fibrin. Thrombin does not exist in normal blood but it may be formed through one of two mechanisms, the intrinsic and the extrinsic coagulation mechanism.

The clotting mechanism is highly complex and its details have not been fully elucidated. Table 14.1 shows the various clotting factors in plasma which have been identified and assigned roman numerals by international convention. A suggested 'cascade' system of interaction of these factors is shown in Figure 14.4.

Intrinsic pathway. All the components of the intrinsic system are present in the blood. Hageman factor (XII) is activated by surface contact; this then leads to a series of enzymatic reactions which act as a biochemical amplifier transforming a small stimulus into effective thrombin production. Two of the reactions steps shown in Figure 14.4 require phospholipid which is provided by the platelets.

Extrinsic coagulation pathway. This is activated during injury when blood comes in contact with tissue. The extrinsic pathway requires a tissue component as well as some, though not all, the clotting factors in plasma (Fig. 14.4).

Table 14.1 Coagulation factors in plasma. (After Mammen in Handbook Exp. Pharm. vol. 27, 1971.)

Factors	
I	Fibrinogen
II	Prothrombin
I	Tissue thromboplastin
IV	Calcium
V	Plasma accelerator globulin, proaccelerin
VII	Proconvertin, serum prothrombin conversion accelerator
VIII	Antihaemophilic globulin (A)
IX	Antihaemophilic globulin (B), Christmas factor
X	Stuart-Prower factor
XI	Plasma thromboplastin antecedent (PTA). Antihaemophilic factor C
XII	Hageman factor
XIII	Laki-Lorand factor, fibrin stabilising factor, transglutaminase

Clot stabilising factor. The action of thrombin on fibrinogen causes fibrinopeptides to be split off and leads to the formation of fibrin monomers which in the presence of calcium form a fibrin gel. Recent work has shown that at this stage a further reaction occurs which leads to a firm fibrin clot. The responsible factor (XIII) is an enzyme, *transglutaminase*, which in the presence of thrombin and calcium forms cross links between fibrin monomers, resulting in an insoluble and firm clot.

Deficiencies of clotting factors cause bleeding disorders of various kinds. Deficiency of antihaemophilic globulin A (factor VIII) is the cause of the most frequent type of hereditary haemophilia and deficiency of factor IX is the cause of the bleeding syndrome of Christmas disease. The incidence of haemophilia B is about 10 per cent of that of haemophilia A. All patients with a congenital coagulation deficiency need the life-long supervision of a designated haemophilia centre and should carry a special medical card. Treatment of these conditions is by the administration of factor VIII or factor IX concentrates. Animal material of high potency is available but it is antigenic. The main risk of human preparations is the serious risk of hepatitis.

Fibrinolysis
When a thrombus is formed its fibrin matrix eventually becomes destroyed by the action of the body's fibrinolytic system. Fibrin formation and fibrinolysis are in dynamic equilibrium and some degree of thrombus formation and destruction may take place continuously in the body. Fibrinolysis is brought about by a protease called *plasmin* or fibrinolysin the precursor of which is called *plasminogen* or profibrinolysin. The agent which converts plasminogen to plasmin in the body is called 'plasminogen activator', a term which refers to an activity rather than to a well-defined single substance. It comprises a 'vascular activator' from blood vessels and a 'tissue activator' which is related to Hageman factor (XII).

Enhancement of fibrinolysis
The concept of fibrinolytic therapy to resolve vascular thrombotic occlusion is an old idea which has recently had some limited practical application. In principle two approaches to fibrinolytic therapy seem possible, the use of preformed plasmin or of a plasminogen activator. Both approaches have been tried but so far the second approach based on activation of intrinsic plasminogen has proved the more successful. Two plasminogen activators have been mainly employed. *Streptokinase* a protein derived from ß-haemolytic streptococci is widely used clinically. It may give rise to pyrexia and severe allergic reactions. *Urokinase* is a plasminogen activator present in human urine. It is non-antigenic in man. Its clinical use has been limited by difficulties of purification and expense.

Fibrinolytic therapy in man
Trials have been carried out on human volunteers which showed that it is possible to lyse artificial thrombi in the veins of the forearm by systemic infusion of streptokinase; in control subject not given streptokinase the veins went on to fibrosis. Streptokinase may be given by intravenous or intra-arterial infusion. A number of small scale trials have been carried out to treat thromboembolic conditions with streptokinase or with urokinase. Good results have been obtained in patients with deep leg vein thrombosis and peripheral arterial occlusion. There is no evidence, so far, that patients with pulmonary embolism or myocardial infarction are benefited by fibrinolytic therapy.

Aminocaproic acid is chemically closely related to lysine. Aminocaproic aicd is an antagonist of plasminogen activation and may be used to antagonise a haemorrhage developing during thrombolytic therapy.

Ancrod (Arvin) is a purified fraction of the venom of the Malayan pit viper. When injected in man, ancrod clots fibrinogen producing intravascular microclots which are subsequently removed by the fibrinolytic mechanism. Ancrod thus produces hypofibrinogenaemia and is claimed to have beneficial effects in thrombotic conditions. This type of action has been referred to as 'therapeutic defibrination'.

Anticoagulants
The coagulation of blood can be inhibited by a variety of substances, many of which though effective *in vitro* are too toxic for use in the general circulation.

Drugs used in vitro
Oxalic acid forms an insoluble calcium salt and 0.1 per cent of oxalate will prevent the coagulation of blood *in vitro* but is too toxic for use in blood transfusion.

Sodium citrate. A 0.4 per cent sodium citrate solution in blood will also prevent coagulation by forming an undissociated calcium citrate complex. Large doses of sodium citrate depress the heart, but the injection of up to 3 pints of citrated blood is safe.

Disodium edetate is a powerful chelating agent which inhibits blood coagulation when present in a concentration of 0.02 per cent by forming an undissociated complex with calcium.

Drugs used in vivo
Drugs which delay blood coagulation are used in the prevention and treatment of intravascular clotting either to reduce the incidence of thrombosis or the extension of a thrombus once it is formed. Two kinds of drugs are used in anticoagulant therapy of which *heparin* and *dicoumarol* are the prototypes. Heparin produces its anticoagulant effect immediately and prevents clotting when added to shed blood or when injected intravenously. By contrast, the coumarins do not prevent clotting when added to shed blood nor do they produce an immediate effect when injected intravenously. Their anticoagulant effect depends on interference with the production of clotting factors in the liver and becomes apparent only after a latent period. The coumarin drugs are usually administerd by mouth.

These two drugs also differ in their action on the clotting mechanism. Heparin lengthens the clotting time by inhibiting thrombin, but it also inhibits earlier stages of the clotting mechanism. The coumarin drugs have no direct effect on the clotting mechanism. They are believed to act by some antagonistic effect on the action of vitamin K in the liver, whereby the production of vitamin K-dependent clotting factors declines.

Heparin

The anticoagulant properties of a fraction prepared from liver were first observed by McLean, a second-year medical student working with Howell at Johns Hopkins University. This substance was later named heparin because, though it occurs in many other tissues, it is most abundant in the liver.

Structure and action. Heparin is a muco-polysaccharide containing several sulphuric acid residues. Heparin from the same species may vary in chain length giving a molecular weight in the range of 12 000 to 25 000. The molecule has a helical structure with the sulphate groups towards the periphery favouring electrostatic interactions with proteins arising from its strong electronegative charge and acidic properties. The interaction of heparin with proteins can be readily prevented by neutralising its electronegative charge with a basic substance such as protamine.

Heparin is contained in mast cells where it is combined with basic substances such as histamine and 5-hydroxytryptamine; it exhibits metachromatic staining giving an intense blue violet colour with the basic dye toluidine blue. Heparin is released alongside with histamine from dog liver during anaphylactic shock, rendering the blood uncoagulable. It has been suggested that the common distribution of mast cells along capillaries may indicate a local function of heparin in preventing capillary thrombosis, though heparin is seldom found in normal blood.

The mechanism of the inhibition of blood coagulation by heparin is complex. One effect is that it acts as an antiprothrombin since, when heparin is added to whole blood, prothrombin conversion to thrombin is prevented. A second action is that it inhibits the thrombin-fibrinogen reaction (Fig. 14.4) by interacting with thrombin. This action of heparin requires the presence of certain plasma components one of which is antithrombin III (heparin cofactor). A third action of heparin is that it inhibits factor Xa by promoting its destruction. The latter effect appears to be of great importance in the application of low-dose heparin. An unrelated property of heparin is its lipotropic action. The intravenous administration of heparin clears the plasma of chylomicra by activating a plasma lipase.

Administration of heparin in man. Heparin may be administered intravenously or subcutaneously. It is not given by intramuscular injection because of the liability to haematoma formation. Heparin is not absorbed from the intestine and does not cross the placenta so that it can be administered to a mother without endangering the foetus. Two aspects of heparin therapy have to be considered: conventional and low-dose heparin.

The object of *conventional heparin therapy* is to achieve adequate anticoagulation without haemorrhage. Heparin is usually given intravenously either by continuous infusion or by injections into an indwelling needle every 4–6 hours. Since the half-life of heparin in the blood is 1–2 hours, the best blood levels are achieved by continuous infusion preferably by a constant infusion pump. No assay exists for the chemical measurement of heparin levels. Its concentration must be measured biologically, the technically simplest test being the whole blood clotting time. Alternatively neutralisation and titration by an antagonist such as protamine may be used. When injected intravenously, heparin has a rapid but transient effect on the clotting of the blood, the effect and duration of effect depending on the dose. The peak effect occurs in about 10 minutes. About 25 per cent of a dose of heparin is excreted by the kidneys in an active form and the remainder is depolymerised and excreted in an inactive form.

Heparin is a valuable agent used in such conditions as deep vein thrombosis and after acute arterial occlusion. Heparin is used for about two days while a loading dose of oral anticoagulant is begun. It is the anticoagulant of choice for the maintenance of extracorporeal circulation. Heparin is often used in the treatment of pulmonary embolism but evidence of heparin's effectiveness in the treatment (as distinct from prophylaxis) of pulmonary embolism is dubious.

Prophylactic use of low-dose heparin. This is a recent development in the prophylaxis of venous thrombosis and pulmonary embolism. Low-dose heparin is given by subcutaneous injection usually into the anterior abdominal wall. It is thought that the action of low-dose heparin is mainly due to inhibition of factor Xa. Several successful trials with prophylactic low-dose heparin have been described of which the following is an example. In a multicentre trial involving more than 4000 surgical patients, 5000 units of heparin were administered thrice daily starting 2 hours before surgery and continuing for 7 days. Fatal pulmonary embolism was significantly reduced (16 in control group, 2 in treatment group). There was a significant reduction in venous thrombosis after treatment as shown by ^{125}I-fibrinogen leg scans. Haemorrhagic complications are infrequent with low-dose heparin.

Protamine sulphate antagonises the anticoagulant and haemorrhagic effects of heparin. It must be given by slow intravenous injection.

Oral anticoagulants

The discovery of the coumarin drugs arose from the observation of Schofield in 1922 that cattle developed a curious haemorrhagic disease after eating spoiled sweet clover hay. The haemorrhagic effect could be counteracted in rabbits by adding alfalfa, a rich source of vitamin K, to the diet. The isolation and identification of the haemorrhagic factor, dicoumarol, was established in 1941 by Link and his colleagues.

In the same year dicoumarol (Fig. 14.5) was introduced for the treatment of thromboembolic diseases. A number of related compounds were subsequently shown to have anticoagulant activity.

Action of oral anticoagulants

The coumarin-type anticoagulants have the common pharmacological action of inhibiting the blood clotting mechanism by interfering with the synthesis of the vitamin K-dependent clotting factors II, VII, IX and X in the liver. The mechanism of action of these drugs may be by interference with the action of vitamin K in the cytochrome oxidase system of the liver. After the administration of a coumarin anticoagulant all four vitamin K dependent clotting factors begin to decline in the plasma at rates corresponding to their biological half-lives. Factor VII has the shortest half-life and is the first to decline but after a week of continuous therapy factors II, VII, IX and X have all declined.

When applying the coumarin drugs clinically it is necessary to keep their activity level under laboratory control so as to achieve adequate anticoagulation without producing undesirable haemorrhage. The best established and most widely adopted control method is the measurement of 'prothrombin' time by Quick's one-stage method. The test consists of mixing equal volumes of citrated or oxalated plasma, tissue extract (usually brain extract) as the thromboplastin source and finally calcium chloride and recording the clotting time. In this test, clotting depends on the extrinsic pathway and therefore on the presence of factors VII, V, X, thrombin and fibrinogen whilst the intrinsic clotting factors XII, XI, IX and VIII are bypassed (Fig. 14.4). The test is thus not strictly a prothrombin test, it measures all the vitamin K-dependent clotting factors with the exception of factor IX. The result of the Quick test is expressed in terms of the clotting-time ratio, derived by dividing the clotting time obtained with the patients plasma by that obtained with normal plasma. Usually a ratio of 2–2.5 is aimed at after oral anticoagulant treatment. A considerable difficulty has been to produce a calibrated thromboplastin reference preparation for the prothrombin test.

Dicoumarol (Bishydroxycoumarin)

The structure of this compound is shown in Figure 14.5. Dicoumarol is slowly absorbed from the gastrointestinal tract and thereafter slowly metabolised. The anticoagulant effect of the drug is not directly related to its blood concentration since after oral administration the maximum increase in clotting time occurs one to two days after the peak level of drug in the plasma. Dicoumarol is strongly bound to plasma proteins and this may explain its slow rate of action and degradation.

The structural resemblance of dicoumarol to vitamin K has led to the suggestion that dicoumarol competes with vitamin K and displaces it from an enzyme system which is required in the synthesis of prothrombin and other

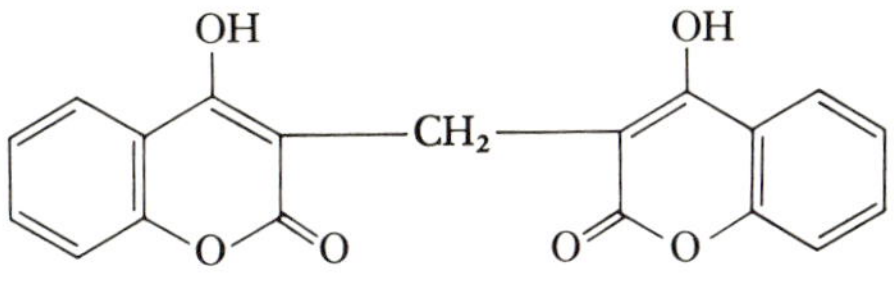

Dicoumarol

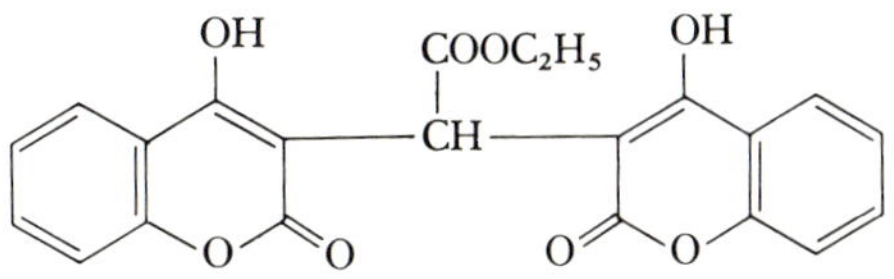

Ethyl biscoumacetate

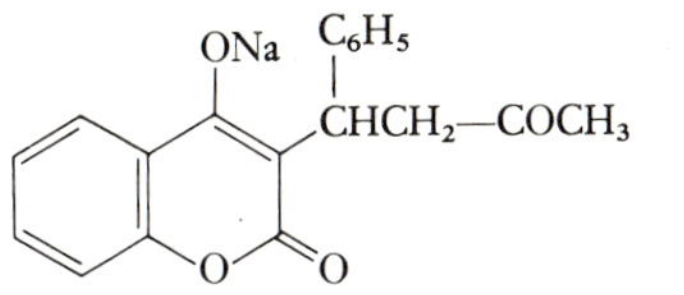

Warfarin sodium

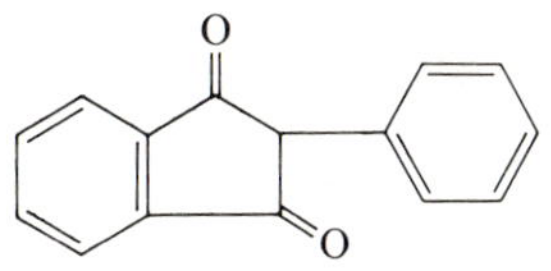

Phenindione

Fig. 14.5 Structural formulae of coumarin anticoagulants.

vitamin-K dependent coagulation factors by the liver. After the administration of a dose of dicoumarol the concentration of factor VII and prothrombin in the plasma declines progressively in the course of two days and, as shown in Figure 14.6, gradually returns to normal in about eight days.

Excessive doses of dicoumarol result in haemorrhage and severe anaemia. Haematuria is one of the commonest forms of bleeding, but this should not occur if control of dosage is gauged by daily estimation of the prothrombin time.

The effects of overdosage with the coumarin drugs can be counteracted by the administration of vitamin K_1 (phytomenadione) (p. 365). This may be given by mouth or intravenously by slow injection.

Dicoumarol has now been largely displaced by other drugs, their choice depending on such factors as rapidity of onset of action, duration of action, ease of control and toxicity.

Warfarin sodium

This is a drug (Fig. 14.5) of intermediate duration of action. After an initial oral dose of 40–50 mg a therapeutic effect may be reached after 36 hours. After prolonged therapy is stopped it takes about three days before the prothrombin time returns to normal. The drug has a

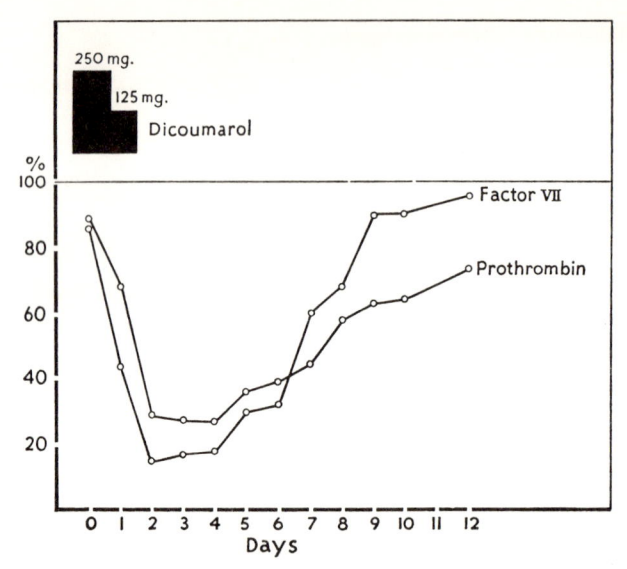

Fig. 14.6 The effect of dicoumarol on the concentration of prothrombin and factor VII in plasma. (After Wright, 1952, in *Blood Clotting and Allied Problems*. Josiah Macy Jr. Foundation, New York.)

cumulative action and after the initial loading a maintenance dose of 5–10 mg may be used and adjusted according to the results of the 'prothrombin' test.

Warfarin sodium is water soluble and can therefore be administered by intravenous injection in patients who do not tolerate oral administration, but the onset of action by this route is no quicker than by oral administration. Warfarin is relatively non-toxic, although rashes occasionally occur.

Phenprocoumon (Marcoumar) has a relatively slow onset of action and produces marked cumulation; hence haemorrhagic manifestations are difficult to control.

Phenindione (Dindevan)
This differs chemically from the coumarin drugs (Fig. 14.5). It is used as an anticoagulant because of the rapid onset and short duration of its action.

Allergic reactions are relatively frequent with this drug including in rare cases severe reactions such as exfoliative dermatitis, kidney and liver damage.

Therapeutic uses of oral anticoagulants
The administration of these drugs should not be attempted unless facilities are available for frequent estimations of the prothrombin time. The aim of treatment is to increase the plasma prothrombin time as measured by the one-stage Quick method to two and a half times the normal value.

It is important that the anticoagulant effects of the coumarin drugs should be checked by laboratory tests since their absorption from the alimentary tract is irregular. Moreover the effects of these drugs are influenced by changes in diet which may affect absorption and by concurrent use of other drugs. For example the effect of anticoagulants is potentiated by salicylates which themselves have an anticoagulant action and by antibiotics which reduce the bacterial production of vitamin K in the intestine.

Drugs which have a higher affinity for plasma proteins than warfarin, for example phenylbutazone and clofibrate, may displace it from its protein binding sites and increase the free concentration of warfarin in plasma and hence increase its anticoagulant effect. Conversely concurrent therapy with sedative and hypnotic drugs such as barbiturates, increases the rate of metabolism of coumarin type drugs by enzyme induction and a higher dose of anticoagulant is necessary to maintain effective control. When the sedative drug is withdrawn, the dose of anticoagulant must be rapidly reduced to avoid dangerous bleeding.

Therapeutic value of anticoagulants and fibrinolytic therapy
There are two main types of thrombosis, venous and arterial. Venous thrombi consist largely of fibrin, whereas arterial thrombi are composed mainly of platelets interspersed with fibrin, red cells and white cells. Although the oral anticoagulants are useful in both types of thrombosis they are generally most useful in prevention of venous thrombosis as they are able to diminish thrombin generation and the subsequent formation of fibrin. Anticoagulants are used solely to prevent the formation of new thrombi or growth of existing thrombi. They do not contribute directly to the lysis or dissolution of an existing thrombus. They may be started after a thrombotic or embolic episode has taken place or alternatively they are given to patients known to be at high risk for thrombotic

complications. It must be appreciated that the use of anticoagulant drugs involves risks to the patient which must be balanced against their benefits. Whilst haematuria and melaena are the commonest complications of treatment, serious and sometimes fatal bleeding may occur in the brain, pericardium, stomach and intestine.

The short-term use of anticoagulants is well established in the treatment of peripheral deep venous thrombosis, in retinal vascular thrombosis and in pulmonary embolism. In deep leg-vein thrombosis treatment may be begun with heparin for the first few days until oral anticoagulants are started. Similarly in pulmonary embolism the patient may be anticoagulated with heparin for the first few days, and then changed over to oral anticoagulants. In acute myocardial infaction anticoagulant therapy has been shown to reduce mortality and decrease the incidence of thromoembolic complications during the first three or four weeks. Opinion is divided about the value of long-term treatment in preventing recurrent infarctions but there is evidence that prolonged therapy is of benefit at least in male patients under the age of 55 years.

The coumarin drugs should not be given to patients with severe liver or kidney disease and they should not be used in pregnancy since they produce severe and fatal haemorrhage of the foetus. In general, anticoagulant drugs should not be used where there is evidence of bleeding from skin or mucous membranes, as in severe anaemia or purpura, in subacute bacterial endocarditis or peptic ulceration.

The object of *fibrinolytic therapy* is to greatly accerate the fibrinolytic process and thus reopen the blood vessels after their occlusion, before necrosis sets in. This approach is fundamentally different from the anticoagulant therapy of thrombosis in which, at best, further clot formation is prevented. Although fibrinolytic treatment has proved effective in lysing clots in human forearm veins, this method of therapy is still in the experimental stage. It holds promise, however, for the future treatment of such conditions as deep vein thrombosis, pulmonary embolism and myocardial infarction.

The control of local haemorrhage

It is frequently necessary to hasten coagulation in order to limit the loss of blood from wounds or during operations.

Physical methods for controlling haemorrhage at the site of bleeding consist in the application of pressure, cold or heat coagulation. An important factor in promoting clotting is the provision of a large surface area of foreign material at the site of haemorrhage, to stimulate fibrin formation and increase the solidity of the clot. This is the basis for the application of cotton wool or gauze to a bleeding surface. The threads of the cotton wool become enmeshed in the new-formed fibrin and thus form an effective haemostatic plug. A disadvantage of these dressings is that they must eventually be removed and this entails fresh tissue damage and a risk of recurrent haemorrhage.

Oxidised cellulose and gelatin sponge can be applied as dressings which are absorbed from the site of application.

Human fibrin foam is a dry artificial sponge-like material which when wetted becomes compressible and can be moulded to the bleeding surface. It is rapidly absorbed by the normal processes of fibrinolysis.

Various drugs can be used to control local haemorrhage. They act (1) by producing vasoconstriction; (2) by precipitating protein at the site of bleeding, and (3) by promoting the natural processes of blood coagulation.

Vasoconstrictor drugs

The use of vasoconstrictor drugs such as adrenaline or noradrenaline is only possible where there is access to the site of bleeding, and cotton wool swabs dipped in a solution of these drugs are often effective in controlling oozing of blood from capillaries.

Astringent drugs

These substances are used to precipitate the blood proteins at the site of bleeding. Ferric chloride, alum or tannic acid are chiefly used, but they are only suitable for controlling capillary oozing and are less effective than the vasoconstrictor drugs.

Coagulant drugs

These may be divided into two groups: (1) substances which promote the transformation of prothrombin into thrombin and (2) substances which clot fibrinogen directly.

A number of snake venoms have thromboplastin activity and cause intravascular clotting.

Russell's viper venom is a very effective local haemostatic and can be used to control prolonged bleeding from a tooth socket in patients with haemophilia. The venom is only stable when dry, and a freshly prepared solution (1 in 10 000) is applied on cotton wool or gauze.

Substances which clot fibrinogen. Preparations of thrombin can be prepared from bovine or human plasma and are applied locally to arrest capillary bleeding. Thrombin can be applied in solution as a spray on in combination with fibrin foam. It must not be injected intravenously since it causes immediate intravascular clotting and embolism.

Persistent haemorrhage can often be arrested by a transfusion of fresh whole blood, which not only contains all the factors required for coagulation, but has the additional advantage of supplying extra fluid.

PREPARATIONS

Iron
Chelating agent
Desferrioxamine mesylate (Desferal) 2 g i.m. 5 g p.o.
Oral iron preparations
Ferric ammonium citrate, up to 6 g daily
Ferrous fumarate, proph 200 mg daily, ther 400–600 mg daily
Ferrous gluconate, 600 mg daily
Ferrous succinate, proph 200 mg daily, ther 400–600 mg daily
Ferrous sulphate, proph 300 mg daily, ther 600–900 mg daily
Iron injections
Iron dextran injection (Imferon) 1–2 ml deep i.m.
Iron sorbitol injection (Jectofer) 1–2 ml (equiv 50–100 mg Fe) deep i.m.

Cobalamins
Cyanocobalamin Injection (Cytamen) 250 μg — 1 mg
Hydroxocobalamin Injection (Neocytamen) 1 mg i.m. 5x, intervals 2–3 days; for maintenance: 1 mg every 2 months

Megaloplastic anaemia
Folic acid 5–20 mg

Platelet aggregation inhibition
Dipyridamole (Persantin) 100 mg 3–4x daily
Sulphinpyrazone (Anturan) up to 800 mg daily

Anticoagulants
Injectable
Heparin 5000–15000 units i.v. or i.m.
Heparin antagonist: Protamine sulphate

Oral
Nicoumalone 2–16 mg daily
Phenindione 300 mg initially; then 50–150 mg daily
Warfarin 15–30 mg initial, then 2–15 mg daily

Vitamin K and analogues
Menadiol sodium diphosphate (Synkavit) 10 mg 1–4x daily
Phytomenadione (Konakion) 5–20 mg p.o., i.m., i.v.

Agents affecting blood clotting and fibrinolysis
Ancrod (from Malayan pit viper): defibrinating agent
Aminocaproic acid: antifibrinolytic agent
Human antihaemophilic protein, Factor VIII (Hemophil)
Oxidised cellulose (Oxycel)
Streptokinase-Streptodornase: fibrinolytic agent
Thromboplastin: initiates conversion of prothrombin to thrombin
Tranexamic acid: antifibrinolytic agent

FURTHER READING

Biggs Rosemary (ed) 1976 Human blood coagulation, haemostasis and thrombosis. Blackwell, Oxford
Biggs R (ed) 1977 The treatment of haemophilia A and B and von Willebrand's disease.
Fletcher J, Huehns E R 1974 Transferrin. In: Advanced haematology. Butterworths, London
Houghie C, Moser K M 1974 Modern concepts of fibrinolysis. In: Advanced haematology. Butterworths, London
Kritchevsky D (ed) 1975 Hypolipidemic agents. Handb. exp. Pharm: 41. Springer, Berlin
Markwardt F (ed) 1978 Fibrinolytics and antifibrinolytics. Handb. exp. Pharm: 46. Springer, Berlin

15. The uterus

Movements of the uterus 217; Innervation of the uterus and drug action 218; Role of neurosecretion 218; Oxytocin 220; Ergot 220; Prostaglandins 222; Use of drugs in labour 222; Analgesia in labour 223; Teratogenic effects of drugs 225.

The physiology of the uterus varies widely in different species, so also does the response of the uterus to drugs. Another general characteristic of the uterus is that its activities show cyclical changes; they are different in dioestrus and oestrus, furthermore profound changes occur during pregnancy. For example, the weight of the human uterus increases during the first pregnancy from about 50 g to 1000 g and its capacity increases from about 5 ml to 5000 ml, whilst the individual muscle fibres increase about 10-fold in length. These changes during pregnancy are accompanied by alterations in the response of the uterus to drugs. After delivery the uterus involutes rapidly, but it does not regain the original virgin size.

Movements of the uterus

The movements of the human uterus can be registered in three ways: (1) by inserting a balloon into the cavity of the uterus and recording the changes in intrauterine pressure when the muscle contracts; (2) by recording externally changes in the shape and consistency of the pregnant uterus which are transmitted to a sensitive recording instrument (tocograph) strapped to the abdomen; (3) by registering the movements of isolated muscle strips of uterus removed during operation. Uterine movements may also be visualised with X-rays after filling the cavity with lipiodol.

The uterus, both *in situ* and when excised, contracts rhythmically. The uterine movements are myogenic in origin, and are not abolished by section of the uterine nerves, and there is no evidence that movements of the uterus are correlated by any local nervous plexus, such as occurs in the gut. The frequency and force of the uterine contractions vary greatly in different conditions of the sex cycle. This variation is due to the complex hormonal control to which the uterus is subject. The hormonal pattern during the menstrual cycle is that in the proliferative phase mainly oestrogen is produced, in the secretory phase oestrogen and increasing amounts of progesterone until, some days before menstruation the production of both hormones decreases. In women the non-pregnant uterus, under the influence of oestrogen alone, shows feeble spontaneous contractions. About midcycle, under the influence of oestrogen and progesterone, these are replaced by larger and more prolonged contractions and the withdrawal of both hormones during menstruation produces powerful co-ordinated contractions resembling those occurring in the pregnant uterus during parturition (Fig. 15.1).

Uterine contractions are depressed during early pregnancy but increase in force towards the end of pregnancy and become fully co-ordinated during parturition.

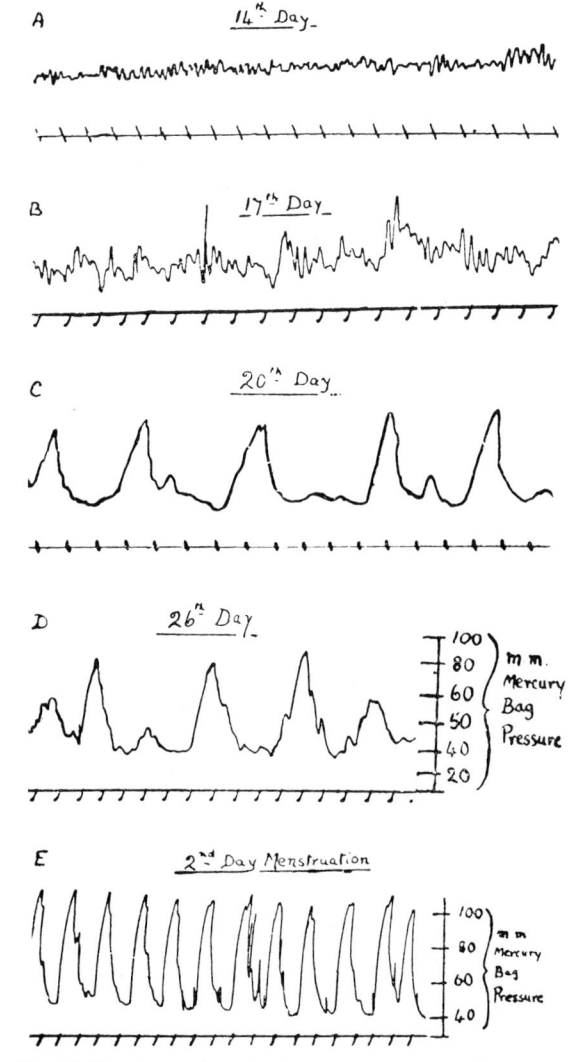

Fig. 15.1 Uterine tracings obtained at various stages of the menstrual cycle (different women). Time marked in minutes. (From Chassar Moir, 1944. *J. Obstet. Gynaec.*)

Co-ordinated uterine contractions originate in the fundus. Myometrial cells in this region act as pacemakers from which conducted action potentials arise. The resulting contraction waves may take 10–20 seconds to travel from fundus to cervix. The electrophysiological parameters of the myometrial cell are dependent on sex hormones. Treatment with oestrogen increases the membrane potential and this can be further raised by treatment with a progestogen. Very high membrane potentials inhibit the electrical activity of the uterus. There is evidence that the local action of endogenous progesterone at the site of placental implantation is responsible for inducing a state of electrical and mechanical quiescence and relative inexcitability in the human myometrium during pregnancy.

Innervation of the uterus and drug action

The uterus receives both excitatory and inhibitory nerves from the sympathetic. The sympathetic outflow to the uterus comes from the second, third and fourth lumbar roots, and passes through the inferior mesenteric ganglion and the hypogastric nerves to the uterus. Nerve fibres also pass to the uterus from the sacral outflow. They would theoretically be expected to stimulate the uterus by their cholinergic action, but there is no clear evidence that these fibres have any motor function in the human uterus.

Stimulation of the sympathetic nerves, therefore, produces a mixed excitatory and inhibitory effect on the uterus, and the relative power of the two sets of fibres varies in different species, and also differs in the same species according to the hormonal state of the uterus. It is an old observation that electircal stimulation of the hypogastric (sympathetic) nerve causes relaxation of the uterus in the virgin cat and contraction in the pregnant cat. This reversal is due to hormonal influences as shown in Figure 15.2; a previous administration of oestrone in an ovariectomised cat causes relaxation of the uterus by adrenaline whilst injection of oestrone plus progesterone causes adrenaline contraction.

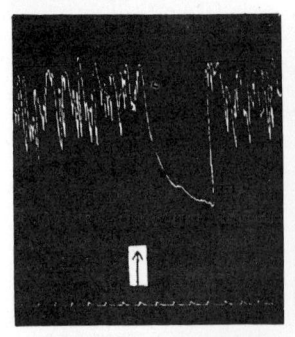

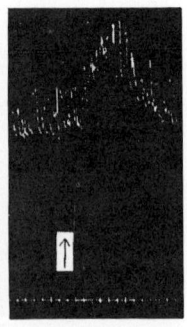

Fig. 15.2 Action of drugs on the movements of the cat uterus *in situ*. (1) The effect of adrenaline in the spayed cat treated with oestrone. (2) The reversal of this effect of adrenaline in the spayed cat treated with oestrone and progesterone. Time interval one minute. (After Robson & Schild, 1938. *J. Physiol.*)

Adrenaline administered systemically inhibits the uterus in pregnant as well as nonpregnant women by virtue of its ß-adrenergic activity. Immediately after the end of an adrenaline infusion there is a rebound increase of uterine activity and tonus which makes adrenaline unsuitable to depress uterine activity clinically in pregnancy.

Noradrenaline stimulates the uterus in both pregnant and nonpregnant women by virtue of its α-adrenergic activity. An intravenous infusion of 2–10 μg/min noradrenaline causes an immediate rise in tonus, amplitude and frequency of myometrial contractions. The contractions are incoordinated and noradrenaline therefore cannot be used clinically to stimulate the uterus in labour.

Isoxsuprine was the first ß-adrenergic drug used clinically in obstetrics. It relaxes the uterus and inhibits spontaneous or oxytocin-induced contractions of the pregnant uterus. It has had limited application in obstetrics. Similar effects are produced by other ß-adrenergic agonists especially those acting preferentially on β_2 receptors, such as salbutamol.

Neither the α-blocker phentolamine nor the ß-blocker propranolol affect the movements of the human uterus. Thus, although the myometrium contains both stimulatory α-receptors and inhibitory ß-receptors, the drugs acting on adrenergic receptors have relatively little application in clinical obstetrics.

Because of the wide species variations in the drug responses of the uterus and the wholly atypical effects obtained with isolated human uterine strips, it is generally agreed that oxytocic drugs can only be adequately assessed by testing their effects on the intact human uterus. An example of the effect of ergometrine on the intact human uterus as assessed by postpartum tocography, is shown in Figure 3.4.

Role of neurosecretion in uterine activity (p. 328)
An important central mechanism for activating the uterus is through the release of oxytocin. The work of Bargman and Scharrer has shown that the neurohypohyseal hormones are synthesised in the hypothalamus and then transported along the hypothalamo-hypophyseal tract to the neurohypophysis for storage and release.

Earlier evidence that oxytocin is synthesised in the paraventricular nucleus and vasopressin in the supraoptic nucleus of the hypothalamus is now doubted; it seems likely that both nuclei can synthesise both hormones. The hormones are bound to neurohypophysin, a cystine-rich carrier protein.

The hypothalamic nuclei can be reflexly activated by certain peripheral stimuli which cause a release of oxytocin; a powerful stimulus for oxytocin release is suckling as shown in Figure 15.3. Other peripheral stimuli such as cervical dilatation may also cause oxytocin release.

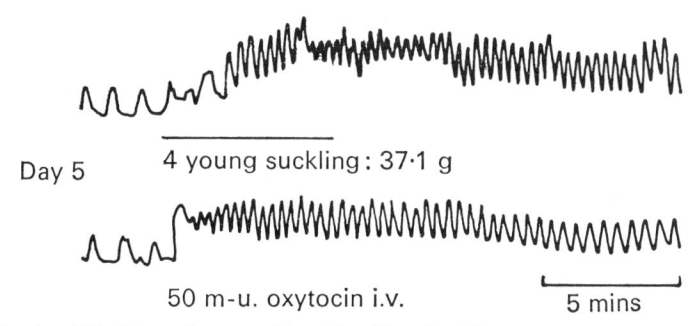

Fig. 15.3 Uterine contractions in rabbits 5 days after parturition. The effect of suckling compared to that of an intravenous injection of oxytocin. The effect of suckling is believed to be due to oxytocin release. After Fuchs, 1966. In Pickles & Fitzpatrick, eds, *Endogenous Substances Affecting the Myometrium*. Cambridge University Press.)

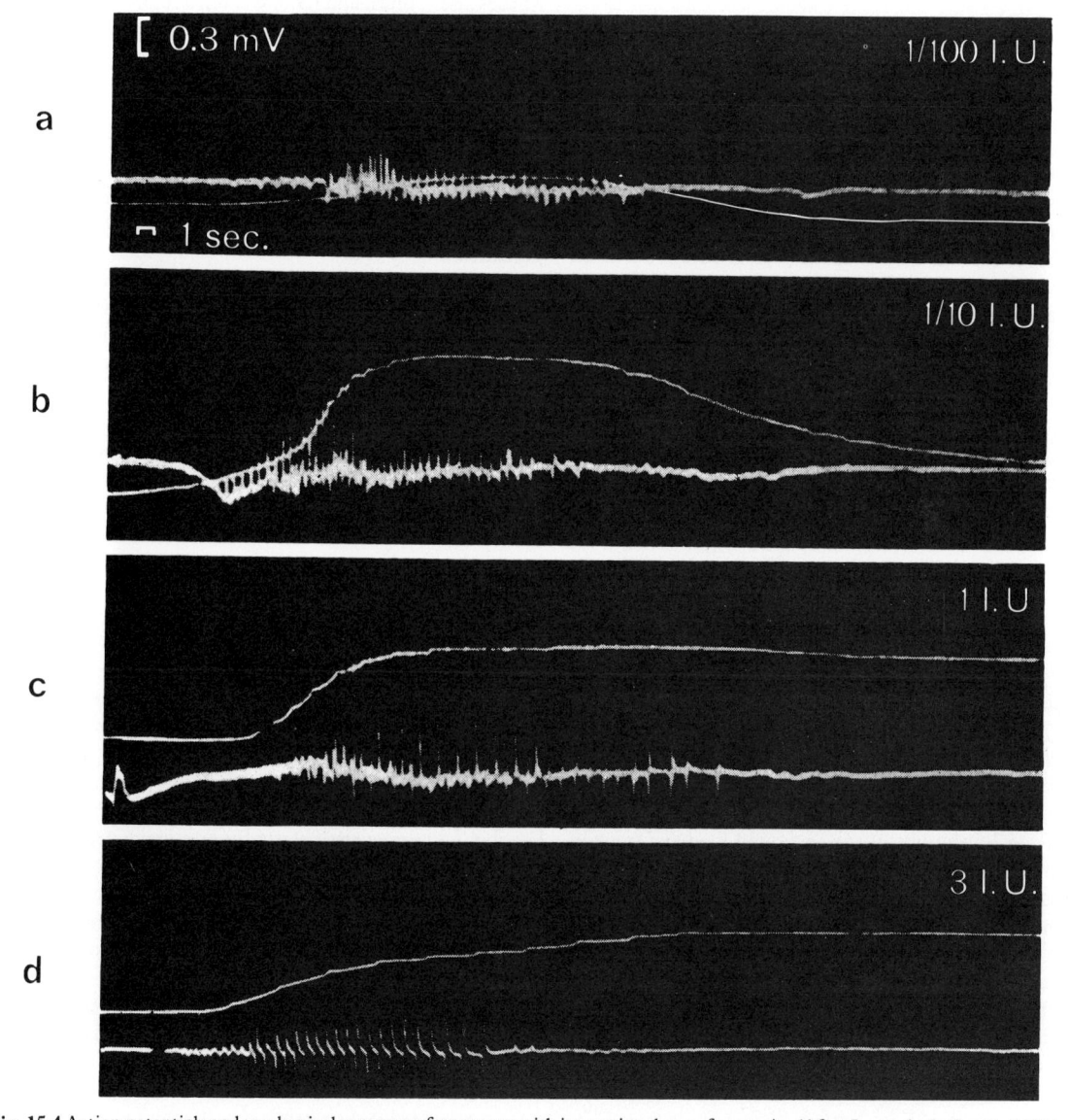

Fig. 15.4 Action potentials and mechanical response of rat uterus with increasing doses of oxytocin. (After Jung, *Arch. Gynäk.* 1957.)

It is uncertain whether oxytocin plays a physiological role in initiating parturition, although the uterus undoubtedly becomes highly sensitive to oxytocin at the time of parturition and the contractions induced by oxytocin infusion at term are closely similar to normal myometrial contractions during labour.

Clinical uses of oxytocic drugs

Three drugs which stimulate the pregnant uterus are of chief clinical importance; oxytocin, prostaglandin and ergometrine.

Posterior pituitary hormones

Dale (1906) found that an extract of the posterior lobe of the pituitary gland had a remarkable effect in stimulating the isolated uterus of animals, and Blair Bell (1909) showed that the extract had a similar effect on the human uterus during labour. It was hoped at first that because the extract was derived from 'natural' sources it would also be 'physiological' in action and free from danger. But reports of uterine rupture following the administration of pituitary extract soon made it obvious that careful dosage was necessary and hence, some form of biological standardisation was essential. Biological assay, based on the response of the guinea-pig uterus showed that the strength of some of the early preparations varied as much as 80-fold.

Later, Kamm separated two fractions from posterior piruitary gland, one of which acts mainly on the uterus (*oxytocin, pitocin*) whilst the other has mainly antidiuretic and vasoconstrictor effects (*vasopressin, pitressin*). Vasopressin was formerly believed to have no action on uterine muscle because it failed to contract the isolated uterus of the guinea-pig. It is now known that vasopressin is by no means without action on the uterus and that its effect depends on the species and the state of the uterus whilst oxytocin also has definite antidiuretic activity if given in a large dose.

The non-pregnant human uterus and the uterus in early pregnancy is more sensitive to vasopressin than to oxytocin. The human uterus becomes more sensitive to oxytocin in the course of pregnancy and at term it is more sensitive to oxytocin than to vasopressin.

Extracts of posterior pituitary gland have been superseded by the use of the separated oxytocic fraction (oxytocin) or its synthetic equivalent (syntocinon) which are less likely to produce pituitary shock. This alarming reaction to the injection of posterior pituitary extract was characterised by a sudden generalised vasoconstriction denoted by an ashy grey appearance of the patient and attributable to the vasopressin content of the extract.

Oxytocin is a polypeptide which can be extracted from the posterior pituitary gland and the hypothalamus and which can also be prepared synthetically. Its chemical structure is outlined in Figure 25.3. Oxytocin can be considered a nonapeptide in which two half-cystine residues constitute together one cystine residue. If the S-S bond of cystine is reduced, the biological activity of oxytocin is completely lost. The serum of pregnant women contains an enzyme, oxytocinase, which destroys oxytocin.

Oxytocin contracts the mammalian uterus. Figure 15.4 shows in a rat uterus that the mechanical responses elicited by oxytocin are accompanied by serial action potentials. In the human uterus at term oxytocin promotes regular co-ordinated contractions proceeding from fundus to cervix which result in steady dilatation of the later; the myometrial contractions are attended by conducted action potentials. The frequency and amplitude of contractions during an intravenous oxytocin infusion is related to dose. At the onset of infusion there is often a slight rise in uterine tonus but this generally subsides and the uterus then relaxes completely between contractions. An overdose of oxytocin leads to excessively frequent contractions with incomplete relaxation between contractions. Very high doses produce tetanic contractions leading to diminished placental blood flow and foetal distress or death. The sensitivity of the uterus to oxytocin increases in the course of pregnancy and becomes maximal near the time of parturition.

Just before the onset of labour a rapid increase occurs in the sensitivity of the uterus to oxytocin and the minimum intravenous dose required to induce a contraction has been used as an index of the nearness of the onset of labour (Smyth's oxytocin-sensitivity test).

Oxytocin also causes contraction of the myoepithelial cells of the mammary gland, which leads to expression of milk from the alveoli and ducts of the gland. The process of 'milk letdown' is essential for the complete evacuation of the gland, which cannot be achieved solely by the mechanical process of suckling or milking.

Oxytocin has a vasodilator effect especially in birds. In man rapid intravenous injection of oxytocin causes an immediate transient fall of blood pressure.

When a large dose of oxytocin (> 20 mU/min) is infused intravenously in man it may cause severe water intoxication with convulsions through the antidiuretic action of oxytocin.

Ergot alkaloids

Ergot (*Claviceps purpurea*) is a fungus which grows on rye and on certain grasses. Extracts of ergot contain an amazing variety of substances with potent pharmacological actions. Histamine, acetylcholine, tyramine and ergosterol were all isolated originally from ergot.

Chronic ergot poisoning due to eating bread made from rye infected with ergot was formerly common in Europe. The 'epidemics' of ergotism were of two types. In one type gangrene of the extremities occurred; whilst in the second convulsions were the chief feature. In both types abortions were a standard occurrence.

Many attempts have been made to isolate the active principles of ergot, and in 1906 Barger and Carr and, independently, Kraft, discovered an alkaloid which was named ergotoxine. It is now known that ergotoxine is a mixture of three alkaloids, ergocristine, ergokryptine and ergocornine, with similar actions. Later, in 1920, Stoll described another alkaloid, ergotamine, which he isolated from ergot. None of these compounds, however, produced the therapeutic effects of the crude drug.

In 1935 four different research teams announced the isolation of a new alkaloid. In Britain, Dudley and Moir named their compound ergometrine. In Switzerland ergobasine was isolated by Stoll and Burckhardt, while in America, ergostetrine was described by Thompson, and ergotocine by Kharasch and Legault. It was subsequently shown that these four compounds are identical in chemical structure and pharmacological properties.

The ergot alkaloids are derivatives of lysergic acid and the chemical structure of ergometrine is shown in Figure 15.5. Ergometrine is soluble in water, while ergotoxine and ergotamine are relatively insoluble in water but soluble in alcohol. Ergometrine is therefore present in aqueous extracts of ergot.

Ergometrine. This alkaloid has a selective action on the uterus. It has little effect on the isolated uterus but produces a rapid stimulant action on the human postpartum uterus *in siut*. If the uterus is contracting normally,

Fig. 15.5 Chemical structures of lysergic acid and ergometrine.

ergometrine produces little effect, but on the quiescent uterus it initiates a long persistent rhythm of powerful contractions (Fig. 15.6). The mechanism of action of ergometrine is not known. It may, like the related drug ergotamine, (p. 127) stimulate α-adrenoceptors or 5-HT receptors of the uterus. The action is rapid in onset and occurs within half to one minute if the drug is given intravenously and two to four minutes after intramuscular injection. When administered by mouth ergometrine is rapidly absorbed and produces contraction of the uterus in four to eight minutes, the effect lasting for three to six hours. The usual dose of ergometrine for parenteral administration is 0.1 to 0.5 mg. Ergometrine occasionally

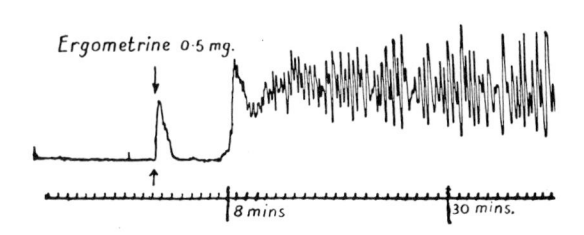

Fig. 15.6 Contractions of the human uterus at the end of the first week of puerperium recorded by intra-uterine balloon.
Ergometrine 0.5 mg by mouth gave a series of rapid uterine contractions after eight minutes. (After Chassar Moir, 1935. *Proc. Roy. Soc. Med.*)

produces vomiting. A more serious, if rare, side effect is a rise of blood pressure which may last several hours.

Methylergometrine has an action similar to ergometrine but is slightly less active weight for weight (Fig. 3.4b).

Prostaglandins
Prostaglandins (p. 91) stimulate both the non-pregnant and the pregnant human uterus *in vivo*. In the pregnant uterus they produce a series of co-ordinated contractions accompanied by relaxation of the cervix; the latter effect may be due to a direct relaxant action of prostaglandin on cervical smooth muscle. The action of prostaglandin on the uterus differs from that of oxytocin. In the uterus at term the two drugs produce similar co-ordinated contractions although prostaglandins have a greater tendency to increase uterine tone. In early and middle pregnancy prostaglandins are capable of developing co-ordinated uterine activity to the point where the uterus expels its contents whilst oxytocin generally cannot produce expulsion at this early stage.

The prostaglandins chiefly used in obstetrics are PGE_2 and $PGF_2\alpha$ or synthetic compounds such as dinoprostone, (prostin E_2) or dinoprost trometamol (prostin $F_2\alpha$). They may be administered intravenously or preferably by the intrauterine extra amniotic route by which they are better tolerated. Prostaglandins are sometimes used in the second trimester of pregnancy for therapeutic abortion and for evacuating the uterus in cases of missed abortion or hydatidiform mole; but they may fail to produce a complete abortion necessitating surgical evacuation of the uterus. During the first trimester surgical methods are altogether quicker and more effective.

Prostaglandins have also been employed for the induction of labour at term by slow intravenous infusion, sometimes in combination with oxytocin. A drawback or prostaglandins is that they may cause nausea and vomiting or diarrhoea. They also often cause erythema along the infusion site. Systemic side effects are particularly prominent when prostaglandins are administered by intravaginal pessary in an attempt to produce abortion.

The clinical course of labour

There are three well-defined stages in the process of normal labour (Fig. 15.7).

The first stage — from the onset of labour pains till complete dilatation of the cervix. The contractions of the uterine muscle occur every 15 to 30 minutes; during this stage the cervix is gradually dilated and the membranes and presenting part of the fetus descend into the cervix, thereby assisting the dilatation.

The second stage — from the time of complete dilatation of the cervix until the birth of the infant. The uterine contractions gradually increase in force, frequency and duration, and are reinforced by contractions of the muscles of the abdominal wall in the attempts to expel the infant through the birth canal. Usually the head of the infant is born first, then the shoulders and the body together with the remaining amniotic fluid.

The third stage — from the birth of the infant until the complete expulsion of the placenta and membranes. The uterus becomes smaller in size, the placenta is gradually detached from its site on the uterus and this is accompanied by bleeding. The amount of blood lost varies from 300 to 600 ml. The placenta and membranes are expelled spontaneously or by pressure on the uterus.

After the third stage the uterus diminishes further in size and becomes firm and hard and this assists in controlling any further haemorrhage from the uterus.

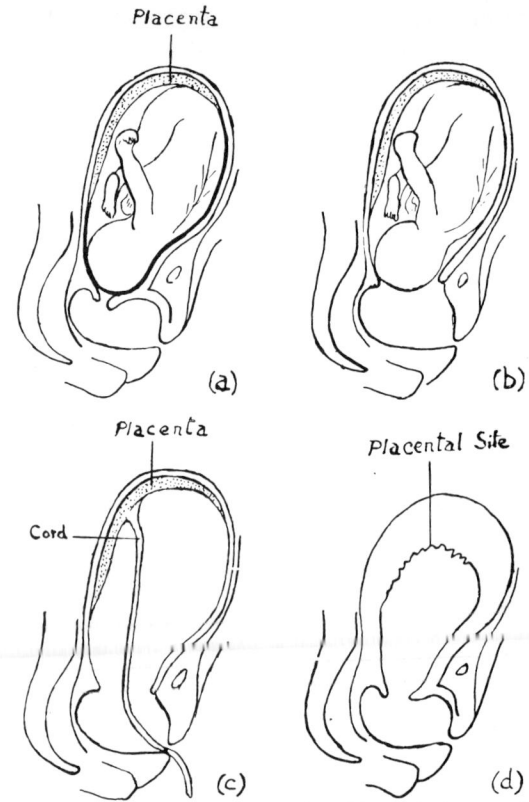

Fig. 15.7 Diagrammatic representation of the clinical course of labour. (a) Beginning of 1st stage; (b) end of 1st stage — full dilatation of the cervix; (c) end of 2nd stage — birth of the fetus; (d) end of 3rd stage — placenta expelled.

Use of drugs in labour

The uterus at full term becomes very sensitive to oxytocin and small doses of this drug are sometimes used to initiate uterine contractions or to reinforce them when the first stage is unduly prolonged. In *uterine inertia* the best method is to administer oxytocin intravenously in a dilute solution containing 2 to 10 units in a litre of 5 per cent dextrose solution. By this method a constant concentration of the drug can be maintained in the blood stream and the rate of infusion can be adjusted according to the uterine response and absence of signs of fetal distress. The injection of larger doses of oxytocin has been shown to give rise to a transient bilirubinaemia in the newborn.

The first essential principle is the use of oxytocin in the first stage of labour is that it must never be used if any mechanical obstruction is present. Stimulating the uterus to contract against an immovable obstacle can produce disastrous effects, amongst which are death of the fetus and rupture of the uterus. Oxytocin should only be used if the following conditions are observed:

1. The uterine contractions are less than average in strength and frequency.
2. There is no mechanical obstruction to easy delivery.
3. The condition of the fetus is good.

The chief use of ergometrine and related drugs is in the prevention and treatment of postpartum haemorrhage. In domiciliary practice by midwives these drugs should not be given till after the delivery of the placenta, since otherwise the placenta may be retained and its manual removal become necessary. In hospital practice it is usual to administer an oxytocic drug in the course of the second stage to expedite the expulsion of the fetus. The drugs most frequently used in the final stages of labour are ergometrine and methylergometrine. These same drugs are also used postpartum with the object to produce firm contractions of the uterus and thus decrease postpartum haemorrhage. They are also used to control haemorrhage associated with abortion. These drugs are very useful when haemorrhage is severe because of their rapid onset and prolonged duration of action. They may be given orally in cases of delayed involution of the uterus.

ANALGESIA IN LABOUR

An obstetric analgesic should give satisfactory relief from pain without interfering with the normal processes of labour and delivery or depressing the infant's respiration. Moreover, it should be easily administered in any environment.

Obstetric analgesia may be achieved by administering analgesic drugs parenterally or by gaseous inhalation analgesia. Alternatively, regional analgesia may be produced by local anaesthetics. General anaesthesia is now rarely used in obstetrics except in some cases when operative delivery is necessary.

Analgesic drugs in obstetrics

An analgesic drug may be required when labour is progressing and painful uterine contractions occur. A first dose is usually given before pain becomes severe and smaller doses may be given to maintain analgesia.

Pethidine (p. 283) is frequently used in labour since it raises the pain threshold without diminishing uterine contractions. It can be given by mouth but more usually 100–150 mg pethidine is administered intramuscularly. Undesirable side effects include vomiting, dizziness and hypotension. Pethidine is transported across the placenta and may cause mild asphyxia in the baby. *Pentazocine* 40 mg has about the same analgesic activity as 100 mg pethidine and is frequently used in childbirth. It does not produce drug dependence. *Morphine* is sometimes employed in childbirth because of its strong analgesic, sedative and euphoriant properties but it frequently causes vomiting in the mother and respiratory depression in the foetus. The use of narcotic antagonists to counteract neonatal asphyxia caused by analgesic drugs is discussed on page 285.

Sedative and tranquillising drugs have no analgesic activity *per se* but they are usefully combined with pethidine, which has little sedative activity, if pain and anxiety coexist. A tranquilliser may by itself exacerbate pain but if a phenothiazine derivative such as promazine or phenergan is administered with pethidine it will often relieve pain more effectively than pethidine alone. Benzodiazepines may be used to combat anxiety; they do not affect uterine activity in clinical doses.

Inhalation analgesia in childbirth

Subanaesthetic concentrations of anaesthetic gases are administered, usually by the patient herself, with the aim of producing analgesia without loss of consciousness.

Nitrous oxide and oxygen mixtures constitute one of the most satisfactory methods of analgesia in labour. N_2O is extremely safe provided that it is administered with a high admixture of oxygen (30 per cent or more) (p. 302). If the proportion of nitrous oxide to oxygen reaches or exceeds 9:1 and is so maintained for more than 5 min, marked fetal anoxaemia and occasionally profound asphyxia neonatorum results. Because of the risk of fetal anoxia, nitrous oxide and air analgesia should no longer be employed in childbirth. Nitrous oxide 50 per cent to 70 per cent with oxygen is powerfully analgesic producing near maximal analgesia after a few breaths and wearing off equally rapidly. Mixtures of 50 per cent oxygen and 50 per cent nitrous oxide administered from a single cylinder are conveniently administered using special apparatus in which the patient inhales from a fitted face mask and herself operates the demand valve.

Trichlorethylene (Trilene) (p. 302) produces strong analgesia in subanaesthetic concentrations. It is administered by special inhalers operated by the patient delivering 0.33 per cent or 0.5 per cent trichlorethylene vapour in air. Trichlorethylene acts more slowly than nitrous oxide and its action persists longer. It does not inhibit normal labour but occasionally produces tachypnoea, cardiac irregularities and nausea or gives rise to drowsiness and confusion. In such cases it is necessary to reduce the inhaled concentration or discontinue inhalation.

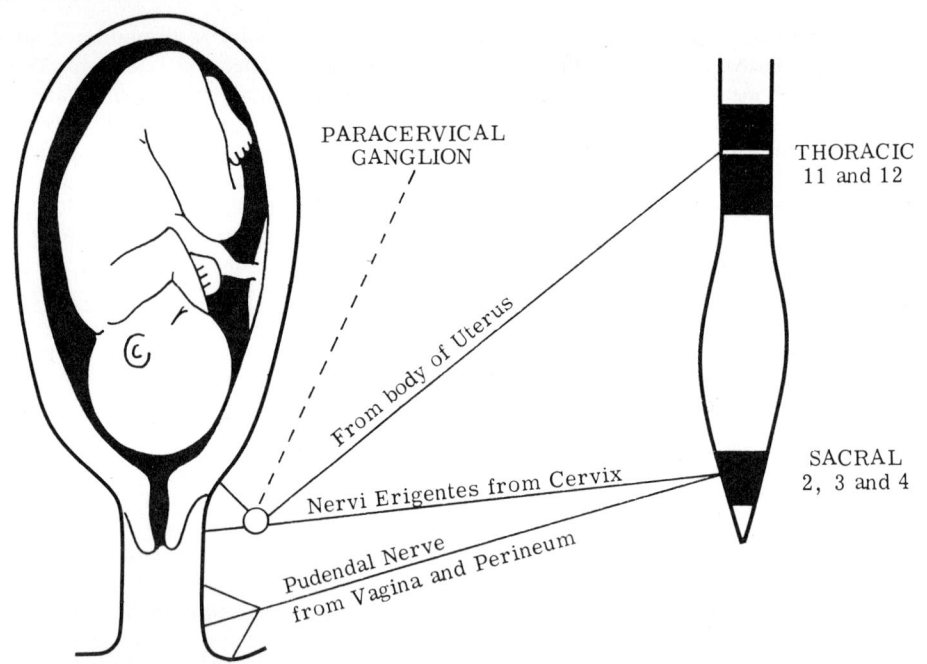

Fig. 15.8 Schematic representation of the sensory innervation of the birth canal. (After Moir, 1974. In Hawkins, ed., *Obstetric Therapeutics*. Baillére, Tindall, London.

Methoxyflurane (Penthrane) 0.35 per cent resembles trichlorethylene in its relatively slow effect. With both agents, the vapour has to be inhaled for some minutes before pain relief is maximal. When methoxyflurane is administered by special, patient-operated inhalers it is a safe analgesic. It is, however, expensive and occasionally produces confusion and loss of patient co-operation.

General anaesthesia
General anaesthesia in childbirth is the domain of the specialist anaesthetist Maternal mortality due to the complications of general anaesthesia remains relatively high in obstetrics and is usually associated with pulmonary aspiration of the stomach contents. The foetus may be put at risk by maternal hypoxia and hypotension. Some general anaesthetics, such as halothane, markedly depress uterine contractions. A relatively safe procedure for obstetric anaesthesia is induction with thiopentone followed by maintenance with nitrous oxide and oxygen.

Regional analgesia
Regional analgesia by local anaesthetics is now frequently used for the relief of pain in labour and for operative delivery. Its advantage is complete pain relief, the patient remaining conscious and able to participate in her labour. Regional analgesia lacks certain risks of general anaesthesia such as aspiration of stomach contents. But it requires specialised techniques, generally only available in hospital, and has the drawback of potential hypotension and on rare occasions neurological sequelae. A safe and effective form of obstetric regional analgesia is epidural anaesthesia in its lumbar or caudal form. Figure 15.8 shows the pathways concerned in the transmission of pain from the uterus and lower birth canal which may be blocked by local anaesthetics. Regional analgesia is further discussed in Chapter 23.

EFFECTS OF DRUGS ON THE FETUS

It has long been recognised that certain drugs when administered during pregnancy may adversely influence the continued development of the fetus and induce expulsion of the contents of the uterus. The production of abortion by ingestion of rye contaminated with ergot and the high incidence of miscarriages in women who worked in the lead industry or lead mining are classical examples. These and other substances such as volatile oils and aloes have often been used with varying success in attempts to produce abortion, but there is little evidence to show that they have any selective action on fetal as distinct from maternal tissues.

The transmission of drugs across the placenta and the resultant effects on the fetus have been frequently reported. A notable example is morphine which when given to the mother a few hours before delivery reduces the ability of the newborn child to breathe spontaneously. In some instances pin-point pupils have been observed in the newborn, and even the occurrence of an abstinence syndrome has been noted in the infant born of a mother addicted to the drug. The administration of antithyroid drugs during pregnancy has resulted in the production of fetal thyroid enlargement and there is well documented evidence that thiouracil and related drugs cross the placental barrier and influence the thyroid-pituitary relationship of the fetus in much the same way as in the adult. Progestational drugs administered during pregnancy may produce a masculinising effect on the female foetus.

Transplacental transmission of sulphonamides, penicillin, streptomycin, tetracycline and other antibiotics has been detected in human and other species, the drug concentration attained in fetal tissues depending on the dose and frequency of administration to the mother. In general, the rate of elimination from the fetus is slower than from maternal tissues because of the general lack of drug metabolising enzymes in the fetus.

Teratogenic effects of drugs

The experimental production of abnormalities in development and growth of the embryo by X-ray irradiation and by a variety of drugs has been studied in the chicken embryo and in various mammalian species. These investigations have included the use of naturally occurring substances, for example an excess of vitamin A or of hormones such as insulin, thyroid, hydrocortisone and progesterone, as well as cytotoxic drugs which are used in the treatment of malignant diseases. In most of these experiments, the fetus was stillborn or prematurely expelled from the uterus and these researches seemed to have little connection with the human congenital abnormalities of the face, skull, central nervous system, heart or alimentary system seen in about three per cent of newborn babies.

A new emphasis was given to this subject by the discovery that thalidomide, an apparently harmless sedative and hypnotic drug, when taken during early pregnancy can cause fetal malformations. In 1961 reports from Western Germany and Australia showed that in some infants born of mothers who had been given thalidomide, the development of the limb buds had been affected so that the hands and feet arose from the trunk in a manner resembling the flippers of a seal, a condition described as phocomelia from the Greek words *phokos*, meaning seal, and *melos*, meaning limb. Although the specific mechanism involved in the arrest in development of the limb buds is not known, it has been established that the embryo is particularly vulnerable to the effects of the drug between 28 and 42 days after conception.

A number of other drugs have since been suspected of producing tetatogenic effects in man; for example the antihistamine meclozine, which is widely used as an antiemetic in the treatment of pregnancy sickness, was withdrawn from sale in Sweden because its use was associated with the occurrence of spina bifida, meningocele and talipes. Later reports of its use in other countries, including the United Kingdom, the United States, Germany and Italy, however, failed to confirm this and no clear-cut evidence of teratogenic effects from this drug has been obtained in a variety of animal species. Amongst drugs suspected to carry some risk to the fetus in early pregnancy are the following: folic acid antagonists such as methotrexate can harm the fetus and since cotrimoxazole (septrin) contains trimethoprim, a folic acid antagonist, this preparation should not be given for urinary infections during pregnancy. Drugs which have been reported to carry a slight risk of causing congenital abnormalities include such standard drugs as aspirin and barbiturates as well as the antiepileptic drug phenytoin sodium. Nicotinamide, which is a common constituent of multi-vitamin preparations, has come under suspicion and even the taking of antacids has been reported to be associated with a higher incidence of congenital abnormalities. Progestogens, oestrogens and androgens can all cause profound effects on the fetus if given in large doses. Fortunately, many of the life-saving drugs such as digitalis and most antibiotics have not so far been shown to harm the fetus but streptomycin and related aminoglycoside antibiotics may cause damage to the eighth cranial nerve in the fetus. The tetracyclines may interfere with bone development and produce discoloration of the primary dentition. Clearly, drugs should be avoided in early pregnancy if at all possible.

Despite much experimental work there is no obvious relationship between chemical structure and teratogenic effect, and drugs with the same type of pharmacological actions produce different types of fetal abnormalities in different species. So far there has been poor correlation between the teratogenic effects of a drug in laboratory animals and in man. Considerable difficulty has been experienced in providing a laboratory test for thalidomide and conflicting reports have been published of its teratogenic effects when tested in the same species. More recently it has been shown that reproducible abnormalities are obtainable with thalidomide in the embryos of subhuman primates. It has become clear that new methods will require to be developed for screening drugs for teratogenic effects and that it will be necessary to test the drugs on a number of species of animals during different stages of fetal development.

Since there are as yet no reliable methods for determinating the safety or danger of drugs in respect to teratogenicity in the human fetus, the current consensus of opinion is that no drug should be prescribed for pregnant women unless drug therapy is essential.

PREPARATIONS

Dinoprost Trometamol (Prostaglandin $F_2\alpha$)
Dinoprostone (Prostaglandin E_2)
Ergometrine maleate (Ergonovine) 0.5–1 mg p.o., 0.2–1 mg i.m. 100–500 μg i.v.
Methylergometrine maleate 100–200 μg s.c., i.m., or i.v.
Oxytocin (Pitocin, Syntocinon) 2–5 U in 1 l by slow i.v. infusion

FURTHER READING

Berde B (ed) 1968 Neurohypophysial hormones. Handb. exp. Pharmacl vol 32

Berde B, Schild H O (ed) 1978 Ergot alkaloids. Handb. exp. Pharmacl vol 49

Berry C L (ed) 1976 Human Malformations Brit med. Bull 32:1-98

Forfar J O 1973 Drugs to be avoided during the first three months of pregnancy. Prescriber's journal 13:130

Fuchs A R 1966 The physiological role of oxytocin in the regulation of myometrial activity in the rabbit. In Pickles, Fitzpatrick (eds). Endogenous substances affecting the myometrium. Cambridge University Press, London

Her Majesty's Stationery Office 1964. Deformities caused by thalidomide

Moir J C 1964 The obstetrician bids, the uterus contracts Br. Med. J. 2:1025.

Moir D D 1974 Drugs used during labour: analgesics, anaesthetics and sedatives. In D F Hawkins (ed) Obstetric therapeutics. Baillere Tindall, London

Robson J M, Sullivan F & Smith R L (eds) 1965 Embryopathic activity of drugs. Churchill London

Saameli K 1979 Effects on the uterus. In Berde, Schild (eds) Ergot alkaloids and related compounds. Handb. exp. Pharm. 49 Springer, Berlin

Sullivan F M 1976 Effects of drugs on foetal development. In Foetal physiology and development. Saunders, London

Utting J E, Gray T C (ed) 1968 Obstetric anaesthesia and analgesia. Br. med. Bull. 24:1

16. The skin

Structure and functions of the skin 227; Pharmacology of the skin 228; Psoriasis 228; Skin infections 229; Animal parasites 230; Acne 230; Hypersensitivity reactions of the skin 230; Mechanism of contact sensitisation 230; Eczema 230; Urticaria 231; Drug reactions of the skin 231; Undesirable effects of topical steroids 231.

Structure and function of the skin

The skin has a complex structure shown in Figure 16.1. It is one of the largest organs of the body, for the weight of the whole human skin amounts to about 4 kg. It is a highly differentiated tissue, with a variety of complex functions. The most obvious of these functions are the protection of underlying tissues and the regulation of heat loss.

The skin contains comparatively large amounts of cholesterol and the activation of 7-dehydrocholesterol by ultra-violet light to form vitamin D is a unique and important function of the skin. The subcutaneous tissues appear to play an important part in inorganic metabolism because they have the power of fixing a considerable quantity of sodium chloride and act as the chief chloride depot in the body.

The sweat glands are estimated to number about two million. Their chief purpose is to secrete water, the evaporation of which permits the rapid loss of heat. The sweat contains about 0.35 per cent sodium chloride and small amounts of urea, uric acid and other constituents of the blood. The sweat glands are constantly active, and the insensible perspiration amounts to about 500 ml a day in a temperate climate and much more in a hot and dry climate. The body can, in extreme cases, excrete as much as 10 litres of sweat a day.

The sweat glands are divided into two classes, the eccrine and apocrine glands. The eccrine glands occur all over the body and secrete only water and water-soluble substances. The apocrine glands are limited to the axillary, mammary and genital regions. These glands are secondary

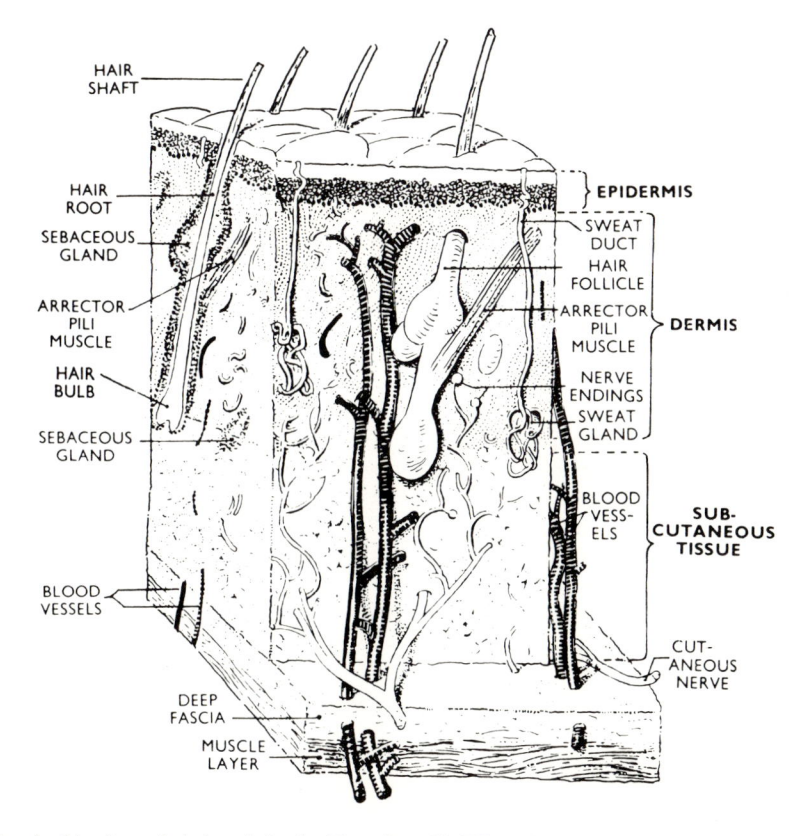

Fig 16.1 The skin, showing blood vessels, hair and glands. (From Ross JS, Wilson KJW 1973 Foundations of anatomy and physiology. Churchill Livingstone, Edinburgh.)

228 APPLIED PHARMACOLOGY

sexual characters which develop at puberty and secrete nitrogenous and fatty substances in addition to water and salt. They are more fully developed in the female than in the male and are believed to undergo cyclic changes in activity coincident with menstruation. In most mammals the apocrine glands are distributed all over the body and are responsible for the odours characteristic of species and sex.

The sebaceous glands are developed in connection with the hair follicles, and their secretory products are formed as a result of the disintegration of the cells forming the lobules of the gland. This secretion is called sebum, and is particularly rich in fatty substances. The sebum acts as a lubricant to the hair and also forms a thin waterproof protective coating over the skin surface. The development of the sebaceous glands is controlled by the sex hormones, and a general increase in the size and number of the glands occurs at puberty, coincident with the sex changes in the hair. The sebacious glands do not appear to be under the direct control of the central nervous system.

Pharmacology of the skin
Powerful drugs including antibiotics, corticosteroids and antimitotics are used in the treatment of skin diseases but clinical trials in which treatments of skin diseases are quantitatively assessed are relatively rare. This is due to the strong empirical traditions of dermatology, as a subject based on observation and experience rather than an experimental science; and also to the protracted and often recurrent nature of skin ailments which renders the quantitative assessment of drug action upon them particularly difficult. Short-term drug effects such as occur in other fields can seldom be obtained in the skin.

In the following pages certain skin diseases of special pharmacological interest will be discussed.

Psoriasis
This is an important skin disease which occurs in about 1 per cent of the population. The sex distribution of psoriasis is about equal and there is a great deal of evidence of familial incidence. The genetical pattern of the disease has not been clarified, it probably depends on a dominant autosomal gene with incomplete expression. Environmental influences modify the degree of gene expression, explaining why, in a person with an inherited predisposition, a skin trauma or a stress situation may cause the appearance of a psoriatic lesion.

Nature and mechanism of psoriasis. The basic defect appears to be one of keratinization resulting in an abnormally high turnover rate of the epidermal cell layer. The normal transit time for an epidermal cell to reach the surface has been estimated as about 27 days while in an active psoriatic plaque this is reduced to three or four days. Figure 16.2 shows characteristic changes seen in a psoriatic epidermis including marked hyperplasia of the keratin

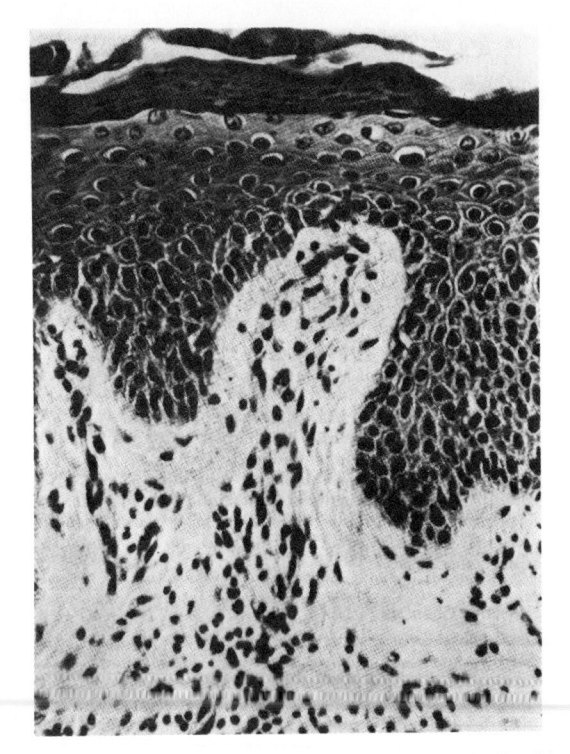

Fig. 16.2 Psoriatic epidermis showing active epidermal cells with prominent nucleoli, acanthotic epidermis and overlying parakeratotic keratin. A granular layer is not formed, and the dermis shows an infiltrate around the capillaries in the dermal papillae. (After Jarrett (1973). The Physiology and Pathophysiology of the skin. Academic Press. London.)

layer and acanthosis characterised by long rete pegs extending deep into the dermis. There is increased cellular activity evidenced by the prominent nucleoli in the nuclei of epidermal cells. The dermal papillae are oedematous and contain dilated blood vessels. When the keratin scales are removed *in vivo* by gentle curettage, pin-point haemorrhages are seen to occur.

Drug treatment of psoriasis
A variety of treatments which reduce the increased keratin cell turnover will reduce the rash whilst they are being applied but it is generally found that when treatment is stopped the psoriatic lesions return although the time taken for their recurrence is variable. The following drugs are chiefly used in psoriasis:

Dithranol (Anthralin), a mixture of dihyroxyanthrone tautomers, or *Tar* (BP) are applied to the lesions as pastes usually in conjunction with ultraviolet light treatment. Applications require technical skill but they are clinically effective although the mechanism of their action is not clear. One theory of the action of dithranol is that it reacts with DNA to inhibit the synthesis of nucleoprotein thus decreasing the proliferation of keratin.

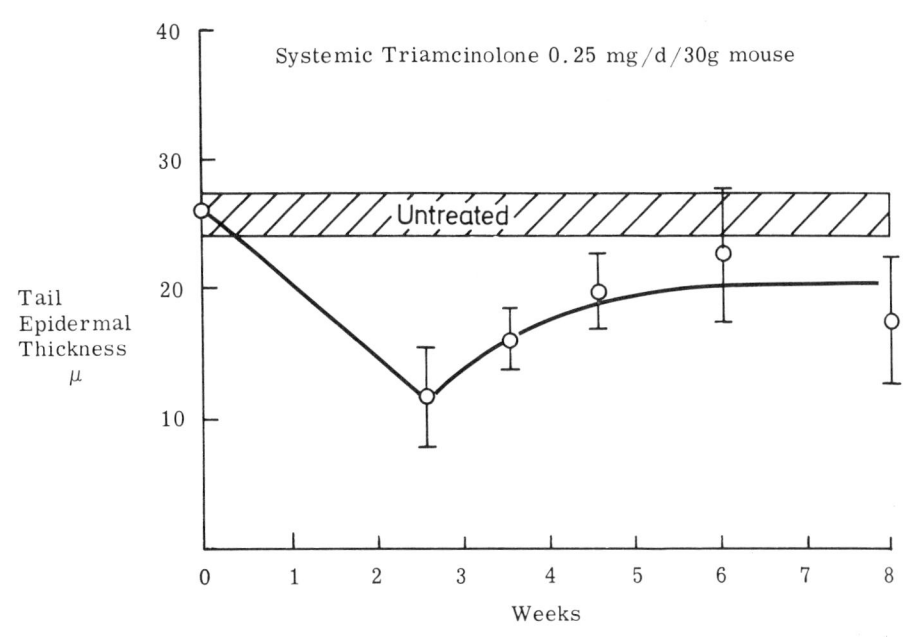

Fig. 16.3 Graph showing the thinning effect of systemic triamcinolone on mouse tail epidermis. The thinning effect of triamcinolone becomes less after about three weeks in spite of continuing systemic application. (After Jarrett, 1973. *The Physiology and Pathophysiology of the Skin*.)

Topical corticosteroids are a useful adjunct in the treatment of psoriasis although they are inadequate alone. Figure 16.3 shows that a fluorinated corticosteroid, triamcinolone, produces a thinning effect on the epidermis of the mouse tail. The mouse tail preparation has been used as a bioassay technique for investigating the effect of steroids on mitosis in the skin.

Methotrexate, hydroxyurea and cyclophosphamide are cytotoxic drugs which are given by mouth or by injection and are effective agents in the treatment of psoriasis. They are capable of improving all types of psoriasis by their action of inhibiting cell turnover in the keratin layer of the skin. Methotrexate (p. 380) is most widely used in psoriasis. All are severely limited by their toxicity which restricts their use to the treatment of severe and progressive cases of the disease. All rapidly proliferating tissues are affected by the cytotoxic drugs, for example it has been found that mouth ulcers frequently occur after their application. A serious complication of methotrexate and similar drugs is liver injury. To guard against it the cytotoxic drugs must be administered intermittently.

Skin infections

They are caused by various species of bacteria, viruses and fungi and can sometimes be treated by specific drugs, although in many cases traditional applications are of proved value.

Bacterial infections may be treated by antibiotics applied topically or systemically.

Impetigo is a superficial skin infection due to staphylococci or streptococci. Vesicles develop in the upper epidermal and keratin layers and soon become incrustated. The natural course of the disease is about three weeks and with modern treatment this is reduced to a few days. Topical antibiotics may be used but those liable to contact sensitisation should not be used in spite of the short period of treatment. A convenient preparation for topical application is 0.1 per cent gentamicin cream.

Erysipelas is a more serious infection which affects the dermis. It is caused by *Streptococcus pyogenes*. The patient is disturbed and has fever. Treatment is by systemic antibiotics such as benzyl penicillin or phenoxymethylpenicillin.

Virus infections of the skin include *Herpes simplex* (cold spot) and *Herpes zoster* (shingles). Both are caused by DNA-containing viruses and can be treated by the antiviral agent *idoxuridine* (p. 396). This acts by blocking the uptake of thymidine into the DNA of the virus and it thus inhibits the replication of certain viruses. Idoxuridine may be applied locally to the skin in a 5 per cent solution in dimethylsulphoxide. There is statistical evidence that repeated applications of idoxuridine may shorten the duration of attacks of both *Herpes simplex* and *Herpes zoster*. Idoxuridine is also used in the treatment of herpes keratitis and herpes encephalitis. It is inactivated by deaminases in the tissues.

Fungus infections of the skin include infections by ringworm and candida. Ringworm fungi, as the name implies, tend to produce discoid or ringed lesions which are erythematous and scaling. They may be symptomless or itching.

Griseofulvin (p. 413) is an antifungal antibiotic which is absorbed from the gastrointestinal tract and deposited in the deeper layers of the skin, the keratin of the nails and the hair thus preventing fungous invasion of newly formed cells. It is metabolised in the liver to 6-demethylgriseofulvin. For superficial forms of ringworm, treatment needs to be continued for 3 to 6 weeks and for infections of the nails it may need to be continued for up to 12 months. Ringworm may also be treated by local applications. Whitfield's ointment containing benzoic and salicylic acid is very successful.

Animal parasites
Scabies. The pregnant female invades the horny layer of the skin laying two or three eggs a day and leaving a fine grey-white line. Burrows are mostly seen in the finger clefts and other creases. Itching begins when the subject has become sensitised to the mite which takes three to six weeks. Should a patient who has previously suffered from scabies catch it afresh he will, because he is already sensitised, itch at once.

In the treatment of scabies the selected drug should be applied to the whole body except the face after a hot bath and left for two periods of 24 hours after which all the Sarcoptes should be killed. All human bedmates must be treated at the same time. The most commonly used drug in scabies is *gamma benzene hexachloride* 1 per cent as lotion or cream applied to the skin. A newer effective drug is *crotamiton*. This also has a marked antipruritic action. *Benzyl benzoate* emulsion is a traditional remedy.

Pediculosis. Louse infestation is more dangerous than scabies, for lice may convey the infective agents of typhus and relapsing fever. The insecticide *dicophane* (DDT) has been most commonly used as a prophylactic and for treatment but since the emergence of DDT-resistant lice the insecticide gamma benzene hydrochloride (p. 467) is being increasingly used in pediculosis. *Malathion* is an organophosphorus insecticide which is highly effective against lice. A 0.5 per cent lotion is sprinkled on to the scalp for head lice and rubbed in well, care being taken to avoid contamination of the eyes. After allowing the hair to dry it must be left untouched for 12 hours and then shampooed and dried. This is repeated one week later.

Acne
Acne vulgaris is a common skin disorder of sebaceous glands. Sebum is retained due to hyperkeratosis of the follicular orifices followed by bacterial activity and inflammation. The sebaceous glands are activated at the time of puberty and hormonal stimulation is an important factor.

A frequently effective form of treatment for acne is by small doses of antibiotic given over long periods, e.g. tetracycline or oxytetracycline 250 mg taken orally once or twice a day. This treatment may take over a month to begin taking effect and it may be continued for a year or more. Oestrogens are sometimes used to reduce androgenic stimulation of sebaceous glands but their use is limited by undesirable side effects. Many topical preparations as well as ultraviolet light are used in acne. *Tretinoin* (Retinoic acid, Vitamin A acid) stimulates the epithelium to give rise to a less cohesive horny layer and produce epidermal sloughing. It has been used topically in the treatment of acne with some success.

Hypersensitivity reactions of the skin
A variety of skin ailments in which an antigen-antibody reaction appears to be involved come under this heading. Allergic phenomena have been discussed in Chapter 8; two types are particularly relevant to the skin: immediate hypersensitivity reactions based on sensitisation by IgE antibodies and delayed hypersensitivity reactions transmitted by sensitised lymphocytes.

Mechanism of contact sensitisation
Contact sensitisation is an example of delayed hypersensitivity of the skin produced by contact with a sensitising agent. A typical example is sensitisation of the skin to primula extract. Topical application of the extract to the shaved skin of a guinea pig gives rise at first to a localised reaction but a few days later the whole skin has become sensitised to primula extract and reacts to it. Contact sensitisation is not due to circulating antibody but to circulating sensitised lymph node cells.

Eczema
This is frequently classed into 'atopic' or constitutional eczema and eczema due to external agents but both may be manifestations of delayed hypersensitivity. Disodium cromoglycate (p. 181) is ineffective in eczema although it is effective in typical immediate hypersensitivity reactions based on histamine release. Eczema is a distinctive reaction consisting of eruptions which are initially pin-head sized and are erythematous, papular, vesicular or weeping. Atopic eczema is seen in its most characteristic form in infants.

Treatment. The treatment of eczema requires clinical knowhow and experience. It is based on topic applications in which a variety of lotions, creams and ointments are applied to the skin. By far the most effective drugs are the corticosteroids which in cases of infection may be combined with an antibiotic. The corticosteroids must be used sparingly. Most active are the *fluorinated corticosteroids* (p. 343) but at each stage the weakest effective corticosteroid at the lowest effective concentration should be used; 1 per cent *hydrocortisone* applications being the least damaging. Systemic corticosteroids should not be employed for the routine treatment of eczema, although they can be most valuable in severe cases.

Urticaria
Urticaria exhibits some of the features of an immediate hypersensitivity reaction although it would be a mistake to equate any naturally occurring disease too closely with an experimental laboratory condition. A point of similarity to the laboratory condition is the involvement of histamine which in laboratory experiments can be shown to originate from sensitised mast cells. The principal human tissue-sensitising antibody is IgE (p. 100).

An acute attack of urticaria presents as itching weals. They are transient, lasting a few hours and leaving no signs afterwards. The weal resembles the 'triple reaction' following intradermal histamine. Urticaria may be caused by an allergen, e.g. some specific food or drug. It sometimes represents an acute emergency if it is accompanied by angioneurotic oedema of the larynx. This can be rapidly alleviated by an injection of adrenaline. In chronic urticaria it is often very difficult to find a definite allergen or cause.

Treatment. Most urticarias respond to oral H_1 *antihistamines* (p. 98) but these are only effective whilst a sufficient concentration is maintained in the bloodstream. Their sedative action is a drawback though it may be beneficial at night. If antihistamines are employed in urticaria they should be given in an adequate dosage and for a sufficient period of time.

Drug reactions of the skin
A wide variety of urticarial or erythematous eruptions or conditions resembling eczema, purpura or acne may be produced by drugs. When a drug reaction is suspected, all drug therapy should be stopped, if possible. A test dose administered after recovery from the reaction may then reliably incriminate a drug.

Skin tests are of limited value in the diagnosis of drug eruptions, since negative skin tests may be found in patients who subsequently experience systemic reactions to the drug. Intradermal, scratch or prick tests may be used. Patch tests are used in the diagnosis of allergic eczematous contact dermatitis.

Peculiar skin reactions produced by certain drugs include the following:

Nalidixic acid, an antibacterial agent for treating urinary tract infections produces a bullous skin reaction after exposure to sunlight.

Practolol, a cardioselective ß-blocker produces a psoriatic rash and conjunctival damage.

Ampicillin produces a morbilliform rash when given to patients with infectious mononucleosis.

Effects of topical corticosteroids on the skin
Topical corticosteroids are widely used in the treatment of skin diseases. There is a theoretical risk of adrenal suppression by corticosteroids applied to the skin, but studies in which blood cortisol levels were measured have shown that adrenal suppression after topical corticosteroids occurs rarely in adults unless occlusive methods of administration are employed. In infants a lowering of plasma cortisol has been demonstrated when powerful corticosteroids were applied to the skin in infantile eczema, but rarely after the topical application of hydrocortisone. A danger of the indiscriminate use of powerful topical corticosteroids such as betamethasone and flucinolone is atrophy of the epidermis. Atrophic striae, due to damage of dermal collagen, may produce persistent scars in children and adolescents.

PREPARATIONS

Psoriasis
Dithranol (Anthralin) 0.01–1% paste or ointmen Prepared Coal Tar

Bacterial Infections
Cetrimide cream 0.5%
Chlorhexidine gluconate solution
Chlortetracycline ointment 3%
Gentamicin ointment 1 mg/g
Neomycin cream 0.5%

Fungal Infections
Amphotericin cream (Fungilin) 3%
Benzoic acid compound ointment (Whitfields')
Candicin, intravaginal 3 mg
Clotrimazole (Canestan) 1% cream
Griseofulvin tablets 500 mg–1 g daily
Miconazole (Daktarin) 2% cream
Natamycin (Pimafucin) 2% cream
Nystatin, oral, cutaneous, ocular candidiasis
Tolnaftate (Tinaderm) 1% cream or solution

Scabies
Benzyl Benzoate (Ascabiol) 25%
Crotamiton (Eurax) 10% lotion or ointment

Lice
Dicophane application 2%; dusting powder 10%
Gamma benzene hexachloride, application 0.1%
Malathion (Derbac) 0.5% application and shampoo

Acne
Benzoyl peroxide gel (Acetoxyl) 5 and 10%
Tretinoin (Retin-A) 0.025% solution or gel

REFERENCES AND FURTHER READING

Hunter J A A 1973 The structure and function of the skin in relation to therapy. Br. med. J. 4: 340, 411
Jarrett A (ed) Physiology and pathophysiology of the skin, vol 1-4. Academic Press, London
Marks Janet 1976 Skin diseases. In: Avery G S (ed) Drug treatment. Churchill Livingstone, Edinburgh
Marks R, Samman P D (ed) 1977 Dermatology. Heinemann, London
Rook A et al 1978 Textbook of dermatology. Blackwell, Oxford
Schild H O 1962 Mechanism of contact sensitisation. J. Pharm. Pharmac. 14: 1–8

SECTION FOUR

Pharmacology of the central nervous system and local anaesthetics

17. Basic neurohumoral and electrophysiological mechanisms

Synaptic transmission in the CNS 235; Acetylcholine 235; Monoamines 235; Amino acids 235; The electroencephalogram and sleep 236; The reticular activating system 237; The hypothalamus 238; The limbic system 238; The extrapyramidal system 239; Tardive dyskinesia 239; Theories of mental disease 240; Amine mechanisms in manic-depressive disease 240; Dopamine hypothesis of schizophrenia 240; Opiate receptors 241; Development of drugs which affect mental activity 242.

Synaptic transmission in the c.n.s.
It is now generally accepted that synaptic transmission in the central nervous system (c.n.s.) is chemically mediated, i.e. a nerve impulse arriving at a nerve terminal within the c.n.s. liberates a chemical mediator which diffuses across a synapse to excite or inhibit another neurone. The actions of drugs which affect the c.n.s. can be explained in terms of interference with these transmission processes. Interference may occur: (1) by blocking, mimicking or potentiating the effects of transmitters at receptor sites on the postsynaptic membrane; (2) by acting on receptor sites at presynaptic nerve terminals to either inhibit or increase the release of transmitter; (3) by unspecific effects on nerve membranes not necessarily connected with receptor action.

The principal substances believed to play a transmitter role in the c.n.s. are as follows.

Acetylcholine. There is much evidence that acetylcholine functions as a central transmitter. It is widely distributed in the c.n.s. together with the enzymes choline acetylase and choline esterase which synthesise and destroy it. Subcellular fractionation studies of brain tissue have demonstrated that acetylcholine is mainly contained in synaptic vesicles present in nerve endings. Neurones which respond to the microiontophoretic application of acetylcholine by electrical excitation or inhibition occur in many regions of the brain and spinal cord, including the Renshaw cells of the spinal cord and neurones in the medulla, pons, thalamus and cortex. Both types of receptors, muscarinic receptors blocked by atropine and nicotinic receptors blocked by beta-erythroidine (a tertiary curare-like substance), occur in the c.n.s. The hypothalamus with its important autonomic connections contains many cholinoceptive neurones, suggesting that acetylcholine is as likely to play a part in the basic mechanisms of action of psychotropic drugs as the monoamines.

Monoamines. Unlike acetylcholine, the monoamines are found mainly in the hypothalamus and brain stem. The brain contains more noradrenaline than adrenaline. The *locus caeruleus* is a group of pigmented neurones in the upper medulla containing high concentrations of noradrenaline and innervating the cerebral cortex, brain stem nuclei and hypothalamus. Dopamine also occurs in the brain but its distribution differs from that of noradrenaline, suggesting that it has an independent role as transmitter in addition to being the metabolic precursor of noradrenaline (p. 75). 5-Hydroxytryptamine (serotonin) is concentrated in the hypothalamus and brain stem and almost certainly plays a role as transmitter. The actions of psychotropic drugs have frequently been interpreted in terms of interfecence with the synaptic functions of noradrenaline, dopamine and 5-hydroxytryptamine.

Specific neurones in the c.n.s. which store dopamine, noradrenaline and 5-hydroxytryptamine have been demonstrated by fluorescence histochemistry. A schematic representation of tracts in the brain and spinal cord as demonstrated by this method is shown in Figure 17.1. Dopaminergic neurones of the nigrostriatal pathway are involved in the extrapyramidal control of skeletal muscle activity. Cell bodies of 5-HT neurones are found particularly in the raphe nuclei of the brain stem. Ascending raphe neurones innervate the hippocampus which is part of the limbic system considered to be important in the control of emotional behaviour. Descending raphe neurones influence spinal motor neurone excitability by an action depending on 5-HT. It has been shown that an increased 5-HT level produces hyperextension and limb tremors in spinal rats.

It is of interest that LSD (p. 265) an ergot derivative which is a peripheral antagonist of 5-HT produces a 5-HT-like action when applied centrally. Both LSD and 5-HT inhibit neuronal activity when applied to raphe nuclei by microionophoresis. Possibly they both stimulate a common central presynaptic 5-HT receptor which causes inhibition of 5-HT release.

Amino acid transmitters
Several amino acids have powerful effects on neurones and there is much circumstantial evidence of their role in transmission processes in the mammalian central nervous system. Four amino acids have been particularly singled out, glycine and GABA as inhibitory transmitters and glutamate and aspartate as excitatory transmitters. Although it is not possible to apply to amino acids the fluorescent histochemical techniques used to trace catecholamine and 5-HT neurones they can be localised by autoradiography following their uptake by specific neuronal uptake mechanisms. It has been shown in this

236   APPLIED PHARMACOLOGY

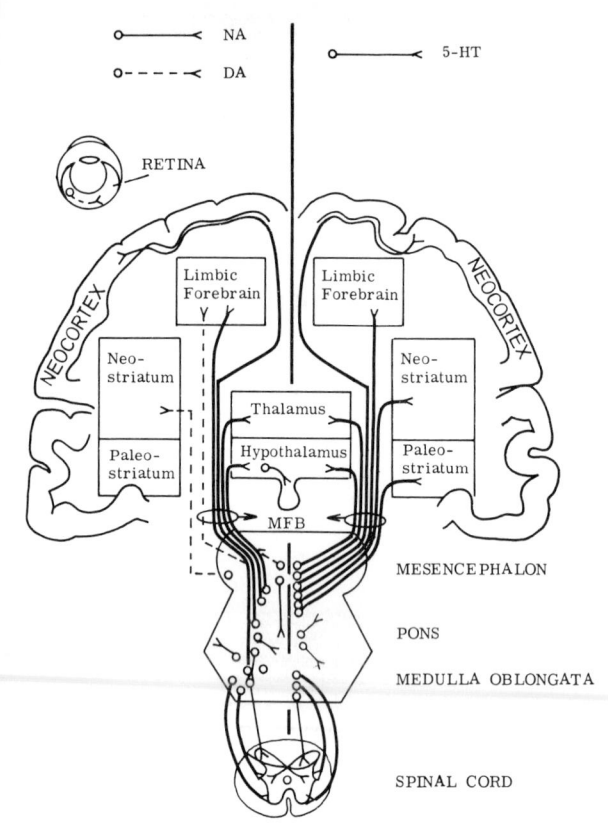

Fig. 17.1 Schematic representation of the bodies and their axonal projections of dopaminergic (DA), noradrenergic (NA), and serotonergic (5-HT, 5-hydroxytryptamine) neurones in the brain and spinal cord, as determined by fluorescence histochemistry. Dopamine and norepinephrine-containing neurones are shown on the left, 5-hydroxytryptamine-containing neurones on the right. (From Andén et al, 1966, *Acta Physiologica Scandinavica*.)

way that ³H-glycine uptake is confined to the spinal cord whereas a more widespread ³H-GABA uptake occurs in the cerebellum, caudate, locus caeruleus and substantia nigra.

Glutamine stimulates a variety of neurones including cortical neurones. *Gamma-aminobutyric acid* (GABA) is chemically closely related to glutamic acid from which it differs only by the removal of a carboxyl group (Fig. 17.2); the presence or absence of a carboxyl group thus determines whether the molecule serves an excitatory or inhibitory function. The formation of GABA in nervous tissue occurs through decarboxylation of L-glutamate by the enzyme L-glutamate decarboxylase (GAD) present in synaptosomes. The degradation of GABA occurs by a pyridoxal-dependent transaminase referred to as GABA-T. When an inhibitor of GABA-T is administered *in vivo* it causes a marked rise of the steady-state concentration of GABA in the brain.

GABA exerts an inhibitory effect in the nerve-muscle preparation of the crayfish where it exerts a presynaptic as well as a postsynaptic action. Its basic effect is an increase in chloride permeability of the cell membrane. In the mammalian central nervous system GABA may act by a presynaptic mechanism to produce inhibition. Inhibition by GABA and *glycine*, which has been proposed as an inhibitory transmitter in the spinal cord, can be distinguished by the action of specific antagonists: the alkaloid bicuculline is a specific antagonist of GABA and the alkaloid strychnine is a specific antagonist of glycine.

The classification of amino acid receptors, as indeed of all central receptors, presents peculiar difficulties since they cannot be investigated, as with peripheral receptors, by applying antagonists under equilibrium conditions. Based on their specific uptake mechanisms it has been suggested that the centrally active amino acids glutamate, aspartate, glycine and GABA may each act on a separate receptor.

Substance P (p. 91) is a pharmacologically active polypeptide which has been proposed as a potential transmitter substance in sensory neurones. Substance P has been synthesised. It is an undecapeptide present in many parts of the c.n.s.

Other tissue hormones are found in central nervous tissue including histamine, prostaglandins and ATP. They have all been suggested as possible transmitters in the c.n.s. but their role in this respect is less well substantiated than the substances discussed above.

The electroencephalogram and sleep

The electroencephalogram (e.e.g.) has been subdivided into frequency bands designated by the letters alpha, beta, delta and theta. The wave bands of the e.e.g. can be resolved into their individual components by means of a mathematical Fourier analysis carried out by computer, but more commonly the simple baseline e.e.g. is used, which can provide considerable information about physiological and pathological (e.g. epilepsy) events. The most important physiological features manifested by the e.e.g. are those of arousal and sleep.

Fig. 17.2 Conversion of glutamic acid to GABA.

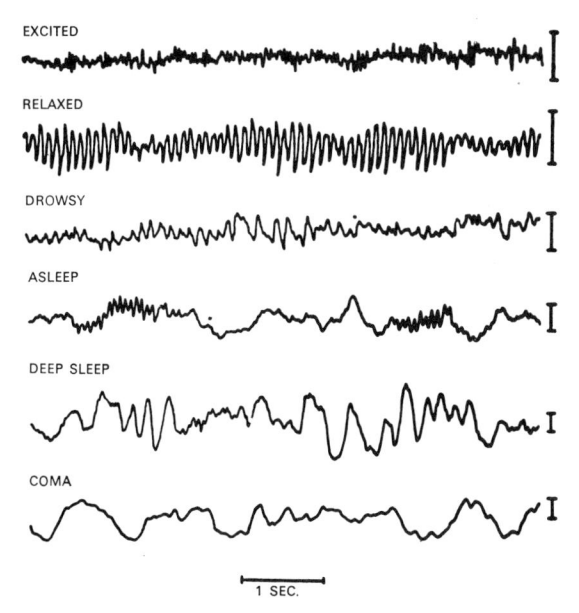

BASIC NEUROHUMORAL AND ELECTROPHYSIOLOGICAL MECHANISMS 237

Fig. 17.3 Examples of electroencephalograms (e.e.g.) of human subjects in various states of arousal, sleep and coma. (After Penfield and Jasper, 1954. *Epilepsy and functional anatomy of the human brain*. Little Brown, Boston.)

Figure 17.3 shows typical e.e.g. patterns in man during various stages of arousal. A relaxed subject, awake but with eyes closed, generally exhibits alpha rhythm of frequency 8 to 13 Hertz (Hz). The alpha rhythm can be made to disappear suddenly when vigilance is raised through eye opening or by concentration on mental arithmetic. The 'excited' asynchronous pattern then appears with dominant frequency of 14 to 25 Hz (beta rhythm). If, on the other hand, drowsiness increases, alpha rhythm is lost and a low voltage e.e.g. appears in which theta (4-7 Hz) and delta ($\frac{1}{2}$-3 Hz) rhythms predominate.

When a subject falls asleep, large slow waves appear in the e.e.g. interspersed with 'sleep spindles' (Fig. 17.3). Gradually the whole e.e.g. becomes dominated by large slow waves. Dement and Kleitman have distinguished four e.e.g. stages of sleep: stage 1, without spindle activity; stage 2, with spindles on a low voltage background; stage 3, with high voltage slow waves and some spindling; stage 4, dominated by high voltage slow waves. An e.e.g. pattern resembling deep (stage 4) sleep may also occur in barbiturate coma or when the blood supply to the brain is reduced as during fainting.

The pathways and mechanisms controlling the sleep-waking cycle are incompletely understood. The cycle seems to involve a diffuse thalamic projection system as well as the reticular activating system. The spindling pattern of the e.e.g. may be generated in thalamic nuclei and this supports the suggestion that the thalamic system and the reticular activating system interact antagonistically in the sleep waking cycle. It seems probable that serotoninergic pathways play an important role in sleep. There is evidence that the raphe nuclei, located along the midline throughout the medulla, pons and midbrain, are involved in sleep. The raphe system is serotoninergic; its surgical or chemical lesion in cats, produced by blocking the synthesis of 5-hydroxytryptamine by p-chlorophenylalanine, leads to permanent insomnia which can be alleviated by administering the 5-HT precursor 5-hydroxytryptophan.

Rapid eye movement sleep
It is well established that normal sleep is interrupted several times each night by phases of *paradoxical* or *rapid eye movement* (REM) sleep lasting some 20 minutes each. During this phase the e.e.g. adopts an abnormal pattern in which slow waves are interspersed by bouts of alpha rhythm and 'saw tooth' waves. Besides rapid jerky eye movements, this phase is characterised by vivid dreams and a loss of muscle tone of which the dreamer becomes aware if he has a nightmare in which he struggles to escape and finds himself unable to move. The reduction in skeletal muscle tone, especially in neck and limb muscles, is due to descending brain stem influences on the spinal motor neurones in the extrapyramidal motor system. Sexual excitation is prominent in this phase.

There is evidence that a small nucleus located in the pons, the *locus caeruleus*, which is composed largely of noradrenergic nerve fibres, is the pacemaker initiating REM sleep. The terminals of these neurones course all the way up to the limbic region and the cerebral cortex. The significance of REM sleep is not fully understood but it can be considered as part of 'normal' sleep. Barbiturates and other hypnotics shorten the relative duration of REM sleep. The tricyclic antidepressants (p. 258) also reduce the intensity and duration of paradoxical sleep. It has been suggested that the benzodiazepines do not cause a reduction of REM sleep but this is disputed. There is evidence that after the withdrawal of barbiturate in an addict a marked rebound with increase in REM sleep occurs.

The reticular activating system
This term refers to an area in the midbrain investigated by Moruzzi and Magoun. In 1949 these authors stimulated the area with high-frequency electrical pulses and found that resting or drowsy animals were aroused behaviourally whilst their electroencephalogram (e.e.g.) changed to a low voltage, high frequency pattern characteristic of an alert animal. Destruction of this area rendered animals stuporous and sleepy. They concluded that this region of the brain contained the centre for wakefulness and alertness, and that when inactive it caused sleep. More recent evidence suggests that these conclusions may have to be modified. Further work including that by Moruzzi

and colleagues has suggested that sleep may not be just a negative state arising from diminished excitement of the reticular formation but that a positive sleep system may exist in the brain whereby the wake-sleep cycle results from the interaction of two mutually antagonistic systems promoting wakefulness and sleep respectively.

The ascending reticular activating system is stimulated by any novel sensory input including visual and auditory inputs. It has been shown that at least some of the multisynaptic pathways in this system contain noradrenergic synapses. Thus the sedative effects of reserpine, which depletes noradrenaline, and of chlorpromazine, which blocks alpha adrenergic receptors, have been attributed to these actions on adrenergic synapses in the reticular activating system. Barbiturates have a marked effect on the reticular activating system; these drugs raise the threshold for e.e.g. arousal if produced by direct electrical stimulation of the reticular activating area.

The hypothalamus
The hypothalamus is an important centre of integration of eating, drinking, sexual behaviour, temperature regulation and other vegetative functions. Some of these functions are mediated by pathways regulating the autonomic nervous system, others are mediated by tracts to the pituitary gland. Thus hypothalamic cholinergic nuclei control the neurones releasing the posterior pituitary hormones (p. 328). The hypothalamus is also the origin of a number of specific polypeptide factors which regulate the activities of the anterior pituitary gland (p. 322).

The hypothalamus plays a key part in the regulation of ovulation. Hypothalmic releasing factors (p. 322) control the release of luteinising hormone (LH) and follicle stimulating hormone (FSH) by the anterior pituitary. There is evidence that these releasing factors themselves are discharged through dopaminergic neurones in the hypothalamus. The hypothalamus is a target organ for oestrogen. It has been found that ^{3}H oestradiol accumulates specifically in the cells of the anterior pituitary and the median eminence of the hypothalamus as well as in the uterus.

The hypothalamus controls a number of physiological functions which may be modulated by drugs. It has been shown by direct injection into the hypothalamus of rats that acetylcholine and carbachol elicit drinking and that adrenaline and noradrenaline elicit eating. The hypothalamus is a key area in the reward system of Olds. This author discovered that rats would continue pressing levers at a high rate to achieve electrical stimulation of the hypothalamus by an electrode implanted in it.

It is probable that amphetamine produces anorexia by a hypothalamic action. Other psychotropic drugs probably exert effects on the hypothalamus.

The limbic system
The limbic system consists of a group of ganglia and associated tracts which have been considered by neuroanatomists as a functional entity. A diagram of the limbic system is shown in Figure 17.4. The word limbic comes from the latin *limbus* meaning border, because these structures, which include the *hippocampus, amygdala* and *septum*, tend to form a border around the brain stem. As shown in Figure 17.4, the structures have many interconnections and it has been suggested that they can form closed circuits or loops so that impulses generated in a particular nucleus may induce activity that feeds back eventually upon the original nucleus. One such suggested reverberating loop is called the circuit of Papez.

The limbic system has been frequently associated with psychotropic drug action although detailed evidence is lacking. The main reason for implicating the limbic system is that it is known that injury to the system in man and in experimental animals causes profound disorders of memory and emotion. Thus damage to the septal area in animals produces viciousness and exaggerated rage; both sympathetic and parasympathetic discharges can be elicited by electrical stimulation of limbic nuclei. Bilateral damage of the hippocampus produces a characteristic disorder of long range memory. Lesions of the amygdala in animals cause hyperphagia, hypersexuality and a characteristic lack of aggression.

The limbic system has many reciprocal connections with the midbrain reticular formation and a close

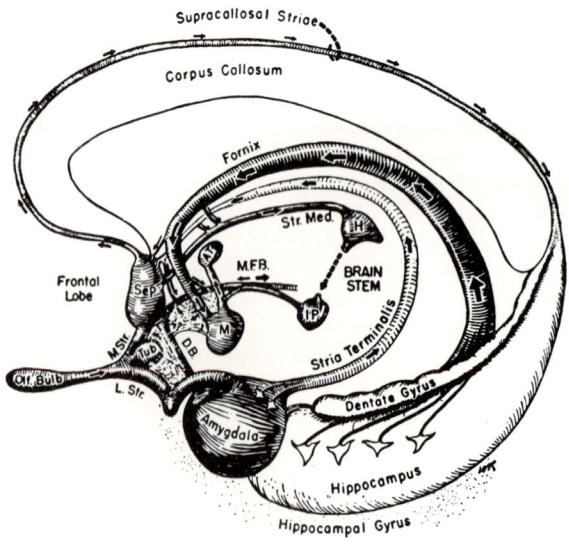

Fig. 17.4 Schematic representation of the relationship of the main subcortical structures and connections of the rhinencephalon, drawn as though all of them could be seen from the medial aspect of the right hemisphere with the intervening tissue 'dissolved away'.
H, habenula; IP, interpeduncular nucleus; M, mammillary body; MFB, medial forebrain bundle; Sep, region of septal nuclei; Olf Bulb, olfactory bulb. (After Maclean, 1949, *Psychosom. Med.*)

relationship with the hypothalamus. Further studies will no doubt show up in more detail its relevance to psychotropic drug action.

The extrapyramidal system
The extrapyramidal system comprises several basal ganglia including the *globus pallidus*, *caudate nucleus* and *putamen*; the latter two are also referred to as the *neostriatum*. Dopaminergic nerves originating in the substantia nigra run to the caudate nucleus. These nigrostriatal pathways are involved in the extrapyramidal control of skeletal muscle tone and coordination.

It has been known that in Parkinsonism, lesions are found in the *substantia nigra* and *corpus striatum*. More recently it has been shown that in Parkinsonism there is a deficiency of dopamine in the brain, and that symptoms can be ameliorated by administering L-dopa, the precursor of dopamine. It thus seems clear that dopaminergic receptors in the striatum are important in controlling the extrapyramidal disturbances of Parkinsonism (p. 273). Formerly, Parkinsonism was treated mainly by means of atropine-like anticholinergic drugs. Their action is explained as follows.

Dopamine and acetylcholine both play an important transmitter role in the basal nuclei and large concentrations of both transmitters are found in the nucleus caudatus. The effects of these transmitters on neuronal activity in the nucleus caudatus may be demonstrated in experimental animals. The effect of administration of L-dopa on the neuronal activity of the mouse caudate is to reduce the rate of firing of these neurones. Thus it appears that the dopaminergic pathway is a predominantly inhibitory pathway. By contrast, acetylcholine appears to have an excitatory effect on the neurones of the caudate nucleus and if acetylcholine is injected into the caudate nucleus in the experimental animal there is an increased rate of discharge of the adjacent neurones. Patients with Parkinsonism are usually made worse by drugs which block the breakdown of acetylcholine. Eserine produces an exacerbation of akinesia, rigidity and tremor in these patients.

It has been suggested that the characteristic disturbance in Parkinsonism is an excessive cholinergic facilitatory bias caused by the lack of a normal dopaminergic inhibitory action on striatal neurones. The atropine-like antimuscarinic drugs can partially restore the bias by damping down the excessive cholinergic facilitation.

Other receptors are dopaminergic and are innervated by the nigrostriatal pathway. The dopaminergic mechanism allows normal muscular activities to take place. This hypothesis could account for various pharmacological effects. Besides explaining the beneficial effects of atropine-like drugs as well as those of L-dopa in Parkinsonism, it can account for extrapyramidal symptoms produced by high doses of neuroleptic drugs such as chlorpromazine and haloperidol. Haloperidol has been shown to be a fairly specific blocker of dopamine receptors. Chlorpromazine is also believed to block dopamine as well as alpha-adrenergic receptors.

Central dopamine receptors. Dopamine receptors in the central nervous system are associated with a dopamine sensitive adenylate cyclase, so that the action of dopamine agonists and antagonists can be screened by their effects on cyclic AMP production in dopamine sensitive brain tissue preparations. Central dopamine receptors have also been investigated by ligand studies measuring the displacement of a labelled high affinity ligand by dopamine agonists and antagonists.

Ungerstedt has introduced a method for testing the effect of stimulation of dopamine receptors in the corpus striatum. The nigrostriatal tract of rats is unilaterally lesioned and made to degenerate by injecting it with 6-hydroxydopamine. Stimulation of supersensitive dopamine receptors on the lesioned side by administering the dopamine receptor stimulant apomorphine induces a circling movement of the animal towards the lesioned side. Amphetamine which stimulates dopamine release in the intact branch induces the opposite turning movement. This behaviour pattern is frequently utilised to analyse the effects of dopaminergic stimulation by drugs used for the treatment of Parkinsonism.

Dopamine receptors are also believed to be involved in a peculiar 'stereotyped' behaviour pattern seen in rats after the administration of apomorphine or of amphetamine. This pattern consists of continuous sniffing, licking and biting of the cage floor or of the animal's own forelegs. The rat sits in a crouched position and normal activities such as grooming, eating and rearing are absent. There is evidence that the abnormal behaviour is mediated by dopamine receptors in the corpus striatum and that apomorphine produces a direct stimulation of the dopamine receptors whilst amphetamine causes stimulation by releasing endogenous dopamine. Evidence that these effects are due to stimulation of dopamine receptors is provided by the finding that they can be reproduced by the administration of dopa and that they are antagonised by haloperidol and chlorpromazine, both of which block dopamine receptors. It has been suggested that 'stereotyped' behaviour in rats may represent an experimental model for the condition of *tardive dyskinesia*.

Tardive dyskinesia. This is a condition seen increasingly in mental hospitals in patients receiving phenothiazines, haloperidol and related antipsychotic drugs. The essential feature of tardive dyskinesia is repetitive involuntary movements of choreo-athetoid type involving the mouth, lips, tongue and extremities. The basic mechanism proposed for this syndrome is the development of dopaminergic hypersensitivity in the nigrostriatal system due to a persistent block of dopamine receptors. The continued block of dopamine receptors may produce (a) supersensitivity of the receptors, (b) increased synthesis of dopamine by a feedback loop.

Tardive dyskinesia is a serious condition caused by neuroleptic drug treatment which is difficult to remedy and may be persistent. It has been suggested that Parkinsonism and chorea can be considered as two poles in a continuum of transmitter disturbances in which dopaminergic function is either decreased or increased.

Amphetamine produces stereotyped behaviour also in primates and in human amphetamine addicts in whom a schizophrenia-like psychosis may occur in which subjects continue for hours with an apparently purposeless activity such as polishing finger nails or dismantling and reassembling clocks and motors.

Theories of mental disease based on amine neurotransmitters

The neurohumoral transmission theory and the associated concepts of drug receptors and competitive drug antagonism have proved extraordinarily fruitful in their clinical applications to the peripheral nervous system. It has been a natural extension to use analogous concepts in the central nervous system. They have been applied particularly to schizophrenic psychosis and manic-depressive disease, two of the most serious human afflictions. It is, however, much more difficult to analyse drug interactions in the central nervous system than in the periphery, partly for technical reasons, since interactions between agonists, antagonists and receptors under equilibrium conditions can seldom, if ever, be obtained in the central nervous system and partly because of the inherent difficulties of quantifying mental processes in terms of measurable responses.

Nevertheless some interesting comprehensive hypotheses have been advanced, which could provide a theoretical framework for the actions of drugs in mental disease.

Amine mechanisms in manic-depressive disease

Brain noradrenergic neurones play a central role in the amine hypothesis of depression. The function of noradrenaline at nerve endings is illustrated schematically in Figure 17.5. The amino acid L-tyrosine is taken up into the noradrenergic neurone by an active transport process. Within the neurone it undergoes ring hydroxylation to dopa (the rate limiting step), followed by decarboxylation to dopamine and uptake into a storage vesicle with associated side chain hydroxylation to form noradrenaline. The storage vesicle content is in equilibrium with intraneuronal noradrenaline accessible to degradation by amine oxidase. As a consequence of a nerve impulse the vesicle is believed to fuse with the neuronal wall releasing its contents into the synaptic cleft. The released noradrenaline may react with presynaptic or postsynaptic receptors, or diffuse away to be inactivated by COMT, or be returned to the neurone by an active uptake process when it is again exposed to amine oxidase.

A functional relationship between amine storage and mental depression was suggested by the finding that reserpine, which depletes the brain of noradrenaline and 5-HT, often caused severe clinical depression. Two relevant further findings were (1) amine oxidase inhibitors increased brain noradrenaline content in animals, elevated the mood of depressed patients and counteracted reserpine depression. (2) Imipramine, which had been shown by clinical observation to have antidepressant activity, inhibited the neural reuptake of noradrenaline and 5-HT. There has also been some evidence that lithium, which is clinically effective in mania, may enhance neural amine reuptake.

These combined findings have given rise to a general hypothesis which in its simplest form states that depression is associated with lack of one or more amine neurotransmitter at specific central synapses, whilst mania is associated with excess amine at these synapses.

Dopamine hypothesis of schizophrenia

Evidence of various kinds has suggested that schizophrenia may be related to faulty cerebral dopaminergic activity. Perhaps the main evidence is that all antipsychotic drugs block dopamine receptors. In laboratory animals the neuroleptics antagonise stereotyped behaviour induced by dopaminergic stimulants such as apomorphine or amphetamine and when used in patients the neuroleptics produce Parkinsonian motor effects attributable to block of dopamine receptors. An overdose of amphetamine (a powerful stimulant of dopamine receptors) in man may produce an apparent psychosis which is indistinguishable from paranoid schizophrenia.

The dopamine hypothesis is at present attracting much attention although it is controversial and its general validity uncertain. Attempts have been made, so far unsuccessful, to find out whether the concentration of the dopamine metabolite homovanillic acid is altered in the cerebrospinal fluid or in autopsied brains of schizophrenic subjects.

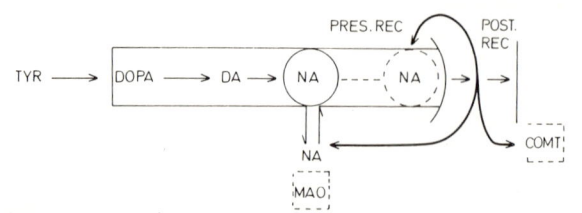

Fig. 17.5 The noradrenergic synapse. TYR L-tyrosine, DOPA dihydroxyphenylalanine, DA dopamine, NA noradrenaline, MAO monoamine oxidase, COMT catechol-O-methyltransferase, PRES. REC presynaptic receptor, POST. REC postsynaptic receptor.

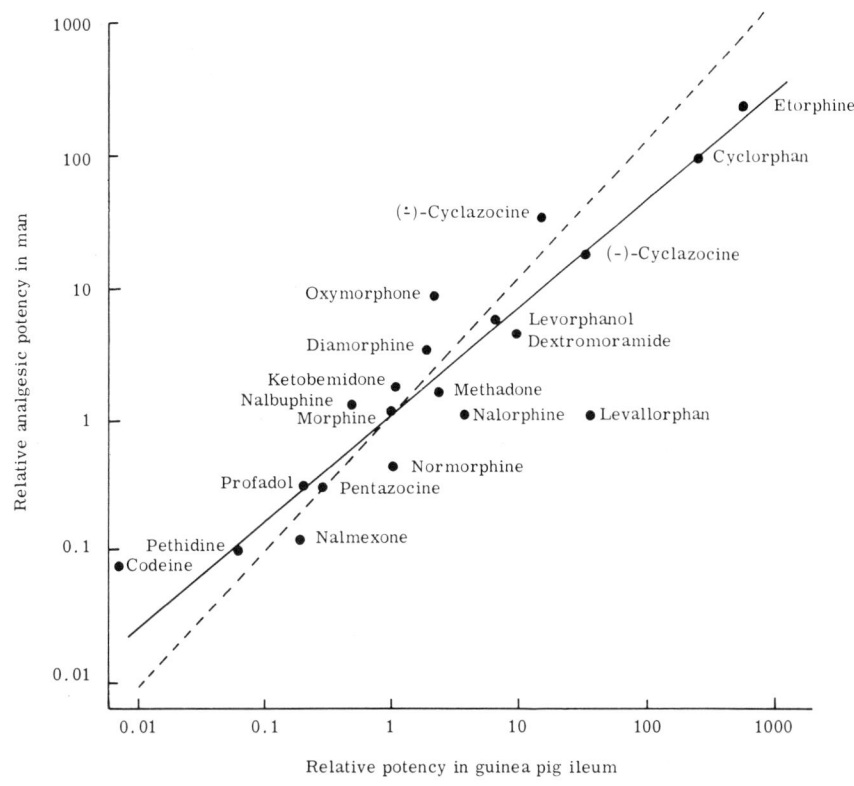

Fig. 17.6 Correlation between the relative agonist potencies in guinea-pig ileum and analgesia in man (morphine=1). Effects on ileum are measured by depression of isometric contraction evoked by electrical stimulation. (After Kosterlitz and Waterfield, 1975, *Ann. Rev. Pharmac.*)

Abnormal metabolism hypothesis. Certain hallucinogenic drugs such as mescaline (p. 266) are O-methylated derivatives of catecholamines and others such as psilocybin (p. 489) are methylated indoleamines. This gave rise to the speculation that schizophrenia may result from brain accumulation of abnormal methylated biogenic amine derivatives. This approach has been followed up for many years, so far without concrete results.

Opiate receptors

The opiate receptor hypothesis has been an interesting new development in the field of central nervous system receptors, linking central and peripheral drug receptors. The following are some of the main experimental findings on which the hypothesis is based.

1. Morphine inhibits the release of acetylcholine from nerve endings of Auerbach's plexus in the isolated guinea pig ileum, elicited by transmural electrical stimulation. Morphine also inhibits contractile responses of the isolated ileum and ductus deferens elicited by electrical stimulation.

2. Other opiate drugs produce analogous effects. Kosterlitz and colleagues have demonstrated a close correlation between the inhibitory effects of opiate analogues in isolated preparations and their analgesic activities in man (Fig. 17.6). Naloxone, a specific morphine antagonist in man, produces a competitive antagonism of morphine in isolated preparations, presumably by competition for the same receptors.

3. Leucine-enkephalin and methionine-enkephalin (Fig. 17.7) two pentapeptides isolated by Hughes from mammalian brain produce morphine-like effects in isolated preparations which are antagonised by naloxone. The enkephalins thus seem to act on the same receptors as morphine.

The role of enkephalins in the body is not understood. They are concentrated in brain areas in which neurones mediating pain pathways occur and it has been suggested

Fig. 17.7 Formula of methionine-enkephalin. Reproduced from Kosterlitz and Hughes, 1977, *Br. J. Psychiat.*, 130.

that they may act as endogenous neurotransmitters involved in analgesic responses. It has recently been discovered that methionine-enkephalin forms part of a larger amino acid sequence in a pituitary polypeptide called ß-lipotropin which has been shown to have analgesic activity in animal experiments. There is presently intense activity in this field. It is not known whether enkephalins or endorphins (a general term employed for endogenous peptides with opioid activity) have a physiological function. Very high amounts of ß-endorphins are present in the intermediate lobe of the pituitary and it has been found that intracerebral injection of these compounds may produce analgesia and a cataleptic action resembling schizophrenia.

Development of drugs which affect mental activity

Drugs which affect mental activity are among the oldest known and have played an important part in the social life of all nations. They are obtained from the most varied botanical sources and include opium, hashish, coca leaves, mescal (peyote), belladonna and alcohol. The active ingredients can be prepared in a variety of forms and are smoked, chewed or incorporated in drinks according to custom. The purpose of taking these drugs has generally been to produce a state of happiness and oblivion by a change in mood and mental activity, without loss of consciousness.

The impetus for the new psychopharmacology has, however, come from a different source, the need to control mental illness. This subject developed rapidly in the nineteen-fifties, largely through clear-sighted clinical observations made when certain new synthetic drugs were used in patients. One of the earliest findings was the beneficial effect produced by chlorpromazine and reserpine in the treatment of psychoses. Even more unexpected was the finding that imipramine, which could not be regarded as a central stimulant from its effects in experimental animals and normal man, nevertheless acted clinically as an antidepressant. Another important development has been the introduction of tranquillisers for the control of anxiety, less liable than barbiturates to cause death when given in an overdose.

It is perhaps significant that in spite of a large amount of animal research carried out by experimental pharmacologists in universities and industrial research laboratories, some of the key advances in psychopharmacology, including some of the most original advances, have come through clinical observation. This is understandable since no valid animal models of human mental illness exist in which the effects of drugs in psychoses can be tested. The pharmacological analysis of drugs acting on the central nervous system is extremely complex and progress continues to be slow. Nevertheless, important advances are being made in the electrophysiological analysis of psychotropic drug action and most fruitfully by studying the interactions of these drugs with central transmitters in the brain.

FURTHER READING

Berger P A, Barchas J D 1977 Biochemical hypotheses of effective disorders. In: Barchas, Berger, Ciaranello, Elliott (eds) Psychopharmacology. Oxford University Press, London
Bradley P B, Dhawan B N (ed) 1976 Drugs and central synaptic transmission. MacMillan, London
Costa E, Trabucchi M (ed) 1978 The endorphins. Raven Press, New York
Cox B, Morris I D, Weston A H (ed) 1978 Pharmacology of the hypothalamus. MacMillan, London
Curtis D R, Johnston G A R 1974 Amino acid transmitters in the central nervous system. Rev. Physiol. 69: 97
Hughes J (ed) 1978 Centrally acting peptides. MacMillan, London
Iversen L L, Snyder S H Handbook of psychopharmacology vol. 1-14. Plenum Press, New York
Jouvet M 1972 The role of monoamines and acetylcholine containing neurones in the regulation of the sleep-waking cycle. Rev. Physiol. 64: 166
Moruzzi G 1972 The sleep-waking cycle. Rev. Physiol. 64: 2
Niewenhujs R, Voogd J, van Huijzen C 1978 The human central nervous system: synopsis and atlas. Springer, Berlin

18. Central depressants: hypnotics and tranquillisers

Barbiturates 243; Other hypnotics 46; Benzodiazepines 248; Meprobramate 251; Phenothiazines 252; Haloperidol 256; Reserpine 256.

The terms central depressant and central stimulant cannot be sharply defined since many centrally acting drugs have both depressant and stimulant actions, the particular effect observed depending on the site and function investigated and frequently on the dose used. Drugs such as chlorpromazine and imipramine have many common pharmacological properties and relatively few qualitatively different properties, yet one is considered a major tranquilliser and the other an antidepressant and they will be discussed in separate chapters. The distinction in this case, between depressant and stimulant, is essentially based on the fact that in clinical use chlorpromazine and imipramine represent drugs with different therapeutic effects.

In the first section of this chapter typical hypnotics, for example barbiturates and related drugs and *minor tranquillisers* such as benzodiazepines and meprobramate will be discussed. Notwithstanding traditional nomenclature, both groups of drugs have hypnotic properties and the benzodiazepines are now frequently used in preference to the barbiturates to induce sleep. There are nevertheless important differences between these drugs in their mechanism of action, which will be emphasised in the course of this discussion. An important practical distinction is that the barbiturates depress strongly the medullary centres of respiration and circulation and in overdose are therefore much more likely to produce lethal effects.

In the second section, a number of compounds which include chlorpromazine and haloperidol are collectively described as *major tranquillisers* and are used for the treatment of psychotic illness, in contrast to the minor tranquillisers used in the treatment of neuroses.

HYPNOTICS

Barbiturates

Barbitone was the first of this series of powerful hypnotics to be used; it was introduced in 1903 by Fischer and v. Mering under the name veronal. The theoretical reaction involved in the formation of barbituric acid from malonic acid and urea is shown below:

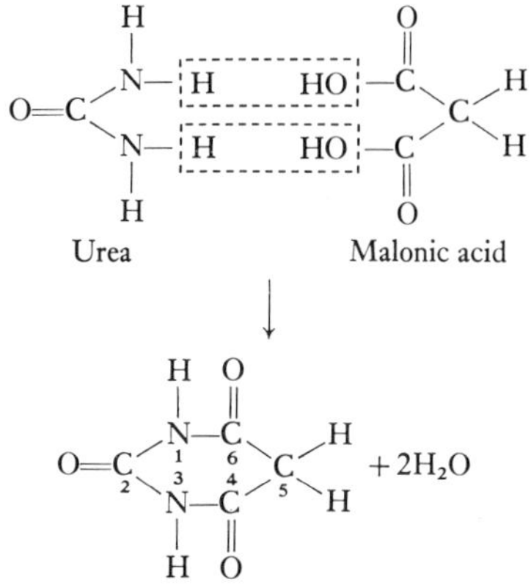

Barbituric acid is not a central depressant. The barbiturate series of drugs arises from substitution of other radicals for hydrogens at the C5 position in the basic barbiturate structure. These compounds are referred to as oxybarbiturates. A further series of compounds, the thiobarbiturates, is formed by substituting the C = O group in position 2 by C = S. The thiobarbiturates are mainly used for intravenous anaesthesia.

Hundreds of derivatives of barbituric acid are known, but this number is a very small fraction of the possible variations. A large amount of research has been carried out to determine the relative merits of the numerous derivatives of barbituric acid. The potency of the barbiturates gradually increases as the length of the alkyl side chain is increased, and reaches a maximum with the amyl compounds. Compounds with longer or branched side chains often have convulsant properties.

Absorption and fate
Barbiturates are readily absorbed from the gastrointestinal tract and they can be administered by mouth or by rectum. A considerable proportion of an oral dose may be destroyed by the liver, hence the same dose of barbiturate produces a much greater effect when given intravenously than when given by mouth. For example, 200 mg pentobarbitone sodium produces anaesthesia when administered intravenously, but when given by mouth it merely produces drowsiness and sleep.

The barbiturates can penetrate the intracellular, as well as the extracellular, fluid compartments of the body. The thiobarbiturates have the peculiarity of accumulating rapidly in the lipid phase. This has two consequences: they penetrate rapidly into brain cells and they also accumulate in fatty tissue; there is no evidence that barbiturates accumulate preferentially in any particular part of the brain.

Duration of action. The barbiturates are broken down by microsomal enzyme systems in the liver and their duration of action depends largely on the ease of oxidation of their side chains. Their rate of breakdown varies: half-destruction of phenobarbitone takes over twenty-four hours whilst half-destruction of hexobarbitone occurs in about five hours. Barbitone is peculiar in that it is not broken down in the body and is excreted unchanged in the urine.

Since barbiturates are weak acids their rate of excretion by the kidney depends on pH. When the urine is acid phenobarbitone is partly undissociated and reabsorbed by the tubules; when the urine is alkaline it dissociates and is excreted.

The barbiturates are often classified into very short, medium and long-acting drugs. The very short-acting barbiturates are used as intravenous anaesthetics (p. 303). For the rest, their classification is based on their known rates of metabolism and on evidence from animal experiments, but it has been difficult to provide reliable quantitative evidence of differences in time course under clinical conditions. It is nevertheless possible to demonstrate differences in time course under standardised experimental conditions in man.

The experiments shown in Figure 18.1 were conducted on normal subjects who received doses of phenobarbitone and quinalbarbitone on an empty stomach. The plan of the assay was balanced so that each subject received two doses of drug on different occasions. The intensity of action of the barbiturates was measured by a method which depends on the property of barbiturates to decrease the smooth tracking response when the eye follows a moving target. Figure 18.1 shows that there is a clear distinction between the two drugs, the effect of phenobarbitone being relatively less intense and more prolonged than that of quinalbarbitone.

Biochemical effects

Since the early work of Quastel which showed that barbiturates inhibit the oxygen consumption of brain tissue *in vitro*, it has been generally considered that these drugs produce their depressant effects by interfering with respiratory enzymes. This is confirmed by *in vivo* evidence that the oxygen consumption of the brain during barbiturate anaesthesia is diminished whilst during normal sleep it is unchanged.

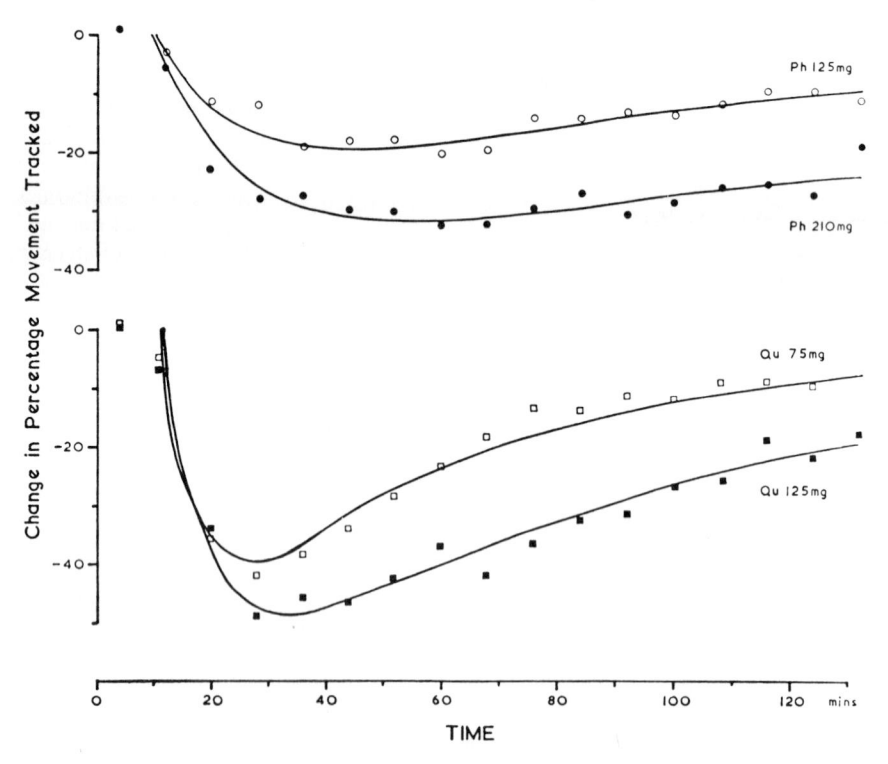

Fig. 18.1 Tissue concentrations of two barbiturates estimated from their effects on eye movements. See text. Note differences in time-action curves of phenobarbitone (Ph) and quinalbarbitone (Qu). (Data kindly supplied by H. Norris.)

Later work has shown that the inhibition of oxygen consumption by barbiturates is not peculiar to brain cells; other cells, e.g. liver cells are similarly affected probably due to inhibition of an early step in the respiratory chain involving coenzyme I and flavoprotein.

Table 18.1 The chemical relationships of the barbiturates and thiobarbiturates

where R is

$$O=C\begin{matrix}N-C\\N-C\end{matrix}C$$

where R^1 is

$$S=C\begin{matrix}N-C\\N-C\end{matrix}C$$

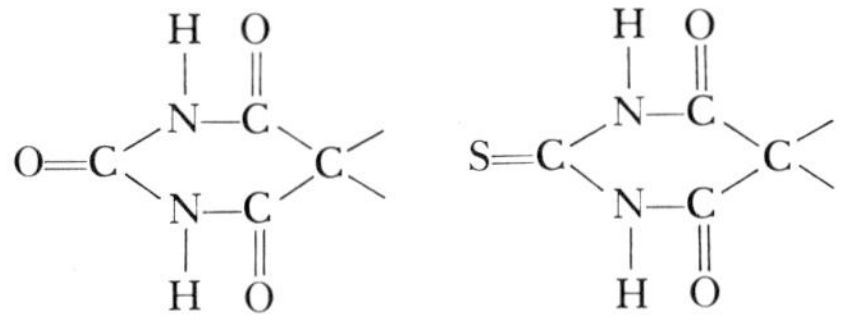

Formula	Name	Hypnotic dose (mg) oral or im	Duration of action
R⟨ethyl, ethyl	Barbitone (Veronal) Barbitone sodium (Medinal)	300–600	Long
R⟨ethyl, phenyl	Phenobarbitone (Luminal) Phenobarbitone sodium (Luminal Sodium)	60–120	Long
R⟨ethyl, phenyl; N—methyl	Methylphenobarbitone (Phemitone)	60–200	Long
R⟨allyl, allyl	Allobarbitone (Dial)	60–200	Medium
R⟨ethyl, isoamyl	Amylobarbitone (Amytal) Amylobarbitone sodium (Amytal Sodium)	100–300	Medium
R⟨ethyl, methyl butyl	Pentobarbitone (Nembutal) Pentobarbitone sodium (Nembutal Sodium)	100–200	Medium
R⟨ethyl, butyl	Butobarbitone Butobarbitone sodium	60–120	Medium
R⟨allyl, methyl butyl	Quinalbarbitone sodium (Seconal Sodium)	100–200	Medium
R⟨ethyl, cyclohexenyl	Cyclobarbitone (Phanodorm)	200–400	Medium
		Anaesthesia induction dose (mg) i.v.	
R⟨methyl, cyclohexenyl; N—methyl	Hexobarbitone sodium (Evipan Sodium)	200–400	Ultra-short
R⟨methyl allyl, methyl pentynyl	Methohexitone sodium (Brevital Sodium)	50–100	Ultra-short
R¹⟨ethyl, methyl butyl	Thiopentone sodium (Pentothal Sodium)	75–150	Ultra-short

Electrophysiological effects

Larrabee has shown that barbiturates act preferentially on synapses, inhibiting ganglionic transmission in concentrations in which total oxygen consumption is unaffected. This suggests a primary effect on excitable membranes, as is also suggested by McIlwain's finding that barbiturates depress the extra oxygen uptake of brain slices produced by electrical stimulation more than their resting oxygen consumption. Bartiturates may interfere with the enzyme processes connected with the transport of cations through cell membranes.

There is evidence that barbiturates have a specific depressant action on arousal mechanisms in the brain stem reticular formation and this is believed to be the basis of their sedative, hypnotic and anasthetic effects. This action of barbiturates on receptors in synapses in the brain stem reticular formation has been demonstrated by applying pentobarbitone iontophoretically to neurones in the reticular formation and thus inhibiting their spontaneous electrical activity.

Although the brain stem reticular formation is particularly sensitive to barbiturates, other neurones are also affected, e.g. neurones in the hypothalamus and in the medulla.

Pharmacological actions

The outstanding action of these compounds is a depression of the central nervous system; any degree of depression may be obtained from mild sedation to complete anaesthesia. These various effects can be produced by almost any barbiturate, depending on dose and method of administration. The barbiturates differ, however, in the onset and duration of their effect and for this reason the choice of a particular compound will depend on the therapeutic action required.

Long-acting barbiturates generally have slow onset of action and pass slowly from blood to brain. Phenobarbitone is uniquely effective for treating epilepsy (p. 269) and is also used for maintaining prolonged sedation, although benzodiazepines are increasingly used for this purpose.

Barbiturates with *short* and *intermediate* duration of action are more rapidly metabolised and much less dependent on renal excretion for elimination. They are used as hypnotics, for preanaesthetic sedation and for obstetric analgesia and amnesia, although increasingly supplanted by benzodiazepines in these various indications.

Some individuals find barbiturate-induced sleep as refreshing as natural sleep, others wake up with a hangover, but in either case mental performance tests indicate some impairment lasting for six to eight hours after a hypnotic dose of a barbiturate.

A characteristic feature of barbiturate-induced sleep in man is that the proportion of REM sleep (p. 237) is reduced, but if the administration of barbiturate is continued tolerance develops and the duration of REM sleep becomes restored. The opposite phenomenon happens when barbiturates are withdrawn from an addict. Withdrawal is followed by an increased duration and intensity of REM sleep and the patient may fall into the paradoxical phase at the very onset of sleep. These changes are not, however, specifically characteristic of barbiturates; similar changes in the sleep pattern occur after the withdrawal of alcohol from an addict.

These drugs are usually prepared as tablets or capsules, and when taken by mouth produce drowsiness within about half an hour. The sodium salts are more rapidly absorbed and act more quickly. Barbiturates are liable to cause confusion in elderly patients.

Analgesia. The barbiturates do not produce experimentally demonstrable analgesia and in severe pain they may aggravate conditions by producing restlessness and delirium. Nevertheless clinical studies have shown that hypnotic doses of barbiturates help to relieve moderate pain, presumably by diminishing the anxiety and fear associated with pain and by inducing drowsiness and sleep.

Intravenous anaesthesia

The ultrashort-acting barbiturates thiopentone and methohexitone given as their sodium salts are powerful intravenous induction agents causing rapid loss of consciousness. Since the barbiturates have little analgesic activity they are seldom used alone for anaesthesia except for brief minor operations. These drugs produce little muscular relaxation and may not abolish superficial reflexes. They cause pronounced respiratory depression after a rapid injection. Transient hypotension, coughing and laryngeal spasm may occur during induction of anaesthesia with barbiturates. Intra-arterial injection of barbiturates may cause tissue necrosis and gangrene. Intravenous barbiturate anaesthesia is further discussed on page 303.

Use in psychotherapy. Doses of barbiturates just short of those which produce complete unconsciousness are often used in psychotherapy. Intravenous administration of amylobarbitone sodium is used for analysis and therapy to allow patients to recall and relate experiences which are normally hidden from consciousness.

Other hypnotic drugs

The chemical structure of some non-barbiturate hypnotics is shown in Figure 18.2.

Paraldehyde

This cyclic ether (Fig. 18.2) is a safe but unpleasant hypnotic. It is used in the treatment of alcohol withdrawal and also as anticonvulsant in status epilepticus. The drug

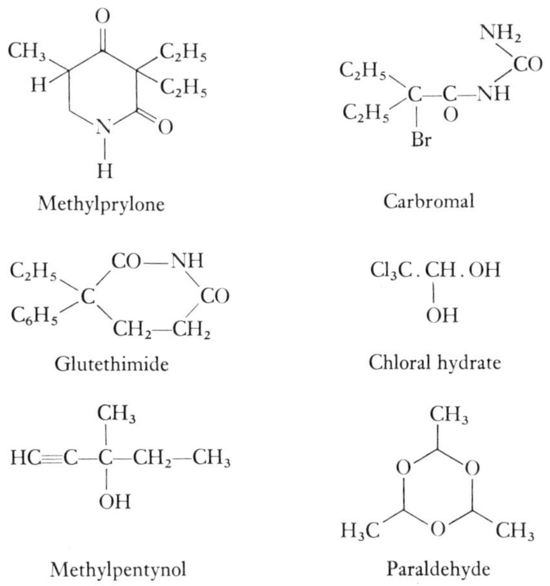

Fig. 18.2 Chemical structures of non-barbiturate hypnotics.

is partly excreted by the lungs, and therefore makes the breath smell, and this limits its use as sedative-hypnotic in general practice.

Chloral hydrate
This drug was the first synthetic hypnotic to be used (Liebreich, 1869) and immediately attained a great popularity. In consequence of a somewhat indiscriminate use, all the possible dangers associated with the drug were rapidly discovered but critical observers consider that chloral hydrate is as safe as, or safer than, most of the new hypnotics. Chloralhydrate is useful as a rapidly acting hypnotic for children.

Chloralhydrate is irritating to the stomach and to avoid vomiting it must be well diluted with water. It is not fully metabolised in the body, but in the liver it is reduced to an alcohol trichloroethanol which is paired with glycuronic acid to form urochoralic acid, an inert compound that is excreted rapidly.

The irritant properties of chloral hydrate have led to the introduction of closely related but less irritant compounds as hypnotics.

Triclofos (tricloryl) is an ester of trichloroethanol, the active metabolite of chloral hydrate. It is a useful hypnotic in doses of 0.5–2 g.

Chloral betain is a chemical complex of chloral hydrate and betaine, whilst *dichloralphenazone* (welldorm) is a complex of chloral hydrate and phenazone (antipyrin). Phenazone is a pyrazolone derivative closely related to amidopyrine, which may in rare cases cause blood dyscrasias.

Carbromal (Adalin)
This compound is a weak hypnotic; it is a monoureide which contains bromine. It was introduced with the idea that it would have the sedative properties of the bromide ion combined with the hypnotic properties of ureides. However, although some inorganic bromide is liberated during its metabolism the amount is too small to play any part in the action of the drug.

Glutethimide (Doriden)
Phenylethyl glutarimide is chemically related to phenobarbitone from which it differs in the structure of the heterocyclic ring (Fig. 18.2) It is a rapidly acting hypnotic which acts for about six hours and has few after-effects. The usual hypnotic dose of glutethimide is 500 mg and this produces about the same hypnotic effect as 200 mg cyclobarbitone.

Glutethimide occasionally produces nausea and skin rashes. Large doses have caused fatal depression of respiration and circulatory collapse. Long-term use may give rise to psychological and physical dependence.

Methylprylone (Nodular) is another sedative drug with an action comparable to that of a short-acting barbiturate. It is used as a sedative and as a hypnotic. It may give rise to dependence.

Methylpentynol (Oblivon). This compound is an unsaturated higher alcohol. It is a colourless liquid with an unpleasant taste which is administered in capsules or as an elixir. Methylpentynol is rapidly absorbed from the alimentary tract and almost completely metabolised in the body. It has sedative and hypnotic actions but, like the barbiturates, methylpentynol has little analgesic action. It is chiefly used as a sedative to allay anxiety in the early stages of labour or in children prior to anaesthesia for tonsillectomy. It is also used to relieve tension in mild anxiety states. The usual dose is 0.25–0.5 g as a sedative and 0.5–1 g as a hypnotic. Large doses produce toxic effects similar to those of an overdose of alcohol. Prolonged use may lead to dependence.

Methaqualone is a quinazolone derivative. It is a hypnotic similar in action to short-acting barbiturates, and the patient wakes free from hangover. Dependence to it has been reported. *Mandrax* is a combination of methaqualone and the antihistamine drug diphen-hydramine (p. 96). It is a hypnotic with a very rapid action which appears to have considerable dependence liability.

Promethazine (Phenergan) and other H_1-anti-histamine drugs (p. 96) have been shown experimentally to prolong barbiturate anaesthesia in animals. In many patients they act as mild hypnotics especially in children and old persons, in whom they produce sound sleep with the minimum of after-effects.

Relative merits of hypnotics

It is difficult to estimate the relative merits of hypnotics; there is a general tendency to overvalue the newer hypnotics and to undervalue the older ones. All the dangers associated with the use of the old hypnotics are well known, and no commercial interest is particularly concerned in pressing their merits. On the other hand, a considerable time is bound to elapse before the possible dangers of a new hypnotic are recognised.

It seems fairly certain that addiction may be formed to any aliphatic hypnotic and the frequency with which this occurs for any particular hypnotic depends chiefly on the frequency with which the drug is used.

Sedative-hypnotic drug dependence
This ranges all the way from patients who use their prescribed hypnotic drug during the day, to reduce anxiety to cases of severe barbiturate addiction with dangerous withdrawal symptoms as discussed on page 484. It is now considered that most sedative-hypnotics may, after prolonged self-administration, induce psychological and physical dependence producing a state of euphoria and intoxication resembling alcohol. Only a few milder sedatives, such as antihistamines, do not seem to produce dependence. The benzodiazepines have in general not been notable as drugs of abuse, although cases of diazepam dependence are becoming more frequent. Amongst barbiturates, the shorter acting drugs with rapid onset of action are most likely to produce dependence whilst phenobarbitone is not. Some non-barbiturate hypnotics such as methaqualone (mandrax) and glutethimide have considerable abuse potential.

Poisoning by sedative-hypnotics
This may arise from an accidental overdose, but most frequently from attempted suicide which is increasing in frequency. It is estimated that over 100 000 cases of self-poisoning requiring emergency admission to a hospital ward have occurred in Great Britain during 1976. The pattern of drugs taken in these suicide attempts has changed: the use of barbiturates is declining whilst that of benzodiazepines, tricyclic antidepressants and paracetamol is increasing. Aspirin intoxication has remained common.

Treatment of sedative-hypnotic poisoning. The 'Scandinavian' method is now generally employed, whilst the use of analeptics has practically ceased. It was previously considered that it is essential to use in an unconscious patient an analeptic such as picrotoxin, bemigride or leptazol which restores consciousness at least temporarily. By contrast the present scheme of treatment relies mainly on adequate ventilation and the administration of oxygen. The patient is intubated with an endotracheal tube and is given 6 to 7 litres of oxygen per minute; when there is dehydration or peripheral circulatory failure 5 per cent dextrose, normal saline or whole blood is administered intravenously. Excretion of drug in the urine can be hastened by administration of a rapidly acting diuretic such as frusemide. Methods of haemodialysis or haemoperfusion may also be used.

The use of tranquillisers to promote sleep
The barbiturates and most of the other hypnotics are depressants of the central nervous system which in small doses cause sedation, in moderate doses sleep and in large doses general anaesthesia. The barbiturates act primarily on the reticular formation but in larger doses cause a profound depression of the vital centres in the medulla and carry the risk of respiratory failure.

An important advance has been the introduction of benzodiazepine compounds such as diazepam and flurazepam which are effective hypnotics but with a different mode of action from the barbiturates. The differences between these two types of drugs are by no means fully understood. One of the most obvious differences is lack of respiratory depression by the benzodiazepines. Another is their relative lack of direct depression of the reticular formation. On the other hand, the benzodiazepines produce marked depression and effects on the limbic system and they have strong muscle relaxing effects. It has been suggested that in contrast to the barbiturates which depress the reticular formation directly, they 'shield' the reticular formation by cutting it off from emotional stimuli, and thus cause sleep.

THE MINOR TRANQUILLISERS

This group comprises a number of drugs used for the treatment of neuroses, particularly pathological anxiety. In their sedative clinical effects they resemble the barbiturates but differ from them in having a wider therapeutic ratio. The various members of this group do not necessarily have a common mechanism of action but they are grouped together because they are employed for similar clinical conditions.

Benzodiazepines
The chemical structures of three representative drugs of this group: chlordiazepoxide (Librium), diazepam (Valium) and nitrazepam (Mogadon) are shown in Figure 18.3. A number of other benzodiazepines have been introduced into clinical practice including oxazepam (Serenide-D) and flurazepam (Dalmane). Although their overall pharmacological actions are similar, they differ in relative potency in regard to particular activities; thus diazepam is more active than chlordiazepoxide in causing muscular relaxation and sleep.

Pharmacological activity
Figure 18.4 shows a comparison of LD50 and ED50 values of diazepam and phenobarbitone in mice, indicating the ED50 values for various parameters. There are striking differences between the two drugs in the much higher therapeutic ratios (LD50/ED50) with diazepam on all parameters.

Muscle relaxant property
This is one of the most readily observable properties of this group of drugs. Figure 18.5 shows this effect in a decerebrate cat during passive stretching of its triceps muscle. The tension-extension diagram shows that the amount of tension for a given degree of stretch is greatly reduced after administration of diazepam. This effect is exerted partly at spinal level since benzodiazepines inhibit polysynaptic spinal reflexes. The main effect, however, is probably due to a depression, exerted at brain stem level, of gamma activity originating from muscle spindles.

This type of relaxant effect also occurs in man and it has been suggested that part of the 'calming' effect of these drugs is brought about by damping the excessive activity of brain stem neurones that exaggerate the discharge of gamma motoneurones in conditions of 'tenseness' and anxiety.

Taming effect
Benzodiazepines have a pronounced effect in reducing aggressive behaviour in animals, as when mice are induced to fight by weak electric shocks applied to the floor of the

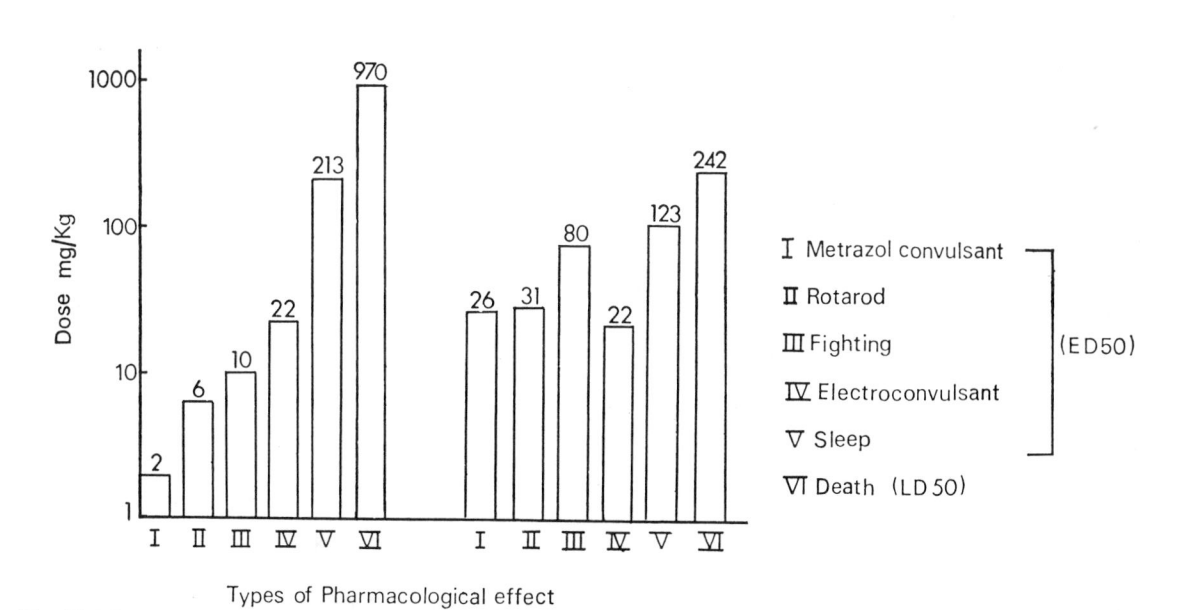

Fig. 18.3 Chemical structures of typical benzodiazepines.

Benzodiazepines are highly lipid soluble and are rapidly absorbed from the gastrointestinal tract. They are largely degraded in the body, in some cases to pharmacologically active metabolites. Their rates of elimination are slow; plasma half lives are of the order of 24 hours. They are strongly bound to plasma proteins.

Fig. 18.4 Comparison of doses (logarithmic scale) required to produce effects in mice with diazepam and phenobarbitone. In each case the LD50 (VI) is shown as well as the ED50 for various parameters (I-IV = antagonism to metrazol convulsion, rotarod, fighting and electroconvulsion; V = hypnotic effect). Note much bigger LD50/ED50 ratios (therapeutic ratio) for diazepam on all parameters. (After Randall and Keppell, 1973. In: The benzodiazepines. Raven Press, New York.)

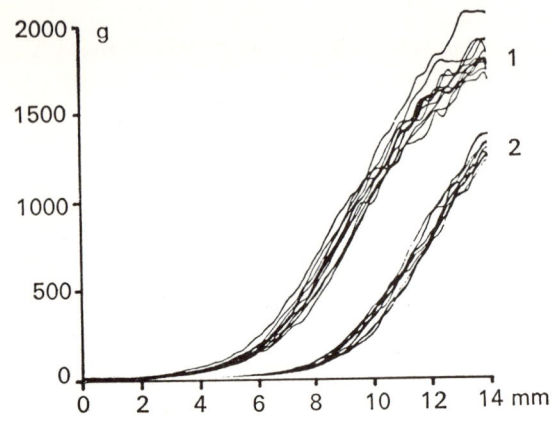

Fig. 18.5 Effect of diazepam on the tension-extension diagram of the triceps surae muscle of a decerebrate cat. Ordinate: active tension (g) abscissa: length of muscle extension (mm). (1) Curves before and (2) after administration of diazepam (0.5 mg/kg). (After Brausch, Henatsch, Student and Takano, 1973. In The Benzodiazepines, Raven Press, New York.)

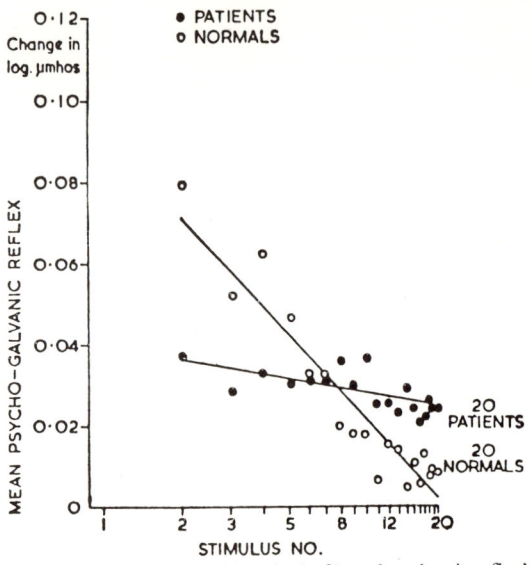

Fig. 18.6 Rate of decline (habituation) of 'psychogalvanic reflex' in patients with anxiety and in normal controls. The reflex was elicited by a brief sound emitted at approximately 1 min intervals. (After Lader and Wing, 1964. *J. Neurolsurg. Psychiat.*, Lond.).

cage or when rats are rendered vicious by septal lesions. The taming effects occur with smaller doses than the muscle relaxant effects.

Another characteristic reaction in animals, of all minor tranquillisers, is that they inhibit conditioned escape responses but not the unconditioned responses unless extremely high doses are used. This discrepancy also applies to the major tranquillisers but it is less pronounced.

Anti-anxiety effect
Whilst reduction of anxiety is probably the main purpose for which these drugs are used clinically, anti-anxiety effects cannot be readily measured in animals. Often indirect approaches are used such as a reduction of gastric ulcer formation in immobilised rats, which is supposed to be due to stress and anxiety.

An attempt to utilise a parameter which is closely related to anxiety in man to measure the effects of anti-anxiety drugs is discussed on page 24. The method is based on the psychogalvanic reflex (PGR) consisting of a transient reduction of the skin resistance following an alerting stimulus. As shown in Figure 18.6, in normal subjects the PGR diminishes on repetition of an alerting stimulus but fails to do so in patients with anxiety states. Drugs which reduce anxiety also increase the rate of habituation of the PGR and this may be used as the basis of a quantitative bioassay of antianxiety drugs (p. 24). In tests of this kind, chlordiazepoxide was found to be about seven times as active, weight for weight, as amylobarbitone.

Whilst the electrophysiological basis of the antianxiety effect of benzodiazepines is not fully understood, it is believed to involve the limbic system of the brain which is supposed to be concerned with the emotions (p. 238). It has been shown that electrical responses in one part of this system, the hippocampus, induced by stimulation of another part, the amygdala, are reduced after the systemic administration of diazepam.

Anticonvulsant activity
Benzodiazepines have strong anticonvulsant effects, particularly against pharmacologically induced convulsions e.g. by metrazol, but also against electrically induced convulsions. They do not act on the seizure focus but inhibit the spread of the seizure.

Benzodiazepines are used in the treatment of epilepsy (p. 273); diazepam is very effective when given by intravenous injection in status epilepticus. Nitrazepam has been used in myoclonic epilepsy. The benzodiazepines are seldom given orally for the control of epileptic seizures, since the blood levels thus achieved are insufficient.

Sedative and hypnotic effects
All benzodiazepines have sedative and hypnotic activities and some, including diazepam and flurazepam, have proved highly effective hypnotics. Their hypnotic activities in man have been studied in specialised 'sleep laboratories' in which subjects are kept for several weeks whilst their sleep patterns are monitored by electroencephalographic, electromyographic and electro-oculographic recording. As a rule, periods of several nights with and without drug are alternated. Normal controls and patients suffering from insomnia are investigated.

These studies have shown the benzodiazepines to be amongst the most satisfactory hypnotics. In common with other hypnotics they shorten the relative duration of REM sleep, but rather less so than the barbiturates, thus preserving a more nearly normal sleep pattern. They also seem to exhibit less REM rebound after withdrawal. Their overall effect is to reduce the delay in falling asleep, diminish waking periods and increase total sleeping time. A characteristic change in sleep pattern appears to be a reduction of the duration of slow wave (stage 4) sleep.

Single doses of 15 mg flurazepam produced a greater hypnotic effect on the second and third night suggesting some carry-over. Patients who complain of insomnia often underestimate their sleeping time. Figure 18.7 shows that only patients who slept less than six hours derived appreciable benefit from hypnotic drugs.

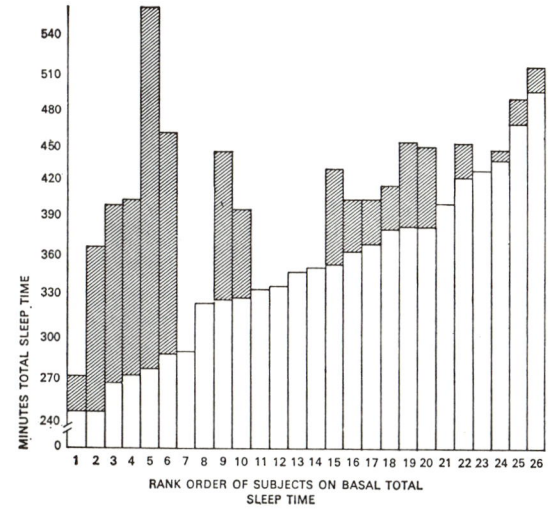

Fig. 18.7 Total sleep times in persons who believed they suffered from insomnia. Control nights: unshaded areas; drug nights (in most cases flurazepam): shaded areas. Only subjects who slept less than six hours derived substantial benefit from the hypnotic drug. (After Dement, Zarcone, Hoddes, Smythe and Carskadon, 1973. In The Benzodiazepines. Raven Press, New York.)

Benzodiazepines are much less addictive than barbiturates. Patients who depend on barbiturates often complain that they cannot sleep without drugs or that they have difficulty in sleeping even whilst they take drugs. In such patients barbiturates should be slowly withdrawn to avoid the serious effects of rapid withdrawal.

Other clinical applications
Benzodiazepines are increasingly used in anaesthesia. Diazepam has been used orally for premedication in children, in whom it produces a calming effect without the drowsiness of conventional sedatives. It has also been used intravenously for the induction of anaesthesia. Although, unlike the intravenous barbiturates, it may not produce full unconsciousness, it causes much less respiratory and circulatory depression. It is now often used by intravenous administration in dentistry.

An important use of benzodiazepines is in the management of alcohol withdrawal symptoms and delirium tremens. These drugs calm the patient promptly and effectively and also have anticonvulsant activity; and they are unlikely to create physical or psychological dependence. The benzodiazepines are thus suited for the type of drug support needed during alcohol withdrawal which must accompany psychotherapeutic and social measures of rehabilitation.

Toxic effects
The benzodiazepines are relatively non-toxic and this is an important reason for their widespread use. They cause relatively little depression of the vital centres of the medulla and instances of successful suicide with these drugs are rare.

Their most common untoward effects are drowsiness, lethargy, muscle weakness and ataxia. Large doses may cause fainting. These effects are particularly likely to occur in elderly patients. When given to psychotic patients chlordiazepoxide may paradoxically cause attacks of rage and confusion. By their sedative effects these drugs are dangerous to drivers, especially when alcohol is also taken. Dependence on benzodiazepines has been reported.

Meprobamate
Anxiety states are generally associated with an increase in muscle tension and this had led to the suggestion that muscle-relaxing drugs may help to allay anxiety. Several attempts have been made to relieve anxiety states with mephenesin, but this drug is not effective because of its short duration of action and irregular absorption from the gastrointestinal tract. Berger, who introduced mephenesin, made a search for other internuncial blocking drugs with longer duration of action and fewer side effect. In 1954 he described meprobamate as the most effective compound amongst a large number of substances investigated.

$$\begin{array}{c} H_3C \\ \diagdown \\ C(CH_2OCONH_2)_2 \\ \diagup \\ C_3H_7 \end{array}$$

Meprobamate

Pharmacological effects
They resemble in some aspects those of the benzodiazepines. Meprobamate is a spinal interneurone blocker and has considerable muscle relaxant activity. It also causes sedation. It has much less animal taming effect than the benzodiazepines: the doses required are higher than those causing muscle relaxation; it has less anticonvulsant activity than benzodiazepines.

Clinical effects
Meprobamate was the first widely used tranquilliser which competed successfully with the barbiturates in the treatment of anxiety and other neuroses. It soon became apparent that it had no place in the treatment of psychoses. It was noted that its antianxiety effect was more closely related to its muscle relaxant action than to its sedative hypnotic action.

Meprobamate diminishes autonomic reflexes and this may be an important facet of its antianxiety effect since one of the physical manifestations of anxiety is an exaggeration of autonomic reflexes.

Meprobamate is used in anxiety states and as a sedative and hypnotic. Patients who are anxious and tense become more relaxed and calmer during the day and sleep better at night, but many patients are disturbed by the muscular weakness and lassitude produced by this drug. It is sometimes used in petit mal epilepsy for its anticonvulsant action and as a central skeletal muscle relaxant.

Undesirable effects. A common untoward reaction is drowsiness. On the other hand cases of extreme excitement have been reported during treatment with this drug. Skin rashes and other hypersensitivity reactions may occur.

The acute ingestion of large doses produces unconsciousness and coma but attempts to commit suicide with meprobamate are rarely successful.

A serious danger of meprobamate and similar drugs is its additive effect with alcohol in impairing driving skills. Another risk is that of drug dependence shown by the compulsive use of the drug and withdrawal symptoms including convulsions when its administration is suddenly discontinued.

Other minor tranquillisers

A variety of drugs other than benzodiazepines or meprobamate have central depressant and antianxiety activities. *Hydroxyzine (Atarax)* which is related to the H_1-antihistamine diphenhydramine has central nervous system depressant and anti-histaminic activities and is frequently used as a minor tranquilliser for surgical premedication.

THE MAJOR TRANQUILLISERS

During recent years a group of depressants of mental activity has been introduced into psychiatric practice, collectively referred to as tranquillisers.

The term is pragmatic, relating to their use in 'tranquillising' patients with psychotic or neurotic illnesses. This group is usually subdivided into major and minor tranquillisers according to whether their main use is for the treatment of psychoses or neuroses.

Chlorpromazine and related phenothiazines

Chlorpromazine (Largactil), like the antihistamine drug promethazine (p. 96) is a phenothiazine derivative (Fig. 18.10). It was discovered in a search for a phenothiazine with strong central and little antihistamine activity. The new drug was given the name largactil because of its large number of pharmacological actions.

The discovery that chlorpromazine is effective in schizophrenia was made by Delay and his colleagues in France in 1952. They noted that it reduced agitation and confusion without causing excessive sedation and called this type of action 'neuroleptic'. Later work has confirmed that chlorpromazine has a distinct central action which is different from that of a merely sedative drug.

Pharmacological effects in animals

In the early stages it was considered that the central activity of chlorpromazine-like drugs could be assessed by their effect in prolonging barbiturate sleeping time, but later work showed that this was a measure of their sedative, rather than their antipsychotic effect, and that derivatives which did not prolong barbiturate sleeping time and which had little sedative action, were nevertheless effective in psychotic patients.

A more relevant measure of the tranquillising effect of these drugs can be obtained by studying their ability to counteract conditioned and unconditioned stimuli. In pole-climbing experiments with rats (Fig. 18.8) chlorpromazine reduces the response to a bell (conditioned stimulus) before reducing that to an electric shock (unconditioned stimulus) whereas barbiturates are more likely to reduce both responses simultaneously.

Chlorpromazine differs from barbiturates in its effect on the brain stem reticular formation. Bradley observed that potentials in the cortex following direct stimulation of the reticular formation are not affected by chlorpromazine,

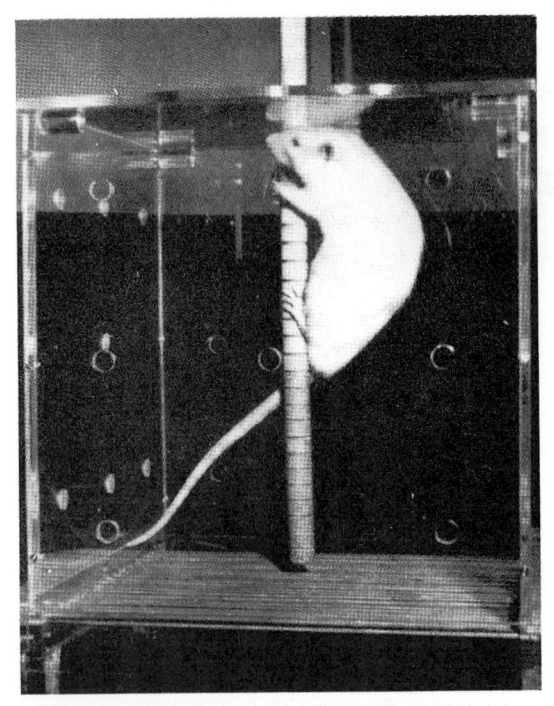

Fig. 18.8 Pole-climbing response. The floor is made of steel rods through which electric shocks are delivered which the animal avoids by climbing up a wooden pole. (After Cook and Weidley, 1957, *Ann. N.Y. Acad. Sci.*)

but depressed by barbiturates. He concluded that chlorpromazine lacks the direct depressant effect on the reticular formation seen with barbiturates. Potentials recorded in the reticular formation following peripheral stimulation are, however, considerably reduced by chlorpromazine. Chlorpromazine may thus have an action related to the inflow of sensory information to the reticular formation. More recent evidence suggests that chlorpromazine blocks central dopamine receptors in the corpus striatum (p. 239) in addition to blocking both peripheral and central alpha-adrenergic receptors. By preventing the normal activity of dopaminergic nerves it can thus produce extrapyramidal distrubances. The actions of phenothiazines on dopamine receptors in relation to the dopamine hypothesis of schizophrenia are discussed on page 240.

The phenothiazines diminish spontaneous motility and in larger doses cause a cataleptic syndrome in which the animals are immobile whilst their limbs can be shaped passively into various postures.

Chlorpromazine produces interneuronal block in the spinal cord by a supraspinal action. It has a powerful effect on the chemoreceptive emetic trigger zone in the medulla, and abolishes vomiting due to apomorphine (p. 194). It also lowers body temperature. Chlorpromazine has a considerable α-adrenergic blocking effect and by virtue of this and also by a central effect it tends to lower blood pressure.

Alterations in animal behaviour by chlorpromazine and related neuroleptics
The following are typical:
1. Inhibition of exploration if an animal is placed in a new environment.
2. Induction of cataleptic immobility.
3. Inhibition of conditioned avoidance response (Fig. 18.8)
4. Inhibition of intracranial self-stimulation in the reward (Olds) areas.
5. Antagonism of stereotyped (bizarre) behaviour induced by apomorphine (Fig. 18.9) or amphetamine. There is a good correlation between the anti-apomorphine and anti-amphetamine activity of neuroleptic drugs and their clinical efficacy in the therapy of schizophrenia. Apomorphine is a powerful stimulant of dopamine receptors and it is now considered likely that a disturbance in dopaminergic activity may be a contributing factor in schizophrenia as discussed further in Chapter 17.

Effects of chlorpromazine in man
When chlorpromazine is administered to man it produces first a feeling of sleepiness which is followed by a condition in which the subject lies quietly and seems indifferent to his surroundings. He does not initiate conversation but if questioned gives an appropriate reply. If submitted to tests

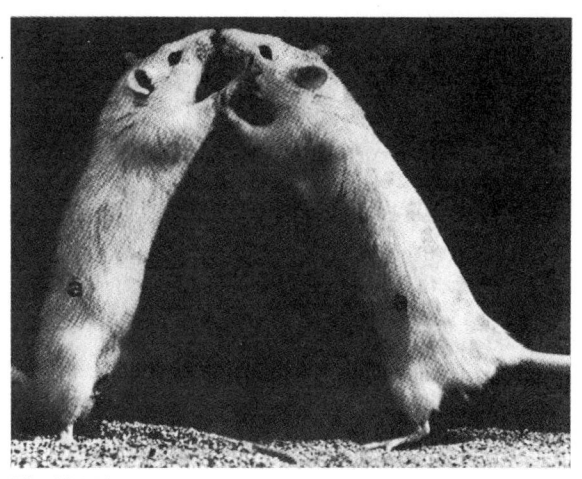

Fig. 18.9 Bizarre social interaction of male Wistor rats following 3.16 μmol/kg (= 1 mg/kg) apomorphine: effect of stimulation of dopamine receptors. (After v. Rossum, 1970, The neuroleptics. Karger, Basel.)

of intellectual function such as digit substitution he may perform normally but tests based on vigilance, such as tracking efficiency are impaired.

Chlorpromazine causes a peripheral vasodilation which increases heat loss and raises skin temperature. The normal vasoconstrictor mechanisms are impaired and the blood pressure falls when the subject is in the upright position.

Treatment of schizophrenic psychoses
The introduction of chlorpromazine and related drugs into psychiatric practice has completely changed the outlook for the treatment of schizophrenia, a disease which affects about 1 per cent of mankind. The other methods available for the treatment of schizophrenic psychoses are as follows.

Psychotherapy. This has severe limitations in this type of illness and many clinicians consider psychoanalytical treatment of a true schizophrenic psychosis to be useless or even harmful.

Treatment by hypoglycaemia. This treatment which was introduced by Sakel in Vienna (1933) consists in the production of hypoglycaemic coma by the intramuscular or intravenous injection of insulin. After about one hour the coma is terminated by an intravenous injection of glucose. This form of treatment has been shown to promote remissions of this disease but is now obsolete.

Electroconvulsion treatment. This is a specific treatment for depressions rather than for schizophrenia where it is regarded mainly as an adjunct.

Prefrontal leucotomy. The neurosurgical treatment of schizophrenia has been largely abandoned since the introduction of neuroleptic drugs and it is now used mainly as a last resort.

Drug treatment

The full effects of a neuroleptic drug given to a schizophrenic patient are seen after one or two weeks of regular medication. These drugs stabilise mood and reduce anxiety, tension and hyperactivity. They are useful in excited patients but may benefit all types of schizophrenia. They are particularly effective in countering stereotyped, repetitive movements and behaviour patterns. The most striking effects are seen in patients with acute psychoses; these drugs control agitation and aggressiveness and enable the patients to enter into activities which were previously impossible.

The basic schizophrenic symptoms of thought distortion, delusions and hallucinations are less affected than tension and excitement and in this sense neuroleptic drugs are not truly curative; nevertheless delusional symptoms are often greatly improved and may even disappear although when medication is stopped the patients frequently relapse within a few weeks.

It is now possible with the help of these drugs to allow patients who would otherwise remain in hospital to carry on with their normal activities; although readmission to hospital may become necessary, the total duration of their stay in hospital is significantly reduced and deterioration due to prolonged stay in hospital is prevented.

Other therapeutic applications of phenothiazines

Besides their use in schizophrenia the phenothiazines are also employed in other psychiatric conditions such as senile agitation and mania in which excitement predominates. The piperazine derivatives have a central stimulant action and may be given to withdrawn psychotics.

Chlorpromazine has a strong antiemetic effect and counteracts vomiting due to drugs, radiation, uraemia and pregnancy but it is relatively ineffective in motion sickness (p. 194). It may relieve an otherwise intractable hiccough. Chlorpromazine is sometimes used in tetanus because of its interneurone blocking effect and in surgery for its body-temperature lowering effects.

Administration and fate

Chlorpromazine is usually given by mouth but it can be administered by deep intramuscular injection and by suppository. Intramuscular injections may cause a fall of blood pressure and fainting. The oral dose varies over a wide range from 30 mg for mild emotional upsets to doses of 1 to 2 g per day in hospitalised psychotic patients.

Chlorpromazine is well absorbed from the gastrointestinal tract and distributed in all tissues. It is excreted in the urine largely as glucuronide or as chlorpromazine sulphoxide. Chlorpromazine is slowly eliminated from the body and in patients medicated for long periods, traces of the drug or its metabolites may be found in the urine up to several months after discontinuing administration.

Related phenothiazines

Following the introduction of chlorpromazine, various other phenothiazine derivatives have been introduced into clinical practice and used in the treatment of psychoses. Most of these newer drugs are more potent than chlorpromazine, weight for weight, but they are not necessarily better drugs since their toxicity is as a rule correspondingly increased.

The chemical structures of some clinically used phenothiazines belonging to the class of 'major tranquillisers' are shown in Figure 18.10. They can be divided into three chemical groups, differing to some extent in their pharmacological and clinical effects.

1. *Dimethylaminopropyl derivatives*. This group includes *chlorpromazine* and *promazine* (Sparine), also the more active *fluopromazine* (Triflupromazine). They have considerable sedative and hypotensive effects. In overdose they produce a Parkinsonian syndrome including tremors, rigidity and salivation.

2. *Piperazine derivatives* include the potent compound *fluphenazine* (Moditen), *perphenazine* (Fentazin) and *trifluoperazine* (Stelazine). These drugs produce rather less sedation in equiactive doses than chlorpromazine.

Because of their relative lack of sedative properties the piperazine derivatives have been used for the treatment of withdrawn apathetic patients with chronic schizophrenia who may be rendered more alert, sociable and communicative. These compounds also have a strong antiemetic action.

In large doses the piperazine derivatives cause, besides typical Parkinsonian symptoms, various dyskinetic reactions. These often involve the muscles of the face and neck including protrusion of the tongue, difficulty in speech and swallowing, oculogyric crises and torticollis. The piperazines may also cause intense motor restlessness (akathisia) with agitation and inability to sit still or sleep.

3. *Piperidine derivatives* such as *thioridazine* (Melleril). This compound rarely produces extra-pyramidal symptoms and it may be substituted for other phenothiazines when such symptoms occur. Thioridazine however causes orthostatic hypotension, dryness of the mouth and other signs of autonomic blockade. In rare cases it has produced a toxic retinitis and patients receiving it should be closely observed for signs of diminished visual acuity. Thioridazine has little or no antiemetic activity.

Untoward effects of phenothiazines

The toxic effects of phenothiazines are of two kinds, normal effects of overdosage and allergic hypersensitivity reactions. A characteristic property of phenothiazines, in which they differ from barbiturates, is their high therapeutic ratio; even very large doses are rarely fatal. In

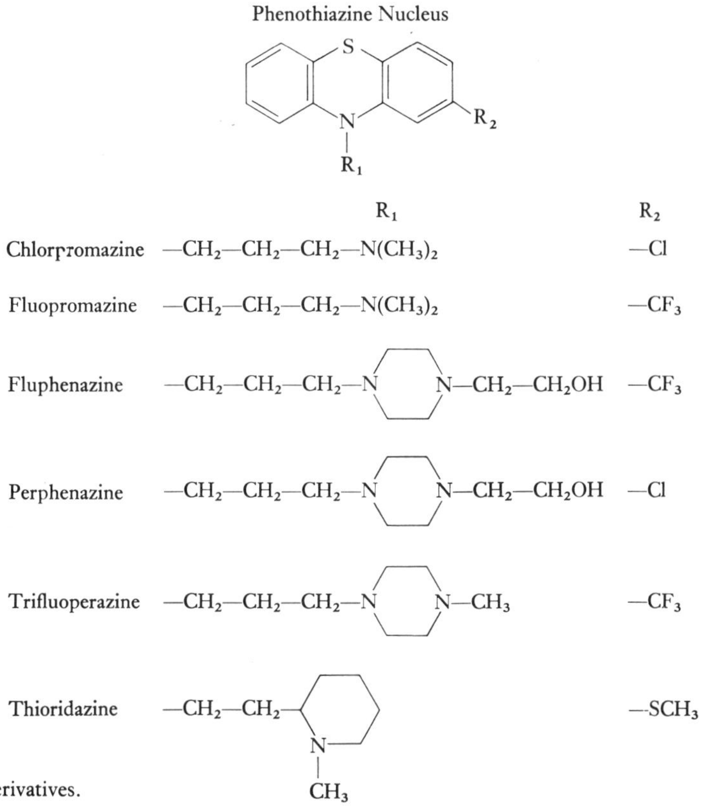

CENTRAL DEPRESSANTS: HYPNOTICS AND TRANQUILLISERS 255

Phenothiazine Nucleus

	R₁	R₂
Chlorpromazine	—CH₂—CH₂—CH₂—N(CH₃)₂	—Cl
Fluopromazine	—CH₂—CH₂—CH₂—N(CH₃)₂	—CF₃
Fluphenazine	—CH₂—CH₂—CH₂—N⟨ ⟩N—CH₂—CH₂OH	—CF₃
Perphenazine	—CH₂—CH₂—CH₂—N⟨ ⟩N—CH₂—CH₂OH	—Cl
Trifluoperazine	—CH₂—CH₂—CH₂—N⟨ ⟩N—CH₃	—CF₃
Thioridazine	—CH₂—CH₂—⟨piperidine⟩ N-CH₃	—SCH₃

Fig. 18.10 Penothiazine derivatives.

further contrast to barbiturates and other sedative-hypnotics they do not give rise to drug dependence. They do not produce ataxia, impairment of consciousness or paradoxical excitement such as may occur after a barbiturate.

The main effects of overdosage with these drugs are sedation, hypotension and extrapyramidal actions. Most patients on phenothiazines experience some degree of drowsiness, but tolerance to the sedative effect develops after a few weeks. The patients usually sleep well at night although they may experience vivid dreams.

The phenothiazines produce a variety of effects on the extrapyramidal system due to block of striatal dopamine receptors. A frequent effect is muscle weakness manifested for example by difficulty in walking. Larger doses especially of the piperazine derivatives produce Parkinsonian symptoms and akathisia. It is important to realise that uncontrollable restlessness may be brought about by a phenothiazine and that this symptom may be wrongly interpreted as an exacerbation of the psychosis and wrongly treated by increasing the dose of the drug.

Mild extrapyramidal symptoms can be controlled by anti-Parkinsonian drugs but severe reactions require a reduction of the dose or replacement by a drug such as thioridazine. The phenothiazine-induced extrapyramidal effects are normally reversible. Due to their adrenergic blocking action the phenothiazines may cause postural hypotension especially after parenteral administration. The hypotensive effect usually diminished with continued use.

Tardive dyskinesia (p. 239)
This is a drug-induced movement disorder which may occur after prolonged neuroleptic treatment and often persists after discontinuing the drug. It is characterised by repetitive pursing of lips and other choreoathetoid movements. Its possible mechanism is discussed on page . The condition occurs in older patients, particularly women and it is not alleviated by antiparkinsonian treatment. Because there are no alternative drugs for the treatment of schizophrenia, tardive dyskinesia may be unavoidable in some patients, but the lowest adequate doses of neuroleptics should be used to lower the risk of this disorder.

Allergic effects. A probably allergic reaction which occurs in a small percentage of patients on phenothiazines, often during the first few weeks of treatment, is obstructive jaundice due to a cholestatic hepatitis. This complication necessitates discontinuance of the drug. It is sometimes possible, after the jaundice has cleared, to resume medication with another phenothiazine derivative. Dangerous blood dyscrasias such as agranulocytosis may occur after chlorpromazine and other phenothiazines, but they are fortunately rare.

Haloperidol

Haloperidol is the prototype of a group of drugs with major tranquilliser or neuroleptic activity which is chemically different from the phenothiazines. Haloperidol is a butyrophenone and its structure is shown below.

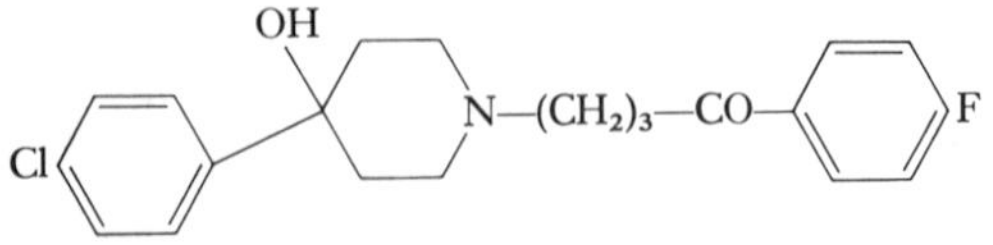

Haloperidol

Pharmacological actions

Haloperidol is a highly active neuroleptic producing all the animal effects described on page 253. Like other butyrophenones it produces a powerful block of dopamine receptors.

Clinical effects. Haloperidol is highly effective in the treatment of psychotic patients but has a relatively high incidence of extrapyramidal side effects. Haloperidol is less sedating than chlorpromazine and causes less hypotension. It also has considerable antiemetic activity. Haloperidol may be used as a substitute for phenothiazines in patients hypersensitive to phenothiazines. Haloperidol is an effective treatment in *Gille de la Tourette's* syndrome manifested by uncontrolled tics and barking cries. It has been shown to improve stuttering.

Reserpine (p. 119)

Reserpine is one of the alkaloids obtained from *Rauwolfia serpentina*, a shrub which grows in India where it has long been regarded as having medicinal properties useful in the treatment of hypertension, insomnia and insanity.

Reserpine was introduced into psychiatric practice at about the same time as chlorpromazine but it is now regarded as less efficacious and is seldom used for the treatment of schizophrenia. It is, however, still extensively studied experimentally because of its remarkable action in causing a depletion of the catecholamine and 5-HT content of the brain.

PREPARATIONS

Hypnotics sedatives and minor tranquillisers

Barbiturates
Amylobarbitone (Amytal) 100–200 mg
Amylobarbitone Sodium (Sodium Amytal) 100–200 mg
Butobarbitone (Soneryl) 100–200 mg
Cyclobarbitone Calcium (Phanodorm) 200–400 mg
Pentobarbitone Sodium (Nembutal) 100–200 mg
Phenobarbitone (Luminal, Gardenal) 30–125 mg thrice daily
Phenobarbitone Sodium (Gardenal Sodium)
Quinalbarbitone (Seconal)
Quinalbarbitone Sodium 100–200 mg

Benzodiazepines
Chlordiazepoxide (Librium) 10–100 mg daily
Diazepam (Valium) 5–30 mg daily
Flurazepam hyd (Dalmane) 15–30 mg
Lorazepam 1–10 mg daily
Medazepam (Nobrium) 15–40 mg daily
Nitrazepam (Mogadon) 2.5–10 mg
Oxazepam (Serenid-D) 10–30 mg

Other sedative-hypnotics
Chloral hydrate mixture 1 g/10 ml 0.5–2 g
Chlormethiazole Edisylate (Heminevrin) 1–2 g
Dichlorphenazone (Welldorm) 0.5–2 g
Gluthethimide (Doriden) 250–500 mg
Hydroxyzine hyd (Atarax) 25–100 mg thrice daily
Methylpentinol (Oblivon) 0.5–1 g hypn
Methyprylone (Noludar) 200–400 mg
Paraldehyde Injection 5–10 ml i.m. or p.o.
Promethazine hyd 20–50 mg (and other H_1-antihistamines)
Triclofos Sodium (Trichloryl) 0.5–2 g

Major Tranquillisers

Key: (but): butyrophenone related cpds, (phen): phenothiazines (dim): with dimethylaminopropyl side chain, (pip): with piperidine side chain, (paz): with piperazine side chain, (thiox): thioxanthenes

Benperidol (Anquil) 250 μg–1 mg but
Chlorpromazine (Largactil) 25 mg 3x daily (phen dim)
Fluphenazine (Moditen) 1–2 mg dl (phen paz)
Droperidol (Droleptan) 5–20 mg (but)
Flupenthixol (Fluanxol) 3–18 mg (thiox)
Haloperidol (Haldol) 3–9 mg daily (but)
Methotrimeprazine (Veractil) 25–50 mg daily (phen dim)
Pericyazine (Neulactil) 15–30 mg daily (phen pip)
Perphenazine (Fentazin) 12–24 mg daily (phen paz)
Prochlorperazine (Stemetil) 15–100 mg daily (phen paz)
Promazine (Sparine) 50–800 mg daily (phen dim)
Thiopropazate (Dartalan) 5–10 mg 3x daily (phen paz)
Thioridazine (Melleril) 30–600 mg daily (phen pip)
Thiothixene (Navane) 10–60 mg daily (thiox)
Trifluoperazine (Stelazine) 2–30 mg (phen paz)
Clozapine (Leponex) 150–600 mg daily (paz)

FURTHER READING

Garattini S, Mussini E, Randall L O (ed) 1973 The benzodiazepines. Raven Press, New York
Jarvik M E (ed) 1977 Psychopharmacology in the practice of medicine. Appleton, New York
Hartmann E 1978 The sleeping pill. Yale University Press.
Hollister E E 1977 Antipsychotic medication and the treatment of schizophrenia. In: Barchas et al. (eds) Psychopharmacology, Oxford University Press, London
Lader M H, Wing Lorna 1966 Physiological measures, sedative drugs and morbid anxiety. Oxford University Press, London
Oswald I 1968 Drugs and sleep Pharmacol. Rev 20:274
van Praag H M 1978 Psychotropic drugs. A guide for the practitioner. MacMillan Press, London
Wynne L C, Cromwell R L, Mathysse S (ed) 1978 The nature of schizophrenia. John Wiley, New York

19. Antidepressants and stimulants of mental activity

Depressive illness 257; Imipramine and related antidepressants 257; MAO inhibitors 260; Lithium 261; Amphetamine and related drugs 262; Amphetamine anorexia 264; Pipradrol 265; Caffeine 265; Cocaine 265; LSD 265; Mescaline 266; Cannabis 266.

Drugs which stimulate the central nervous system are used by the great majority of inhabitants of the world. The drinking of infusions of tea, coffee and maté leaves, or the chewing of guarana paste or of coca leaves have this in common that they are taken for their stimulant action on the higher centres.

Some of the most active cerebral stimulants belong to the group of sympathomimetic amines.

Although the amphetamine group of sympathomimetic drugs increase alertness and allay fatigue in normal human beings they have been found to be of little value in the treatment of clinical depression; they tend to make the depressed more restless and agitated without lifting his lowered mood. A remarkable transformation in the field of antidepressive drug treatment has occurred with the introduction in the 1950s of the monoamineoxidase (MAO) inhibitors and the imipramine-like drugs.

The newer antidepressants, particularly the 'tricyclic' imipramine-like drugs produce little overt stimulation in experimental animals and yet they have been shown, in controlled clinical trials, to counteract depressive illness in man. The analysis of the pharmacological effects of imipramine in animal experiments has proved unrewarding, their most characteristic effects occur on a biochemical level: inhibition of synaptic reuptake mechanisms for catecholamines and indoleamines. The MAO inhibitors cause central stimulation in animals particularly after the injection of the catecholamine precursor, dopa. They also cause an increase of the amine content of the brain.

Depressive illness which is sometimes classified as endogenous or reactive, though a sharp distinction cannot be made, is clinically manifested as one of the poles of manic-depressive disease. The disease may be bipolar with alternating mania and depression, or unipolar with recurrent episodes of mania or depression. The two main groups of drugs used to treat depression both facilitate central noradrenergic transmission: the tricyclics by inhibiting reuptake of NA and 5HT at neuronal nerve endings; the MAO inhibitors by increasing amine concentrations at central nerve terminals. Both drug actions fit into a unified working hypothesis according to which depressive illness represents a malfunction of central noradrenergic transmission (p. 240).

Electroconvulsive therapy
Although there is statistical evidence that drug treatment of depression, particularly by tricyclic antidepressants, is effective compared to placebo, considerable clinical evidence shows that electroconvulsive therapy (e.c.t.) is even more effective and acts more rapidly. Electroconvulsive therapy has not been subjected to double-blind trial, as it came into widespread use before the days of modern clinical trials and there are ethical objections to withholding an established treatment for a serious illness. But in a number of less strict randomised trials in Great Britian and USA a greater proportion of depressed patients showed greater improvement with e.c.t. than with antidepressive drugs. Electroconvulsive therapy is particularly indicated in patients with severe endogenous depression who do not respond to other drugs. Drug therapy is sometimes cautiously combined with e.c.t. to increase the duration of remissions.

The mechanism of e.c.t. is unknown; it is not known whether, like antidepressive drugs, it affects central adrenergic transmission. There are few experimental studies of e.c.t. but it has been shown that when administered for 10 days to rats, e.c.t. enhances behavioural responses mediated by dopamine. Effects similar to e.c.t. are produced in patients by a convulsant ether, fluorothyl (Indoklon). Electroconvulsive therapy remains effective if given to patients anaesthetised with thiopentone.

Electroconvulsive therapy is remarkably safe. It produces a brief period of postictal confusion, but otherwise its main drawback is a disturbance of memory.

IMIPRAMINE AND RELATED ANTIDEPRESSANTS

These compounds are also called tricyclic antidepressants in view of their chemical structure. They have also been referred to as monoamine re-uptake inhibitors because of their postulated principal mode of action.

The antidepressive effect of imipramine was discovered by clinical observation. Because of its structural and pharmacological resemblance to phenothiazines, imipramine was tested for activity in schizophrenia. The Swiss psychiatrist Kuhn who conducted the clinical trial could find no antischizophrenic effect, but discovered that the drug had a hitherto unknown antidepressive activity in patients with endogenous depression. The clinical effectiveness of imipramine in depressive illness was soon confirmed. Various related compounds have since been synthesised and introduced into practice.

Chemistry

Imipramine is an iminodibenzyl derivative and its nucleus bears a close structural similarity to the phenothiazine nucleus, the difference being that the sulphur atom in phenothiazines has been replaced by the CH_2—CH_2 group (Fig. 19.1). The related dibenzocycloheptene nucleus forms the basis of another group of antidepressive compounds which includes amitriptyline.

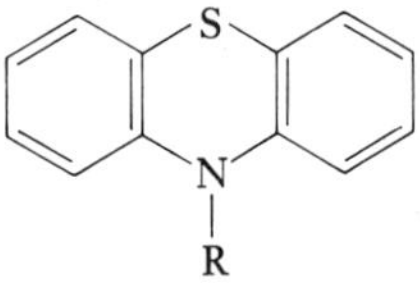

Phenothiazine

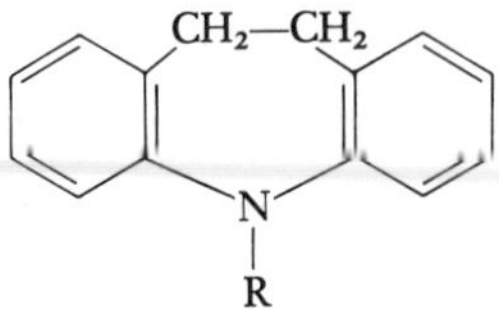

Iminodibenzyl

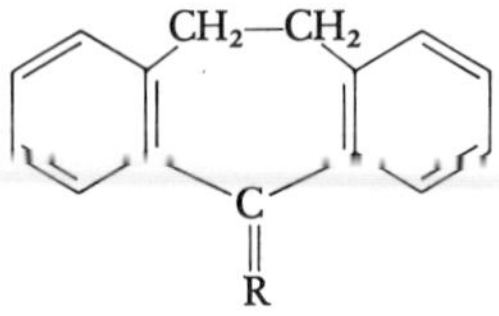

Dibenzocycloheptene

Fig. 19.1 Chemical relationship between the phenothiazine nucleus and the basic structures of tricyclic antidepressants.

Iminodibenzyl derivatives

Imipramine (Tofranil) and *desipramine* (Pertofran) are the most important. Desipramine is a demethylation product of imipramine and has been considered to be the pharmacologically active form of imipramine. It is, however, not certain whether this is so and clinically desipramine is rather less active than imipramine.

Dibenzocycloheptene derivatives

Amitriptyline (Tryptizol, Laroxyl) is widely used clinically. *Nortriptyline* (Allegron, Aventyl), its demethylated derivative, is more potent weight for weight. *Doxepin* is chemically and pharmacologically related to amitriptyline from which it differs in the structure of the central nucleus.

Pharmacological actions of imipramine

The effect of imipramine in experimental animals bears a superficial resemblance to chlorpromazine; for example imipramine depresses the spontaneous activity of mice and prolongs barbiturate sleeping time. It has strong antimuscarinic actions.

The main differences between phenothiazines and imipramine relate to their interactions with other drugs. Imipramine antagonises the psychomotor depressant effect of reserpine whilst chlorpromazine is synergistic with reserpine. In animals in which the brain catecholamines have been depleted, imipramine no longer antagonises reserpine, suggesting that the presence of catecholamines is required for its action. Imipramine potentiates the vasoconstrictor effects of noradrenaline whereas chlorpromazine antagonizes them. Imipramine potentiates the stimulant effects of amine oxidase inhibitors in animals.

Mode of action

Imipramine is a powerful blocker of the reuptake mechanism of noradrenaline at peripheral nerve endings and there is evidence that it produces a similar effect at adrenergic nerve endings in the central nervous system. The resultant increase of noradrenaline at receptor sites in the brain is believed to be the basic mechanism of the antidepressant effect of imipramine.

Amitriptyline, as well as imipramine, was initially reported to inhibit the uptake of noradrenaline in rat brain, but in later studies the uptake of noradrenaline by rat brain

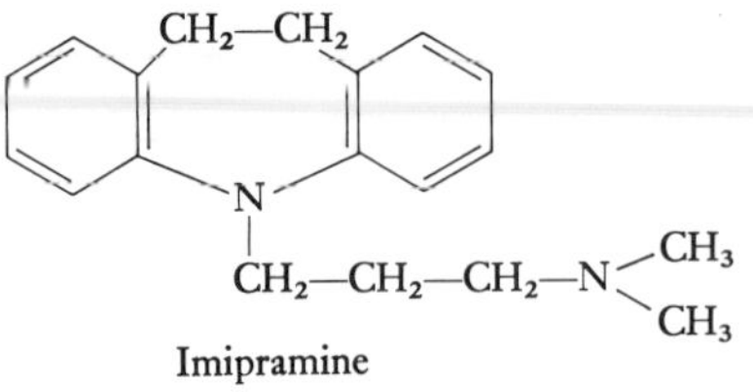

Imipramine

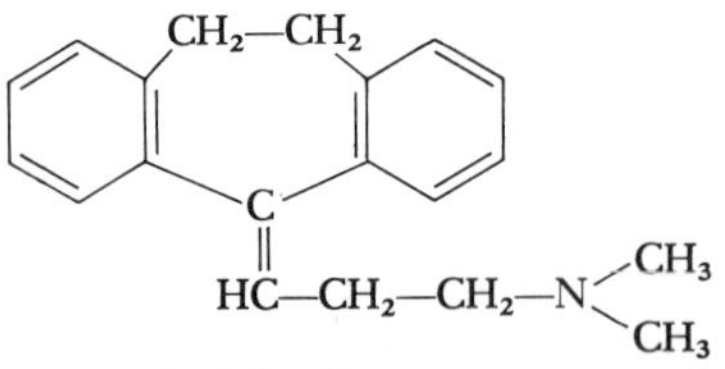

Amitriptyline

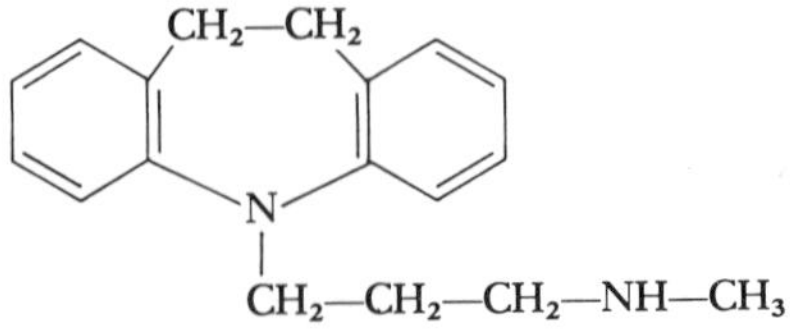

Desipramine

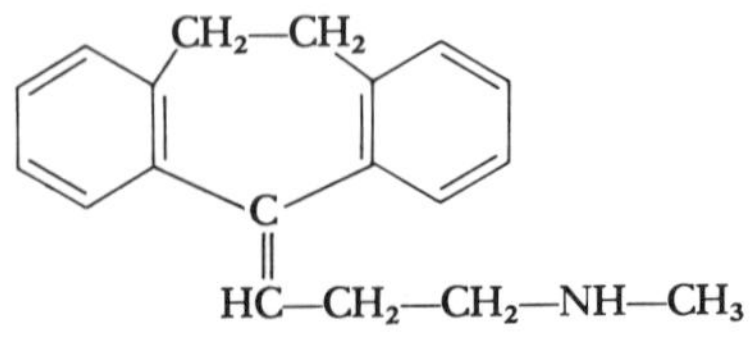

Nortriptyline

Fig. 19.2 Chemical structure of imipramine and related compounds.

did not seem to be inhibited by amitriptyline. On the other hand it has been shown that 5-hydroxytryptamine uptake is inhibited by amitriptyline. It has therefore been suggested that the antidepressant effects of amitriptyline may be due to increased serotonin activity at receptor sites in the brain. The role of noradrenergic and serotoninergic neurones in antidepressant effects remains contrversial. It has been suggested that both are important, perhaps in different clinical types of depression. *Chlorimipramine* is a strong inhibitor of 5HT uptake. Intravenous injections of this drug produce a rapid antidepressant effect in some patients.

Attempts have been made to distinguish between two types of depression, depending respectively on a defect in NA or 5HT uptake, by means of the urinary excretion of the noradrenaline metabolite MHPG (3-methoxy-4-hydroxyphenyl glycol, Fig. 6.5). Depressed patients with a low baseline excretion of MHPG were found to respond to imipramine and are considered to have a defective central noradrenergic system. Patients with a high baseline excretion of MHPG responded to amitriptilyine and are considered to have a defective serotoninergic system.

Effects in man
Imipramine causes neither euphoria nor addiction in normal subjects. It produces sedation and atropine-like effects such as dryness of the mouth and blurring of vision.

The clinical antidepressant effects of oral tricyclics show a characteristic latency. Effects in depressed patients resemble a natural remission of disease which may be complete or incomplete. Patients receiving imipramine may begin to improve after a few days or after a few weeks of continuous treatment; their response is shown by a definite change in the symptomatology of depressive illness such as less frequent early morning waking or absence of suicidal thoughts. One of the great difficulties in assessing the beneficial effects of imipramine is that they are indistinguishable from effects which can occur in the natural course of depressive illness.

Adverse effects
Common side effects of imipramine include dry mouth, tachycardia, difficulties of visual accommodation, severe constipation and bladder retention; besides these atropine-like effects imipramine paradoxically also causes increased sweating. It may produce postural hypotension.

Imipramine causes excitement in a small proportion of patients. It also causes a fine tremor which differs from the extrapyramidal tremors due to phenothiazines. Allergic jaundice sometimes occurs. Blood dyscrasias have been reported but are rare.

The tricyclics can be dangerous drugs when taken in an overdose. They are particularly toxic to the heart and severe cardiac abnormalities may be produced in tricyclic poisoning. Anticholinergic signs progressing to delirium and coma may occur.

Imipramine potentiates the effects of amine oxidase inhibitors and when these drugs are administered together or in close succession toxic effects may be produced.

Clinical effectiveness of tricyclic antidepressants
In assessing antidepressant drugs it is especially important not to rely on overall improvement rates but to judge the result against a placebo; depression is a cyclic disease in which patients improve spontaneously and in which the psychological effects of drug taking may be particularly powerful.

When comparative trials of the drugs are carried out it is desirable to give more than one dose level of each drug but this is seldom done. An alternative is to base the comparison on flexible dose schedules by which each patient receives an 'optimum' dosage from the point of view of effectiveness and side-effects. This is particularly indicated with a drug such as imipramine whose rate of metabolism and therefore effective dosage varies considerably between individuals.

Antidepressant drugs may differ qualitatively besides differing quantitatively; for example amitriptyline has more sedative effect than imipramine and it is therefore more effective in patients who are agitated besides being depressed. In such cases the choice of the patient population may determine the outcome of the trial. Even the choice of doctor may be important; it has been shown, in statistically controlled trials, that doctors who believe in drugs obtain better results than those who are excessively sceptical.

Uncontrolled trials almost always give overoptimistic results. This was the case in early trials with imipramine; but a number of controlled trials have since shown that imipramine is more effective than placebo though not as effective as e.c.t. treatment. On the other hand its undesirable actions are less than those of e.c.t. which, besides very occasionally causing fatal accidents, frequently produces impairment of memory which may be long lasting or persistent. Both imipramine and amitriptyline may bring about either partial or complete remissions of depression; in trials in which the two drugs have been compared amitriptyline has generally been found to be slightly superior in respect of the percentage of patients improved.

The doses of imipramine and amitriptyline are similar, 75 to 125 mg per day for outpatients and 100 to 200 mg for hospital patients. Larger doses lead to a high incidence of side effects; the dose range is thus much narrower than that of the phenothiazines.

Imipramine has been shown to be clinically effective in behaviour disorders in children such as enuresis and night terror.

APPLIED PHARMACOLOGY

New antidepressants
Since the introduction of the prototype tricyclics imipramine and amitryptiline, one of the aims of pharmaceutical industry has been to discover new antidepressants preferably not of the MAO inhibitor type. A number of new antidepressants have been introduced, mostly closely related in structure to the original tricyclics and, like them, blocking the reuptake of monoamines at nerve terminals. Some of the new antidepressants such as *mianserin* which is a powerful 5HT antagonist, seem to have a different mode of action from the imipramine-like drugs. Mianserin is less likely than these to produce anticholinergic effects, but it causes drowsiness in a proportion of patients. Attempts are being made to find new ways of testing compounds with antidepressant activity for example by establishing social behavioural models in animals. *Nomifensine* is an antidepressant with c.n.s. stimulant activity.

MONOAMINE OXIDASE INHIBITORS

Historically the monoamine oxidase (MAO) inhibitors were the first of the new antidepressants to be introduced but they have become largely displaced by the tricyclic antidepressants which are less toxic and whose clinical effectiveness is better substantiated. Although the tricyclics are frequently used in the initial treatment of depression, there remains a place for MAO inhibitors to be used in patients who do not respond adequately to tricyclics and in some cases even to e.c.t. The MAO inhibitors should not be employed unless patients can be closely supervised.

The first of these drugs, iproniazid (Fig. 19.3) was intended for the treatment of tuberculosis. When it was discovered to cause euphoria and excitement in patients its use as an antituberculosis drug was abandoned and it was applied to the treatment of depressive disease. The use of iproniazid has been discontinued in the United States because of its toxicity but elsewhere it is still employed because it is one of the most effective MAO inhibitors known. Iproniazid contains the toxic hydrazine group and attempts to produce less toxic derivatives have followed two lines, less toxic hydrazine derivatives and non-hydrazine MAO inhibitors.

The fundamental action of MAO inhibitors
As previously discussed (p. 76) the destruction of catecholamines is brought about by two enzymes, monoamine oxidase and catechol-*O*-methyl transferase. MAO is an intracellular enzyme contained mainly in the mitochondrial fraction which catalyses the oxidative deamination of the side chain of catecholamines and 5-hydroxytryptamine.

Neural noradrenaline is believed to be stored in at least three cell compartments: a stable pool contained in granules combined with ATP, a more labile pool in granules uncombined with ATP and a non-granular pool near the cell membrane from which noradrenaline is released by nerve stimulation (Fig. 17.5). Noradrenaline is actively accumulated in the storage granules but it also continuously leaks out into a pool where it is exposed to destruction by MAO. MAO inhibitors are powerful enzyme inhibitors which produce an irreversible inactivation of MAO. When administered to experimental animals they produce changes in their catecholamine metabolism: the noradrenaline and dopamine content of their brain is increased, at the same time the normal urinary degradation product 3-methoxy-4-hydroxymandelic acid (VMA) is diminished whilst urinary metanephrine increases.

Corresponding changes occur in 5-hydroxytryptamine metabolism. The content of 5-HT in the brain is increased, the urinary excretion of 5-hydroxyindoleacetic acid is diminished, whilst that of tryptamine is increased.

Actions in man
The MAO inhibitors are slow-acting drugs and it may take about a week before their effects are fully developed. They produce an elevation of mood and a central stimulation in both normal and depressed subjects. Although early enthusiastic reports of the beneficial effects of MAO inhibitors in depressive disease have not been fully confirmed by controlled trials these drugs are clearly effective when compared with placebo.

The MAO inhibitors lower the blood pressure and have been used in the treatment of hypertension (p. 120). These drugs sometimes have a beneficial effect in Parkinsonism, possibly because they increase the midbrain dopamine stores which are decreased in Parkinsonism.

The MAO inhibitors produce wide-ranging biochemical effects in the body and some of their pharmacological effects may be due to interference with enzymes other than monoamine oxidase.

Toxic effects
The MAO inhibitors are more toxic than the imipramine-type drugs and are not now regarded as drugs of first choice for the treatment of depression. They produce a variety of toxic effects either alone or in combination with other drugs and this constitutes the main limitation to their use.

The acute toxic effects of an overdose are agitation, convulsions and collapse. A serious toxic reaction which may occur either early or late in the course of administration is hepatocellular jaundice. The reaction may be allergic and it occurs particularly with the hydrazine derivatives. Other untoward effects include excessive stimulation, tremors and insomnia, and orthostatic hypotension.

Because MAO inhibitors interact with a variety of enzymes in addition to MAO, they prevent the normal destruction of drugs and may give rise to dangerous interactions. Coma and death after normal doses of pethidine or barbiturates have occurred in patients receiving MAO inhibitors. Hypertensive crises in patients receiving MAO inhibitors have been reported after the ingestion of certain foodstuffs such as cheese. The hypertension has been traced to the presence of tyramine in food, the pressor effects of which are greatly potentiated by MAO inhibitors (p. 44).

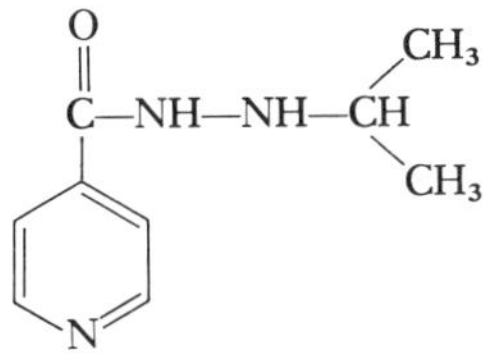

Fig. 19.3 Chemical structure of monoamine oxidase inhibitors.

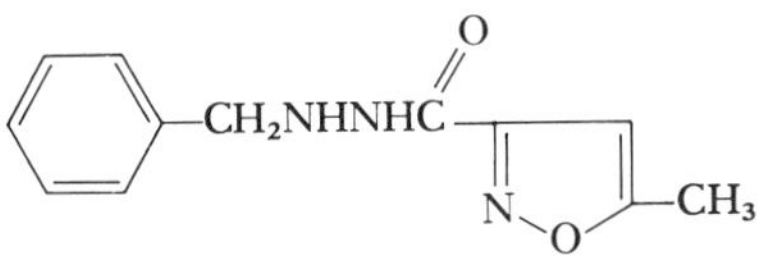

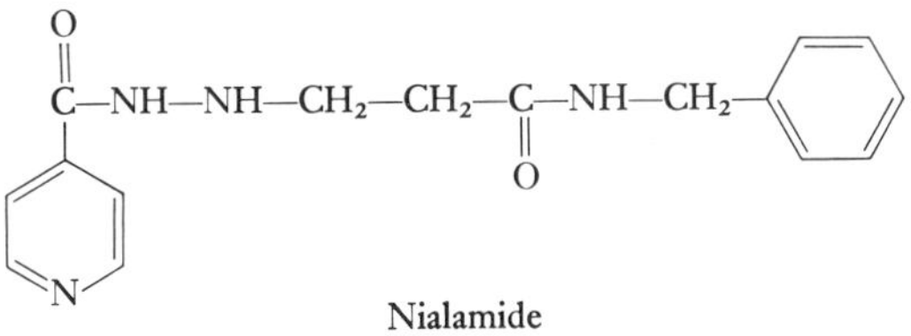

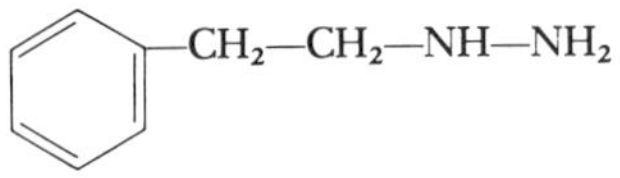

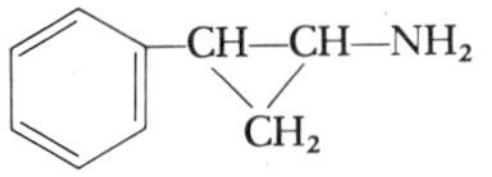

MAO inhibitory drugs. Hydrazine derivatives include *iproniazid* (Marsilid), *isocarboxazid* (Marplan), *nialamide* (Niamid) and *phenelzine* (Nardil) whose structural formulae are shown in Figure 19.3. All hydrazine derivatives are potentially toxic and may produce hepatocellular damage. As mentioned iproniazid has been withdrawn in the United States because of its toxicity.

Tranylcypromine (Parnate) is a non-hydrazine amine oxidase inhibitor. Its actions are intermediate between those of the other MAO inhibitors and amphetamine. It has a direct stimulant effect on the central nervous system and acts more quickly than the hydrazine derivatives.

LITHIUM

The term 'bipolar' affective disease (p. 257) is used for a condition first characterised by the nineteenth century German psychiatrist Kraepelin who called it *manic-depressive psychosis* distinguishing it from *dementia praecox*, a form of schizophrenia. Kraepelin considered that depression and mania were manifestations of a cyclic disease occurring in the same individual at different times. More recently it has been emphasised that patients may also suffer from recurrent 'unipolar' mania or depression. Lithium is considered the only specific antimanic agent presently available but it may also be effective in cyclic depression. The psychiatric effects of lithium were discovered by Cade in Australia in 1949 and fully substantiated by Schou in Denmark in 1965.

Mode of action

The mechanism by which lithium exerts its therapeutic effect is not understood. Lithium is chemically closely related to sodium and can replace it in some of its physiological functions. The effect of lithium cannot, however, be ascribed simply to sodium lack since a therapeutic concentration of lithium would replace only 1 per cent of extracellular sodium. Lithium affects various physiological parameters such as action potentials of heart and muscle. It may affect central amine metabolism; it enhances NA uptake by synaptosomes and inhibits NA and 5HT release in brain slices. A difficulty in the analysis of lithium actions is its slow time scale since its clinical effects may take weeks to develop and may not be detectable in acute experiments.

Clinical uses of lithium

Lithium is completely absorbed from the gastrointestinal tract and excreted by the kidneys with a half-life of about 24 hours. Lithium excretion varies with sodium intake. The addition of salt to the diet increases lithium excretion whilst patients on a low sodium diet retain lithium.

Lithium treatment is mainly indicated in patients with recurrent manic episodes. In frank mania it may be necessary to administer initially an antipsychotic drug such as a phenothiazine before, or together with, the slower acting lithium, which must reach a threshold level in tissues before becoming effective. This may take up to 10 days. In the early hypomanic phase, lithium may be employed in daily oral doses when a therapeutic effect may begin within days or weeks. When lithium is given prophylactically small doses may be administered over long periods under continuous control of lithium serum levels. Although lithium was originally introduced for the treatment of recurrent mania it is now frequently used for maintenance therapy in chronic manic-depressive disorders. However, the agent is not effective in all patients.

Blood levels and toxic effects
A feature of lithium treatment is its narrow therapeutic range. Whilst a maintenance serum level of 0.8–1.2 mEq/l lithium (measured by flame photometry) is considered clinically optimal, a serum level of 2 mEq/l may produce severe toxic effects.

Minor side effects of lithium are mild tremors particularly of the upper extremities which can be controlled by small doses of propranolol. Some degree of initial nausea, lethargy and fatigue need not prevent persevering with the drug. The more serious side effects of lithium treatment are neurological, including blurred speech, vertigo and exaggerated reflexes. Long-term complications include hypothyroidism and goitre. A frequent consequence of lithium treatment is an excessive weight gain. Renal lesions occur with long use.

AMPHETAMINE AND RELATED DRUGS

Amphetamine is racemic phenylisopropylamine. It belongs to the group of sympathomimetic amines but differs from the standard catecholamines in lacking hydroxyl groups in its ring structure and also in possessing an isopropylamine instead of an ethylamine side chain (p.125). It is therefore not destroyed by the enzymes which inactivate catecholamines and is stable and absorbed when taken by mouth.

Amphetamine has peripheral and central actions. Its peripheral sympathomimetic effects are of both the α and β type; thus it produces nasal vasoconstriction and contraction of the sphincter of the bladder but it can also dilate bronchial muscle. Its peripheral mechanism of action is not completely elucidated, its action is partly indirectly mediated through the release of noradrenaline from nerve endings and partly direct through interaction with adrenergic receptors.

There is evidence that the central action of amphetamine is largely indirect, involving the release of noradrenaline and dopamine. It is probable that the 'stereotyped' behaviour produced by amphetamine in experimental animals (p. 239) is associated with the action of released dopamine and the central stimulation with noradrenaline release. Both effects of amphetamine can be prevented by pretreating animals with alpha-methyl tyrosine which inhibits the formation of dopa, the precursor of dopamine. The effects can be restored by the administration of dopa.

The structural formulae of amphetamine and methylamphetamine are shown in Figure 19.4. The drugs are available as the free bases (for example in amphetamine inhalers, now withdrawn from the market) or as salts.

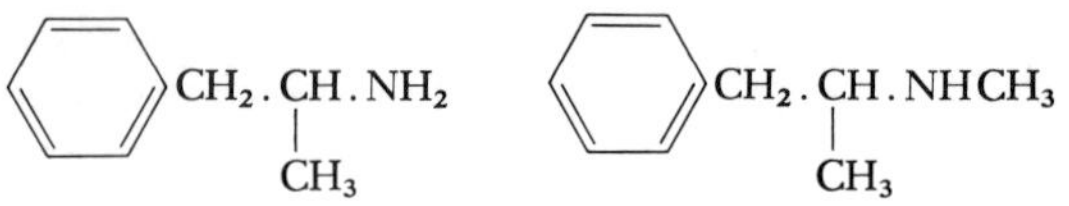

Fig. 19.4

Central stimulation
Amphetamine lowers the threshold for the arousal response in the electroencephalogram.

When amphetamine is injected into mice it produces excitement characterised by great restlessness, frequent and rapid co-ordinated movements and rapid respiration. These effects are very evident if one animal is kept alone in a cage, but the excitement becomes striking when several animals are together in the same cage.

Amphetamine also facilitates more complicated behaviour patterns in animals such as 'goal-directed' behaviour which is either positively reinforced by reward or negatively reinforced by avoidance of punishment. It has been suggested on the basis of self-stimulation experiments in rats that amphetamine facilitates goal-directed behaviour by enhancing the release of noradrenaline from terminals of the medial bundle in the forebrain.

A characteristic effect of *d*-amphetamine seen particularly in rats has been referred to as stereotyped behaviour (p. 239). This type of behaviour is specifically antagonised by chlorpromazine and haloperidol. Antagonism of amphetamine stereotypy has been used as a test for neuroleptic activity.

Effects in man
When amphetamine is given in doses of 5 to 20 mg by mouth to normal individuals, they usually become talkative and active and report that they feel alert, interested and pleased; some, however, report opposite effects and feel depressed and irritable. The effects of amphetamine on the performance of many different tasks have been studied, and improvements have been reported in some, especially arithmetic, speed in reading, motor co-ordination and other relatively simple tasks for which speed is important. In tests which have continued for a long period of time it has been found that whereas control subjects became tired and their performance fell off, those who had been given amphetamine were able to maintain their efficiency (Fig. 19.5). Amphetamine does not usually facilitate new learning nor improve ingenuity or the power to reason, and it may even make these worse. It has been suggested that its beneficial effects may be primarily due to an influence on mood, and that the inclination rather than the ability to perform work may be improved. It has often been reported that under the influence of amphetamine time appears to pass more quickly and this drug is said to be prized for this purpose by prisoners.

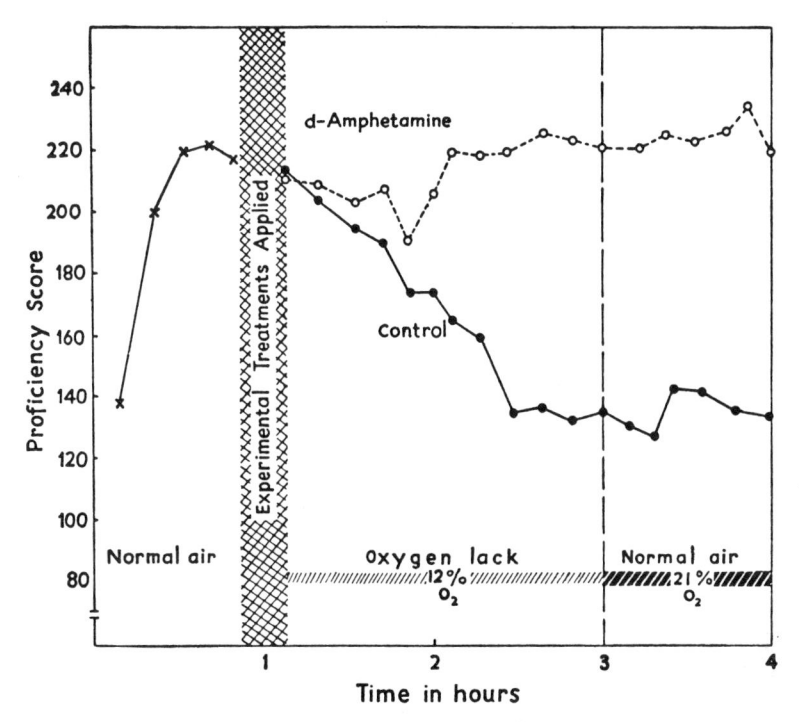

Fig. 19.5 Effect of *d*-amphetamine (5 mg orally) in normal subjects when performing prolonged skilled work under conditions of oxygen lack. The drug prevented the decline in performance brought about by oxygen lack. When the subjects resumed breathing normal air their performance was maintained whilst that of the control group did not return to the level reached before oxygen lack. These results suggest that amphetamine prevented the decline in efficiency brought about by oxygen lack and fatigue. (After Hauty, Payne and Bauer, 1957, *J. Pharmac. exp. Ther.*)

Amphetamine sulphate when administered to normal and obese subjects causes a loss of body weight which is associated with a reduction of voluntary food intake. The weight reduction is not due to an increase in fluid output or to an increase in basal metabolic rate.

Amongst the chief compounds which have been studied in man for their stimulant effects on the central nervous system are *amphetamine sulphate* (benzedrine), *dexamphetamine sulphate* (dextroamphetamine sulphate, dexedrine), *methylamphetamine hydrochloride* (methedrine) and *ephedrine hydrochloride*. The actions of these drugs have been investigated in normal subjects, in patients with narcolepsy, and in states of exhaustion and fatigue. The psychological effects produced are distinct from the analeptic and sleep-disturbing properties of the compounds and they are not related to changes in blood pressure. Methylamphetamine is slightly more active as a central stimulant than dexamphetamine and about one and a half to two times more active than the racemic compound amphetamine, but it gives rise to more side effects.

Absorption, distribution and fate
Amphetamine and related compounds are rapidly absorbed from the gastrointestinal tract. They penetrate the blood-brain barrier readily in contrast to the more polar catecholamines which enter the brain slowly from the blood stream.

As already pointed out amphetamine is not destroyed by amine oxidase or catechol-*O*-methyltransferase; about one-third to one-half of an ingested dose is excreted in the urine the rest is destroyed mainly by microsomal enzymes in the liver. Excretion of unchanged drug is increased in acid urine and decreased in alkaline urine.

Therapeutic uses
Amphetamine is used chiefly for its central stimulating action in the treatment of reactive depression due to acute or chronic illness, misfortune or bereavement and in the treatment of psychopathic states. Psychopathic individuals of the aggressive type, treated with this drug, may become better integrated personalities. Amphetamine sulphate is nearly three times as effective as ephedrine in preventing attacks of sleep in narcolepsy and is used for the diagnosis and treatment of this condition.

Rather paradoxically, the amphetamines may be beneficial in the treatment of the 'hyperkinetic' syndrome in children. These children seem to indulge in much purposeless physical activity and their ability to focus attention is impaired. Such children, mainly boys, are often highly intelligent but they may nevertheless have learning or reading difficulties and occasionally exhibit a degree of physical clumsiness.

Treatment with d-amphetamine has been reported effective in about 50 per cent of such children, rendering them *less* excited and more amenable to educational infuences. The main undesirable effects are insomnia and loss of appetite. On the other hand, the treatment is claimed to involve no risk of toxicity or drug dependence.

There is considerable individual variation in the response to these sympathomimetic amines. The usual optimum dose of amphetamine sulphate is 10 to 20 mg, while that of dexamphetamine sulphate and of methylamphetamine hydrochloride is 5 to 10 mg. A small dose (5 mg) of the drug should be given initially to test for undue sensitivity. Narcoleptic patients appear to tolerate larger doses (20 to 60 mg amphetamine daily). Patients with coronary disease or hypertension should not be treated with these drugs.

Amphetamine anorexia

There is experimental evidence that hunger and thirst are controlled, at least partly, by centres in the hypothalamus. It has been shown that crystals of noradrenaline implanted in the hypothalamus of rats induce voracious eating and crystals of acetylcholine induce drinking. This control system is highly complex and not understood in detail. For example, if noradrenaline is administered systemically it produces the opposite effect, namely a reduction of food intake.

Amphetamine has marked effects on appetite and reduces the spontaneous food intake in animals. Dogs given amphetamine refuse to take their food and may die from starvation.

In man, dexamphetamine reduces appetite and may be used in conjunction with a reducing diet to treat obesity. This action of dexamphetamine is partly, but not entirely, due to a central stimulant effect which makes it less unpleasant for the co-operative patient to deny himself food. After a time, tachyphylaxis to the anorexic effect develops, doses have to be increased and the danger of psychic drug dependence then arises. For these reasons dexamphetamine is now employed with great caution for the treatment of weight reduction and, if so, is used only as a short time adjunct of treatment by reduced calorie intake.

Several drugs have recently been developed which are claimed to have amphetamine-like properties in reducing appetite without its addiction liability.

Diethylpropion is an anorexiant related to amphetamine which has been found to produce less cardiovascular side effects than dextroamphetamine, but it must be used with caution in patients with hypertension or angina.

Fenfluramine is a fluorine containing amphetamine derivative with anorexic activity. It causes drowsiness, in contrast to other amphetamine derivatives, and is claimed to have little or no dependence-inducing liability.

Mazindol is an effective anorexic drug which is structurally unrelated to amphetamine. It is non-addictive, producing, if anything, dysphoria rather than euphoria.

Phenmetrazine (Preludin) is chemically related to amphetamine. It has an appetite suppressant action and is employed for this purpose in doses of 25 mg three times daily before meals.

Although it produces less central stimulation than amphetamine, phenmetrazine abuse and dependence have been described. The general features of phenmetrazine dependence are similar to amphetamine dependence except that the doses of phenmetrazine used by addicts are larger.

Toxic effects

The individual susceptibility to amphetamine varies greatly and signs of severe intoxication may appear after doses varying from 50 to 500 mg. Two kinds of effects are prominent:

1. Signs of sympathetic stimulation including tachycardia, mydriasis, hypertension and central excitation.

2. A transitory psychotic reaction which occurs some 24 hours after ingestion of the drug. The patients are usually not disorientated but suffer from delusions of persecution and visual and auditory hallucinations. The condition may be mistaken for schizophrenia but can be distinguished from it by its subsidence in about a week after cessation of administration of the drug. This is about the time required for the elimination of the drug from the body.

Although amphetamine psychosis may occur after a single large dose it occurs more frequently after prolonged administration. Other effects of chronic administration of amphetamine and related drugs are anorexia and weight loss, tremors and insomnia.

Amphetamine dependence

Amphetamine addiction is becoming an increasingly important social phenomenon and is discussed in Chapter 41.

Amphetamine-barbiturate mixtures. Several mixtures with barbiturates have been introduced clinically with the purpose of mitigating any unpleasant effect of amphetamine excitement. Pharmacological investigation has shown that the two drugs may under certain circumstances potentiate each other; for example when they are mixed in certain proportions they produce greater spontaneous activity in rats than can be obtained with any dose of one drug alone. Similarly in man amphetamine-barbiturate mixtures may produce a greater elevation of mood than each separate ingredient which may help to explain the popularity of these mixtures amongst teenagers.

Pipradrol (Meratran)
When this compound is injected into mice it produces effects which resemble those of amphetamine. The animals become excited, move about rapidly and their normal activities of licking, scratching and eating are carried out with excessive speed. In contrast to amphetamine, doses of pipradrol which produce hyperactivity do not affect the blood pressure and heart rate.

Pipradrol has been reported to benefit patients with depression whilst patients with anxiety are often made worse. Unlike amphetamine it does not inhibit appetite.

Methyl phenidate (Ritalin) is a compound with a central action similar to that of amphetamine. It produces a mild rise in blood pressure and an increase in heart rate in both animals and man. This agent is useful in the management of children with the hyperkinetic syndrome.

Caffeine

The world-wide popularity of drinks containing caffeine or theophylline depends on their action in stimulating mental processes. Therapeutic doses of these drugs in man affect chiefly the higher centres and to a lesser extent the medullary centres. Pavlov and his pupils have shown that caffeine augments conditioned reflexes and diminishes inhibitory processes. After full doses of caffeine it is difficult or impossible to extinguish a conditioned reflex. In man caffeine reduces reaction times and, like amphetamine, can counteract the effects of fatigue on simple prolonged tasks; its effects on new learning and on simple tasks when subjects are not fatigued are probably negligible, any improvements being small and unreliable.

Toxic doses of caffeine produce sleeplessness, tremor, hallucinations and delirium; stimulation of the spinal cord by large doses of the drug in animals results in tetanic convulsions resembling those due to strychnine.

Cocaine (p. 309)

Cocaine was one of the earliest drugs used as a cerebral stimulant; the Spaniards found it in general use for this purpose in Peru at the time of their conquest. The indigenous peoples believed that chewing of coca leaves greatly increased their power of endurance of fatigue.

Nasal insufflation is the most widely practiced mode of cocaine administration, since cocaine is rapidly destroyed in the gastrointestinal tract and metabolised in the liver.

Cocaine increases general locomotor activity, enhances physical and mental endurance, and decreases appetite. Tolerance does not develop to cocaine's excitatory effects. Physiological addiction does not appear to occur with cocaine and abrupt withdrawal in either man or animals does not lead to an abstinence syndrome. Psychological addiction, however, can be a serious problem (p. 484).

Cocaine is believed to exert most of its behavioural and psychological effects through central catecholaminergic mechanisms. Cocaine is a potent inhibitor of neuronal uptake mechanisms for noradrenaline, but it differs in various ways from the tricyclic antidepressants and is not itself an effective antidepressant. There are considerable similarities between the central effects of cocaine and amphetamine.

DRUGS WHICH PRODUCE HALLUCINATIONS

These drugs have also been called psychotogenic or psychotomimetic drugs because they produce or mimic psychotic behaviour.

Lysergic Acid Diethylamide (LSD)

Lysergic acid is the common nucleus of all ergot alkaloids and the mental effects of lysergic acid diethylamide were discovered accidentally by Hofmann in 1943 while using this compound in the synthesis of ergometrine. He reported that he was forced to stop laboratory work in the middle of the afternoon because he had been overcome by a peculiar restlessness associated with dizziness. After reaching home he lay in a delirious state during which he experienced a stream of phantastic images of extraordinary vividness and colour. He suspected some connection between these peculiar symptoms and the substance with which he had been working and this was borne out by a systematic investigation of the effects of lysergic acid diethylamide.

This drug is extremely potent; when 0.05 mg is taken by mouth it produces within an hour characteristic disturbances in perception and changes in mood and thought processes, akin to schizophrenia, which last for several hours. The subject remains conscious, but has the illusion of being detached from his body and of losing contact with his environment which seems to him unreal. His sense of time is distorted so that time seems to pass much more rapidly or more slowly. Objects appear to be changed in form and colour and a progressive distortion of visual perception may occur. The subject may experience phantasies and hallucinations and see complex patterns of faces and eyes as shown in Figure 19.6. The change in mood may be of elation, anxiety or profound depression and is often expressed in an exaggerated form. Efficiency in the performance of various laboratory tasks may not be much impaired, however.

The mode of action of LSD in producing these bizarre effects is not known. The chemical structure of LSD is shown in Figure 41.2.

The action of LSD in the periphery is exerted on 5-HT receptors; LSD is a powerful antagonist of 5-HT (serotonin) on smooth muscle (p. 93). There is evidence that the central actions of LSD are likewise exerted on 5-HT receptors. Electrical recordings have been made from single units in serotoninergic midbrain raphe nuclei. Very

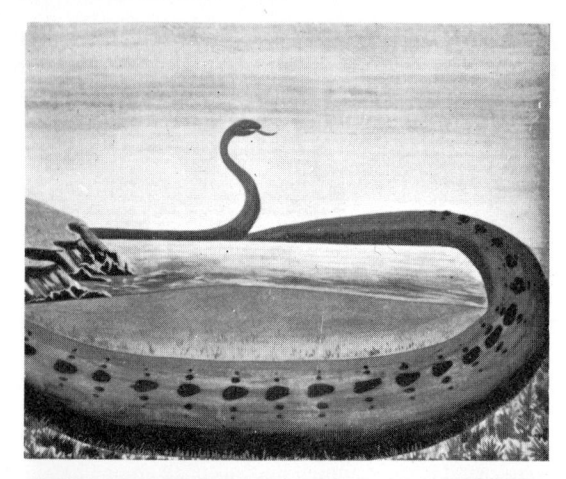

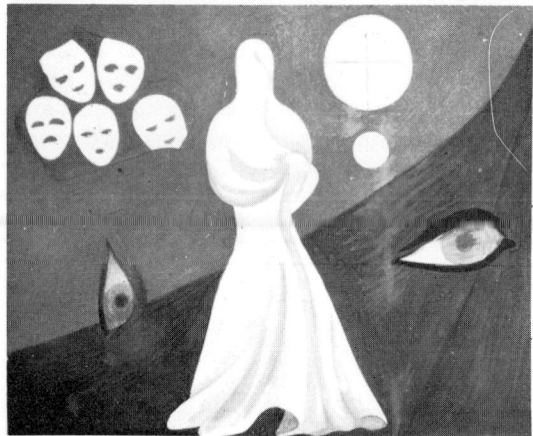

Fig. 19.6 Phantasies and hallucinations experienced by a patient whilst under the influence of LSD. The paintings were executed a few hours after recovery from the drug.

(a) Phantasy of a world-encircling snake; the patient was unable to paint anything like this unless she had had LSD the day before. Normally she was unable to find a subject to paint and her execution was poor whereas in this picture the draughtsmanship is good.

(b) The complex pattern of faces and eyes frequently seen after taking LSD. The fully cloaked figure is a hallucination of the ward sister.
(By courtesy of Dr R A Sandison.)

small doses of LSD inhibit firing from these neurones, presumably through an action on presynaptic neuronal 5-HT receptors.

Psilocybin, an active principle of the 'magic' mushroom, *Psylocybe mexicana*, is an indoleamine which produces a similar clinical syndrome as LSD. The chemical structure of various hallucinogens is shown in Figure 41.2.

Mescaline

This is an alkaloid obtained from a Mexican cactus plant, the dried tops of which are called peyote or mescal buttons. Its chemical structure resembles that of the sympathomimetic amines and is shown in Figure 41.2.

Peyote has long been used by certain American Indian tribes during religious ceremonies. It produces mental changes which resemble those of lysergic acid diethylamide. An oral dose of 400 mg of mescaline causes vivid hallucinations consisting of brightly coloured pictures usually accompanied by distortion of time and space perception. Consciousness is retained and the ability of the subject to solve simple mathematical problems may not be impaired. Mescaline produces dilatation of the pupil and other sympathomimetic effects; it also causes nausea and dizziness.

Cannabis

Preparations derived from the hemp plant *Cannabis sativa* are marihuana, the dried flowering tops of plants and hashish, a resin derived from the flowering top. Cannabis contains a number of pharmacologically active constituents belonging to the class of tetrahydrocannabinols (THC). One of these, Δ^9 THC, is the major pharmacologically active constituent of hashish and marihuana.

Pharmacological effects. The acute effects of cannabis ingestion are partly physical and partly psychological. Characteristic physical findings are tachycardia and injected conjunctival vessels. Tremor of the tongue and mouth, nystagmus and ataxia may also occur. The psychological effects include euphoria, excitement, changes in the appreciation of time and space, raised auditory sensitivity, emotional upheaval and illusions and hallucinations.

The first signs of intoxication, appearing about three hours after consuming the drug by mouth, may be nausea and vomiting and severe disorders of thinking so that conversation becomes disjointed and unintelligible. After smoking hashish resin, acute anxiety and restlessness may come on within half an hour followed later by pleasant sensations with visual imagery.

Cannabis dependence is discussed in Chapter 41.

PREPARATIONS

Tricyclics and related antidepressants
Amitriptyline hyd (Tryptizol) initial 30–150 mg dl,
  maint 20–100 mg dl
Butriptyline hyd (Evadyne) initial 25 mg 3x dl then up
  to 150 mg dl
Clomipramine hyd (Anafranil) 30–150 mg dl
Dibenzepin hyd (Noveril) 240–560 mg dl
Desipramine hyd (Pertrofan) initial 25–75 mg dl,
  maint to 150 mg dl
Dothiepin hyd (Prothiaden) 25–50 mg 3x die
Doxepin hyd (Sinequan) 75–150 mg dl
Imipramine hyd (Tofranil) 75–150 mg dl
Iprindole hyd (Prondol) initial 45–180 mg dl, maint 45–90 mg dl
Maprotiline hyd (Ludiomil) 25–150 mg dl
Mianserin hyd (Bolvidon) initial 10 mg 2–3x die,
  maint 30–60 mg dl

Nomifensine hydrogen maleate (Merital) 50–200 mg dl
Nortriptyline hyd (Aventyl) 10–25 mg 3–4x die
Opipramol hyd (Insidon) 100–300 mg dl
Protriptyline hyd (Concordin) 15–60 mg dl
Tofenacin hyd (Elamol) 80 mg 3x die
Trimipramine maleate 25–125 mg dl
Viloxazine hyd (Vivalan) 50–100 mg 3x die

Monoamine oxidase inhibitors
Iproniazid phosph (Marsilid) initial 100–150 mg dl, maint 25–150 mg dl
Isocarboxazid (Marplan) initial up to 30 mg dl, maint 10–20 mg dl
Phenelzine sulph (Nardil) 15 mg 3x die
Tranylcypromine sulph (Parnate) initial 20 mg dl

Lithium
Lithium Carbonate (Camcolit) 0.25–1.6 g dl

Amphetamine and related drugs
Amphetamine sulphate 5–20 mg dl
Dexamphetamine sulphate (Dexedrine) 5–20 mg dl
Diethylpropion hyd 25 mg 3x die
Fenfluramine hyd (Ponderax) 40–120 mg dl
Mazindol (Teronac) 1–2 mg dl
Methylamphetamine hyd 2.5–10 mg p.o., 10–30 mg i.m. or i.v.
Methylphenidate (Ritalin) 20–30 mg dl
Pemoline (Ronyl) 20 mg
Phentermine 15–30 mg

FURTHER READING

Brimclecombe R W, Pinder R M 1975 Hallucinogenic agents. Wright-Scientechnica, Bristol
Costa E, Garattini S (ed) 1970 Amphetamine and related compounds. Raven Press, New York
Hoffer A, Osmond H 1967 The hallucinogens. Academic Press, New York
Klerman S, Cole J O 1965 Clinical pharmacology of imipramine and related antidepressant compounds. Pharmac. Rev. 71: 101
Paykel E S, Coppen A (ed) 1979 Psychopharmacology of affective disorders. Oxford University Press, London

20. Central depressants of motor function

Epilepsy 268; Methods of assessing antiepileptic drugs 268; Phenobarbitone 269; Primidone 270; Phenytoin 270; Ethosuximide 271; Troxidone 271; Carbamazepine 272; Sodium valproate 272; Acetazolamide 273; Bromides 273; Diazepam in status epilepticus 273; Parkinsonism 273; Levodopa 273; Carbidopa 274; Amantadine 274; Bromocriptine 274; Anticholinergic drugs 274; Centrally acting muscle relaxants 275; Baclofen 276.

The activity of voluntary muscle can be reduced by drugs which act on the central nervous system or at the neuromuscular junction; drugs which block neuromuscular transmission are discussed elsewhere (p. 65). In this chapter, three types of centrally acting motor depressant drugs are described:

(1) anticonvulsant drugs which are used in the treatment of epilepsy, (2) drugs which are used to control tremors and muscular rigidity in Parkinsonism and (3) spinal cord depressant drugs.

EPILEPSY

Epilepsy is a disease characterised by paroxysmal abnormal electrical activity in the brain (Fig. 20.1), often accompanied by loss of consciousness and convulsions. The epileptic attack is initiated by an abnormal focus of electrical discharge originating either in the grey matter or some other part of the brain which then spreads to other parts of the brain and results in convulsions or other manifestations of epilepsy.

There are several types of epilepsy. In *grand mal* or *major epilepsy* the fit is often preceded by a premonitory aura which may consist of a feeling of strangeness or fear or of epigastric discomfort; this is followed by loss of consciousness and tonic and clonic convulsions. *Petit mal* or *minor epilepsy*, which is commonest in children, is characterised by brief periods of clouding or loss of consciousness during which the patient stops activities and after a moment or two resumes them without being aware of the interruption. The attack may be so brief as to show itself only by a vacant stare but frequent attacks of this kind seriously handicap the patient.

Psychomotor (temporal lobe) epilepsy consists of bouts of abnormal sensations or behaviour: for example the patient may have a fit of rage of which he is afterwards oblivious. *Focal or Jacksonian epilepsy* is normally associated with a gross organic lesion of the cerebral cortex. It is characterised by convulsive twitching of isolated muscle groups and may remain localised or progress to generalised convulsions with loss of consciousness.

Each type of epilepsy has a characteristic encephalographic pattern (Fig. 20.1), and may respond to some anticonvulsant drugs but not to others. Whereas phenobarbitone benefits most types of epilepsy, some of the newer drugs act primarily on one or other type.

Mode of action of anticonvulsant drugs
Hughlins Jackson, some hundred years ago, put forward the theory that epileptic seizures were caused by 'occasional, sudden, excessive local discharges of grey matter' and that generalised epileptic convulsions developed when normal brain tissue became invaded by the electrical currents generated in the abnormal focus. Hughlins Jackson's theory has been substantially confirmed by electroencephalographic investigations.

Antiepileptic drugs could thus act (1) by inhibiting or damping the seizure focus itself or (2) by preventing the spread of the abnormal activity to normal brain tissue. Most experimental evidence suggests that antiepileptic drugs generally act by the second mechanism and this is supported by the finding that these drugs can prevent epileptiform convulsions artificially induced by electrical stimulation of the brain.

Methods of assessing anticonvulsant drugs
Anticonvulsant drugs can be assessed in animals by their ability to prevent or modify convulsions produced by electrical stimulation of the brain. These drugs can also be tested by their power to prevent convulsions produced by leptazol and other substances which stimulate the central nervous system.

Estimates of anticonvulsant activity by the two tests do not always agree, possibly because the disturbances produced by electrical stimulation originate in the cortex whilst those produced by drug stimulation arise in subcortical areas. Leptazol convulsions are antagonised more specifically by drugs such as ethosuximide and troxidone which are particularly effective in petit mal. Phenytoin sodium, which acts mainly in grand mal, does not prevent leptazol convulsions but alters the response to electrical stimulation. Phenobarbitone antagonises both electrical and leptazol convulsions.

For many years the only compounds used in the treatment of epilepsy were sedative drugs, mainly bromides and phenobarbitone, but after the introduction of phenytoin sodium in 1938, a large number of compounds have been tested for anticonvulsant activity. Although tests in animals are useful in selecting new compounds, the therapeutic value of an antiepileptic drug can be assessed only by extensive clinical trial in patients with different types of epilepsy.

CENTRAL DEPRESSANTS OF MOTOR FUNCTION 269

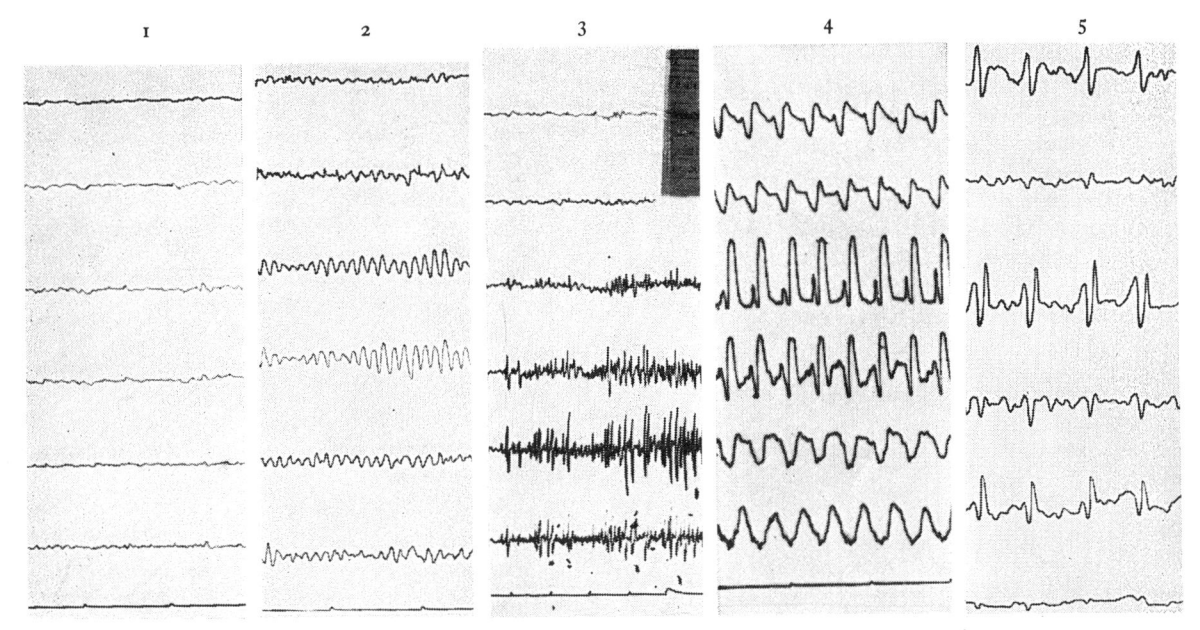

Fig. 20.1 Examples of electroencephalograms (e.e.g.) in normal subjects and patients with epilepsy. 1 and 2. Normal subjects — poor and good alpha rhythms. 3. Epilepsy, grand mal attacks — high amplitude spikes. 4. Epilepsy, petit mal attacks — spike-and-wave-pattern. 5. Jacksonian epilepsy — focal spikes. (By courtesy of Dr R.R. Hughes.)

Drugs used in the treatment of epilepsy

Patients with epilepsy are severely handicapped unless their attacks are completely prevented by means of drugs, and in order to maintain an adequate concentration of drug in the tissues, medication must be continuous. It is important, therefore, that the drug should not produce disturbing side-effects such as dizziness, drowsiness or nausea. It is also important that the drug should not produce allergic skin reactions or dangerous blood dyscrasias, although some of these risks cannot be entirely avoided.

The choice of drug for any individual patient is determined by the type of seizure and the severity of side effects. It is often found that treatment with more than one drug is necessary, either because the patient has epilepsy of a mixed type or because by using two or more drugs the incidence of side effects is reduced. In determining the effective dose it is usual to start with a small dose and to increase it gradually until either attacks are completely prevented or toxic reactions occur. In the latter case administration of the drug must not be abruptly discontinued but the dose is reduced and a second drug is given in gradually increasing doses.

The measurement of plasma drug concentration of anticonvulsant drugs is assuming increasing importance in the treatment of epilepsy. An undue frequency of seizures is often associated with suboptimal plasma drug concentrations and before deciding to change to another drug it may be advisable to increase the dose to try to obtain an optimum plasma level for the patient.

A drug which is effective in a particular type of epilepsy usually also changes the abnormal electro-encephalographic record as shown for example in Figure 20.4.

Most of the important drugs in the treatment of epilepsy are derivatives of barbituric acid, hydantoin and succinimide (Fig. 20.2).

Barbiturates and related compounds

Phenobarbitone (Luminal)
This drug has been used extensively in the treatment of epilepsy since 1915 and remains one of the most important drugs for the treatment of this disease. Animal experiments have shown that it has a specific anticonvulsant action, when compared with other barbiturates; it gives protection both against electroshock- and leptazol-induced convulsions.

Phenobarbitone is the drug of choice for the initial treatment of most types of epileptic seizures. It is effective against grand mal and focal epilepsy and sometimes against petit mal but is ineffective against psychomotor epilepsy. Phenobarbitone may be used alone or in conjunction with other antiepileptic drugs. The usual dose is 100 mg daily by mouth but doses up to 300 mg daily can be given. Phenobarbitone is slowly eliminated from the body. In man its half-life of elimination from the plasma ranges from about 50 to 150 hours.

The toxic effects of phenobarbitone are seldom serious and can usually be controlled by reducing the dose.

Drowsiness and lethargy frequently occur at the beginning of treatment but these symptoms generally disappear with continued use of the drug. Large doses produce vertigo and ataxia. Amphetamine sulphate may be given in doses of 5–20 mg daily to alleviate drowsiness. A disadvantage of phenobarbitone is that it occasionally produces allergic skin rashes.

Methylphenobarbitone (Prominal, Phemitone) is absorbed from the gastrointestinal tract and is broken down to phenobarbitone in the liver. Its actions and side effects are similar to those of phenobarbitone.

Primidone (Mysoline)
This compound can be considered as a derivative of phenobarbitone in which the oxygen in the urea grouping of the barbituric acid is replaced by two atoms of hydrogen. It is partially metabolised in man to phenobarbitone. Primidone is more effective in grand mal than in petit mal and is particularly effective in focal epilepsy. It causes marked sedation. It is given by mouth in daily doses of 0.75–1.5 g, and is often administered together with phenytoin sodium. Combined treatment with primidone and phenobarbitone is undesirable since the two drugs have similar side effects.

Hydantoin derivatives

Phenytoin sodium (Epanutin)
Merrit and Putnam investigated the activity of a number of barbiturates and allied drugs in preventing the convulsions produced in cats by electrical stimulation of the brain. They found that diphenylhydantoin was particulary active. It is probably the most effective drug in the treatment of grand mal and completely prevents attacks in about 60 per cent of patients. It is also useful in the treatment of psychomotor epilepsy but ineffective in petit mal where it may even increase the frequency of attacks. The adult daily dose is 300–600 mg by mouth. Phenytoin sodium has little hypnotic effect and in this respect differs from the barbiturates; it may even cause sleeplessness, proving that a sedative action is not an essential property of an antiepileptic action.

The toxic effects of phenytoin sodium may be divided into those which require only a reduction of the dose and those which are so dangerous that administration of the drug must be discontinued. Amongst the former are insomnia and gastric disturbances; nystagmus frequently occurs and when this is associated with diplopia and ataxia the dose must be reduced. Hypertrophy of the gums is a

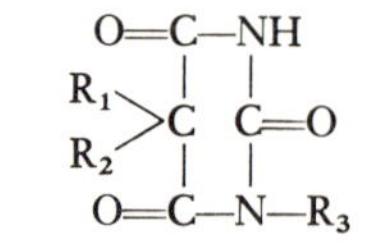

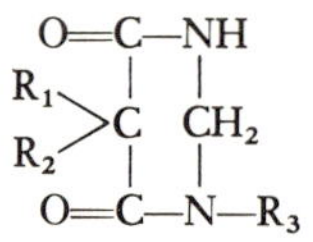

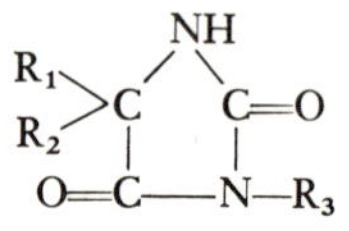

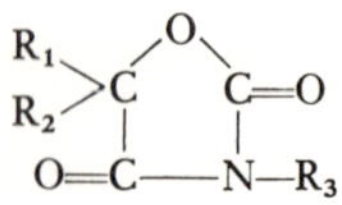

Nucleus	Drug	Substituents		
		R_1	R_2	R_3
1. Barbiturate	Phenobarbitone	C_6H_5	C_2H_5	H
	Methylphenobarbitone	C_6H_5	C_2H_5	CH_3
2. Hexahydropyrimidinedione	Primidone	C_6H_5	C_2H_5	H
3. Hydantoin. Phenytoin sodium	C_6H_5	C_6H_5	H	
	Methoin	C_6H_5	C_2H_5	CH_3
4. Oxazolidine-dione	Troxidone	CH_3	CH_3	CH_3
	Paramethadione	C_2H_5	CH_3	CH_3
5. Succinimide	Ethosuximide	C_2H_5	CH_3	H
	Phensuximide	C_6H_5	H	CH_3

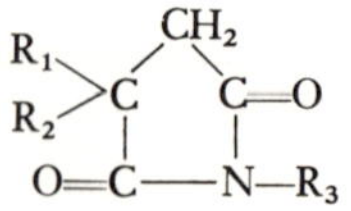

Fig. 20.2 Chemical structures of antiepileptic drugs.

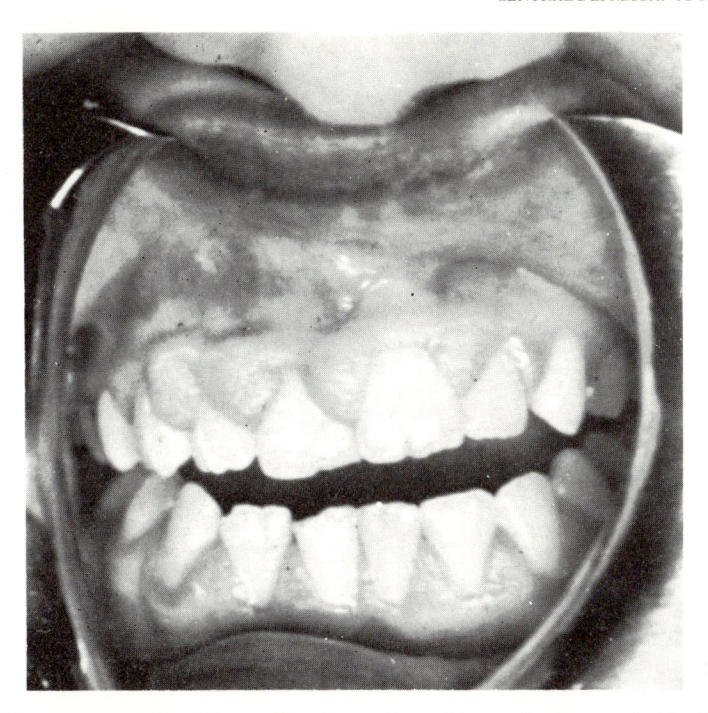

Fig. 20.3 Enlargement of the gums especially of the papillae, in a patient with grand mal, treated with phenytoin sodium. (By courtesy of Professor E. D. Farmer.)

peculiar side effect which is seen particularly in young patients after several months of treatment with phenytoin sodium (Fig. 20.3). The cause of this condition is not known; its development can be retarded by careful attention to the teeth. More serious toxic effects are skin reactions which include a morbilliform rash with fever and exfoliative dermatitis. The use of phenytoin for the treatment of cardiac arrhythmias is discussed on p. 146.

Methoin (Mesontoin) a closely related compound, is more sedative than phenytoin sodium but less so than phenobarbitone. Its actions and uses are similar to those of phenytoin sodium but it is less liable to cause gingivitis. Methoin may produce skin eruptions and more rarely agranulocytosis or aplastic anaemia.

Succinimides

Ethosuximide (Fig. 20.2) is the drug of choice for true petit mal absences with 3 per second wave and spike discharges in the electroencephalogram. The condition is shown in Figure 20.4 as well as the effect of the drug troxidone upon it. Ethosuximide produces similar e.e.g. effects as troxidone but is less toxic; it has been the outcome of a systematic search for an effective and relatively non-toxic drug in petit mal. Experimentally it is most active against leptazol-induced convulsions. Clinically it is ineffective in grand mal and psychomotor epilepsy.

Ethosuximide often causes gastrointestinal upsets and drowsiness but some degree of tolerance to these effects occurs. Serious reactions of the haemopoietic system and skin are rare.

Phensuximide (Fig. 20.2) was the first succinimide used in petit mal. It is less active than ethosuximide.

Oxazolidinediones

Trimethadione (Troxidone) (Fig. 20.2) was the first effective agent used in the control of petit mal showing that drugs could act selectively on different types of epilepsy. In laboratory animals its main action is to prevent leptazol convulsions whilst it is inferior to phenytoin in preventing electroshock convulsions. Whilst highly active in petit mal it may even aggravate grand mal. Its main drawback is its toxicity.

Drowsiness and nausea frequently occur in the early stages of treatment with troxidone but later disappear. A frequent side effect is photophobia, which is disturbing but does not lead to permanent damage and can be relieved by wearing dark glasses. When morbilliform or urticarial skin rashes develop the drug must be temporarily withdrawn. Other dangerous complications, fortunately rare, are agranulocytosis and aplastic anaemia. It is therefore necessary to pay special attention to the development of sore throat or fever and to make periodic white cell counts. Treatment must be stopped when the neutrophil counts falls below 2000.

Paramethadione (Paradione) (Fig. 20.2) This drug is closely related to troxidone and has similar

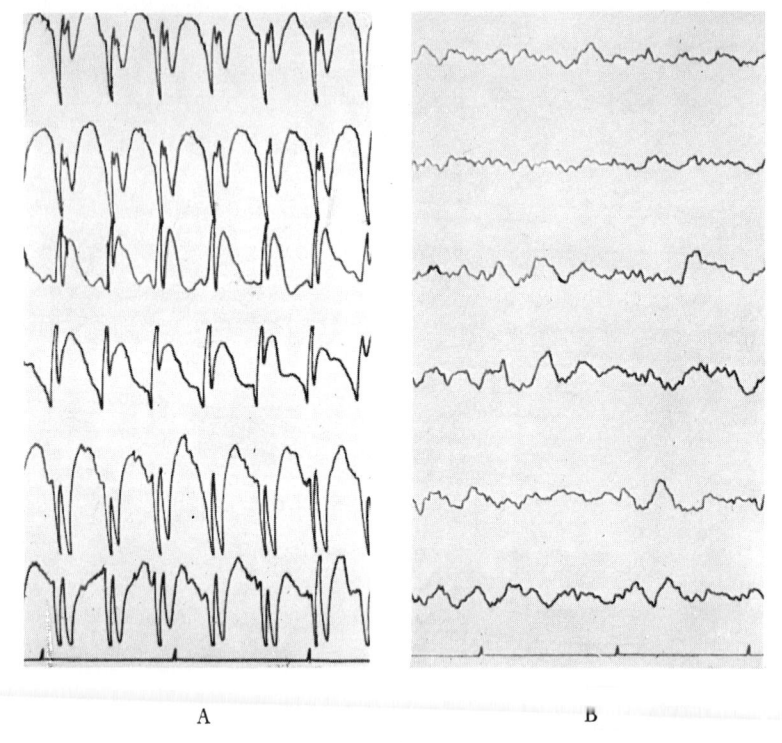

Fig. 20.4 Electroencephalograms of a child with petit mal. A, before treatment; B, three months after treatment with troxidone showing absence of typical spike and wave activity. (By courtesy of Dr R. R. Hughes.)

pharmacological properties. It may be used in patients who are refractory to treatment with troxidone or develop toxic reactions to it.

Carbamazepine

Carbamazepine (Tegretol) differs chemically from other antiepileptic drugs. It is a tricyclic compound (Fig. 20.5) chemically related to imipramine. Carbamazepine is an anticonvulsant, clinically effective in psychomotor epilepsy and in grand mal, though ineffective in petit mal. It is also used as a highly specific analgesic for *trigeminal neuralgia* and other forms of neuralgia.

The anticonvulsant effects of carbamazepine in animals resemble those of phenytoin. It antagonises electroshock but not leptazol convulsions. Clinically carbamazepine is particularly effective in psychomotor (temporal lobe) epilepsy including the secondary generalisation of the focal activity into tonic-clonic seizures. It is less effective against the generalised grand mal seizures alone. When treatment of epilepsy with phenytoin is ineffective a change to carbamazepine may be made, or phenytoin may be combined with carbamazepine. Neither drug produces the sedative effects of phenobarbitone or primidone both of which are often poorly tolerated in children.

Adverse reactions to carbamazepine occur relatively frequently. Neurological effects, generally reversible, include ataxia, dizziness and diplopia. Blood dyscrasias have been described on rare occasions. Carbamazepine is reported to have a psychotropic effect in improving mood and alertness in epileptic patients.

Sodium valproate

Valproate (dipropylacetate) inhibits GABA metabolism raising GABA concentrations in the brain. Sodium valproate has been used in epileptic children and has been found to reduce the number of fits. Sodium valproate may be added to an existing antiepileptic treatment. It is particularly effective in treating myoclonic jerks in children. The side effects of sodium valproate are mild drowsiness and nausea.

Clonazepam is a recently introduced benzodiazepine used in various types of epilepsy. It produces marked drowsiness.

Fig. 20.5 Carbamazepine.

Acetazolamide

This carbon anhydrase inhibitor (p. 164) has been used in many forms of epilepsy, particularly in petit mal in children. It is often combined with other antiepileptic drugs. Its anticonvulsive action may decline with continuous administration owing to the acid-base disturbance produced.

Sulthiame is a carbonic anhydrase inhibitor sometimes used as an anticonvulsant.

Bromides

Bromides were the first effective antiepileptic drugs. They have a low therapeutic index and for this reason are now seldom used except occasionally for the treatment of grand mal seizures. They are of pharmacological interest because of their peculiar distribution in the body which is closely similar to, though not entirely identical with, that of chloride.

The bromides are effective anticonvulsant drugs and when present in a sufficient concentration in the brain may completely prevent epileptic attacks. The blood concentration of bromide which is required to check convulsions is about 125 mg/100 ml; this usually also produces considerable drowsiness and mental depression.

Bromism. Excessive accumulation of bromide produces mental depression, deficient memory, general stupidity and muscular weakness. Skin eruptions of various forms are a usual feature of bromide poisoning. The most typical form of eruption consists of large bullae, while in other cases acne and sometimes erythema occur. In severe bromism the mental symptoms already mentioned are exaggerated, the patient's gait is unsteady, and he cannot speak without stammering.

Status epilepticus

This is a condition in which generalised convulsive seizures occur with such frequency that the patient does not recover consciousness between attacks, and which may lead to exhaustion and death. Status epilepticus is treated by the intravenous administration of 0.4-0.8 g of phenobarbitone sodium or amylobarbitone sodium.

More recently the administration of *diazepam* (Valium) by intravenous injection of doses of 10 mg, repeated as required, has been found to control seizures in status epilepticus.

The patient requires constant nursing attention and measures must be taken to prevent hyperthermia and dehydration and to ensure an adequate airway and oxygenation.

PARKINSONISM

The extrapyramidal system (p. 239) comprising the basal ganglia and related structures plays an important part in the regulation of muscle tone and movement. Parkinsonism is a symptom-complex which is due mainly to lesions of the basal ganglia. A characteristic pathological feature of Parkinsonism is the occurrence of atrophy and depigmentation of the *substantia nigra* and of degeneration of the nigrostriatal tracts.

Biochemically the brains of patients who have suffered from idiopathic or postencephalitic Parkinsonism show a marked depletion of the dopamine content of the striatum which can account for the extrapyramidal symptoms seen in these patients. Dopamine acts as an inhibitory transmitter within nigrostriatal pathways of the extrapyramidal motor system while acetylcholine has excitatory activity. The aim of treatment in Parkinson's disease is enhancement of the dopaminergic system by replenishing striatal dopamine and inhibition of the cholinergic system by blocking central cholinergic receptors (p. 239).

Parkinsonism is characterised by slowing and weakening of voluntary movements, muscular rigidity and tremors. In paralysis agitans, tremors and muscular rigidity are the main features, whilst in post-encephalitic Parkinsonism excessive salivation and painful spasm of the ocular muscles (oculogyric crises) may also occur. The symptoms usually progress slowly for many years but eventually the patient becomes completely disabled by the disease. The condition can be considerably improved by treatment with drugs in conjunction with physiotherapy and psychotherapy.

The alkaloids of belladonna and other solanaceous plants as well as certain synthetic anticholinergic compounds, were formerly the only drugs known to be effective in alleviating the symptoms of Parkinsonism. During recent years, however, an important new compound, levodopa, has been added, and is now the most effective drug in the treatment of Parkinsonism.

Levodopa

The use of L-dopa in Parkinsonism is a remarkable application of rational pharmacotherapeutics. As has been pointed out Parkinson's syndrome results from any pathological or drug-induced disorder which entails a reduction of activity of the dopaminergic system in the striatum with consequent dominance of the cholinergic system. Therapy may be directed either towards decreasing cholinergic activity or restoring dopaminergic activity.

Although in idiopathic Parkinsonism the function of the degenerated dopaminergic tracts cannot be restored, their effects can be mimicked by increasing the dopamine content of the striatum. Dopamine itself does not penetrate the blood-brain barrier, but it is possible to raise the level of dopamine by administration of its immediate precursor L-dopa (Fig. 6.3) which does enter the brain.

Early clinical trials with dopa in Parkinsonism involved relatively short-term administration with doubtful results but when dopa was administered in large doses for long periods there was substantial neurological improvement.

Clinical effects. The therapeutic effect of levodopa may take up to four weeks to appear. The clinical features most likely to improve are bradykinesia, disturbances of gait and rigidity. Oculogyric crises are relieved in most patients. Tremor is helped only in a minority of patients. About 50 per cent of patients with Parkinsonism will obtain some relief from treatment with levodopa. The dose is 0.5–4.0 g per day.

Adverse effects. L-Dopa often causes anorexia and nausea and should therefore be administered with food. The emetic effect is due to an action of dopamine on the medullary chemoreceptor trigger zone. If necessary an antihistamine, such as cyclizine, may be given to diminish nausea and vomiting. Hypotension may occur, as well as nausea and sweating. The most troublesome side effects are choreoathetoid movements, usually starting in the face. Psychiatric disturbances such as delusions may also occur.

Some of the side effects, such as hypotension, may be largely peripheral due to the action of dopamine formed in the blood stream, and attempts have been made to prevent the peripheral but not the central formation of dopamine by the concurrent administration of a dopa decarboxylase inhibitor which does not penetrate the c.n.s.

Carbidopa inhibits the peripheral decarboxylation of levodopa to dopamine and since it does not cross the blood-brain barrier, effective brain concentrations of dopamine are produced with lower doses of levodopa. At the same time peripheral side effects due to dopamine are reduced.

It is given with levodopa to enable a lower dosage to be used.

Benserazide produces similar effects to carbidopa.

Bromocriptine

This is a semisynthetic ergot derivative which is a stimulant of dopamine receptors. By virtue of this action it produces (1) a beneficial effect in Parkinsonism, (2) inhibition of lactation by suppressing prolactin secretion. It also suppresses growth hormone secretion in acromegaly.

When given to patients with Parkinsonism treated with levodopa it produces a further improvement in gait and rigidity and alleviation of tremor. Adverse effects, particularly dyskinetic movements are similar to those produced by levodopa.

Amantadine

Amantadine is an antiviral agent which has been found to have a therapeutic action in Parkinsonism similar to that of dopa. It is, however, less effective than dopa and the therapeutic response although more rapid tends to be less lasting.

The mode of action of this drug is unknown. It is mainly used in patients who cannot tolerate levodopa. It is possible to combine the two drugs.

Anticholinergic drugs (p. 70)

Charcot introduced atropine for the treatment of Parkinsonism, and both atropine and hyoscine have been traditional remedies in the treatment of this condition. They have now been substantially replaced by synthetic antimuscarinic drugs. Many of these drugs also have antihistamine activity, but there is no clear evidence that their antihistamine activity contributes to their therapeutic effect in Parkinsonism.

The anticholinergic drugs benefit particularly patients whose symptoms are mild. They may be profitably combined with levodopa. Rigidity responds best to this type of drug, but bradykinesia and tremor are also improved.

Adverse effects. These may be considered in two groups; central and peripheral. Central side effects include giddiness and confusion which may be severe and lead to hallucinations. The peripheral side effects include atropine-like effects of blurring of vision, dryness of the mouth, tachycardia, difficulty with micturition and constipation. Acute glaucoma may be precipitated owing to the mydriatic effects and acute urinary retention may occur in the presence of prostatic hypertrophy.

Indications. The anticholinergic drugs are particularly useful in drug-induced Parkinsonism occurring in patients treated with chlorpromazine or haloperidol. In these conditions L-dropa is not particularly effective since the dopaminergic receptors are already blocked by the psycholeptic drugs and little benefit can be achieved by increasing the levels of striatal dopamine. Many psychiatrists indeed prescribe anticholinergic drugs as routine prophylaxis when treating psychotic patients with phenothiazines.

Benzhexol (Artane) has peripheral actions similar to those of atropine but is only one half to one tenth as active when compared with it by various pharmacological tests. The effects of benzhexol in the treatment of Parkinsonism are similar to those of atropine, and in therapeutically effective doses (2.5–10 mg daily) the side effects are similar. Excessive doses may give rise to dizziness and mental confusion.

Benztropine (Cogentin) *and caramiphen* (Parpanit) also have atropine-like actions and are used in treatment of Parkinsonism.

Diethazine (Diparcol) is a derivative of phenothiazine and is thus chemically related to the antihistamine compound promethazine. Diethazine has relatively little antihistamine activity. It improves the control of movements but does not diminish excessive salivation in patients with Parkinsonism. It produces drowsiness and dizziness, especially in the early stages of treatment.

Ethopropazine (Lysivane) is chemically closely related to diethazine and has similar pharmacological and clinical effects.

Orphenadrine (Disipal) is a derivative of diphenhydramine with weak antihistamine properties and seems to be useful as a supplementary drug in the treatment of postencephalitic patients. It has more effect in controlling secretion than severe tremors and often produces euphoria which is probably its most useful property.

CENTRALLY ACTING SKELETAL MUSCLE RELAXANTS

Many diseases of the brain and spinal cord result in rigidity and spasm of voluntary muscles. This condition may arise from a lesion of the extrapyramidal motor system as in Parkinsonism or it may be due to disease of the pyramidal motor system affecting either the cortex, the internal capsule, pons, medulla or spinal cord. These crippling conditions are widespread and occur as a result of injury at birth, cerebral haemorrhage or thrombosis, or focal disease of the central nervous system as in multiple sclerosis. Muscular spasm and stiffness also occur as a consequence of infectious disease of the muscles or their disuse in arthritis. These patients suffer much inconvenience from pain and limited muscular movement and there is a great need for drugs which will reduce the spasticity. Unfortunately, drugs which do so, also tend to increase the weakness of the muscles so that although the discomfort of the patient is lessened, his ability to use his muscles is not improved.

Control of muscle tone
The tone of a muscle is its tension at rest. Both smooth and striated muscle have an intrinsic tone which is a property of the muscle itself, but striated muscle receives in addition tonic impulses through its motor nerve.

These impulses are regulated by two superimposed control systems. The first is centered in the reticular formation of the brain which sends both facilitatory and inhibitory impulses to the spinal motor neurones. For example, if a cat is decerebrated muscle rigidity develops due to the removal of inhibitory influences, but if in addition certain centres in the midbrain which initiate facilitatory impulses are destroyed rigidity ceases and the muscles become flaccid.

The second control system comprises (1) the alpha efferents to the motor endplate, (2) the gamma efferents to the muscle spindles, and (3) afferents from the muscle spindles. Together they form a control system which may become deranged. It has been suggested that overactivity of gamma (fusimotor) efferents may play an important role in rigidities in man and that the relaxation which follows the injection of procaine into a muscle may be due to a block of gamma activity.

Effects of central relaxant drugs
Most spinal cord reflexes involve interneurones. If a drug depresses polysynaptic reflexes without depressing a monosynaptic reflex, such as the stretch reflex, it can be inferred that part of its action, at least, is on interneurones. This is one of the most characteristic effects of centrally acting relaxant drugs.

In experimental animals these drugs produce diminished motility, ataxia, loss of the righting reflex, flaccid muscular paralysis and in large doses death due to respiratory failure. The safety margin between the doses which produce muscular relaxation and those which produce death is relatively large.

Although these drugs can produce complete muscular paralysis similar to that produced by neuromuscular blocking drugs they are not used as adjuncts in general anaesthesia because of their widespread effects on the central nervous system. Apart from their selective action on internuncial neurones of the spinal cord they also produce depression of brainstem neurones.

Most of the centrally acting relaxants have a general sedative effect and prolong the sleeping time produced by barbiturates. Their sedative and anti-anxiety effect is an important facet of their clinical use.

Mephenesin (Myanesin)
Gilbert and Descomps observed in 1910 that a phenolic ether of glycerol produced transient paralysis in guinea pigs and rabbits. Berger and Bradley in 1946 investigated a series of compounds of this type and, finding that most of these had a similar paralysing action, chose methylphenoxypropanediol (mephenesin) for further investigation.

Mephenesin has a selective depressant effect on interneurones of the spinal cord. This effect is illustrated in Figure 20.6 which shows that mephenesin does not abolish a simple reflex arc such as the knee jerk, but that it depresses the flexor reflex which involves more than one internuncial neurone. The figure also shows that mephenesin does not produce a neuromuscular block, like tubocurarine.

Mephenesin antagonises spinal convulsions and is a powerful antagonist of strychnine and, when injected intravenously, it abolishes spasm in tetanus. Although mephenesin, when administered intravenously, reduces muscular spasm and rigidity caused by lesions of either the pyramidal or extrapyramidal system its practical uses are limited by its toxicity and its short duration of action; attempts have therefore been made to synthesise other less toxic compounds with similar and more prolonged actions. The drugs which have been investigated include derivatives of propanediol (meprobamate, carisoprodol)

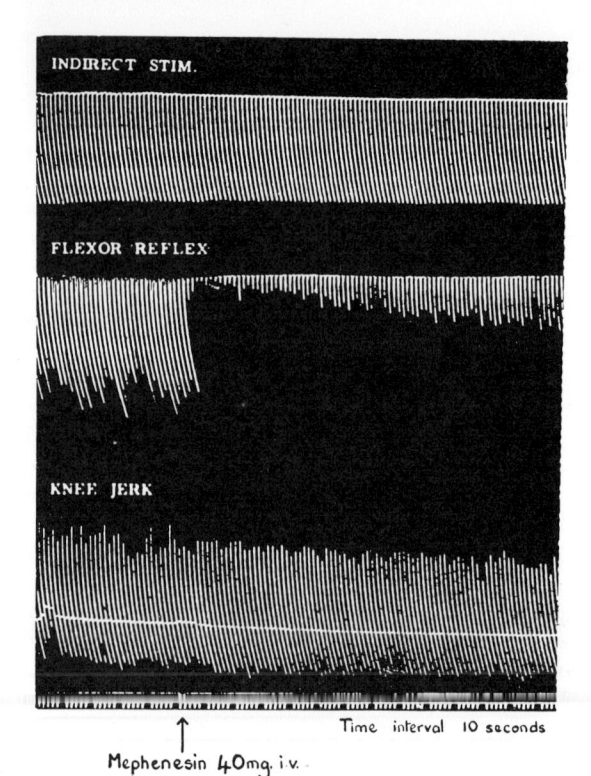

Fig. 20.6 The effect of mephenesin on indirect excitability of skeletal muscle, the flexor reflex, and the knee jerk of the anaesthetised cat. At the arrow 40 mg mephenesin was injected intravenously. (After Berger, 1949. *J. Pharmac.*)

and compounds of the benzodiazepine group, e.g. chlordiazepoxide and diazepam (p. 249).

Meprobamate (Equanil, Miltown)
The chemical structure of this compound is shown on page 251. In experimental animals the action of meprobamate on the spinal cord resembles that of mephenesin in inhibiting reflexes which involve several internuncial neurones and thus diminishing muscle tone. Meprobamate is more effectively absorbed than mephenesin and when administered by mouth to monkeys it produces at first a sedative effect which is followed by incoordination and muscular paralysis. The therapeutic response to meprobamate seems to be closely related to its effects in relaxing anxiety and tension, discussed on page 251.

Carisoprodol (Carisoma) is structurally related to meprobamate which it also resembles in its depressant action on spinal interneurones. It has some analgesic and considerable sedative properties. Carisoprodol has been found effective when administered in children with cerebral palsy in whom it reduces spasticity and improves general performance.

Chlordiazepoxide (Librium)
This compound (Fig. 18.3) has been shown in experimental animals to inhibit the polysynaptic pathways in the spinal cord. Its effectiveness as a skeletal muscle relaxant in man is closely associated with the relief of anxiety and agitation. It is used for its tranquillising properties which are discussed on page 249.

Diazepam (Valium) is closely related in structure and pharmacological actions to chlordiazepoxide. In experimental animals it is more active than the latter in depressing spinal reflexes. Diazepam reduces anxiety and like chlordiazepoxide is extensively used for this purpose.

Other muscle relaxants
Baclofen (Lioresal) is chemically closely related to GABA and produces GABA-like effects in various test systems. In man it is a muscle relaxant acting on the spinal cord particularly on the gamma-efferent system. It has been used with success in patients with multiple sclerosis and severe spinal spastic conditions. Side effects include dizziness and confusion as well as depression or euphoria.

Dantrolene is a muscle relaxant reported to act at the stage of excitation-contraction coupling. It is used clinically in cases of painful muscle spasm.

Clinical usefulness of central relaxant drugs
The pathophysiology of spasticity is complex and as yet poorly understood. It is now realised that drugs affecting muscle tone produce effects not only on spinal interneurones but also on centres in the midbrain which are influenced by muscle spindle afferents and which regulate the activities of alpha and gamma motoneurones.

Although a great deal of research has gone into the development of these drugs they have so far proved rather disappointing in practice. There can be no doubt that they can cause relaxation and a reduction of spasm of skeletal muscle to the point of producing extreme muscle weakness and ataxia. They have been used for the treatment of various types of muscle rigidity and spasm but many clinicians consider that in the cases where they have been clinically effective in alleviating 'tension' their sedative actions are as responsible as their relaxant effects on muscles.

PREPARATIONS

Anticonvulsants
Beclamide (Nydrane) 0.5–1 g 3–4x die
Carbamazepine (Tegretol) 200 mg–1.2 g dl
Chlormethiazole (Ch. 18)
Clonazepam (Rivotril) 4–8 mg
Ethosuximide (Emeside) 500 mg dl
Ethotoin (Peganone) 1–3 g dl
Methylphenobarbitone (Prominal) 100–600 mg dl
Methoin 50 mg–max 600 mg dl
Paramethadione (Paradione) 900 mg–1 g dl
Pheneturide (Benuride) 600 mg–1 g dl

Phenobarbitone
Phenobarbitone Sodium p.o. 30–125 mg 3x die
Phenytoin Sodium (Epanutin) 100 mg 2–4x die
Primidone (Mysoline) 500 mg–max 2 g dl
Sulthiame (Ospolot) 100–200 mg 2–3x die
Troxidone (Tridione) 900 mg dl
Valproate Sodium (Epilim) init 200 mg 3x die, maint 0.8–1.4 g dl

Drugs used in Parkinsonism
Amantadine hyd (Symmetrel) 200 mg dl
Benserazide hyd 50–250 mg dl
Benzhexol hyd (Artane) 2–20 mg dl
Benztropine mes (Cogentin) 500 µg–max 6 g dl
Biperiden hyd (Akineton) 1–2 mg 2–3x die
Bromocriptine mes (Parlodel) 40–300 mg dl
Carbidopa 25–200 mg dl
Chlorphenoxamine hyd (Clorevan) 50–100 mg 3–4x die
Ethopropazine hyd (Lysivane) 50–200 mg dl
Levodopa init 250 mg dl, maint 2.5–8 g dl
Methixene hyd 2.5 mg 3–6x die

Orphenadrine (Disipal) 200–400 mg dl
Procyclidine hyd (Kemadrin) 7.5–30 mg dl
Tigloidine hyd (Tyglissin) 1–2 g dl

Centrally acting skeletal muscle relaxants
Baclofen (Lioresal) 5–20 mg 3x die
Carisoprodol (Carisoma) 350 mg 4x die
Chlordiazepoxide (Ch. 18)
Dantrolene Sodium (Dantrium) 25–100 mg 4x die
Diazepam (Ch. 18)
Mephenesin (Myanesin) 1–3 g dl
Meprobramate (Equanil) 0.4–1.2 g dl
Methocarbamol (Robaxin) 1.5–2 g 4x die

FURTHER READING

Boissier J R, Hippius H, Pichot P (ed) 1975
 Neuropsychopharmacology. Excerpta Medica, Amsterdam
Laidlaw J, Richens A (ed) 1976 A textbook of epilepsy. Churchill Livingstone, Edinburgh

21. Analgesic drugs

Measurement of analgesic activity 278; Opium analgesics 279; Actions of morphine 279; Codeine 282; Heroin 282; Oxymorphone 282; Levorphanol 283; Pentazocine 283; Pethidine 283; Fentanyl 283; Methadone 284; Nalorphine 285; Naloxone 285; Antipyretic analgesics 285; Salicylates 286; Non-steroidal anti-inflammatory agents 289; Ibuprofen 289; Phenylbutazone 290; Indomethacin 290; Para-aminophenol analgesics 290; Paracetamol toxicity 291; Colchicine 292; Probenecid 292; Allopurinol 293.

One of the most important purposes for which drugs are used is the relief of pain, but the manner in which analgesics act is only imperfectly understood. Simple depressants such as alcohol or aliphatic hypnotics dull the perception of pain to a certain extent, but their action in this respect is surprisingly limited since they do not produce well marked relief until a semicomatose condition is reached.

Morphine, on the other hand, can relieve pain in doses which do not produce marked mental confusion. The essential action of morphine appears to be diminution of attention and anxiety and it is particularly effective in relieving chronic pain of moderate intensity. Thus, distress caused by a painful stimulus is largely due to its persistence in the memory and is usually augmented by fear of its recurrence.

Analgesic drugs can be divided into two main groups.

The opiate analgesics including morphine, its derivatives and other related synthetic compounds; all the most potent analgesics belong to this group. These drugs are effective in pain arising from superficial structures such as skin and mucous membranes, in the more deep seated pain arising from joints, periosteum and muscles and also in visceral pain due to distension of hollow viscera. Both the naturally occurring and the synthetic drugs of this group appear to have a fundamentally similar mode of action; they also have this in common that they are specifically antagonised by the compound naloxone.

The *antipyretic* or *anti-inflammatory analgesics* such as aspirin, phenacetin and amidopyrine and related compounds, e.g. phenylbutazone. These substances are not only less effective as analgesics than those in the former group but they are also much more selective in their action. Whilst they are effective, and sometimes surprisingly so, in pain arising from the teeth and joints and in headache and neuralgia, they have little effect on visceral pain.

In addition to these drugs which have a specific action on pain perception, many drugs are capable of alleviating pain by influencing the cause of the pain. Ergotamine relieves migraine because it acts as a vasoconstrictor of the blood vessels of the external carotid bed and the nitrites relieve angina by relaxing blood vessels. The severe pain and oedema of acute gout can be rapidly and effectively controlled by the oral administration of colchicine but the explanation of this action is not known.

Measurement of analgesic activity
Various methods have been used for measuring analgesic activity. These methods are usually designed to determine the activity of drugs in preventing or alleviating artificially induced pain. The following pain stimuli may be used: (a) radiant heat applied to the tail or feet of small animals or by a lamp shone on the skin of the forehead or finger of human subjects; (b) electrical stimulation of the tooth pulp of suitably prepared dogs or of human subjects; (c) mechanical pressure applied to the nail bed or a superficial bony surface, or an artery clip applied to the tail of a mouse; (d) inflation of a sphygmomanometer cuff on the arm to produce pain from muscle ischaemia.

It is important to measure not only the intensity but also the duration of effect of drugs and to avoid producing permanent damage to the tissue since this will prevent repeated observations. Preferably the test method should provide a graded relation between intensity of pain stimulus and dose of analgesic needed to suppress the pain. In this way a quantitative assessment of analgesic activity may be obtained.

Drugs differ in their ability to suppress various types or qualities of pain. Certain qualities of pain are not easily reproduced experimentally and analgesics such as aspirin which are useful in many clinical conditions often fail to show analgesic activity by experimental tests.

It is generally agreed that the effectiveness of an analgesic drug cannot be adequately assessed by testing its activity in relieving experimentally produced pain in healthy subjects. For this reason clinical methods of assessing analgesic activity have been devised. In order to obtain a quantitative measure of analgesic activity, patients with cancer or postoperative wounds and other painful conditions are instructed to assign to their pain a numerical score. Patients are selected with pain of sufficient intensity to require a powerful analgesic drug and they must be sufficiently intelligent to discriminate between pain of various grades, such as very severe, severe, moderate, slight or no pain. The scores can then be recorded on 'pain charts' of the type described by Keele and his colleagues.

Another procedure involves the use of trained observers who interview patients as to the degree of pain relief after the administration of a dose of analgesic drug. The relief is scored on an arbitrary scale. Neither patient nor observer should be aware of the nature of the drug administered.

A comparative assay in which the analgesic effects of morphine and codeine were tested in subjects with chronic pain is shown in Figure 3.7. A sequential procedure was used in this assay. Two doses of the standard drug, morphine, and two doses of the test drug, codeine, were administered to a number of patients. In the second part of the test, two doses of each drug were again used but adjusted in the light of the previous results so as to bring them into the same range of effectiveness. The regression lines of Figure 3.7 plotted on a logarithmic dose scale, indicate that morphine is 13 times as active as codeine.

Although the information derived from an assay of this kind is useful, it is incomplete. There are other relevant points to be considered such as whether the two drugs have the same maximum analgesic effects. For example there is evidence that when still higher doses are used the codeine curve levels off before the morphine curve so that the maximal relief obtainable with codeine is less than with morphine.

Another important point is whether equianalgesic doses of the two drugs differ in their side effects. For example the respiratory depressant actions of two analgesic drugs can be measured by their effects on alveolar CO_2, and related to their analgesic effects (p. 30) in order to find out whether the two drugs differ in their therapeutic ratios.

Tests of drug dependence
In the past the only way to assess the addictive properties of analgesics was from evidence of their clinical use, so that any dependence-producing liability of a new drug may have become apparent only after a considerable time. More recently, methods have been developed, based on observations on drug addicts, which enable dependence liability to be assessed in a relatively short time.

Tests in man. Addicts are stabilised by the regular administration of daily doses of morphine. When morphine is suddenly withdrawn from such individuals they exhibit an abstinence syndrome manifested by tremor, restlessness and fever (p. 483). The symptoms may be evaluated numerically by a point-scoring system. About 30 hours after withdrawal, when the morphine-abstinence syndrome reaches its peak, the new compound is administered at a predetermined dosage level. The suppression, if any, of the abstinence syndrome is compared in degree and duration with that achieved by a standard dose of morphine.

The new compound is considered to cause drug dependence if it can successfully substitute for morphine under these circumstances. A quantitative estimate of its relative physical dependence producing activity may be obtained by determining a dose equivalent to a standard dose of morphine. It has been shown in this way that heroin is more effective in causing physical dependence than morphine, equivalent doses being 18 mg heroin and 50 mg morphine.

Tests in animals. Since tolerance and addiction liability are closely linked it can usually be assumed that a drug which produces rapid tolerance in animals is addictive. The degree of tolerance may be assessed quantitatively from the increase in the ED50 value in analgesic tests after prolonged administration of the drug, mixed with food or water, to rats or mice.

OPIOID ANALGESICS

Opium is the dried latex or milky exudation obtained by incising the unripe capsules of *Papaver somniferum*. It contains variable amounts of alkaloids which can be classified into two groups.

Phenanthrene   Isoquinoline

1. Morphine, codeine, and thebaine, which are derivatives of phenanthrene.
2. Papaverine, narcotine, narceine, laudanosine, etc., which are derivatives of isoquinoline.

Powdered opium BP is standardised to contain 10 per cent of morphine.

Morphine, the structure of which is shown in Figure 21.1, contains two hydroxyl groups, one of which is a phenolic hydroxyl, and the other an alcoholic hydroxyl. Codeine has the phenolic hydroxyl replaced by the methoxyl group. Thebaine has both hydroxyl groups replaced by methoxyl groups.

Codeine has much less analgesic activity than morphine and is practically free from any liability to produce addiction. Thebaine is a powerful convulsant but has no clinical uses. Papaverine has no analgesic activity; its only important pharmacological action is relaxation of all smooth muscle including that of the arterioles (p. 123).

Pharmacological actions of morphine

The action of morphine on the central nervous system is a curiously irregular one, for it depresses some centres much more than others, and has a distinct stimulant action on certain functions.

The action of morphine in different animals depends in part on the degree of development of the central nervous system; much larger doses of morphine are required in lower animals than are required in the higher animals to produce the same effects. The analgesic dose of morphine in the mouse is 2 mg/kg, whilst in man it is about 0.2 mg/kg, and the lethal dose for a 20 g frog is the same as for a 70 kg man. The action of morphine on different species of animals also varies greatly; it produces depression in the dog, whilst in the cat it often causes excitement, but if the cat is kept perfectly quiet a hypnotic action is seen similar to that in the dog. The action of morphine in the dog is complicated; the first effects observed are salivation, vomiting and defaecation, but the animal then becomes lethargic, drowsy and falls asleep. The action of morphine on the central nervous system is therefore much more complicated than is that of the aliphatic narcotics which produce depression in all animals.

Analgesic effect

The most important pharmacological effect of morphine is analgesia. Analgesics are drugs which reduce pain without producing unconsciousness. Morphine belongs to the group of central analgesics, in contrast to the local analgesics or local anaesthetics (Ch. 23) which produce their effects by blocking conduction in nerves. The morphine-like analgesics are often referred to as narcotic analgesics in contrast to another class of analgesics, the anti-inflammatory or antipyretic analgesics which will be discussed later.

Wolff, Hardy and Goodell consider that the analgesic action of morphine has three basic components: (1) elevation of the pain threshold; (2) dissociation of pain perception from reaction to pain in such a way as to free pain from its implications; and (3) production of lethargy and sleep.

The precise site of the analgesic action of morphine-like drugs is not known. There is evidence that painful stimuli reach the cortex by two different pathways. The primary pathway reaches the cortex by way of the thalamus to provide perception and localisation of the stimulus. The secondary pathway reaches the cortex by way of collaterals through the reticular formation and allows stimuli to be modified and integrated. Previous experience plays an important role in pain sensation and one of the main effects of morphine is to diminish the effect of previous experience by distracting attention and diminishing anticipation of pain. Morphine-like drugs are more effective against dull constant pain than against sharp intermittent pain, and in contrast to the antipyretic analgesics they also relieve visceral pain.

A subcutaneous injection of 10 mg of morphine in man produces an inclination to sleep and dims sensations. The subject becomes introverted and pays little attention to feelings of hunger or cold. Psychological tests show that such doses of morphine produce very little depression of the higher mental functions. After small doses of morphine, subjects do mental work as well as normally but the ability to concentrate continuously is impaired. In some long established addicts, however, memory and other mental functions appear to be well preserved.

The effect of morphine on mood varies from euphoria to dysphoria. The latter is mainly due to side effects; morphine derivative such as diacetylmorphine (heroin) which have fewer unpleasant side effects are particularly likely to cause euphoria and addiction. In some individuals morphine can cause marked excitement or even delirium.

Other effects on the c.n.s.

Morphine constricts the pupil by an action on the oculomotor nucleus. A 'pin point pupil' is a characteristic sign of morphine administration in man. In species which are depressed by morphine such as man and the dog it constricts the pupil, but in the cat and mouse in which it causes excitement, morphine dilates the pupil.

Morphine affects various hypothalamic centres; thus it lowers body temperature and it produces antidiuresis by causing a release of antidiuretic hormone.

Doses of 10 mg of morphine in man depress the respiratory centre in the medulla slightly. The centre becomes less sensitive to CO_2 (Fig. 12.2) and the pressure of carbon dioxide in the blood rises. The rate of respiration is usually more affected than depth and after an initial period of depression of both, the depth of respiration may increase again thus compensating for the decreased rate. Large doses of morphine cause irregular periodic breathing and apnoea. The rise in arterial pressure produced by morphine causes an increase in cerebrospinal fluid pressure.

The cough centre is very sensitive to the morphine-like drugs (p. 173); doses as small as 4 mg morphine or 12 mg codeine suppress coughing. This action is useful in unproductive cough, but when morphine is used for premedication, care must be taken not to depress the cough reflex unduly during the postoperative period.

Nausea and vomiting often occur after morphine, due to stimulation of the chemoreceptor trigger zone in the area postrema of the medulla. Nausea occurs in about 30 per cent of subjects and vomiting in about 10 per cent. Nausea is more likely to occur in the upright position due to the additive effect of vestibular stimulation. Morphine also stimulates the vagal centre in the medulla and causes slowing of the pulse.

Effects on smooth muscle

The main effect of morphine on the gastrointestinal tract is an increase of tone of the pyloric, ileocoecal and anal sphincters and a diminished rate of propulsive movements of the intestine. Intestinal secretions are diminished. These actions, combined with a decreased sensory response to the stimulus of defaecation, lead to constipation (p. 200).

Morphine increases the pressure in the common bile duct and may also cause a spasm of the sphincter of the bladder leading to distension and a constant but ineffective desire to micturate. It has some constrictor effect on bronchial muscle which has been attributed to histamine release. Normally the bronchoconstrictor effect is not prominent but it may become dangerous when morphine is used in asthmatic patients.

Effects on the skin. When morphine is injected intradermally it produces a triple response which is due to histamine release. Systemic administration of morphine often causes itching and sweating.

Mode of action
In contrast to the unspecific depressant action of general anaesthetics morphine has selective pharmacological actions which can be explained in terms of interactions with specific receptors. Recent studies which have greatly clarified the notion of morphine or opiate receptors discussed on page 241. A consequence which follows from the receptor approach is that the distinction between agonists and antagonists in the opiate field becomes less sharp. Thus, whilst naloxone (p. 285) can be regarded as a pure antagonist acting on morphine receptors without any agonist activity, the overall action of nalorphine (p. 285) is of a partial agonist capable of both activating and blocking receptors. Naloxone and nalorphine antagonise not only morphine derivatives but also the synthetic analgesics pethidine and methadone which presumably act on the same receptors. They do not antagonise structurally unrelated drugs such as the anti-inflammatory analgesics.

Fate in the body
Morphine is absorbed from the gastrointestinal tract, but is usually administered subcutaneously or intramuscularly. It is partly broken down in the body and partly excreted in the urine in a conjugated form as the glucuronide. Small amounts of morphine are excreted in the gastrointestinal tract and, after subcutaneous injection, traces of the drug appear in the intestine in a few minutes.

Tolerance to morphine is very rapidly established, and after regular administration for 10 to 20 days the body becomes more resistant to its action. Tolerance is more marked to the depressant effects of morphine, such as analgesia, respiratory depression and sedation than to its stimulant effects. Little or no tolerance develops to the miotic and constipating effects of morphine. The tolerance that can be acquired for morphine is greater than that acquired for other drugs, for the ordinary lethal dose of morphine is about 300 mg, and morphine addicts have been known to take up to 5 g per day.

Therapeutic uses of morphine
Until recently morphine and its derivatives have been the chief drugs used to relieve severe pain, but new synthetic analgesic drugs have been introduced which are equally or more effective than morphine. The opium alkaloids, however, have also a sedative action which makes them particularly effective drugs when sleeplessness is associated with severe pain.

These properties make morphine one of the most indispensable and important drugs used in therapeutics.

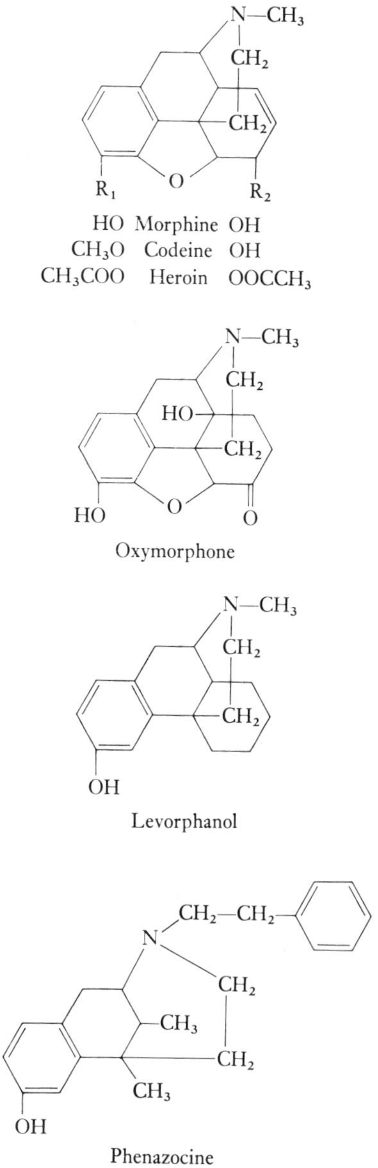

	R_1		R_2
	HO	Morphine	OH
	CH_3O	Codeine	OH
	CH_3COO	Heroin	$OOCCH_3$

Oxymorphone

Levorphanol

Phenazocine

Fig. 21.1 Structural formulae of morphine and related analgesic drugs.

The aphorism of Sydenham that without the help of opium few would be sufficiently hardhearted to practise medicine is still true today because no other type of drug can completely replace the morphine group as regards relief of pain. Unfortunately, morphine often causes nausea and vomiting; its also depresses the respiratory centre and produces constipation, actions which are very undesirable in conditions in which the drug is most needed.

A dose of 15 mg morphine hydrochloride is usually required to relieve pain but to relieve severe pain larger doses are necessary. The chief limiting factor is the depressant action of the drug on the respiratory centre.

Infants and the aged are very susceptible to this action of morphine: it cannot be given to infants with safety, and only small doses should be given to the aged.

Morphine is used to depress the cough centre and to relieve irritable cough. It has a powerful depressant action on the cough centre, but has an equally powerful action on the respiratory centre, and must be used with great caution in patients with dyspnoea due to pulmonary oedema in left-side heart failure.

The use of morphine in the symptomatic control of diarrhoea is discussed on page 200.

One of the main disadvantages of morphine is its liability to produce addiction or drug dependence. This is discussed on page 482.

Morphine poisoning

Doses of morphine above 100 mg produce toxic effects which are often fatal. The patient sinks into a deep sleep, from which he cannot be awakened. The circulation is at first not greatly affected, but there is great depression of the respiratory centre, periodic or Cheyne-Stokes breathing often occurs, leading to complete respiratory failure. When the respiration is insufficient to oxygenate the blood adequately, heart failure and death occur. The occurrence in a patient of deep coma, pin point pupils and slow respiration strongly suggest poisoning by a morphine-like drug and this can be confirmed if there is a sudden improvement in respiration after the intravenous administration of naloxone or nalorphine.

Morphine derivatives

The structural formula of morphine and some derivatives is shown in Figure 21.1. By substitution of the alcoholic or phenolic groups it is possible to synthesise various ethers and esters of morphine. It is also possible to make oxidation products of morphine and allied alkaloids. Many attempts have been made to provide derivatives of morphine without its undesirable properties of depression of the respiratory centre, liability to addiction and its constipating effect.

Codeine

Codeine is the methyl ether of morphine; it is a normal constituent of opium but is usually prepared by methylation of the phenolic group of morphine. After absorption most of the codeine is excreted in the urine in a conjugated form, small amounts are excreted as unchanged codeine or as morphine.

The pharmacological actions of codeine resemble those of morphine but are weaker. The analgesic activity of codeine in man has been variously estimated as one sixth to one fifteenth that of morphine (Fig. 3.7). Codeine has greater stimulant actions on the central nervous system than morphine and this limits the administration of very large doses of codeine. Partly for this reason it is of little use in severe pain.

It is about ten times less active than morphine in depressing the respiratory and cough centres, but even very large doses of codeine do not produce death by respiratory paralysis. Therefore, codeine is much the safer drug to use for the treatment of cough and it has the further advantage that its continued use seldom produces dependence. Codeine is less constipating than morphine and much less liable to produce nausea and vomiting.

Diamorphine (heroin)

When both hydroxyl groups are acetylated the morphine ester diacetylmorphine (diamorphine, heroin) is formed (Fig. 21.1). The differences between heroin and morphine are related to their physicochemical properties. Heroin is more water soluble and more rapidly absorbed than morphine. It is also more lipid soluble and penetrates the blood brain barrier more readily. Heroin is rapidly converted in the body to monoacetylmorphine and then to morphine (p. 43). It has been suggested that heroin acts as a carrier which is transported to the brain more readily than morphine and is converted there to the active compound morphine. This could explain why heroin has less peripheral and more central effects than morphine.

Heroin resembles morphine in its general effects and is two to three times more potent as an analgesic drug. It is very effective in checking cough, but since it acts more strongly on the respiratory centre, it is in no way safer than morphine. It is also claimed that heroin has less tendency to produce vomiting and constipation which is an important advantage in postoperative treatment. It is, however, a powerful drug of addiction and the effects of heroin dependence are usually considered to be worse than those of morphine dependence.

Oxymorphone (Numorphan)

This compound, dihydrohydroxymorphinone, is a semisynthetic derivative of morphine in which the alcoholic group is replaced by a ketonic group. Its chemical structure is shown in Figure 21.1. The analgesic activity of oxymorphone in man is five to ten times that of morphine; when given in equianalgesic doses its duration of action is about the same but it is less constipating. It has little antitussive action.

Oxymorphone can be used for the relief of severe pain in which its sedative and euphoric effects are also valuable. Like morphine it causes nausea and may produce alarming respiratory depression. This can be antagonised by naloxone. As with morphine, addiction and tolerance also occur.

Oxycodone pectinate is administered intramuscularly or by suppository to produce a more prolonged analgesic effect than morphine.

ANALGESIC DRUGS

Levorphanol (Dromoran)
This compound, 3-hydroxy-N-methylmorphinan, belongs to the morphinan series which differ in structure from the morphine group by the absence of an oxygen bridge (Fig. 21.1). It has about four times the analgesic activity of morphine but in equianalgesic doses the side-effects of these two drugs are similar.

The absorption of levorphanol from the alimentary tract is more reliable than that of morphine and the usual oral dose of levorphanol tartrate is 1.5–4.5 mg. Its liability to produce addiction is similar to that of morphine.

Phenazocine and pentazocine
Phenazocine (Narphen) (Fig. 21.1) is a benzmorphan derivative with a potency similar to oxymorphone. In equianalgesic doses it produces less sedation than morphine but similar respiratory depression. It is also liable to produce addiction.

Pentazocine (Fortral) is a derivative of phenazocine which has approximately one third the analgesic potency of morphine when given by injection. It is also a weak narcotic antagonist and may induce withdrawal symptoms if given to a morphine addict. Its principal advantage is that true dependence is almost unknown with it. It causes relatively little respiratory depression and is used in obstetrics where 40 mg gives good pain relief for about two hours with a low incidence of sickness.

Other synthetic analgesics
A number of compounds with morphine-like analgesic activity have been synthesised which are chemically quite distinct from the opium alkaloids. The most important of these compounds are pethidine and methadone.

Pethidine (Meperidine)
This substance (Fig. 21.2) was prepared in 1939, in a search for an antispasmodic drug with atropine-like properties. During the routine testing of the compound in mice, it was found to produce an erection of the tail similar to that produced by morphine (Straub reaction) and this chance observation led to the discovery of its analgesic action.

The analgesic activity of pethidine is only about one-tenth that of morphine and of shorter duration; it has little sedative action compared with the latter drug. Pethidine has no appreciable depressant action on the cough centre in man and, although it has some depressant action on the respiratory centre (Fig. 12.2), it does not depress the respiration of the new-born infant in doses which produce analgesia during labour. Although pethidine has a weak atropine-like action on isolated smooth muscle preparations it may contract the smooth muscle of the intestine in the intact animal. In man, pethidine, like morphine, produces spasm of the duodenum and contracts the sphincter of Oddi. In this way it may precipitate an attack of biliary colic. Unlike morphine it does not contract the colon and does not cause constipation.

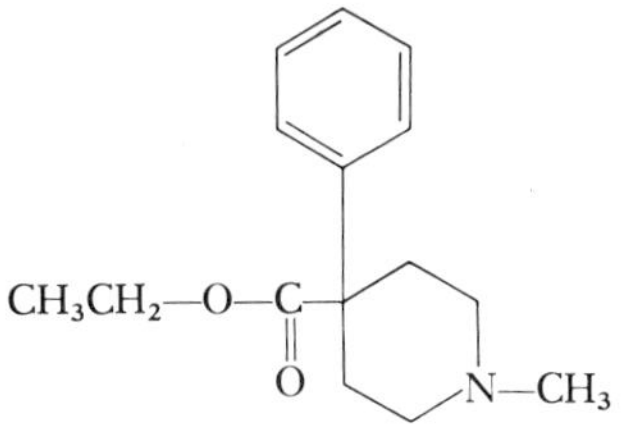

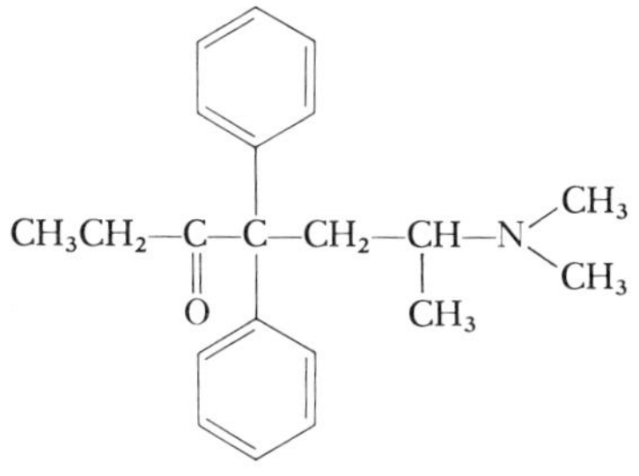

Fig. 21.2 Structural formulae of pethidine and methadone.

The chief side effects of pethidine are vertigo, dryness of the mouth, nausea and vomiting, and euphoria, which occur more often in the ambulant than in the resting subject. Tolerance and addiction to pethidine occurs but is less severe than with morphine.

The main therapeutic use of pethidine is in the relief of visceral pain arising from contraction of certain types of smooth muscle, for example renal colic and labour pains. It is less effective than morphine in controlling severe postoperative pain. Pethidine hydrochloride in doses of 50 to 100 mg by intramuscular injection acts in about 15 minutes and its effects last for about three hours; in the relief of chronic pain pethidine administered by mouth is as effective as when it is injected intramuscularly.

Nausea and vomiting by pethidine may be lessened by the addition of chlorpromazine which also provides the missing central sedation.

Phenoperidine and Fentanyl
Both these potent analgesics are related to pethidine; 2 mg phenoperidine and 0.2 mg fentanyl are about equivalent to 10 mg morphine in analgesic potency and respiratory depression. Both are used in conjunction with droperidol for neuroleptanalgesia (p. 305). Their respiratory depression may take several minutes to develop fully after intravenous injection and may be countered by nalorphine.

When fentanyl is administered intravenously in surgery it produces profound analgesia and when it is combined with a neuroleptic drug such as droperidol a state is brought about in which the patient is calm and indifferent to his surroundings and is able to co-operate with the

Methadone (Physeptone)
This compound possesses many of the characteristic actions of morphine. It is readily absorbed from most routes of administration and is metabolised to a considerable extent in the body; about 20–30 per cent is excreted in the urine. Its chemical structure is shown in Figure 21.2.

The actions of methadone resemble those of morphine in producing analgesia, respiratory depression, vomiting, tolerance and addiction. The activity of the L-isomer is much greater than that of the D-isomer. In animals the analgesic potency of methadone is about equal to that of morphine and ten time greater than that of pethidine. When tested on human volunteer subjects by applying radiant heat, methadone is about one to three times as active as morphine and about thirty times as active as pethidine (Fig. 21.3).

Clinical trials of methadone have shown that it relieves post-operative pain, pain due to dysmenorrhoea and to renal colic. The respiratory depressant action of methadone contraindicates its use for controlling labour pain. In contrast to morphine, methadone is much less sedative. It is very effective against cough even when given by mouth, but this route of administration is less satisfactory for the relief of pain. The incidence of side effects is lower than with morphine and is greater in ambulant than in non-ambulant patients. The chief side effects are nausea, vomiting, headache, drowsiness or euphoria, and dryness of the mouth.

Marked tolerance to the analgesic, sedative and respiratory depressant actions of methadone has been observed in dogs and in man, and there is little doubt that this drug causes addiction. This is also shown by the fact that methadone when given to morphine addicts completely alleviates the symptoms of morphine withdrawal. The withdrawal symptoms of methadone are, however, milder and of shorter duration than those of morphine.

Methadone-supported withdrawal. When methadone is administered to patients after withdrawal from heroin or morphine it satisfies their craving for the narcotic without producing euphoria. If withdrawal from the opiate is gradual, methadone may thus be administered in its place at first, followed by gradual reduction of the methadone dose. An alternative procedure, advocated by some clinicians, is to continue giving methadone in a single daily oral dose to these patients thus helping their rehabilitation (p. 491).

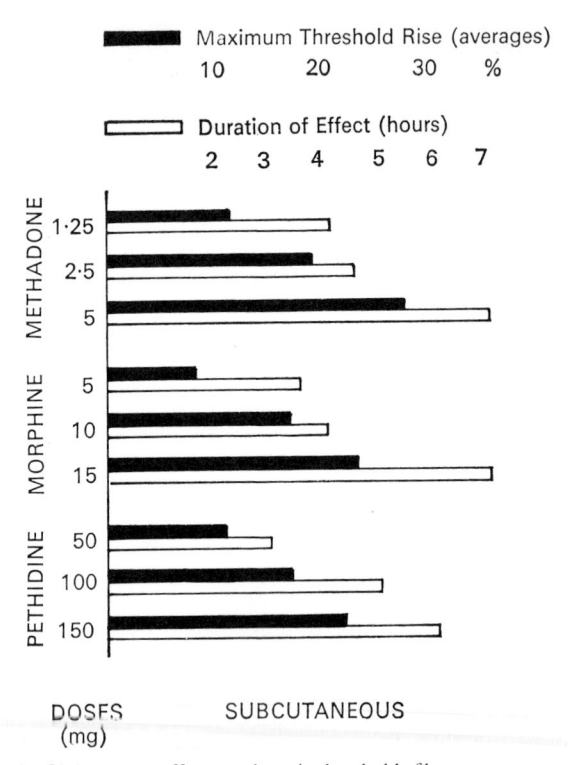

Fig. 21.3 Average effects on the pain threshold of human volunteers of methadone, morphine and pethidine. The stimulus used was a graded amount of radiant heat applied by a beam of light on a blackened area of the forehead. (Wolff, Hardy, Goodell method). The figure shows the maximum percentage rise in the threshold stimulus and the duration of the analgesic effect. (After Christensen and Gross, 1948, *J. Amer. med. Ass.*)

Dextromoramide resembles methadone with about twice its analgesic potency. It is a powerful drug used for pain of great intensity. It causes less drowsiness and constipation than morphine but produces marked respiratory depression and may induce persistent nausea and vomiting. It is liable to produce drug dependence.

Dipipanone is a methadone analogue and a moderately potent analgesic. It is effective by the oral route and is frequently prescribed together with an antiemetic such as cyclizine.

Dextropropoxyphene is an analgesic related to methadone with activity of the order of codeine. Dependence on it has been reported. *Distalgesic* is a proprietary preparation containing dextropropoxyphene and paracetamol which is increasingly used for self-poisoning in Great Britain.

Morphine antagonists

In 1915, Pohl reported that N-allylnorcodeine antagonised the depression of respiration produced by morphine and awakened a dog from deep sleep due to morphine. Many years later the structure of morphine was modified by removing the N-methyl group to form normorphine; normorphine base was then made to react with allyl bromide to form N-allylnormorphine hydrobromide (nalorphine Fig. 21.4) which was found to be a powerful antagonist of morphine.

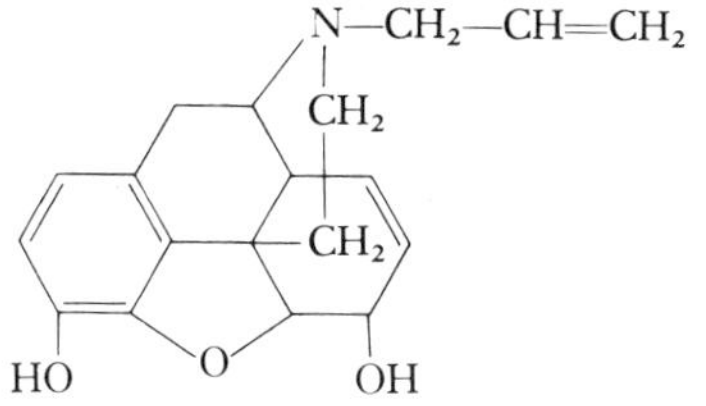

Fig. 21.4 Structural fomulae of morphine antagonists.

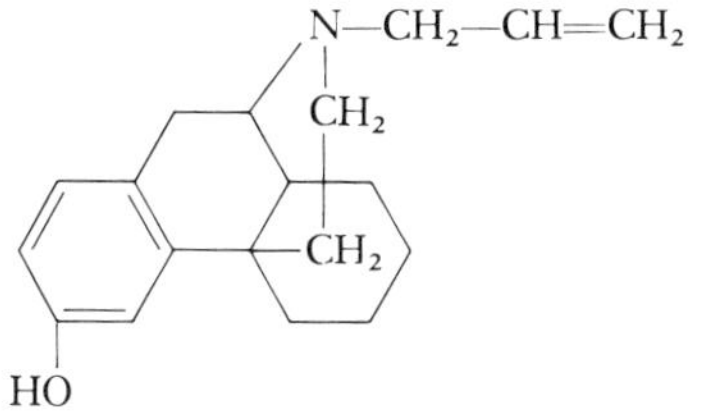

Nalorphine has a number of morphine-like actions of its own. Its main difference from morphine is that (1) it does not produce euphoria but causes unpleasant mental effects, (2) it is non-addictive and (3) it produces withdrawal symptoms when administered to morphine addicts. The most important property of nalorphine is its ability to counteract the respiratory depression caused by morphine and related drugs.

Nalorphine (Lethidrone)
Nalorphine (N-allylnormorphine, Fig. 21.4) can be regarded as a partial agonist acting on morphine receptors (p. 15). Such substances may be expected to have both agonist and antagonist properties.

It was formerly believed, on the basis of animal experiments, that nalorphine had no analgesic effect but it is now known that in man it has weak analgesic activity. Nalorphine is non-addictive and does not give rise to tolerance or physical dependence. It cannot be used as an analgesic, however, owing to its unpleasant central effects including anxiety and visual hallucinations.

Although nalorphine produces some respiratory depression, it can antagonise respiratory depression produced by morphine and related analgesic drugs. Nalorphine has little or no effect in mild respiratory depression but where this is severe it may produce a dramatic increase in respiratory rate and minute volume. It has been shown that a prerequisite for the antagonistic effect of nalorphine is a high blood pCO_2. Nalorphine antagonises the respiratory depressant actions of pethidine, methadone, and other analgesic drugs related to morphine, but not those due to barbiturates, cyclopropane or ether.

Another example of nalorphine antagonism is the development of typical signs of withdrawal in monkeys and dogs addicted to morphine and related analgesic drugs, within five minutes of an injection of nalorphine. Acute abstinence syndromes are also observed when nalorphine is injected into patients addicted to morphine or methadone. These withdrawal symptoms may be very severe and cannot readily be relieved by injections of morphine or methadone. When nalorphine is given to a morphine addict it causes dilatation of the constricted pupil and this has been used as a test of opiate addiction.

Nalorphine is used to prevent neonatal asphyxia when there is a risk that this may be due to obstetric analgesic drugs. It can also be administered intravenously to the mother in doses of 10 mg ten minutes before delivery.

Naloxone is chemically related to nalorphine but is a pure antagonist lacking agonist activity. Kosterlitz has shown by quantitative measurements that it is a competitive antagonist of the inhibitory effect of morphine on guinea pig ileum. Naloxone used as antagonist gave similar pA_2 values when tested with morphine, levorphanol and codeine suggesting that these drugs all act on the same receptor.

Naloxone may be used to decrease neonatal respiratory depression arising from the administration of a morphine-like analgesic to the mother.

Levallorphan (Lorfan) is more active, weight for weight, than nalorphine but its actions and uses are similar. Levallorphan is a very effective antagonist of opiate-induced respiratory depression.

ANTIPYRETIC ANALGESICS

The antipyretic analgesics were originally introduced because they reduced body temperature in fever. Several of these drugs, notably aspirin, were developed by the German pharmaceutical industry during the late nineteenth century and they are still widely used. Their clinical emphasis has shifted, however, and they are now employed much less as antipyretics than for their analgesic, antirheumatic and anti-inflammatory effects. Indeed, these drugs are now considered primarily as analgesics and anti-inflammatory agents and although their action in severe pain is not as powerful as that of the morphine-like drugs they also lack their undesirable properties of causing euphoria, tolerance and drug dependence.

Chemically the antipyretic analgesics can be divided into:

1. Salicylates such as aspirin.
2. Aniline derivatives such as phenacetin.
3. Pyrazole derivatives such as amidopyrine and phenylbutazone.
4. Indomethacin and other newer drugs.

Analgesic action of antipyretic analgesics

The function of the pain sense is protective; in Sherrington's classification of the senses, pain is termed 'nociceptive', which means sensitive to noxious agents.

Pain fibres have bare nerve endings which are distributed in the skin and in deeper structures. Pain arises from mechanical injury of these fibres through compression, deformation, stretching and cutting or by the action of chemical agents on them. Various substances which are liberated in the body during injury such as bradykinin, 5-hydroxytryptamine and histamine have been shown to cause pain when applied to the base of a blister which has been denuded of skin.

Pain sensation is conveyed by (1) fast medullated fibres of 2–4 μm diameter which conduct at a rate of about 20 m per second (A delta fibres) and (2) slow non-medullated fibres of about 1 μm diameter conducting at a rate of 1–2 m per second (C fibres). There is evidence that the former relay sharp pain and the latter dull aching pain. These neurones synapse in the posterior horns of the spinal cord with a set of neurones whose dendrites cross to the contralateral side to form the spinothalamic tracts. Their central connections are discussed on page 280.

It is usual to distinguish between three main types of pain: (1) superficial or cutaneous pain, (2) deep somatic pain originating from muscles, joints, tendons and fasciae, (3) deep visceral pain.

The antipyretic analgesics do not counteract appreciably cutaneous pain and do not raise the cutaneous threshold to pricking or heat; they are inactive in visceral pain. They are mainly effective in pain originating from muscles and joints, in headache resulting from distension of blood vessels and meninges, and in pain originating from nerve trunks. They are particularly active against pain originating from inflamed swollen structures. Thus, it has been shown in experiments in which the pain threshold in rats was measured by applying pressure to a foot, that antipyretics raised the threshold when pressure was applied to a swollen inflamed foot but not when applied to a normal foot. These findings suggest that, in addition to their centrally exerted effects on pain perception the antipyretic analgesic exert a peripheral action in diminishing 'inflammatory pain' by decreasing inflammation and capillary permeability and that a peripheral effect contributes substantially to their overall analgesic activity.

Anti-inflammatory effect of antipyretic analgesics

The anti-inflammatory effect of the antipyretic analgesics is fundamental both to their analgesic action and to their antirheumatic effect. The latter is particularly important in relation to rheumatoid arthritis which is one of the most crippling diseases of modern industrial society.

In testing drugs for anti-inflammatory activity various empirical models of inflammation are made use of. Activity in one or more models of inflammation is then compared with clinical effectiveness. This is necessary since the underlying mechanisms of rheumatism are only imperfectly understood. Some of the inflammatory models against which antirheumatic drugs such as phenylbutazone or indomethacin can be tested are as follows:

1. Oedema and swelling of the rat hind paw after the local injection of substances such as the seaweed extract carrageenin.
2. Erythema after applying ultraviolet radiation to the depilated skin of the guinea pig.
3. Granuloma pouch. The dorsal subcutaneous tissue of the rat is injected with 25 ml of air. The resultant sac is injected with a chemical irritant resulting in the formation of a sterile abscess. Alternatively cotton pellets may be implanted subcutaneously.
4. Adjuvant arthritis. There is much evidence that the inflammation associated with rheumatic diseases has an immunological basis. An inflammatory reaction, based on sensitisation, may be produced in certain strains of rats by injecting them intradermally with mycobacteria in mineral oil. When an injection is made into the footpad the injected foot swells rapidly during the first 4–6 days. Thereafter the swelling subsides until the 8th day and then resumes. Approximately 9–10 days after inoculation the other foot becomes swollen and inflammatory nodules may be found on the ears and tail. Drugs can be evaluated by their effect in inhibiting either the early inflammatory phase or the later phases.
5. Inhibition of prostaglandin synthesis. Potential antirheumatic drugs may be tested for this effect based on the hypothesis that antirheumatic activity is correlated with inhibition of prostaglandin synthesis (p. 92).

Salicylates

Natural products which contain precursors of salicylic acid such as willow bark which contains the glycoside salicin, and oil of wintergreen, which contains methylsalicylate, have long been used for the treatment of rheumatism. Salicylic acid and acetylsalicylic acid (aspirin) were synthesised in the 1850s and sodium salicylate soon became the treatment of choice in rheumatic disease. Aspirin was introduced into medicine in 1899 because it was considered to be less irritant to the stomach than salicylate.

The chemical structure of salicylates is shown below.

Sodium salicylate — COONa, OH

Methyl salicylate — COOCH$_3$, OH

Acetylsalicylic acid (aspirin) — COOH, OCOCH$_3$

Salicylic acid and methylsalicylate are highly irritant and are used only in local applications. Sodium salicylate is administered by mouth sometimes combined with sodium bicarbonate (p. 288).

Aspirin is obtained by substitution of the phenolic group of salicylic acid. Acetylsalicylic acid is relatively insoluble but its sodium and calcium salts are readily soluble; aluminium acetylsalicylate is even less soluble than aspirin. Tablets of soluble salts of acetylsalicylic acid are hygroscopic and must be protected from moisture. Effervescent aspirin (e.g. Alka Seltzer) and buffered aspirin are buffered, neutralised forms of acetylsalicylate.

Absorption of aspirin

Aspirin is largely absorbed from the intestine, but to some extent also from the stomach, as the undissociated acid. Absorption of aspirin from the stomach is important because this leads to its rapid appearance in the bloodstream, but it also causes damage to the gastric mucosa which may result in occult blood appearing in the faeces and sometimes in frank gastric haemorrhage.

Undissolved particles of aspirin given on an empty stomach are particularly liable to produce localised inflammatory reactions of the gastric mucosa because they act as a source of concentrated acetylsalicylic acid. Soluble buffered aspirin preparations are transported more rapidly through the stomach into the intestine. Enteric coated tablets do not damage the stomach but their absorption is considerably delayed as shown in Figure 21.5.

Fate of salicylate in the body

When a single dose of sodium salicylate is given by mouth appreciable concentrations of salicylate are found in the plasma within 30 minutes, peak levels are reached in approximately 2 hours and thereafter the concentration declines slowly over a period of 8 hours or more (Fig. 21.6).

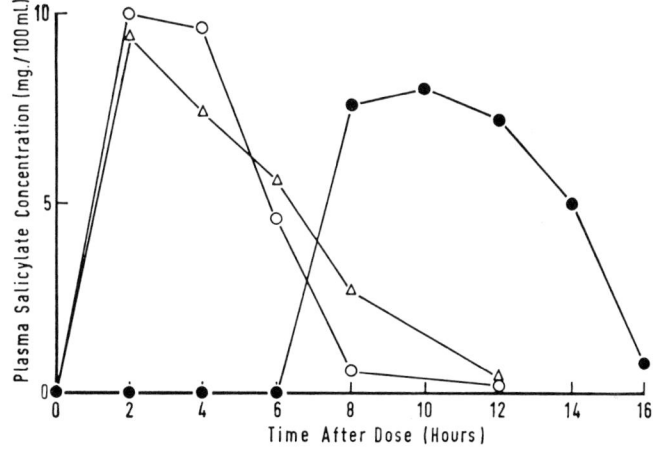

Fig. 21.5 Plasma salicylate concentrations after a single dose of various aspirin preparations.

1.0 g of an aspirin preparation was administered to the same subject in the fasting state on three occasions. Each point represents the mean of these three sets of observations. Plain aspirin is depicted by open circles, enteric-coated aspirin by closed circles, and aspirin-glycine by open triangles. (After Ansell, 1963, *Salicylates*, Churchill.)

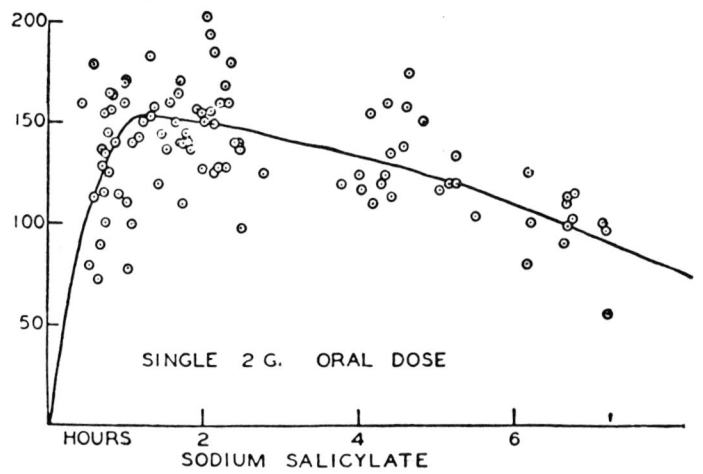

Fig. 21.6 Concentration of salicylate in plasma after single oral doses of 2 g sodium salicylate. (After Smith, reproduced by Gross and Greenberg, *The Salicylates*, 1948).

Most of the salicylate in plasma is combined with plasma proteins and is therefore non-diffusible. Serum containing sodium salicylate loses practically none of the salicylate to isotonic saline on prolonged dialysis, whilst serum dialysed against isotonic saline containing salicylate rapidly gains salicylate. As the concentration of salicylate in plasma increases, relatively less of it is in the bound form and the proportion of ultrafiltrable salicylate is raised.

Approximately 25 per cent of salicylate in the body is oxidised, the rest is excreted in the urine as compounds containing salicylic acid. Of the total amount of salicylate eliminated in the urine approximately one quarter is present as salicyluric acid, one quarter as the sulphuric or glucoronic acid conjugates of salicylic acid and one half as free salicylate.

The rate of urinary excretion of salicylate is higher in alkaline than in acid urine. This is due to the fact that salicylic acid is a weak acid of which the unionised lipid soluble fraction is highly diffusible whereas diffusion of the ionised fraction is negligible. When the urine is acid the tubules contain a high proportion of unionised salicylate which diffuses back into the blood whereas in alkaline urine the unionised fraction is small and salicylate clearance is increased. When salicylate is given by mouth it is sometimes combined with an equal quantity of sodium bicarbonate to reduce toxicity. The decreased toxicity is largely due to the fact that the administration of sodium bicarbonate increases the renal clearance and reduces the blood level of salicylate as shown in Figure 21.7.

Acetylsalicylic acid is hydrolysed partly in the gastrointestinal tract and partly after absorption into the blood stream; very little unchanged ester is excreted in the urine. After the ingestion of 0.6 g acetylsalicylic acid, free salicylate persists in the plasma for many hours, but the concentration of the acetyl ester declines rapidly and it cannot be detected after two hours. Since the persistence of the acetyl ester in blood corresponds approximately to the duration of analgesia it is probable that the unhydrolysed ester is the effective therapeutic agent.

Pharmacological actions of aspirin

Aspirin has analgesic, anti-inflammatory and antipyretic actions. It is used for the relief of less severe types of pain such as headache, rheumatic pain, myalgia and toothache, but it is also often effective in certain types of severe pain, such as pain associated with nerve compression or uveitis.

Some, at least, of the effects of aspirin can be attributed to interference with prostaglandin metabolism. Thus the administration of relatively small doses of aspirin in man results in an increase in bleeding time. This effect is believed to be due to inhibition by aspirin of the formation of aggregation-promoting thromboxane (p. 209) intermediates in the formation of prostaglandins from arachidonic acid. It has also been suggested that the antirheumatic and anti-inflammatory effects of aspirin and 'aspirin-like' drugs such as indomethacin may be due to interference with prostaglandin biosynthesis.

Toxic effects of salicylates

Salicylates may produce local and systemic toxic effects. Aspirin taken on an empty stomach is irritant and in animals and man may cause focal gastric erosions and bleeding. Aspirin frequently causes slight gastric bleeding; in a group of over 200 individuals with normal digestive tracts receiving aspirin the majority lost between 2 and 6 ml of blood per day and a small proportion a good deal more. Soluble aspirin caused as much bleeding as plain aspirin.

In the treatment of rheumatoid arthritis large doses of salicylates are administered and may give rise to a condition called salicylism. Typical signs are tinnitus followed by deafness, nausea and vomiting. Salicylates interfere with carbohydrate metabolism and in large doses they may produce ketosis; this leads to a systemic acidosis followed later by alkalosis through overbreathing and a consequent loss of carbon dioxide.

Aspirin poisoning. Attempted suicide by means of aspirin is not uncommon, but is often unsuccessful since large doses tend to produce severe vomiting. The fatal dose of aspirin in an adult is of the order of 30 g. Aspirin poisoning in small children is generally due to the accidental swallowing of tablets.

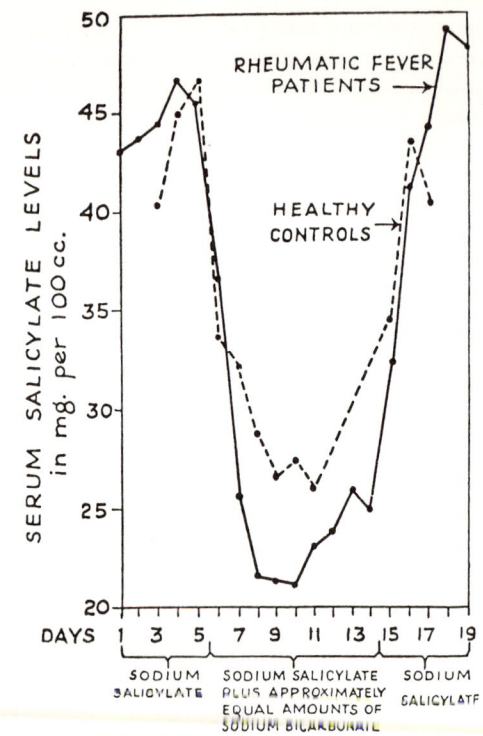

Fig. 21.7 Effect of sodium bicarbonate on the serum salicylate levels of four rheumatic patients and four healthy subjects. (After Smull, Wégria and Leland, *J. Amer. med. Ass.*, 1944.)

Treatment of aspirin poisoning consists in trying to eliminated the drug from the body and in correcting the disturbance of the acid-base balance. Apart from gastric lavage, bicarbonate may be administered systemically in order to promote the renal excretion of salicylate and to combat acidosis, but it is important to avoid producing a dangerous alkalosis. The use of peritoneal exchange dialysis or of an artificial kidney may be life-saving in aspirin poisoning.

Aspirin allergy. Aspirin sometimes becomes antigenic by combining with plasma proteins and it then provokes the formation of antibodies (p. 103). Aspirin allergy is usually severe but fortunately rare; it tends to occur particularly in middle-aged women. The allergic condition may manifest itself by an attack of asthma or angioneurotic oedema or a skin rash following ingestion of the drug.

Aspirin allergy resembles penicillin allergy in that it cannot be predicted by skin tests but only by the clinical history. These patients must be strictly enjoined not to take aspirin in any form.

Antirheumatic drugs

Aspirin and salicylates are the basic drugs used in rheumatoid arthritis. The theory that the antirheumatic effect of aspirin is closely related to its action in inhibiting prostaglandin synthetase is discussed on page 286. Large doses of aspirin need to be employed in rheumatic fever, dosage being determined by the severity of the disease and the occurrence of side effects such as tinnitus and gastric intolerance. Aspirin reduces the fever. It relieves pain and stiffness in patients with rheumatoid arthritis. Figure 21.8 shows the effect of sodium salicylate in a patient with acute rheumatic fever.

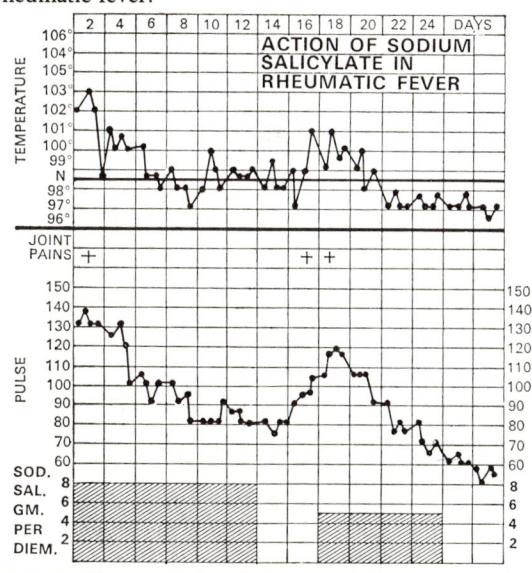

Fig. 21.8 Effect of sodium sacicylate in case of acute rheumatic fever. When the drug was stopped for two days there was recurrence of pains and a rise in temperature. (*From case of Prof. Murray Lyon.*)

Action of corticosteroids in rheumatic diseases

The rheumatic diseases consist of a group of disorders including rheumatic fever, rheumatoid arthritis, ankylosing spondylitis, osteoarthritis, and some non-articular forms of rheumatism in which there are fibrinoid changes in the connective tissues of the body. These changes are believed to arise from allergic tissue reactions as a result of which the extracellular components of connective tissue are altered and the collagen fibres disintegrate and disappear. Such lesions are usually accompanied by localised pain and oedema of tissues and generalised signs of an inflammatory reaction. The term *collagen diseases* has been used to describe these and other related disorders of the blood vessels and skin such as periarteritis nodosa, disseminated lupus, and scleroderma.

Administration of corticosteroids to patients with rheumatic fever and rheumatoid arthritis produces remarkable clinical relief but the signs and symptoms recur when the treatment is withdrawn. The mechanism of this action is not known. A corticosteroid does not eliminate the cause of the disease although it appears to modify the tissue response to the causative agent. Since it has been known for many years that salicylates and other antipyretic analgesic drugs also relieve pain and swelling in rheumatic disorders, attempts have been made to determine whether this effect is due to an increase in the output of adrenal cortical hormones by these drugs, but there is no clear-cut evidence of an action of this nature.

Several attempts have been made to compare the effectiveness of salicylates and corticosteroids in the management of rheumatic fever. There is general agreement that treatment with either type of drug does not prevent the complication of valvular heart disease. These drugs diminish pain and may be lifesaving in severely ill patients by their anti-inflammatory effects, but in this respect the corticosteroids are probably superior to the salicylates. At the beginning of an attack penicillin is usually also given for about ten days in order to destroy any haemolytic steptococci present in the nose and throat.

Non-steroidal anti-inflammatory agents

Many patients cannot tolerate large doses of aspirin for long periods and in view of the prevalence of rheumatoid and related conditions the need has arisen to find other drugs for use in their treatment. Most of these drugs are inhibitors of prostaglandin synthetase and they are generally liable to produce gastrointestinal disturbances and peptic ulceration.

Ibuprofen and fenoprofen

Both these drugs are derivatives of phenylpropionic acid. They have anti-inflammatory and analgesic activity and are effective in rheumatoid arthritis and other forms of joint disease. These drugs produce gastrointestinal upsets but they are claimed to produce untoward reactions less frequently than aspirin.

Mefenamic acid produces similar actions.

Phenylbutazone and oxyphenbutazone
These drugs, both pyrazolones (p. 291), have strong anti-inflammatory and analgesic properties.

Metabolism of phenylbutazone
Phenylbutazone is converted to two metabolites in man. One of these is oxyphenylbutazone, which is as active as an antirheumatic agent as the parent compound. Phenylbutazone is much more slowly metabolised by man than by various animal species: thus in rats and dogs its half-life is about 6 hours but in man about 72 hours. The prolonged retention of phenylbutazone in the body is responsible for its sustained effects but may lead to cumulation after repeated daily doses and consequent toxicity. Phenylbutazone is strongly bound to plasma proteins.

Clinical uses of phenylbutazone
Because of its antirheumatic and analgesic properties, phenylbutazone is effective in countering the inflammatory reactions of rheumatoid arthritis and acute gout; it also has considerable activity in other rheumatic conditions including osteoarthritis and ankylosing spondylitis.

The chief drawback of phenylbutazone is its toxicity. It may cause gastric irritation, haematemesis and occasionally other types of bleeding. It can also produce allergic skin rashes, leucopenia and rarely agranulocytosis.

Indomethacin
Indomethacin (indocid) is an indole derivative of the following structure:

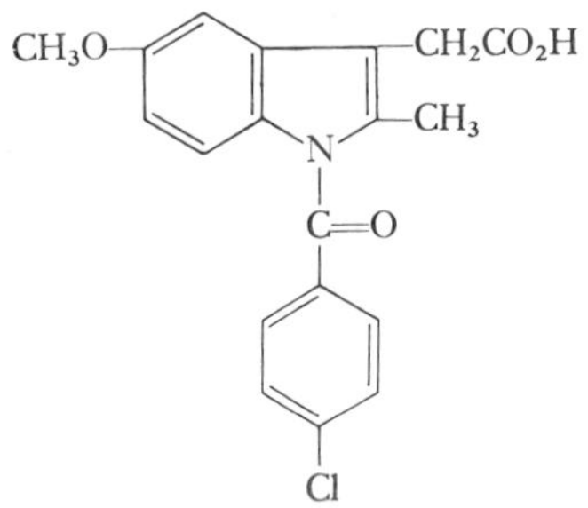

Indomethacin

Following oral ingestion it is almost completely absorbed within one hour and peak plasma volumes are reached within one to two hours. In the blood it is strongly bound to plasma proteins. It is relatively rapidly cleared from the body with a half-life of less than 20 hours. It is recovered in the urine mainly as indomethacin glucuronide.

Anti-inflammatory activity
Indomethacin has strong anti-inflammatory activity when tested in chronic inflammatory processes such as the cotton pellet granuloma pouch. It also inhibits carrageenin-induced oedema in the rat hindpaw. When tested in adjuvant arthritis (p. 286) it has activity comparable to that of the corticosteroid prednisone.

Clinical effects
Indomethacin is used clinically for its anti-inflammatory, antirheumatic and antipyretic effect. Its analgesic effect is seen particularly when pain is due to inflammation. It is effective in rheumatoid arthritis in which it reduces pain and tenderness of the joints. It is also useful in controlling the pain and stiffness of osteoarthritis and to control acute attacks of gout.

Like other non-steroid anti-inflammatory agents, indomethacin is not as effective in rheumatic conditions as the corticosteroids but it lacks their unavoidable side effects. Furthermore indomethacin may be combined with corticosteroids whose dosage can thus be reduced.

Toxic effects
Toxic effects of indomethacin have become apparent with its wider use. Frequent adverse reactions are headache, dizziness, nausea and diarrhoea. A serious complication is the occurrence of gastric and duodenal ulcers and the drug should be discontinued when there is evidence of occult bleeding.

Other antirheumatic agents
Several different essentially empirical approaches have also been used in the management of rheumatoid arthritis.

Gold compounds
Preparations such as *sodium aurothiomalate* are mainly indicated in active juvenile or adult rheumatoid arthritis. Their mode of action is not known, but they exert an anti-inflammatory effect in these disorders. They are administered by deep intramuscular injection.

The usefulness of gold treatment is limited by toxicity. Toxic reactions are liable to occur in up to 50 per cent of patients but in some 5 per cent of patients these reactions may be severe and on rare occasions fatal.

Other agents which have been found to be clinically successful in some cases of severe rheumatoid arthritis are: *penicillamine*, a chelating agent used in Wilson's hepatolenticular degeneration (p. 274); *azathioprine*, a cytotoxic and immunosuppressive drug (p. 381); and *chlorquine* an antimalarial (p. 440).

Para-aminophenol analgesics
Acetanilide, phenacetin and paracetamol have antipyretic and analgesic properties and are particularly effective in relieving the pain of headache, toothache and neuralgia.

All the aniline derivatives are liable to produce methaemoglobinaemia.

Acetanilide was synthesised in 1863 and introduced into medicine in 1886 as 'antifebrin' when its antipyretic activity was discovered by accident after its administration to a febrile patient. If it is administered repeatedly in large doses, acetanilide produces cyanosis due to the conversion of haemoglobin into methaemoglobin or sulphaemoglobin.

Phenacetin (acetophenetidine) largely replaced acetanilide in practice because it was less liable to produce methaemoglobinaemia.

Phenacetin is often used in combination with aspirin and caffeine (aspirin compound tablets) or with aspirin and codeine (codeine compound tablets). The latter contain 8 mg codeine phosphate; this amount of codeine is enough to cause constipation but does not contribute appreciably to the analgesic effect of the tablet, which is mainly due to its high content of aspirin and phenacetin.

In recent years it has become apparent that individuals who consume large amounts of mixtures of antipyretic analgesics (such as aspirin compound tablets) may show evidence of kidney damage which in some cases takes the form of interstitial nephritis and papillary necrosis. Since analgesic mixtures generally contain phenacetin this drug has been considered to be the chief cause of kidney damage although other ingredients, such as aspirin, may contribute to it. Although the connection between antipyretic analgesics and kidney damage has not been entirely clarified, it is now considered inadvisable for patients to consume large amounts of analgesic mixtures over long periods of time.

Paracetamol (N-acetyl-p-aminophenol, panadol) is the chief metabolite of acetanilide and phenacetin. It is formed rapidly in the body from each of these drugs and probably accounts largely for their analgesic activity; when tested in man the analgesic activity of paracetamol is about equal to that of the parent compounds. It is the least likely of the three aniline derivatives to produce methaemoglobinaemia and is now frequently used clinically either alone or in combination with other drugs.

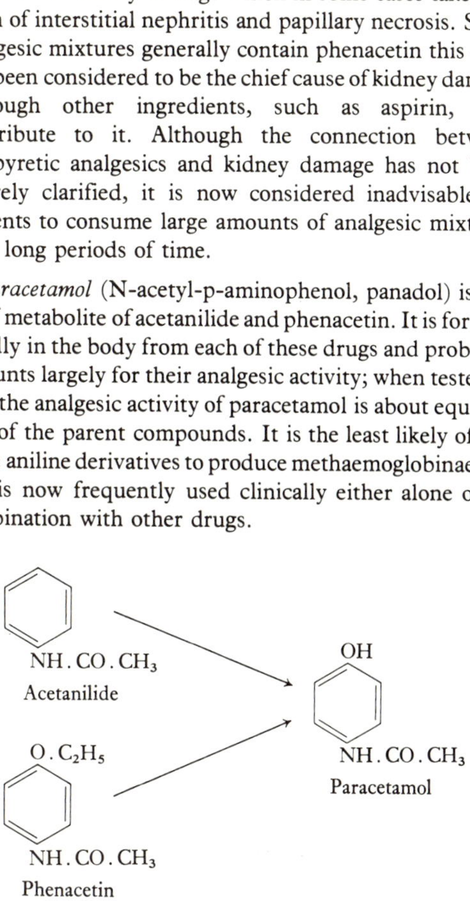

Paracetamol toxicity. In view of increasing restrictions on the use of phenacetin due to its nephrotoxic effects and its substitution by paracetamol, the possible toxic effects by the latter are assuming importance.

The main advantage of paracetamol over aspirin is that it does not cause gastric irritation and gastrointestinal bleeding. In contrast to phenacetin it does not cause methaemoglobinaemia and other haematological disturbances. In further contrast to phenacetin, there have been few cases of kidney damage clearly attributable to paracetamol, which is surprising in a metabolite of phenacetin. The main hazard of an overdose of paracetamol is hepatic necrosis which may be fatal. A subject who takes 50 tablets of aspirin will suffer from acute salicylate intoxication, as discussed, but will probably recover if he is correctly treated. By contrast a person taking 50 tablets of paracetamol may show no immediate effects but within a few days he may be severely ill with hepatic failure against which no effective form of treatment is at present available.

Pyrazole derivatives

The first clinically used pyrazolone compound was antipyrine introduced in 1884, followed soon by amidopyrine (pyramidon). Another important pyrazole derivative, phenylbutazone, was introduced much later, in 1948 and is discussed on page 290. These compounds are effective antipyretics, analgesics and antirheumatics, but they may on rare occasions produce agranulocytosis. For this reason antipyrine and amidopyrine are now seldom used in Great Britain whilst courses of treatment with phenylbutazone are usually restricted to limited periods of time.

The chemical structure of these compounds is shown below.

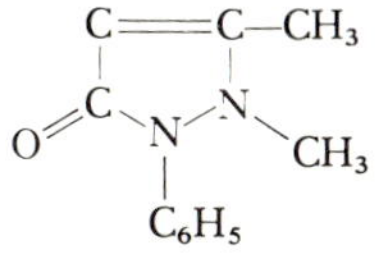

Phenazone
(antipyrine)

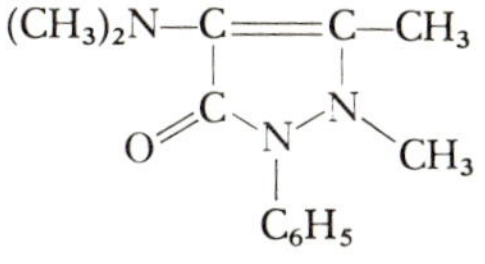

Amidopyrine
(pyramidon)

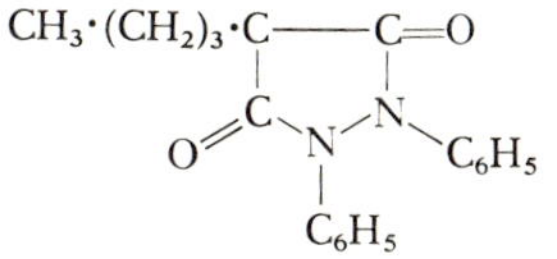

Phenylbutazone
(butazolidin)

Acetanilide

Phenacetin

Paracetamol

DRUGS USED IN GOUT

Gout is a metabolic disorder caused be derangement of purine metabolism. The end product of purine metabolism in man is uric acid. Whilst in birds and reptiles uric acid is the main product of all protein metabolism, the uric acid excreted by the human kidney is derived mainly from nucleoprotein.

The metabolic disorder of gout could be due either to an increased production of uric acid or to a decreased rate of elimination. Experiments with tracers suggest that in primary gout the main defect is an endogenous overproduction of uric acid. Uric acid is relatively insoluble and in patients with gout it becomes deposited in various parts of the body, particularly the joints. This gives rise to acute attacks of arthritis and finally to a chronic form of gouty arthritis in which the uric acid level of the plasma becomes chronically elevated.

The excretion of uric acid by the kidneys is not fully understood but a possible mechanism is indicated in Figure 21.9. According to this scheme uric acid is normally almost completely reabsorbed by the proximal tubules, whilst the portion which appears in the urine is secreted by the distal tubules. Certain drugs may interfere with reabsorption by the proximal tubules and in this way increase urate elimination.

Three kinds of drugs may be used in gout: (1) those such as colchicine which counteract the pain and swelling of the acute attack, (2) those like probenecid which promote renal excretion of uric acid, and (3) those like allopurinol which interfere with its metabolism.

Colchicine

Extracts of the autumn crocus *Colchicum autumnale* have been used for centuries in the treatment of gout. The alkaloid colchicine derived from this plant was first isolated in 1820 by Pelletier and Caventou.

Action in gout. The action of colchicine was previously considered to be entirely specific for gout, but it is now realised that certain related conditions (pseudogout) may also respond to it. Colchicine has no effect on serum uric acid levels and does not seem to promote the excretion of uric acid by the kidneys.

In the treatment of an acute attack of gout, colchicine is administered orally in doses of 0.5 to 1 mg hourly until the pain and swelling are relieved or toxic symptoms develop. No more than 10 tablets should be given altogether, since colchicine is toxic and may produce severe nausea and diarrhoea. Colchicine should be given at the earliest appearance of symptoms, when it may abort an attack, rather than after the full attack has developed; it can also be administered intravenously.

Colchicine treatment may be given in conjunction with phenylbutazone which is also very effective in acute gout. Indomethacin is also effective.

Action on cell division. Colchicine has a remarkable effect on cell division by arresting cellular mitosis in the metaphase. The antimitotic action has been the subject of much experimental work but has not, so far, found useful clinical applications.

Sulphinpyrazone (Anturan)

This compound is chemically related to phenylbutazone. It is a highly active uricosuric agent which is used in the treatment of chronic gout.

Another action of sulphinpyrazone is to inhibit platelet aggregation (p. 209).

The main side effect of sulphinpyrazone is nausea and abdominal pain; it may also activate a latent gastric ulcer.

Probenecid (Benemid)

Probenecid was introduced with the object of retarding the renal excretion of penicillin (p. 401); it is now seldom used for this purpose but is employed in gout since it promotes the renal excretion of uric acid.

The mechanism of this interference is considered to be as follows. Penicillin excretion and urate reabsorption probably involve the same carrier in the proximal tubule. The transport system for penicillin (P) can be formulated as

$$\text{plasma} \quad P + X \rightleftharpoons PX \rightarrow P + X \quad \text{tubule}$$

where X is an intracellular carrier. Substances which compete reversibly for X such as para-aminohippurate

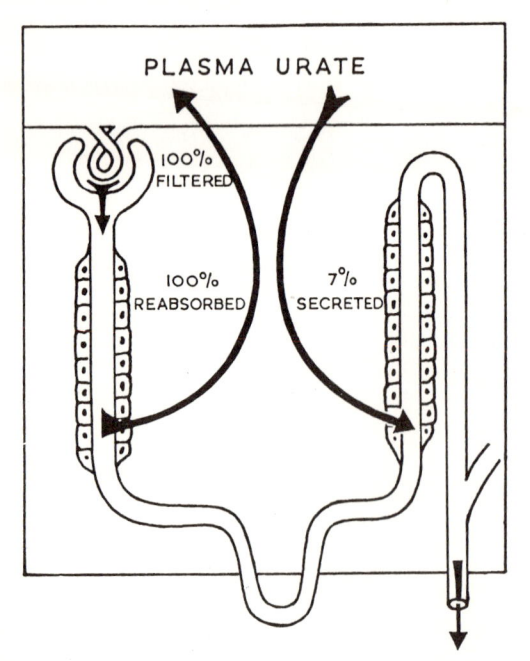

Fig. 21.9 Circulation of urate in the kidney. (After Dixon, 1963, *Salicylates*, Churchill.)

(PAH) would be expected to inhibit penicillin excretion but would not necessarily inhibit the reverse process of uric acid reabsorption since free carrier remains available at the tubular end. Probenecid, however, has a high affinity for X and therefore does not dissociate from it readily, so that the carrier is no longer available for the transport of uric acid.

Use of probenecid in gout. Patients with chronic gout usually have a raised blood uric acid and if they are treated with a uricosuric agent such as probenecid during intervals between attacks, the blood uric acid level falls and they are less likely to have another attack. The dose of probenecid is regulated on the basis of symptomatic response and blood uric acid levels.

Probenecid is of no use in an acute attack of gout and may even aggravate it. Patients receiving probenecid should have plenty of fluids since the increased urinary excretion of urates may lead to the formation of uric acid stones especially if the urine is acid.

Probenecid may be given together with small doses of colchicine. Probenecid should not be used in conjunction with salicylates which interfere with its uricosuric action.

Allopurinol (Zyloric)

This compound (Fig. 21.10) is chemically related to uric acid. It inhibits the enzyme xanthine oxidase which catalyses two essential steps in the formation of uric acid from hypoxanthine. Allopurinol inhibits the formation of uric acid, acting by a different mechanism from the uricosuric drugs probenecid and sulphinpyrazone, which promote the excretion of uric acid. As a result of allopurinol action, the uric acid level in plasma is lowered and its urinary excretion diminished.

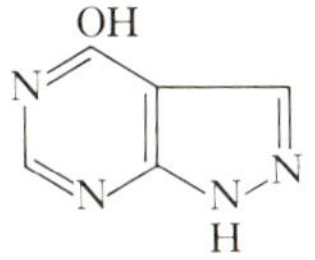

Fig. 21.10 Allopurinol

By lowering the uric acid concentration in the plasma the dissolution of tophi is facilitated and the incidence of attacks of gout is reduced.

Clinical uses. Allopurinol does not interfere with the clinical effectiveness of colchicine or the uricosuric drugs and since it sometimes causes attacks of acute gout at the beginning of treatment, colchicine is often used when treatment with allopurinol is begun.

The main indication for allopurinol is the treatment of patients with chronic hyperuricaemia whether in cases of gout or in certain blood dyscrasias. It may also be administered to prevent the increase in blood uric acid produced by thiazide diuretics.

Allopurinol therapy is generally effective in severe chronic gout exhibiting nephropathy, tophi and renal urate stones. When given in effective doses of 200 to 300 mg per day or above, over long periods, it decreases blood uric acid levels, produces resorption of tophi and an improvement in joint function.

Allopurinol is well tolerated by most patients, although occasionally it may cause allergic manifestations such as skin rashes.

PREPARATIONS

Opioid and related analgesics
Codeine phosph 10–60 mg
Dextromoramide tart (Palfium) 5–15 mg
Dextropropoxyphene hyd (Doloxene) to 260 mg dl
Diamorphine (Heroin) 5–10 mg po, s.c., i.m.
Dihydrocodeine tart 30–60 mg
Fentanyl citr 0.05–0.1 mg for short duration pain for
   neuroleptanalgesia 0.05mg/ml fentanyl + 2.5 mg/ml
   droperidol 1 ml/15 kg slow i.v. inf
Levorphanol tart (Dromoran) 1.5–4.5 mg
Methadone hyd (Physeptone) 5–10 mg po, s.c.
Morphine sulph 10–20 mg po, s.c., i.v.
Pentazocine 30–60 mg s.c., i.m., i.v.
Phenazocine hyd 5–20 mg po, 1–3 mg i.m.
Pethidine hyd 50–100 mg po, 25–100 mg s.c.
Phenoperidine hyd 0.5–5 mg i.v.

Narcotic antagonists
Cyclazocine 4–6 mg
Levallorphan tart (Lorphan) 200 μg–2 mg i.v.
Nalorphine hyd 5–10 mg i.v.
Naloxone hyd (Narcan) 400 μg s.c., i.m., i.v.

Antipyretic analgesics
Aspirin 0.3–1 g
Compound Aspirin Tablets (aspirin 225 mg, phenacetin 150 mg,
   caffeine 30 mg)
Paracetamol (Panadol) 500 mg–1 g up to 4x die

Non-steroid anti-inflammatory drugs
Alcofenac (Prinalgin) 500 mg–1 g 3x die
Aurothiomalate Sodium 1–50 mg i.m.
Azapropazone (Rheumox) 300 mg 4x die
Chloroquine phosph 150–900 mg dl
Diclofenac Sodium (Voltaren) 25 mg 3x die
Benorylate (actylsalicylic ester of paracetaml) 1–1.4 g up to 4x die
Fenoprofen Calcium (Fenopron) 300–600 mg 3–4x die
Flufenamic acid (Arlef) 600 mg dl
Feprazone (Methrazone) 200 mg 2x die
Flubiprofen (Froben) 100–150 mg dl
Hydroxychloroquine sulph (Plaquenil) 0.2–1.2 g dl
Ibuprofen (Brufen) 0.6–1.2 g dl
Indomethacin (Indocid) 50–150 mg dl
Mefenamic acid (Ponstan) 500 mg 3x die
Naproxen (Naprosyn) 250 mg 2x die
Oxyphenbutazone (Tandacote) 200–400 mg dl
Penicillamine hyd 0.5–1.5 g dl
Phenylbutazone (Butazolidin) 200–400 mg dl
Sulindac (Clinoril) 100–300 mg dl

Drugs used in gout
Allopurinol (Zyloric) 200–400 mg dl
Colchicine init 1 mg then 500 μg every 2 h
Probenecid (Benemid) 1–2 g dl

FURTHER READING

Braude M C et al (ed) 1973 Narcotic antagonists. Raven Press, New York

Harcus A W, Smith R B, Whittle B A 1977 Pain — new perspectives in measurement and management. Churchill Livingstone, Edinburgh

Kelley W N, Weiner I M (ed) 1978 Uric acid. Handb. exp. Pharm. 51

Vane J R, Ferreira S H (ed) 1979 Anti-inflammatory drugs. Handb. exp. Pharm. 50 (I & II)

22. Anaesthetics

Mode of action of anaesthetics 295; Stages of anaesthesia 296; History of anaesthetic drugs 298, Effect of solubility on uptake of inhalation anaesthetics 299; Ether 300; Vinyl ether 301; Halothane 301; Methoxyflurane 302; Enflurane 302; Nitrous oxide 302; Cyclopropane 303; Intravenous barbiturates 303; Non-barbiturates for intravenous anaesthesia 304; Ketamine 304; Neuroleptanalgesia 305; Premedication 305; Neuromuscular blockers 305; Choice of anaesthetics 306.

Mode of action of anaesthetics

The fundamental action of anaesthetic drugs consists of an unspecific and reversible depression of cell function. A very large number of aliphatic compounds can produce this type of action, and these drugs have many common properties. They are generally chemically inert substances which are more soluble in lipids and in lipid solvents than in water. Moreover, among these substances, homologous series can be found whose members possess anaesthetic powers of graded intensity. The aliphatic anaesthetics are therefore, a very favourable field for the investigation of the relationship between pharmacological action and chemical or physical properties, and a large amount of work has been done of these lines. The following are a few points of special interest.

Overton (1901) and Meyer (1899) made the first systematic study of this problem, and measured the minimum concentrations of drugs required to immobilise tadpoles. They also measured the relative solubility of drugs in oil and in water by dividing the solubility of the drug in oil by its solubility in water. This quotient is termed the oil/water distribution coefficient of the drug. Overton and Meyer investigated hundreds of compounds, and came to the conclusion that the activity of aliphatic anaesthetics varied as their oil/water distribution coefficient; that is to say, the greater the relative solubility of a drug in oil as compared with water, the greater its anaesthetic power. This hypothesis is of interest, because it represents the first attempt to correlate the pharmacological actions of drugs with their physical properties. The hypothesis also agrees very well with the theory that cells are surrounded with a lipoprotein membrane, for, if this be the case, it is natural that the lipid soluble drugs should enter the cells most easily.

A further generalisation was proposed by Ferguson who suggested that the anaesthetic action of a substance is related to its chemical potential.

The chemical potential or thermodynamic activity is a fundamental parameter related to other physicochemical properties such as surface activity and lipid solubility. The thermodynamic activity of a substance can be measured by its relative saturation, i.e. its effective anaesthetic concentration in a medium relative to the saturated concentration in that medium.

According to the above theory substances which exert an unspecific depressant action should be present at the same relative saturation when they exert equal anaesthetic effects. Table 22.1 shows indeed that although the vapour pressures of different substances required for anaesthesia in mice vary a great deal, their relative saturation is comparatively constant.

An example of unspecific depressant drug action is provided by the homologous straight-chain alcohols. In this series the thermodynamic activity increases with each additional carbon atom in the molecule and there is a corresponding increase in pharmacological activity as shown in Figure 22.1.

Table 22.1 Isonarcotic concentrations of gases and vapours for mice at 37°C (After Ferguson, 1939. Proc. Roy. Soc., *B*.)

Substance	Pressure at saturation 37°C.(p_s) mmHg	Pressure at narcotic conc.(p_t) mmHg	Relative saturation $\frac{p_t}{p_s}$
Nitrous oxide	59 000	760	0.01
Acetylene	51 700	494	0.01
Methyl ether	6100	91.2	0.02
Methyl chloride	5900	106	0.02
Ethylene oxide	1900	43.1	0.02
Ethyl chloride	1780	38.0	0.02
Diethyl ether	830	25.8	0.03
Methylal	630	21.3	0.03
Ethyl bromide	725	14.4	0.02
imethylacetal	288	14.4	0.05
Diethylformal	110	7.60	0.07
Dichlorethylene	450	7.22	0.02
Carbon disulphide	560	8.36	0.02
Chloroform	324	3.80	0.01

Mullins extended the work of Ferguson and concluded that equal anaesthetic effects occurred when a certain volume fraction of the membrane was occupied by the anaesthetic agent. The fraction was calculated to be about 1/100th of the membrane volume. One interpretation is that this represents a fraction of lipid 'pores' in the membrane through which ion movements can occur.

The action of anaesthetics resembles a physical rather than a chemical effect, for when the drug reaches a certain concentration it paralyses the cells, but this action is rapidly and completely reversed by lowering the concentration of the drug. The use of anaesthetics is entirely dependent on the fact that their action is rapidly and completely reversible.

Anaesthetics have a well-marked selective action, since the higher centres of the brain are paralysed by

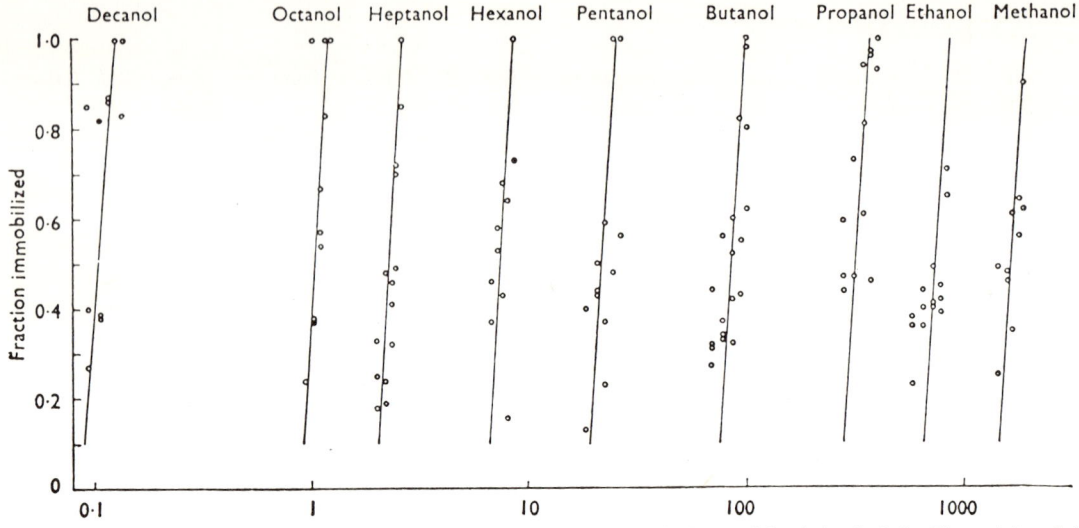

Fig. 22.1 Example of an unspecific depressant action (on motility of paramaecia) by straight chain alcohols. The activity of the alcohols increases about three-fold with each additional carbon atom in the molecule. (After Rang, 1960. *Brit. J. Pharmacol.*)

concentrations which produce little action on the other organs of the body. This selective action does not appear to be due to any selective concentration of anaesthetics in the brain, and it is not markedly specific, for these drugs in higher concentrations will paralyse any living cell. The simplest explanation of the mode of action of anaesthetics is to suppose that they produce a similar action on all cells. It would be possible to account for the apparent specific action by assuming that the functions of the brain are more readily disturbed than those of other tissues because they depend on a network of neuronal pathways with multiple synapses; a slight impairment of each link of a complex network may, by an additive effect, disrupt the whole system.

There is evidence that anaesthetics act selectively on synaptic transmission. Thus Larrabee has shown that transmission in the superior cervical ganglion is blocked by a considerably lower concentration of anaesthetic than that required for block of conduction along the axons leading to and from the synapses.

Stages of anaesthesia

All anaesthetics produce in the central nervous system a basically similar sequence of events. As a general rule the most complex and most recently established functions are depressed first, and there is no marked selective action on any particular type of function.

The important difference between the action of anaesthetics and that of alcohol is that the former cause loss of consciousness much more rapidly than the latter. Alcohol often produces great excitement prior to loss of consciousness, but as soon as consciousness is lost the patient passes into a comatose condition. Anaesthetics, when they are inhaled, produce an early loss of consciousness, which is followed by a stage of excitement. This difference is partly due to the mode and rate of administration, for ether, when it is drunk, produces an excitement stage more violent than that produced by alcohol.

Progress of ether anaesthesia. Although ether is now seldom used as the sole anaesthetic the development of ether anaesthesia represent a prototype of the stages of inhalation anaesthesia. Due to its slow onset, the development of anaesthesia with diethylether can be clearly divided into four stages: (1) induction; (2) excitement; (3) surgical anaesthesia; (4) commencing bulbar paralysis. In cases uncomplicated by premedication, these stages are characterised by the following signs and symptoms:

1. *Stage of induction.* The patient is conscious and experiences feelings of warmth, giddiness, and frequently of suffocation. The anaesthetic produces a marked hypnotic effect, and the patient may go to sleep; in this stage there is a progressive decrease in reaction to painful stimuli.

2. *Stage of delirium.* This stage begins when consciousness is lost and primitive emotions control behaviour. The auditory sense is usually last to disappear and first to recover. The reflex responses to stimuli are usually exaggerated, because the normal inhibitory influence of the higher centres is removed. Different individuals behave very differently during this stage, for some pass through it tranquilly, whilst others show great excitement; excitement is particularly common with muscular men or heavy drinkers. In this stage the breathing is irregular, and frequently the breath is held for some time, and then a deep breath is taken. The pulse is rapid and strong. All reflexes are present; for instance,

coughing, vomiting, the conjunctival reflex, and the reaction of the pupil to light. The pupils are dilated, owing to the excitement causing an increased secretion of adrenaline.

3. *Stage of surgical anaesthesia.* Breathing is regular and slow and abdominal in type, and the pulse becomes slow and regular; the pupils are contracted as in sleep. During this stage the various reflexes disappear in an irregular order and the patient becomes quiet.

The ordinary postural reflexes which maintain muscle tone disappear early, the muscles of the limbs and of the abdominal wall relax, and cutting of the skin or of the muscle does not produce reflex muscular contractions. The coughing, vomiting and conjunctival reflexes disappear a little later than the muscular reflexes. The last peripheral reflexes to disappear are the spasmodic movements of the diaphragm, which are provoked by irritation of the abdominal viscera, and in order to completely abolish these it is necessary to increase the depth of anaesthesia. Guedel introduced a useful subdivision of the stage of surgical anaesthesia into four planes; this scheme which is based on the effects of ether anaesthesia is shown in Figure 22.2. The first plane is characterised by roving movement of the eyeballs and full respiratory movements. In the subsequent planes central fixation of the eyeballs occurs and there is a progressive diminution in the movements of the intercostal muscles and the diaphragm. With anaesthetics other than ether the reduction in respiratory movements is less pronounced since ether, in addition to its central action, also has a peripheral neuromuscular blocking action.

The hypothalamic centres are paralysed during surgical anaesthesia. The most important consequence of this effect is that the heat regulating mechanism is paralysed and hence exposure to cold evokes no protective responses such as shivering, and the patient's temperature tends to fall to the temperature level of his surroundings.

4. *Stage of bulbar paralysis.* The paralysis produced by an anaesthetic becomes dangerous as soon as the vital centres of the medulla begin to be seriously affected, and as a general rule the anaesthetic should be reduced as soon as there is evidence that the patient is approaching this condition. The respiratory centre is the most sensitive of the vital centres and the chief feature of this stage is progressive depression of the respiration. The respiration becomes shallow and irregular and as a result the

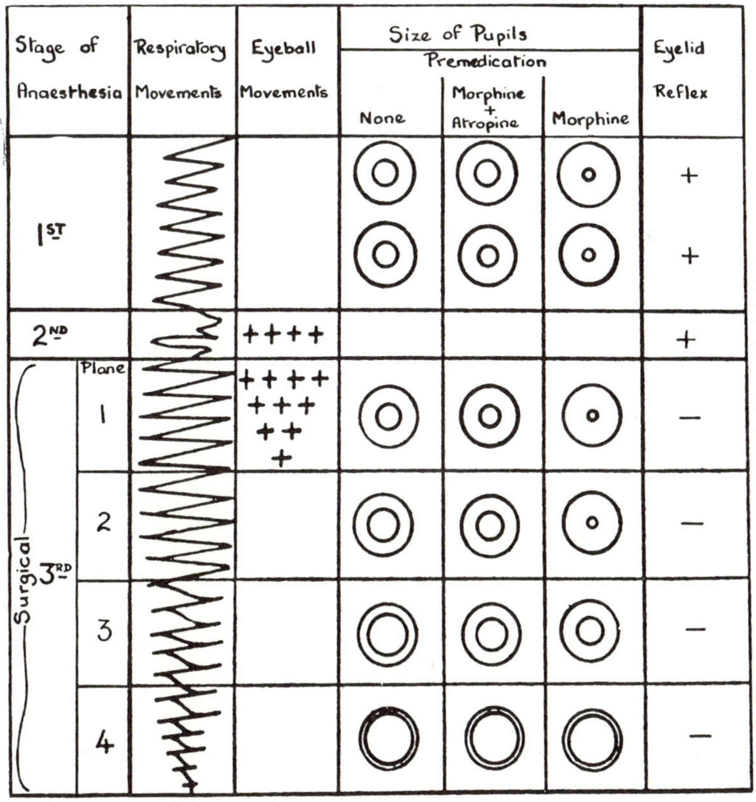

Fig. 22.2 Chart showing certain typical signs as they occur during ether anaesthesia. Transition from the second to the third stage is characterised by the appearance of full rhythmic respiration and the disappearance of reflex closure of the eyelids when the upper eyelid is gently raised with the finger. The chart shows that in order to assess the pupillary changes the anaesthetist must know what premedication has been used. (Guedel, 1937, *Inhalation Anaesthesia.*)

oxygenation of the blood becomes imperfect. The anoxaemia causes dilatation of the pupils, which is one of the first signs of danger. The pulse becomes rapid and feeble and the blood pressure falls. These effects are partly due to the deficient oxygen supply to the heart and partly to depression of the vasomotor centre.

During recovery the patient passes through the same stages as during induction, only in the reverse order. The first signs of recovery are usually dilatation of the pupil and return of the conjunctival reflex, and the coughing and vomiting reflexes return shortly afterwards. A short stage of excitement often precedes the return of consciousness, but after consciousness has returned the patient usually feels drowsy and may sleep for some hours.

Progress through various stages with other inhalation anaesthetics. The progression through various stages is not so well defined during anaesthesia with other agents, particularly when a combination of anaesthetics is employed. The pattern of depression may vary according to the anaesthetic agent used. For example whilst ether anaesthesia is characterised by marked analgesia, minimal autonomic cardiovascular impairment and good muscular relaxation, halothane anaesthesia is characterised by poor analgesia, unreliable muscular relaxation and considerable impairment of cardiovascular reflexes.

Certain effects of inhalation anaesthetics are common. Thus involuntary eye movements generally indicate absence of deep anaesthesia, whilst lack of the pupillary light reflex indicates deep anaesthesia, unless this is due to premedication by an atropine-like drug. All the inhalation anaesthetics depress temperature reflexes and during deep anaesthesia cortical electrical activity is depressed. All anaesthetics affect the e.e.g., but earlier suggestions that the e.e.g. might be used to measure the depth of anaesthesia have not been borne out by more recent investigations which have shown that the effects of anaesthetics on the e.e.g. differ widely. For example cyclopropane causes progressive synchronisation of the e.e.g. whilst enflurane produces spike-dome complexes of the e.e.g. resembling seizure activity.

Development of anaesthetic drugs

In 1798 Humphry Davy, aged 20, started investigating the chemistry and pharmacology of nitrous oxide and published his results in 1800. These brilliant researches showed that it was possible to anaesthetise human beings with nitrous oxide. Davy suggested its use for operations, but no notice was taken of this for more than 40 years.

In 1842 Crawford Long used ether as an anaesthetic in operations but did not publish his results. In 1844 Wells used nitrous oxide as an anaesthetic but, when he attempted to demonstrate his method in Boston, the demonstration was a failure. This caused a temporary setback in the use of nitrous oxide and 20 years elapsed before it was reintroduced and successfully used. In 1846 Morton used ether for the extraction of teeth, and on October 16th of that year he demonstrated the use of ether as a surgical anaesthetic with complete success at the Massachusetts General Hospital. The discovery was taken up with amazing speed; ether was used for surgical operations in London in December 1846, and in January 1847 Simpson used it in Edinburgh to relieve the pains of labour. Within a few months ether had revolutionised surgical practice in Great Britain and France. On November 15th 1847, Simpson used chloroform for an operation at the Royal Infirmary of Edinburgh. Chloroform was easier to give and easier to take than ether, and at once achieved great popularity. A brisk controversy regarding the merits of the two drugs, largely conducted on national lines, continued for the next 50 years until finally the superior safety of ether was generally recognised.

The anaesthetic effects of ethyl chloride were also discovered in 1847 but after that no other general anaesthetic drugs were discovered for about 80 years, although the method of administering volatile anaesthetics was greatly improved by the introduction of apparatus to control their rate of administration. In 1922, Brown and Henderson showed that ethylene was a more powerful anaesthetic gas than nitrous oxide and in 1928 Lucas and Henderson demonstrated the anaesthetic properties of the gas cyclopropane.

Although intravenous anaesthesia by chloral hydrate was reported as early as 1872, successful clinical anaesthesia by intravenous injection of non-volatile drugs became possible only after the discovery in 1932 of hexobarbitone (Evipan), a barbiturate which is rapidly destroyed in the body and produces a short-lasting depression of the central nervous system.

At present anaesthesia is produced either by the inhalation of a volatile anaesthetic or by the intravenous injection of a non-volatile drug. Some anaesthetics can also be administered rectally but this method is seldom used to produce surgical anaesthesia.

INHALATION ANAESTHESIA

The inhalation anaesthetics fall into two groups: (1) those which are liquids at room temperature and atmospheric pressure and must be volatilised before they are inhaled, and (2) those which are gases at normal pressure and temperature. These drugs are absorbed and excreted very rapidly through the lungs and hence the depth of anaesthesia can be rapidly altered. These properties also favour quick recovery when the administration has ceased.

The whole of the blood in the body passes through the lungs every 30 seconds, and hence a drug can be introduced into the blood stream more rapidly by inhalation than by any other method of administration, except of course, intravenous injection. Furthermore a volatile drug is excreted more rapidly than a non-volatile drug.

Effect of solubility on the uptake of inhalation anaesthetics

The extent to which a given gas will dissolve in a liquid can be expressed by its solubility coefficient. The Ostwald solubility coefficient is the volume of gas at ambient pressure and temperature taken up by a unit volume of liquid. This coefficient is shown for various anaesthetics in blood in Table 22.2. The coefficients vary over an almost hundredfold range. The solubility of an anaesthetic has an important effect on its pattern of distribution in various tissues. Basically, the more soluble an anaesthetic is in blood the longer it will take to reach equilibrium between alveolar air and blood and *vice versa*. Thus, cyclopropane and nitrous oxide, which are relatively insoluble in blood, will reach equilibrium with it rapidly and produce their full anaesthetic action in a short time, whilst ether which is highly soluble in blood will reach equilibrium and its full action very slowly if it is administered at a constant concentration.

Table 22.2 Ostwald solubility coefficients of various inhaled anaesthetics in blood at 37°C

Ethylene	0.14
Cyclopropane	0.46
Nitrous oxide	0.47
Halothane	2.3
Trichloroethylene	9
Chloroform	10.3
Di-ethyl ether	12
Methoxyflurane	13

Figure 22.3 shows two analogue schemes devised by Mapleson in which the distribution patterns of inhalation anaesthetics of low solubility (cyclopropane, nitrous oxide) and of high solubility (ether) are compared. The tissues are divided into three groups: (1) viscera, which includes the heart, brain, liver and kidneys, represent a small fraction of the body volume but a large fraction of the cardiac output because of their rich blood supply; (2) muscle (including skin), forming a large fraction of the body volume, but having a small blood supply at rest; (3) fat, which constitutes a relatively small fraction of the body volume with a poor blood supply, but is more soluble for anaesthetics than blood.

Figure 22.3 shows that a low solubility anaesthetic, e.g. cyclopropane, reaches rapid equilibrium in tissues such as brain with its good blood supply whilst its distribution in muscle and fat is slow. It follows that the brain gets close to equilibrium with inspired air, long before equilibrium with body tissues is reached. Figure 22.3 also shows that a high solubility anaesthetic such as ether reaches equilibrium more slowly. Because of the greater solubility of such an anaesthetic, neither the arterial blood in the lungs nor the brain becomes rapidly saturated whilst at the same time the anaesthetic gets distributed in muscle and fat. It follows that the brain can only reach equilibrium with inspired air at a time when the whole body is nearly equilibrated with the anaesthetic.

The above considerations show why anaesthetists do not administer a highly soluble anaesthetic, such as ether, at a constant rate until equilibrium occurs but administer it first at a concentration which is much higher than that required to anaesthetise the brain, and then reduce the concentration to prevent the patient becoming too deeply anaesthetised.

The account given above explains certain difficulties in the administration of anaesthetics. Owing to the rich blood supply of the brain any sudden increase in the concentration of anaesthetic inhaled may produce a depression of the central nervous system out of proportion to the actual amount of anaesthetic taken up by the body, and similarly cessation of administration of the anaesthetic

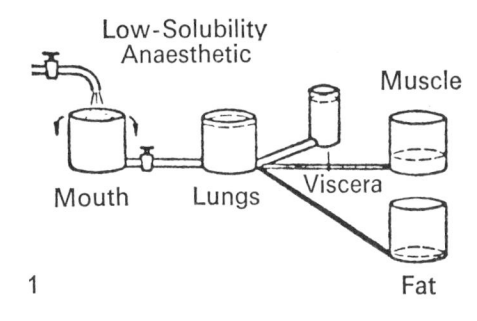

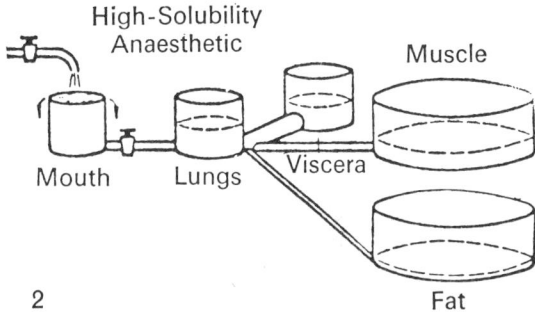

Fig. 22.3 Water analogue representing the distribution of inhalation anaesthetics of (1) low and (2) high solubility. The tissues are divided into 3 groups (see text); 'viscera' includes the brain. The cross section of each vessel is proportional to the capacity of the tissue to store anaesthetic, i.e. to its volume multiplied by the solubility of the anaesthetic in the tissue. The quantity of fluid in each vessel corresponds to the amount of anaesthetic present in it at a certain moment of time after beginning administration at a constant rate. The bore of the pipe leading to each vessel represents the blood flow to that tissue multiplied by the solubility of the anaesthetic in blood. (After Mapleson, 1972, *Heffter's Handbook*, vol. 30, Springer.)

causes a rapid fall in the concentration of anaesthetic in the brain.

In practice the safety of general anaesthesia is greatly increased through the use of drugs for premedication. These drugs are intended to diminish the amount of anaesthetic required and to reduce the undesirable side effects of anaesthetics.

Methods of administration

Inhalation anaesthetics may be administered in the following ways:

The open method consists of dropping a volatile liquid, e.g. ether, on a loose fitting mask covered with several layers of gauze.

The semi-closed method. A tight-fitting mask with an expiratory valve is applied to the face. A constant stream of oxygen or a mixture of oxygen and nitrous oxide is supplied to the patient either directly or after passing through a bottle of volatile anaesthetic.

The closed method. The patient breathes in and out of a bag containing the anaesthetic mixture, and provision is made for a continuous supply of oxygen and absorption of CO_2 (Fig. 22.4).

For the maintenance of anaesthesia closed methods are more economical. With a closed circuit the risk of explosion is lessened and body heat is better conserved since the anaesthetic gases are kept warm and moist by the patient's breath and there is no heat loss through evaporation.

Volatile liquids

Ether (diethyl ether)

$$CH_3-CH_2-O-CH_2-CH_3$$

This volatile liquid boils at 35°C; its vapour is highly inflammable and when mixed with air forms an explosive mixture. The vapour of pure ether will ignite at 190°C, whilst vapour, if contaminated by peroxides, may ignite at 100°C. The low boiling point of ether renders it difficult to administer in the tropics.

Ether when exposed to light and air forms various peroxides, and dioxyethyl peroxide has been shown to be a powerful irritant in low concentrations. The impurities in ether are of importance because they increase the irritant action of the gas. Anaesthetic ether should therefore be kept in small well-closed containers, and should not be used if the container has been opened for more than 24 hours.

Ether on evaporation reduces the temperature of the surrounding air, and, unless precautions are taken, the patient inhales very cold vapour which greatly increases the irritation of the respiratory passages. A concentration of ether which can be breathed without discomfort at 30°C is irrespirable at 10°C. The irritant ether vapour produces discomfort to the patient and for this reason ether should not be employed in the induction stage.

Pharmacological effects of ether

Ether stimulates sympathetic activity by a central action and produces a rise of blood pressure and an acceleration of the heart rate. It also causes a rise in the blood sugar. In man, ether anaesthesia does not depress the heart and does not tend to induce ventricular fibrillation. Ether has a neuromuscular blocking effect and potentiates the effects of tubocurarine.

The chief troubles associated with the use of ether as an anaesthetic arise from its irritant properties. It causes a free secretion of bronchial mucus which may interfere with respiration.

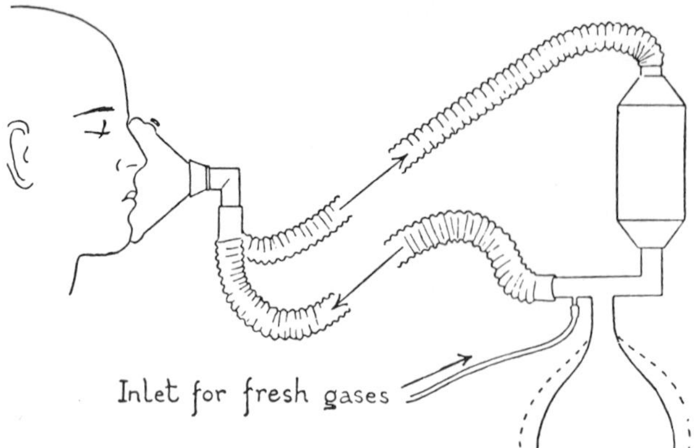

Fig. 22.4 Closed method. In this type of closed circuit method (circle method) valves must be used to direct the flow of gases through the soda-lime canister. Oxygen is added to the system at a rate of about 250 ml/min. Ether (or another inhalation anaesthetic) is added gradually into the circuit until the required degree of anaesthesia is reached. After that only small quantities of anaesthetic need to be added to compensate for leakages. (After Macintosh & Bannister, 1952, *Essentials of General Anaesthesia*, Blackwell.)

Ether anaesthesia produces some impairment of liver and kidney functions and, after ether anaesthesia, acetone and diacetic acid may be present in the urine as well as albumin and casts. Nevertheless, in spite of the current decline of its use, ether remains one of the safest anaesthetics.

Postoperative lung complications of volatile anaesthetics. A variety of lung complications may occur after operations. These are most likely to occur after prolonged administration of ether, but they may also occur after other inhalation anaesthetics, and even after operations with intravenous anaesthetics. The main factor is the development of localised collapsed areas due to imperfect ventilation of the lungs.

Massive collapse or atelectasis involving the lower lobes of the lungs is the most serious lung complication. This is probably due to deficient drainage of the bronchial tree during any prolonged period of unconsciousness which causes viscid mucus to accumulate and to block the finer bronchi. The impacted bronchi are invaded by micro-organisms and pneumonia results.

The most important method of preventing postoperative collapse is the removal of bronchial secretions by suction and by encouraging the patient to cough and to change his position in bed frequently.

Vinyl ether (divinylether)

$$CH_2=CH-O-CH=CH_2$$

This anaesthetic was introduced in 1933 by Leake. Its boiling point is 28.3°C and it is therefore more volatile than ether, is less irritant, and more rapid in its anaesthetic action. It is used in similar concentrations as ether and it also forms an explosive mixture with air. Vinyl ether is very unstable and decomposes rapidly when exposed to the air and to light. It must therefore be stored in tightly sealed coloured bottles. Vinesthene is a preparation of vinyl ether which contains in addition 3.5 per cent of absolute alcohol in order to render it less volatile.

Vinyl ether is a powerful anaesthetic and care is required in its administration since the various stages of anaesthesia are rapidly passed. It is now rarely used except for very short operations.

Chloroform

$$Cl-\underset{\underset{Cl}{|}}{\overset{\overset{Cl}{|}}{C}}-H$$

This is a volatile liquid which boils at 62°C. The liquid is irritant and if it remains in contact with the skin it may produce burns, if it enters the eye it will produce severe injury to the conjunctiva.

Chloroform is a powerful anaesthetic but has now become obsolete because of its toxicity.

The dangerous symptoms, or deaths, which have occurred under chloroform anaesthesia fall into three groups: (1) sudden heart failure occurring in the stage of induction; (2) dangerous symptoms or deaths occurring in the later stages of prolonged anaesthesia; and (3) delayed chloroform poisoning due to liver damage.

Halothane (Fluothane)

$$F-\underset{\underset{F}{|}}{\overset{\overset{F}{|}}{C}}-\underset{\underset{Br}{|}}{\overset{\overset{Cl}{|}}{C}}-H$$

This is a potent inhalation anaesthetic, first described by Raventos in 1956. It is a clear non-explosive and non-inflammable liquid with a chloroform-like smell; its boiling point is 50°C.

Anaesthesia may be induced with 1.5 to 3 per cent v/v halothane given with oxygen or with mixtures of nitrous oxide and oxygen. More usually anaesthesia is induced with intravenous thiopentone before giving halothane with oxygen. Anaesthesia is maintained with 0.5 to 1.5 v/v halothane and recovery is usually rapid. Halothane is non-irritant to the respiratory tract.

Muscular relaxation with halothane is moderately good but it may be necessary to use a neuromuscular blocking drug such as suxamethonium or gallamine to achieve complete relaxation. The cardiac output, arterial pressure and pulse rate are reduced by halothane in proportion to the depth of anaesthesia. Halothane dilates the bronchioles and reduces salivation and bronchial secretions and is a suitable anaesthetic for patients with bronchial asthma.

Halothane is a useful anaesthetic which is employed a great deal in thoracic surgery and, because of its non-inflammability, whenever electrocauterisation is required. It is not used in obstetrics since it inhibits uterine contractions.

Signs of halothane overdosage are respiratory depression, bradycardia and profound hypotension. Cardiac arrhythmias may occur. Halothane sensitises the heart to catecholamines.

Post-halothane jaundice is a serious but rare occurrence. The effects of acute and chronic exposure to anaesthetic doses of halothane were extensively studied in various species of experimental animals but no significant functional and morphological changes in the liver were observed.

In the early 1960s a number of clinical reports of postoperative hepatic damage in patients who had been anaesthetised with halothane led to a re-examination of this problem. In Great Britain, the evidence obtained from post mortem reports showed that the incidence of fatal hepatic necrosis in patients who had halothane anaesthesia twice within a month was about 1 in 6000. Retrospective surveys were also carried out in the United States and the collective evidence suggest that there is a significant association between the occurrence of post-halothane jaundice and two halothane anaesthetic exposures repeated within four weeks. When the interval between repeated halothane anaesthesia is greater than four weeks the risk is much smaller. Present evidence suggests that hypersensitivity to halothane resulting in liver damage may occur in some individuals after repeated administration.

Methoxyflurane (Penthrane)

$$\begin{array}{cc} Cl & F \\ | & | \\ HC & - COCH_3 \\ | & | \\ Cl & F \end{array}$$

This is a non-inflammable volatile liquid with a fruity smell which boils at 104°C. Because of its low vapour pressure at room temperature the maximum achievable concentration of the anaesthetic in air is only about 3 per cent. It may be used in a concentration of 0.35 per cent for obstetric analgesia and in a concentration of 1.5 per cent or more for general anaesthesia.

Methoxyflurane is seldom used alone as an anaesthetic, partly because induction with this agent is slow (10 to 20 min). It is a potent anaesthetic, however, and is suitable for maintaining anaesthesia during long operations. When used in high concentrations it tends to depress respiration and blood pressure and cause sinus bradycardia.

High doses of methoxyflurane have been shown to cause kidney damage, presumably due to the fact that the anaesthetic is metabolised in the liver to free fluoride and oxalate both of which are nephrotoxic.

Enflurane (Ethrane) and its isomer *isoflurane (Forane)* are both fluorinated ethers with basic characteristics resembling halothane. Both are powerful non-explosive anaesthetics said to be less liable than methoxyflurane to undergo metabolism to fluoride and to produce kidney damage. Enflurane produces muscular relaxation sufficient for abdominal surgery. It is often given with nitrous oxide. Enflurane is a respiratory depressant. A potential drawback is that it may produce electroencephalographic dysrhythmias.

Trichloroethylene (Trilene)

$$\begin{array}{c} H \\ \diagdown Cl \\ C = C \\ Cl \diagup \diagdown Cl \end{array}$$

This is a non-inflammable liquid which boils at 87°C. Owing to its low volatility it cannot be administered by an open mask and is unsuitable for administration by closed circuit methods since it interacts with soda lime to form the highly toxic substance dichloracetylene. It must therefore be given by a special inhaler in which a mixture of trichloroethylene and air is inspired by the patient through a non-return valve and exhaled through an expiratory valve on the face-piece. One of the characteristic actions of trichloroethylene is that it produces marked analgesia in low concentrations, and inhalation of 1-2 ml produces dizziness and analgesia lasting for a few minutes without loss of consciousness. Trichloroethylene is used mainly as an obstetric analgesic and as an anaesthetic for minor surgery of short duration.

Anaesthetic gases

Nitrous oxide

N_2O is the only inorganic gas used clinically to produce anaesthesia in man. It is a colourless gas with a faint smell and is one and half times as heavy as air. Nitrous oxide is not explosive and non-inflammable but it supports combustion. The tissue cells, however, cannot use it as a source of oxygen. Nitrous oxide is stored in cylinders as a liquid under 40 atmospheres pressure.

Nitrous oxide in concentrations which do not produce anoxia has only a weak anaesthetic action. This can be demonstrated by administering a mixture of 20 per cent oxygen and 80 per cent nitrous oxide. This mixture has the same oxygen content as air and it produces analgesia and unconsciousness but does not cause surgical anaesthesia in a normal adult unless he has received premedication; even so, full muscular relaxation cannot be achieved. The inhalation of a mixture of 80 per cent nitrous oxide and 20 per cent oxygen produces no change in blood pressure, no depression of respiration or postoperative shock. In order to produce anaesthesia for surgery with this mixture it is necessary to give in addition another anaesthetic such as halothane and a neuromuscular blocking drug.

Full anaesthesia can be obtained with nitrous oxide by reducing the concentration of oxygen inhaled and thus causing anoxaemia. This method, however, can be dangerous in unskilled hands because, to produce full anaesthesia, it is necessary to restrict the oxygen supply to a point where serious injury may be caused to the brain. For this reason pure nitrous oxide can be given only for very brief periods.

Indeed, most anaesthetists consider that oxygen restriction below 20 per cent oxygen with 80 per cent nitrous oxide is never justified whilst others would allow lower percentages of oxygen for short periods followed by 20 per cent oxygen.

Nitrous oxide is widely used and more techniques of general anaesthesia are based upon it than any other agent despite its low intrinsic potency. The highest concentration of nitrous oxide that can be given safely for maintenance of anaesthesia ranges from 75 to 80 per cent and for prolonged anaesthesia a 65:35 mixture of nitrous oxide and oxygen is considered to be necessary to completely avoid anoxia.

To produce surgical anaesthesia it is usual to induce anaesthesia by an intravenous barbiturate followed by the inhalation of nitrous oxide in oxygen, anaesthesia can then be continued by adding small amounts of halothane or another volatile anaesthetic to the inspired mixture. Nitrous oxide has a marked analgesic effect even in low concentrations which is made use of in childbirth (p. 223). Nitrous oxide with oxygen, sometimes together with halothane, is widely used in dental surgery.

Untoward effects of nitrous oxide. Apart from the serious dangers of anoxia they are small. It has been shown that 80 per cent nitrous oxide has a slight depressant action on cardiac contractility. Nausea and vomiting sometimes occur after nitrous oxide. A peculiar sequel of nitrous oxide anaesthesia is diffusion hypoxia. Nitrous oxide diffuses more rapidly through the alveolar wall than oxygen. Hence during induction with nitrous oxide it diffuses preferentially into the blood leaving relatively more oxygen in the alveoli, whilst during recovery the opposite happens and alveolar oxygen concentration is diminished. Oxygen should therefore be administered during emergence from prolonged anaesthesia with nitrous oxide.

In summary, apart from its fundamental drawback of low potency, which can be remedied by combination with other drugs, nitrous oxide is an excellent anaesthetic which is non-inflammable and non-irritant, acts rapidly and also has marked analgesic activity.

Cyclopropane (Trimethylene)
This gas has the formula $(CH_2)_3$ or

$$\begin{array}{c} CH_2 \\ \diagup \diagdown \\ H_2C\!-\!CH_2 \end{array}$$

It is one and half times as heavy as air and forms with air a mixture that is inflammable and explosive.

Cyclopropane is a powerful anaesthetic with a rapid action (Fig. 22.3), which produces anaesthesia in 1 to 3 minutes. A concentration between 10 and 20 per cent is usually sufficient for anaesthesia whilst 4 per cent produces analgesia. High concentrations (45 per cent) rapidly produce respiratory arrest.

Cyclopropane is administered by rebreathing in a closed system into which oxygen and cyclopropane are introduced as required and from which carbon dioxide is removed by soda lime. It should be administered by an experienced anaesthetist, since the stages of anaesthesia are passed very rapidly. Induction by cyclopropane is very rapid but marked excitement and even delirium may occur during this stage. Recovery from the anaesthetic is equally rapid and may be also accompanied by excitement. Satisfactory muscular relaxation can usually be obtained with the additional use of neuromuscular blocking drugs. Cyclopropane often produces cardiac irregularities such as ventricular extrasystoles and tachycardia. Capillary oozing may be troublesome during operation. In contrast to anaesthesia with nitrous oxide, the tissues are well oxygenated and the skin remains pink owing to the high concentration of oxygen used in the closed circuit.

Cyclopropane is not irritant to the mucous membrane of the respiratory tract. Cyclopropane depresses the respiratory centre and for this reason assisted ventilation is generally used during cyclopropane anaesthesia.

Cyclopropane is an excellent anaesthetic with a wide range of safety between anaesthetic and lethal dose. Its main drawback is the danger of explosion and for this reason it is being increasingly abandoned in favour of the non-explosive halogenated hydrocarbon anaesthetics.

INTRAVENOUS ANAESTHESIA

Barbiturates (p. 243)
Certain barbiturates and thiobarbiturates which are inactivated relatively quickly in the body can be used by intravenous injection to produce general anaesthesia. Their elimination from the body is, however, much slower than that of a volatile anaesthetic, hence it is much more difficult to reverse the effects of an overdose.

These ultra-short acting barbiturates produce a rapid onset of unconsciousness but they are relatively ineffective analgesics and do not completely abolish responses to painful stimuli. They are used mainly for three purposes.

1. To produce brief general anaesthesia for minor operations and diagnostic procedures, for example, cystoscopy.

2. For the pleasant and rapid induction of anaesthesia which is then continued with other anaesthetics.

3. As basal anaesthetics in doses which are insufficient to produce full anaesthesia but which enable the amount of the main anaesthetic to be reduced.

The drugs which are chiefly used for intravenous anaesthesia are the oxybarbiturates: hexobarbitone sodium (evipan sodium) and methohexitone sodium (brevital sodium), and the thiobarbiturates: thiopentone sodium (pentothal) and thiamylal sodium (Surital). The chemical formulae of some of these compounds are shown in Table 18.1.

Thiopentone sodium (Pentothal)
This drug produces a fuller relaxation, less twitching and a longer anaesthesia than does hexobarbitone sodium and is preferred to it by most anaesthetists.

The effect of an intravenous dose of one of these drugs depends not only on the total quantity but also on the rate of injection. For example a rapid injection of 0.3 g thiopentone sodium may produce unconsciousness followed by rapid recovery whilst a slow injection of the same dose produces only drowsiness. In the latter case the drug diffuses away into the tissues before the blood level necessary for anaesthesia is reached. In the former case a high concentration of drug in the blood is produced and a corresponding rapid accumulation of drug in the brain with its rich blood supply. The blood level soon falls because the drug becomes distributed in other tissues, especially the body fat, and is also destroyed in the liver; in consequence the concentration of the drug in the brain is reduced and the patient reawakens. Thiopentone which is present in the body fat eventually re-enters the blood stream and is destroyed in the liver. Only a small fraction of the drug is excreted unchanged in the urine. Thus, although the anaesthetic effect of an injection of thiopentone may last for only 5 or 10 minutes, the drug is only slowly eliminated and complete recovery of the patient may not occur for several hours.

The general aim of administration is to produce a high concentration of drug in the brain and to prevent this concentration from falling too rapidly. One method recommended is to give 0.3 g thiopentone sodium in about 10 seconds and then wait for 30 seconds during which time the patient usually falls asleep. After this safety pause, the injection is continued until the desired degree of anaesthesia is produced. More drug may be then injected from time to time if the depth of anaesthesia is to be maintained. The essential condition is that the dose is determined for each individual during the injection by careful observation. Figure 3.10 shows the degree of individual variation in response to another barbiturate, amylobarbitone sodium (sodium amytal), and in the case of hexobarbitone the dose needed to produce anaesthesia in patients of the same age and sex may vary from 0.4 g to 1.5 g.

Thiopentone can be used alone either for short anaesthesia or for prolonged anaesthesia by continuous intravenous infusion. It is more usual however to use in addition nitrous oxide or some other inhalation anaesthetic since thiopentone is a poor analgesic. Furthermore the maintenance of a prolonged anaesthesia of constant depth with thiopentone is difficult and the rate of recovery is slow. Usually the patient regains consciousness within 10 to 15 minutes of the last injection but after prolonged thiopentone anaesthesia recovery may take an hour or more.

Methohexitone sodium or *thiamylal sodium* are frequently used for anaesthesia in outpatient departments because of the rapid recovery from their effects.

Dangers of barbiturate anaesthesia. The chief danger of these drugs is that an overdose depresses respiration and if this happens during operation mechanical ventilatory support becomes necessary. Soluble hexobarbitone is liable to produce clonic twitchings. Barbiturates sometimes produce laryngospasm and are therefore not suitable as anaesthetics for operations involving the larynx and respiratory passages. These drugs are also contraindicated in patients with respiratory obstruction.

Solutions of thiopentone sodium are very irritant and must not be injected unless it is certain that the needle is in the vein. A particularly serious complication is the accidental intra-arterial injection of the solution; this causes a violent and prolonged contraction of the blood vessels which usually results in gangrene and may necessitate amputation of the limb. The spasm of the arterioles can sometimes be relieved by an injection of 3–5 ml of a 2 per cent solution of procaine hydrochloride into the artery.

Intravenous anaesthesia is very pleasant for patients since the operation of introducing the needle is negligible; the induction is very rapid and there are few if any aftereffects. The method has attained great popularity but it also involves certain risks and must only be used if measures have been prepared for dealing with respiratory depression.

Non-barbiturates for intravenous anaesthesia

Diazepam (p. 249)

An aspect of the action of diazepam and related benzodiazepines is its ability to produce amnesia. Intravenous diazepam may be used as an anaesthetic for minor procedures such as reduction of fractures in which total immobility of the patient is not necessary, merely the abolition of the memory of a painful procedure. It is used in dental surgery. Diazepam causes slight respiratory depression but compared with thiopentone induction it causes less hypotension and bradycardia.

Ketamine

This new type of drug is said to produce 'dissociative anaesthesia' because during induction the patient feels dissociated from his environment. He appears to be awake, in that movement may occur and the eyes remain open, but he is apparently unconscious and unresponsive to pain which he cannot afterwards recollect.

Intravenous ketamine may be used as the sole anaesthetic agent for short diagnostic or surgical procedures that do not require skeletal muscle relaxation and it is also used for induction of anaesthesia by other agents.

Untoward effects include blood pressure rises and psychological effects during emergence from anaesthesia varying from a pleasant dream-like state to hallucinations and in rare cases delirium. A potential disadvantage in children is a long awakening time and postoperative vomiting.

Ketamine hydrochloride

Neuroleptanalgesia
This is a state of calm mental detachment with mild sedation, accompanied by a high degree of analgesia, which may be induced prior to anaesthesia by nitrous oxide and oxygen. Neuroleptanalgesia is usually produced by combining a drug of the haloperidol group such as droperidol with a short acting opiate drug such as fentanyl (p.283). They may be administered either separately or as a combined slow intravenous infusion (innovar). When the droperidol-fentanyl mixture is combined with nitrous oxide-oxygen it is referred to as neuroleptanaesthesia.
The droperidol-fentanyl mixture without nitrous oxide can be used for diagnostic procedures such as bronchoscopy and to provide sedation and analgesia for burn dressings.

Althesin
Selye discovered in 1941 that certain steroids would produce anaesthesia in laboratory animals. Hydroxydione is a steroid which was used at one time clinically as an anaesthetic but has been abandoned because it caused thrombosis. Althesin consists of a mixture of two steroids, alphaxolone and alphadolone, which produce rapid anaesthesia when injected intravenously in man. Althesin is a clean anaesthetic without after-effects which may be used for the induction of anaesthesia or in anaesthesia for short procedures. In some patients it causes twitchings and involuntary movements. Severe cardiovascular and respiratory reactions to althesin have been reported.

Propanidid is a very short acting intravenous anaesthetic. It is prone to produce allergic reactions.

PREMEDICATION

This term refers to the use of drugs before administration of an anaesthetic. Its purposes are to calm the patient and allay anxiety, thus facilitating induction. Another purpose especially of opioid administration is to diminish the amount of general anaesthetic subsequently required. Other purposes are more specific; to diminish pain present before operation, to decrease salivation and to antagonise vagal action on the heart. A variety of drugs have been used for premedication and no generally acceptable unique approach has emerged.

Opiate analgesics and their derivatives. A combination of morphine and an anticholinergic drug (atropine, scopolamine) was almost universally used in conjunction with ether anaesthesia to diminish both secretions and apprehension. Opiates and derivatives are still considered essential when preoperative pain is present. All the opiates produce sedation but they also increase the incidence of pre- and postoperative nausea and vomiting. Pentazocine or fentanyl are now frequently employed for premedication in place of morphine or pethidine.

Sedatives and hypnotics. Relatively short-acting barbiturates such as quinalbarbitone and pentobarbitone are now frequently used for preoperative medication. They cause less nausea and vomiting than the opiate drugs although postoperative restlessness and pain are greater.

Anti-anxiety drugs. Diazepam does not reduce pain but when given preoperatively it produces sedation and lessens apprehension. The absence of nausea and vomiting is a considerable advantage of the benzodiazepines when used for preoperative medication.

NEUROMUSCULAR-BLOCKING DRUGS IN ANAESTHESIA

To produce deep muscular relaxation by means of a general anaesthetic, it is usually necessary to establish a depth of anaesthesia in which the medullary centres of respiration and circulation are depressed. Under such conditions many of the physiological mechanisms for maintenance of the circulation and resistance to injury are impaired and the patient is liable to develop surgical shock. The advantage of using the neuromuscular blocking drugs is that they produce muscular relaxation by their peripheral action, and make it possible to obtain full surgical anaesthesia with a much smaller amount of general anaesthetic. The mode of action of these drugs and their classification into two types, those which prevent depolarisation of the motor endplate and those which depolarise it are discussed in Chapter 5. These drugs are used in conjunction with various anaesthetic agents such as nitrous oxide and oxygen, halothane and thiopentone sodium.

Tubocurarine chloride was the first neuromuscular-blocking drug introduced into clinical practice (p. 66) and is still one of the most widely used. This drug tends to increase salivation and atropine or hyoscine premedication should be given to avoid this troublesome effect. It is usual to induce anaesthesia with thiopentone sodium and to follow this with an intravenous injection of 10–30 mg of tubocurarine chloride. This may be given in two stages; first a test dose of 5 mg is administered to determine whether the patient is unduly sensitive to the drug followed by a second dose of 10–20 mg. Endotracheal intubation is performed to maintain a clear airway. This enables intermittent positive pressure ventilation to be safely given and also prevents aspiration of regurgitated stomach contents. Anaesthesia may then be maintained with nitrous oxide and oxygen or any other suitable general anaesthetic. When ether is used only about one third of the usual dose of tubocurarine is required, since ether itself produces some neuromuscular block.

It is customary to assist recovery from tubocurarine at the end of the operation by administration of neostigmine. To prevent the muscarine actions of this drug, atropine (1 mg) is given intravenously at least 5 minutes before the intravenous injection of 2 to 5 mg neostigmine methylsulphate.

Gallamine triethiodide (Flaxedil) although weaker than tubocurarine has the advantage that it does not produce ganglionic block. It may however produce tachycardia.

Pancuronium is a bisquaternary ammonium steroid that is about five times as active as tubocurarine. It is a competitive neuromuscular blocking agent with little action on the cardiovascular system.

Suxamethonium chloride (Scoline) *and*
Suxamethonium bromide (Brevidil M)
Suxamethonium (p. 68) is the chief depolarising muscle relaxant drug in clinical use. Its outstanding property is the short duration of its action which makes it suitable for a procedure such as the the introduction of a bronchoscope which requires brief relaxation of the muscles of the larynx. Suxamethonium is also extensively used in conjunction with thiopentone to reduce muscular movements during electroconvulsive therapy. An intravenous injection of 50 mg suxamethonium produces half a minute by complete muscular relaxation which lasts approximately 5 minutes.

Respiratory depression and even apnoea may occur immediately after the injection and in some patients with a genetic deficiency of cholinesterase (p. 29) the apnoea may be prolonged. Muscle pains are a frequent after-effect of suxamethonium administration.

CHOICE OF ANAESTHETIC

This is a complex problem. At one extreme there is the question of the best method for use by a specialist anaesthetist in a large institution, and at the other extreme the question of the safest method for use in an emergency operation in a cottage by a practitioner who seldom administers anaesthetics.

Nitrous oxide and oxygen, halothane and thiopentone and under conditions where special equipment is lacking, ether, are the anaesthetic drugs most frequently employed and current practice is to use two or more of these or other general anaesthetics for induction and maintenance of anaesthesia.

Depending on the type of operation, the anaesthetist must produce analgesia, anaesthesia and muscular relaxation to a varying extent. Whereas formerly these three actions were obtained rather indiscriminately by the use of a single drug, it is now possible to produce each of these effects in a graded fashion. By a combination of analgesic, local and general anaesthetic and neuromuscular blocking drugs a balanced anaesthesia may be achieved which provides the optimum conditions for the surgeon and the minimum disturbance for the patient.

In spite of many advances in the use of anaesthetics the death rate from anaesthesia is by no means negligible. In a large scale investigation of the deaths associated with anaesthesia and surgery in United States hospitals it was estimated that 1 in 1500 patients dies from the anaesthetic. The mortality rate from individual anaesthetics could not be accurately determined since they were seldom used alone. In a survey of anaesthetic deaths occurring in British hospitals, the most frequent causes of death were inhalation of regurgitated stomach contents and circulatory failure, especially in the course of intravenous barbiturate anaesthesia. Another frequent cause of death was respiratory obstruction or respiratory depression in the immediate postoperative period.

PREPARATIONS

Inhalation anaesthetics

Anaesthetic gas
Cyclopropane, induct 25–50% with oxygen, maint 10–20% with oxygen
Non-halogenated volatile fluid
Ether (Diethylether), induct 10–30%, surg anaesth 5–15%
Halogenated volatile liquids
Halothane (Fluothane) induct 1–4%, maint 0.5–2%
Fluroxene (Fluoromar) induct 6–12% maint 3–8%
Methoxyflurane (Penthrane) analges 0.5%, anaesth 1.5–3% for short time with nitrous oxide, anaesth mainten 0.5%
Trichlorethylene (Trilene) analges 0.25–0.75%

Intravenous anaesthetics

Barbiturates
Methohexitone Sodium (Brietal) 30–120 mg slow i.v. infus
Thiamylal Sodium (Surital) 3–6 ml 2.5% sol
Thiopentone Sodium (Penthotal) 100–150 mg i.v.

Non-barbiturates (short acting)

Alphadolone acet and Alphaxalone (Althesin) 50–75 μg/kg slow i.v.
Etomidate sulph 300 μg/kg i.v.
Ketamine hyd (Ketalar) 2 mg/kg i.v.
Propanidid (Epontol) 5–10 mg/kg i.v.

Neuromuscular blocking drugs

Competitive blocking agents
Alcuronium Chloride (Alloferin) init 0.6–1.1 mg/kg i.v.
Fazadinium Bromide (Fazadon) 0.75–1 mg/kg i.v.
Gallamine Triethiodide (Flaxedil) 2–2.5 mg/kg i.v.

Pancuronium Bromide (Pavulon) init 0.02–0.08 mg/kg, subseq 0.01–0.02 mg/kg i.v.
Metocurine Iodide (Metubine, Dimethyltubocurarine init 0.11–0.14 mg/kg subseq 0.02–0.03 mg/kg i.v.
Tubocurarine Chloride 0.2–0.4 mg/kg i.v.

Depolarising blocking agents
Suxamethonium Chloride (Anectine) init 0.6–1.1 mg/kg i.v.
Suxethonium Bromide (Brevidil E) (short duration of action)
Hexafluorenium bromide (Mylaxen) 0.3–0.4 mg/kg (prolongation of suxamethodium action by inhibition of plasma cholinesterase)

FURTHER READING

Adriani J 1970 The pharmacology of anaesthetic drugs. Charles Thomas, Springfield
Attia R R, Grogono A W (ed) 1978 Practical anaesthetic pharmacology. Appleton, New York
Chenoweth M B (ed) 1972 Modern inhalation anaesthetics. Handb. exp. Pharm. 30. Springer, Berlin
Dripps R D, Eckenhoff J E, Vandam L D 1977 Introduction to anaesthesia. Saunders, Philadelphia
Dundee J W, Wyant G M 1974 Intravenous anaesthesia. Churchill Livingstone, Edinburgh
Gray T C, Nunn J F (ed) 1979 General anaesthesia. Butterworths, London
Macintosh R et al (4th edn in prep.) Physics for the anaesthetist. Blackwell, Oxford
Paton W D M, Speden R N 1965 Anaesthetics and their action on the central nervous system. Br. Med. Bull. 21. 44
Vickers M D, Wood Smith F G, Stewart H C 1978 Drugs in anaesthetic practice. Butterworths, London

23. Local anaesthetics

Methods of producing local anaesthesia 308; The nerve impulse 308; Mode of action of local anaesthetics 309; Cocaine 309; Procaine 310; Lignocaine 311; Prilocaine 311; Bupivacaine 311; Cinchocaine 311; Amethocaine 311; Butacaine 311; Methods of application and testing 311; Therapeutic index 312; Local anaesthesia of mucous membranes 312; Terminal anaesthesia 313; Conduction anaesthesia 313; Epidural anaesthesia 313; Spinal anaesthesia 313; Dangers of local anaesthesia 315.

Methods of producing local anaesthesia
Local anaesthesia may be produced in the following ways:
1. By the application of cold
2. By pressure on nerve trunks
3. By rendering tissues anaemic
4. By paralysing sensory nerve endings or sensory nerve fibres with drugs.

The last of these methods is by far the most important.

The application of cold by means of a spray of some volatile liquid, such as ethyl chloride, is a very convenient method of producing anaesthesia of a small area of skin for a few seconds, but a more lasting effect cannot be produced, because prolonged freezing kills the tissues. Refrigeration is a possible method of anaesthesia in patients in whom an injured limb has to be amputated. The circulation to the limb is occluded by a tourniquet and the limb is surrounded by ice. After a few hours it is completely analgesic and may be amputated without causing shock to the patient. In this method the tissues are not frozen but are cooled sufficiently to prevent conduction of nerve impulses.

The production of local anaesthesia by pressure upon nerve trunks was practised in pre-anaesthetic surgery, but is of no importance nowadays. Partial anaesthesia is produced by depriving any part of its blood supply, as can be done by means of a tourniquet, and this effect is of some importance, because the local anaesthesia induced by the hypodermic injection of drugs is often assisted by the injected fluid producing a local anaemia.

Many drugs can paralyse nerve endings, but only a few paralyse the sensory nerve endings without injuring the surrounding tissues. Phenol, for example, kills all forms of protoplasm, and if a dilute solution of phenol is applied to a wound it produces a preliminary irritation, which is followed by a partial anaesthesia. This anaesthesia is due to the phenol destroying a thin film of tissue on the surface of the wound, and with it killing the exposed sensory nerve endings. Phenol has no specific action on nerve endings, but destroys them together with all the surrounding tissues. This action of phenol is used in relieving toothache, for phenol, if applied in concentrated form to the surface of a tooth cavity, will anaesthetise any sensitive dentine that is exposed.

The true local anaesthetics produce a temporary interruption of nervous conduction in concentrations much lower than those required to act upon other tissues.

Nature of the nerve impulse
In order to understand the action of local anaesthetic drugs it is necessary to consider briefly the nature of the nerve impulse, which depends on a complex series of changes in permeability of the nerve membrane to ions.

In the resting state there is a difference of potential between the interior and the exterior of the membrane of 70 to 90 millivolts. This potential difference is due to concentration gradients of potassium and sodium inside and outside the nerve fibre. The concentration of potassium inside the fibre is much greater than outside and the opposite is the case for sodium; since the resting permeability to sodium is much smaller than to potassium, the resting membrane potential of nerve is determined mainly by its potassium gradient.

Local anaesthetics do not affect the resting membrane potential of nerve in a systematic way but they abolish its ability to initiate and conduct an action potential. Conducted nerve impulses are based on a regenerative process of point to point excitation which enables signals to be conveyed over long distances without attenuation. The regenerative process can be demonstrated experimentally by applying currents to the nerve which lower the potential difference between inside and outside. At a potential difference of about 50 millivolts, the relation between current and potential suddenly changes. The displacement of the membrane potential increases out of proportion to the applied current and at a critical level the membrane potential flares up into a propagated spike, the nerve impulse.

The basis of the regenerative process by which a partial depolarisation of the membrane potential becomes automatically amplified, is a sudden increase in the sodium conductance g_{Na}. As a consequence sodium ions enter the fibre at an increasing rate and by carrying their positive charge across the membrane reinforce the initial lowering of the membrane potential. Due to this explosive rise of sodium conductance the membrane potential first falls to zero and then becomes temporarily reversed. Hodgkin and Huxley have shown that the opening of the sodium gate is a transient event: immediately afterwards the sodium permeability becomes greatly reduced and an outflow of potassium occurs which restores the original polarised state of the membrane.

The ionic composition of the nerve fibre is subsequently restored by the re-entry of potassium and extrusion of sodium. Sodium extrusion takes place against an electrochemical gradient; it is an active secretory process (sodium pump) at the expense of an energy requiring metabolic reaction in which the breakdown of ATP plays an important role.

Mode of action of local anaesthetics

The fundamental action of local anaesthetics is the abolition of the regenerative entry of sodium during conduction of the nerve impulse. The exact cellular mode of action of these drugs is unknown. They almost certainly act on the cell membrane, changing its physiochemical characteristics. As has been mentioned (p. 17), local anaesthetics affect isolated surface layers of lipids in proportion to their activity.

As their action is produced the threshold for electrical excitability of the nerve rises and complete conduction block eventually ensues. Local anaesthetics often paralyse sensory nerve fibres before motor fibres; this is not due to a specific affinity for sensory fibres but can be accounted for by the smaller size of these fibres which allows a more rapid penetration by the local anaesthetic drug.

Local anaesthetic drugs can be divided into two main groups, water-soluble and water-insoluble compounds. The latter have only limited uses. The water soluble compounds are usually tertiary or secondary amines which are capable of forming hydrochlorides and are administered as such. The effective moiety of the molecule is the undissociated base. This is shown by the fact that local anaesthetic activity increases when the pH is made more alkaline and also by the fact that the most active local anaesthetic drugs are weak bases, a substantial proportion of which is present in the undissociated form at the pH of the body fluids. It is believed that only the free base can penetrate the tissues and reach the site of local anaesthetic action in the cell membrane. There is a difference of opinion as to which form is active once the local anaesthetic has reached its site of action. There is evidence that it is the cation rather than the free base which combines with receptors.

The classical water-soluble local anaesthetic drugs are tertiary amino esters of an aromatic acid of the following general structure:

$$\text{>N-C}\cdots\text{C-O-}\overset{\overset{\displaystyle O}{\|}}{\text{C}}\text{-}\bigcirc$$

To this group belong procaine, amethocaine and butacaine; cocaine has the same general structure but is a more complex molecule.

Another group of water-soluble local anaesthetics are not esters but substituted amides. To this group belong lignocaine, prilocaine and bupivacaine. The older local anaesthetic cinchocaine is also an amide.

The water-insoluble local anaesthetic drugs are simple esters of aminobenzoic acid; owing to their low solubility they are used only in dusting powders or ointments. The chief compounds in this group are benzocaine (ethyl aminobenzoate) and butyl aminobenzoate (butesin).

An interesting new category of powerful local anaesthetics are tetrodotoxin and saxitoxin contained in the tissues of some fish and clams. These toxins are amongst the strongest poisons known and their main action is to block the sodium channels in the cell membrane producing an irreversible block of nerve conduction.

Cocaine

The alkaloid cocaine is obtained from the leaves of a South American plant, *Erythroxylon coca*. Coca leaves have been used by the natives of Peru as a cerebral stimulant from time immemorial, and were first introduced into Europe for this purpose. In a paper published in 1884 on the central effects of cocaine, Sigmund Freud referred to its local anaesthetic effects in the following words: 'The capacity of cocaine and its salts when applied in concentrated solutions to anaesthetise cutaneous and mucous membranes, suggests a possible future use especially in cases of local infections.' He suggested that cocaine might be used as an anaesthetic in the eye and later that year Koller introduced it as a local anaesthetic in ophthalmic work; its use spread quickly to laryngology, and later to general surgery.

Cocaine is a derivative of the base ecgonine, and is benzoyl ecgonine-methyl-ester (Fig. 23.1).

Cocaine blocks sensory nerve endings without producing initial stimulation. It produces this effect at a dilution of 1 in 5000, and its action is selective, for at this concentration it does not injure other tissues. The sensation of pain is abolished before that of touch, but at a sufficiently high concentration cocaine blocks all sensory endings. Cocaine also blocks nerve trunks when injected into their neighbourhood. The sensory fibres are affected before the motor fibres. Cocaine is well absorbed from mucous membranes and its clinical use as a local anaesthetic depends on this property.

Cocaine potentiates the action of adrenaline. It produces a marked vasoconstriction by a potentiation of noradrenaline released at sympathetic nerve endings. The most probable explanation is that cocaine occupies the re-uptake sites for noradrenaline at sympathetic nerve endings (p. 77) and in this way increases its concentration at the receptor sites.

When a 1 per cent solution of cocaine hydrochloride is applied to the conjunctival sac, it anaesthetises the cornea. In addition it causes blanching of the conjunctiva, dilatation of the pupil and retraction of the upper eyelid, but these effects do not occur after removal of the superior cervical ganglion and degeneration of the sympathetic nerve supply to the eye. Local application of cocaine also causes vasoconstriction and shrinking of the mucous membrane of the nose and the larynx.

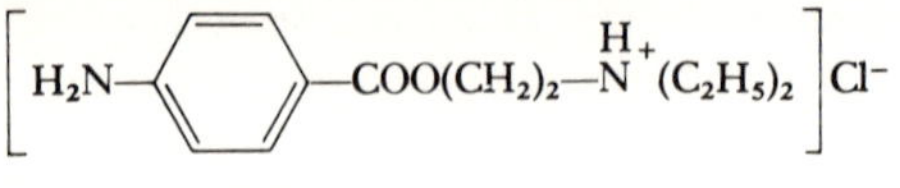

Procaine hydrochloride

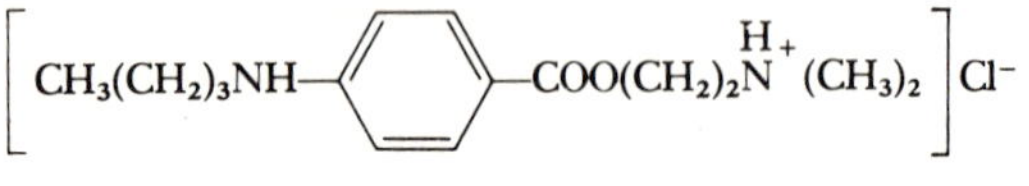

Amethocaine hydrochloride

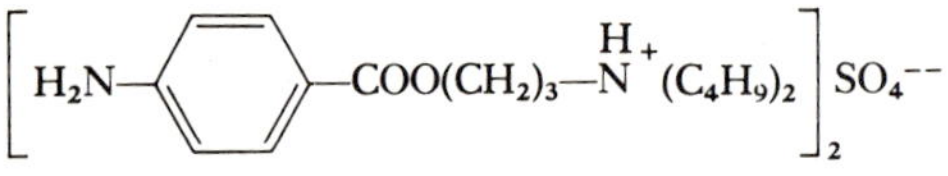

Butacaine sulphate

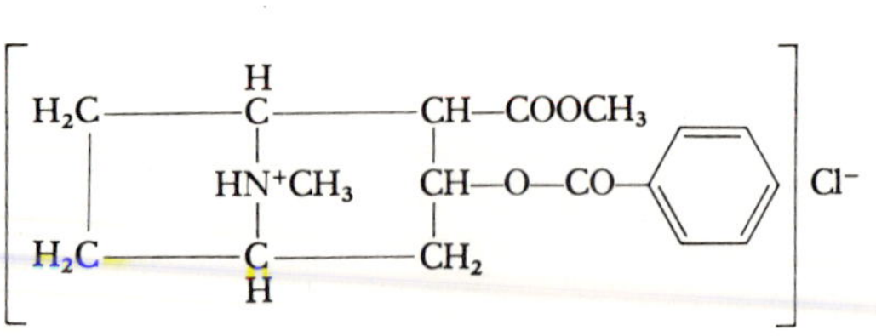

Cocaine hydrochloride

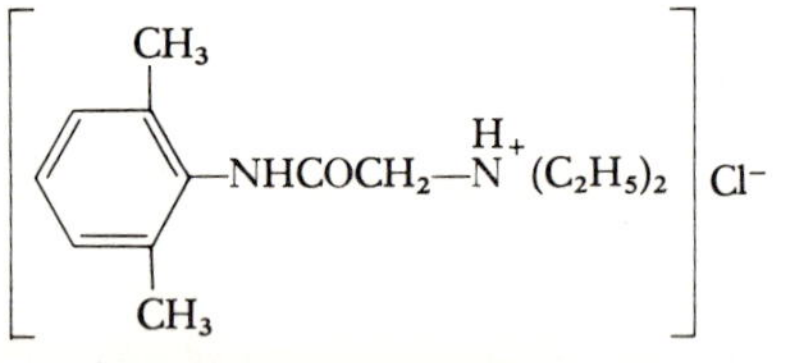

Lignocaine hydrochloride

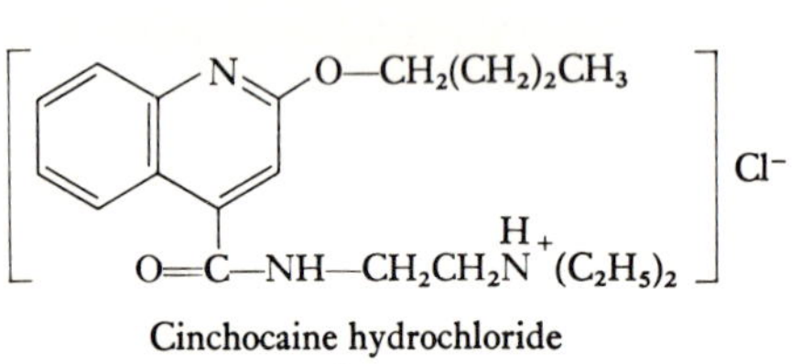

Cinchocaine hydrochloride

Fig. 23.1 Structural formulae of local anaesthetic drugs.

Cocaine has a powerful central stimulant action it causes increased wakefulness, a greater power of endurance of hunger and fatigue and motor excitement. These effects are due to actions on central aminergic systems. Cocaine is an inhibitor of neuronal uptake mechanisms for noradrenaline, dopamine and 5-hydroxytryptamine. Psychological addiction to cocaine occurs and can be a serious problem (p. 484).

Toxic effects. The chief symptoms of mild cocaine poisoning are confusion and motor excitement, quickened pulse and irregular respiration, pallor, vomiting and dilatation of the pupils, and occasionally a rise of temperature. The cerebral excitement may manifest itself in several different ways, and erotic manifestations are reported to occur in women. Clonic convulsions, unconsciousness and collapse occur in the severer cases of poisoning. Diazepam is used in the prevention and treatment of these central effects.

Cocaine also has a toxic action on the heart which may be responsible for the sudden collapse sometimes produced by overdosage of cocaine.

Death has been reported to have followed the subcutaneous injection of 50 mg of cocaine, but the minimal lethal dose for an ordinary individual is probably above 200 mg.

Procaine (Fig. 23.1)

The undesirable actions of cocaine when administered as a local anaesthetic have led to a search for less toxic substitutes. Einhorn found that esters of aminobenzoic acid have local anaesthetic activity when brought into contact with nerve endings and that their water-soluble tertiary amino derivatives are effective substitutes for cocaine. In 1905 he introduced procaine (novocain) as a much less toxic local anaesthetic. This compound differs from cocaine in several respects. Procaine hydrochloride is poorly absorbed from mucous membranes and it therefore produces local anaesthesia only if it is injected so as to bring it into contact with nerve trunks or nerve endings. In contrast to cocaine, procaine does not produce vasoconstriction but vasodilation, hence it is rapidly carried away by the blood stream from the site of injection and in order to localise and prolong its local anaesthetic action, it is necessary to administer it along with a vasoconstrictor drug such as adrenaline.

Toxic effects. Procaine is much less toxic than cocaine but the relative toxicity of these two compounds depends on the method of administration. Animal experiments have shown that when given by rapid intravenous injection the lethal dose of procaine is only about three times that of cocaine, but when administered subcutaneously the lethal dose of procaine is about fifty times that of cocaine. This is due to the fact that procaine is rapidly broken down in the tissues and bloodstream to p-amino-benzoic acid and diethylaminoethanol by an enzyme, procainesterase, which is closely related to cholinesterase.

The safety of procaine depends on the fact that when it is absorbed slowly, the liver can destroy it as rapidly as it is absorbed. Provided that the drug is absorbed slowly, large doses can be given without producing central effects. When injected intravenously at the rate of 10-20 mg per minute it causes flushing of the skin of the face and neck and a sensation of warmth but no toxic central effects.

The following toxic effects may occur when the drug is rapidly absorbed: convulsions which may be followed by respiratory paralysis; a sudden fall of blood pressure, during which the patient becomes cold and clammy. Sensitisation to procaine may occur and procaine dermatitis is sometimes seen in nurses and dentists who frequently handle solutions of this drug.

Amides

Lignocaine (Lidocaine, Xylocaine) (Fig. 23.1)
Lignocaine was introduced as a local anaesthetic by Löfgren in 1948. This compound is not an ester and is much more stable than procaine in aqueous solution.

Lignocaine is not irritant to the tissues; it is readily absorbed from mucous membranes and is used for surface and infiltration anaesthesia. Figure 23.2 shows that lignocaine is about two and a half times as active as procaine when tested intradermally.

Lignocaine is probably the most popular local anaesthetic used at present. The main reasons are its stability, rapidity of onset and good tissue penetration. It has no effect on blood vessels and the addition of a vasoconstrictor such as adrenaline prolongs its effects and delays systemic absorption but the added adrenaline may also give rise to severe complications. Lignocaine is effective by all routes of administration.

Lignocaine has central sedative qualities which may be quite marked. Serious systemic effects such as convulsions and cardiovasular collapse occur rarely and are usually due to accidental overdosage or inadvertent intravascular injection. This can be prevented by careful aspiration of the needle before injection.

Lignocaine has antiarrhythmic activity as discussed on page 145.

Prilocaine (Citanest) is an amide related to lignocaine. It is less toxic and cumulative than lignocaine and is more rapidly metabolised. A disadvantage of the use of prilocaine is the possibility that cyanosis due to the formation of methaemoglobin may occur if large doses (over 600 mg) are administered. The methaemoglobinaemia usually disappears in 24 hours and has little clinical significance.

Bupivacaine is highly lipid-soluble and is approximately four times as active as lignocaine. Its main feature is its long duration of action and in contrast to lignocaine, its lack of tachyphylaxis. It is used for epidural anaesthesia in childbirth.

Cinchocaine (Nupercaine) (Fig. 23.1)
This amide is the most active local anaesthetic in clinical use; it is also the most toxic. Its action is very prolonged. It is well absorbed from mucous membranes and is used for surface anaesthesia either in aqueous solution or as an ointment. It has also been used as a spinal anaesthetic. Cinchocaine is extremely active and when injected it must be used in very dilute solutions (0.05 to 0.1 per cent); if cinchocaine is injected in the concentrations appropriate for procaine it produces cardiac arrhythmias and convulsions which may be fatal.

Esters

Amethocaine (Tetracaine) (Fig. 23.1)
This compound is closely related in chemical structure to procaine. It is about 10 times more active than procaine but correspondingly more toxic; when used in equiactive concentrations amethocaine has a more prolonged action than procaine. Amethocaine is readily absorbed from mucous membranes and can be used for surface as well as for conduction and infiltration anaesthesia.

Butacaine (Butyn) (Fig. 23.1)
This drug is closely related chemically to procaine but differs from it in penetrating mucous membranes readily. Unlike cocaine it does not cause vasoconstriction or dilatation of the pupil when applied to the eye.

Methods of applying and testing local anaesthetic drugs

Local anaesthesia with drugs can be produced in the following ways:
1. By application to mucous surfaces to produce paralysis of nerve endings: surface anaesthesia.
2. By intradermal or hypodermic injection to produce paralysis of nerve endings: terminal or infiltration anaesthesia.
3. By injection around nerve trunks to produce block of nerve fibres: conduction anaesthesia.
There are various forms of conduction anaesthesia:
   a. Nerve block anaesthesia. A localised perineural injection is made along the course of a nerve at a point distant from the operative site.
   b. Field block anaesthesia. The solution is injected close to the nerves around the area to be anaesthetised.
   c. Epidural anaesthesia. The local anaesthetic solution is injected into the epidural space. Its site of action is at the epidural sections of the spinal nerves.
4. By injecting drugs subdurally in the lumbar region to produce conduction block of the posterior roots: spinal anaesthesia.

In assessing the activity of local anaesthetic drugs it is necessary to take into account the fact that these drugs differ in their power to penetrate mucous membranes. It is important therefore that their activity should be assessed not only when they are injected, but also when they are applied to the surface of a mucous membrane. Local anaesthetic drugs do not act when they are applied to the unbroken skin but are very effective when the skin is scarified or when the epidermis is removed to expose the nerve endings in the dermis. Local anaesthetics can be tested as follows.

Surface anaesthesia
A standard solution of cocaine is dropped into one eye of a rabbit or guinea pig and a solution of the substance under test in the other eye. The corneal reflex is tested at intervals by touching the cornea with a light object a number of times and determining what proportion of stimuli are effective.

Infiltration anaesthesia

Intracutaneous wheals are made in the human skin or the shaved guinea pig skin. The response to a light pin prick is tested at intervals as in the preceding test. The results of a test in which the activity of lignocaine and procaine was compared in man are shown in Figure 23.2. In this experiment each subject received on the flexor surface of the forearm four intradermal injections of 0.2 ml of saline containing two different concentrations of each of the two drugs. At intervals of five minutes each wheal was pricked six times with a pin and the anaesthetic activity was scored by the number of pricks not felt.

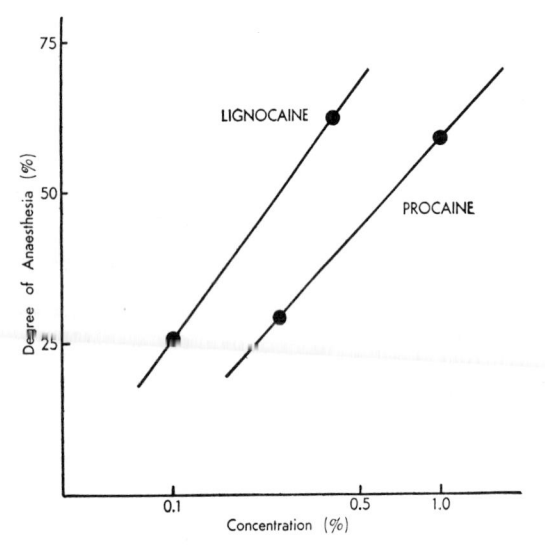

Fig. 23.2 Comparison of the local anaesthetic activity of lignocaine and procaine by intradermal injection in human skin. The figures plotted are the mean results obtained in an experiment on 52 medical students with 0.1 and 0.4 per cent of lignocaine and 0.25 and 1 per cent of procaine. The intradermal wheals containing the four different doses were made in a random order to allow for differences in the sensitivity along the flexor surface of the forearm. To avoid subjective errors of assessment the wheals were identified with letters until testing had been completed. Each wheal was tested for anaesthesia by pricking with a pin six times in different parts of the wheal using a stimulus just great enough to elicit pain on normal skin near the wheal. The test was repeated every five minutes for half an hour and the total number of pricks not felt gave a measure of the anaesthetic activity. Lignocaine was found to be 2.6 times more active than procaine. (After Mongar, 1955, *Brit. J. Pharmacol.*)

Conduction anaesthesia

This may be tested on the nerve muscle preparation or the sciatic plexus of frogs. In the latter method the solution is poured into the abdominal cavity of an eviscerated frog and the concentration is determined at which the frog fails to withdraw its legs when the feet are dipped in acid.

Spinal anaesthesia

This may be produced in rabbits or cats by injecting local anaesthetic drugs into the spinal subarachnoid space, and this method may be used for testing, in a preliminary fashion, the activity of a compound as a spinal anaesthetic.

Toxicity tests and therapeutic index

Macdonald and Israels measured both the activity and toxicity of local anaesthetics and constructed a form of therapeutic index for various local anaesthetics. To measure toxicity in their procedure the local anaesthetic is slowly infused into a cat until spontaneous respiration ceases. At this point artificial respiration is instituted and the animal is allowed to recover. Within a few hours the drug has for practical purposes been eliminated and spontaneous respiration is resumed. Another drug may now be infused in the same way and the relative toxicity of the two local anaesthetic drugs may thus be tested on the same animal.

These authors have compared the relative efficiency of various local anaesthetics which was expressed as:

$$\text{relative efficiency} = \frac{\text{relative efficacy}}{\text{relative toxicity}}$$

The relative efficacy was determined by the intradermal wheal test in man and also by the corneal reflex test in the rabbit. Values relative to cocaine are shown in Table 23.1. It is seen that cinchocaine is more efficient than cocaine as a surface anaesthetic and slightly more efficient than procaine as an infiltration anaesthetic.

The Uses of local anaesthetic drugs

Local anaesthetics are used for a number of different purposes and their relative merits depend largely on the conditions under which they are used.

Local anaesthesia of mucous membranes

Local anaesthesia of mucous membranes can be readily produced by the application of certain local anaesthetics such as *amethocaine* or *lignocaine*. The activity of these

Table 23.1 Relative Efficiency of Local Anaesthetics (After Macdonald and Israels, 1932. *J. Pharmac.*)

Drug	Relative toxicity (Respiratory arrest in cat)	Relative efficacy Intradermal wheal (man)	Relative efficacy Rabbit cornea	Relative efficiency Intradermal wheal (man)	Relative efficiency Rabbit cornea
Cocaine	100	100	100	1	1
Procaine	17	100	6	6	$\frac{1}{3}$
Cinchocaine	200	2000	5000	10	25

drugs depends upon two factors; their ability to penetrate mucous membranes, and their power of anaesthetising nerve endings. The chief mucous membranes to which local anaesthetics are applied are those of the eye, nose, throat, urethra and bladder.

The quantity of drug employed in the eye is small, and hence there is less danger of central toxic effects. The drug should penetrate freely and should not produce irritation or corneal injury. In operations on the eye it is of vital importance that the drug employed should be absolutely reliable as regards the depth of local anaesthesia produced, because any hitch in the operation may endanger the eye. Many ophthalmic surgeons consider that no other drug is as reliable as cocaine, and it is still widely used for this work. Cocaine may, however, prevent regeneration of the corneal epithelial cells and damage the cornea causing it to become opaque. For these reasons other drugs such as *amethocaine* or *benoxinate* are now frequently used to anaesthetise the cornea. These drugs cause some irritation of the cornea but do not cause permanent damage. In contrast to cocaine they do not produce vasoconstriction or dilatation of the pupil. Procaine can be employed in eye surgery but subconjunctival injections must be given.

The following concentrations are commonly used for surface anaesthesia in the respiratory tract: lignocaine 2–4 per cent, amethocaine 1–2 per cent.

Terminal anaesthesia by hypodermic injection
A local anaesthetic, when injected hypodermically, is brought into immediate contact with the nerve endings, and therefore its power of penetration is not important. The points of chief importance are that the drug should act for a sufficient length of time, that it should not produce an initial irritation, and that it should not produce toxic effects, for when it is necessary to anaesthetise a large area, a considerable quantity of drug must be injected.

The action of local anaesthetics is greatly increased by the addition of adrenaline. The presence of 1 in 250 000 to 1 in 100 000 adrenaline produces vasoconstriction, delays the absorption of the drug and therefore prolongs its action; it reduces the minimal concentration required to produce local anaesthesia and also reduces the chance of toxic central effects being produced.

Another advantage of the use of adrenaline is that the local anaemia reduces bleeding during the operation. The action of adrenaline in increasing the action of a local anaesthetic is very marked; the injection of 0.5 ml of 2 per cent procaine alone produces a partial local anaesthesia which lasts for about 20 minutes, but the addition of 1 in 100 000 adrenaline enables the same amount of procaine to produce a local anaesthesia which does not completely disappear for an hour. Adrenaline containing solutions of local anaesthetics should be avoided in the digits, penis and ear because they may cause gangrene.

Large areas can be anaesthetised by infiltration anaesthesia. In this method a dilute solution of a local anaesthetic is injected in sufficient quantities to render the tissues rigid. A suitable solution for infiltration contains lignocaine 0.25–0.5 per cent with adrenaline at a concentration of 1 in 200 000. The anaesthesia is produced partly by the solution producing local anaemia and partly by the specific action of the local anaesthetic.

Conduction anaesthesia
Higher concentrations of local anaesthetic are needed to block nerve trunks than suffice for nerve endings; moreover, conduction block of nerve trunks usually involves the injection of the drug into the neighbourhood of moderate-sized veins. Hence it is particularly important not to use a toxic drug, for there is always the risk of rapid absorption even though adrenaline be added to the solution.

Procaine 2 per cent or lignocaine 1–2 per cent are usually employed.

For *dental anaesthesia* lignocaine 2 per cent is widely used ready mixed with adrenaline 1:50 000 or 1:80 000 in 2 ml cartridges. Prilocaine 3 per cent may also be used with a lower concentration of adrenaline (1:300 000) because of its prolonged action. Prilocaine may also be used with felypressin 0.03 iu/ml (p. 329) in patients in whom the administration of adrenaline is undesirable.

Caudal anaesthesia is a type of conduction anaesthesia in which the solution is injected extradurally into the caudal space in order to anaesthetise the nerves running in the sacral canal. Continuous caudal anaesthesia has been used particularly in child birth (p. 224).

Epidural anaesthesia. In this method the local anaesthetic drug is injected into the epidural or interdural space, between the parietal and the medullary layers of the dura. The position of the needle in the epidural space is shown in Figure 23.3; the anaesthetic diffuses through the intervertebral foramina along the perineural sheaths and thus blocks the nerve roots. The advantages of epidural over spinal anaesthesia are that spread to the brain cannot occur since the epidural space ends at the foramen magnum and there is no risk of spinal headache or meningeal irritation. The total quantity of drug that must be used for epidural anaesthesia is about five times greater than that needed for spinal anaesthesia and hence it is most important to guard against accidental injection of the anaesthetic solution into the subarachnoid space.

Spinal anaesthesia
Spinal anaesthesia was introduced into surgical practice by Bier in 1889, but the anaesthetic employed was cocaine, and the accidents which occurred were so numerous that the method soon fell into disrepute. When procaine was later used as a spinal anaesthetic much better results were obtained. The method is confined mainly to operations on the lower half of the body. The sequence of events in spinal

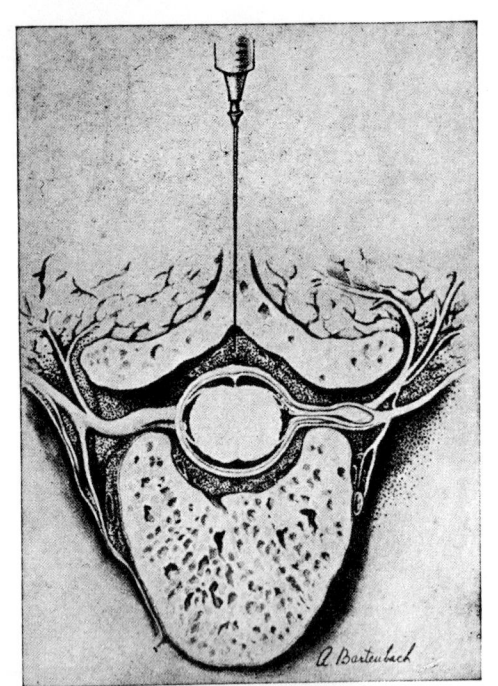

Fig. 23.3 Position of needle for the injection of a drug to produce epidural anaesthesia. (From Harger et al., 1941, *Am. J. Surg.*)

anaesthesia is illustrated in Figure 23.4. The sensory nerves are paralysed first and pain sense is lost before the sensation of touch. The sympathetic vasoconstrictor fibres are paralysed at approximately the same time as the sensory fibres, as shown by a marked rise of skin temperature. Motor function is paralysed last and recovers most rapidly. The motor paralysis may involve the respiratory muscles.

The spinal anaesthetics chiefly in use are procaine, amethocaine, lignocaine and cinchocaine.

The spread of anaesthesia in the spinal canal depends on many factors including the site, quantity and force of injection, the posture of the patient and the specific gravity of the solution. Solutions are usually made either hyperbaric or hypobaric in order to control their spread. Solutions of procaine are usually heavier than cerebrospinal fluid and with the patient in the sitting position these hyperbaric solutions travel to the lowest part of the dural canal. Cinchocaine being extremely potent can be injected in a dilute solution of lower specific gravity than cerebrospinal fluid. When the patient is sitting, this hypobaric solution rises in the spinal canal. Methods have been worked out for controlling the spread of anaesthesia, by keeping the patient sitting for a certain number of seconds, and then placing him in a head-down position.

Dangers of spinal anaesthesia. The chief immediate dangers of spinal anaesthesia are paralysis of respiration, and a sudden fall of blood pressure. The latter effect is largely due to splanchnic paralysis and for this reason ephedrine or methedrine are usually administered beforehand. It has also been suggested that the fall of blood pressure in spinal anaesthesia is of cardiac origin due to a reduction of respiratory movements and a consequent damming back of the venous blood in the right side of the heart.

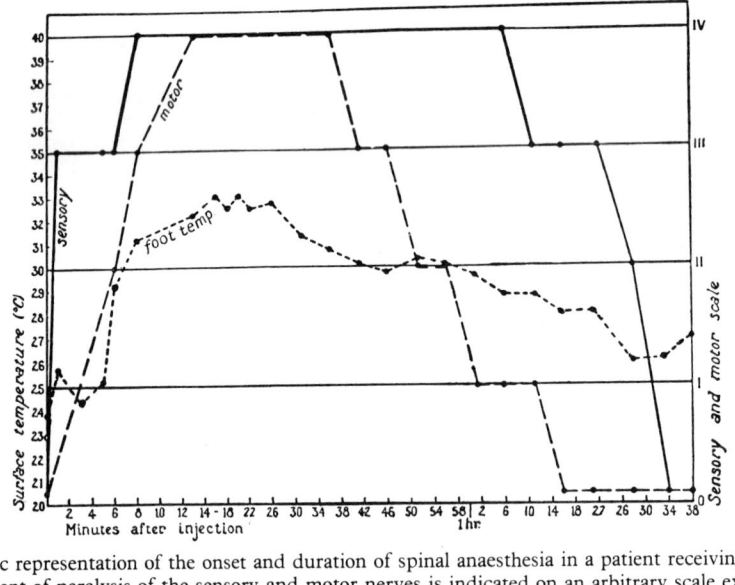

Fig. 23.4 Diagrammatic representation of the onset and duration of spinal anaesthesia in a patient receiving 100 mg procaine hydrochloride. The extent of paralysis of the sensory and motor nerves is indicated on an arbitrary scale extending from I to IV. Sensory loss was graded from complete loss of sensation (IV), through loss of pain but not of touch (III), to incomplete analgesia (II and I). Motor function was graded from complete loss of function (IV), through limited movement of toes (III), and of feet (II), to moderate weakness of legs (I). Paralysis of the sympathetic vasoconstrictor fibres was assessed by measuring the skin temperature. (After Emmett, 1934, *J. Am. med. Ass.*)

The results obtained with spinal anaesthesia vary greatly. Minor unpleasant after-effects such as headache, urinary retention, transient paraesthesias and loss of reflexes occur relatively frequently, but the more serious after-effects are largely due to faulty technique. They include severe headache, lasting for a week or more, prolonged paralysis of nerve roots and meningitis.

Prolonged local anaesthesia can be produced with ointments or dusting powders containing the relatively insoluble compounds, benzocaine and butesin. These are often used in painful wounds and ulcers, and to relieve itching.

Dangers of local anaesthesia

Systemic reactions by local anaesthetics with symptoms referable to the central nervous and cardiovascular system may result from absorption into the blood stream of toxic amounts of drug. The manifestations may be convulsions or drowsiness and unconsciousness. Any excitatory responses are enhanced by metabolic or respiratory acidosis. Local anaesthetics have direct actions on heart muscle affecting conduction and excitability. Procainamide and lignocaine are employed as antiarrhythmic agents as discussed on page 145.

Because the circulating blood level of local anaesthetics is responsible for their toxicity intravenous injection is the most dangerous, but application to the pharyngeal, tracheal and bronchial mucosa may also lead to high blood levels because of the vascularity of these areas and the rapid absorption of the drug from the lungs. Most instances of sudden cardiovascular collapse have involved local anaesthesia of the respiratory tract.

A second factor responsible for the occurrence of systemic reactions is the rapidity of hydrolysis of the local anaesthetic. Local anaesthetic esters which are destroyed by cholinesterases in blood and liver are likely to be less toxic than the more slowly destroyed amides. An important cause of untoward reactions is the amount of adrenaline absorbed. This should be minimised and in cases of extensive infiltration anaesthesia 1:200 000 adrenaline is a sufficient and effective concentration.

If convulsions develop an intravenous injection of thiopentone or pentobarbitone has been used in the past but since barbiturates may add to circulatory or respiratory depression intravenous diazepam is now increasingly used.

PREPARATIONS

Amethocaine hyd (Tetracaine) 0.5–1% cream, max 1 oz
Bupivacaine hyd (Marcaine) infil 0.25%, caud 0.25%
Cinchocaine hyd (Nupercaine) urethr 0.1%
Cocaine hyd surf 1–4%
Lignocaine hyd (Lidocaine, Xylocaine) surf 2–4%
Mepivicaine hyd (Carbocaine) infil block epid 0.5–2%
Oxybuprocaine hyd (Benoxinate) surf eye 0.4%
Prilocaine hyd (Citanest) infil block caud 1–2%q;
Procaine hyd (Novocain) infil 0.25–0.5% + adren 1:200 000, nerve block caud epid 1–2% spin 10%

FURTHER READING

Covino B G, Vassallo Helen G 1976 Mechanism of action and clinical use. In local anaesthetics. Grune Stratton, New York
Hunter A R 1975 Neurosurgical anaesthesia Blackwell, Oxford
Katz B 1966 Nerve, muscle and synapse McGraw Hill, New York
Lechat P (ed) 1971 Local anaesthetics. Int. Enc. Pharm. Ther. Sect 8:1
Mongar J L 1959 Use of randomised blocks in local anaesthetics assays. In quantitative methods in human pharmacology. Pergamon, Oxford
Ritchie J N, Greengard P 1966 Ann. Rev. Pharma: 6:405

SECTION FIVE

Hormones and vitamins

24. Fundamental aspects of hormone action

Formation and metabolism of cyclic AMP 319; Mode of action of adenylcyclase 319; Hormones affecting adenylcyclase 320; Second messenger concept 320; Cyclic GMP 320; Oestrogen receptors 321; Androgen receptors 321; Hypothalamic control of anterior pituitary 322; TRH 322; LHRH 322; GHRIH 323; Other hypothalamic factors 323; Significance of hypothalamic hypophysiotropic hormones 323.

CYCLIC NUCLEOTIDES AND HORMONE ACTION

Since the discovery of cyclic AMP by Sutherland, in 1956, a great deal of information has accumulated indicating that this cyclic nucleotide and possibly others (cyclic GMP) play a key role in modulating the action of certain hormones.

Formation and metabolism of cyclic AMP (p. 79)
Cyclic AMP (cAMP) can be considered as a regulatory agent which controls the rates of a variety of cellular processes. It is formed from adenosine triphosphate (ATP) by the enzyme adenyl cyclase present in the cell membrane through the following reaction.

Cyclic AMP is rapidly degraded within the cell by a second enzyme system, cyclic nucleotide phosphodiesterase (PDE), which transforms cyclic AMP to adenosine monophosphate (5'-AMP). PDE is a highly complex enzyme and most mammalian tissues contain multiple forms of this enzyme. Adenyl cyclase and PDE are in a state of dynamic equilibrium which controls the level of cAMP within the cell. Many hormones affect cyclase activity whilst many synthetic drugs act on PDE. It has been known since the early work on cyclic AMP that xanthine derivatives, such as theophylline, and papaverine inhibit PDE thereby raising the concentration of cyclic AMP. Prostaglandins are powerful inhibitors of PDE. Attempts have been made to produce tissue-specific PDE inhibitors, e.g. inhibitors of platelet PDE to prevent platelet aggregation or of lung PDE to produce bronchodilatation.

Mode of action of adenylcyclase (adenylylcyclase)
Many hormone receptors are believed to be closely linked to adenyl cyclase. According to a nomenclature introduced by Sutherland and his colleagues the hormone is considered as the *first messenger* which brings about an increase in the intracellular level of cyclic AMP called the *second messenger*. The latter then triggers off a series of reactions which vary according to the type of cell stimulated. Whether a given hormone stimulates adenyl cyclase in a given tissue would depend on whether the tissue contains receptors for the hormone. A highly simplified scheme of the minimum interaction postulated

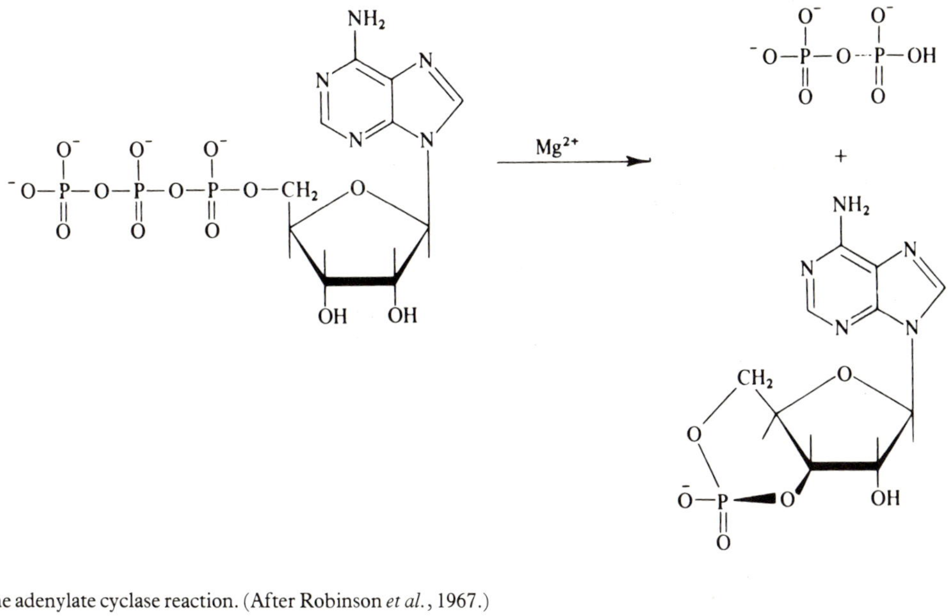

Fig. 24.1 The adenylate cyclase reaction. (After Robinson *et al.*, 1967.)

is shown in Figure 24.2. According to this model, the protein component of the system consists of two subunits, a regulatory subunit (R) facing the extracellular fluid and a catalytic subunit (C) with its active centre directed towards the interior of the cell. In this scheme the receptor is regarded as part of the regulatory subunit, in other more complex schemes receptor and regulatory subunit are regarded as separate.

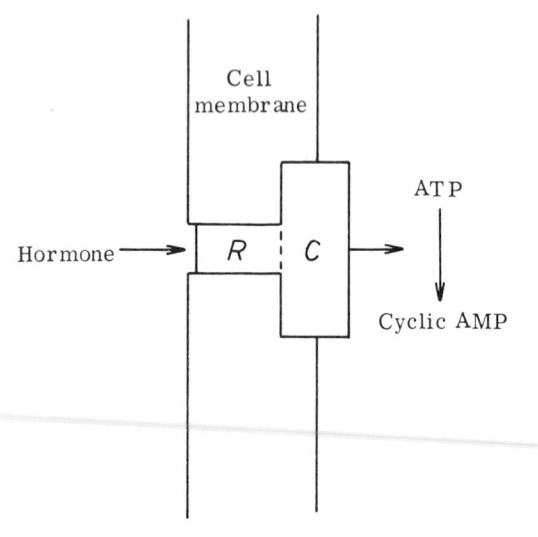

Fig. 24.2 Possible model of the protein component of the membrane adenyl cyclase system. (From Robinson et al., 1967.)

The reactions initiated by cyclic AMP vary according to the effector system. One of the earliest systems investigated has been the stimulation of phosphorylase by cyclic AMP following the action of adrenaline on striated muscle. In the series of reactions started by cyclic AMP the first is the activation of a protein kinase leading to a phosphorylation reaction. This causes a sequence of events leading to the breakdown of muscle glycogen and the formation of lactic acid. It has been shown that many reactions promoted by cyclic AMP start with a phosphorylation reaction.

Hormones affecting adenyl cyclase
A variety of hormones increase cAMP levels in target tissues whilst producing their characteristic hormonal effects. The following are examples of hormones which increase cAMP formation, and their respective target organs and actions.

Catecholamines (ß-adrenergic stimulants). Liver (glycogenolysis, gluconeogenesis), striated muscle (glycogenolysis, lactic acid formation) heart muscle (increased contractility), smooth muscle (usually relaxation), fat cells (lipolysis).
Glucagon. Liver (glycogenolysis, gluconeogenesis), pancreas (insulin release).
ACTH. Adrenal cortex (glucocorticoid synthesis), fat cells (lipolysis).
LH and *FSH.* Gonads and corpus luteum (steroid hormone formation).
Parathyroid hormone. Bone (calcium mobilisation), kidney (phosphaturia).
Hypothalamic hypophysiotropic stimulant hormones. Anterior pituitary (release of six main anterior pituitary hormones and increase of cAMP in specific pituitary cell types). Hypothalamic inhibitory hormones reduce cAMP levels in anterior pituitary target cells.
Vasopressin. Kidney (increased water permeability).
Gastrin. Gastric mucosa (acid secretion).
Histamine. Brain.
Prostaglandin PGE_1. Platelet (aggregation inhibition).
Hormones may decrease cAMP levels. A notable example is insulin which reduces cAMP levels in adipose tissue, causing decreased lipolysis. Another example is inhibition of cAMP by hypothalamic inhibitory hormones.

Second messenger concept
Whilst the second messenger concept has gained wide acceptance it has become apparent that the interaction with cAMP is frequently more complicated than was at first believed. The basic idea has been that the first messenger (hormone) carried information to the cell and the second messenger transferred this information to the cell's internal machinery. Evidence that cAMP represents the second messenger was generally based on (1) increased cAMP levels after hormone stimulation, (2) qualitative reproduction of the hormone effect by external addition of cAMP or its dibutyryl derivative. Recent work has shown that other 'second messengers' particularly Ca^{++} may play an important role as for example in the action of catecholamines on cardiac contractility.

It is believed that Ca^{++} plays a central role in cardiac excitation-contraction coupling and that during the cardiac action potential a major Ca^{++} influx into the myocardial cell takes place in the form of a slow intard Ca^{++} current during the plateau phase of the action potential. Whilst an increase in Ca^{++} available to the contractile protein is central to the inotropic action of catecholamines there is evidence that cAMP contributes to the Ca^{++} movement in the myocardial cell. Thus it has been shown that dibutyryl cAMP can increase the inward Ca^{++} current. It is not known precisely how this effect is brought about but it has been suggested that it may be connected with the phosphorylation of a protein kinase which promotes the transport of Ca^{++} by the cardiac sarcoplasmic reticulum.

Cyclic GMP
The finding that cyclic AMP is involved in many hormone actions has stimulated interest in other cyclic nucleotides. Of these, cyclic guanine 3',5'-monophosphate (cGMP) has

been detected in many mammalian tissues and its effects have been intensively studied. Other cyclic nucleotides such as cyclic cytidyl phosphate, have been detected in tumour cells.

Concentration of cGMP in mammalian tissues are generally lower than those of cAMP but a variety of agents are known to elevate cGMP levels in tissues without raising cAMP levels, including drugs which elicit contraction in smooth muscle. Levels of cGMP in the smooth muscle of the isolated ductus deferens are elevated by acetylcholine, noradrenaline and potassium chloride all of which cause contraction of the muscle. The increase in cGMP is abolished by specific antagonists, e.g. by atropine in case of acetylcholine and by phentolamine in case of adrenaline.

The basic role of cGMP is not fully understood. Some workers have suggested that the increase in cGMP is a secondary effect, following an increase in intracellular calcium brought about by the smooth muscle stimulants. Others have suggested that cAMP and cGMP are biological effectors with contrary actions involved in regulating certain cellular functions which are bidirectionally controlled.

OESTROGEN RECEPTORS

The term *oestrogen receptor* has been applied by Jensen and his colleagues to intracellular oestradiol-binding proteins found in cells of the uterus and other oestrogen-sensitive 'target' tissues. When labelled oestradiol is injected into immature female rats, it rapidly accumulates in the cells of the endometrium and myometrium where it binds to certain protein constituents in the cytosol and the nucleus. Oestradiol-binding cytosol protein has been detected in cells of the uterus, vagina, mammary gland and hypothalamus in relatively high concentration whilst it is lacking in tissues such as striated muscle which do not respond to oestrogen stimulation. An interaction of oestradiol with a protein in the cell *nucleus* takes place as a secondary reaction step following its initial binding to cytosol protein. There is evidence that other steroid hormones including progesterone, dihydrotestosterone, cortisol and aldosterone also react by two stage processes involving first the cytoplasm and subsequently the nucleus.

The binding of oestradiol to cytosol protein in the uterus is highly specific. The closely related hormone oestrone fails to bind unless it is first transformed to oestradiol in the body. Ethinyloestradiol is strongly bound but the related compound mestranol is not bound unless it is first demethylated to ethinyloestradiol by the liver.

The question arises whether the uterine cytosol protein can be regarded as a pharmacological *receptor* for oestradiol. Bearing in mind our previous definition of drug receptors as specific cellular recognition sites with which drugs react when they produce their effects (p. 10), the cytosol protein seems to fulfil the requirement of specificity. The second requirement, a clear link between receptor binding and hormonal effect, cannot as yet be fully substantiated. It is an attractive hypothesis, however, that the binding of oestradiol to cytosol protein and its subsequent translocation to the nucleus are integral stages of the action of the hormone. If so, they must represent very early stages in the cycle of events initiated by oestradiol, since actinomycin D and puromycin fail to inhibit its binding to cytosol and nuclear protein although they arrest the early hormonal effects of oestradiol such as stimulation of RNA and protein synthesis.

Mode of action of oestrogenic steroids

There is experimental evidence that steroid hormones stimulate the biosynthesis of proteins in their respective target cells causing the appearance of new ribosomes in the cytoplasm. This evidence and the finding that steroid hormones accumulate in the nucleus suggests that oestrogens, and steroid hormones in general, may act on the nuclear genetic apparatus which controls protein synthesis. The sex hormones may thus produce their effects by stimulating activity in previously quiescent genes.

Hormones produce their primary effects at rate limiting metabolic steps from where their actions are subsequently amplified. There has been some controversy whether the primary action of oestradiol occurs at the level of formation of messenger RNA on a template of DNA (*transcription*) or at the ribosome level of *translating* the mRNA message into specific instructions for building up new amino acids for protein synthesis. Most investigators have concluded that the primary site of action of oestrogen is probably at the transcriptional or genomic level.

Steroid hormones frequently produce an increase in cell permeability in their target organs. It has been suggested that this might result from the production of permeability-increasing enzymes (permeases) as a manifestation of increased protein synthesis.

Androgen receptors

Work in this field is of special clinical interest because of the involvement of androgens in prostatic hypertrophy and carcinoma. The main androgen, testosterone, is transported in the plasma in the form of a stable complex with plasma proteins. When testosterone enters the prostatic androgen 'target' cell it is metabolised, the principal product being *5-α-dihydrotestosterone* which is itself a powerful androgen. This is selectively bound to a cytoplasmic receptor protein forming an androgen-receptor complex. The activated complex is translocated into the nucleus where it stimulates processes such as genetic transcription. Evidence for a specific receptor interaction is provided by blocking it by anti-androgen steroids such as *cyproterone*.

HYPOTHALAMIC CONTROL OF ANTERIOR PITUITARY

An important advance in our understanding of hormone action has been the discovery of a set of central co-ordinating mechanisms relating the functions of the brain and the anterior pituitary. A vascular plexus connecting the anterior pituitary and the hypothalamus was described by Popa and Fielding in 1930. It is now believed that these vessels represent a portal vascular system which transports hormones released by the hypothalamus, which control the various secretory functions of the anterior pituitary. These hormones are referred to as hypophysiotropic hormones or as pituitary stimulating and inhibiting hormones and they mediate effects of the central nervous system on the pituitary gland.

There has been intensive activity in this field. Several hypothalamic hypophysiotrophic factors have been characterised and synthesised and their biological activities established. Each is named for what was initially postulated to be its sole biological activity although it was soon found that each hypothalamic factor might have more than one action. The amino acid sequence of three established hypothalamic *factors* (now referred to as *hormones*) are shown in Figure 24.3. They are:

1. TRH, thyrotrophin-releasing hormone. It stimulates the synthesis and release of thyrotrophin (TSH) by the anterior pituitary and in many species, including man, the release of prolactin (PRL).

2. LHRH, luteinising hormone-releasing hormone which regulates the release of both luteinising hormone (LH) and follicle-stimulating hormone (FSH).

3. GHRIH, growth hormone release-inhibiting hormone, called *somatostatin*. It *inhibits* the release of growth hormone (GH) by the anterior pituitary. It also inhibits the secretion of insulin and glucagon by direct action on the pancreas.

Thyrotrophin-releasing hormone (TRH)

Thyrotrophin-releasing hormone (Fig. 24.3) is a tripeptide (L-pyroglutamyl, L-histidyl, L-proline amide) which was the first hypothalamic peptide synthesised. It is isolated from pig and sheep hypothalamus and is biologically active in all species tested. TRH induces the release of TSH and PRL from pituitary glands *in situ* and from isolated pituitary cells.

Activity by TRH in man after intravenous injection may be demonstrated by radio-immunoassay of TSH. TRH does not stimulate the release of corticotrophin, luteinising and follicle-stimulating hormone. It does not stimulate growth hormone release in normal subjects but stimulates its release in acromegalics.

Clinically TRH is used mainly for diagnostic purposes in thyroid disease. In one test a rapid intravenous injection of TRH is given and the consequent raised TSH level in blood is measured by radioimmunoassay. Patients with hyperthyroidism fail to respond to TRH by a raised blood level of TSH because of the inhibitory effect of increased circulating T_3 and T_4 (p. 331) on the thyrotroph cells.

Injections of TRH in man may produce nausea, flushing and a desire to micturate. There has been some evidence that TRH affects mood and may be beneficial in depression, but this is controversial.

Luteinising hormone-releasing hormone (LHRH)

This hormone is a decapeptide synthesised in 1971. It releases both luteinising hormone (LH) and follicle-stimulating hormone (FSH). Current evidence suggests that there is only one gonadotrophin-releasing hormone in man; this is now frequently referred to as LH/FSH-RH (*gonadorelin*). It has been found that in adults, LH release predominates over FSH whilst before puberty the release of FSH is greater.

LHRH has potential clinical applications, there is evidence that in certain forms of pituitary-hypothalamic

Thyrotropin releasing factor (TRF)

(Glu)–(His)–(Pro)—NH$_2$

Luteinising hormone releasing factor (LRF)

(Glu)–(His)–(Trp)–(Ser)–(Tyr)–(Gly)–(Leu)–(Arg)–(Pro)–(Gly)—NH$_2$

Somatostatin

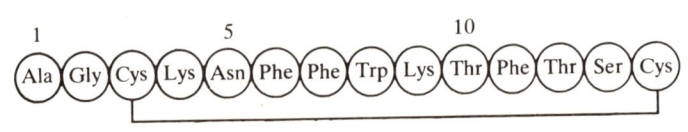

(Ala)–(Gly)–(Cys)–(Lys)–(Asn)–(Phe)–(Phe)–(Trp)–(Lys)–(Thr)–(Phe)–(Thr)–(Ser)–(Cys)

Fig. 24.3 Amino acid sequences of thyrotropin releasing factor, luteinising hormone releasing factor and somatostatin. (After Fleischer and Guillemin, 1976. In Parsons, ed., Peptide Hormones *Biological Council*.)

disease injections of LHRH can restore ovulation in women and spermatogenesis in men. A variety of analogues of LHRH have been synthesised some with greatly increased activity. Other synthetic analogues inhibit the action of endogenous LHRH.

Growth hormone release-inhibiting hormone (GHRIH)
This factor, also called *somatostatin*, is a polypeptide consisting of 14 amino acids isolated from hypothalamic tissue. Its structure is shown in Figure 24.3. The naturally occurring form has a cyclic structure but a non-native linear form of the molecule is also active. It is a potent inhibitor of growth hormone (GH) release in the whole animal and from isolated pituitary cells. Somatostatin infusions in man acutely inhibit GH secretion induced by hypoglycaemia or sleep. The effect is immediate and there is a rapid rebound on ending the infusion. In acromegalic patients the plasma GH level falls suddenly during somatostatin infusion.

Injections of somatostatin in conscious baboons, besides producing a fall in circulating growth hormone, also cause a fall in the plasma levels of insulin and glucagon. There is evidence that these effects of somatostatin are due to a direct action on the alpha- and beta-cells of the pancreas. Somatostatin also inhibits TRH-induced TSH release but has apparently no effect on the secretion of prolactin, luteinising hormone, follicle-stimulating hormone or corticotrophin.

The clinical applications of somatostatin are not yet fully explored. It has been suggested that its action in lowering growth hormone and glucagon secretion might be employed in the treatment of juvenile diabetes.

Other postulated hypothalamic hypophysiotropic factors
There is evidence that the hypothalamus contains additional polypeptide substances which may be involved in promoting or inhibiting the secretion of anterior pituitary hormones. In some cases the existence of such factors has been supported by strong circumstantial evidence although they have not, so far, been obtained in pure form.

Corticotrophin releasing factor (CRF) was the first of these substances recognised but it was never obtained in pure form.

Growth hormone releasing factor (GRF) has been postulated but has not so far been satisfactorily characterised.

Prolactin release inhibitory factor (PRIF) has been demonstrated in crude hypothalamic extracts but it has not yet been characterised.

In some cases the action of a postulated factor may be explained in terms of a known hormone with more than one type of activity. Thus the postulated *prolactin releasing factor (PRF)* may be identical with TRH. A postulated specific *follicle stimulating releasing factor (FRF)* may be identical with LRH. It has been suggested that PRIF acts on dopamine receptors and may possibly be dopamine itself.

Significance of hypothalamic hypophysiotropic hormones
The discovery that the secretion of anterior pituitary hormones is itself controlled by a set of hypothalamic hypophysiotropic-releasing hormones is of fundamental physiological significance. It has revealed a means by which the hypothalamus can regulate the feedback control of anterior pituitary hormones such as thyrotrophin, corticotrophin and gonadotrophins. Although the detailed mechanisms of feedback control are not understood it now seems likely that the level of circulating thyroid hormones determines the output of TSH from the pituitary by control mechanisms which may operate at hypothalamic level. Circulating cortisol may control adrenocortical output by control mechanisms in the hypothalamus and perhaps also in the anterior pituitary, and oestrogens may act on the hypothalamus to regulate pituitary output of FSH and LH.

The pharmacological implications of the newly discovered hypothalamic hormones are beginning to be evaluated. So far they have been largely diagnostic but therapeutic applications are gradually evolving. Both the hypothalamic hormones themselves and their synthetic and semisynthetic derivatives may be important. For example the semisynthetic ergot derivative bromocriptine (p. 274) which has been shown to inhibit prolactin secretion may operate by a mechanism which mimics the hormonal control of prolactin release.

PREPARATIONS

Gonadotrophin Releasing Factor (LH/FSH-RF, Gonadorelin) 500 μg 2x die i.m.
Growth Hormone Release Inhibiting Hormone (GHRIH, Somatostatin)
Thyrotrophin Releasing Hormone (TRH, Protirelin) 200 μg i.v.

25. Pituitary, thyroid and parathyroid

The pituitary gland 324; Hormones of the anterior pituitary 324; Growth hormone 324; Prolactin 325; Gonadotrophic hormones 325; Chorionic gonadotrophin 325; Thyrotrophic hormone 326; LATS 327; ACTH 327; Hormones of posterior lobe 329; Action of vasopressin 329; Actions of oxytocin 329; Thyroid gland 330; Thyroxine and tri-iodothyronine 331; Thyroid function tests 332; Thyroid secretion and iodine metabolism 332; Endemic goitre 332; Cretinism 333; Myxoedema 333; Antithyroid drugs 333; Potassium perchlorate 334; Radioactive iodine 334; Parathyroid hormone 335; Calcitonin 336.

The endocrine system
Endocrine secretions constitute part of the system of chemical control of body functions and are a particular group of agents for which a centralised form of production has been evolved. They have one common property of practical importance, namely, that the centralisation involves the risk of the centre being deranged by disease.

THE PITUITARY GLAND

The activities of the pituitary gland are of a unique character, since the posterior lobe and the hypothalamic centres together constitute a mechanism which regulates the activity of the autonomic system and salt and water metabolism, whilst the anterior lobe which is itself regulated by hypothalamic-releasing *factors* or *hormones* (p. 322) is largely concerned with regulating the activity of the other endocrine organs.

The two lobes of the pituitary gland, although closely associated anatomically, differ completely in their origin, structure and function. The posterior lobe, or *pars nervosa* originates as a diverticulum of the brain.

The rest of the gland is developed from Rathke's pouch, a diverticulum from the upper portion of the buccal cavity. The posterior wall of the pouch forms the *pars intermedia* and the anterior wall forms the anterior lobe or *pars glandularis*.

Hormones of the anterior pituitary
The anterior pituitary or adenohypophysis has been called the 'dictator' or 'master' gland, for it produces a large number of hormones which regulate the activity of other endocrine glands. Removal of the anterior lobe causes a wide variety of deficiency symptoms which can be corrected by administration of hormones extracted from the gland.

The anterior pituitary hormones are protein in nature and are therefore difficult to separate or purify. The following hormones have been clearly demonstrated:

(1) Growth, (2) Lactogenic, (3) Gonadotrophic, (4) Thyrotrophic, and (5) Adrenocorticotrophic.

The mammalian anterior pituitary also contains certain other physiologically active peptides the function of which is not clearly established. Several of these peptides are chemically related to adrenocorticotrophin with which they share a common heptapeptide sequence. They include alpha- and beta- melanocyte-stimulating hormones and two separate lipotrophins.

Growth hormone (Somatotrophin. Human growth hormone, HGH)
In 1909 Aschner showed that, after hypophysectomy, young dogs failed to grow. Later, Evans and Long (1921) demonstrated that injection of anterior pituitary gland extracts restored the arrested growth of hypophysectomised animals and that giant rats could be produced by injecting such extracts into normal young rats.

Growth hormone promotes skeletal, visceral and general body growth. It stimulates protein production and affects mineral metabolism. There is a complex interaction between growth hormone and insulin. Insulin secretion by the pancreas is stimulated by growth hormone, but under some circumstances growth hormone antagonises insulin action and when given to diabetic subjects it causes an increase in blood sugar and produces ketosis.

Growth hormone is a water-soluble protein with molecular weight about 22 000. Its complete amino acid sequence has been determined. Human growth hormone is present in the pituitary in greater abundance than any other hormone accounting for 10 per cent of the dried weight of the gland. Its concentration in blood can be measured by radioimmunoassay, its release is controlled by a hypothalamic growth hormone-releasing factor (GRF). Growth hormone release is stimulated by sleep and hypoglycaemia.

Several clinical conditions are associated with disturbances of secretion of the anterior pituitary gland, involving the growth hormone. The signs and symptoms depend upon whether the derangement occurs before or after puberty. Diminished secretion at an early age results in pituitary dwarfism, a condition which may respond in a limited fashion to injections of human growth hormone. Hypersecretion, which is often associated with enlargement of the pituitary gland, produces gigantism if it occurs before puberty, and acromegaly if it begins after normal growth has ceased.

It is recognised that growth hormone extracted from the pituitary glands of different species varies and that only human growth hormone and possibly primate hormone is effective in man. Human growth hormone has been administered with good effects for the long-term treatment of patients with hypopituitary dwarfism.

Lactogenic hormone, Prolactin
Chemistry. It has proved difficult to separate chemically human prolactin from growth hormone but it is now clear that they are separate, though closely related, proteins. Both are single chain polypeptides of almost identical length, though differing in respect of several constituent amino acids. The striking similarities between the two hormones suggest that they arose from a common ancestral precursor. They can be sharply differentiated by radioimmunoassay which is now the standard method of measuring the prolactin content of human plasma. Biological assays, such as measurement of milk secretion in tissue culture, may also be used. The molecular weight of prolactin is about 21 500.

The turnover of prolactin in the pituitary is much faster than that of growth hormone. The total gland content of prolactin is turned over several times in a single day.

Action and blood level. The characteristic action of prolactin in the human female is:

1. Growth and differentiation of the breast during pregnancy. This action requires the presence of other hormones, particularly oestrogen and progesterone needed for the proliferation of the mammary ducts and alveoli.
2. The induction of milk secretion during late pregnancy and the puerperium. In animals, prolactin is an essential luteotrophic hormone in rats, it causes crop sac stimulation in doves and it produces behavioural changes in birds and mammals centred around caring for their offspring.

Present evidence is that prolactin secretion by the anterior pituitary is controlled by a hypothalamic prolactin release *inhibiting* factor (PRIF) whereas growth hormone secretion is regulated by hypothalamic growth hormone release *stimulating* factor (GRF) (p. 323). Neither has so far been identified. Prolactin levels in blood exhibit pronounced diurnal variations; they are highest at the end of a period of sleep. The strongest stimulus for prolactin release in postpartum women is the act of nursing.

Prolactin secretion is affected by a variety of agents. It is increased by TRF and is inhibited by dopamine and dopaminergic stimulants such as apomorphine. *Bromocriptine,* a semisynthetic ergot derivative (p. 274) inhibits prolactin secretion and lowers circulating prolactin levels. It can be used to suppress both puerperal and non-puerperal galactorrhoea.

Placental lactogen is a protein with similar actions as prolactin which is found in human placenta.

Gonadotrophic hormones
The anterior pituitary gland is the timekeeper that regulates the sexual cycle of female mammals and this is effected by the secretion of two hormones. The follicle-stimulating hormone (FSH) causes ripening of the ovarian follicles in the female. The follicle responds to FSH by the secretion of liquor folliculi, proliferation of the granulosa cells and development of the thecal layers resulting in a general enlargement of the structure. It is not certain whether FSH alone can cause oestrogen secretion by the follicle; it is more probable that full maturation of the follicle and optimal oestrogen secretion require the concerted action of both FSH and LH.

In the male, FSH acts on the germinal epithelium of the seminiferous tubules, where it promotes full spermatogenesis.

The luteinising hormone (LH), also called interstitial cell stimulating hormone, acts on the ovarian follicle after it has been under the prior influence of FSH. Under the synergistic action of these two hormones the follicle rapidly reaches full maturation, secretes maximal quantities of oestrogen, and ovulation occurs by the formation of a corpus luteum. LH has a specific effect in inducing the synthesis and secretion of progesterone by the corpus luteum. Whether the regressive changes in the ovary which occur with luteinisation are due to LH is uncertain.

In the male the principal action of LH is on the interstitial cells of Leydig, promoting the secretion of androgen which secondarily stimulates the accessory organs of reproduction and may also play a role in spermatogenesis in conjunction with FSH.

Chemistry. Luteinising hormone and follicle-stimulating hormone are glycoproteins. Each is composed of two dissimilar sub-units held together by non-covalent bonds. One, termed the alpha sub-unit, is common to both hormones whilst the beta sub-unit is characteristic of the particular hormone. The same alpha sub-unit linked to different beta sub-units also occurs in chorionic gonadotrophin and in thyrotrophin.

An unspecific biological assay of both luteinising hormone and follicle-stimulating hormone is based on the weight of the immature mouse uterus. More specific bioassays which distinguish the two hormones have been introduced but they have now been largely superseded by radioimmunoassays based on the respective beta sub-units which are highly specific for LH and FSH. Immunological techniques can be used to measure human chorionic gonadotrophin in pregnancy urine. They provide a simple reliable pregnancy test. Peak levels of urinary chorionic gonadotrophin occur about the ninth week of pregnancy.

Chorionic gonadotrophin. At the onset of pregnancy in women, there is a large excretion of gonadotrophic activity in the urine which is mainly luteinising (Fig. 25.1). The similarity of this gonadotrophic factor to that obtained from the pituitary originally led to some confusion but it is

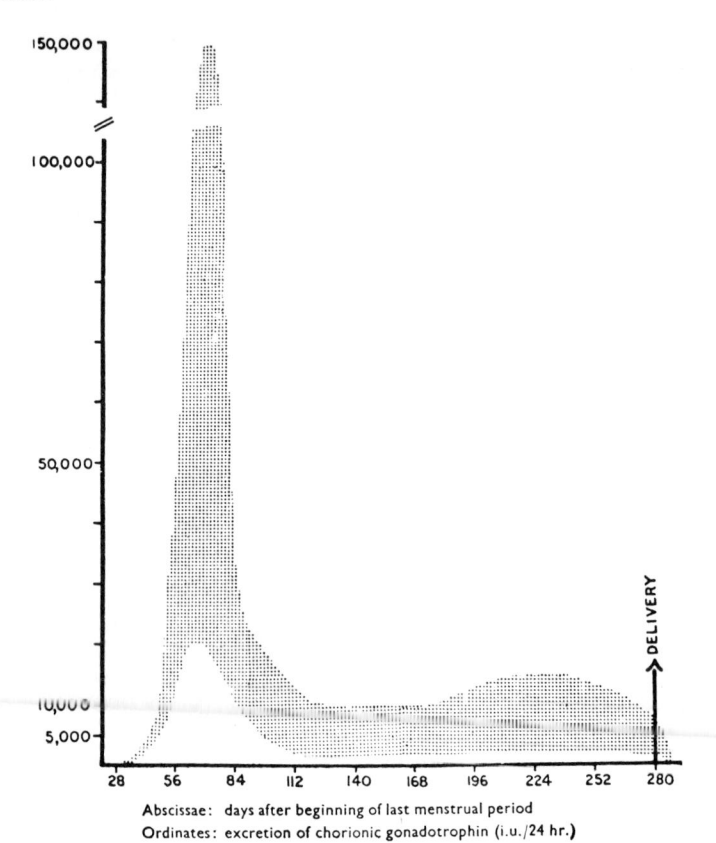

Fig. 25.1 Range of excretion of chorionic gonadotrophin in normal pregnancy. The assay was based upon the production of a full squamous response in the vaginal smear of 21-day-old rats. (After Venning, 1955, *Brit. Med. Bull.*)

now established that it is produced in the placenta. It is also present in the blood, urine and tissues of patients with certain malignant tumours of the reproductive system. It is known as chorionic gonadotrophic hormone or chorionic gonadotrophin. The presence of this substance in urine provides an extremely useful test for early pregnancy.

Therapeutic uses. Pituitary and chorionic gonadotrophic hormones are used in the treatment of menstrual disorders and of sterility in women. Since chorionic gonadotrophic hormone stimulates the interstitial cell tissue it may be used in the treatment of cryptorchidism to produce descent of the testes. Delay or failure of the testicles to descend into the scrotal sac may be due to mechanical obstruction or other unknown causes. Although the testes in most cases descend spontaneously into the scrotal sac at puberty, it is now recognised that for normal development the testes should be in the scrotal sac by the age of ten years. In the majority of cases of undescended testicles in boys, preparations of human chorionic gonadotrophin (HCG) will cause descent of the testes but it is necessary to avoid too rapid development of the external genitalia and secondary sex characteristics; it is seldom desirable to begin treatment before the tenth year.

Thyrotrophic hormone

This is known as thyroid stimulating hormone (TSH). It stimulates the activity of the thyroid, increasing iodide trapping, the formation of thyroid hormones (p. 331) and their release. The processes of intermediary metabolism within the gland such as glucose oxidation, ribonucleic acid synthesis and phospholipid formation are stimulated. Hypophysectomy causes thyroid atrophy in mammals and injection of TSH causes hypertrophy and hyperplasia of the thyroid. TSH is a glycoprotein of molecular weight 28 000. It consists of α- and ß-sub-units which can be separated by gel filtration. The separated sub-units have little or no biological activity. Pituitary TSH is secreted by specific basophilic cells.

The TSH receptor. When TSH, labelled with ^{125}I, is incubated with thyroid membranes a small amount of the label will bind specifically to 'receptors' in the membrane. This forms the basis of a convenient receptor assay for TSH. Scatchard plots of TSH are heterogenous indicating several TSH binding sites with different affinities. The interaction of TSH with its receptors has been shown to cause calcium entry and the activation of adenylylate cyclase which is probably followed by phosphorylation of several key enzymes.

Biological assays of TSH involving the release of radioiodine are difficult and imprecise. Radioimmunoassays of TSH are now available and have made a major contribution to the diagnosis and management of thyroid disease. In general the more severe the thyroid failure, the higher the serum TSH level. TSH measurements after the administration of TRH (p. 322) show that patients with hypothyroidism due to primary thyroid disease show an exaggerated and prolonged TSH response to TRH, whilst patients with hyperthyroidism fail to respond to TRH because of the action of increased circulating T_3 and T_4. The interference by circulating thyroid hormones with the action of TRH and TSH release represents a negative feedback loop tending to maintain circulating thyroid levels constant.

Long-acting thyroid stimulator (LATS) is an immunoglobulin found in patients with Graves' disease which blocks the binding of TSH to human thyroid membranes. LATS also has a prolonged stimulant effect on TSH causing stimulation of the thyroid gland. The precise role of LATS in thyrotoxicosis is not known.

Adrenocorticotrophic hormone

When an animal is hypophysectomised the adrenal cortex atrophies and this can be prevented by the injection of an extract of anterior pituitary gland. If such an extract is injected into a normal animal the adrenal cortex enlarges and there is an increased secretion of adrenal steroids. The pituitary hormone which causes this effect is called adrenocorticotrophic hormone (corticotrophin, ACTH) and was isolated in 1943 by Sayers and his colleagues and by Li and his co-workers.

Chemical structure. Human ACTH is a single chain polypeptide of 39 amino acids with molecular weight approximately 4500. ACTH has been completely synthesised and the amino acid sequences required for its physiological action have been identified. The first 24 amino acids of the amino terminal are required for activity whilst the function of the carboxy terminal 25-39 is not known. The core of the molecule consist of the heptapeptide sequence 4-10 which retains reduced corticotrophin activity.

Actions and release. The main target organ of ACTH is the adrenal cortex on which it has at least two actions: (1) Maintenance of the weight of the adrenal gland; (2) Steroidogenesis. Stored cholesterol esters in adrenal cortical cells are enzymatically converted to cortisol and adrenal androgens. ACTH also has extra-adrenal actions. It may be responsible for pigmentation in patients with Addison's disease, although some workers consider that the pigmentation is due to melanocyte secreting hormone secreted together with ACTH.

Pituitary ACTH secretion exhibits marked spontaneous diurnal variations. In consequence cortisol levels reach a maximum in the early morning hours from 4-8 a.m. and then fall gradually to reach the lowest point around midnight. The circadian effect depends on the individual's sleep-walking cycle and is controlled by CRF release from the hypothalamus. A second control mechanism for ACTH is negative feedback whereby high circulating cortisol levels inhibit ACTH release by an action of cortisol on CRF release from the hypothalamus and probably also by a direct action on the pituitary. Conversely, low or absent circulating cortisol stimulates ACTH release through overproduction of CRF. A further important control mechanism operates in stress. Under moderate stress cortisol release may be markedly increased whilst very severe stress, e.g. during surgery, may cause a sudden cessation of ACTH secretion and cortisol release. Patients who have recently been treated with corticosteroids are particularly at risk because their ACTH secretion is already impaired.

Concentration of ACTH in blood may be measured by radioimmunoassay. An extremely sensitive biological assay for ACTH based on a cytochemical method has recently been described.

Actions on the adrenal cortex. Under normal resting conditions there is a continuous secretion of hydrocortisone from the adrenal cortex; this may be increased tenfold after an injection of ACTH. The effects of ACTH depend on the ability of the adrenal cortex to secrete hydrocortisone and other steroids and an injection of 100 units ACTH causes about a threefold increase in the excretion of 17-ketosteroids in the urine. The secretion of aldosterone is not significantly increased. ACTH also causea a marked decrease in the number of circulating eosinophils and lymphocytes and an increase in the number of neutrophils. The excretion of potassium in the urine is increased and there is a retention of sodium and chloride.

Clinical uses. The biological activity of commercial preparations of ACTH varies and their corticotrophin activity can be determined by a biological assay which depends on measuring the depletion of ascorbic acid in the adrenal glands of hypophysectomised rats after injection of the hormone. One of the main uses of corticotrophin is as a diagnostic agent in the investigation of disorders of the pituitary and the adrenal cortex.

The therapeutic uses of ACTH are based mainly on the fact that it is capable of releasing hydrocortisone (cortisol). Compared with cortisol itself, the administration of ACTH has the advantage of stimulating the release of several other cortical steroids, but its effects are less reliable than those of cortisol administration since the response of the adrenal glands to a standard dose of ACTH varies.

ACTH is not absorbed when taken by mouth and must be given by intramuscular or intravenous injection. The effect of ACTH on the adrenals is very rapid but short lasting. When a single dose is injected intravenously its effects last for only about six hours as judged by the increase in 17-ketosteroid excretion. For this reason ACTH is mainly indicated when a rapid maximal release of hydrocortisone is required, as, for example, in the treatment of severe asthma. When a prolonged action is desired ACTH must be injected at frequent intervals, or it may be administered intramuscularly once or twice daily as a gel from which it is slowly released; in these circumstances it is sometimes better to give cortisol or a synthetic glucocorticoid which have a more reliable action and can be taken by mouth.

On the other hand, ACTH has the advantage that it tends to preserve the functional integrity of the patient's own adrenal cortex, the function of which may be completely suppressed, even to the point of adrenal atrophy, by prolonged administration of exogenous corticosteroids.

Side effects of corticotrophin are hypertension, pigmentation, hirsutism and acne. The side effects are dose-dependent and, provided corticotrophin is given intermittently twice weekly, the dose can be so adjusted that side effects are not serious.

Tetracosactrin. This is a synthetic compound with ACTH activity containing the first 24 of the 39 amino acids of the peptide chain of natural corticotrophin. Tetracosactrin is a pure substance which can be prescribed on a weight basis and may be used in the presence of hypersensitivity to natural ACTH. It is available as short acting *cortrosyn* or *synacthen* or as a depot compound combined with zinc phosphate for prolonged action.

Long acting tetracosactrin may be used where long-acting corticotrophins are indicated as in the collagen diseases of rheumatoid arthritis and systemic lupus erythematosus. A dose of 1 mg intramuscularly elevates plasma cortisol for up to 48 hours. It is used intermittently on alternate days for collagen disease and once weekly for severe bronchial asthma. Short-acting tetracosactrin is used mainly as a diagnostic tool in assessing adrenocortical function.

POSTERIOR LOBE OF THE PITUITARY

The posterior lobe of the pituitary and the hypothalamus together form a functional unit — the neurohypophysis — which controls some of the most important vital functions, in particular the water balance of the body. This unit comprises the supraoptic and paraventrical nuclei of the hypothalamus which are connected to the posterior lobe by nonmyelinated fibres in the stalk. When these fibres are cut, secretion of antidiuretic hormone is stopped as effectively as by removal of the gland, and the condition of diabetes insipidus ensues. It is now believed that the posterior pituitary hormones are elaborated in the hypothalamic nuclei and are conveyed along the nerve fibres of the neurosecretory cells to the posterior lobe of the pituitary gland where they are stored.

Mechanism of release of posterior pituitary hormones
Figure 25.2 shows a diagram of the neurosecretory pathways in the hypothalamus and the neurohypophysis in man. It has been suggested that the supraoptic nucleus is concerned with the synthesis of vasopressin and the paraventricular nucleus with that of oxytocin but evidence on this point is conflicting and, on the whole, does not support such a simple dichotomy. The neurosecretory hypothesis of Bargmann and Scharrer postulates that the hormones are transported from the cell bodies in the hypothalamus to the nerve endings in the neural lobe by axoplasmic flow. Secretion of the hormones into the blood stream probably involves the generation of an elecrtrical impulse in the cell body which travels towards the nerve terminal, and brings about release of the hormone. Douglas and Poisner have shown that the release of posterior pituitary hormones requires calcium and have suggested that a depolarising electrical stimulus may induce neurosecretion by promoting the entry of calcium into the nerve terminal.

The supraoptic and paraventricular nuclei are themselves innervated by both cholinergic and adrenergic nerves.

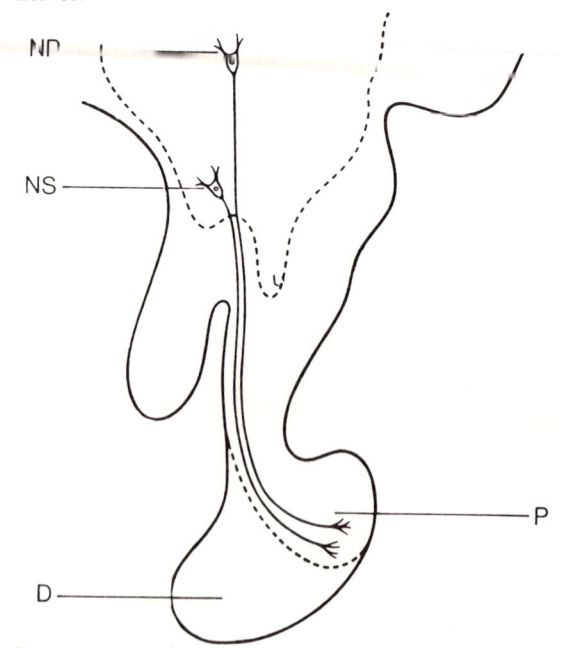

Fig. 25.2 Diagram of the neurosecretory pathways in the hypothalamus and the neurohypophysis in man; NP and NS neurosecretory cells in the paraventricular and supraoptic nucleus of the hypothalamus, P neurohypophysis, D adenohypophysis. (After Berde, 1959. *Recent Progess in Oxytocin Research.* C. Thomas, Springfield.)

Physiological stimuli causing release of posterior pituitary hormones
There is evidence that various physiological stimuli can cause release of oxytocin and vasopressin. Release of

vasopressin by a hypertonic solution is illustrated in Figure 11.5. It has also been shown that haemorrhage causes vasopressin release and that changes in blood volume as well as changes in blood osmolarity may affect vasopressin release thus subserving its fundamental physiological role in the homoeostatic control of the extracellular fluid volume.

Suckling causes a reflex secretion of oxytocin (Fig. 15.3) and of prolactin. Milk ejection in women can be inhibited by local anaesthesia of the teat. Oxytocin plays an essential role in lactation by producing milk ejection. The role of oxytocin in parturition is less clear and there is now considerable evidence against the earlier hypothesis that the onset of parturition is brought about by oxytocin release from the neurohypophysis. For example it has been shown that in women, in whom milk ejection pressure from the breast and intra-amniotic fluid pressure were recorded simultaneously, the increased uterine activity during delivery was not accompanied by increases in milk ejection pressure.

Hormones of the posterior lobe

The human neurohypophysis contains oxytocin and arginine-vasopressin. In the pig arginine vasopressin is replaced by lysine vasopressin. Several related neurohypophysial peptides have been found in other vertebrates. The hormones are contained within neurosecretory granules bound to a carrier protein called neurophysin. The hormone-neurophysin complexes are formed by electrostatic bonds between the carboxyl group of neurophysin and the free terminal NH_2 group in the peptides. There is evidence that a separate neurophysin is combined with oxytocin and another with vasopressin, both complexes have been crystallised.

The chemical structure of vasopressin and oxytocin is known and they have been synthetised by du Vigneaud and his colleagues. Each of these hormones is a polypeptide composed of eight amino acids, one of which is cystine. The activity of the hormones depends on the disulphide bridge of cystine remaining intact. Oxytocin and vasopressin have six amino acids in common and differ from each other in regard to two as shown in Figure 25.3.

Actions of vasopressin

Vasopressin plays a crucial role in the concentrating mechanism of the kidney by increasing the permeability to water of the distal part of the nephron (p. 159). A morphologically demonstrable effect produced by applying ADH (vasopressin) to the non-luminal surface of a renal collecting duct is shown in Figure 25.4. The cells are seen to swell and vacuoles appear within them which are presumably filled with water. Apart from increasing the permeability of the lumen cells to water, ADH also

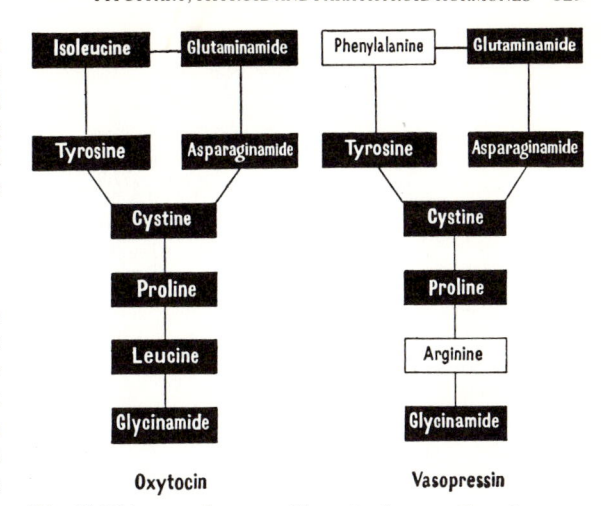

Fig. 25.3 Diagram of structural formulae for oxytocin and vasopressin. In vasopressin from swine glands arginine is replaced by lysine. (After Triangle, 1958.)

increases their sodium resorption. These effects are mediated by cyclic AMP.

Somewhat larger doses of vasopressin constrict blood vessels. A well-known phenomenon is pallor of the human skin after the administration of vasopressin. This effect is produced by relatively small doses which do not alter blood pressure and cardiac output, indicating a special affinity of vasopressin for skin vessels. Microcirculatory studies with vasopressin have shown that it acts primarily on venules in contrast to adrenaline which acts primarily on arterioles.

Vasopressin decreases myocardial blood flow; as a consequence of this, when a high dose of vasopressin is administered there is an increase in systemic blood pressure associated with a decrease in cardiac output.

Clinical uses. The use of vasopressin and synthetic analogues with greater antidiuretic activity for antidiuretic action in diabetes insipidus is discussed on page 156. *Felypressin* (octapressin) (2-phenylalanine-lysine vasopressin) is sometimes used with local anaesthetics since it has relatively little antidiuretic activity, compared to its vasoconstrictor activity (p. 313).

Actions of oxytocin

Oxytocin stimulates the uterus, especially at term (p. 220) and if administered in labour produces a pattern of co-ordinated contractions which closely resembles normal spontaneous uterine contractions. Its actions on the uterus are discussed on page 223. It has been found that different S-S polypeptides of this series vary in their uterine stimulant and antidiuretic activities. Oxytocin has particularly strong uterus stimulating activity. De-amino-oxytocin has comparable activity to oxytocin on rat uterus but greater activity than oxytocin on human uterus. Lysine

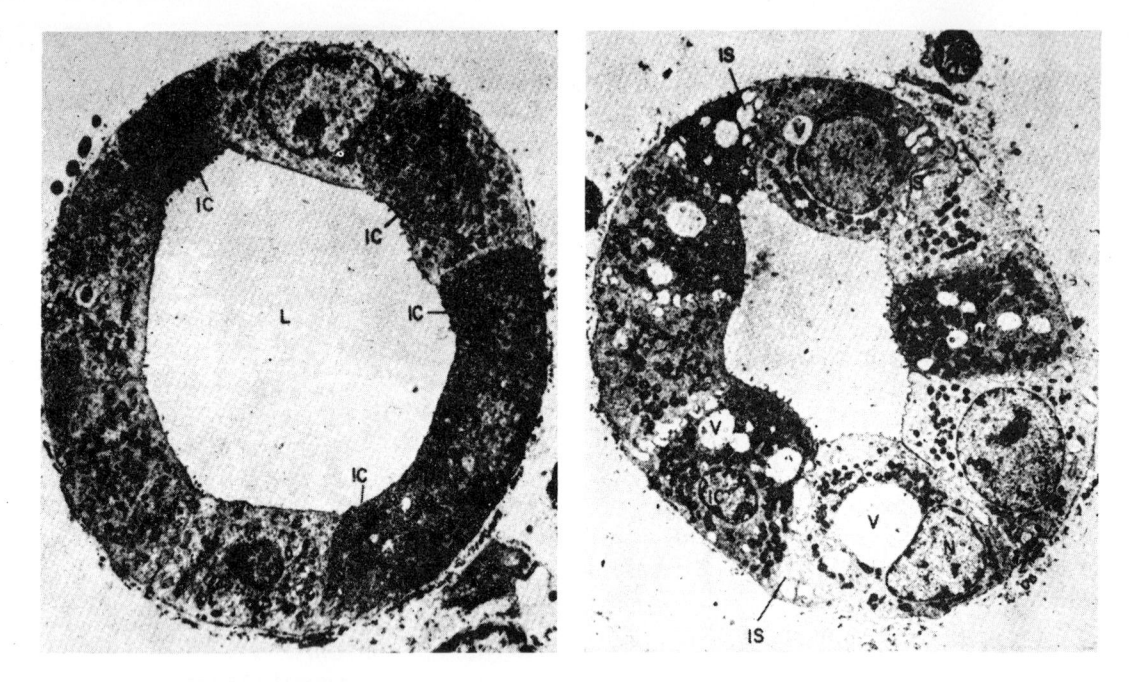

Fig. 25.4 Effect of ADH on renal collecting duct (rabbit). Left: without ADH, right: with ADH. Note that with ADH the cells swell, the lumen becomes smaller because of bulging of the cells and within the cells themselves there are large vacuoles presumably filled with water. (After Ganote, Grantham, Moses, Burg and Orloff, 1968. *J. Cell. Biol.*)

vasopressin has strong antidiuretic but only weak oxytocic activity. Nevertheless it can be shown that the various S-S polypeptides all act on the same uterine receptors since they produce the same pA_2 values when tested with the same competitive antagonist (p. 13).

Oxytocin causes a contraction of the myoepithelium of the mammary gland, which leads to expression of milk from the alveoli and ducts of the gland. The process of 'milk let down' is essential for the complete evacuation of the gland, which cannot be achieved solely by the mechanical process of suckling or milking. Oxytocin has some vasodilator effect in man (though less so than in birds) and rapid intravenous injections may cause a transient fall of blood pressure.

Biological assay. Several official methods for the standardisation of extract of posterior pituitary gland are described. One of these depends on estimating the oxytocic activity of the extract on the isolated rat uterus and comparing this effect with that produced by the international standard posterior pituitary powder. Oxytocin produces a fall in blood pressure in the chicken and another official method of assay depends on this property. A bioassay method by which oxytocin in plasma extracts can be estimated is by recording milk ejection pressure form a cannulated teat duct in a lactating rat. A bioassay method for vasopressin in body fluid extracts is by intravenous injection in rats under ethanol anaesthesia maintaining a constant water load. Radioimmunoassays for vasopressin and oxytocin have been developed.

THE THYROID GLAND

Goitre is a deformity that has been well known since classical times, and it is interesting to note that the Greeks treated this condition with the ashes of sponges, which contain iodine. In 1820 Coindet instituted iodine therapy for goitre and Chatin published a series of papers between 1850 and 1870 in which he proved conclusively that goitre was associated with a deficiency of iodine in the soil. This brilliant work was, however, too far ahead of contemporary knowledge for its importance to be recognised.

It was not until 1882 that Sir Victor Horsley proved the thyroid to be a gland of internal secretion, deficiency of which caused cretinism and myxoedema. In 1891 Murray showed that injection of a glycerine extract of thyroid could cure myxoedema and it was soon found that an equally good result could be obtained by oral administration of dry thyroid. Finally, in 1895, Baumann proved that the thyroid contained an iodine compound, and this discovery at last explained the fact established by Chatin, that iodine deficiency caused disordered thyroid function. Thirty years later Kendall isolated an active crystalline compound from the thyroid gland which he named thyroxine. The structural formula of thyroxine was shown by Harington to be

$$HO-C_6H_2I_2-O-C_6H_2I_2-CH_2CH(NH_2)COOH$$
Thyroxine

Harington and Barger synthesised thyroxine in 1927. In 1952 Gross and Pitt-Rivers showed that the thyroid contains in addition triiodothyronine, the metabolic activity of which is three to five times greater than that of thyroxine. The thyroid also contains two inactive precursors of these hormones, monoiodotyrosine and diiodotyrosine.

Iodide is taken by the thyroid from the circulating blood and in the thyroid it is oxidised to iodine. In the presence of iodine a conversion of tyrosine to monoiodotyrosine and diiodotyrosine occurs. This conversion takes place within the protein thyroglobulin which is present in the thyroid. By the coupling of two molecules of diiodotyrosine, thyroxine is readily formed as follows:

$$HO-C_6H_2I_2-CH_2.CH(NH_2)COOH + H \quad O-C_6H_2I_2-CH_2.CH(NH_2)COOH$$

One molecule of diiodotyrosine combines less readily with one molecule of monoiodotyrosine to form triiodothyronine. These reactions result in the formation of a thyroglobulin that contains the four amino-acids monoiodotyrosine, diiodotyrosine, thyroxine and triiodothyronine.

The thyroid contains proteolytic enzymes which act on thyroglobulin to form a pool of free amino acids in the thyroid. Of these thyroxine and triiodothyronine escape into the circulation. In the plasma, thyroxine is strongly bound to two proteins called thyroxine-binding globulin and thyroxine-binding prealbumin. A small fraction of thyroxine is bound to serum albumin. Triiodothyronine is likewise protein-bound, though not as strongly as thyroxine.

Thyroxine and triiodothyronine

The fundamental action of these substances usually referred to as T_4 and T_3 is to increase the oxygen consumption of cells, probably by an action on mitochondria. A further primary action may be an increase in protein synthesis.

Only the free fraction of the thyroid hormones is biologically active; the ratio of T_4 to T_3 is normally about 8:1. Only a relatively small amount of T_3 is secreted as such by the thyroid gland, most of it is formed from T_4 in the tissues. The metabolic activity of T_3 is about 4 times greater than that of T_4. The thyroid hormones are metabolised at different rates, the half life of T_4 is 6–7 days and that of T_3 is $1\frac{1}{2}$ days.

The circulating level of thyroid hormones is regulated through a feedback system which comprises thyroid, anterior pituitary and hypothalamus. As the blood level of free thyroid hormones increases, the secretion of TSH is inhibited and thyroid secretion decreases, conversely low thyroid hormone levels caused increased release and blood levels of TSH with increased secretion of thyroid hormones. Secretion of TSH is brought about by thyrotrophin releasing hormone (TRH) of the hypothalamus but the controlling mechanisms for TRH release are not fully understood.

Thyroxine

This is a stable compound the sodium salt of which (L-thyroxine sodium) is soluble in alkaline solution. It is absorbed when given by mouth. It may also be administered parenterally, but because of its strong alkalinity must be injected intravenously and not subcutaneously. The activity of preparations containing thyroxine may be estimated biologically or chemically by determining the proportion of iodine in combination as thyroxine.

When tested on tadpoles and rats, L-thyroxine has about three times the physiological activity of D-thyroxine. On patients measured by thyroid function tests L-thyroxine has about eight to ten times the activity of D-thyroxine.

The action of thyroxine is characterised by two peculiarities. Firstly, a series of small doses produces a much greater effect than does a single dose, however large. Secondly, the onset of the action is delayed, for example, a single dose of 0.1 mg levothyroxine when given to a patient with thyroid deficiency, takes from six to eight days to produce its maximum effect. This is shown by an increase in basal metabolic rate, which does not return to its original level for four or five weeks. When administered in repeated doses, the rise in basal metabolic rate is accompanied by a general increase in fat and carbohydrate metabolism; the blood sugar level is raised, glycogen storage in the liver is decreased and glycosuria may occur. The excretion of nitrogen and calcium in the urine is also increased. These changes result in a loss in body weight which is associated with the signs of increased excitability of the tissues innervated by the sympathetic system.

The initial dose of thyroxine sodium should not be greater than 0.1 mg daily. In elderly patients and those with cardiac diseases, the initial dose should be 0.05 mg on alternate days because of the danger of precipitating angina or myocardial infarction if the cardiac oxygen consumption is suddenly increased. Doses may then be increased gradually at intervals of 2–3 weeks until the desired effect is obtained.

Liothyronine (triiodothyronine). In patients with myxoedema the effects of liothyronine are qualitatively similar to those of thyroxine but it has a much quicker action. Intravenous administration of liothyronine sodium produces a response in the myxoedematous patient within 24 to 48 hours, whilst a similar response to thyroxine is seen only after 7 to 10 days. Liothyronine is used in the treatment of thyroid-deficiency states, particularly when a rapid effect is required. Mixtures of thyroxine and liothyronine in a 4:1 proportion are sometimes used clinically to simulate the effects of thyroid extract.

$$HO-\underset{}{C_6H_3I}-O-\underset{I}{C_6H_3}-CH_2CH(NH_2)COONa$$

Liothyronine Sodium

Use of thyroid hormones in euthyroid subjects
Thyroid preparations are sometimes given in order to reduce weight, but this practice is dangerous. If a normal person uses thyroxine or liothyronine in a dosage which is equivalent to his daily endogenous hormone secretion, his pituitary will cease to secrete TSH, and the net results will be to leave him in the same metabolic state as he was before starting medication. If he uses larger doses, they may produce weight reduction at the expense of causing hyperthyroidism.

Thyroid hormones have been shown to reduce blood cholesterol, but their use in this context is particularly dangerous since patients with elevated blood cholesterol are apt to have coronary atherosclerosis, and hyperthyroidism in such patients may cause angina and heart failure. Attempts have been made to use D-thyroxine for this purpose since it has a relatively greater effect on blood cholesterol than on oxygen consumption.

Thyroid function tests
The levels of both T_3 and T_4 in serum can now be measured by radioimmunoassay. Serum TSH levels can also be measured by radioimmunoassay and are useful in the diagnosis of thyroid disease. Patients with hypothyroidism generally have a raised serum TSH level particularly after the application of TRH. In hyperthyroidism, TSH secretion is lowered through the inhibiting effect of circulating thyroid hormones. A particularly sensitive test in hyperthyroidism is the absence of TSH elevation after the injection of TRH.

Toxic effects of thyroxine. The fact that a single excessive dose of thyroxine produces less toxic effects than the same quantity given in divided doses, indicates that any large excess of thyroxine is cleared relatively quickly. In the case of moderate overdosage it is probable that about one-tenth of the drug present is cleared daily and this slow excretion coupled with the delayed action favours the production of cumulative toxic effects. It may be assumed that the full effect of any particular rate of administration will not be seen before several weeks, and hence the dosage of thyroxine should be increased cautiously.

Overdosage of thyroxine causes the following symptoms: palpitation with a rapid and often irregular pulse, nervousness with insomnia, headache and muscular tremors, dilatation of the skin vessels, increased sweating, a temperature above normal, and occasionally disturbance of digestion with vomiting and diarrhoea. At the same time there is loss of weight. Exophthalmus rarely, if ever, is produced by thyroxine overdosage.

The mechanism of production of exophthalmus, which is a characteristic sign of Graves' disease, is not fully understood. In animals, exophthalmus can be produced by the injection of pituitary thyrotrophic hormone, but in man such injections cause thyroid enlargment and increased secretion of thyroid hormone without significant exophthalmus. Some workers have postulated the production of an 'exophthalmus-producing substance' by the pituitary which is related to, but not identical with, thyrotrophic hormone.

Thyroid secretion and iodine metabolism
The normal thyroid contains an average of 15 mg iodine of which about 15 per cent can be isolated as thyroxine. Only traces of iodine are found in other tissues of the body. The iodine content of the thyroid depends upon the amount of iodine taken in the food. This quantity is very minute, and the human body does not require more than a fraction of a milligram per day.

The thyroid gland provides an example of an endocrine activity which is dependent on an adequate supply of a particular element. The human body probably does not require more than a total of 2 g of iodine during life, unfortunately this element is so scarce in certain regions, that this minimum quantity is not supplied in the normal diet.

Endemic goitre. Enlargement of the thyroid gland is frequent in certain countries, e.g. Switzerland and New Zealand, and much rarer in others, e.g. Japan. The prevalence of simple goitre depends chiefly on the iodine intake, but other factors are also concerned.

Prophylactic administration of iodides in goitrous districts has been practised with success both in America and Europe. Marine showed that iodide medication not only prevents the occurrence of goitre but also causes a reduction in the size of moderately enlarged glands. In addition to this action in inhibiting goitre the prophylactic treatment with iodide has been found to produce marked beneficial effects, both on the rate of growth, and on the mental development of the children.

If iodides are added to cooking and table salt in a concentration of 0.001 per cent this would supply about 0.1 mg daily. Recommendations have been made that all salt used in Great Britain should contain between 15 and 30 parts of iodide per million parts of salt.

Cretinism. Congenital deficiency in thyroid secretion produces cretinism. The whole development of a cretin is abnormal and stunted, but the development of the skeleton and the nervous system is particularly affected. It is important to recognise the signs of cretinism at as early an age as possible. If treatment with thyroid hormone is begun at four months or so, the improvement, both physically and mentally, is usually spectacular and within a few months the individual is almost unrecognisable. When treatment is delayed, though there is satisfactory physical growth, the child remains backward and simple minded.

Myxoedema. Deficiency of thyroid secretion causes a reduction in the basal metabolism, and a general depression of the mental and physical activities. The condition is termed myxoedema on account of an accumulation of mucoprotein in the tissues whereby the subcutaneous tissues are thickened by a non-pitting oedema. The skin is dry and scaly and the hair tends to fall out. The patient lacks energy, is slow, deaf and stupid and cannot maintain any mental effort. He often complains of constipation. The skin temperature is subnormal and the patient cannot tolerate cold weather. The heart is enlarged, the pulse is slow and signs of congestive heart failure may further complicate the picture.

The administration of thyroid hormone produces a remarkable change in such patients; there is an increase in basal metabolism, improvement in the mental and physical condition, and a rapid disappearance of the myxoedema. In the treatment of myxoedema large doses of thyroxine may be required but in the initial stages small daily doses (0.1 mg) are used since a sudden increase in metabolism of the heart may give rise to angina pectoris or even sudden death.

Antithyroid drugs

Mode of action

In order to understand the effects of antithyroid drugs it is necessary to consider in further detail the reactions which lead to the synthesis of thyroxine discussed on page 331.

The iodide concentrating mechanism of the thyroid gland, sometimes referred to as *iodide pump* or *trap*, concentrates plasma iodide about 25 times, incorporating it in protein. This step is extremely fast; iodine-labelled protein has been demonstrated within 11 seconds of the intravenous injection of ^{131}I in mice. The uptake step is followed by a second step involving the iodination of tyrosine to monoiodotyrosine, followed more slowly by subsequent reactions leading to thyroxine. It has been shown that these reactions take place in the colloid of the thyroid gland and involve its principal constituent, the giant molecule (M.W. 680 000) of thyroglobulin.

This sequence of events has been considerably clarified by means of two types of specific inhibitors: (1) drugs which block the iodide pump such as potassium perchlorate and (2) drugs such as thiourea, thiouracil and carbimazole which, whilst permitting iodide concentration by the gland, prevent its incorporation into organic compounds. Both types of drug have been used clinically for the treatment of thyrotoxicosis, although the less toxic thiourea derivatives are generally preferred.

Antithyroid drugs

When rabbits are fed on a diet of cabbage or rape seed the thyroid gland becomes enlarged. Kennedy showed in 1942 that these goitrogenic effects are due to thiourea contained in brassica seed. It was subsequently shown that thiourea, thiouracil and related goitrogenic drugs affect the thyroid gland, increasing its size and weight whilst diminishing production of thyroid hormone. It is now known that these substances act by interfering with the combination of iodine with tyrosine thus preventing the formation of triiodothyronine and thyroxine. In the absence of the thyroid hormones the production of TSH by the pituitary gland is increased, causing an enlargement of the thyroid gland. At the same time the peripheral effects of thyroid hormone deficiency become apparent. Patients with hyperthyroidism can be controlled by antithyroid drugs.

Chemical structure. The chemical structure of some antithyroid agents is shown in Figure 25.5. Methimazole

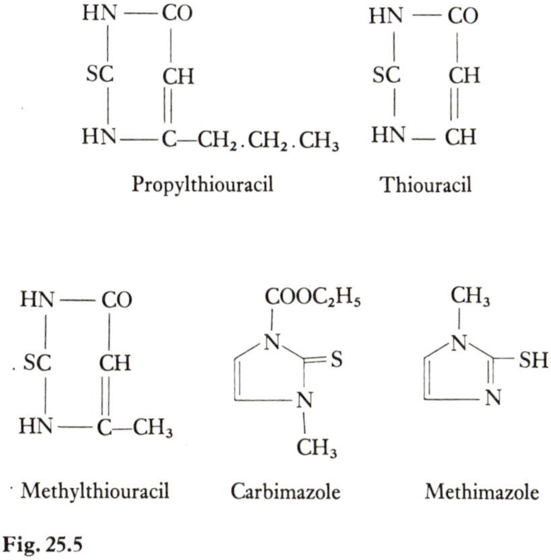

Propylthiouracil   Thiouracil

Methylthiouracil   Carbimazole   Methimazole

Fig. 25.5

and carbimazole are closely related and it is probable that the latter is transformed to methimazole in the body.

Clinical effects. The thiouracil compounds are readily absorbed from the alimentary tract and are excreted in the urine. They are distributed in all tissues and are present in the milk of lactating animals.

When an antithyroid compound is given to a patient with thyrotoxicosis there is a delay in response; this delay is due to the continued action of T_4 and T_3 already stored in the gland. When this store is depleted and the output of thyroid hormones has diminished the patient shows marked subjective improvement with diminished sweating and tremor, a drop in pulse rate and fall in the basal metabolic rate.

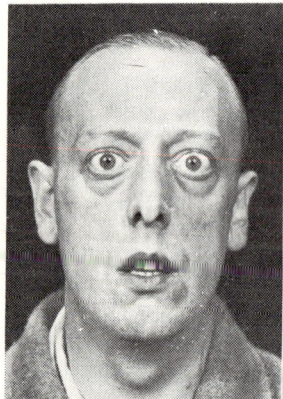

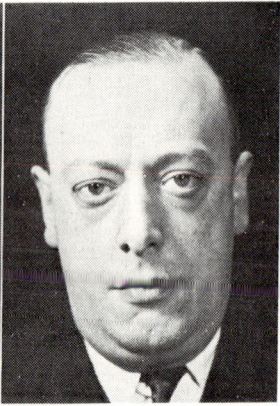

Fig. 25.6 Patient aged 33 years with 10 months history of thyrotoxicosis: (a) before treatment; (b) after 54 days treatment with thiouracil. During this period his weight increased from 10st 13lb (69.4 kg) to 13st 7lb (85.7 kg), and the pulse rate fell from 120 to 88 per minute. (After Wilson, 1946. *Lancet.*)

Since the release of TSH is dependent on the blood level of the thyroid hormones, the pituitary gland is stimulated to produce more TSH when the output of thyroid hormones has ceased. This in turn acts on the thyroid gland producing hyperplasia of the cells and enlargement of the gland. The aim of treatment with antithyroid drugs should therefore be to diminish but not to inhibit completely the output of hormone.

Dosage and duration of treatment. The dosage of these drugs depends on the severity of the thyrotoxicosis. The average initial daily dose of the drug propyl thiouracil is 300 mg and that of carbimazole 20 to 30 mg. Carbimazole is at present the main antithyroid drug used in Great Britain. These drugs are given by mouth, three or four times daily. When the symptoms have been controlled, the dose can be reduced and adjusted according to the clinical condition of the patient. Subjective improvement, some relief of sweating, tremor and tachycardia, and an increase in weight usually become apparent within a fortnight, but the basal metabolic rate does not usually return to normal until two to three weeks after beginning treatment.

When the thyrotoxicosis has been satisfactorily controlled, treatment may be continued on a daily maintenance dose of an antithyroid drug and in some patients there is complete remission and drug treatment can be discontinued. Alternatively, the patient may be prepared for sub-total thyroidectomy. During prolonged maintenance therapy with antithyroid compounds small doses of liothyronine or thyroxine are sometimes also administered in order to prevent the occurrence of myxoedema and to reduce the risk of enlarging the goitre through excessive secretion of TSH.

Toxic effects with carbimazole are rare. They usually occur within the first few weeks of treatment, maculopapular and urticarial eruptions and nausea being the most common. Agranulocytosis is a potential serious complication although unusual. Patients who develop a sore throat and fever must stop the drug and at once seek medical advice.

Beta-adrenoceptor blocking drugs such as propranolol are increasingly used in hyperthyroidism to reduce tachycardia and anxiety. They may be given preoperatively to prepare patients rapidly for thyroidectomy and they are highly effective in the management of hyperthyroid crisis.

Potassium perchlorate

This drug acts by a different mechanism since it inhibits the uptake of iodide (iodide pump) by the thyroid. Its effect can be overcome by raising the iodide level of the plasma.

Although it is clinically effective, potassium perchlorate is seldom used because of the risk of aplastic anaemia. It is sometimes used in patients who are allergic to the thiourea group of drugs.

Action of iodine

The administration of small doses of iodine produces a remarkable remission of symptoms of hyperthyroidism. The effect is transient and cannot be sustained for long periods by continued administration of iodine. This method of treatment should, therefore, be reserved for preparing patients for subtotal thyroidectomy.

Radioactive iodine

Of the 12 radioactive isotopes of iodine that have been described only ^{131}I with a half-life of 8 days is used extensively in the diagnosis and treatment of thyroid disease.

The diagnostic use of radioactive iodine depends on the fact that the rate of accumulation of iodine in the thyroid is related to the activity of the gland. When a dose of radioactive sodium iodide is given by mouth the rate of uptake in the gland can be measured by placing a Geiger counter over the neck; the amount excreted in the urine can also be estimated. In a patient with hyperthyroidism most of the dose of radioactive iodine is taken up by the thyroid and only a small amount of radioactive material appears in the urine, whilst in a normal person accumulation by the thyroid is much less and a large proportion of the dose is excreted in the urine (Fig. 25. 7). In hypothyroid patients the amount taken up by the thyroid is less than normal and the amount excreted in the urine is greater.

Parathyroid hormone

Human parathyroid hormone (PTH) is a single chain polypeptide of 84 amino acids. It differs slightly from ox and beef PTH both of which have been completely synthesised. Existing radioimmunoassays are based on animal PTH which differs slightly in immunological reactivity from the human hormone.

The principal function of PTH is raising the calcium concentration in plasma and extracellular fluid and

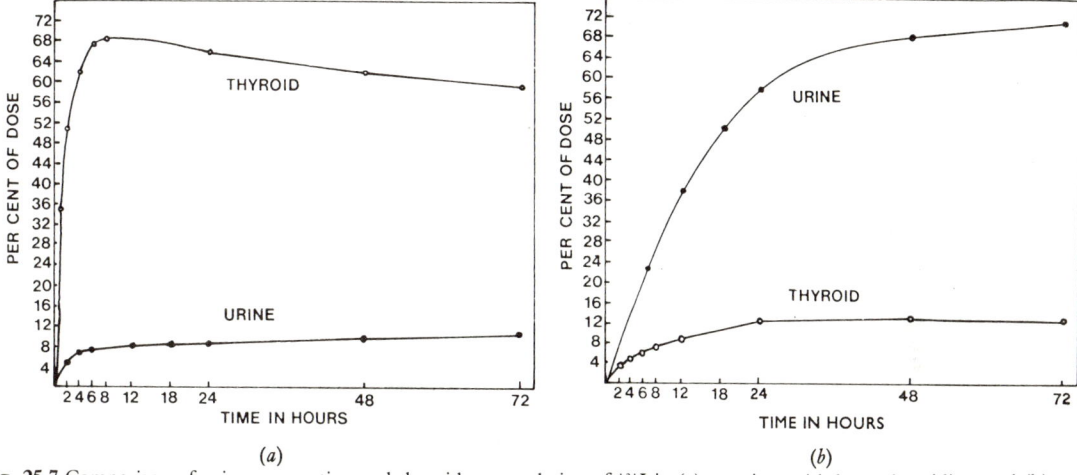

Fig. 25.7 Comparison of urinary excretion and thyroid accumulation of ^{131}I in (a) a patient with hyperthyroidism and (b) a patient with normal thyroid function. (Keating and Albert, 1949. *Recent Progress in Hormone Research.*)

The therapeutic use of radioactive iodine is based on the fact that it is selectively taken up and highly concentrated by the thyroid gland. The isotope emits ioising radiations which interfere with mitosis and destroy cell function. A disadvantage of the method is the difficulty in determining the dose necessary to control symptoms without producing myxoedema. A serious disadvantage is the potential danger of producing malignant changes in the thyroid; for this reason this treatment is often restricted to patients of over forty years of age.

Radioactive iodine is also used for the treatment of cancer of the thyroid and its metastases, but the success of this method depends on the uptake of iodine by the malignant cells. Unfortunately, this is often low and attempts have been made to increase the uptake of ^{131}I by the metastases by surgical removal of the thyroid gland.

THE PARATHYROID GLANDS

The parathyroid glands are small vascular glands about the size of an apple seed which are situated near the dorsal surface of the thyroid gland. In man there are usually four glands, each weighing 25-40 mg. The parathyroid glands are a development of terrestrial animals; they do not exist in fishes. It has been suggested that they may have evolved when the bony structure became solid, to regulate calcium metabolism in bone.

decreasing the plasma phosphate concentration. PTH accelerates bone breakdown and increases renal calcium retention and intestinal calcium absorption. It inhibits renal tubular reabsorption of phosphate which leads to phosphaturia and hypophosphataemia. The effects of PTH on bone and the kidney are mediated by cyclic AMP. The action of PTH in promoting intestinal calcium absorption resembles that of vitamin D but it is not known whether the two effects are in any way connected.

The secretion of parathyroid hormone by the anterior pituitary is controlled by the concentration of ionised calcium in the blood, a low level of calcium leading to increased output of the hormone. PTH is rapidly eliminated in the circulation with a halftime of about 20 minutes.

Hypoparathyroidism. The main clinical features of hypoparathyroidism are due to hypocalcaemia. Hypoparathyroidism may occur as a result of faulty thyroid surgery but more frequently it occurs as a consequence of defective parathyroid function in infants and is characterised by exaggerated reflexes and tetany. The condition is seldom treated by parathyroid extracts which are expensive and must be given by parenteral injection. Most patients respond to vitamin D preparations combined with large oral calcium supplements.

Calcitonin (thyrocalcitonin)

This hypocalcaemic hormone produces effects which are opposite to those of the parathyroid hormone, namely a decrease of the plasma calcium level. There has been some initial doubt whether calcitonin is produced by the parathyroid or the thyroid; present opinion is that it is a secretion of the thyroid gland produced by special cells known as parafollicular or C cells. Hence its alternative name, thyrocalcitonin.

Calcitonin is a polypeptide hormone of 32 amino acids. The potency of calcitonin is estimated by comparing its hypocalcaemic effect in rats with that of a standard preparation. The B.P. preparation is pork calcitonin; salmon calcitonin (*salcatonin*) differs in amino acid sequence from human calcitonin. Salcatonin is frequently used and is highly effective in man.

Calcitonin is released from the thyroid in response to hypercalcaemia. In this respect it is the opposite of parathyroid hormone (PTH) which is released in response to hypocalcaemia. Calcitonin lowers blood calcium by two separate mechanisms: (1) it decreases bone resorption; (2) it increases renal calcium excretion. Calcitonin increases renal phosphate excretion and in this respect its overall renal effect resembles that of PTH. Overall, calcitonin produces a fall in serum calcium and phosphate.

Clinical uses. Calcitonin and salcatonin are used in the treatment of idiopathic hypercalcaemia in infancy and in hypercalcaemia due to overdose of vitamin D. Their best established indication is in osteitis deformans (Paget's disease of bone) when injections of calcitonin or salcatonin may relieve bone pain and return calcium balance to normal. The biochemical abnormalities of Paget's disease, i.e. increased levels of serum alkaline phosphatase and of urinary hydroxyproline are also corrected.

PREPARATIONS

Anterior pituitary and placental hormones

Adrenal cortex
Corticotrophin (ACTH, Acthar) 20–80 u i.m., s.c. or by slow i.v. infus
Tetracosactrin (Synacthen) 250 µg i.m. i.v.

Growth
Human growth hormone (HGH, Somatotrophin)
Mammary gland
Prolactin (PRL)
Gonads
Human chorionic gonadotrophin (HCG, Pregnyl) 500–5000 u twice weekly i.m.
Human follicle stimulating hormone (FSH, Follitropin)
Human luteinising hormone (LSH, Lutotropin)
Menotropins (Pergonal) human menopausal gonadotrophin
Thyroid
Thyrotrophin (TSH, Thyroid stimulating hormone) 10 i.u.

Posterior pituitary hormones
Desmopressin (DDAVP) 10 –20 µg intranasal
Felypressin (Octapressin)
Oxytocin Ch. 15
Vasopressin (ADH, Antidiuretic hormone)

Thyroid hormones
Liothyronine Sodium (L-triiodothyronine) (Tertroxin) 5–100 µg dl
Thyroxine Sodium (Levothyroxine, Eltroxin) 50ß300 µg dl

Antithyroid agents
Carbimazole (Neomercazole) 30–60 mg dl
Methimazole (Tapazole) 15–60 mg dl
Propylthiouracil 300–400 mg dl, maint 100–300 mg dl
Iodine aqueous solution (iodine 5 g, potassium iodide 10 g aq ad 100 ml) (Lugols' sol 1% w/w iodine)
Potassium perchlorate 200–800 mg dl
Sodium iodide I^{131} 4–10 millicurie

Parathyroid and calcitonin
Calcitonin (Thyrocalcitonin) Pork 40–160 u dl, Salcatonin (Salmon calcitonin, Calcynar)
Parathyroid Injection 40–300 u dl

FURTHER READING

Berde B (ed) 1968 Neurohypophysial hormones and similar polypeptides. Handb. exp. Pharm. 23. Springer, Berlin
Evered D 1976 Disease of the thyroid. Pitman, London
Hall R, Anderson J, Smart G A, Besser M 1974 Fundamentals of clinical endocrinology. Pitman, London
Macintyre I 1969 Calcitonin. Heinemann, London
Parsons J A (ed) 1976 Peptide hormones. MacMillan Press, London
Pitt-Rivers R, Trotter W R (ed) 1964 The thyroid gland (2 vols) Butterworths, London
Williams R H (ed) 1974 Textbook of endocrinology. Saunders, Philadelphia

26. Insulin and corticosteroids

Insulin 337; Actions of insulin 337; Chemistry 339; Insulin receptors 339; Soluble and slow acting insulin 339; Insulin standardisation 340; Oral hypoglycaemic drugs 340; Insulin coma 342; Glucagon 342; The adrenal cortex 343; Aldosterone 345; Fludrocortisone and deoxycortone 345; Glucocorticoids 346; Actions of cortisol 346; Therapeutic uses of corticosteroids 347; Complications of glucocorticoid therapy 349; Metyrapone 349.

INSULIN

v. Mering and Minkowski demonstrated in 1889 that removal of the dog's pancreas produced a persistent glycosuria; pancreatic grafts abolished the glycosuria. Subsequent work led to the view that the pancreas was a gland of 'internal secretion' and that certain histologically identifiable cell groups in it, called islets of Langerhans, were probably responsible for the secretion.

Knowledge of the internal pancreatic secretion, called *insuline* by de Meyer, made little advance until Banting and Best, in 1921, produced extracts from the pancreas which decreased the level of sugar in the blood and urine of pancreatectomised animals and human diabetics. Crystalline insulin was produced by Abel in 1926 and the complete chemical structure of insulin was established by Sanger in 1955 (Fig. 26.1).

There is histochemical evidence that insulin is present in special cells within the islets of Langerhans, called ß cells. The ß cells can be selectively destroyed by specific cytotoxic agents such as alloxan or streptozotocin, a toxic antibiotic derived from a strain of *streptomyces*. Injection of these agents produces a form of 'chemical' diabetes which closely resembles diabetes due to surgical removal of the pancreas. Another type of cell contained in islet tissue is called α cell and has been shown to store the hyperglycaemic polypeptide glucagon (p. 342). A third type of islet cell has been identified which probably stores the polypeptide gastrin (p. 186).

Experimental diabetes mellitus
Surgical removal of the pancreas in the dog produces a grave condition which is fatal in one to two weeks. If the animal is kept on a mixed diet it excretes large amounts of glucose whilst its blood sugar is raised; it drinks and eats excessively and suffers from polyuria, hyperlipaemia, hypercholesterolaemia, ketonaemia and ketonuria. Administration of glucose leads to a prolonged elevation of blood sugar and any administered sugar is lost in the urine. Such animals rapidly lose weight in spite of a voracious appetite; they exhibit progressive acidosis and dehydration and finally die in coma. Their liver and muscle glycogen stores are greatly depleted, but the glycogen stores of heart muscle remain normal. All these symptoms are promptly relieved by the administration of insulin.

Human diabetes mellitus
Human diabetes mellitus is a disease of glucose metabolism which is usually due to an insufficient output of endogenous insulin, as a result of which the blood sugar is abnormally high and sugar appears in the urine. The commonest symptoms of the disease are polyuria, polydipsia, tiredness and loss of weight. The disturbance in carbohydrate metabolism is due to the fact that the liver and skeletal muscles cannot store glycogen and the tissues are unable to utilise glucose. When the kidney threshold for glucose is exceeded, glucosuria occurs with consequent increase of water excretion and disturbances of electrolyte and water balance. Protein metabolism in the liver is also deranged and an excessive amount of protein is transformed into carbohydrate. In addition, the amount of fat metabolised by the diabetic patient is excessive, and since normal fat catabolism can only proceed at a limited rate, ketone bodies are present in the blood and the urine in much larger amounts than normally. These substances are excreted in the urine as ß-hydroxybutyric acid and acetoacetic acid and as acetone in the breath. Accumulation of these acids in the blood produces acidosis; furthermore acetoacetic acid has a toxic effect which leads to coma and circulatory collapse.

Actions of insulin
The most obvious effect produced by insulin is a rapid fall in blood sugar as shown in Figure 26.2. This effect is produced by small doses in the diabetic whilst much larger doses are needed in the normal subject. The reduction of blood sugar is mainly due to the formation and storage of glycogen in the liver and in the skeletal muscles. Lack of insulin prevents, or at any rate greatly retards, the formation of glycogen in the liver and the muscles, and in consequence glucose accumulates in the blood.

The conversion of glucose into glycogen involves the formation of glucose-6-phosphate: this reaction, which occurs by the interaction of glucose and adenosine triphosphate (ATP), is catalysed by the enzyme hexokinase. Glucose-6-phosphate can be readily metabolised; it may be deposited as glycogen or oxidised to carbon dioxide and water; it may also be converted to fat.

Mechanism of action of insulin
The mechanism of action of insulin has been investigated since the early work of Banting and Best but in spite of a

variety of hypotheses it is still uncertain whether the effects of insulin can be reduced to a single basic mechanism. A number of effects of insulin on glucose, fat and protein metabolism have been described.

Glucose metabolism. There is evidence that in the absence of insulin, glucose transport across the cell membrane is reduced. This applies particularly to striated muscle cells, causing a lack of glycogen build-up in muscle. In addition, insulin stimulates the enzyme glycogen synthetase which promotes the conversion of glucose into glyogen in skeletal muscle and the liver.

Fat metabolism is profoundly deranged in diabetes. Insulin is involved in both fat synthesis and breakdown. Defective fat synthesis results in the accumulation of beta-hydroxybutyric acid and acetoacetic acid, the latter giving rise to acetone on decarboxylation. Insulin inhibits free fatty acid mobilisation, possibly due to inhibition of a specific lipase. In the absence of insulin the action of lipolysis-promoting hormones, including catecholamines, corticosteroids, growth hormone and thyroid, is unopposed and this tends to raise the free fatty acid level of the blood.

Protein metabolism. The observation that diabetes is accompanied by loss of body weight, depletion of tissue protein and a rise in the rate of nitrogen excretion has led to the idea that insulin plays a part in stimulating protein synthesis, in spite of the fact that insulin administration in normal animals has no significant effect on protein deposition. Experimental evidence that insulin affects protein synthesis has come from experiments on the isolated rat diaphragm. Manchester and Young have shown that in this preparation insulin stimulates the incorporation of radioactive amino acids into protein, perhaps by influencing the activity of ribosomes which are intimately concerned in the mechanism of protein biosynthesis.

Control of insulin secretion and blood sugar
The rate of secretion of insulin is mainly determined by the amount of glucose in the blood passing through the islets of Langerhans.

The standard oral glucose tolerance test indicates the response of the islet cells to raised blood glucose. After a 12-hour fast the subject receives 50 or 100 g glucose and the effect on blood glucose concentration is measured at half-hourly intervals.

When the blood sugar level is decreased sufficiently to cause hypoglycaemia, the central nervous system becomes excited and stimulates the adrenal glands to produce adrenaline which causes a liberation of glucose from the glycogen in the liver. This insulin-adrenaline balance is probably the mechanism whereby the blood sugar level is rapidly regulated. Other endocrine mechanisms involved in the control of blood sugar are the anterior pituitary growth hormone and corticosteroid secretion. Cortisol has a pronounced hyperglycaemic effect. The effect of glucagon secretion on the regulation of blood sugar is discussed on page 342.

Nervous effects on insulin secretion. Characteristic cholinergic and adrenergic nerve endings are found in close association with pancreatic islet cells and their selective activation can be shown to influence insulin secretion. It has been found in animal experiments that vagus stimulation causes insulin release which can be blocked by atropine. Beta adrenergic stimulation also causes insulin release which is blocked by propranolol. Alpha adrenergic stimulation inhibits insulin release and this effect is blocked by α-adrenoceptor blockers such as dihydroergotamine. It is not known whether these autonomic effects are important clinically in insulin secretion which appears to be basically controlled by the glucose level of blood.

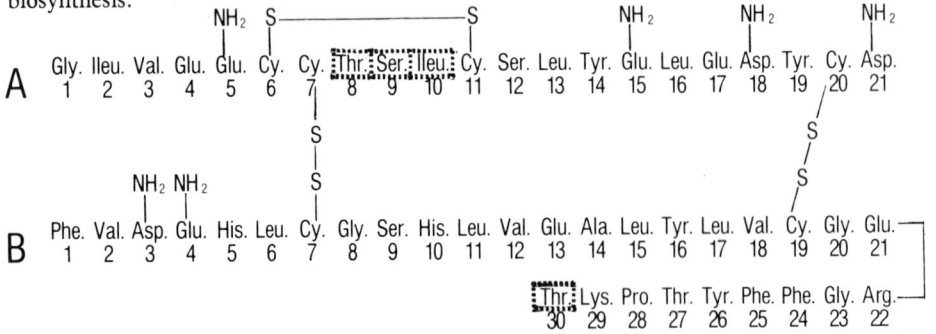

Fig. 26.1 Structure of human insulin. The structures of insulin from certain animal spaces differ only as follows:

| | Chain A || Chain B ||
	8	9	10	30
Man	Thr	Ser	Ileu	Thr
Pig	Thr	Ser	Ileu	Ala
Rabbit	Thr	Ser	Ileu	Ser
Beef	Ala	Ser	Val	Ala

Chemistry

Insulin is a protein the structure of which has been completely elucidated by Sanger and his colleagues in Cambridge. The three-dimensional structure of insulin has been elucidated by X-ray crystallography. The insulin molecule contains two unbranched peptide chains linked by two disulphide bridges. One chain (*A chain*) has four free amino groups and a disulphide bridge of its own; the other (*B chain*) has two free amino groups (Fig. 26.1). There are minor differences in the amino acid composition of insulins from different species such as the cow, whale, sheep, horse and man, but they all appear to be physiologically active in man. Differences are mainly apparent by immunological methods, e.g. by radioimmunoassays. The molecular weight of the insulin monomer is about 6000; the naturally found insulins are probably dimers or polymers of this unit.

It is now known that insulin *in vivo* is first sythesised as a single polypeptide chain, named *pro-insulin*. Pro-insulin folds allowing the regions of the molecule that subsequently become A and B chains to lie in close proximity and thus favour the formation of the S-S bridges linking the A and B chains. The active insulin is then formed by splitting off a connecting peptide (C-peptide) linking the A and B chain. Proinsulin has greatly reduced biological activity.

Administration and preparations of insulin

Insulin cannot be given by mouth since it is destroyed by the gastric secretion; it must be administered parenterally. Insulin rapidly leaves the blood stream and becomes bound by tissues. An enzyme, insulinase, which inactivates insulin has been found in liver, muscle and kidney.

Insulin receptors

The first step of insulin action is believed to be an interaction between hormone and specific receptors situated on the cell membrane. Insulin receptors have been inferred by (1) measuring the binding and dissociation rates of radioactive insulin; (2) inhibition of binding by unlabelled insulin; (3) electron microscopy of freeze-etched preparations making visible the attachment to receptors of insulin labelled with a large prosthetic group. It has been found that when fat cells are treated with labelled insulin the quantity of insulin required to give half-maximal inhibition of binding is approximately 100-fold in excess of that required to give a half-maximal biological effect suggesting the presence of a large proportion of 'spare' receptors.

Soluble insulin

Injection of insulin B.P. is a clear solution of crystalline insulin which has a pH of 2.5 to 3.5 and is standardised to contain 20, 40 or 80 units per ml. This preparation, which is referred to as Soluble Insulin is usually injected subcutaneously but can also be given intravenously. When administered subcutaneously it produces its full effect in two to three hours and the action lasts for five to eight hours. Injected intravenously, insulin has a quicker, stronger but short-lived action, which reaches a maximum in half to one hour and ceases in three to four hours. An important use of soluble insulin is in the treatment of emergencies such as diabetic ketosis and of conditions in which the insulin requirements of the patient change rapidly as in acute infections or after operations. Its main disadvantage for routine maintenance therapy is its short duration of action which makes it necessary to give two or three injections per day.

Continuous intravenous infusion in depancreatised animals indicates that the probable human production of insulin is not more than 20 units a day. On the other hand, a severe diabetic may need 100 units daily of soluble insulin. This difference can be explained by the fact that intermittent subcutaneous injections form a very inefficient substitute for the natural method of regulated continuous intravenous infusion carried out by the islet tissue. It is obviously desirable to use a preparation of insulin which will avoid wide fluctuations in the level of blood sugar.

Slow-acting insulins

Various slow-acting preparations have been introduced to enable insulin to be administered less frequently. Differences in the time course of action on the blood sugar

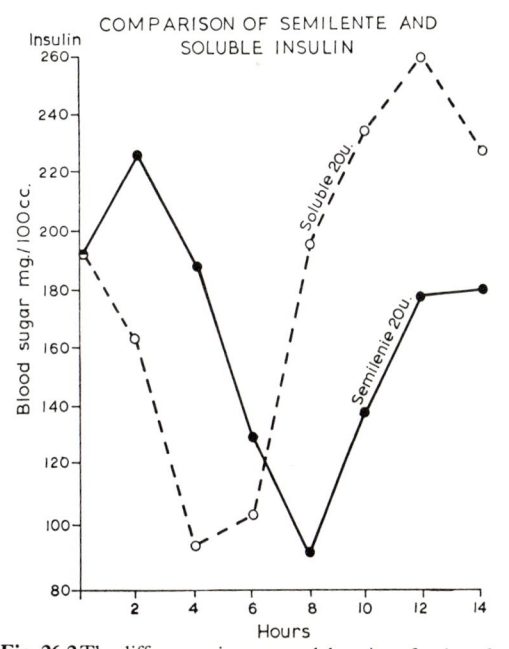

Fig. 26.2 The differences in onset and duration of action of soluble insulin and amorphous insulin zinc suspension (semilente) studied under identical circumstances. (After Duncan, 1959, in *Diseases of Metabolism*, W. B. Saunders Co., Philadelphia.)

between a preparation of soluble insulin and a more slowly acting preparation of an amorphous insulin zinc suspension (semilente) are shown in Figure 26.2. It was discovered early that insulin formed a precipitate with protamines prolonging its action and that zinc further prolonged the action of protamine insulin. The duration of action of an insulin injection can also be controlled by combining crystalline and amorphous insulin in the same syringe. *Novo* insulins are available in a variety of forms corresponding to different durations of action:

Actrapid. Short acting neutral insulin solution; twice or more daily; pig insulin.

Semitard. Amorphous insulin zinc suspension; twice daily; pig.

Rapitard. Insulin crystals (ox) and solution (pig); once or twice daily.

Monotard. Insulin zinc suspension; usually once; pig.

Lentard (lente). Insulin zinc suspension; usually once; pig and ox.

Ultratard (ultralente). Insulin zinc suspension; once daily; ox.

Immunological responses to insulin

Since all preparations of commercial insulin are foreign proteins to man, they may produce immunological reactions. This is true even of the most highly purified insulins. For example beef insulin differs from human insulin in respect of at least three amino acids whilst pork insulin, which is closest to human insulin, nevertheless differs from it in respect of the C-terminal amino acid in the B-chain.

Although the introduction of porcine insulin has been an advance over earlier ox preparations, even porcine insulin has resulted in the formation of insulin binding antibodies, and it is now believed that antibody formation is generally stimulated not by the insulin molecule itself but by impurities. If commercial crystalline insulin is subjected to gel filtration, impurities can be separated into three fractions. A large molecular fractions (a) is found only in very impure preparations. Fraction (b) consists essentially of proinsulin and is the most important antigenic component. Fraction (c) is virtually non-antigenic.

Purified proinsulin-free preparations (monocomponent (MC) insulins) have been introduced by Scandinavian firms. Antigenicity affects particularly the long-acting insulins and can be largely avoided by using highly purified preparations. The main manifestations of antigenicity are as follows:

1. Insulin allergy. Itchy lumps may develop during the first few weeks of insulin treatment, occurring several hours after injection.

2. Lipoatrophy. Some degree of fat atrophy at injection sites frequently occurs and is probably due to an immunological reaction.

3. Insulin resistance. This rare phenomenon may sometimes be due an immunological reaction. The patient should change to a highly purified preparation.

Insulin standardisation

The factor of safety in insulin therapy is relatively small, for the amount of insulin which produces hypoglycaemia is fairly close to the amount needed to produce the desired therapeutic effect. The clinical use of insulin would indeed be beset with great difficulties were it not possible to standardise the drug biologically with considerable accuracy. The general principle of standardisation is to determine the amount which will produce hypoglycaemia in rabbits or convulsions in mice, and to compare it with the dose of a standard preparation of insulin necessary to give the same effects. The details of these methods have been worked out very carefully, and the accuracy obtainable is remarkable. When international tests were carried out in different laboratories on a single preparation, the results agreed within 10 per cent. The international standard preparation is a quantity of pure dry crystalline insulin hydrochloride, 1 mg of which contains 24 units of activity.

Determination of insulin levels in blood. Sensitive biological and immunological methods have been developed which are capable of measuring the concentration of circulating insulin in serum. The biological methods mainly used are based on: (1) the effect of insulin in stimulating $^{14}CO_2$ production from ^{14}C labelled glucose by the epididymal fat pad of the rat, and (2) insulin stimulation of glucose uptake by the isolated rat diaphragm.

A sensitive radioimmunoassay of insulin has been developed and is increasingly used, but it is difficult to separate insulin from pro-insulin.

Oral hypoglycaemic drugs

In 1942 Janbon and his colleagues in Montpellier discovered that a substituted sulphonamide which they used for the treatment of typhoid fever, produced severe hypoglycaemia in undernourished patients. This observation was followed up by Loubatières who showed that when the drug was administered intravenously or by mouth to normal dogs, it produced a hypoglycaemia which was related to the concentration of the sulphonamide in the blood.

Since 1953 a number of sulphonylurea derivatives have been introduced as oral hypogylcaemia drugs of which *tolbutamide* (Rastinon) and *chlorpropamide* (Diabinese) are used in the treatment of diabetes mellitus. Other orally effective hypoglycaemic drugs are the diguanides, *phenformin* (Dibotin) and *metformin* (Glucophage) which differ from the former group chemically and in their mode of action (Fig. 26.3).

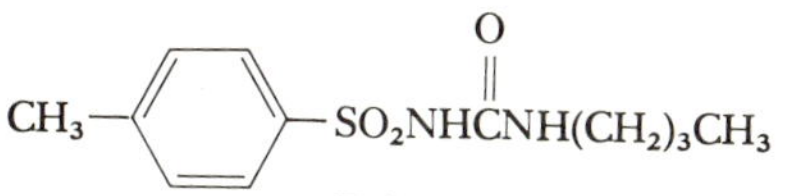

INSULIN AND CORTICOSTEROIDS 341

Tolbutamide

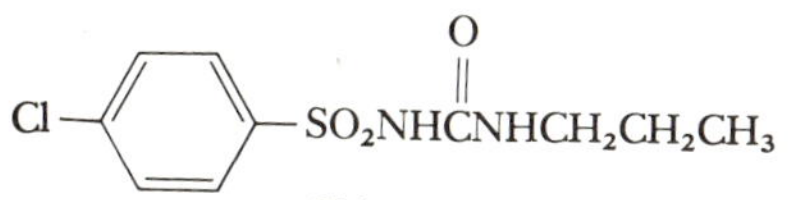

Chlorpropamide

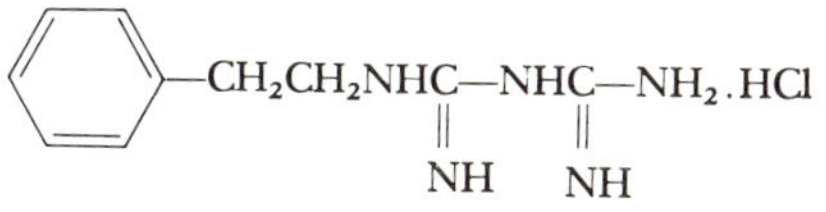

Phenformin

Fig. 26.3 Structure of oral hypoglycaemic drugs.

Mode of action
When sulphonylureas are administered to animals from which the pancreas has been completely removed, no fall in blood sugar is observed. If however, a small remnant of pancreatic tissue is present, there is a fall of blood sugar. Loubatières concluded that these drugs probably stimulate the ß-cells of the pancreas to secrete more insulin, and depress the secretion of the hyperglycaemic hormone glucagon by the α-cells. The diguanide derivatives lower the blood sugar in experimental animals in the absence of pancreatic islet cells; their action is probably directly on the tissues since they increase the glucose uptake of the isolated diaphragm.

Therapeutic uses
Clinical usage of these drugs has shown that they lower the blood sugar of patients with diabetes mellitus. They are particularly indicated in elderly mild diabetics in whom dietary measures have failed to control the blood sugar and they should be given in addition to a strict diet. The development of ketosis is an indication for insulin treatment. In general, young diabetics and those requiring large doses of insulin show little or no response to the oral drugs and when administration of insulin is a vital necessity, any attempt to replace this by administration of sulphonylureas is likely to result in a serious relapse.

Tolbutamide which has an effective half-life of about four hours is given in initial daily doses of 0.5 to 1.0 g and its effects can usually be maintained in doses of 0.25 g two or three times daily. *Chlorpropamide* has a longer duration of action (24-36 hours). Treatment with *phenformin* is usually begun with much lower doses of 12.5 mg daily gradually increased.

Glibenclamide is a more recently introduced oral hypoglycaemic drug belonging to the sulphonylurea group. It is a very potent hypoglycaemic agent in that 5 mg glibenclamide has about the same effect as 250 mg chlorpropamide. It appears to be well tolerated.

Toxic effects
The sulphonylureas carry some of the risks associated with sulphonamides. Severe reactions have occasionally been reported including blood dyscrasias but these are rare and in general these drugs are safe and remarkably free from side effects. Biguanides achieve their hypogylcaemic action by causing widespread metabolic abnormalities and are more liable to produce severe side effects. They produce rises in blood lactate and pyruvate; several cases of lactic acidosis, some fatal, have been reported after phenformin. Other adverse reactions of biguanides are referable to the gastrointestinal tract. All oral hypoglycaemic drugs may cause severe hypogylcaemia. A curious side effect, seen particularly with chlorpropamide, is flushing after taking alcohol.

Place of oral hypoglycaemic drugs
Although oral hypoglycaemic drugs have been in use for 25 years, their place in the treatment of diabetes is not definitely established. Many specialists regard them as highly satisfactory drugs with an excellent record of safety, particularly the sulphonylureas. They are not indicated in the young or in severe diabetes or ketosis, but they are effective in maturity-onset diabetes when patients cannot be controlled by diet alone. The oral hypoglycaemics can be safely withdrawn after some months, continuing treatment by diet alone, in contrast to insulin which can seldom be withdrawn without causing acute deterioration.

A recent large-scale trial in USA indicated that tolbutamide treatment might be responsible for an excess of cardiovascular deaths. This trial has been criticised on statistical ground, but it has initiated a more cautious approach to oral hypoglycaemics. It is considered that treatment with these drugs should not be unduly prolonged, and strenuous attempts at proper dieting should always be made.

Dietary therapy
In the treatment of diabetes mellitus dietary therapy plays a key role differing in insulin-requiring and in maturity-onset diabetes. Maturity-onset diabetics, particularly those with obesity, can frequently be controlled by diet alone provided that carbohydrate restriction is strictly adhered to. Many standard diabetic diets are available; some of the weight-reducing diets are relatively easy to follow. Obese diabetics may lose one to two pounds weight in a week on a strict diet. In maturity-onset diabetics who are not overweight, the aim of antidiabetic dieting should be to keep the patient's weight at slightly below normal levels. Failure of dietary treatment, requiring additional treatment, usually with oral hypoglycaemic drugs, is defined as persistence of glycosuria with postprandial blood glucose levels of more than 150 mg per 100 ml.

In insulin-requiring diabetics the diet should be based on the energy requirements of the patient. A frequent method, when insulin is used, is to restrict only carbohydrate in the diet allowing freedom of choice as regards proteins and fat. Young insulin-dependent diabetics generally require between 120 and 300 g of carbohydrate daily. Once the total daily carbohydrate allowance is decided this may be apportioned to various meals as convenient, with most carbohydrate given during meals following an insulin injection. The diet must contain an adequate amount of protein. The fat allowance depends on the carbohydrate and protein components.

Coma in diabetic patients

A diabetic patient under routine treatment with insulin is subject to two opposite dangers, namely, coma due to ketosis and hypoglycaemic coma. It is essential to determine immediately which form is present and the history of the mode of onset of coma may be of considerable help in this respect.

Coma due to ketosis. This is due to derangement of metabolism from such causes as omission of the usual insulin, infection or febrile illness. The most obvious signs are dehydration shown by the dry shrunken tongue and the smell of ketone bodies in the breath. Analysis of the urine will indicate the presence of ketone bodies and of sugar, thus proving that the coma is due to ketosis. Large amounts of fixed base are lost by vomiting and by excretion with the ketone bodies, and the alkali reserve is usually reduced by 50 per cent or more. The treatment of ketosis consists in replacing the electrolytes and fluids as quickly as possible and administering insulin at frequent intervals according to the effect produced on the blood sugar level. Large amounts of insulin may be necessary since dehydration, infection, and acidosis increase the resistance to insulin. An initial dose of 80 units of soluble insulin intramuscularly and 20 units intravenously may be injected, thereafter further doses of 40 to 80 units are injected intramuscularly at intervals of about an hour.

The loss of extracellular fluid leads to circulatory collapse and must be corrected by the intravenous infusion of a solution containing either 0.9 per cent sodium chloride or 1.85 per cent sodium lactate or a combination of one volume of sodium lactate injection and two volumes of sodium chloride injection. Opinions vary as to whether glucose should be administered in the early stages, since the blood sugar level is already abnormally high. The present tendency is to reserve glucose for the later stages of treatment.

There is a severe disturbance of potassium metabolism in ketosis: large amounts are lost from the cells, the potassium content of the extracellular fluid is temporarily raised and potassium is rapidly lost in the urine. It is necessary to make good this loss, but intravenous administration of potassium may produce toxic effects on the heart. For this reason potassium chloride is usually given by mouth when the patient recovers consciousness.

Coma due to hypoglycaemia. This results from excess of insulin. It may be caused by a patient taking a full dose of insulin and then omitting to take the usual subsequent meal, or by a mistake in the dose of insulin. Vigorous physical activity also diminishes the insulin requirements of the patient.

Hypoglycaemia may occur at night due to the action of a slow-acting insulin. The subjective symptoms are less obvious to the patient and the usual warning may be missed.

The initial symptoms of hypoglycaemia are hot flushes, faintness, sweating, tremulousness and a vague feeling of apprehension. Sometimes the subject becomes violently excited and aphasia, delirium, collapse and coma may ensue. Some of these symptoms are due to overproduction of adrenaline caused by the low blood sugar.

Fortunately, these symptoms can be relieved quickly by the oral administration or intravenous injection of glucose. A subcutaneous injection of adrenaline or glucagon will cause glycogenolysis and an immediate rise in blood sugar.

GLUCAGON

Injections of impure pancreatic insulin sometimes produce a transient rise of blood glucose before the expected drop. This led to the identification of a hyperglycaemic factor in pancreatic extracts by Kimball and Murlin, which they named 'glucagon'. Glucagon has now been synthesised and shown to be a polypeptide with 29 amino acid residues. Pancreatic glucagon is found in the α cells of the islets of Langerhans. In addition to pancreatic glucagon, other hyperglycaemic polypeptides which are chemically distinguishable from pancreatic glucagon have been detected in the duodenum and jejunum and are collectively referred to as gastrointestinal glucagon or enteroglucagon.

Glucagon concentrations in blood can be detected by radioimmunoassay, although difficulties have arisen due to inhomogeneity of different glucagons.

Actions

The principal action of glucagon is to raise blood glucose. The hyperglycaemia is accompanied by a rapid transient fall of the glycogen content of the liver. Glucagon has also been shown to increase the rate of new sugar formation from protein whilst decreasing the activity of glycogen synthetase, in contrast to insulin which augments it. Thus the total effect of glucagon is to increase the hepatic output of glucose.

An interesting effect of glucagon is a powerful stimulation of cardiac contractility.

Glucagon is rapidly destroyed in the body.

Mode of action. There is good evidence that glucagon produces its effects through cyclic AMP. In the liver it stimulates adenylcyclase; this in turn increases the amount of active phosphorylase which catalyses the breakdown of glycogen to glucose. These effects are potentiated by cortisol.

Physiological function. The occurrence of glucagon in the pancreas was at first considered to be a curiosity with no functional significance, but this attitude has changed since it was discovered that glucagon normally circulates in the blood. Its main function is probably to counteract hypoglycaemia; low blood sugar has been shown to stimulate glucagon secretion.

Clinical uses

The main clinical use of glucagon is for the treatment of insulin hypoglycaemia in cases where the intravenous administration of glucose is impracticable. Glucagon must be given early in the attack, since it becomes ineffective once liver glycogen is exhausted. If administered parenterally to patients in hypoglycaemic coma, it acts in 5–20 minutes. Oral dextrose should also be administered to prevent a relapse.

The cardiotonic effect of glucagon can be made use of in cardiac surgery and during intensive care treatment. Glucagon must be administered intravenously in such cases owing to its transient action.

Adverse reactions to glucagon include nausea and vomiting.

THE ADRENAL GLANDS

Adrenaline (epinephrine) was isolated in 1901 in crystalline form from the adrenal medulla by von Fürth who named it suprarenin and by Takamine who named it adrenalin. Within a few years its structure was determined and its synthesis accomplished. This was the first example of the full chemical identification of an endocrine secretion. The activity of the adrenal medulla is not essential for survival and the secretion of adrenaline appears to be a mechanism for facilitating the rapid preparation of the body for violent exertion. The actions of adrenaline are discussed in Chapter 6.

The adrenal cortex

In 1855 Addison showed that destruction of the adrenal glands produced a syndrome, which is now known as Addison's disease. This is characterised by great muscular weakness, bronzing of the skin, arterial hypotension and gastrointestinal disturbance which may be manifested by vomiting or diarrhoea.

Subsequent experiments on animals showed that removal of the adrenal cortex rapidly produces muscular weakness, dehydration and a fall in blood pressure. The animals usually die 6–48 hours after the operation. Characteristic changes occur in the salt content of the blood after adrenalectomy. There is a decrease in plasma chloride, bicarbonate and particularly in plasma sodium; associated with this is an increase in plasma potassium. The glycogen stores in the liver and muscles are decreased and the blood sugar level may also be reduced. The normal tone of the blood vessels is also dependent on the activity of the adrenal cortex for when this is removed experimentally or destroyed by disease, as in Addison's disease, a progressive fall in blood pressure occurs.

Animal experiments and clinical observations on Addison's disease indicate that reduction of potassium intake coupled with a high sodium chloride intake produces striking benefit. Many attempts have been made to isolate an active principle from the adrenal cortex and in 1931 Swingle and Pfiffner prepared an extract of the adrenal cortex. They showed that this extract was able to restore to almost normal health, animals which were dying after adrenalectomy.

Over 40 steroid hormones have been isolated from extracts of the adrenal cortex but only about 7 have appreciable activity in increasing the survival time of adrenalectomised animals and in influencing mineral, carbohydrate and protein metabolism. No one compound can reproduce all the physiological effects of the gland.

There are two main types of activity in adrenal cortex extracts. One is concerned with inorganic metabolism and the maintenance of renal function; the other with glycogen and protein metabolism. The chief compounds with the first type of activity are desoxycorticosterone and the highly active, naturally occurring, compound aldosterone. The most important compounds in the second group are hydrocortisone, cortisone and corticosterone. It is convenient to classify the adrenal cortical steroids into mineralocorticoids and glucocorticoids, but it is now appreciated that the hormones have an action in varying degree on both mineral and carbohydrate metabolism.

Synthetic corticosteroids

In addition to these naturally occurring compounds several new steroids with glucocorticoid activity have been synthesised (Fig. 26.4). By the introduction of a double bond between carbon atoms 1 and 2 of cortisone and hydrocortisone, prednisone and prednisolone respectively are produced, which are about five times more active as glucocorticoids without a corresponding increase in mineralocorticoid activity. When a fluorine atom is substituted in the 9α position of prednisolone together with modifications in the 16α position by the addition of a hydroxyl group (triamcinolone) or a methyl group (dexamethasone), compounds with strong glucocorticoid and little or no mineralocorticoid activity are produced. The compound fluocinolone acetonide (synalar) contains a second fluorine atom and is very effective if applied topically in eczema, contact dermatitis and some other skin conditions.

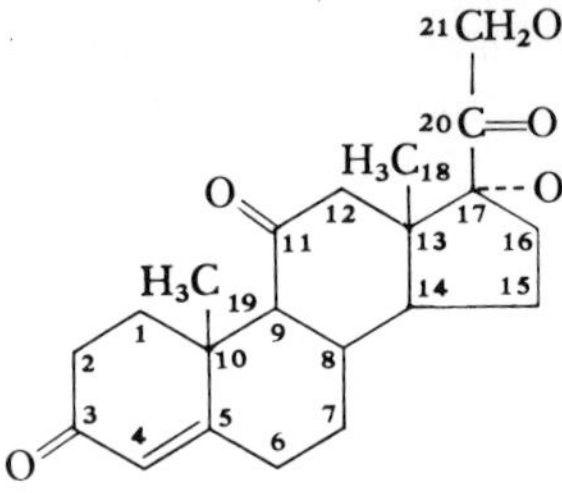

Cortisone

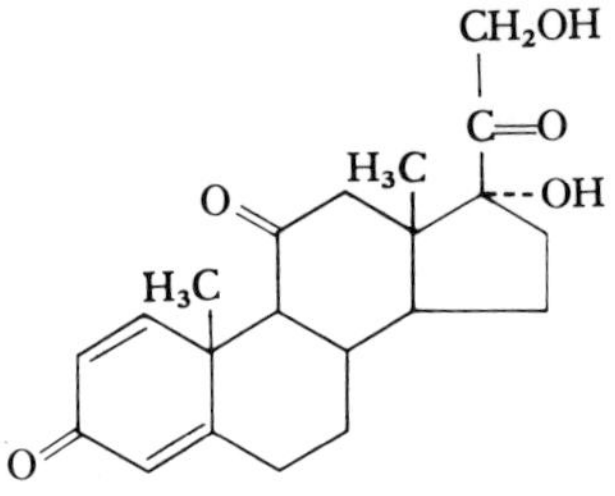

Prednisone

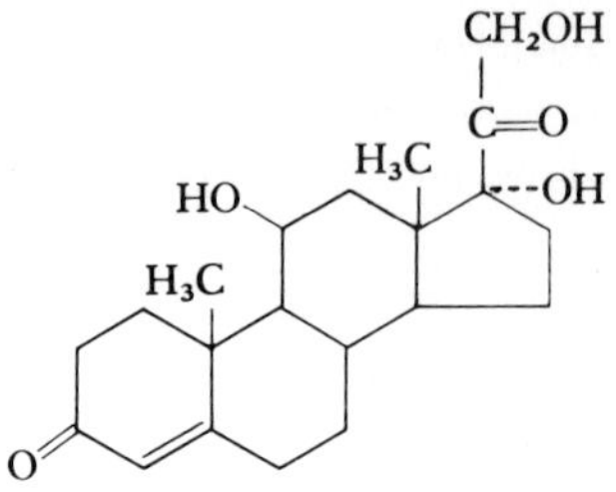

Hydrocortisone (Cortisol)

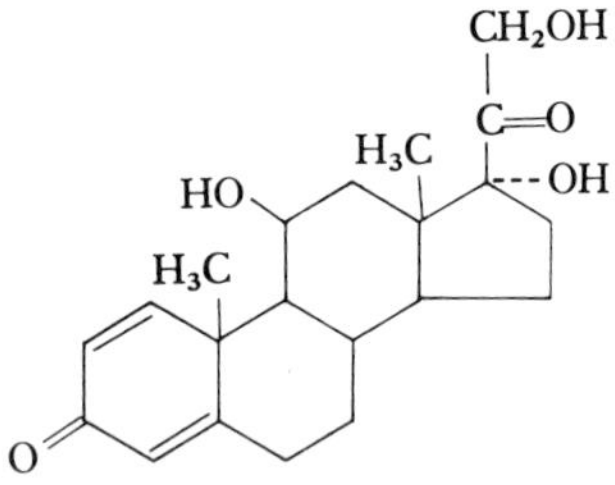

Prednisolone

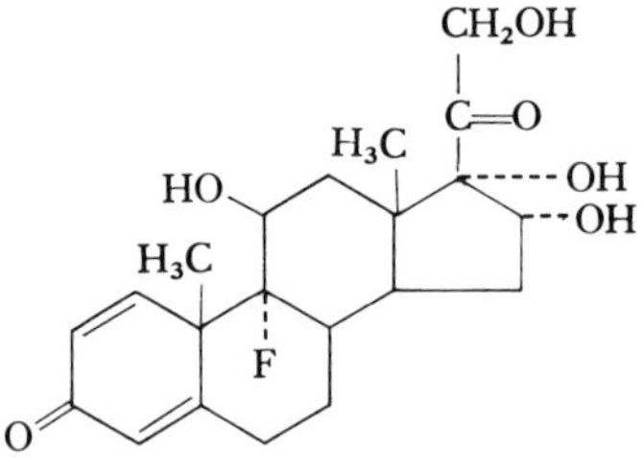

Triamcinolone

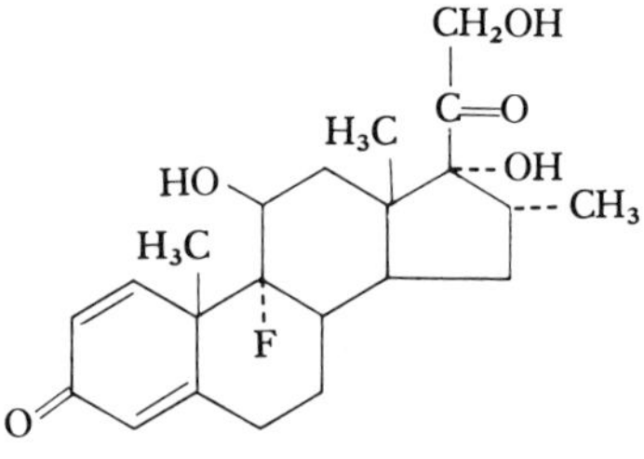

Dexamethasone

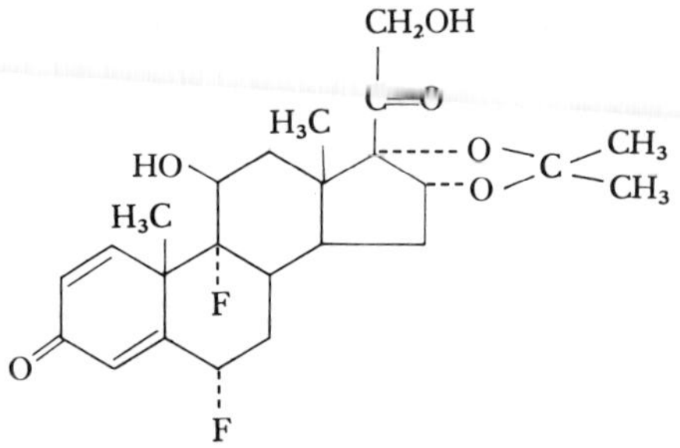

Fluocinolone Acetonide
(Synalar)

Fig. 26.4 Structure of natural and synthetic glucocorticoids.

The relative activities of some of these compounds when tested experimentally are shown in Table 26.1.

Control of secretion of corticosteroids

There is evidence that aldosterone is produced in the outer part of the adrenal cortex, the zona glomerulosa, whilst hydrocortisone and corticosterone are produced in the inner zona fasciculata-reticularis. The two zones respond differently to hypophysectomy; the glomerulosa is not markedly changed whereas the fasciculata-reticularis rapidly atrophies. This is due to the fact that the cells concerned with secretion of glucocorticoids are under the influence of the pituitary adrenocorticotrophic hormone ACTH. The factors which control the regulation of cortisol levels by ACTH are discussed on page 327. The secretion of aldosterone on the other hand appears to be regulated independently. It is controlled partly by the electrolyte composition of the blood and it has been shown that the octapeptide angiotensin II (p. 127) stimulates aldosterone secretion from the adrenal cortex. There is evidence that the production of angiotensin through the action of the enzyme renin released from the kidney may constitute a physiological mechanism by which aldosterone secretion is regulated. Renin is produced by cells of the juxtaglomerular apparatus of the kidney in the wall of the afferent arteriole and is released into the circulation where it acts enzymatically on angiotensinogen to form the decapeptide angiotensin I (p. 127). This is converted to the octapeptide angiotensin II by converting enzyme.

Aldosterone, hydrocortisone and corticosterone have been isolated not only from adrenal gland extracts but also from human adrenal venous blood.

Table 26.1 Relative potencies of glucocorticoids (after Nabarro, 1961, *Prescr. J.*)

Glucocorticoids	Relative potency by weight	Salt retaining action
Cortisone	1	Marked
Hydrocortisone	1.2	Marked
Prednisone	5	Slight
Prednisolone	5	Slight
Methyl prednisolone	6	None
Triamcinolone	6	None
Dexamethasone	35	Very slight
Betamethasone	35	Very slight

Mineralocorticoids

The mineralocorticoids, particularly aldosterone, are the most potent adrenal steroids in maintaining life after adrenalectomy. When given in small doses to adrenalectomised animals they apparently maintain health, growth and reproductive capacity. The primary action of the mineralocorticoids, with which their life-maintaining effect can be most closely associated, is that of preventing the excessive excretion of sodium and retention of potassium by the kidneys after adrenalectomy. Adrenalectomised animals maintained in this way, however, are unable to respond adequately to stressful situations and require the additional administration of glucocorticoids.

The structural formulae of some compounds with mineralocorticoid activity are shown in Figure 26.5.

Aldosterone

This compound is the main mineralocorticoid secreted by the adrenal glands. It was isolated from extracts of adrenal glands by Simpson and Tait in 1954. In experimental animals administration of aldosterone produces a retention of sodium, a progressive depletion of potassium and an increase in arterial blood pressure. Primary aldosteronism in man may arise from adrenal cortical adenoma, or hyperplasia of the adrenal glands. It is characterised by arterial hypertension, polyuria, and muscular weakness due to a progressive deficiency of potassium.

Excessive secretion of aldosterone probably contributes to the oedema of patients with hepatic cirrhosis and the nephrotic syndrome and this is the basis for the therapeutic use of antagonists of aldosterone such as spironolactone (p. 163).

The regulation of aldosterone secretion appears to be largely mediated through the renin-angiotensin system. The primary stimulus is probably a decrease in intrarenal arteriolar pressure which causes a release of renin by the kidney. The resulting angiotensin then stimulates the adrenal cortex to secrete aldosterone. Other factors may be involved in regulating aldosterone secretion including plasma sodium and potassium concentrations and probably also ACTH although its role is not as clear as in the regulation of cortisol secretion.

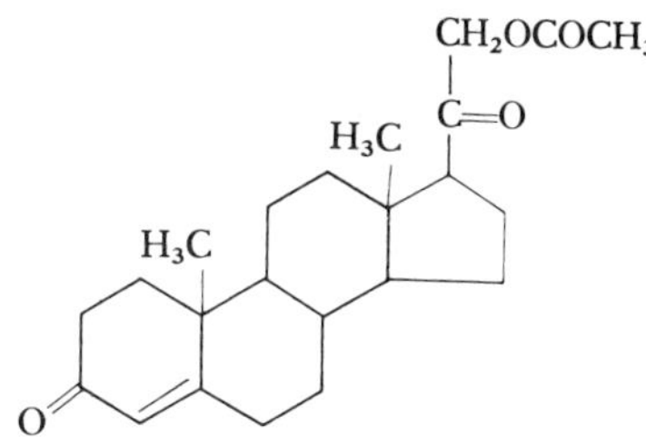

Deoxycortone acetate
(Desoxycorticosterone acetate)

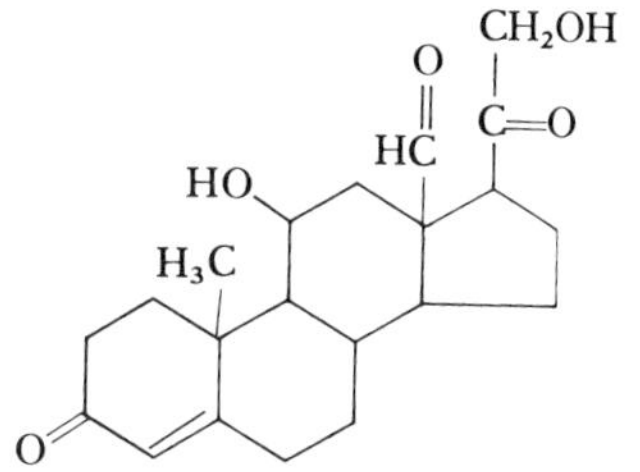

Aldosterone

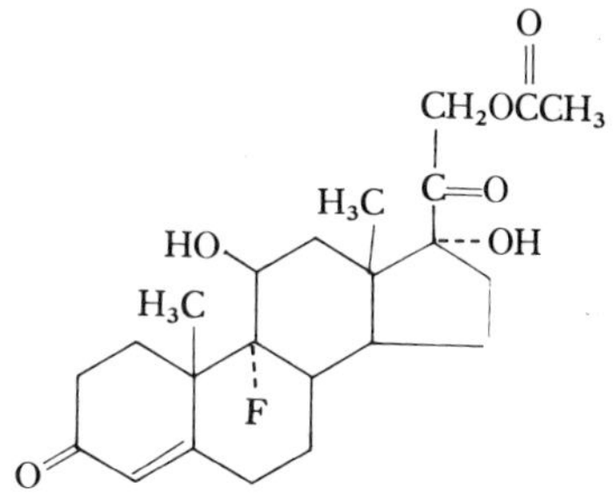

Fludrocortisone Acetate

Fig. 26.5 Compounds with mineralocorticoid activity.

Fludrocortisone

This compound has strong mineralocorticoid and glucocorticoid activity and is effective when given by mouth. It is about 10 times more active than DCA in producing retention of sodium and is used in the treatment of Addison's disease. Its methyl derivative, 2 methly-9α fluorohydrocortisone, has been synthesised and is even more active than aldosterone.

Deoxycortone acetate (DOCA, DCA) is available as an oily solution containing 5 mg in 1 ml. The main action of deoxycortone acetate is on electrolyte and water metabolism; it causes marked retention of sodium and of water and an increase in potassium excretion. It has been used for the maintenance treatment of patients with Addison's disease in the chronic phase of adrenal insufficiency and the dose may vary from 5 to 10 mg per day to 5 mg per week, depending on the severity of the case. When pellets of 50 to 300 mg of DCA are implanted into the subcutaneous tissue of such patients the duration of effect varies from three to six months.

A disadvantage of deoxycortone acetate is that it has very little effect on carbohydrate metabolism and on the maintenance of muscle efficiency. Much better results have been obtained when in addition a compound with glucocortical activity is given daily by mouth.

Glucocorticoids

The term glucocorticoid is applied to a group of adrenal cortical steroids which originally were considered to be concerned with influencing the blood sugar level, glycogen storage and carbohydrate turnover. Their activity was measured in terms of liver glycogen deposition in the adrenalectomised animal. By contrast the activity of mineralocorticoids was measured in terms of sodium retention in the adrenalectomised animal. It was found that the activity of compounds in promoting liver glycogen deposition was correlated with their activity in maintaining the capacity of skeletal muscle to perform work and also with their capacity to cause involution of lymphoid tissue and their anti-inflammatory effects. The separation of a glucocorticoid class of steroids therefore seemed well founded. It is nevertheless now recognised that the separation of the two classes of steroids is arbitrary and that all possess to a greater or lesser extent both types of action.

The prototype of glucocorticoids is cortisone which was isolated from the adrenal cortex in 1936 and independently identified by workers in America and Switzerland. Shortly afterwards the closely related compound hydrocortisone (cortisol) was also isolated. It is believed that these two compounds are interconvertible in the body since both are present in the urine but only hydrocortisone has been detected in adrenal venous blood.

Cortisol binding and measurement

Most of the cortisol in the blood stream is bound to protein especially to the alpha-globulin transcortin which has a high affinity for cortisol. Albumin which is present in much greater amounts in blood has a lower affinity for cortisol. Normally, more than 95 per cent of cortisol present in the circulation is bound to protein. Only the free cortisol fraction which is in equilibrium with the bound fraction exerts physiological effects and can be filtered by the glomerulus.

Because of the high degree of protein-binding, injected cortisol is eliminated relatively slowly with a halftime of about 100 minutes. If the blood level of cortisol is raised the cortisol binding capacity of transcortin may be exceeded and the free fraction may then reach 25 per cent of the total. Cortisol is broken down in the liver where it is conjugated with glucuronic acid in a form suitable for renal excretion.

The urinary excretion of 17-hydroxycorticoids is often used as an index of adrenal function. A more revealing assay is the measurement of the corticosteroid concentration in plasma which enables dynamic test procedures with frequent samplings to be carried out.

Actions of cortisol (hydrocortisone)

This compound has widespread effects in the organism that can be summarised as follows:

1. Effects on carbohydrate metabolism. It raises the blood sugar level and may cause glycosuria.

2. Effects on protein metabolism. Hydrocortisone inhibits protein synthesis but not protein breakdown so that a negative nitrogen balance results. The excretion of aminoacids and uric acid in urine is increased.

3. Fat metabolism is affected in a complex way. Prolonged administration of hydrocortisone in man causes a redistribution of fat; fat is deposited in the face and neck and is lost from the limbs.

4. Hydrocortisone affects salt and water exchanges in a different way from aldosterone. Whilst the latter acts mainly on sodium reabsorption by the kidney and the tubular clearance of potassium, hydrocortisone has an action on water diuresis which is not fully understood. It is known, however, that the inability of adrenalectomised animals to respond by diuresis to a water load can be corrected by hydrocortisone but not by aldosterone. Both types of action are required for the maintenance of normal kidney function in patients with Addison's disease. Hydrocortisone increases calcium excretion.

5. Hydrocortisone has marked effects on tissues derived from the embryonic mesenchyma including connective tissue, lymphoid tissue and bone marrow. It causes involution of lymphoid tissues and the thymus. When corticotrophin (ACTH) is injected in man a marked fall in the lymphocyte and eosinophil count occurs due to the action of the released hydrocortisone.

Hydrocortisone has an anti-inflammatory and antiallergic effect which is unspecific. Every type of inflammatory response is inhibited, whether due to a bacterial toxin, to a primarily toxic chemical agent or an immunological response. The sequence of the allergic reaction including histamine release may be inhibited; the growth and histamine forming activity of mast cells is markedly inhibited.

From the clinical point of view the action of hydrocortisone is symptomatic since the cause of the inflammatory or allergic disturbance is not affected; nevertheless the drug is often of the greatest therapeutic value when applied in the critical stages of inflammatory, allergic or 'collagen' diseases.

6. Hydrocortisone produces definite psychological effects. It corrects the depressive mood of patients with Addison's disease and when administered to others it may produce restlessness accompanied by euphoria. Sometimes a psychotic reaction is precipitated.

7. Hydrocortisone inhibits the release of endogenous ACTH.

Hydrocortisone has appreciable 'mineralocorticoid' activity manifested by sodium retention. Some of the newer synthetic glucocorticoids which are more active as anti-inflammatory agents produce no appreciable sodium retention; they are therefore clinically more useful where a glucocorticoid action is desired. On the other hand their effects on carbohydrate and protein metabolism parallel their anti-inflammatory effects.

Administration of corticosteroids

The systemic effects of corticosteroids can be produced by oral, intramuscular or intravenous administration of suitable preparations of these hormones.

Corticosteroids with the exception of deoxycortone are absorbed from the gastrointestinal tract. For oral administration cortisone acetate, hydrocortisone, prednisone and prednisolone, betamethasone and dexamethasone or their acetates are readily absorbed. For many purposes prednisone or prednisone acetate are satisfactory. Prednisone and prednisolene are interconvertible in the body.

Cortisone acetate suspension when injected intramuscularly is only slowly absorbed and this route of administration is used when a slow prolonged effect is required. When a rapid action is needed in the treatment of life-threatening conditions such as acute leukaemia, status asthmaticus or pemphigus, hydrocortisone sodium succinate or prednisolone 21-phosphate can be injected intravenously in aqueous solution.

Hydrocortisone acetate is much less soluble than hydrocortisone in body fluids and for this reason has a particularly long-lasting action when applied locally to mucous membranes. It may be applied in solution or in an ointment in 1 per cent concentration to the skin or mucous membranes or injected into joints. Fluocinolone acetonide (synalar) is applied as cream or ointment to the skin in 0.025 per cent concentration. Beclomethasone is used as an aerosol. Triamcinolone acetonide may be used topically as a cream (aristocort) or injected into joints. Corticosteroids are frequently combined with an antibiotic for topical use which should be non-sensitising.

Therapeutic uses

The therapeutic uses of corticosteroids can be divided into two groups. (1) Replacement therapy for patients with adrenocortical insufficiency owing to disease of the adrenal glands or of the pituitary. (2) Supplementary therapy for patients whose endogenous production of hydrocortisone is presumably insufficient; it has been found that a variety of disease processes can be improved by increasing the hydrocortisone level of the blood or tissues either by the administration of a corticosteroid, or by increasing the endogenous production of hydrocortisone by means of ACTH. In certain disorders such as autoimmune haemolytic anaemia or systemic lupus erythematosus the corticosteroids produce a dramatic improvement whose mechanism is not understood.

Replacement therapy. In the treatment of acute Addison's disease (crisis), an intravenous infusion of glucose saline containing hydrocortisone sodium succinate may be life-saving. The hormone is administered at a rate of 10 to 40 mg hourly for several hours, after which cortisone acetate can be given by mouth in doses of 100 mg daily.

Patients with chronic hypoadrenalism require permanent maintenance treatment with a glucocorticoid. Since the physiological hormone, hydrocortisone, is available it can be employed in a schedule mimicking the normal circadian rhythm. Most patients are well controlled on oral cortisol 20 mg each morning and 10 mg each evening. Cortisone acetate is an alternative but it is sometimes poorly absorbed. It has to be converted to cortisol before it is effective. Patients with primary hypoadrenalism generally also require addition of a mineralocorticoid. The mineralocorticoid of choice is fludrocortisone starting with 0.05mg per day and increasing if necessary. Evidence of overdosage with mineralocorticoid are signs of sodium retention such as oedema and hypertension. A sign of potassium depletion is hypokalaemic alkalosis and muscular weakness.

Supplementary therapy. Corticosteroids or ACTH are used in the treatment of a number of conditions which have been collectively described by the term collagen diseases. These diseases include rheumatic fever, rheumatoid arthritis, periarteritis nodosa and certain skin diseases such as lupus erythematosus and dermatomyositis.

The corticosteroids are amongst the most effective drugs used in clinical medicine but discussion of the detailed use of corticosteroids and corticotrophin in various clinical indications including conditions such as rheumatism and the collagen diseases is beyond the scope of this treatise. These drugs produce relief in many of the rheumatic disorders but their side effects are formidable. The dosage appropriate to the different diseases varies widely and it is a matter of clinical judgment whether in some conditions large doses are justified and in others the risk of adverse effects from high doses is greater than the prospect of long term benefit.

Hench, Kendall and their colleagues first showed that following the administration of cortisone to patients with rheumatoid arthritis, there was rapid relief of pain and a marked increase in the movements of the joints. The symptoms of rheumatoid arthritis can usually be controlled by the oral administration of 7.5 to 15 mg of prednisone daily or and equivalent drug; the effect of a dose lasts about 6 to 12 hours, and it should, therefore, be given three or four times a day. These drugs have a palliative but no curative effect, since improvement is not maintained when medication is stopped. In a controlled clinical trial it has been shown that the clinical improvement of 30 patients with rheumatoid arthritis who were treated with cortisone was no greater after 1 year than that of 31 treated with aspirin.

Corticosteroids have a striking action in acute rheumatic fever which is illustrated in Figure 26.6. Whilst the effect of corticosteroids on fever and joint pain and swelling is probably no greater than that of large doses of salicylates, many authorities consider that corticosteroid therapy reduces the incidence of permanent cardiac damage in this disease. Most clinicians consider that corticosteroids should only be used in rheumatoid arthritis when the disease is rapidly progressive and not usually in the initial stages. Once treatment with corticosteroids has begun it has to be continued for a prolonged time and undesirable effects frequently follow. Maintenance therapy should be kept at the lowest effective dosage level.

Intra-articular injections of hydrocortisone acetate or a related corticosteroid are beneficial in the treatment of rheumatoid arthritis. They are also sometimes used in cases of osteoarthritis, where they may benefit the juxta-articular lesions commonly found in this condition. An important contraindication to the intra-articular use of a steroid is the possibility of infection of the joint.

Corticosteroids rapidly control the symptoms of allergic diseases such as asthma, hay-fever, and drug rashes. In the treatment of status asthmaticus ACTH is particularly effective since it causes a rapid rise in the blood level of hydrocortisone. The use of corticosteroids given systemically or by aerosol in bronchial asthma is discussed on page 182.

Local application of a corticosteroid to the nasal mucous membrane may abort attacks of hay-fever and vasomotor rhinitis. Hypersensitivity reactions to drugs which cannot be controlled by antihistamine compounds are often amenable to treatment with ACTH or oral corticosteroids.

Corticosteroids have an important place in the treatment of ocular diseases; many types of inflammatory reactions of the eye are suppressed by these drugs, irrespective of whether the reaction is caused by infection, allergy or trauma. Most diseases of the outer eye can be effectively treated by local application of glucocorticoids in solution or as an ointment, often combined with an antibiotic. For the treatment of diseases of the inner eye, subconjunctival injections of the hormones or systemic administration may be required.

The corticosteroids are effective in the treatment of many skin diseases, some of which do not respond to any other form of treatment. The usually lethal conditions of pemphigus or generalised exfoliative dermatitis have been successfully treated with large doses of corticotrophin or of various glucocorticoids. The prognosis of systemic lupus erythematosus has greatly improved since corticosteroids have been regularly used for its treatment.

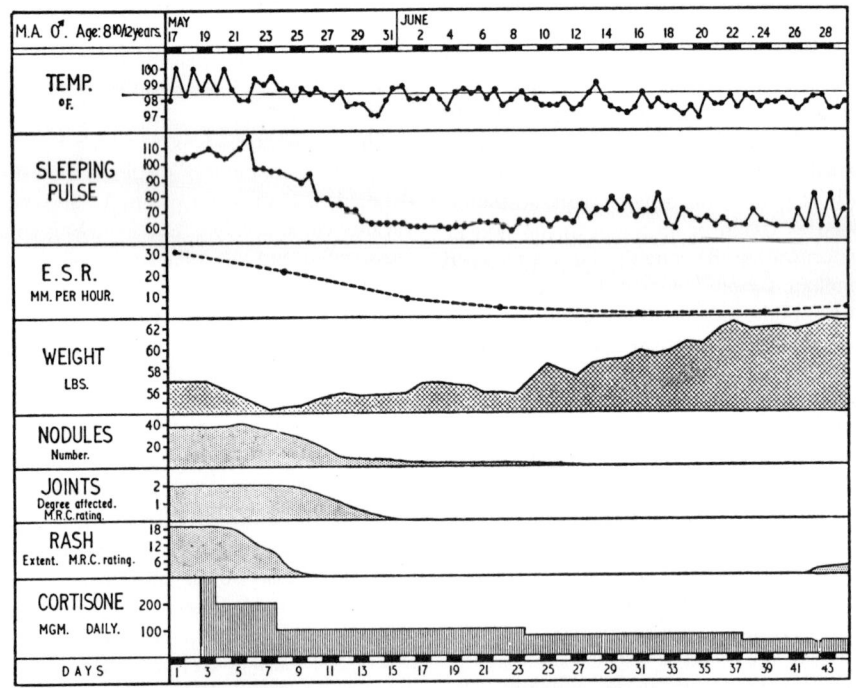

Fig. 26.6 Showing rapid beneficial effect of cortisone on the temperature, pulse and sedimentation rate in a boy with rheumatic fever and a rash of five weeks duration. Nodules which had been present for a fortnight disappeared rapidly. Carditis was present at the beginning of treatment associated with a loud apical systolic murmur. Three years later the heart was normal. (After Schlesinger, 1955. *Practitioner.*)

The corticosteroids are frequently used in the treatment of various diseases of obscure pathology on the grounds that their application has proved empirically beneficial. An example is the use of prednisolone in treating patients with the nephrotic syndrome.

Complications of glucocorticoid therapy
The undesirable effects of the therapeutic use of the glucocorticoids are of two types: (1) those due to overdosage of the hormone which represent an exaggeration of its physiological actions, (2) those which occur mainly after hormone withdrawal and which reflect a state of adrenal insufficiency due to suppression of the endogenous production of corticosteroids.

Although the basis of treatment is the supplementation of a deficient endogenous production of hormone, it is necessary in order to achieve a satisfactory therapeutic effect, to administer doses which are substantially greater than would be required simply to correct the deficiency. Thus efficient steroid therapy usually involves a temporary state of hormone overdosage. As a consequence it is almost inevitable that alterations in the normal pattern of metabolism will occur. If the treatment is prolonged, manifestations of overdosage will appear. The most common are an accumulation of fat, especially in the face, usually termed 'moon-face', mental disturbances and retention of salt and water. In association with this there may arise acute exacerbation of an underlying quiescent disease. By inhibiting the normal tissue response to infection and injury, glucocorticoids may activate latent tuberculosis or promote the spread of localised pyogenic infections; the healing of wounds or of peptic ulcers is delayed and gastric haemorrhage or perforation may occur; latent diabetes may also become apparent. Prolonged steroid therapy often leads to a negative calcium balance which may cause osteoporosis and possibly vertebral collapse.

In contrast to the effects of overdosage which occur during treatment, sudden withdrawal or curtailment of corticosteroids produces symptoms of hormone deficiency due to persistent depression of endogenous secretion of hormones. This state of adrenal insufficiency may lead to an acute exacerbation of the disease for which treatment was given and, if accompanied by an intercurrent infection, may be disastrous to the patient. For this reason it is desirable to reduce gradually the dosage of the glucocorticoids and even to use ACTH to stimulate the adrenals.

Metyrapone (Metopirone)
Metyrapone inhibits beta-hydroxylation at carbon 11 of the basic steroid ring by inhibiting a hydroxylating enzyme in the adrenal cortex. It thus blocks the formation of hydrocortisone. As a consequence an increased ACTH secretion occurs which causes the adrenal to release a number of corticosteroid precursors which can be determined in the urine.

The compound can be used to test pituitary function. In patients with hypopituitarism there will be no increased excretion of steroid precursors since no ACTH is released, whilst in patients with Cushing's syndrome the output of these steroids will be abnormally high.

PREPARATIONS
Effects on blood sugar
Insulins
Biphasic Insulin Injection. Crystals of bovine insulin in a solution of porcine insulin. Insulin Novo Rapitard (pro-insulin freed)
Globin Zinc Insulin Injection
Insulin Injection (Soluble Insulin) 20, 40, 80 u/ml
Insulin Zinc Suspension (Amorphous or Crystalline). Novo Semilente amorph pro-insulin freed. Lentard mixture of beef and pork insulin. Monotard MC monocompon pork insulin. Semitard MC suspension amorphous pork ins. Ultratard susp cryst beef insul
Isophane Insulin Injection. Insul susp with protamine and zinc
Neutral Insulin Injection. Buffered bovine or porcine insulin, pH 6.6–7.7

Oral hypoglycaemic drugs
Acetohexamide (Dimelor) 250 mg–1.5 g dl
Chlorpropamide (Diabenese) 250 mg–500 mg dl
Glibenclamide (Daonil) 2.5–20 mg dl
Glibornuride (Glutril) 12.5–50 mg dl
Glipizide (Glibenese) 2.5–30 mg dl
Glymidine (Gondafon) 0.5–1.5 g dl
Metformin hyd (Glucophage) init 1–1.5 g dl, subs up to 3 g dl
Phenformin hyd (Dibotin) 50–200 mg dl
Tolazamide (Tolanade) 50 mg–1 g dl
Tolbutamide (Rastinon) 0.5–1.5 g dl

Hyperglycaemic drugs
Diazoxide up to 1 g dl
Glucagon (HGF) 0.5–1 mg s.c., i.m., i.v. (1 mg = 1 u)

Corticosteroids
Glucocorticoids
(a) Tablets
Betamethasone 0.5–5 mg dl
Cortisone Acetate 12.5–400 mg dl
Dexamethasone 0.5–10 mg dl
Hydrocortisone 10–40 mg dl
Methylprednisolone 8–80 mg dl
Paramethasone acetate init 4–12 mg dl
Prednisolone 10–100 mg dl
Prednisone 10–100 mg dl
Triamcinolone init 4–48 mg dl, maint no more than 6 mg dl

(b) Injections
Betamethasone sod phosph (Betnesol)
Dexamethasone sod phosph (Decadron)
Hydrocortisone sod succ (Efcortelan) 100–130 mg i.v.
Methylprednisolone acetate 10–80 mg intra-articular or i.m.
Prednisolone pivalate (Ultracortenol) 25 mg intra-articular
Triamcinolone acetonide 2.5–40 mg intra-artic, 1 mg intraderm, 60 mg i.m.

(c) Topical
Beclomethasone diproprionate (Propaderm) 0.025% oint, 0.5% cream

Clobetasol proprionate (Dermovate) 0.05% cream, oint
Desonide (Triseldon) 0.05% cream
Diflucortolone valerate (Nerisone) 0.1% cream
Flurandrenolone (Haelan) 0.0125-0.05 cream oint lot
Flucloronole acetonide (Topilar) 0.025% cream oint
Fluocinolone acetonide (Synalar) 0.01-0.25% cream oint lot
Fluocinonide 0.05% cream
Fluprednidene acetate 0.1% cream
Halcinonide (Halciderm) 0.1% cream
Hydrocortisone acetate 0.5-2.5% oint
Triamcinolone acetonide 0.025-0.5% oint

Mineralocorticoids
Aldosterone (Electrocortin, Aldcorten) 500 μg i.v. i.m.
Deoxycortone Acetate (Doca) 2.5 mg dl i.m.
Fludrocortisone Acetate (Florinef) 1-2 mg, maint 100-200 μg dl

Test of pituitary function
Metyrapone (Metopirone) 250-750 mg 6x every 4 h

FURTHER READING

Azarnoff D L (ed) 1975 Steroid therapy. Saunders, Philadelphia
Christy N P (ed) 1971 The human adrenal cortex. Harper & Row, New York
Lefebvre P J, Ungar R H (ed) 1972 Glucagon. Pergamon, Oxford
Maske H (ed) 1971 Oral wirkende antidiabetica. Handb. exp. Pharm. Springer, Berlin
Petrides P, et al. 1978 Diabetes mellitus: theory and management. Urban & Schwarzenberg, Baltimore
Volk B W, Wellmann K F (ed) 1977 The diabetic pancreas. Plenum Press, New York

27. Sex hormones

Regulation of the ovarian cycle 351; Hormonal control of pregnancy 351; Oestrogens 353; Clinical uses of oestrogens 355; Progestogens 355; Androgens 357; Anabolic steroids 358.

The sex hormones are steroids produced by the ovary and the testes and also by the adrenal cortex and the placenta. They are concerned with the development of the secondary sex characteristics and with reproduction. In addition to these specific effects they also have a general metabolic action and deficiency or overproduction of these hormones results in a severe impairment of general health.

HORMONAL CONTROL OF OVARIAN CYCLE

The functions of the female sex organs are regulated by a very complex system of endocrine control. The subject is one of unusual difficulty, because there is a wide variation in the sexual functions in different species of animals. The fundamental work has been carried out chiefly on mice, rats and rabbits, and human reproductive functions are being interpreted in the light of principles established by these experiments.

Regulation of the ovarian cycle
In most mammals, including women, the ovaries show cyclical activity which is correlated with changes in the uterus and vagina. The anterior pituitary gland controls the activities of the ovaries by means of two gonadotrophic hormones (p. 325): the follicle stimulating hormone (FSH) which causes ripening of the ovarian follicles and liberation of oestrogenic hormones from the ovary, and the luteinising hormone (LH) which acts on the corpus luteum and causes liberation of progesterone. A further anterior pituitary hormone, prolactin (PRL) (p. 325), is involved in the growth and function of the mammary gland. Prolactin is essential for maintaining the corpus luteum of rats, mice and ferrets and some other species in which it acts as a 'luteotrophic' hormone. There is, however, no evidence of a luteotrophic role of prolactin in other species, including monkeys and primates.

In rats and mice, ovulation, liberation of oestrogens and certain typical changes in uterus and vagina all occur together, and this series of changes is termed 'oestrus'. The alteration of oestrus with quiescent periods termed 'dioestrus' constitutes the 'oestrus cycle'. The oestrus changes in the uterus and vagina in rats and mice are as follows: the blood vessels of the uterus dilate, the endometrium swells, and the organ increases two- or threefold in weight. At the same time typical changes occur in the vaginal epithelium. These vaginal changes offer a suitable method of determining the occurrence of oestrus in rats and mice, and have been very useful in experimental work.

Ovulation is followed by the development of the corpus luteum, and this is associated in the majority of mammals with the changes which are produced by luteal hormone secreted by the corpus luteum. These changes are hypertrophy of the uterus and development of the mammary glands. If pregnancy does not occur the corpus luteum retrogresses, and a fresh cycle commences.

The menstrual cycle
The periodic menstrual flow which occurs in monkeys, apes and women differs essentially from the oestrus of rodents. The latter phenomenon occurs at the same time as the maturation of the ovum and the outpouring of oestrogens by the ovary. In women, however, ovulation usually occurs in the middle of the menstrual cycle, that is, about 14 days before the onset of the ensuing menstrual period (Fig. 27.1).

The chain of events is that the periodic activity in the anterior pituitary gland results in the secretion of follicular stimulating hormone which excites ovulation, and the secretion by the ovary of oestadiol. Oestradiol causes enlargement of the uterus and proliferation of the uterine endometrium. Following upon this, secretion by the anterior pituitary of a luteinising hormone supports the development of the corpus luteum which secretes progesterone; progesterone, by causing an increase in complexity of the glandular structure, prepares the endometrium for implantation of the fertilised ovum. After about 10 days, if the ovum is not fertilised and implanted, the corpus luteum regresses and the supply of ovarian hormone is cut off. As a result the uterine endometrium breaks down and menstruation occurs. The duration of menstrual flow varies considerably, but normally lasts from 3 to 5 days.

The sequential secretion of gonadotrophins by the anterior pituitary is itself under the influence of hypothalamic hypophysiotropic factors (p. 322).

Hormonal control of pregnancy
The presence of the developing fertilised ovum maintains and augments the secretory activity of the anterior pituitary gland. In consequence the corpus luteum does not regress, but increases both in size and in activity.

The human placenta, when it develops, assumes important endocrine functions and secretes ovarian and also gonadotrophic hormones. Consequently, although removal of the ovaries before placental development causes abortion in women, yet this does not always do so later on in pregnancy.

Factors influencing conception
In a woman with a normal cycle of 28 days, ovulation usually occurs between the 13th and 15th day before the commencement of the menstrual flow. The life of spermatozoa in the genital tract is probably not more than 48 hours, and the unfertilised egg does not survive longer than 24 hours after ovulation. These data indicate that conception may normally occur between the 11th and 17th days of the menstrual cycle. Knaus concluded that the optimum period for conception is 14 to 16 days, and that conception does not occur before the 11th or after the 17th day. The question of whether a 'safe period' really exists has been the subject of considerable controversy. It is now generally believed that the limits mentioned above express only probabilities, and that in exceptional cases conception may occur at any period in the menstrual cycle. The fertilised ovum is implanted in the uterus about ten days after fertilisation.

It is possible to inhibit ovulation by the administration of a variety of sex hormones and of these progesterone and related compounds are the most effective. During prolonged treatment of infertile women with oestrogen and progesterone, Rock, Garcia and Pincus found that these patients had amenorrhoea. The hormones were later given from the 5th to the 25th day of the cycle and it was found that in this way ovulation and conception could be prevented. The use of oral contraceptives is discussed on page 476.

Tests for pregnancy
Urinary tests for pregnancy are of great antiquity. The Berlin medical papyrus (c. 1250 B.C.) states that the urine of a pregnant woman stimulates the growth of seeds, whilst that of a non-pregnant woman inhibits growth. Since oestrogens have a stimulant action on plant growth this test would probably give fair results.

A number of pregnancy tests in animals have been introduced following the discovery by Aschheim and Zondek in 1927 that the implantation of the fertilised ovum in the uterus was accompanied by the excretion of large quantities of gonadotrophic hormone in the urine. However, the original Aschheim-Zondek test using immature female mice, the Friedman test using the immature female rabbit and the Hogben test using the

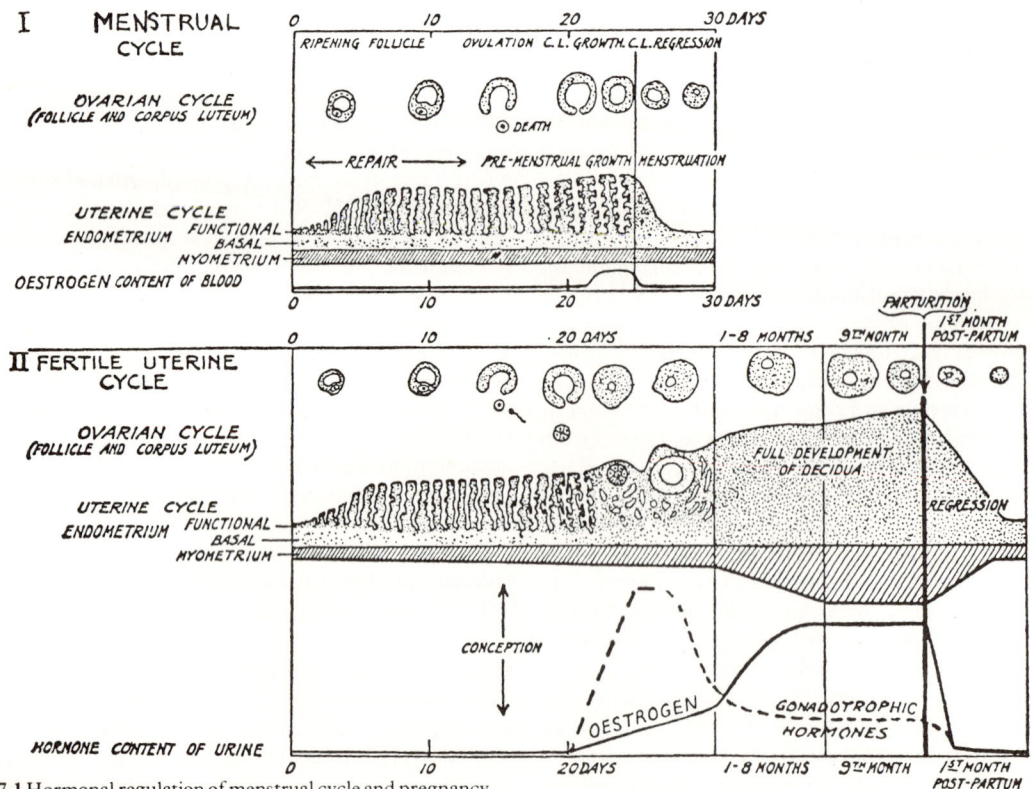

Fig. 27.1 Hormonal regulation of menstrual cycle and pregnancy.

female South African toad, *Xenopus laevis*, have now been almost entirely superseded by immunological test methods for pregnancy urine based on human chorionic gonadotrophin immunoassay.

False positives are obtained when there is a cause other than pregnancy for large amounts of gonadotrophin in urine as in hydatidiform mole and chorionepithelioma both of which give strongly positive results. Positive results may also be obtained with the urine of menopausal women. The tests can be of value in the diagnosis of ectopic pregnancies, but in 25 per cent of ectopic pregnancies false negative results are obtained.

OESTROGENS

There are two types of ovarian hormones; oestrogens and progestogens. Oestrogens produce oestrus or heat in ovariectomised animals. Of the three main human oestrogens *oestradiol* is the most active, and is the major secretory product of the ovary. *Oestrone* is an oxidation product of oestradiol and *oestriol* is a reduction product of oestrone. Oestradiol, together with the other oestrogens, has an unsaturated terminal steroid ring (Fig. 27.2) containing a phenolic hydroxyl which facilitates purification and separation.

Actions of oestrogens

The basic aspects of the interaction of oestrogen and oestrogen receptors are discussed on page 321.

In rodents oestradiol causes directly the changes of oestrus. The most easily recognisable effect is a proliferation of the vaginal epithelium which causes the appearance of cornified epithelial cells in vaginal smears. Associated with these changes in the vagina, there is enlargement of the uterus with proliferation of the endometrium.

In women the oestrogens act on the vaginal mucosa, the endometrium, the uterine muscle and the mammary glands. In the vagina they cause growth and cornification of the epithelium and an increase in the number of papillae. In the cervix there is an increase in cell height of the mucosa and cervical secretions are stimulated. Oestrogens cause a thickening of the endometrium and increased mitosis of the cells of the glands. However the growth of the endometrium is limited and the cells remain straight and tubular; the endometrium thus becomes prepared for the glandular proliferating action of progesterone. Prolonged administration of oestrogen maintains the growth of the endometrium without producing bleeding, but when the oestrogen is suddenly withdrawn, bleeding usually occurs within 48 hours. The activity of the uterine musculature is increased by oestrogens and its responsiveness to oxytocin is enhanced.

Oestrogens also promote the growth of the ducts and nipples of the mammary glands. Oestrogens also have widespread metabolic effects on cells and influence their energy turnover and water distribution. They have a general sodium chloride and water retaining effect.

Two methods are mainly used for the biological assay of oestrogenic activity: (1) estimation of cornified cells in vaginal smears of ovarectomised mice, and (2) the increase in uterine weight of ovariectomised rats. Plasma levels of oestrogens can now be measured by radioimmunoassay.

The naturally occurring oestrogens are rapidly metabolised by the liver and are excreted in the urine as inactive glucuronides or sulphates.

Several long-acting preparations of oestradiol have been prepared. The benzoic and propionic esters of this compound are more stable and act for a longer time than the parent compound. Hence oestradiol monobenzoate and dipropionate are used clinically by intramuscular injection, the effect of a single injection lasting about three to four days. More prolonged effects of oestradiol can be obtained by injection of a microcrystalline suspension of the compound or by subcutaneous implantation of fused pellets.

Synthetic oestrogens

Synthetic oestrogens have been introduced which are less readily metabolised, have a more prolonged action and can be administered by mouth. These compounds are either steroids with ester groups or other substituents which delay their metabolic inactivation, or they are relatively simple non-steroid compounds such as stilboestrol (Fig. 27.2). Another way of prolonging the action of oestrogens is to administer compounds which are not themselves active but are slowly metabolised in the body to oestrogens or to use compounds like chlorotrianisene which are taken up in the body fat and slowly released into the circulation.

Ethinyloestradiol is a derivative of oestradiol in which the hydrogen atom in the 17 carbon position is replaced by an ethinyl group. It is highly active by mouth because the ethinyl group protects the compound from inactivation in the liver.

Mestranol is the methyl ether of ethinyloestradiol, and like the latter is used as the oestrogenic component of oral contraceptives (p. 476).

Stilboestrol. In 1938 Dodds and his co-workers synthesised diethylstilboestrol, a relatively simple compound of stilbene which has been shown to possess all the physiological activities of the naturally occurring oestrogens and in addition is nearly as active when given by mouth as by injection. This substance is commonly known as stilboestrol and has the same therapeutic effects as the natural oestrogens.

Stilboestrol should not be administered during pregnancy because of the American evidence that vaginal adenomas and adenocarcinomas may occur in young

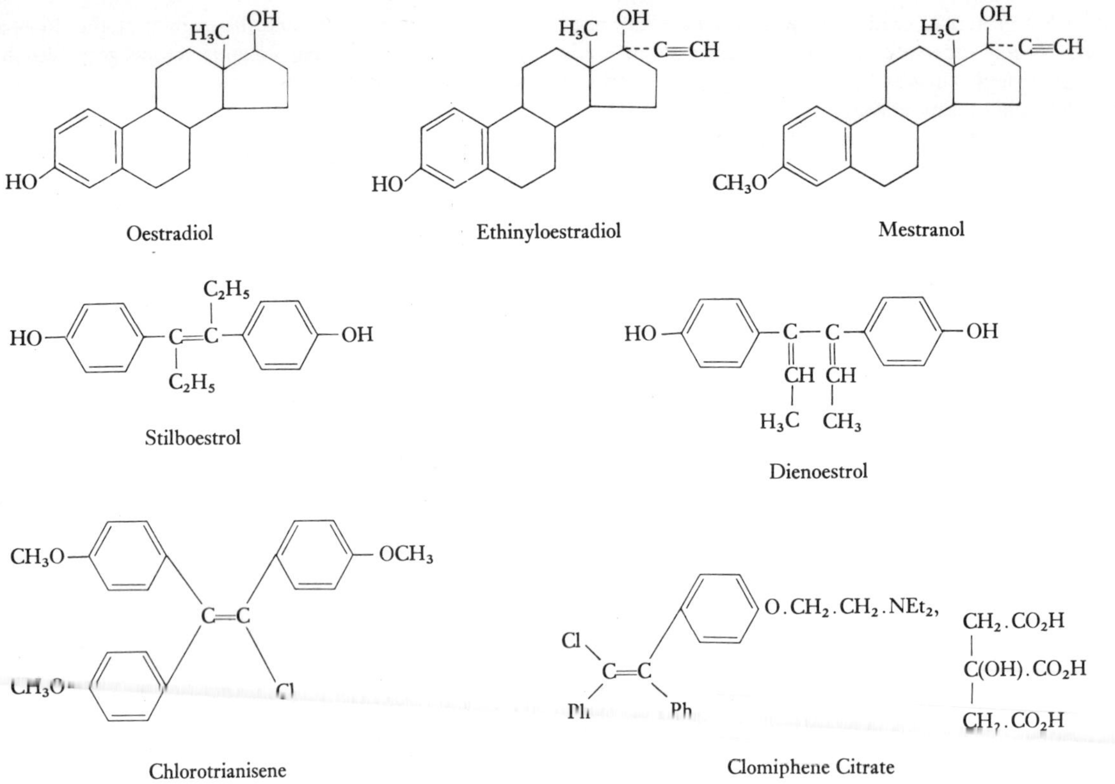

Fig. 27.2 Chemical structure of oestrogens.

females whose mothers received stilboestrol during pregnancy.

Dienoestrol, another synthetic oestrogen, is related to stilboestrol. It is less active than stilboestrol, but produces less nausea, and for this reason is more useful than stilboestrol for the suppression of lactation.

Chlorotrianisene (TACE). This compound is a pro-oestrogen and is converted in the liver into a metabolite which has oestrogenic activity. The prolonged action of chlorotrianisene is due to its storage in the body fat from which it is slowly released and then metabolised. It is used for the palliative treatment of prostatic carcinoma.

Clomiphene. This compound is chemically related to chlorotrianisene (Fig. 27.2). In the rat it has slight mixed oestrogenic and antioestrogenic activity, but its most striking clinical effect is to produce an enlargement of the ovaries and to induce ovulation in patients with amenorrhoea. A likely explanation of the ovulatory effect of clomiphene is that it competes with oestrogen at the hypothalamic level thereby causing increased secretion of LH—FSH—RH (p. 322) and a consequent increase in LH and FSH levels with resultant ovarian stimulation.

Clomiphene citrate has been used to induce ovulation in subfertile women. The main untoward effect is enlargement of the ovary and occasional development of ovarian cysts. A significant increase in the incidence of multiple births has been reported in women who have become pregnant after the administration of clomiphene.

Clinically the administration of clomiphene in subfertile women is sometimes combined with the administration of *menotropins* (human menopausal gonadotrophins).

Comparative activity of oestrogens

It is impossible to make any clear-cut statement regarding the relative activity of different oestrogens, since this depends on the species, method of administration and the effect which is taken as an index of activity. For example in rats ethinyloestradiol is less active than stilboestrol yet clinically it is much more active (Table 27.1). In man the relative activity of different oestrogens seems to depend on the therapeutic endpoint chosen. Consistent results can be obtained by recording the occurrence of 'withdrawal bleeding' after a fortnights administration of a daily dose of oestrogen to amenorrhoeic women.

Toxic effects of oestrogens

The most frequent side effect of oestrogen therapy is nausea. Some degree of nausea is experienced by many patients but this rarely progresses to vomiting. The salt and water retaining action of oestrogens may give rise to headache, tension in the breasts and an increase in body weight. Bleeding from the endometrium may occur after

Table 27.1 Relative clinical potencies of some oral oestrogens (after Swyer, 1965, *Pharm. J.*)

Oestrogen	Potency ratio	Approximate equivalent dose (mg)
Stilboestrol	1	1
Dienoestrol	0.26	4
Hexoestrol	0.05	20
Oestrone	0.04	25
Ethinyloestradiol	25	0.05

withdrawal or even during administration of the oestrogen. If oestrogens are used in the male they may cause breast engorgement, loss of libido and impotence.

Clinical uses of oestrogens

The chief clinical uses that have been established for these compounds are as follows:

Alleviation of menopausal disorders. The majority of women during the menopause suffer from unpleasant symptoms such as hot flushes, heavy perspiration, headaches, nausea and dizziness. Considerable relief is produced in most cases by oral administration of stilboestrol or ethinyloestradiol. This treatment is continued for interrupted periods of 21 days for about 6 or 9 months and the daily dosage needed to produce relief varies widely.

Similar treatment also relieves pathological conditions associated with the menopause such as kraurosis vulvae and leucoplakia.

Treatment of amenorrhoea. Oestrogens have been used to replace the ovarian hormone secretion in patients with amenorrhoea. Some clinicians employ only oestrogens or only progestogens but in most cases a combination of oestrogen and progesterone therapy is used.

Vulvovaginitis. In children, administration of oestrogens improves the nutrition of the infected area and assists in terminating the infection. In senile atrophy of the vaginal mucosa there is often intense itching of the vulva which can be relieved by a short intensive course of oestrogen therapy.

Inhibition of lactation. A single dose of 5 mg stilboestrol will usually suppress lactation if given within 24 hours of birth. The effect is due to inhibition of prolactin secretion by the pituitary. Satisfactory results have been obtained with stilboestrol, hexoestrol or dienoestrol. Dienoestrol may be given in an initial daily dose of 1 mg which is diminished by 0.1 mg each day until the dose is 0.3 mg daily.

Contraception. The use of oestrogens and progestogens in the control of fertility is discussed in Chapter 40.

Control of carcinoma of the prostate. It has been known for some time that castration is a useful method of controlling malignant disease of the prostate. The beneficial effects of oestrogens in the treatment of carcinoma of the prostrate are probably due to feedback inhibition of the anterior lobe of the pituitary. This depresses LH secretion with consequent reduced secretion of testosterone. The diminished amount of dihydrotestosterone (p. 358) formed leads to atrophy of the prostatic glandular epithelium. Oestrogens are sometimes used for the treatment of metastasizing breast cancer but although in some patients remissions are produced, in others the growth of the tumour is accelerated (p. 382).

Atrophic rhinitis. Thus uncommon condition can be relieved both in men and women by oestrogen therapy.

Seborrhoea and acne. These conditions are probably associated with an unbalanced secretion of male hormone and they can generally be relieved temporarily by the administration of oestrogens.

PROGESTOGENS

Progesterone is produced by the corpus luteum, the placenta, the testis and the adrenal cortex. It is distributed rapidly in the body fat and is metabolised by the liver. The main excretion product found in the urine is pregnanediol but this corresponds only to a small fraction of the total production of progesterone in the body. By the use of radioactive progesterone it has been shown that the total amount of this hormone produced daily by the body during the luteal phase of the cycle is approximately 30 mg whilst at the end of pregnancy it is about 200-300 mg. Progesterone has been synthesised but its short duration of action and its ineffectiveness when given by mouth make it unsuitable as a therapeutic agent. A number of compounds with progesterone-like activity have been synthesised which are much more active than progesterone and are effective by oral administration. These compounds are referred to as progestogens.

Actions of progesterone

The chief function of progesterone is concerned with the preparation of the uterus for implantation of the fertilized ovum and it acts only on the uterus which has already been sensitised by oestrogens. In the vagina, progesterone decreases the thickness of the epithelium with loss of the cornified zone. The secretions of the cervix are altered and the crystalline pattern of ferning of the cervical mucus disappears. In pregnancy the cervix, due to the action of progesterone, becomes soft and thin-walled.

Progesterone transforms the endometrium from the proliferative to the secretory stage and increases the complexity of its glandular structure. It causes marked dilatation and spiralling of the glands; the stromal cells differentiate to form the decidua and the secretion of glycogen is increased. The excitability and contractility of the myometrium is reduced by progesterone and the

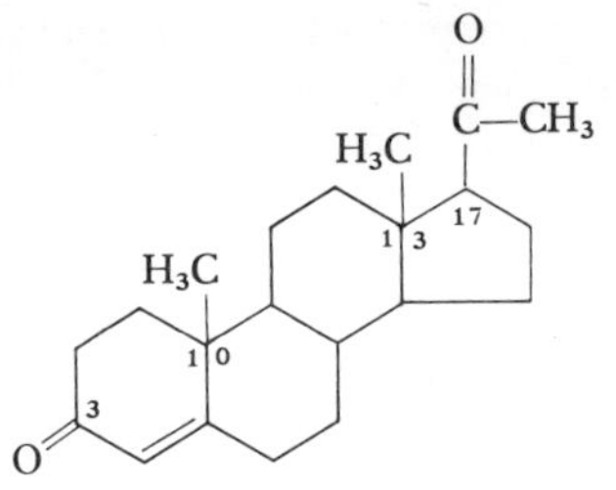

Fig. 27.3 Chemical structure of progestogens.

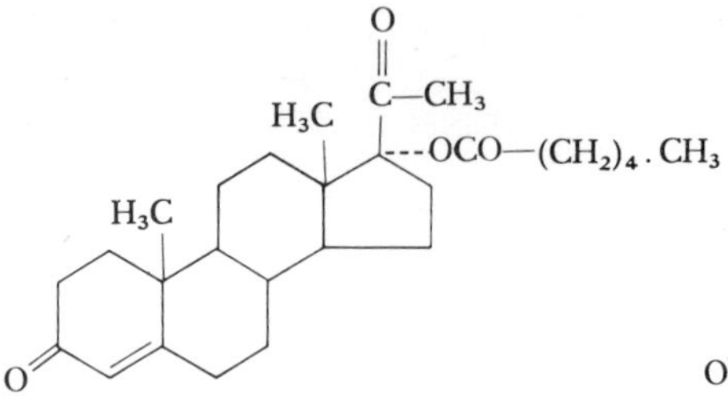

uterine muscle becomes less sensitive to oxytocin. Follicular development and ovulation is suppressed by progesterone, probably by inhibition of gonadotrophin secretion by the anterior pituitary gland.

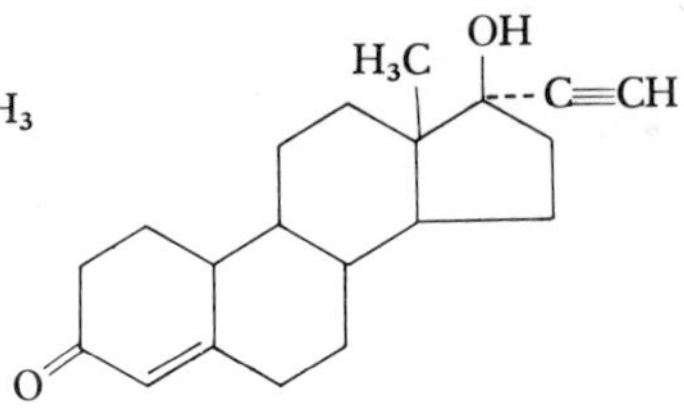

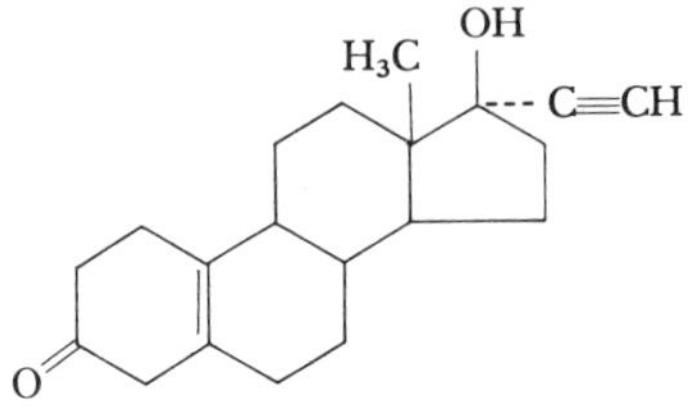

Assay of progestogens. Progesterone activity may be assayed by determining the endometrial changes which it produces in immature or ovariectomised rabbits (Clauberg test). The animals are first given a series of injections with an oestrogen and then the progestational compound is administered. The amount of progestational proliferation of the endometrium is determined by histological examination.

The assessment of human progestogen activity may be carried out by the histological examination of endometrial biopsy after administration of the progestogen. Another method is to assess the ability of the compound to inhibit ovulation. This can be determined indirectly by the absence of a rise in the urinary excretion of pregnanediol during the second half of the menstrual cycle. A third method is to determine the minimum dose of the progestogen necessary to postpone menstruation; in this test the drug is administered for 20 days after the 20th day of the cycle, and menstruation should not occur until administration of the drug is discontinued. Progesterone secretion in the body may be assessed by the estimation of its breakdown product pregnanediol in a 24-hour urine specimen. Plasma progesterone levels can be measured by radioimmunoassay.

Synthetic progestogens
A number of steroids with progestational activity have been synthesised. They are all derivatives of progesterone, testosterone or 19-nortestosterone and with one exception,

17-hydroxyprogesterone, are active by mouth (Fig. 27.3).

Progesterone-3-cyclopentynol ether. This compound probably owes its activity to a slow release of progesterone in the body. 17-*Hydroxyprogesterone caproate* is a depot preparation which is administered intramuscularly and exerts a prolonged action lasting for up to 10 days.

Ethisterone. This is the ethinyl derivative of testosterone and was the first progestogen to be used clinically but it is now mainly of historical interest. In contrast to progesterone it is active by mouth but its activity is much less than that of the newer progestogens.

Norethisterone is the ethinyl derivative of nortestosterone. It is a potent orally active progestogen which also has some androgenic and oestrogenic activity.

Norethynodrel is chemically closely related to norethisterone from which it differs only in the position of the double bond in the A-ring. It also is a potent progestogen active by mouth with rather more oestrogenic and less androgenic activity than norethisterone.

Clinical uses of progestogens
The chief clinical uses of these compounds are as follows:

Threatened and habitual abortion. The maintenance of pregnancy is dependent on a supply of progesterone which may come from either the corpus luteum or the placenta. The chief use of progestogens is in the treatment of habitual or threatened abortion. It is generally agreed that administration of a progestogen is a rational form of treatment although considerable doubts have been expressed as to its efficacy. In threatened abortion progestational therapy is indicated only in patients who show evidence of progesterone deficiency by the cervical mucus test. Treatment may be by oral administration of a

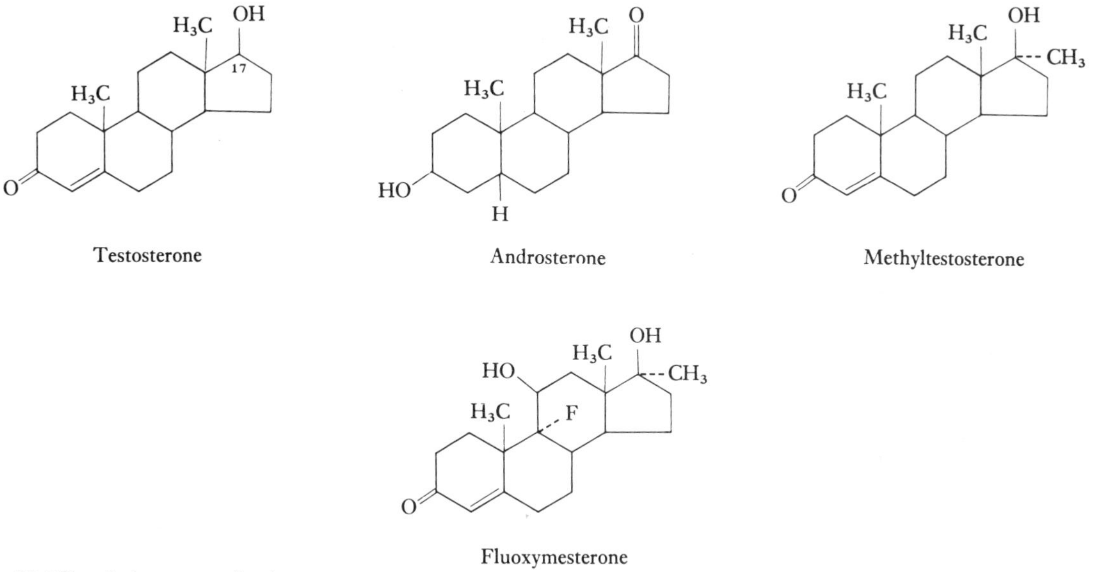

Fig. 27.4 Chemical structure of androgens.

progestogen or intramuscular injection of 17-hydroxyprogesterone caproate at weekly intervals in doses of 125 to 500 mg.

Infertility. This is sometimes due to deficiency of progesterone secretion. In such cases oral administration of norethisterone or norethynodrel 5 to 10 mg daily for 10 days from the 15th day of the cycle may lead to a full secretory response.

Control of uterine bleeding. Norethisterone or norethynodrel given daily for 20 days in doses of 10 to 20 mg will usually arrest dysfunctional bleeding. A few days after treatment is stopped, a withdrawal bleeding occurs. After several cycles of treatment, regular spontaneous menstruation may result.

In the treatment of endometriosis it is usual to give a continuous course of treatment with a progestogen and a small dose of an oestrogen.

Dysmenorrhoea. It is known that the painful irregular uterine contractions of dysmenorrhoea can be prevented by inhibiting ovulation. Stilboestrol has been used to inhibit ovulation in dysmenorrhoea and more recently progestogens administered from the 5th to the 25th day of the menstrual cycle have been used for the same purpose.

Oral contraceptives. The daily administration of a progestogen alone or in combination with a small dose of an oestrogen from the 5th to the 25th day of the cycle will prevent conception. These contraceptive uses are discussed in Chapter 40.

Toxic effects. The androgenic activity associated with progestogens given for the treatment of threatened abortion may occasionally produce virilization of the female foetus.

ANDROGENS

The effects produced by castration of males have been known since the dawn of history. In 1849 Berthold discovered that grafting of the testis produced growth in the capon's comb and Brown-Sequard stated in 1885 that the injection of testicular extracts produced various beneficial effects in old men. The results he described were undoubtedly due to suggestion, but the interest they excited helped to start the modern science of endocrine therapy. Voronoff claimed that remarkable rejuvenation could be produced by grafting anthropoid testicles into elderly gentlemen. Although testicular grafts were considered to produce beneficial effects on castrates these effects were transitory since the grafts were quickly absorbed.

Actions of androgens

The activities of the testes are under the control of the anterior pituitary gland. The follicle stimulating hormone (FSH) in the male, after puberty, produces a continuous stimulation of the testis which results in a steady output of spermatozoa by the germinal epithelium. The luteinising hormone (LH) stimulates the interstitial cells to produce the androgenic hormone testosterone.

Testosterone promotes the development of the secondary sex characteristics. It promotes the growth and development of the external genitalia, the prostate and the seminal vesicles. It also determines the growth of the facial hair, enlargement of the larynx and thickening of the vocal cords which occur at puberty. Testosterone is probably also required for the stimulation of normal spermatogenesis in conjunction with FSH.

Another important property of testosterone is its ability to stimulate protein synthesis; this anabolic effect is associated with the retention of nitrogen, potassium and calcium and is important in determining the muscular development of the growing male. Androgens increase libido both in the male and female.

Androgenic activity may be assayed by the ability of the substance to promote the growth of the capon's comb or to increase the weight of prostrate and seminal vesicles of immature rats.

Testosterone is the main androgen produced by the Leydig cells of the testis. Small amounts of testosterone are also produced by the adrenal cortex and by the ovary. Testosterone is converted in some of the target cells in the body to the compound 5α-dihydrotestosterone. Testosterone is transported in the blood bound to 'testosterone-binding globulin'. The concentration of testosterone in blood is very low and its determination in blood requires special techniques. It has been shown that hypogonadism is usually correlated with low testosterone blood levels.

Testosterone is metabolised in the liver to the weakly androgenic androsterone which has been isolated from male and female urine.

Synthetic androgens
Like the naturally occurring oestrogens, *testosterone* is rapidly metabolised. It is relatively inactive when given by mouth and must be administered by intramuscular injection. For prolonged action testosterone crystals may be implanted subcutaneously. Esters of testosterone have a more prolonged action than the parent compound. Testosterone propionate and other esters such as the cyclopentylpropionate and phenylpropionate are injected in oily solution or in a microcrystalline aqueous suspension.

Oral preparations are also available such as *methyltestosterone* and its more active fluorinated derivative *fluoxymesterone*; the former is usually given by sublingual administration.

Therapeutic uses of androgens
Hypogonadism in the male, when associated with testicular failure, responds well to the administration of the long-acting androgens which cause development of the secondary sex characteristics and increased potency. They are also used together with oestrogens in the treatment of menopausal complaints but excessive doses must be avoided since they may cause hirsutism.

Androgens are also used in the treatment of metastasizing carcinoma of the breast; their beneficial effect is probably due to inhibition of secretion of the gonadotrophic hormones of the anterior pituitary. Patients treated in this way may develop signs of virilization and become oedematous due to sodium and water retention.

Testosterone must not be used in patients with carcinoma of the prostrate since it promotes the growth of this type of malignant tumour.

ANABOLIC STEROIDS

Testosterone has a strong nitrogen-retaining effect which promotes protein synthesis and preparations containing it have been used in conditions in which an anabolic rather than an androgen effect was required. In view of their virilizing effects, particularly in women and children, a search has been made for compounds in which the anabolic activity was not associated with androgenic activity.

In screening compounds of this type it is usual to use castrated rats. The animals are injected with the compound; the weight of the levator ani is a measure of its anabolic activity and that of the seminal vesicles of its androgenic activity. Several compounds have been synthesised with predominantly anabolic activity.

The structure of two of these compounds is shown in Figure 27.5. Nandrolone phenylpropionate (Durabolin) is injected intramuscularly whilst norethandrolone (Nilevar) can be given by mouth.

Side effects. The therapeutic use of anabolic steroids is still in the experimental stage, and the full range of toxic effects which they may produce is not known. They should not be used in pregnancy because of the risk of serious damage to the foetus, nor should they be used in patients with prostatic carcinoma because of their androgenic activity. Another toxic hazard is the occurrence of jaundice and liver damage when used for long periods. All anabolic steroids produce some virilizing effects and may also depress gonadotrophin production by the pituitary. Continuous treatment with anabolic steroids may lead to sodium and water retention with resultant oedema.

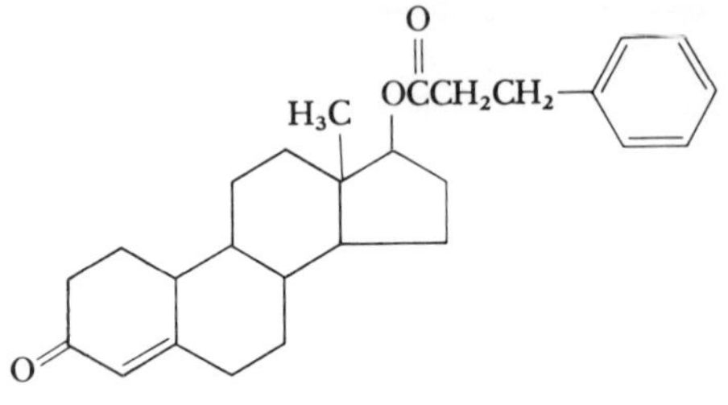

Nandrolone phenylpropionate

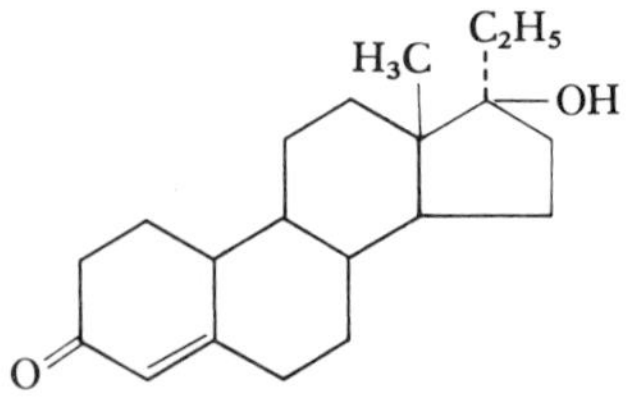

Norethandrolone

Fig. 27.5 Chemical structure of anabolic steroids.

Therapeutic uses of anabolic steroids. The main use of anabolic steroids is in the treatment of severe debilitating illness or during convalescence after major surgery or severe injury. They have also been used in the treatment of osteoporosis because of their protein and calcium retaining properties. Anabolic steroids have also been used in the treatment of acute renal failure and of retarded growth in children but their place in the treatment of these conditions is not established. Anabolic steroids stimulate erythropoietin production by the kidney. They have been found effective in increasing haemoglobin levels in patients with aplastic anaemia.

PREPARATIONS

Oestrogens
Steroidal
Ethinyl oestradiol 0.05 mg 1–3x die p.o.
Oestradiol, Oestradiol benzoate 0.5–1.5 mg i.m.
Oestriol
Oestrone 0.1–2 mg i.m.
Nonsteroidal
Chlorotrianisene (Tace) (pro-oestrogen) 12–25 mg dl in carc of prostate
Dienoestrol 0.01% vag cream
Diethylstilboestrol 1 mg dl
Hexoestrol 2–3 mg dl p.o.
Methallenoestril (Vallestril) 6 mg dl for 6 w (menop)

Progestogens
Dydrogesterone 5–30 mg dl
Hydroxyprogesterone hexanoate 250–500 mg i.m. 1–2x weekly
Medroxyprogesterone acetate 2.5–20 mg dl p.o.
Megestrol acetate 160 mg (carc of breast)
Norethisterone acetate (Norethindrone) 5–20 mg dl (amenorrh)

Androgens
Fluoxymesterone (Ultandren) 10–20 mg dl p.o. bucc
Mesterolone (Proviron) 50–100 mg dl
Testosterone Enanthate 200–400 mg i.m. every 4 w

Anabolic steroids
Ethyloestrenol (Orabolin) 2–4 mg dl
Methandienone (Dianabol) 2.5–10 mg dl
Nandrolone phenylproprionate (Durabolin) 25–50 mg weekly
Oxymetholone (Anapolon) 5–10 mg dl

Ovulatory agent
Clomiphene citr 50–100 mg die for 5 days

Antigonadotrophic agent
Danazol 800 mg dl (endometriosis, reduces serum FSH and LH)

Antiandrogenic agent
Cyproterone acet 100–200 mg dl

FURTHER READING

Brotherton J 1976 Sex hormone pharmacology. Academic Press, London
Carey H M 1979 Clinical uses of female sex steroids. Butterworths, Sidney
Kochakian C D (ed) 1976 Anabolic-androgenic steroids. Handb. exp. Pharm. 43. Springer, Berlin
Tausk M (ed) 1972 Progesterone, progestational agents and antifertility drugs. Int. Enc. Pharm. Ther. Sect. 48: 2 vols
Voss H E, Oertel G 1973 Androgene I. Handb. exp. Pharm. 35 Springer, Berlin
Voss H E, Oertel G et al 1973 Androgene II und Antiandrogene. Handb. exp. Pharm. 35. Springer, Berlin

28. The vitamins

Discovery of vitamins 360; Causes of vitamin deficiency 360; Fat-soluble vitamins 361; Vitamin A 361; Vitamin D 362; Vitamin E 364; Vitamin K 365; Water-soluble vitamins 366; The vitamin B complex 366; Thiamine 366; Riboflavine 367; Nicotinic acid 368; Pyridoxine 368; Folic acid 369; The cobalamins 369; Ascorbic acid 369; Vitamin content of diets 370.

In addition to proteins, carbohydrates and fats which provide metabolic energy, the body needs a variety of substances for its maintenance; some of these it can manufacture but others it has to obtain ready made. The latter substances fall into two groups, namely, those which are inorganic and stable and those which are organic and more easily destroyed. Iodine and iron are examples of inorganic substances. Deficiency occurs unless the diet contains a few milligrams of these per week, and preserved foods supply them just as well as fresh foods. The second group of organic substances, which are present in fresh food and some of which may be destroyed by the processes used in the preservation or cooking of food, are termed vitamins. Vitamins are constituents of the diet, other than protein, carbohydrate, fat and inorganic substances, which are essential for the normal metabolic functioning of the body.

Discovery of vitamins

The discovery of vitamins represents an advance of great practical importance, since it has revealed a means of preventing and curing some of the commonest diseases of nutritional origin. The fact that an adequate supply of fresh vegetable food is essential for the maintenance of health, and even of life, was discovered as soon as mankind acquired sufficient skill in navigation to make long voyages, and the history of early ocean navigation is very largely a history of struggles against scurvy. Early in the eighteenth century it was recognised that green vegetables or the juice of citrus fruits were the only cure or preventative of scurvy. As early as 1600 lemon juice was used with success at sea as an antiscorbutic, and Lind showed in his book on scurvy, which was published in 1757, that the disease could be prevented and cured by administration of lemon juice. He also showed that dried vegetables were useless for this purpose. Captain Cook at once realised the importance of this work, and, by applying it, was able to maintain his crews in perfect health during voyages that lasted for years — a fact that had never before been accomplished. Improvements in agriculture and the advent of steam transport greatly reduced the incidence of scurvy in the nineteenth century.

Beri-beri is a disease which spread rapidly in the East in all rice-eating countries during the latter half of the nineteenth century, and between 1878 and 1882 nearly 40 per cent of the personnel of the Japanese navy were affected. Takaki was convinced that the disease was caused by errors in the dietary, and in 1885 he reformed the naval diet. The most important changes were an increase in the meat ration and the substitution of barley for a part of the rice, which had previously been the principal article of food. As a result of these changes beri-beri practically disappeared from the Japanese navy. In 1890 Eijkman found that by feeding fowls on polished rice he could produce a polyneuritis closely resembling beri-beri. He also showed that this polyneuritis could be prevented or cured by giving the fowls small quantities of rice polishings or extracts of rice polishings. These results explained the great increase in beri-beri in the latter half of the nineteenth century, for the indigenous populations had always prepared rice in the unpolished form with the seed coats intact, but the Europeans introduced machinery to produce polished rice, in which the seed coats are removed, and it was the introduction of this polished rice which caused the spread of beri-beri. Funk introduced the term 'vitamine' in attempting to isolate the active principle present in rice polishings.

As a result of efforts to rear animals on diets of highly purified or synthetic substances Lunin showed in 1881 that mice could not live on a seemingly complete diet of protein, fats, carbohydrates and salts. Pekelharing made similar investigations and concluded 'that there is a still unknown substance in milk which even in very small quantities is of paramount importance in nutrition'. Hopkins later showed that while rats failed to grow and died when fed on purified diets, they grew and flourished if a little milk was added to the diet. The experiments of Osborne and Mendel indicated the existence of a fat-soluble factor and by 1918 it was recognised that at least three separate accessory food substances or vitamins existed, and that the presence of all of these in the diet was essential for the maintenance of life. More than 30 vitamins and pro-vitamins are now known and practically all of these have been isolated as definite chemical compounds. This advance, however, has revealed the fact that the substances grouped under the term 'vitamin' differ very widely both as regards chemical constitution and physiological function.

Causes of vitamin deficiency

It is easy to recognise and describe the effects of gross vitamin deficiency; advanced avitaminoses such as rickets, scurvy and beri-beri are relatively rare in this country. The effects of partial deficiency however are very important as they are believed to be a common cause of chronic ill-health, and mild forms or 'subclinical' manifestations of rickets and of scurvy are still evident, especially in children.

Deficiency of vitamins may result from one or several of the following factors.

1. *Deficiency of vitamins in food.* Inadequate amounts of food may be the simple cause of vitamin deficiency. This may occur in patients who are maintained for some time on special restricted diets. Lack of variety may also be a cause. This was formerly seen in people who lived on a monotonous diet of tea, white bread and margarine. The processes to which food is subjected may also influence the vitamin content of the diet.

2. *Failure to absorb vitamins from food.* This is a common complication of diseases of the alimentary tract. Achlorhydria, gastritis or diarrhoea may prevent the absorption of components of the vitamin B complex and the neuritis which often accompanies chronic alcoholism is probably due to deficient absorption of vitamin B_1. The prolonged use of liquid paraffin may interfere with the absorption of vitamin A by dissolving carotene which is then excreted in the faeces. As a rule, failure to absorb fat involves failure to absorb fat-soluble vitamins, e.g. in patients with steatorrhoea. A further example of this is the fact that in obstructive jaundice the absorption of vitamin K is prevented and this results in a delay in the clotting of the blood.

3. *Increased vitamin needs.* In infants and children and in women during pregnancy and lactation the vitamin needs are high. In prolonged febrile illness and in thyrotoxicosis increased supplies of vitamins are often necessary. The adequacy of the vitamin supply therefore depends on two variable factors, namely, the amount absorbed and the needs of the body.

Ascorbic acid is stored in high concentrations in the suprarenal cortex and other tissues. Most animals do not require any food supply of this vitamin because they can synthesise it, the exceptions being the guinea pig and the monkey. The human body probably does not produce any ascorbic acid and can only be maintained in good health when the food contains an adequate quantity of this compound.

In the case of the vitamins of the B group it has been shown that aneurine, riboflavine and nicotinic acid can be synthesised in the intestine of animals and of human beings. It has been estimated that as much as 80 per cent of the estimated human requirements of nicotinic acid may be synthesised by bacteria in the human intestine. Under favourable conditions of an open-air life in a sunny climate, vitamin D is formed in the skin by irradiation of dehydrocholesterol by the ultraviolet light from the sun, but under urban conditions in winter in northern latitudes, the vitamin has to be obtained from the food.

The role of vitamins in metabolism can be appreciated most easily if they are regarded as part of the mechanism of the chemical control of body functions. Vitamin A for example, plays an essential part in the biochemical processes required for rod vision in the retina. Thiamine (aneurine, vitamin B_1) and riboflavine (vitamin B_2) are cofactors which form part of the enzyme mechanisms by which the normal metabolism of the cell is carried out. The nomenclature of the vitamins, which, owing to the fact that they were discovered one by one were termed A, B, C, D, is tending to break down; the original vitamin B, for example, is now known to contain at least 20 substances most of which have been chemically identified. The vitamins are often classified according to whether they are fat-soluble or water-soluble.

FAT-SOLUBLE VITAMINS

Vitamin A

Vitamin A is an unsaturated alcohol which is easily oxidised. It occurs only in animal tissue where it is chiefly present in liver, fatty fish, milk and eggs. The main precursors of vitamin A are α- and ß-carotenes and these occur in plants as the yellow coloured pigments which are

$$\text{Retinol (Vitamin A}_1\text{)}$$

present in carrots, turnips, spinach and broccoli tops. As far as is known, animals depend to a large extent on plant carotenes for their source of vitamin A. The name vitamin A is applied to a number of substances of very similar structure found in animal tissues. The principal and most active substance is all-*trans* retinol which may be prepared synthetically while material prepared from natural sources is accompanied by several isomers. Retinol is generally used in the form of esters such as the acetate, palmitate or proprionate. Preformed vitamin A which is present in milk, eggs, butter and liver, is almost completely absorbed. Butter and milk however, are not wholly reliable because their content of vitamin A depends on the food of the cow. Grass-fed cows obtain adequate amounts of carotenes, but the food of stall-fed animals contains very little because carotene is destroyed when grass is dried to form hay. Vitamin A is stored in the liver, and liver oils — particularly fish liver oils — provide the vitamin in a relatively concentrated form.

The activity of preparations containing vitamin A may be determined by physical or by biological methods. The spectrographic method consists in determining the ultraviolet absorption of a solution of the preparation at a wave length of 328 nm. The antimony trichloride test depends on the fact that this reagent develops a blue colour with vitamin A, the intensity of which is related to the amount of the vitamin present. Concentrations of vitamin A in blood may be determined by radioimmunoassay.

Vitamin A activity is usually expressed in terms of units. The activity of 1 i.u. vitamin A is contained in 0.3 μg all-*trans* retinol.

Vitamin A deficiency
Vitamin A has at least two important physiological functions: (1) it combines as a chromophore with a specific protein called opsin to form visual purple, a substance in the rods of the retina which is concerned with dark adaptation; (2) it is an essential factor for the normal metabolism of epithelial cells. Signs of vitamin A deficiency have been described in animals and in man.

Effects in animals. The chief effect of vitamin A deficiency is an atrophy of epithelial tissue which is followed by proliferation of the basal cells with subsequent keratinisation of the new cells. This change reduces the power of the epithelium to resist bacterial invasion. One of the first obvious effects of severe vitamin A lack is a purulent conjunctivitis. The trachea and bronchi are similarly affected and hence bronchopneumonia often results. In the genitourinary tract calculi frequently form either in the kidney pelvis or in the bladder. Injury to the gums and the enamel-forming cells in the teeth causes pyorrhoea alveolaris and defective formation of dental enamel.

Complete deprivation of vitamin A causes arrest of growth and death in a few weeks in young rats. Adult animals are less affected because they have a considerable store of vitamin A in their liver fat.

Clinical effects. Night blindness is one of the earliest manifestations of human vitamin A deficiency. The ability to see in a dim light is dependent on the presence of visual purple. Vitamin A is necessary for the formation of this retinal pigment and even a partial deficiency of the vitamin delays the rate of regeneration of visual purple after exposure to light. Thus the impairment in the rate of dark adaptation is used as a measure of vitamin A deficiency. It has been shown that the administration of vitamin A will increase the sensitivity to dim light, but although very large doses (100 000 units) of vitamin A have been used, the improvement of vision is not greater than that produced by doses of 5000 units daily. This test is not specific for vitamin A as night blindness is also caused by other conditions, e.g. retinitis pigmentosa.

As in animals, keratinisation of epithelium may be seen in the human subject. Most usually it occurs in the conjunctiva when the surface may be dry and wrinkled (xerophthalmia), or the cornea may ulcerate (keratomalacia); Bitot's spots are the small yellowish areas which appear in the conjunctiva. The skin becomes rough and dry. Round sharply defined papules due to hyperkeratosis of the pilosebaceous follicles appear on the side of the forearms and thighs. These skin changes may also be seen in subjects who are deficient in other vitamins.

The fact that vitamin A deficiency makes animals highly susceptible to respiratory infections, suggests that this effect may occur in man, but whether vitamin A administration can reduce the incidence of infections of the respiratory tract in man is a matter of dispute. Many experiments have been made to solve the simple problem whether administration of cod liver oil during the winter reduces the incidence of colds in groups of employees. Unfortunately the results obtained have been contradictory. In a study in which 16 adults were given a diet deficient in vitamin A and carotene for periods of 6½ to 25 months, the earliest definite signs of depletion were defective night vision with a raised rod threshold and a fall in the value for vitamin A in the blood plasma. The only clinical signs and symptoms which were commoner in this group compared with a control group receiving a supplement of vitamin A were dryness of the skin and eye discomfort. There was no significant difference in the incidence of coughs and colds in the two groups.

Daily requirements. It has been estimated that the following amounts will meet the average needs:

Children	1500–5000 units
Adults	3000–5000 units
Women, lactating or pregnant	6000–8000 units

The average daily requirements (4500 units) may be obtained in 1½ teaspoonfuls of cod liver oil or 1 halibut liver oil capsule (BP).

Therapeutic uses. Many therapeutic uses for this vitamin have been suggested, but the present position is that, although partial deficiency of the vitamin is probably common, its value as a curative agent for any definite pathological condition except in frank vitamin A deficiency, is not firmly established. The chief aim should be to obtain sufficient intake of vitamin A in the form of natural foodstuffs, as these are not only cheaper but also provide other vitamins of which we know little.

Prolonged administration of very large amounts of vitamin A to infants produces anorexia, pruritic rashes, and painful soft tissue swellings accompanied by radiological evidence of thickening of the long bones. These effects disappear rapidly when the intake of vitamin A is reduced.

Vitamin D

In 1924 Hess and Steenbock showed independently that certain inactive food substances when exposed to ultraviolet light acquired antirachitic properties. Similar exposure of cholesterol and other sterols caused the production of an antirachitic factor. It was subsequently demonstrated by Rosenheim that the substance activated by irradiation was ergosterol, and in 1930 Bourdillon and co-workers isolated from irradiated ergosterol a crystalline substance which was named calciferol. Subsequent research has shown the existence of a group of sterols with antirachitic properties possessing the same ring structure as cholesterol. Although several sterols have antirachitic properties, the term Vitamin D is used to designate two of clinical importance: *ergocalciferol* (calciferol, vitamin D_2), from yeast and fungal ergosterol sources, is the active ingredient supplied commerically, while *cholecalciferol* (vitamin D_3) is formed in the skin by conversion of the

Cholecalciferol (Vitamin D_3)

provitamin, 7-dehydrocholesterol, to cholecalciferol upon exposure to the sun's ultraviolet rays. Cholecalciferol can also be formed by irradiation of food.

Metabolic activation of vitamin D. Recent studies have shown that vitamin D undergoes metabolic activation in the liver and kidney. It is metabolised in the liver to *25-hydroxycholecalciferol (25-HCC)* which is an intermediary in the synthesis of several hydroxylated forms in the kidney, principally *1,25-dihydroxycholecalciferol (1,25-DHCC)* which is believed to be the active agent promoting the intestinal absorption of calcium and perhaps also the mineralisation of bone. This compound which is also referred to as $1,25(OH)_2D_3$ is the most highly active vitamin D metabolite. It has been isolated and chemically synthesised.

Physiological function of vitamin D

Normal absorption of calcium and phosphorus from the intestine can only occur if there is an adequate supply of vitamin D. The mechanism by which vitamin D promotes calcium absorption is not known with certainty, but it has been shown that it stimulates the synthesis of a calcium-binding protein which may be involved in the absorption of calcium. The increased phosphate absorption is probably an indirect consequence of calcium absorption.

The absorption of dietary calcium is essential for the maintenance of a level of extracellular calcium sufficient to lead to deposition of bone. In the absence of vitamin D the blood level of calcium becomes inadequate, causing a compensatory release of parathyroid hormone (p. 335).

Parathyroid hormone raises plasma calcium and phosphate at the expense of bone, which becomes demineralised whilst renal excretion, particularly of phosphate, increases.

Vitamin D deficiency

The effects produced by vitamin D deficiency in both growing animals and children are uniform and definite. The formation of bone is deranged so that the epiphyses become swollen and radiological examination shows that the normal clear line of calcification has disappeared. Microscopic examination shows disorganisation of the calcifying tissue. The bones laid down under such conditions are soft and spongy, and bend under the weight of the body. The dentition is also deranged and the teeth have defective enamel and dentine. This derangement constitutes the condition of rickets that can be produced in most mammals, and even in birds.

Experiments on rats have shown that the development of rickets is influenced not only by the amount of vitamin D present but also by the calcium/phosphorus ratio in the food.

In rickets there is disturbance of phosphorus metabolism whereby the blood phosphates are reduced while the blood phosphatase is increased. In the presence of adequate amounts of vitamin D the level of blood phosphates is restored to normal.

Daily requirements. The needs are greatest in growing children and in nursing and pregnant mothers. It has been estimated that the following average daily intake of vitamin D will ensure the maximum rate of growth in children and prevent the onset of rickets.

Infants and children
400–800 units
Adults 200–400 units
Women, lactating or pregnant
400–800 units

In the curative treatment of rickets about two to three times these amounts are necessary.

Calcium absorption and vitamin D

The bare maintenance intake of calcium in an adult is about 0.75 to 1 g daily. Calcium is absorbed with difficulty even by healthy persons, and it is usually assumed that only about 25 per cent of the calcium in the food is absorbed. Hence the amount of calcium that must be absorbed by an adult in order to maintain equilibrium is about 0.25 g daily. The percentage of calcium absorbed from food depends on the nature of the diet: subjects fed on brown bread which is rich in phytic acid, require about twice the amount of calcium in their diet to maintain calcium balance, than persons fed on more completely extracted white bread. During the period of growth and bone formation much larger quantities of calcium are needed. Growing boys between 6 and 14 years store from 0.2 to 0.4 g calcium a day, and require a daily food content of from 1 to 2 g.

Similarly, the need for calcium is high during pregnancy and lactation. In the last three months of pregnancy the foetus stores the equivalent of 66 g of ash, and this corresponds to a calcium storage of about 0.3 g a day. During lactation the increased calcium demand persists, for a child after six months takes a litre of milk daily and this contains 1 g calcium. During these periods a food content of at least 1.5 g calcium daily is needed.

Calcium absorption cannot be adequate unless the diet contains a sufficient quantity, but even when there is plenty of calcium in the food the absorption may still be inadequate. The estimation of calcium absorption is difficult, because calcium is partly excreted into the colon, and hence a high calcium content in the faeces may be due either to deficient absorption or to excessive excretion. The reason for the defective absorption of calcium from the gut is that calcium, carbonates and phosphates are all present. The physical chemistry of such a mixture is obscure, but the important practical fact is that only under certain conditions will the calcium remain in an absorbable condition, either in true solution or in colloidal suspension, and it is easily converted into the completely insoluble compounds, calcium carbonate, calcium phosphate or calcium phytate. Excess of calcium, excess of phytic acid, or alkalinity, all favour the precipitation of calcium in an insoluble and non-absorbable form.

The simplest method of increasing the calcium content of the diet is to increase its milk content. One litre of cow's milk contains 1 g of calcium, which is about equal to the normal daily requirement of an adult, but rickets in children is usually due to a deficiency in vitamin D, and not to a deficiency of calcium in the diet.

Therapeutic uses
Vitamin D is of chief importance in the prevention and treatment of rickets. Natural sunlight is seldom available in sufficient amounts in Great Britain and exposure to ultraviolet light is often used as an alternative. Vitamin D is essential for persons of all ages. Vitamin D_3 is present in animal fats, egg yolk, fish liver oils, milk, margarine and cereals; infant food is often fortified with vitamin D. The daily requirements of vitamin D in adults are very small. The supply need not come directly from the diet if there is an adequate exposure to sunlight. Supplementation is needed for infants, particularly premature infants, children throughout the growth years and adults, especially elderly persons who are not exposed to sunlight. Pregnant and lactating women may need vitamin D supplementation if 400 iu daily is not provided by the diet. However, excessive amounts during pregnancy are potentially dangerous for the foetus.

Osteomalacia, or adult rickets, also requires vitamin D treatment. This condition may arise in more or less severe form in elderly people or in the presence of absorption defects as in steatorrhoea. The place of vitamin D in the treatment of senile osteoporosis is uncertain.

A liberal supply of vitamin D is necessary whenever it is desired to increase the absorption of calcium, and large doses of the vitamin have been given to promote the healing of fractures, and in the treatment of hypocalcaemic tetany arising after thyroidectomy.

Toxic effects. Gross excess of irradiated ergosterol produces severe intoxication and death in rats. These effects may be produced by the toxic by-products of irradiation, but it is now known to be produced also by pure calciferol in excess. Toxic effects are produced by feeding animals with moderate excess (e.g. 20 times the therapeutic dose) of either calciferol or of cod liver oil. Hypercalcaemia and renal calcinosis has occurred in children where the daily intake of vitamin D has exceeded 1000 units (25 μg).

In the treatment of lupus vulgaris large doses of 7.5–10 mg of calciferol daily have been claimed to give successful results but the value of this application is now doubted. Prolonged treatment with large doses may cause abnormal deposition of calcium in various parts of the body, particularly in the arteries and kidneys. The toxic symptoms include anorexia, loss of weight, headache, abdominal pain and vomiting or diarrhoea. These may be associated with a rise in blood calcium from the normal value of 10 mg to 15 mg per 100 ml.

Vitamin E (Tocopherol)
Evans showed in 1921 that when rats were fed on a diet containing the vitamins then known as A, B, C and D they appeared to be perfectly normal but were unable to

α-Tocopherol

reproduce. This failure to reproduce was attributed to the absence from the diet of a substance, 'factor X', later named vitamin E. In 1936 Evans, Emerson and Emerson isolated from wheat germ oil an alcohol with a high vitamin E activity which they called tocopherol from the Greek word for child-bearing. The chief natural source of vitamin E is wheat germ oil, but green vegetables, fats, eggs and meat are also good sources. α-, ß- and γ-Tocopherol have been synthesised; ß-and γ-tocopherols are isomers and contain one methyl group less than α-tocopherol. It has been shown that α-tocopherol possesses the highest vitamin E activity. Vitamin E is not destroyed by cooking.

Effects of vitamin E deficiency

In the female animal a deficiency of vitamin E results in abortion. Implantation of the ovum occurs in a normal manner but, following placental changes, the foetus dies. In the male, degeneration of the germinal epithelium occurs and this is followed by spermatozoal inactivity, and later azospermia, sterility and impotence result.

The anterior pituitary glands of these animals undergo degenerative changes and it has been suggested that vitamin E deficiency not only affects the production of the gonadotrophic hormones but also the production of prolactin. When young rats are suckled by mothers fed on a vitamin E-deficient diet they develop a nutritional muscular dystrophy. Degenerative changes in the renal tubules have also been shown in rats fed on a similar diet. These changes are prevented but not cured by the addition of α-tocopherol to the diet. Vitamin E is an antioxidant and some of the effects of deficiency of this vitamin, for example tubular degeneration, can be prevented by the administration of a redox dye such as methylene blue.

Therapeutic use

Clear evidence of a deficiency of vitamin E in man, requiring treatment, is rare. Such evidence is sometimes found in infants with fat absorption defects who may exhibit muscle changes resembling those seen in vitamin E deficient animals. Vitamin E levels are low in the newborn and it is important that this deficiency should not be aggravated by artificial diets low in vitamin E.

It is difficult to assess clinical evidence of vitamin E therapy. Since 1933 there have been numerous reports of the successful treatment of women with histories of habitual abortion. For example, Currie treated 37 women who in 130 pregnancies had only produced 16 viable infants. After treatment there were 37 pregnancies which resulted in 37 viable infants (2 pairs of twins), and there were only 2 abortions. These reports have been subject to criticisms.

An extensive literature has accumulated on the beneficial effects of intensive tocopherol therapy in coronary, rheumatic and hypertensive heart disease and peripheral vascular disease but there is no evidence of vitamin E deficiency in these patients. The present view is that a deficiency of vitamin E can occur in patients in whom fat absorption is impaired. These patients show systemic disturbances which can be remedied by the administration of vitamin E.

Vitamin E may be administered orally in capsules containing 0.2 ml of wheat germ oil concentrate or tablets containing 3 mg α-tocopherol. The daily requirements of vitamin E are not known.

Vitamin K

Vitamin K (koagulations-vitamin) was shown by Dam and Schonheyder in 1934 to be a fat-soluble vitamin, deficiency of which causes spontaneous haemorrhages and prolongation of the blood clotting time in chickens.

Chemistry

The term vitamin K is applied to a group of quinone compounds with antihaemorrhagic effects. They are all related to menadione, also called vitamin K_3. The two main vitamin K forms in nature are vitamin K_1 (phytomenadione) and the closely related vitamin K_2. Both are fat-soluble and almost insoluble in water.

Several related compounds with vitamin K activity have been synthesised, some of which are water-soluble, for example *menadiol* (synkavit). The coumarin anticoagulants antagonise vitamin K (p. 213).

Occurrence and metabolism

Vitamin K occurs in a high concentration in certain vegetables such as spinach and cabbage and in lower concentrations in tomatoes, peas and pig liver. It is doubtful whether healthy adults are dependent on the dietary intake of vitamin K since it is synthesised by bacteria of the normal intestinal flora. Babies during the first days of life, when the intestinal flora is undeveloped, cannot synthesise the vitamin.

Menadione (Vitamin K_3)

Phytomenadione (Vitamin K_1)

Like all fat soluble vitamins, vitamin K is absorbed with dietary fat and requires the presence of bile salts for adequate uptake. After absorption the vitamin is utilised in the liver. It is rapidly metabolised so that rapid depletion occurs if absorption is reduced.

The main physiological function of vitamin K is to promote the formation of certain factors essential for blood coagulation by the liver. The various factors concerned are discussed on page 210. Vitamin K may act as a co-factor in their synthesis.

Vitamin K deficiency
Vitamin K deficiency can cause haemorrhagic disease in animals and man. The main causes of deficiency in man are as follows.
  1. Reduced dietary intake, especially in the newborn. Milk is a poor source of vitamin K.
  2. Inhibition of synthesis of the vitamin by intestinal bacteria, e.g. after giving sulphonamides.
  3. Deficient absorption of the vitamin as in sprue or obstructive jaundice.
  4. Impaired utilisation of the vitamin through liver damage or by the action of the coumarin group of anticoagulant drugs.

Therapeutic uses
Vitamin K_1 is the most effective compound as an antidote to haemorrhage due to overdosage of coumarin anticoagulant; in conditions in which poor absorption is the cause of deficiency, various analogues may be substituted for the natural vitamin K_1.

In haemorrhage due to anticoagulant drugs 10 mg vitamin K_1 is administered intramuscularly or by slow intravenous injection. The prothrombin level should be estimated after 3 hours and a further dose given if necessary. A low prothrombin level alone may be treated by giving 5–10 mg vitamin K_1 by mouth.

For the prophylaxis or treatment of haemorrhagic disease of the newborn a single dose of vitamin K_1 (0.5–1 mg) may be given intramuscularly to the infant or a synthetic substitute by mouth to the mother before delivery.

In haemorrhagic disease associated with poor absorption or utilisation, either vitamin K_1 or a synthetic analogue such as menadiol (synkavit) may be used.

WATER-SOLUBLE VITAMINS

Vitamin B complex
In 1890 Eijkman showed that rice polishings contained a water-soluble substance which was essential to life and distinct from the antiscorbutic vitamin. This substance was found to be widely distributed in the germ of seeds and in many other vegetable and animal foods. Subsequent work has shown that the term vitamin B covers a large group of different substances. At least eleven crystalline compounds have been separated and are associated with some specific function in animal nutrition. The chief factors identified are as follows:
  1. Thiamine or aneurine (vitamin B_1).
  2. Riboflavine (vitamin B_2).
  3. Nicotinic acid and nicotinic acid amide.
  4. Pyridoxine (vitamin B_6).
  5. Folic acid (pteroylglutamic acid).
  6. Cyanocobalamin (vitamin B_{12}).
  7. Pantothenic acid or filtrate factor which prevents dermatitis in chickens.
  8. Biotin (vitamin H_1). Prevents egg-white dermatitis.
  9. Choline. Essential for growth of rats, chickens and dogs.
  10. Para-aminobenzoic acid.
  11. Inositol.

Thiamine, aneurine (vitamin B_1)
The chief natural sources of this vitamin are the outer layers of grain, e.g. wheat and rice; good supplies are also available in bacon and yeast. Thiamine and other B group vitamins are synthesised by the bacteria of the intestine

Thiamine hydrochloride

and this endogenous supply may partly make good a deficient intake of these vitamins in the diet. Thiamine is essential for the normal intermediate metabolism of carbohydrate; thiamine pyrophosphate (cocarboxylase) acts as a coenzyme required in the decarboxylation of pyruvic acid to acetaldehyde. Cocarboxylase prevents the accumulation of pyruvate which is toxic to the organism. Vitamin B_1 plays a role in the synthesis of acetylcholine in nerves.

Thiamine deficiency
A deficiency of vitamin B_1 affects particularly functions of the nervous system and the heart involving metabolism of carbohydrates. The liver, gastrointestinal tract and muscle are also affected.

After about twenty days on a vitamin B_1 deficient diet, pigeons develop polyneuritis. Thiamine lack arrests the growth of young rats and their heart rate falls from about 520 to 350 per minute (bradycardia).

Beri-beri occurs chiefly amongst the rice-eating peoples of the East, and its incidence has increased since the introduction of polished rice. White bread, which contains no thiamine, is the staple article of diet during the winter months in parts of Newfoundland and Labrador, and several epidemics of beri-beri have appeared there.

Infantile beri-beri was at one time a fearful scourge in the Philippine Island and in 1909 it was found that this disease was causing a mortality of 56 per cent. The Philippine Government in 1914 arranged for the free distribution of rice polishings to infants suffering from this disease, and this extract was found to produce a complete cure in a few days.

The chief feature of beri-beri is peripheral neuritis, and there are two forms of this disease; in the dry form the nervous lesions are accompanied by great wasting, while in the wet type there is oedema associated with heart failure.

Partial deficiency of thiamine is likely to occur in persons who are on a restricted diet for a long time. Experiments on human subjects have shown that thiamine deficiency may develop in from one to three months on a diet limited to 0.22 mg of thiamine per 1000 calories. The symptoms disappear after the intake is raised to 0.5 mg per 1000 calories. Other observers have reported signs of deficiency after four to nine weeks on diets supplying 0.64 mg of thiamine per day. Certain individuals fail to become thiamine deficient even on diets containing only 0.1 mg per day and indeed continue to excrete large quantities of thiamine in the faeces. It must be concluded that in these subjects thiamine is synthesised by the bacteria in the intestine.

Partial vitamin B_1 deficiency in man leads to mental symptoms including depression, irritability and failure to concentrate. Peripheral symptoms include tenderness and weakness of the calf muscles, paraesthesia and hyperaesthesia and reduced tendon reflexes. Electrocardiographic changes show the development of cardiomyopathy. General complaints include weakness, anorexia and stomach upsets and loss of weight. Most of these changes are reversed by the administration of thiamine, but changes due to peripheral neuritis are sometimes irreversible.

Daily requirements
An adult requires about 1 to 1.5 mg thiamine hydrochloride daily. Nursing and pregnant women usually require more than this amount. If diets contain a high proportion of carbohydrate, an adequate allowance of aneurine should be available for metabolism of glucose; a ratio of 0.6 mg aneurine per 1000 calories is adequate.

Therapeutic uses
Thiamine has been used with success in the treatment of progressive polyneuritis and alcoholic neuritis. It has also been found to increase appetite in patients recovering from chronic diseases. Some types of heart disease, e.g. in chronic alcoholism, are due to insufficient absorption of thiamine from the gastrointestinal tract and are benefited by administration of this vitamin.

Thiamine is usually taken by mouth but it may also be given intramuscularly or intravenously when absorption from the gastrointestinal tract is deficient. The dose required for the treatment of beri-beri is about 25 mg daily.

Riboflavine (vitamin B_2)
This substance is the colouring matter present in skimmed milk. It also occurs in considerable quantities in meat, liver and young green vegetables. It can also be synthesised by bacteria in the intestine. Riboflavine is a stable compound

Riboflavine

which is not destroyed by the normal processes of cooking unless the food is cooked whilst exposed to light or the medium is strongly alkaline. Riboflavine phosphate acts as the prosthetic group of the yellow respiratory enzyme which Warburg has shown to constitute a portion of the normal oxidative mechanism of living cells and which plays an essential role in the oxidation of carbohydrate. Several other enzyme systems in the body have been shown to contain riboflavine as a coenzyme.

Riboflavine may be assayed by the intensity of its fluorescence in aqueous solution or by its effect on the growth rate of rats or microorganisms.

Riboflavine deficiency
Animals fed on a riboflavine deficient diet fail to grow and develop inflammatory lesions of the mucous membrane and skin.

Riboflavine deficiency in man is characterised by lesions of the lips, tongue, skin of the face, eyes and scrotum or vulva. The usual manifestations are redness and soreness of the lips along the lines of closure, and fissures at the angles of the mouth, seborrhoeic accumulation on the alae nasi and nasolabial folds and on the ears. The tongue is often sore and magenta coloured. Scrotal dermatitis is one of the easiest signs of riboflavine deficiency. The eyes may be affected and photophobia, impairment of visual acuity, congestion of the sclera and interstitial keratitis occur. Examination of the eyes with the slit-lamp microscope shows an invasion of the cornea by capillaries. Deficiency of riboflavine during pregnancy may cause skeletal deformities in the foetus.

The probable human requirement of riboflavine is about 2 mg per day. For the treatment of riboflavine deficiency 3 to 10 mg daily either orally or parenterally may be used.

Nicotinic acid (niacin)

This compound has a curious history. In 1913 Funk claimed that it was vitamin B. This was disproved and no further interest was taken in the compound until 1935, when Elvehjem showed that it was the curative factor for pellagra. It has also been called the PP or pellagra-preventing factor.

Nicotinic acid amide (Nicotinamide)

Nicotinic acid

Nicotinic acid occurs in meat, liver and yeast and can be synthesised by the bacteria of the human intestine. Nicotinamide, the amide of nicotinic acid, is a constituent part of the coenzymes, diphosphopyridine nucleotide and triphosphopyridine nucleotide, which are present in all living cells. These coenzymes when attached to specific proteins function in oxidation-reduction systems by virtue of their ability to accept hydrogen atoms from certain substrates and transfer them to other hydrogen accepting substrates such as the flavine enzymes. Nicotinic acid is thus required for a number of reactions which are essential for the survival of the cell.

Nicotinic acid deficiency

When dogs are fed on a diet deficient in nicotinic acid, the resistance of the oral cavity to infection is lowered and necrotic areas swarming with Vincent's organisms appear. This condition is known as 'black tongue' which is believed to be analogous to human pellagra. Experimental 'pellagra' has been produced in monkeys and in other animals. These conditions can be cured by the administration of nicotinic acid.

Pellagra is a multiple deficiency disease which occurs in countries where the population is poorly nourished and often maize is the staple diet. Although nicotinic acid deficiency is one of the main factors in pellagra, a lack of other B vitamins is also involved. Pellagra is characterised by disturbances of the skin, gastrointestinal tract and central nervous system: dermatitis, diarrhoea and dementia. Loss of weight, asthenia, digestive disturbances and infections of the mouth and throat are characteristic of the prodromal stage of pellagra and may be due to a deficiency of nicotinic acid. Pellagrous dermatitis is usually confined to parts of the body exposed to light. Pellagra is probably not a simple nicotinic acid deficiency disease, but also involves deficiency of other members of the vitamin B complex.

The daily requirement of nicotinic acid is difficult to assess and is probably about 15 to 20 mg.

Therapeutic uses

In the treatment of pellagra, nicotinic acid or nicotinamide is given by mouth in doses of 100 mg three times daily; or 20 mg may be administered intravenously in normal saline two or three times daily. Nicotinic acid produces a marked transient vasodilation of the face, trunk and upper extremities, without causing a fall of blood pressure. Dilatation occurs mainly in the vessels of the skin and of the pia arachnoid. Nicotinic acid has been found to relieve headache, an injection of 100 mg intravenously being usually effective within 2 to 3 minutes. It is also used in the treatment of Menière's disease. Nicotinic acid, but not nicotinamide, is used in the treatment of certain types of hyperlipidaemias.

Pyridoxine (vitamin B_6)

The activity of naturally occurring 'vitamin B_6' is due to several closely related derivatives of pyridine, the most important of which are pyridoxine, pyridoxal and pyridoxamine. The physiological function of vitamin B_6 is concerned with the metabolism of protein. Like other vitamins, pyridoxine acts in the form of coenzymes called pyridoxal-5-phosphate and pyridoxamine phosphate. These coenzymes help to catalyse a number of reactions involved in the metabolism of amino acids. As a coenzyme for decarboxylation of amino acids, pyridoxine plays an important part in brain metabolism, particularly in the formation of brain amines required for synaptic transmission.

Pyridoxine hydrochloride

Deficiency of vitamin B_6 in animals can be produced either by feeding a diet lacking the vitamin or by administering an analogue such as desoxypyridoxine or the tuberculostatic drug isoniazid, which antagonise the action of the vitamin by preventing the attachment of the coenzyme pyridoxal-5-phosphate to the apoenzyme of the various amino-acid decarboxylases. The signs of vitamin B_6 deficiency in animals are retarded growth, anaemia, epileptiform fits and lesion of the skin. Although vitamin B_6 deficiency in man is rare, several cases of this deficiency have been observed in infants who developed convulsions when fed with canned autoclaved milk. Convulsions following the administration of isoniazid have also been reported which were counteracted by the administration of pyridoxine.

Pyridoxine has been found to prevent peripheral neuritis in patients receiving large doses of isoniazid without significantly interfering with its therapeutic action (p. 423).

A group of inherited defects have recently been discovered, collectively referred to as *vitamin B_6-dependent states,* which include various inborn errors of metabolism. In these patients the tissue levels of pyridoxine are normal but its binding to the apoenzyme appears to be impaired. They are benefited by the administration of additional amounts of pyridoxine.

The daily requirement for vitamin B_6 has been estimated to be about 2 mg.

Folic acid (pteroylglutamic acid) (p. 207)

This is a factor essential for the growth of *lactobacillus casei* and certain other micro-organisms and for haematopoesis in animals. It has a complex chemical structure which is built up of glutamic acid, *p*-aminobenzoic acid and a substituted pteridine. It is converted in the body to a formyl derivative folinic acid which is its physiologically active form. Folic acid is necessary for the synthesis of compounds such as purines, pyrimidines and certain amino acids. It is present in a combined form or 'conjugate' in liver, yeast, milk and green vegetables.

Folic acid

Folic acid deficiency

Lack of this vitamin prevents the normoblastic process of blood formation from the megaloblastic stage. This deficiency may arise either from diminished intake of foodstuffs containing the conjugated vitamin or from failure to break down or utilise the conjugate. In man folic acid is formed by bacterial action in the intestine; destruction of the bacterial flora by administration of sulphaguanidine causes anaemia which can be cured by the administration of folic acid. The cytotoxic effects of folic acid analogues are discussed on page 380.

In patients with nutritional macrocytic anaemia and the macrocytic anaemias of sprue, pellagra or pregnancy, folic acid produces a favourable blood response and remarkable clinical improvement. In the treatment of Addisonian pernicious anaemia, folic acid improves the blood picture, but the neurological symptoms are not controlled and may even be aggravated (p. 207).

The daily requirements of folic acid in the non-pregnant person are about 100 micrograms but during the last three months of pregnancy the daily requirement may be about 500 micrograms. Prophylactic administration of folic acid to poorly nourished women who have frequent pregnancies is advocated by many clinicians especially during the last trimester.

Cyanocobalamin (vitamin B_{12})

This is a red crystalline substance which has been isolated from liver and from cultures of the organism *streptomyces griseus*, which also produces streptomycin. It has a very complex structure built round an atom of cobalt. In addition to cyanocobalamin a number of other closely related cobalamins with vitamin B_{12} activity have been isolated. Vitamin B_{12} is a factor essential for the growth of micro-organism *lactobacillus lactis Dorner* and stimulates growth in rats and pigs. Small amounts of cyanocobalamin or hydroxycobalamin (vitamin B_{12a}) when injected intramuscularly in patients with pernicious anaemia produce a characteristic reticulocyte response and remission of the disease. These actions are discussed on page 206.

Other members of vitamin B group

Pantothenic acid (vitamin B_5), biotin (vitamin H), choline, para-aminobenzoic acid and inositol are essential growth factors and experimentally induced deficiency of these factors produces characteristic changes in animals. They all seem to be present in adequate quantities in foodstuffs or are formed by bacterial action in the intestine. It is not known if deficiency of these substances occurs in man and their therapeutic uses have not been established.

Ascorbic acid (vitamin C)

This substance, formerly known as the anti-scrobutic vitamin, was shown by Svirbely and Szent-Györgi to be a carbohydrate of relatively simple structure. Ascorbic acid

Ascorbic acid

is a strong reducing agent and plays a part in cellular oxidation-reduction reactions. It appears to be particularly important for the formation of bone, teeth, and collagen tissues. High concentrations of ascorbic acid are present in the adrenal cortex from which it can be released by the administration of ACTH.

The most important natural sources of ascorbic acid are fresh fruit and green vegetables. Blackcurrants, lemons and oranges contain large amounts of the vitamin and preparations of these fruits in the form of juice or syrup are extensively used. Rose-hip syrup is specially rich in vitamin C (200 mg per 100 ml). Dried grain contains little ascorbic acid but it is formed in large quantities during germination and hence it can be obtained by allowing dried peas or grain to germinate. Potatoes do not contain large amounts but are an important source of the vitamin, since they are eaten in large quantities.

Ascorbic acid is now synthesised on a commercial scale. L-Ascorbic acid is the active form whilst the D-isomer is inactive. It is stable in the pure crystalline form and is fairly stable in acid solutions but disappears rapidly from foods when these are cooked or preserved at room temperature. The vitamin C content of cow's milk is not significantly decreased when it is pasteurised or dried.

Ascorbic acid may be estimated biologically on guinea-pigs fed on a scurvy producing diet. A chemical method is commonly used in which the reducing power of ascorbic acid can be detected by an indicator, 2:6 dichlorphenol indophenol.

Vitamin C deficiency

Deprivation of ascorbic acid causes in the guinea pig a decrease in weight in about two weeks, with the onset of scurvy in about three weeks, and death from acute scruvy in about four weeks. The chief signs are tenderness and swelling of the joints, tenderness of the gums and loosening of the teeth. Post-mortem haemorrhages are found all over the body, and rarefaction of the long bones is also present.

Deprivation of ascorbic acid affects the cardiovascular system causing injury to the capillary endothelium. It appears to be of importance also in regard to the normal development of the gums, teeth and skeleton, processes which were formerly believed to be entirely dependent on vitamin D. In experiments made on scorbutic guinea pigs it was found that wounds do not heal firmly owing to disorganised arrangement of fibroblasts. Ascorbic acid appears to be necessary for the formation of firm scar tissue and in its absence fractures do not unite because callus is not formed.

Clinical effects. In the classical descriptions of scurvy great prominence was given to the effect produced on the cardiovascular system, especially the diminished power of the capillary walls to resist pressure. The earliest clinical manifestation of vitamin C deficiency is follicular hyperkeratosis followed by perifollicular haemorrhage. The chief symptoms in adults are sore and bleeding gums, diarrhoea, oedema and haemorrhages, which may occur in any part of the body; there is also great muscular weakness. Scurvy develops in infants fed on a scorbutic diet at about the age of eight months. The growth is not affected and the disease may occur in large, fat children. The most striking symptoms are sore gums, pain and tenderness in the limbs associated with periosteal haemorrhages, especially in the lower limbs.

The earliest evidence in infants are skeletal changes in the ankles and wrists which can be demonstrated radiologically. Capillary fragility is increased as shown by an increase in the number of petechiae formed when a blood pressure cuff is inflated above the elbow.

The adequacy of the daily supply of ascorbic acid has been tested quantitatively by measuring the amount which is excreted in the urine. Daily test doses of ascorbic acid are given by mouth until the vitamin can be detected in the urine; the lower the past intake of vitamin the poorer the degree of saturation of the tissues and hence the greater the delay until it appears in the urine. In this way the vitamin C status of the patient can be assessed.

Daily requirements

Whilst many mammals can synthesise vitamin C the human organism cannot do so. An adult requires from 25 to 75 mg ascorbic acid daily; in the absence of infection or pregnancy a daily intake of about 20 mg is probably the minimum requirement.

The requirements of infants as advocated by various authorities range from 20 to 50 mg daily. These amounts can usually be supplied by the nursing mother. Cow's milk however has only one-sixth to one-half the ascorbic acid content of human milk and for artificially fed infants a supplementary intake of ascorbic acid is necessary.

In common with other vitamins, ascorbic acid requirements are increased during periods of metabolic strain such as pregnancy and infection. An adequate intake of the vitamin is also necessary to ensure the normal healing of wounds and fractures.

Therapeutic uses

The only absolute indication for vitamin C is in the prevention and relief of symptoms associated with scurvy. In the treatment of adult scurvy it may be necessary to administer up to 500 mg daily.

In addition to its use in scurvy, the administration of vitamin C has been suggested as an aid to recovery or for prevention in a variety of diseases. These suggestions are supported by common individual experience although controlled data are lacking.

It has been shown that in many infectious diseases the level of ascorbic acid in the body becomes very low and on this basis large doses of vitamin C have been advocated to hasten recovery from infections, or to prevent the common cold. Vitamin C is frequently given to promote wound healing after surgery or dental extractions. Vitamin C supplements are frequently given to artificially fed babies since cow's milk is not a reliable source of the vitamin.

VITAMIN CONTENT OF DIETS

The raw materials of man's diet, before they are finally consumed, may be subjected to several processes. Since vitamins are unstable substances and are present in relatively small amounts, it follows that as a result of these processes, the vitamin content of the end product may be much less than that of the raw material. Modern milling removes germ and seed coverings thus enhancing the keeping properties of flour which is important in days of long distance transport. But in the process most of the vitamins are also removed. Drummond estimated that the intake of thiamine in the early nineteenth century was 700–800 units daily but that when the new methods of milling emerged, this was reduced to 200–300 units. 'Bread, the staff of life, has been reduced by roller mills to a broken reed.'

Most vitamins except vitamin C are stable at the temperatures used in domestic cooking and the diminished vitamin content of cooked foods is due to the loss of the vitamins by extraction or to their destruction when food is kept hot for prolonged periods or reheated. Since the water-soluble vitamins are extractable, their availability depends on whether the cooking liquor plus extractions is retained and used along with the solids. Storage of raw food results in loss of vitamin C; this applies particularly to apples and root vegetables. Modern methods of canning have shown that it is possible to preserve most of the vitamin content of foods. This is important in the case of fruits which cannot be kept long in a raw state. Experiments have shown that animals can be maintained in health on a diet consisting entirely of canned foods.

Owing to the synthesis on a commercial scale of several of the vitamins it is now possible to restore lost vitamins to foodstuffs or to fortify them with additional ones. The former is of great value with respect to the grain foods which provide the commonest and cheapest source of food energy. Vitaminised margarine, containing additional vitamins A and D, is a further contribution, so that a bread and margarine diet to-day is greatly improved.

There is still a gross difference in health between the poor and the rich, a difference due in part to deficient vitamin supply, which can be seen in the slower rate of growth of poor children and the higher incidence of disease.

The proper combination and use of natural foods is a prime factor in the prevention of diseases and in increasing resistance to infection. Information derived from animal experiments only provides a limited guidance as regards the effects of vitamin lack in human malnutrition. Animal experiments are designed to demonstrate as rapidly as possible the effects of a total lack of a single factor from an otherwise adequate diet. In human malnutrition there is usually a partial deficiency of most of the vitamins. A balanced diet offers the maximum security. Towards this end many attempts have been made to lay down standards of food requirements which would ensure a high level of health and vitality. The Food and Nutrition Board of the National Research Council, U.S.A., recommended standard daily levels of intake for adult men and women (including pregnant and nursing) and children. These recommendations are shown in Table 28.1.

Table 28.1 Recommended daily vitamin allowances

		Infants 0-6 months	Children 1-4 yr	Adults male	fem	preg	lact
Vit A activity	iu	1400	2000	5000	4000	5000	6000
Vit D	iu	400	400	400	400	400	400
Vit E activity	iu	4	5	12-15	12	15	15
Ascorbic acid	mg	35	40	45	45	60	80
Folic acid	ug	50	100	400	400	800	600
Niacin	mg	5	9	16-20	16	14-18	16-20
Riboflavin	mg	0.4	0.8	1.5-1.8	1.4	1.4-1.7	1.6-1.9
Thiamin	mg	0.3	0.7	1.2-1.6	1.2	1.3-1.5	1.3-1.5
Vitamin B_6	mg	0.3	0.6	1.6-2.0	2.0	2.5	2.5
Vitamin B_{12}	ug	0.3	1.0	3.0	3.0	4.0	4.0

Adapted from *Report of Food and Nutrition*, 1974. US Nat. Acad. Sci. 8th rev.ed.

PREPARATIONS

Vitamin A (Retinol) proph 1.5–2.5 mg dl ther 3–15 mg dl
Vitamin B_1 (Thiamine, Aneurine) proph 2–5 mg dl, ther 25–100 mg dl
Vitamin B_2 (Riboflavine) proph 1–4 mg dl, ther 5–10 mg dl
Vitamin B_6 (Pyridoxine, Pyridoxal and Pyridoxamine) pyridoxine deficiency 10–20 mg dl
Vitamin B_{12} (Cyanocobalamin) (Hydroxocobalamin). B_{12} defic:hydroxocobalamin 30–50 μg dl for 7–10 d followed by 100 μg/week until remiss; maint 100 μg/month
Vitamin C (L-Ascorbic Acid) proph 25–75 mg dl; ther 200–600 mg dl

Vitamin D
Calciferol (Ergocalciferol, Vitamin D_2, Irradiated Ergosterol) prevent 20 μg (100 u) dl, treatm rickets osteomalacia 0.125–1.25 mg dl; treatm hypoparathyr 1.25–5 mg dl
Cholecalciferol (Activated 7-Dehydrocholesterol, Vitamin D_3) same dose as calciferol
Calcifediol (25-Hydroxycholecalciferol) active metabolite of calciferol or cholecalciferol 1,25-Dihydroxycholecalciferol, active metabolite of calcifedol by hydroxylation in the kidneys
Vitamin E (α-Tocopherol) 5–30 u
Vitamin K_1 (Phytomenadione) 5–20 mg slow i.v. infus

FURTHER READING

De Luca H F, Paaren H E, Schnoes H K 1979 Vitamin D and calcium metabolism. Topics in current chemistry 83. Springer, Berlin

Irving J T 1973 Calcium and phosphorus metabolism. Academic Press, New York

Metzler D E 1977 Biochemistry. The chemical reactions of living cells. Academic Press, New York

Paul A A, Southgate D A T 1978 The composition of foods. Medical Research Council Special Report. Her Majesty's Stationery Office, London

Sebrell W H, Harris R S (ed) 1967 The vitamins (vol I–VII). Academic Press, New York

SECTION SIX

Chemotherapy of tumours and infections

29. Cytotoxic drugs in the treatment of cancer

Genetic makeup of the cancer cell 375; Role of immunological factors in cancer 375; Tumour-specific antigens 375; Immunosuppressive effects of anticancer drugs 376; Cancer due to immunosuppressive drugs 376; Chemical induction of cancer 376; General principles of anticancer therapy 376; The cell cycle 377; Drug resistance 377; Testing anticancer drugs 377; Alkylating agents 378; Antimetabolites 379; Antitumour agents of natural origin 381;!u Hormones in the treatment of cancer 382; Unwanted effects of cytotoxic drugs 383; Choice of anticancer drugs 383; Treatment of cancer 384.

Genetic make-up of the cancer cell

It is generally assumed that cancer cells originate from normal cells by a genetic mutation involving the suppression or abolition of growth control. The mechanism by which this is brought about is beginning to be understood through studies of certain virus-induced cancers in animals.

Although no true cancers of man have as yet been definitely proved to be caused by viruses, several animal tumours, including monkey tumours and breast cancer in mice, have been produced in this way. Of special interest are those tumour viruses, such as the polyoma virus of mice which are composed essentially of the genetic material desoxyribonucleic acid (DNA). If a tissue culture of fibroblastic cells is exposed to polyoma virus, the virus may grow vegetatively destroying the cell and releasing large numbers of newly synthesised virus particles; alternatively some cells may survive and transform into cancer cells showing new hereditary characteristics. The operative transforming unit is viral DNA which becomes associated with the DNA of the host chromosomes altering the hereditary make-up (genotype) of the cell. The new genotype is retained by all the descendants of the transformed cell.

The change in the genotype alters the behaviour (phenotype) of the cell which acquires the ability to grow unrestrictedly in the tissues of a host, giving rise to a tumour. A genetic change leading to tumour growth is called 'neoplastic transformation'. Other factors which can initiate tumour growth through changes in the DNA apparatus, as demonstrable by chromosome abnormalities, are X-rays and certain mutagenic chemicals such as alkylating agents.

It is now recognised that in addition to enzymes necessary for DNA replication and recombination, cells also possess mechanisms that can repair DNA damaged by radiations or mutagenic chemicals and thus help to maintain normal cell viability. The function of these mechanisms is to repair DNA strands that have been damaged by exposure to sunlight or the carcinogenic chemicals in the environment; without their protective function the incidence of malignancies due to environmental damage would be much greater.

Role of immunological factors in cancer

The occurrence of some form of immunological control of tumour growth has been suggested by the finding that although complete regression of proved cancer is rare, some tumours regress partially or grow unusually slowly and only a small fraction of tumour emboli probably manifest themselves as metastases. It is probable that immunological mechanisms are responsible for the elimination of small clusters of malignant cells but it seems unlikely that these mechanisms are very powerful since the invading cells are not foreign to the body.

The absence of a powerful immune response has therapeutic implications which distinguish cancer chemotherapy from the chemotherapy of infections. A drug which inhibits the growth of a micro-organism without destroying it may nevertheless be curative since the defence mechanisms of the body can ultimately eliminate the invader, but in order to cure a malignant growth, a drug must eliminate all or nearly all the malignant cells. It has been shown that the administration of a single malignant cell may kill an animal; thus one leukaemic cell injected into a compatible mouse can multiply and ultimately cause death of the animal from leukaemia.

Tumour-specific antigens

Tumour-specific transplantation antigens were first demonstrated in 3-methylcholantrene-induced sarcomas in inbred (syngeneic) mice and shown to produce immunity against subsequent challenges with the same tumour. Tumour rejection antigens have also been detected in polyoma virus-induced mouse tumours. These antigens are present on the cell surface and they may be detected by *in vivo* rejection of transplanted tumour cells or by *in vitro* serological tests such as membrane immunofluorescence.

Evidence for tumour-specific immune reactions in human cancer is scarce and confined to only a few types of malignant growth. In *Burkitt's lymphoma*, which occurs most frequently in African children, the patient's serum contains antibody reacting with the surface of lymphoma cells. The antibody also reacts with a herpes group virus referred to as the Epstein-Barr virus suggesting a possible viral aetiology of the lymphoma. In *acute leukaemia* antibodies against their own leukaemic cells are found in the serum of some patients. There is some evidence of a host immunological reaction in *malignant melanoma* and in *neuroblastoma* a condition in which spontaneous regressions may occur.

Immunosuppressive effects of cytotoxic drugs

Cytotoxic drugs have been shown to suppress the immune response in experimental animals by inhibiting the proliferation of antibody forming cells. This has been demonstrated, for example, by the induction of tolerance to skin homografts by cytotoxic drugs. The drugs 6-mercaptopurine and azathioprine (Imuran) are particularly effective in this respect (see below). This property of cytotoxic drugs is made use of in tissue transplantation but increases its hazards by making the patient less able to deal with intercurrent infections.

Cyclosporin is a recently introduced immunosuppressive drug which appears to affect specifically reactions dependent on lymphocyte proliferation. It has been found effective in inhibiting transplantation immunity reactions.

Immunosuppression and cancer

It is believed that cell-mediated delayed hypersensitivity reactions may contribute to immunosurveillance suggesting that factors which cause defects in the immune system will facilitate tumour growth. This appears, indeed, to be the case. Thus patients receiving drugs such as azathioprine (Imuran) to control immune reactions during transplantation surgery show an increased incidence of malignant disease, especially of the lymphoreticular system. Patients receiving anti-lymphocyte serum during transplantation surgery also tend to develop lymphoreticular malignancies.

The chemical induction of cancer

The occurrence of cancer amongst tar workers led to experiments which showed that when certain tar products are applied to the skin of rats and mice they produce cancer. Kennaway synthesised the first chemical carcinogen, 3:4 benzpyrene, after isolating it from coal tar.

Several other chemical carcinogens were discovered through investigations into environmental cancer in man. Some examples of these are shown in Table 29.1. Industrial carcinogens are further discussed on page 472.

It is not known whether any normal body constituent can cause cancer. It has been claimed that large doses of oestrogens are carcinogenic but this has not been substantiated. Boyland has shown that metabolites of the amino acid tryptophan are carcinogenic; this finding may have clinical significance since abnormalities of tryptophan metabolism have been detected in human bladder cancer patients. A derivative of desoxycholic acid which occurs in bile, methylcholanthrene, is carcinogenic.

The relationship between smoking and cancer is discussed on page 490.

GENERAL PRINCIPLES OF CANCER CHEMOTHERAPY

The aim of cancer chemotherapy is to damage some vital mechanism in the neoplastic cell without vitally endangering the host. This aim would be easier to accomplish if some fundamental metabolic difference could be established between normal and cancer cells. Warburg considered that tumour cells differed from normal cells by their higher rate of glycolysis relative to respiration but this is now not believed to constitute a fundamental distinction.

The essential difference between malignant and non-malignant cells is the ability of the former to grow progressively. Studies on pure cell lines have revealed a number of differences in the cell membranes of malignant and non-malignant cells but it has been difficult to distinguish clearly a particular cell component which is invariably associated with malignancy. Based on studies of genetic cell segregation it has recently been suggested (Harris) that malignant cells may contain a characteristic membrane glycoprotein which has not so far been chemically identified. Such studies are of interest because they might eventually lead to an immunological basis for the diagnosis and treatment of malignant tumours.

The main characteristic of cancer cells is their immaturity and rapid growth. All cytotoxic drugs with

Table 29.1 Extrinsic carcinogenic chemicals discovered by their action in man. (After Clayson, 1966. In Ambrose & Roe, eds, *The Biology of Cancer*. Van Norstrand, London.)

Tissue of election of human cancer or related condition	People affected	Class of carcinogens	Example
Skin	Chimney sweeps Pitch and tar workers Mule-spinners	Hydrocarbons	3:4-Benzpyrene
Bladder	Chemical workers Rubber workers Dyestuffs workers	Aromatic amines	2-Naphthylamine
Lung (nose)	Metal refiners (nickel processers)	Metals	Chromium Nickel
Liver	Chemical workers (liver cirrhosis)	Tannic acid Chlorocarbons Dialkylnitrosamines	—
Bone and leukaemia	Dial painters Radiochemical workers	Radiochemicals	Radium

antitumour activity probably exert their effects by impairing the synthesis or function of nucleic acids which are intimately involved in the processes of cell division and growth. Many of the cytotoxic drugs also inhibit specific enzyme systems other than those associated with nucleic acid function, but it is the attack on nucleic acids, particularly DNA, that is likely to cause the most significant biological damage.

Drugs which interfere with nucleic acid function are likely to affect cells in all rapidly dividing tissues. Since the mitotic index of tumour cells is usually higher than that of surrounding normal tissue, this property could provide a basis for a specific action of cytotoxic drugs on tumour cells, were it not for the fact that certain normal tissues have a growth rate as rapid and a metabolic rate as high as tumour tissue. The turnover rate of intestinal mucosa and bone marrow cells is of the order of days, even hours, and these tissues are as susceptible to the action of cytotoxic drugs as are neoplastic tissues.

Anticancer drugs and the cell cycle

The concept of anticancer drug activity during a phase of the life cycle of proliferating malignant cells has theoretical and practical importance for cancer therapy. The life cycle of a cell is illustrated in Figure 29.1. Mitosis occupies a discrete phase of the life cycle designated as D (division). After the cell has completed division it enters the G_1 (gap 1) phase the length of which varies markedly in different tumour cells. Emerging from G_1 the cell begins a phase of active DNA synthesis, the S phase. After completing DNA synthesis the cell enters a short phase of apparent rest, the G_2 (gap 2) phase, before initiation of mitosis.

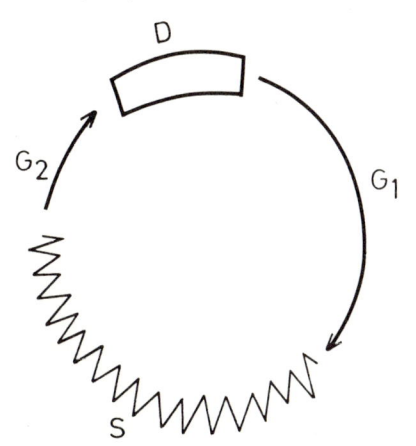

Fig. 29.1 The cell cycle: D, cell division: G_1, the phase preceding active DNA synthesis: S, the phase of DNA synthesis; G_2 the premitotic resting phase. (After Cline, 1971, *Cancer Chemotherapy*, Saunders.)

Cytotoxic drugs have been divided into phase-specific and phase-non-specific agents; the distinction, although not absolute, is of practical value. Rapidly proliferating tumours such as acute lymphoblastic leukaemia are likely to respond to agents which affect the phase of cellular DNA synthesis such as methotrexate and cytarabine. On the other hand, slowly proliferating tumours such as myeloma, in which cells divide rarely, respond to alkylating agents which damage the helical structure of DNA independently of the phase of the cell cycle.

Drug resistance

The success of cancer treatment by cytotoxic drugs is severely limited by the emergence, in the course of treatment, of cells which are less susceptible to the particular drug in use. The probable explanation for this phenomenon is the emergence, by mutation, of resistant cell variants with alternate metabolic pathways which can bypass the selective action of the cytotoxic drug. Since the toxicity of the drug for the host remains unimpaired the slight but essential margin of greater toxicity for the neoplastic cell is thus lost.

Drug resistance extends only to a particular class of anticancer agents, so that a tumour which has become resistant to one type of drug may remain fully susceptible to another. It is considered that the simultaneous use of two or more cytotoxic drugs delays the emergence of resistant cells for reasons analogous to those discussed in connection with the combined use of antituberculosis drugs (p. 419). A further advantage of the use of combinations of anticancer drugs is that their therapeutic effects tend to be additive or potentiating whilst their toxic effects may not be additive.

The testing of anticancer drugs

In a large investigation carried out by the American Cancer Society a variety of methods of screening anticancer drugs was examined. Seventy-four biological systems were studied including experimental tumours, embryonic tissues, bacteria, viruses and enzyme systems. It was concluded that tumours could not be replaced as screening tools for anticancer agents by any other biological test and that tests in a variety of animal tumours provided the best indication of activity, short of human trials which are impracticable in the initial stages.

The types of animal tumours used for drug screening may be prepared by transplant, or induced spontaneously by chemicals or viruses; they may take the form of solid tumours, ascites-producing tumours or leukaemias. A measure of chemotherapeutic activity in solid tumours which is frequently used is the ratio T/C of the weight of treated (T) and untreated control (C) tumours. The toxicity of the anticancer drug is usually determined first from dose-mortality curves and a dose at which say four out of six animals survive is then injected into the treatment group of animals.

When large numbers of potential anticancer drugs are being screened sequential methods of analysis may be adopted in order to eliminate the less promising compounds consistently. An example of a two-stage sequential procedure is shown in Table 29.2.

After the initial screening procedure has been completed, the selected drugs are submitted to further testing. The activity of the new compound is compared with that of known anticancer drugs by tests on a wider range of animal tumours. The ability of the compound to induce drug resistance is examined and more extensive studies are made of its acute and delayed toxicity before evaluation in human tumour therapy is undertaken.

Table 29.2 Two-stage sequential procedure for accepting or rejecting a potential anticancer drug during initial screening. (After Schneiderman, 1961. In de Jonge, ed., *Quantitative Methods in Pharmacology*. North Holland Publ., Amsterdam.)

Test number	Critical value for cumulative T/C*	Action if critical value is Exceeded	Not exceeded
1	$(T/C)_1 = 0.44$	Reject	Test again
2	$(T/C)_1 \times (T/C)_2 = 0.19$	Reject	Accept

*See text for definition of T/C

DRUGS USED IN THE TREATMENT OF NEOPLASTIC DISEASE

The systematic use of drugs, other than radioisotopes, for the treatment of neoplastic disease began during, or shortly after, the second world war. Several groups of such drugs can be distinguished.

1. Alkylating agents

Alkylating agents are compounds capable of introducing an alkyl group into another chemical molecule. They are highly reactive and interact with a variety of functional groups found in tissues; their reactions take place under physiological conditions of temperature and hydrogen ion concentration. Most cytotoxic alkylating agents are bifunctional, i.e. they possess two reactive groups. It is believed that the bifunctional alkylating agents are highly effective because they join two adjacent functional groups on cells, a property known as 'cross-linking' which has some similarity to the cross-linking of fibres in textile processing. Although these compounds can attack many chemical groupings in the cell, their major biological effect is believed to be due to their interaction with the DNA of the cell nucleus which results in growth inhibition. Amongst widely used biological alkylating agents are *nitrogen mustards* containing the group — $N(CH_2CH_2Cl)_2$. In neutral or alkaline solution the tertiary amines undergo an intramolecular transformation with release of chloride ion to form a highly reactive cyclic ethyleneimmonium derivative as follows:

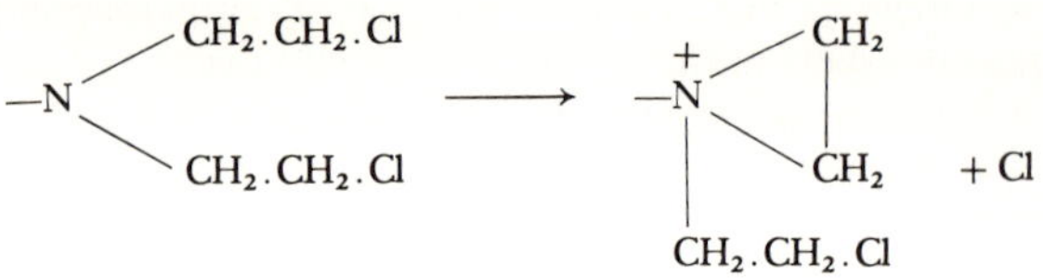

The biological activity of nitrogen mustards is related to their chemical reactivity as measured by the rate of hydrolysis of their chlorine atoms.

Pharmacological actions

The pharmacological actions of alkylating agents resemble those of ionising radiations in affecting particularly the cell nucleus. They inhibit cell division and produce genetic mutations and they also inhibit antibody formation. As already mentioned, the cytotoxic action of alkylating agents on neoplastic tissue is unspecific and related to its rapid growth rate.

Amongst body tissues the haemopoietic system is particularly affected. Within a few hours of administration of a nitrogen mustard to an experimental animal, mitosis of the bone marrow and lymph node cells ceases and disintegration of the formed elements becomes apparent. In patients lymphocytopenia may occur within a day and granulocytopenia within a few days of administration. Other tissues damaged are the reproductive organs in the male and female and the germinal epithelium of the intestine and cornea.

Clinically the alkylating agents frequently cause nausea, anorexia and vomiting, which may be decreased by the administration of a phenothiazine.

Mustine (Mechlorethamine)

This compound (Fig. 29.2) was studied as a potential war gas and the finding that it caused profound depression of the haemopoietic system led eventually to its clinical trial in the treatment of leukaemias. It was the first of the nitrogen mustards to be used in the treatment of malignant disease. Mustine is now not widely used because it is a dangerous vesicant which has to be administered by careful intravenous injection. It is however rapidly and highly effective and is still employed clinically in the initial treatment of Hodgkin's disease.

Chlorambucil (Leukeran)

This nitrogen mustard (Fig. 29.2) can be administered orally. It is a slow acting and relatively non-toxic alkylating agent. Chlorambucil is of most use in the treatment of conditions associated with proliferation of white blood cells, particularly lymphocytes.

Cyclophosphamide (Endoxana)

This compound was introduced with the aim that it should

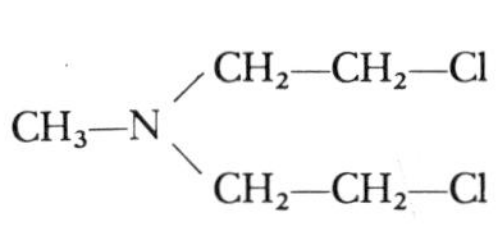

Fig. 29.2 Chemical structure of nitrogen mustards.

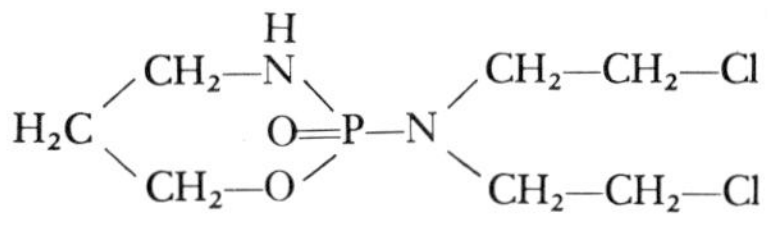

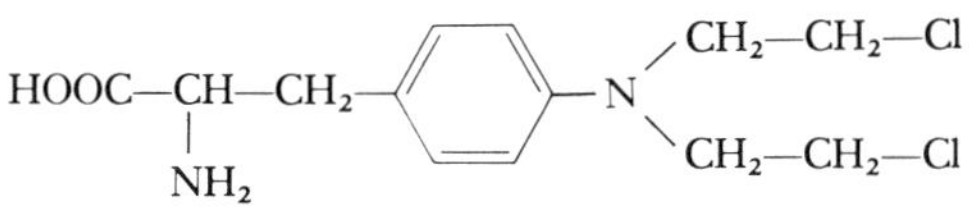

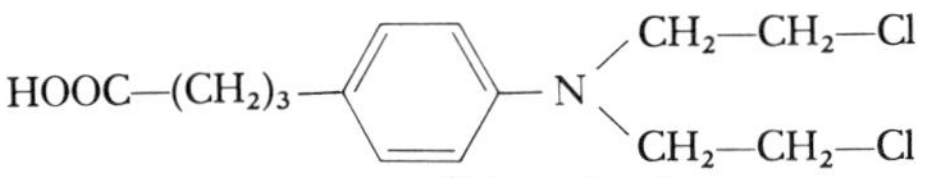

remain inert until it becomes activated by the tumour tissue thus making it more effective as an antitumour agent and less toxic to the host. In fact tumour tissue does not as a rule activate cyclophosphamide, but it becomes activated by the liver where the P–N bond of the molecule is split (Fig. 29.2).

An advantage of cyclophosphamide is that it can be administered orally in repeated small doses. Its clinical effects resemble those of nitrogen mustard and it is used in the treatment of Hodgkin's disease, lymphosarcoma and multiple myeloma. It is also used in the treatment of carcinoma of the breast. It is less liable than other alkylating agents to produce thrombocytopenia but frequently causes nausea and vomiting and often results in temporary alopecia. It may produce a haemorrhagic cystitis.

Melphalan (Alkeran) is another orally absorbed nitrogen mustard which embodies the amino acid phenylalanine in its structure (Fig. 29.2). Both the L- and D-isomers have been made, and the form containing the natural L-amino acid has been found to be five times as active biologically as the D-isomer although their chemical reactivities are identical. This illustrates the importance of the carrier molecule for cytotoxic activity.

Melphalan has been shown to produce an increase in the duration of survival of patients with multiple myeloma, particularly when given in combination with prednisolone.

Busulphan (Myleran)
This compound is a dimethanesulphonate. In low doses it selectively depresses the granulocyte count and its chief use is in the treatment of chronic myeloid leukaemia.

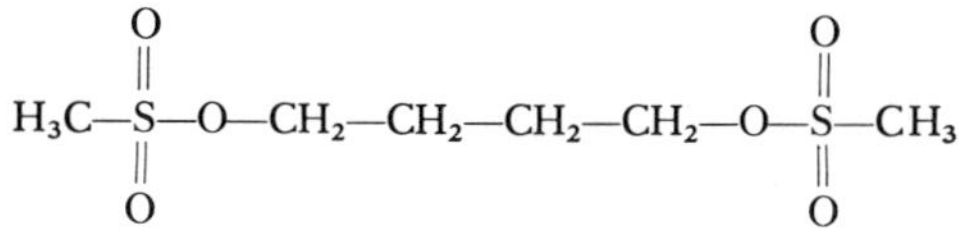

Busulphan is administered by mouth and is well absorbed; it is excreted in the urine as methanesulphonic acid. The leucocyte count usually shows a decrease within two to three weeks of starting treatment. Pigmentation of the skin frequently occurs. The drug may cause vomiting and general malaise like other alkylating agents, but its chief toxic effects are due to depression of the bone marrow with resultant granulocytopenia and thrombocytopenia.

Tretamine (triethylenemelamine, *TEM*) and *thio-TEPA* triethylene thiophosphoramide) are cytotoxic alkylating agents belonging to the ethyleneimine class.

Choice of alkylating agent
In general, alkylating agents all have the same spectrum of antitumour activity, but because of their differential effects on bone marrow cells in toxicity studies, some of them have become associated with the treatment of particular diseases. However, cross-resistance exists between the drugs and when resistance has developed to one, another alkylating agent given in comparable dose, is seldom effective.

In addition to the classical alkylating agents some newer antineoplastic compounds of different chemical structure may be functionally classified with this group.

Procarbazine (Natulan) is an antineoplastic agent which suppresses mitosis. It probably reacts directly with the DNA molecule. It is well absorbed orally. Its main use is in the treatment of Hodgkin's disease.

Dacarbazine is a recently introduced antineoplastic agent which has been found effective in the treatment of malignant melanoma and sarcomas. It may function as an alkylating agent after metabolism in the liver.

2. Antimetabolites

Antimetabolites are substances with a molecular structure similar to that of a natural metabolite which interfere with the function of the latter. These compounds were introduced for the treatment of malignant growth by

380 APPLIED PHARMACOLOGY

Farber and his colleagues who demonstrated in 1948 that the folic acid analogue aminopterin (Fig. 29.3) produced complete though temporary remissions of acute leukaemia in children.

Folic acid analogues
Folic acid (p. 369) is a vitamin which is concerned with 'one carbon' transfers, i.e. the insertion of groups containing single carbon atoms into molecules. Folic acid is enzymatically reduced in the body to tetrahydrofolic acid and related compounds such as folinic acid which are coenzymes for many essential biosynthetic reactions including the synthesis of the DNA constituent thymidylic acid. In the absence of folic acid the formation of both DNA and RNA is inhibited.

Folic acid is activated in the body by the enzyme folic reductase, and its analogues such as aminopterin and the more active methotrexate (Fig. 29.3) combine so strongly with the active site of this enzyme that the true substrate, folic acid, cannot replace them to any significant extent. The strong binding of the analogues accounts for their prolonged action and retention in the body. Early work on folic acid antagonists was carried out by Hitchings and his colleagues, who studied the interactions of folic acid and various analogues in cultures of *Lactobacillus casei* and this was followed later by their clinical use for the treatment of malignant growth.

Methotrexate (Amethopterin)
This compound is chemically closely related to folic acid (p. 369) from which it differs in two respects: by the substitution of the hydroxyl group in the 4-position in the folic acid molecule with an amino group and by an additional methyl group. Methotrexate was found to be clinically more useful than the earlier compound aminopterin in which the additional methyl group is lacking (Fig. 29.3).

When a lethal dose of methotrexate is given to an experimental animal the main lesions occur in the intestinal tract and bone marrow. The intestinal tract exhibits a severe haemorrhagic enteritis and in the circulating blood there is a progressive reduction in the leukocyte and to a lesser extent the lymphocyte count.

In children with acute lymphoblastic leukaemia methotrexate is administered by mouth in daily doses until either a remission is obtained or signs of toxicity appear such as ulceration of the mouth or diarrhoea. Resistance to methotrexate by the tumour cells develops rapidly and is usually associated with an increase in folic reductase activity.

A high percentage of favourable responses has been observed in choriocarcinoma and related trophoblastic diseases with methotrexate alone or combined with other agents. This type of tumour can be considered a partial homograft and it seems likely that the favourable results obtained in this instance are due to the combined effects of the drug and an immune reaction by the patient. In choriocarcinoma intensive courses of methotrexate may be given by intramuscular or intra-arterial injection and after each course folic acid may be used to prevent toxic side effects.

Methotrexate has also proved useful in the treatment of psoriasis and mycosis fungoides.

Purine and pyrimidine analogues
DNA and RNA are polynucleotides consisting of nucleotide subunits. Four ribonucleotides and four deoxyribonucleotides are arranged in a special sequence to form the RNA and DNA strands respectively. Each nucleotide consists of purine or pyrimidine bases attached to ribose or 2-deoxyribose. The bases in RNA are the purines adenine and guanine and the pyrimidines cytosine and uracil; in DNA uracil is replaced by thymine. The structures of purine, pyrimidine and adenylic acid, a typical nucleotide, are shown below.

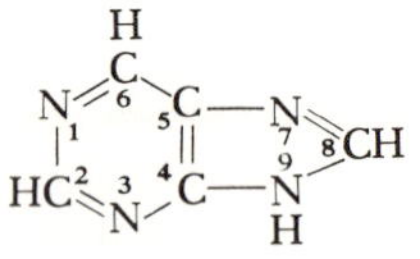

Purine

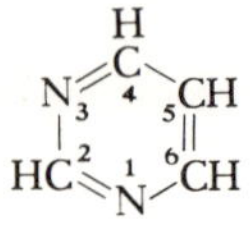

Pyrimidine

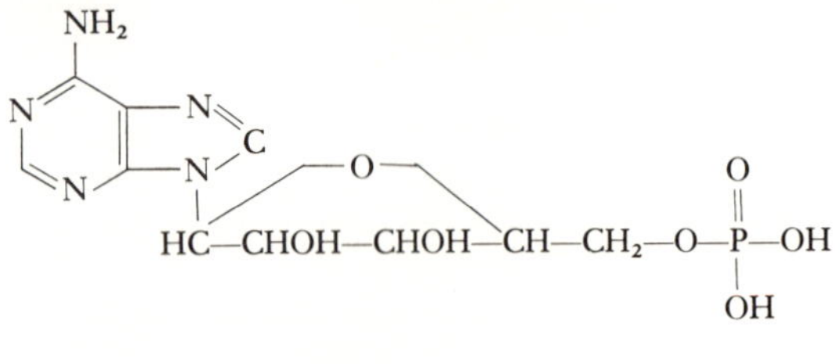

Adenylic acid

The use of purine and pyrimidine analogues as antitumour agents is based on the idea that they will

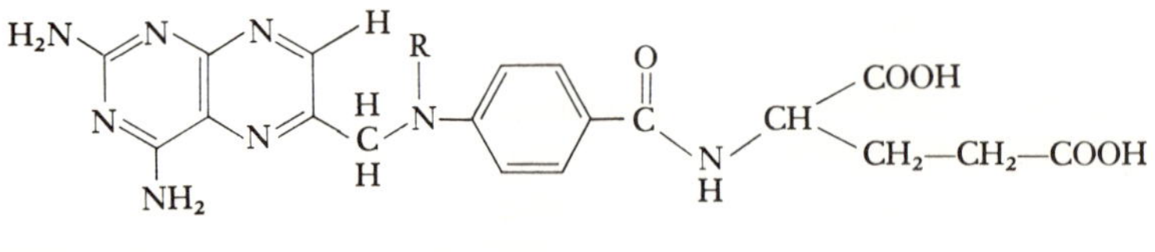

Fig. 29.3 Aminopterin (R = H), methotrexate (R = CH$_3$).

interfere with the normal synthesis of the nucleic acids of the rapidly growing tumour tissue.

Mercaptopurine (Puri-nethol)

Mercaptopurine

This compound can be considered an analogue either of adenine which is 6-aminopurine or of hypoxanthine which is 6-hydroxypurine. Its main biological effect is due not to the base itself but to its ribotide formed by the cell. The cell thus performs a 'lethal synthesis' by transforming a relatively harmless substance into one which can interfere with essential metabolic processes. It has been found that cells which have become resistant to 6-mercaptopurine have lost the enzyme required to convert the base to its ribotide.

The cellular mode of action of mercaptopurine is complex; its main actions are twofold: (1) it interferes with the conversion of inosinic acid into adenylic and guanylic acid; (2) it inhibits biosynthesis of purine by 'feedback inhibition', i.e. the excess concentration of the false metabolite inhibits an earlier stage of biosynthesis.

Mercaptopurine is usually administered by mouth. It is readily absorbed and rapidly metabolised. Clinically the drug has proved most useful in the treatment of lymphocytic leukaemia in children.

An important application of mercaptopurine is for the suppression of immune responses particularly in connection with tissue transplantation. Suppression occurs only if the drug is administered during the early period of induction of the immune response.

The initial dose of mercaptopurine is usually 2.5 mg/kg daily. Dosage must be controlled by frequent blood counts so as to avoid excessive depression of the bone marrow and it is adjusted according to the response. Resistance to the drug often develops but there is no cross resistance to other types of cytotoxic agents. Treatment with mercaptopurine is frequently combined with other cytotoxic drugs.

Thioguanine has actions and uses similar to mercaptopurine. There is cross-resistance between them.

Azathioprine (Imuran) is a related drug with actions similar to those of mercaptopurine. Its main application is as an immunosuppressive drug in tissue transplantation or in autosensitisation diseases. In organ transplantation the use of azathioprine has become almost universal. It is used in preference to mercaptopurine from which it is derived because it produces less liver damage. Its main toxic effect is bone marrow depression.

Fluorouracil is a pyrimidine derivative which has been shown to inhibit experimentally produced tumours in animals. One of its actions is to interfere with the formation of thymidylic acid which is a component of DNA. Its mode of action in this respect is analogous to that of the folic acid antagonists which produce a similar effect but by a different mechanism.

Fluorouracil is administered intravenously. It has been shown to produce improvement in about 20 per cent of patients with carcinoma of the breast, the gastrointestinal or the female genital tract. It is a highly toxic drug with a small therapeutic margin. Its initial toxic effects are anorexia and nausea followed by stomatitis and diarrhoea. It may produce severe leukopenia with attendant risk of generalised infection.

6-Azauridine is a less toxic pyrimidine analogue used in the treatment of leukaemias.

Cytarabine (Cytosine arabinoside) is an antimetabolite which inhibits the synthesis of DNA by blocking a step in pyrimidine interconversions. It inhibits the synthesis of DNA and also has antiviral properties. It is used in the treatment of acute myeloblastic leukaemia, frequently in conjunction with other antineoplastic agents such as daunorubicin, vincristine and prednisone. White cell counts should be determined regularly during treatment with cytarabine. Cytarabine is also used in the treatment of herpes infection (p. 397).

3. Antitumour agents of natural origin
A number of naturally occurring substances have been found to inhibit the growth of experimentally produced tumours in animals and some of them have been introduced into clinical practice.

Vinca alkaloids
The plant *Vinca rosea*, the periwinkle, was traditionally believed to have antidiabetic properties but this claim could not be confirmed. It was found, however, whilst investigating extracts of periwinkle, that they produced depression of the bone marrow and inhibition of tumour growth. Four alkaloids of Vinca have so far been shown to have antitumour activity and the structures of two of them, *vinblastine* (Velbe) and *vincristine* (Oncovin), have been fully elucidated.

Mechanism of action. The vinca alkaloids have been shown to exert a specific action on the mitotic cycle which is arrested at the metaphase. They are thus particularly effective in tumours undergoing frequent cell division. They produce this effect by combining with protein of intracellular microtubules causing them to be disrupted.

Clinical uses. Vinblastine has been found effective in the treatment of Hodgkin's disease and of choriocarcinoma. Successful results have been reported with vincristine for acute lymphoblastic leukaemia in children. The alkaloids may cause neurological manifestations including paraesthesias and nerve pain, and leukopenia. Drug resistance may develop but there appears to be no cross resistance between the two alkaloids. Treatment with them is often combined with other cytotoxic drugs.

Colchicine and demecoline. Colchicine, which is used clinically as a specific treatment for gout (p. 292), has long been known to be a powerful inhibitor of cell division. Concentrations of colchicine of $1:10^8$ are sufficient to produce metaphase arrest in a culture of fibroblasts. The mitotic apparatus of the cell is made of fibrous protein and colchicine may interfere with its function of mechanically separating the duplicated chromosomes.

Colchicine affects all dividing cells but in doses in which it produces antitumour effects it is too toxic for clinical use. *Demecolcine* is a less toxic derivative which has been used in place of busulphan for the treatment of myeloid leukaemia in patients who have become resistant to the latter drug.

Actinomycin. Several antimicrobial substances with antitumour activity have been isolated from species of *Streptomyces*. Various mixtures of these substances are designated by a terminal letter. Actinomycin D is a powerful antitumour and immunosuppressive agent which probably produces its effects by a direct physicochemical combination with DNA. Clinically it has been used mainly in the treatment of Wilms' kidney tumours in children in which it produces regression of pulmonary metastases.

Daunorubicin (rubidomycin) is an antibiotic which has been found successful in producing remissions in childhood lymphatic leukaemias.

Doxorubicin (adriamycin) is effective in leukaemias but also in a number of solid tumours including sarcomas.

Colaspase (asparaginase)
The development of L-asparaginase followed the observation that a substance present in normal guinea pig serum inhibited the growth of transplanted tumours in mice. This effect was found to be due to L-asparaginase, which destroyed L-asparagine on which certain tumours are dependent. In contrast, normal cells which are capable of synthesising their own asparagine are not influenced by the presence of asparaginase.

This observation is of interest since it demonstrates a specific biochemical difference between normal cells and certain neoplastic cells. In clinical trials, L-asparaginase has produced temporary remissions in patients with acute lymphoblastic leukaemia.

4. Hormones in the treatment of cancer

Hormones have been used for the treatment of tumours arising from tissues such as mammary gland, uterus and prostate whose normal growth is dependent on hormones. In addition the corticosteroid hormones are used because of their ability to suppress cell division particularly in lymphocytes.

Androgen control of prostatic cancer
Prostatic cancer cells retain many of the qualities of their normal antecedents; in particular, they respond to testosterone and more particularly its reduced metabolite 5-α-dihydrotestosterone (p. 358) by growth and production of the enzyme acid phosphatase, whilst in the absence of testosterone they shrivel. Huggins suggested in 1941, on the basis of animal experiments, that patients with prostatic carcinoma might benefit from bilateral orchidectomy. This was found to be the case and similar effects were also produced by the administration of oestrogens.

The treatment of inoperable prostatic cancer often consists in surgical removal of the testes and the administration of an oestrogen such as stilboestrol in doses of 1 mg daily. Larger doses of stilboestrol should not be used in these patients since 1 mg daily is as effective as 5 mg in reducing tumour size whilst their cardiovascular mortality has been shown to be increased by oestrogen.

Treatment of mammary cancer by oestrogens and androgens
This is based on the apparently contradictory experimental evidence that the growth of mammary cancer in women can be slowed by (1) removal of the ovaries (Bateson, 1896) and (2) treatment with oestrogens (Haddow, 1944).

In premenopausal women the treatment of choice is removal of the ovaries because the administration of oestrogen to these patients may potentiate tumour growth. On the other hand a proportion of postmenopausal women with mammary cancer are benefited by treatment with large doses of oestrogens. Androgens are given to premenopausal patients with inoperable mammary carcinoma in conjunction with removal of the ovaries. Androgens probably produce their effects by inhibiting the function of the anterior pituitary gland and also by antagonising the growth-promoting effects of natural oestrogens on malignant cells.

Corticosteroids
Corticosteroids such as prednisone are often valuable in the treatment of leukaemia and allied disorders. The characteristic effect of these drugs in producing shrinkage of lymphatic tissue is the basis of their use in the initial treatment of acute lymphatic leukaemia in childhood. Large doses of prednisone, 40 to 80 mg given daily for about four weeks, usually produce remissions which can be maintained thereafter by treatment with antimetabolite drugs. A particularly successful combination appears to be that of prednisolone and vincristine which may cause complete remissions in children with acute lymphoblastic leukaemia. Spontaneous haemorrhage associated with thrombocytopenia is a common feature of acute leukaemia and of bone marrow damage produced by X-ray treatment

or cytotoxic drugs; this complication can often be controlled by high doses of prednisone or prednisolone. Corticosteroids are also sometimes useful in suppressing the haemolytic anaemia which may occur in chronic leukaemia or malignant reticuloses.

Unwanted effects of cytotoxic drugs

Cytotoxic drugs are used not only for the treatment of malignant growth, but increasingly for other purposes such as suppression of transplantation immunity and the treatment of non-malignant conditions such as psoriasis and, on an experimental basis, rheumatoid arthritis. It is thus important to emphasise their many and serious side effects.

The effects of cytotoxic drugs can be compared to those of ionising radiations. Irradiation damage becomes manifest at the stage of mitosis when irradiated cells fail to divide and die. Rapidly dividing cells such as the epithelial cells lining the gastrointestinal tract and bone marrow cells are thus the first to show evidence of radiation injury and the first symptoms of which patients complain are anorexia, nausea and occasionally vomiting. Leucopenia soon develops accompanied by thrombocytopenia and signs of multiple bleeding.

Similar effects occur after cytotoxic drugs. There is also hair loss and ovarian and testicular function is impaired. The immune responses of the body are damaged, infections spread and mild infections may become severe or fatal. Higher doses of both radiation and cytotoxic drugs produce severe pathological changes including pneumonitis, nephritis and hepatitis.

A particular danger of cytotoxic drugs is that they may induce cancer, for example patients on immunosuppressive drugs tend to develop malignant lymphomas. Since all cytotoxic drugs are mutagenic and teratogenic they should not be used in pregnancy.

Dose-reponse curve of anticancer drugs

As illustrated in Figure 29.4 the dose-response curve of cytotoxic drugs is very steep; although this figure refers to experimental leukaemia in mice there is evidence that dose response curves of cytotoxic drugs in man are likewise steep both in respect of their chemotherapeutic action and toxicity. It follows that any increase in dosage will produce a sharp increase in toxicity but the risk may have to be taken if the aim of maximal eradication of malignant cells is to be achieved. If a remission has been accomplished, e.g. in the treatment of acute leukaemia, the patient may be maintained on a lower dosage schedule but the complete withdrawal of cytotoxic drug therapy usually leads to a rapid relapse.

Choice of anticancer drug

Antineoplastic agents do not all act on the same sites and at the same stage of the mitotic cycle. Treatment with several

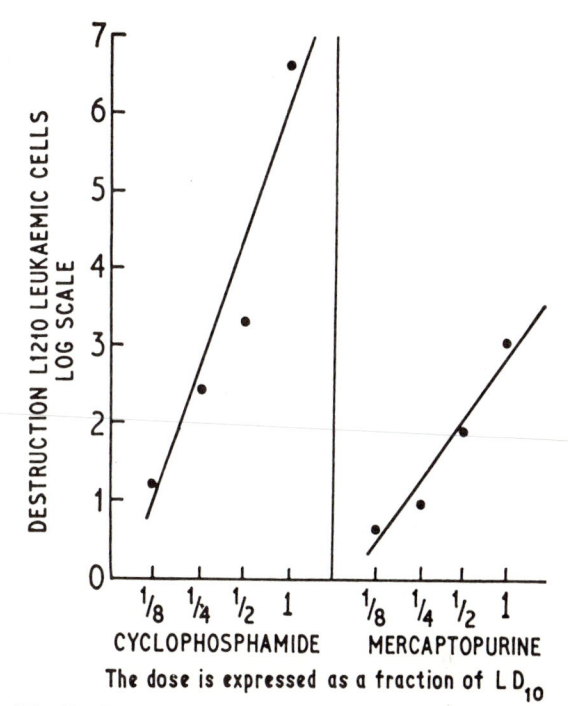

Fig. 29.4 The dose-response curve of two cytotoxic drugs (expressed as a fraction of LD_{10}) on the destruction of leukaemic cells in mice. (After Frei and Freireich, 1965, *Advances in Chemotherapy*.)

agents together or in sequence, with interruptions in the treatment to allow for recovery of function of normal cells, is usually more effective than treatment with a single agent. Also, combination therapy reduces the severity of side effects compared to those obtained with high doses of single agents.

Clinical experience with these drugs has resulted in some of them being particularly frequently used for the treatment of special forms of cancer. For the treatment of *choriocarcinoma*: methotrexate, actinomycin D and vinblastine are often used. In *Burkitt's lymphoma*: cyclophosphamide, methotrexate and vincristine. In *melanoma*: dacarbazine. In *myeloma*: melphalan and cyclophosphamide. In *neuroblastoma*: cyclophosphamide, daunorubocin and vinca alkaloids. In *Wilms' tumour*: actinomycin D and vincristine. In *Hodgkin's disease*: combination chemotherapy using alkylating agents, procarbazine, a vinca alkaloid and prednisone.

Treatment of leukaemias. Co-operative studies involving large numbers of patients have given the following results. *Acute lymphoblastic leukaemia* is best treated with cyclic or sequential regimens. To induce a remission: vincristine and prednisone are used. To maintain remission: methotrexate, mercaptopurine and cyclophosphamide. In *acute myeloid leukaemia* remissions may be induced with combinations of several of the following drugs: cytarabine, daunorubicin, thioguanine, vincristine and prednisone.

For maintenance of remission these same and other drugs may be used. In *chronic lymphatic and myeloid leukaemias* in adults palliative effects may be obtained with chlorambucil and busulphan respectively.

Administration of antineoplastic drugs. Apart from routine methods of administration their effectiveness may be increased by special techniques. Cytotoxic drugs may be injected directly into the tumour or body cavity or they may be administered by intra-arterial infusion. Isolated regional perfusion entails isolation of the blood supply of the tumour in an extracorporeal circulation so that the cytotoxic agent can be given at a high dosage. This is most easily carried out in the limbs.

Treatment of cancer
This has become a matter for the specialist. The current proven methods of treating malignant disease are by surgery, radiotherapy and chemotherapy. Immunotherapy is not yet an established method of treatment, although immunotherapy, e.g. of leukaemias, is practiced with some success in certain centres, notably in France. Various combinations of treatment are used and specialised centres have been set up in which different forms of treatment can be applied.

All the antimitotic cytotoxic drugs, including the alkylating agents, antimetabolites and naturally occurring cytotoxic agents, are sufficiently toxic to normal cells to limit seriously the doses that can be safely administered. Even colaspase, which prevents cancer cells from growing but is believed not to interfere with cell division of normal cells, produces toxic effects. The possibility of killing a sufficiently high percentage of cancer cells by chemotherapy to produce a clinical cure can be achieved only with certain exceptional neoplastic growths including choriocarcinoma, Burkitt's lymphoma and some tumours of young children such as neuroblastoma and Wilms' tumour.

Combination treatment with radiotherapy and chemotherapy is effective in Hodgkin's disease. In acute lymphoblastic leukaemia in children prognosis has now greatly improved and in some treatment centres up to 50 per cent of patients have been reported alive after 5 years. In addition to standard chemotherapy these patients must be treated for involvement of the central nervous system by leukaemic cells and for infections due to depression of the immune apparatus.

PREPARATIONS

Alkylating agents
Busulphan (Myleran) init 2–4 mg p.o. dl, maint 0.5–2 mg dl
Chlorambucil (Leukeran) 5–10 mg p.o. dl, maint 2–4 mg dl
Cyclophosphamide (Endoxana) 100–150 mg dl p.o. i.v.
Dacarbazine (DTIC) 2–4.5 mg/kg dl i.v. ia
Estramustine Phosphate (Estracyt) 15–450 mg dl by slow i.v. inj
Ethoglucid (Epodyl) 1% v/v for bladder inst
Lomustine 130 mg/m^2 p.o. every 6 w
Melphalan (Alkeran) 2–15 mg p.o. dl
Mitorbronitol (Myelobrom) 250 mg dl
Procarbazine hyd (Natulan) 50–250 mg dl
Thiotepa 15–30 mg i.v.

Antimetabolites
Axathioprine (Imuran) 100–150 mg dl p.o.
Colaspase (L-Asparaginase) 200 u/kg dl
Cytarabine (Citosine arabinoside, Cytosar) up to 2 mg/kg i.v. for 10 d
Fluorouracil (5-Fluorouracil) init 12 mg/kg i.v. for 4 d
Hydroxyurea (Hydrea) 20–30 mg/kg dl
Mercaptopurine (Puri-Nethol) 100–200 mg dl
Methotrexate (Aminopterin) 5–100 mg p.o.; also i.m. i.v.
Thioguanine (Lanvis) init 2 mg/kg p.o. dl

Antitumour agents of natural origin
Actinomycin D (Dactinomycin) 500 µg i.v. for 5 d
Daunorubicin hyd (Rubidomycin) 2 mg/kg every 4–7 d
Doxorubicin (Adriamycin) 1.2–2.4 mg/kg every 3 w
Vinblastine sulph (Velbe) 100–500 µg/kg i.v. once weekly
Vincristine sulph (Oncovin) 25–75 µg/kg i.v.

Oestrogens and progestogens
Drostanolone prop
Gestronol hexan 200 mg/w
Medroxyprogesterone acet 300 mg/d
Nandrolone phenylpropr
Norethisterone ac
Stilboestrol diphosph (Fosfoestrol)

Oestrogen antagonist
Tamoxifen citr (Nolvadex) 10–20 mg 2x die (mamm malign)

FURTHER READING

Becker F F (ed) 1977 Cancer. A comprehensive treatise. 6 vols. Plenum Press, New York
Sartorelli A C, Johns D G (ed) 1974 Part I. 1975 Part II. Antineoplastic and immunosuppressive agents. Handb. exp. Pharm. 38, I; 38, II. Springer, Berlin

30. Basic aspects of antibacterial chemotherapy

Development of chemotherapy 385; Targets for chemotherapeutic attack in the bacterial cell 386; Competition for an essential metabolite 386; Interference with DNA function 388; Inhibition of ribosome function 388; Impairment of the bacterial wall 389; Mechanism of bacterial resistance 390.

Development of chemotherapy

The name 'chemotherapy' was used by Ehrlich to define a particular type of study having as its aim the discovery of synthetic chemical substances acting specifically on infective organisms. Ehrlich believed that synthetic chemical substances could never be ideal therapeutic agents because they would always damage the host as well as the parasite, in contrast to the antitoxic sera which attacked the parasite like 'magic bullets'. The most that could be hoped for was to produce substances which were maximally 'parasitotropic' and minimally 'organotropic'. Ehrlich could hardly have foreseen that within less than 50 years of his discovery of salvarsan, penicillin would be discovered which kills micro-organisms without damaging the host. The development of chemotherapy during the present century is one of the most important therapeutic advances made in the history of medicine.

Antiprotozoal drugs. The earliest discoveries of the use of drugs to destory parasites in the body were the action of mercury in syphilis (Marcus Cumanus, 1495) and of quinine in malaria (1630). No further advances of importance were made until the first decade of this century.

Modern antiprotozoal chemotherapy was founded by Ehrlich, who commenced in 1904 a systematic search for an effective remedy for syphilis. Since that date specific drug cures have been discovered for most of the diseases caused by protozoal parasites. Although most of these important advances have been introduced by means of systematic laboratory researches, yet the methods have been essentially empirical, and remarkable practical successes have often been achieved in the absence of any definite theoretical knowledge regarding the mode of action of the drugs used.

Antibacterial drugs. Towards the end of the nineteenth century Koch attempted to cure septicaemia in animals by means of intravenous injection of drugs and tried most of the disinfectants then known without success. Research on these lines was continued for forty years, but, although powerful disinfectants were discovered, which were relatively non-toxic to animals, the results were uniformly disappointing. For example, it was found possible to inject quantities of optochin and acriflavine sufficient to render the blood of experimental animals bactericidal, but such treatment did not protect them against lethal doses of bacteria. This long history of failure was terminated by the discovery that members of the sulphonamide group, although feeble disinfectants *in vitro*, produced a remarkable antibacterial action *in vivo*.

It is of interest to note that sulphanilamide was synthesised in 1908 and sulphonamide dye in 1909. Their bacterial action was investigated by German and American workers in the years 1914-18. The dye prontosil was synthesised in 1920 and in 1933 its clinical action in curing a boy of peritonitis was reported by Foerster. In February 1935, Domagk published the results of experimental work on prontosil carried out in 1932 and of clinical investigations obtained since 1933. This publication caused immediate world-wide interest and appeared to be a sudden and revolutionary discovery, but the history outlined above shows that it had been preceded by many years of preparatory work. The introduction of the sulphonamides was the beginning of an era of effective antibacterial chemotherapy. This development has been of the utmost importance and has led to the introduction of powerful antibiotics with antibacterial action such as penicillin, streptomycin and the tetracyclines and to powerful synthetic antituberculosis drugs such as isoniazid.

Development of antibiotics

It has been known for more than 50 years that certain micro-organisms can produce substances which inhibit the growth of other micro-organisms. Such substances are termed *antibiotics*. Antibiotic substances are produced by a wide range of bacteria, fungi and actinomycetes.

The older biological work on antibiotics was rarely supported by adequate biochemical examination, and quantitative assay methods were lacking. Experience has shown that little real knowledge of an antibiotic can be expected before a quantitative method of bioassay has been devised and the substance has been isolated in a relatively pure form.

In 1936 glyotoxin was purified and isolated in a crystalline form. Glyotoxin is an antibiotic substance obtained from fungi which has a strong inhibitory action on plant pathogens. The great impetus to antibiotic research, however, arose from the discovery of the chemotherapeutic action of penicillin and its isolation in a pure form.

Antibiotics are by definition selective since they harm foreign micro-organisms without harming the organism that synthesises them; they are also selective in attacking only certain micro-organisms and in being able to differentiate between micro-organism and host. Selectivity is thus a key to the understanding of the mode of action of antibiotics.

Progress in the understanding of the mode of action of antibiotics has depended on a knowledge of bacterial morphology and biochemistry. It is now known that bacteria are surrounded by a rigid wall which can withstand considerable pressures and which contains a thin cytoplasmic membrane acting as an osmotic barrier. If the cell wall becomes weakened, the cytoplasmic membrane is unable to withstand the high osmotic pressures in the cytoplasm and it bursts. The cytoplasm itself is morphologically undifferentiated, unlike that of animal or plant cells, but it contains a variety of substances including nucleoprotein.

TARGETS FOR CHEMOTHERAPEUTIC ATTACK IN THE BACTERIAL CELL

Figure 30.1 shows various possible targets for attack by an anti-bacterial chemotherapeutic agent. Target (1) represents an active enzyme centre which a chemotherapeutic drug occupies, competing with an essential nutritive metabolite as is the case with sulphonamides. Target (2) represents an altered conformation of the enzyme, e.g. by an allosteric mechanism such as might occur in feedback inhibition. Target (3) is an effect on the DNA apparatus of the cell; target (4) is on the ribosome system responsible for protein synthethis. Target (5) represents the bacterial cell membrane; target (6) the bacterial cell wall. Targets 4–6 apply especially, though not exclusively, to antibiotics. Most antibiotics probably affect several targets and only in a few cases is the intimate molecular mechanism of their action understood. It is nevertheless possible now, to attempt a classification of some of the main antibiotics according to their principal site of action (Table 30.1). Some important mechanisms of chemotherapeutic action are discussed below.

Competition for an essential metabolite (Target 1)

Fildes suggested that many antibacterial compounds produce their effects by interfering with substances that are essential for bacterial growth. Bacteria may be deprived of essential metabolites by antibacterial compounds which interfere with the metabolite itself or block the enzyme system of the micro-organism which normally deals with the metabolite.

Woods showed in 1940 that extracts from yeast inhibit the bacteriostatic action of *sulphonamides* and that the substance responsible for this inhibition was *p*-aminobenzoic acid.

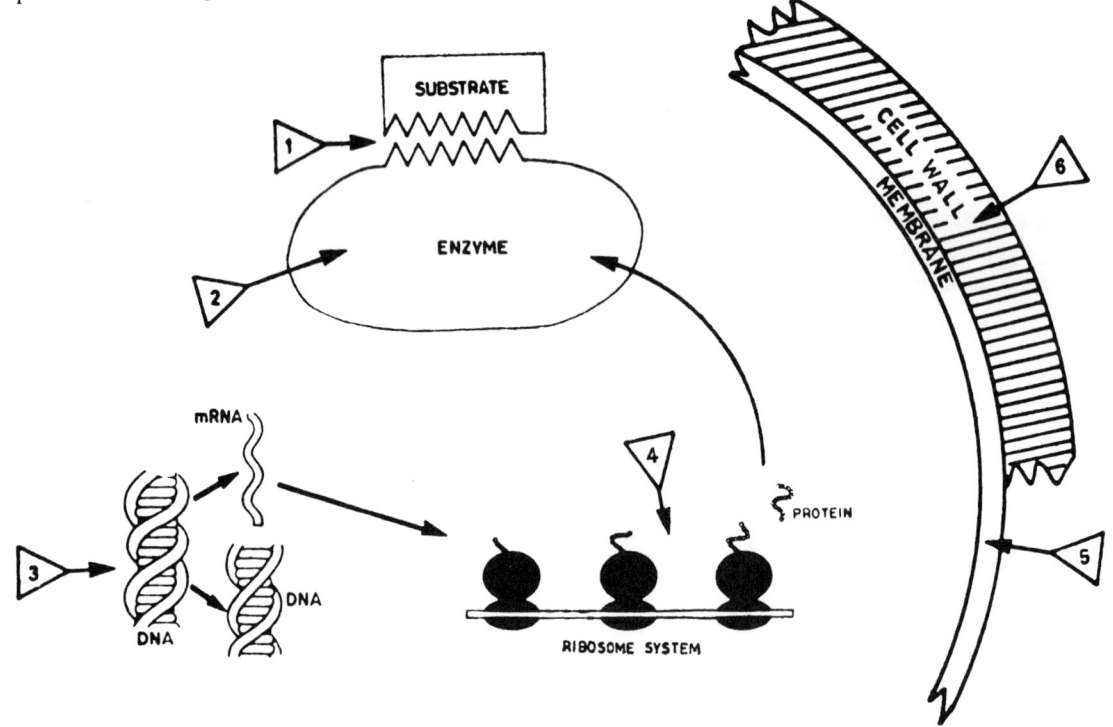

Fig. 30.1 Targets for chemotherapeutic attack in the bacterial cell (see text). (After Gale, 1972. *The Molecular Basis of Antibiotic Action*. University of Hull.)

Table 30.1 Classification of some antibiotics according to mechanism of action.

Inhibition of DNA dependent RNA polymerase	Interference with protein synthesis	Impairment of cytoplasmic membrane	Impairment of cell wall
Rifampicin	Streptomycin Tetracyclines Chloramphenicol Erythromycin	Polymyxin Amphotericin B Nystatin	Penicillin Cephalosporin Cycloserine Bacitracin

He suggested that *p*-aminobenzoic acid was an essential metabolite of bacterial cells and that the structurally related compound sulphanilamide competed for the bacterial enzymes responsible for the metabolism of *p*-aminobenzoic acid. It was later shown that sulphanilamide and *p*-aminobenzoic acid compete for the same enzyme receptors and that the bacteriostatic action of sulphanilamide is reversed by an excess of *p*-aminobenzoic acid.

p-Aminobenzoic acid   Sulphanilamide

The hypothesis of Woods and Fildes that *p*-aminobenzoic acid is an essential metabolite has been confirmed and its synthesis by many bacteria has been demonstrated.

p-Aminobenzoic acid is a constituent part of the folic acid molecule and is necessary for its synthesis by bacteria. In some cases the function of *p*-aminobenzoic acid in bacterial metabolism appears to be concerned in making folic acid available to the bacteria, since folic acid is capable of overcoming sulphonamide inhibition of bacterial growth. In contrast to *p*-aminobenzoic acid, which is a competitive antagonist of sulphonamides, the antagonism of folic acid and sulphonamides is non-competitive. In the presence of a sufficient concentration of folic acid all concentrations of sulphonamide are inactive, as folic acid provides the product of the enzyme reaction which the sulphonamide inhibits.

Structure-activity relations in sulphonamides
Bell and Roblin have suggested that the activity of substituted sulphonamides depends on their physico-chemical properties, notably their ionisation and the electron density of the SO_2 group. They predicted that antibacterial activity in a series of sulphonamides with increasing acid dissociation constants, would increase to a maximum and then decrease. Figure 30.2 taken from their work, shows that there is indeed a close correlation between the acid dissociation constant and the bacteriostatic activity of sulphonamides. This is a remarkable instance of correlation between physical properties and pharmacological activities in a series of compounds.

Control of microbial enzymes (Targets 1 and 2)
Competitive inhibition of an essential metabolite would not in itself produce a marked inhibitory effect unless the affinity of the inhibitor for the enzyme was extremely high. A compound may inhibit an isolated purified enzyme *in vitro*, but in the living cell new substrate is continuously supplied by the previous enzyme in the metabolic pathway, so that in time the concentration of natural substrate would become sufficiently high to reverse the effect of the inhibitor. Other mechanisms which could contribute to inhibition are as follows:

1. *Feedback inhibition.* This is a control mechanism by which the accumulating product inhibits the activity of an enzyme in a previous stage of the metabolic pathway, possibly through an 'allosteric' interaction with the enzyme. This mechanism could set a limit to further accumulation of the substrate and thus prevent reversal of the inhibitor.

2. *Repression.* Accumulation of the product may activate 'repressor genes' which inhibit the formation of new enzyme.

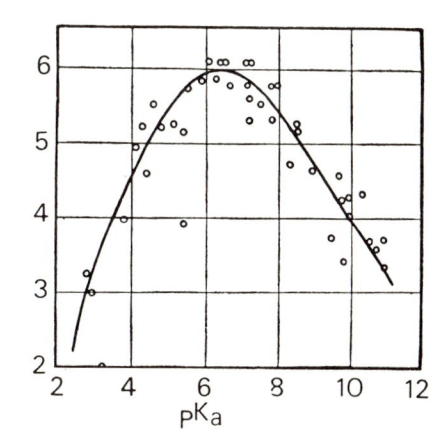

Fig. 30.2 The relation of *in vitro* activity to the acid dissociation constant (pK_a) of sulphonamides. (After Bell and Roblin, 1942. *J. Am. Chem. Soc.*)

3. *Two-step inhibition.* Inhibitory effects may be greatly increased by blocking two successive stages in the same reaction pathway, a principle made use in the development of *co-trimoxazole*, a mixture of a sulphonamide and trimethoprim, a folic acid antagonist (p. 395).

Interference with DNA function (Target 3)
Cellular information is encoded in DNA and for the continued existence of the bacterial cell progeny, this information must be replicated, *transcribed* and *translated.* Transcription is the technical term used for the synthesis of RNA on a template of DNA; translation is the term used for the synthesis of peptide chains containing specific sequences of amino acids which are determined by the nucleotide sequence in messenger RNA molecules and primarily by those in DNA.

A number of drugs have been shown to impair the function of bacterial or protozoal DNA. The acridine disinfectants (p. 460) interfere with the template function of DNA by intercalation of the DNA strand. The acridine compound, proflavine, binds to DNA *in vitro* and X-ray studies show evidence of intercalation of the DNA helix by proflavine molecules causing a partial unwinding of the double helix structure. Several important chemotherapeutic drugs are believed to bind to DNA by intercalation including the antiprotozoal agents lucanthone (p. 453) and chloroquine (p. 440). The carcinogen 3-4 benzpyrene (p. 376) causes DNA intercalation, although for carcinogenic activity *in vivo* the physically bound (intercalated) hydrocarbon must presumably be converted to a chemically bound (covalently linked) state. The antitumour agent actinomycin D (p. 382) is a specific inhibitor of DNA-directed RNA synthesis which probably intercalates the DNA strand.

Substances which bind to DNA do not discriminate between forms of naturally occurring DNA and exhibit little selective toxicity. Greater selectivity can be achieved by employing drugs which inhibit the next reaction step by inhibiting the enzyme transcriptase (DNA-dependent RNA polymerase) which catalyses the synthesis of RNA on a DNA template. The semisynthetic antibiotic *rifampicin* inhibits bacterial transcriptase without affecting this enzyme in body cells (p. 423).

Inhibition of ribosome function (Target 4)
Ribosomes are concerned with protein synthesis: the assembly of polypeptide chains is carried out on intracellular polyribosomes or polysomes by the interaction of transfer RNA and messenger RNA. Many antibiotics inhibit bacterial protein synthesis by interfering with ribosomal function.

It has been shown that *streptomycin* binds to a specific ribosomal subunit in bacteria, affecting their capacity to synthesise protein. In streptomycin-sensitive bacteria protein synthesis is altered or abolished, whilst in bacteria which have been rendered streptomycin-resistant by chromosome mutation, protein synthesis is unaffected by streptomycin, either because it fails to bind to ribosomes or because of a change in configuration which renders the drug ineffective even when it is bound. An opposite genetic change is that ribosomes actually become streptomycin dependent so that the bacterial organism cannot survive in the absence of streptomycin. Analogous effects on bacterial ribosome function are produced by other aminoglycoside antibiotics including *neomycin*, *kanamycin* and *paromomycin*. *Tetracyclines* are classical wide spectrum antibiotics which produce a variety of effects in growing cultures. They chelate calcium and other divalent cations and it has been suggested that chelation may play a part in their inhibitory effects. Present evidence, however, indicates that their main effect is on bacterial protein synthesis by an action on ribosomes.

The bacterial ribosome is composed of a smaller (30 S) and a larger (50 S) subunit. Streptomycin and the tetracyclines bind to the smaller subunit. Several other antibiotics believed to act through inhibition of bacterial protein synthesis, including *chloramphenicol* and the *macrolides*, bind to the larger ribosomal subunit.

Increased permeability of the cytoplasmic membrane (Target 5)
The cytoplasmic membrane acts as an osmotic barrier and as a medium for the selective transport of nutrients into the cell. Certain surface active antibiotics, mostly basic polypeptides such as the *polymyxins* and *gramicidin* exert their bacterial effect by increasing the permeability of the membrane. In contrast to the antibiotics which affect cell wall synthesis, these compounds exhibit no lag phase and their activity does not depend on growth and division of bacteria.

Addition of polymyxin to sensitive bacteria produces a rapid release of small molecules from their interior due to disorganisation of the structure of the cytoplasmic membrane. These effects are relatively unspecific and resemble those of surface active detergents (p. 458) with antibacterial activity.

By contrast, *amphotericin B* and related polyenes have a selective action against organisms whose cytoplasmic membrane contains sterols. They are effective against yeast and fungi but ineffective against bacteria whose cytoplasmic membrane does not contain sterols. It has been shown experimentally that polyenes, e.g. *nystatin*, readily penetrate monolayers of sterols such as cholesterol or ergosterol.

An interesting way of affecting the cytoplasmic membrane is by means of ionophores. For example, the antibiotic *valinomycin* is an ionophore which specifically binds potassium, transporting it through the cytoplasmic membrane. Ionophore antibiotics are highly toxic since

BASIC ASPECTS OF ANTIBACTERIAL CHEMOTHERAPY 389

they affect ions which are essential to all cells and they have so far no useful clinical application.

Impairment of the bacterial cell wall (Target 6)
Cell walls of different bacteria vary in their composition but all possess a common ground substance, a peptidoglycan, which has great strength and provides the bacterial surface with the rigidity necessary to protect the underlying cytoplasmic membrane from osmotic shock. Any drug which impairs the structure or synthesis of this peptidoglycan will permit membrane damage and consequent loss of function and even lysis of the cell. Peptidoglycan is unique to the bacterial cell so that specific inhibition of its production should have a highly selective effect.

The structure of cell wall peptidoglycan from *Staph. aureus* is shown in Figure 30.3. It consists of a polysaccharide backbone made of alternating N-acetylglucosamine and N-acetylmuramic acid with peptide chains attached to the muramic acid units. The

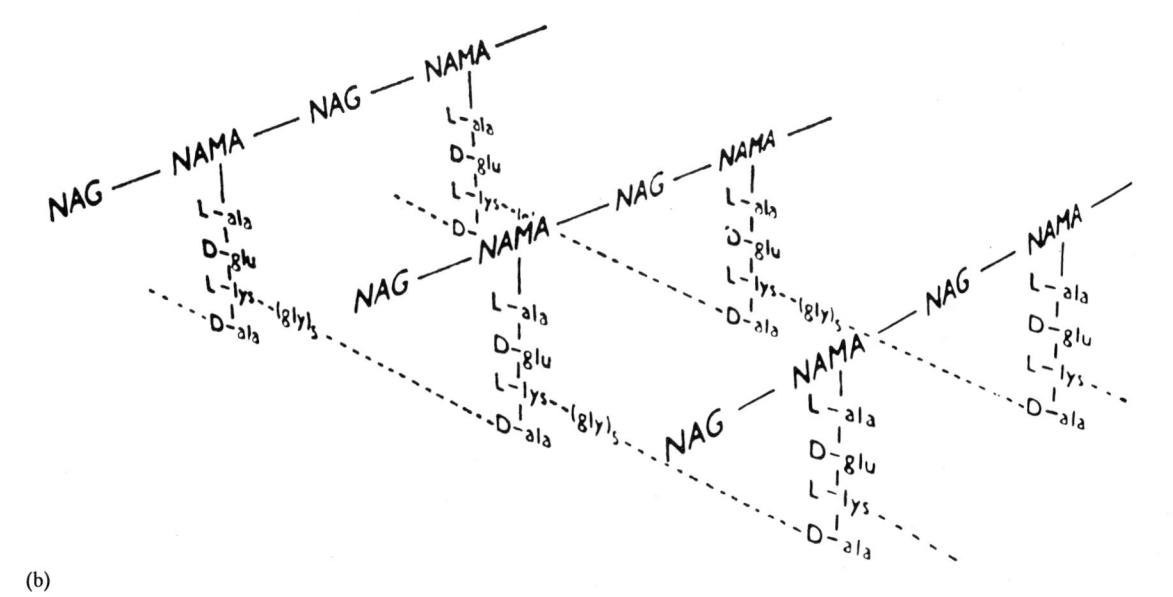

Fig. 30.3 (a) Peptidoglycan structure in *Staph. aureus*. Lower figure (b) shows nature of cross linking. NAG = N-acetyl-glucosamine. NAMA = N-acetyl-muramic acid. (After Gale, 1972. *The Molecular Basis of Antibiotic Action*. University of Hull.)

peptide chains are crosslinked to provide a strong three-dimensional net. The cell walls of other bacteria have a similar basic structure with minor chemical differences.

Mode of action of penicillin. Park showed in 1952 that in staphylococci treated with penicillin there occurs an accumulation of the uridine phosphate derivative of N-acetylmuramic acid. This compound can be considered as the biosynthetic starting point of peptidoglycan to which the side chain amino acids (Fig. 30.3a) are sequentially added, each addition being brought about by a separate enzyme and requiring ATP. In the final stage the cross link between side chains, shown in Figure 30.3(b), is formed by the action of a transpeptidase enzyme.

Penicillin prevents the cross linking reaction. It has been shown to block the active centre of the transpeptidase, presumably by virtue of a structural analogy between the penicillin molecule and the D-ala (Fig. 30.3b) side chain which the transpeptidase normally affects. Penicillin reacts covalently with the enzyme centre so that its effect is irreversible and the possibility of overcoming the inhibition competitively does not arise.

Another antibiotic which inhibits bacterial cell wall synthesis is *cycloserine*. D-Cycloserine is an analogue of D-alanine which forms part of the peptidoglycan structure and in contrast to pencillin its effects can be antagonised by an excess of D-alanine. The antibiotics *cephalosporin* and *bacitracin* also impair cell wall synthethis.

MECHANISM OF BACTERIAL RESISTANCE

When penicillin was introduced it soon became clear that some bacterial strains became resistant to it. Furthermore, whilst some previously sensitive strains became merely insensitive to penicillin others were capable of actively destroying it.

This problem has become of great importance in relation to most antibiotics, and as each new agent has been introduced a period of maximum effectiveness has generally been followed by the appearance of increasing proportions of resistant strains. The appearance of penicillin-resistant staphylococci over the years is illustrated in Figure 30.4. There are some exceptions to this general rule; for example spirochaetes seem to have retained their sensitivity to penicillin over many years.

Biochemical basis of resistance
It is now widely agreed that resistance to chemotherapeutic agents is due to genetic bacterial selection and that development of resistance by a slow process of adaptation is unlikely to be very relevant; hence the present tendency to explain resistance formation in terms of selection rather than adaptation.

The main biochemical mechanisms of bacterial resistance are as follows.

1. *Chromosomal mechanisms* such as modification of the target enzyme. For example, in the case of sulphonamides

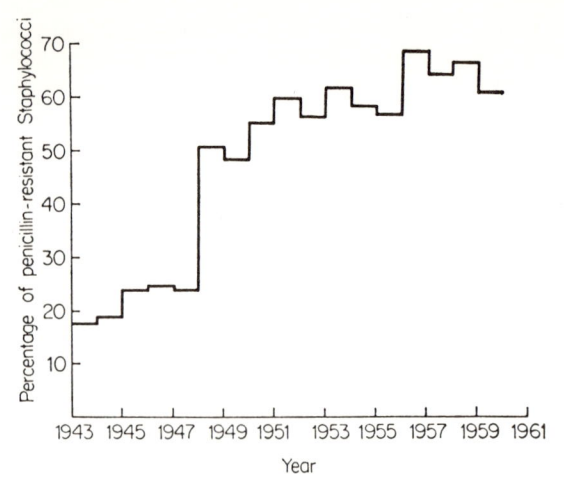

Fig. 30.4 The incidence of penicillin resistant staphyloccoci during the period 1943-1959. (After Munch-Petersen and Boundy, 1962. *Bull. Wld Hlth Org.*)

the target enzyme (tetra-hydropteroic acid synthetase) may lose its affinity for the drug whilst retaining affinity for its substrate PABA. The organism will then continue to grow in a sulphonamide medium. Another possible chromosomal mechanism is a permeability change. For example it has been shown that tetracycline-sensitive cells accumulate tetracycline but resistant cells cannot accumulate it. The location of the genes affected in these cases is likely to be on the chromosome.

2. *Extra-chromosomal mechanisms* affecting bacterial *plasmids*. These changes are likely to consist in the production of one or more enzymes capable of inactivating the antibiotic. There are two main types of inactivating enzymes: (a) destroying enzymes such as penicillinase which opens the ß-lactam ring of penicillin:

(b) substituting enzymes which inactivate by acetylation, phosphorylation or adenylylation. Substitution reactions are responsible for resistance to the aminoglycoside antibiotics streptomycin, neomycin and kanamycin.

Plasmid location of resistance genes
The importance of extrachromosomal bacterial genetic elements, called plasmids, for resistance development has only recently been recognised. Plasmids can be perceived by electronmicroscopy. They are much smaller than chromosomes and hence carry less genetic 'information'. They carry specialised genes which enable the bacterial cell to destory antibiotics and hence to survive in a milieu rich in antibiotic. Plasmids occur in staphylococci and

enterobacteria (where they are called R-factors) and they may carry resistance determinants for one or more antibiotics including ampicillin, streptomycin, tetracycline, chloramphenicol and neomycin.

In addition to being genetic entities which multiply with the cell, plasmids are also capable of being transferred to other bacterial cells. Transfer occurs by two main mechanisms called transduction and conjugation. *Transduction*, which occurs in staphylococci and enterobacteria, involves the passing of DNA from cell to cell by means of a bacterial virus (bacteriophage). *Conjugation* involves physical contact between two bacteria during which plasmid DNA passes unidirectionally using hair-like processes (sex-pili) to affect transfer. Transference of self-replicating (infectious) genes occurs by conjugation.

In this way resistance may spread in enterobacteria, especially since one bacterial cell may carry multiple plasmids. The factor responsible for promoting conjugation and survival as a self-replicating element in the recipient is called resistance transfer factor (RTF) or sex factor. Such factors may also be carried from one bacterial species to another e.g. from *E. coli* to *shigellae*.

Importance of extrachromosomal resistance factors

It is clear that selection plays a major part in the process of emergence and survival of resistant bacterial populations following the use of antibiotics. The bacterial cell may not be able to evolve effective chromosomal mutations to protect it from highly efficient antibiotics, but additional extrachromosomal genes, which give rise to inactivating factors, may protect it and assure its survival.

The main importance of extrachromosomal resistance factors probably does not lie in the emergence of resistant pathogens during the treatment of an individual, but in the emergence of resistant bacterial populations in a community following the introduction of a new antibacterial agent. For example only about one in one million enteric organisms may carry R-factors which confer resistance against tetracycline, but during treatment, provided that these rare organisms survive, resistant organisms are likely to spread and may affect not only the individual himself but also others in the hospital ward.

FURTHER READING

Bull A T, Meadow P M (ed) 1979 Companion to microbiology. Longman, London

Gale E F, Cundliffe E, Reynolds P E, Richmond M H, Waring M J 1972 The molecular basis of antibiotic action. John Wiley, London

Newton B A 1970 Chemotherapeutic compounds affecting DNA structure and action. Adv. Pharm. Chemoth. 8: 150

Volk W A 1978 Essentials of medical microbiology. Lippincott, Philedelphia

31. Synthetic compounds for the chemotherapy of infections

Chemistry of the sulphonamide drugs 392; Antibacterial activity 393; Absorption, distribution and excretion of sulphonamides 393; Toxic effects 394; Relative merits 394; Therapeutic uses of sulphonamides 395; Trimethoprim and cotrimoxazole 395; Nitrofurantoin 396; Nalidixic acid 396; Antiviral agents 396; Methisazone 396; Idoxuridine 396; Interferon 397.

THE SULPHONAMIDES

In 1935 Domagk published his observations showing that the red dye named prontosil could protect mice against several thousand times the usual lethal dose of haemolytic streptococci, and that it had a very valuable curative action in clinical cases of such infections. In the same year Bovet and his colleagues showed that the simpler compound p-amino-benzenesulphonamide produced a similar action to prontosil, and concluded that the latter was an inert substance which was broken down in the body to the simpler and active form. Subsequent work has confirmed this conclusion, and this simple derivative has been named sulphanilamide.

Chemistry of the sulphonamide drugs

The spectacular therapeutic success of these drugs led to the synthesis and investigation of a large number of related compounds and the chemical structures of some of the more important of these antibacterial sulphonamides are shown in Table 31.1.

Two types of compound can be derived by substitution of (1) the amide (SO_2NH_2) group (R_2) and (2) the amino (NH_2) group (R_1).

The most active sulphonamides belong to the first type in which the amide group is substituted. The substituent group is usually a heterocyclic ring. The first heterocyclic sulphonamide used was sulphapyridine (M & B 693),

Table 31.1 Structural formulae of sulphonamide drugs.

Amino Group = R_1	Sulphanilamide H_2N—⟨ ⟩—SO_2NH_2	R_2 = Amide Group
	R_1—⟨ ⟩—R_2	
Sulphadiazine	H_2N	$SO_2.NH$—(pyrimidine)
Sulphadimidine	H_2N	$SO_2.NH$—(dimethylpyrimidine with CH_3 groups)
Sulphafurazole	H_2N	$SO_2.NH$—C(=C-CH_3)—O—N=C-CH_3
Phthalysulphathiazole	⟨ ⟩—CO.NH / COOH	$SO_2.NH$—(thiazole)

which was introduced in 1937. It had a greater therapeutic range than sulphanilamide, but had the disadvantage of frequently causing intense vomiting and other severe toxic symptoms. Other compounds have since been introduced, which though not much more active than sulphapyridine, are considerably less toxic. They include, amongst others, sulphadiazine, sulphadimidine, and sulphafurazole (Table 31.1).

Compounds of the second type, in which the amino group is masked, must be activated in the body by removing the substituent group, since a free amino group is essential for antibacterial action. An example is phthalylsulphathiazole. As with the diazo group of prontosil which is broken down in the body and the free amino group restored, so too the phthalyl substituent is split off in the intestine and the active compound is slowly liberated.

The sulphonamides were the first effective systemic antibacterial drugs introduced and although their therapeutic uses have now somewhat declined they are of considerable historical and theoretical interest.

Related compounds
Several important therapeutic advances have resulted from the development of other sulphonamide derivatives. The sulphone, dapsone, is a sulphonamide derivative found to have tuberculostatic activity and is now used mainly in the treatment of leprosy (p. 428). The heterocyclic sulphonamide, acetazolamide has a highly specific inhibitory effect on carbonic anhydrase and reduces the reabsorption of sodium bicarbonate in the renal tubules, resulting in diuresis. This discovery led to the further development of powerful oral diuretic drugs such as chlorothiazide and related thiadiazine derivatives (p. 160). Another group of substituted sulphonamides, the sulphonylureas were shown to produce severe hypoglycaemia and this observation gave rise to the development of the oral hypoglycaemic drugs, tolbutamide and chlorpropamide (p. 340).

Antibacterial activity
The sulphonamides were first believed to be effective only against haemolytic streptococci but in 1936, Buttle and his colleagues showed that sulphanilamide protected mice against both meningococci and pneumococci. Further work established that these drugs are also effective against a wide variety of bacteria including *E. coli*, *N. gonorrhaeae*, *Str. pyogenes*, *Str. pneumoniae*, *Brucella abortus*, and to a variable extent against *Kl. aerogenes* and *pneumoniae*, *Proteus vulgaris*, *Staph. aureus*, *H. influenzae* and *pertussis* and the organisms causing bacillary dysentery. The sulphonamides produce no effect on viruses, spirochaetes, trypanosomes or other protozoal parasites.

It is generally agreed that the different sulphonamide compounds differ in antibacterial activity in a quantitative rather than a qualitative manner. The most active compound against one type of micro-organism is likely to be the most active against all other types.

Comparative activity. In assessing the relative activity of different sulphonamides a convenient method has been devised which makes use of the functional relationship and antagonism between sulphonamides and *p*-aminobenzoic acid. Wood found that the bacteriostatic activity of each sulphonamide is proportional to its ability to counteract the antibacteriostatic action of *p*-aminobenzoic acid (PABA). He therefore used the term 'bacteriostatic constant' (K) where:

$$K = \frac{M\text{-PABA}}{M\text{-sulphonamide}} \text{ preventing bacteriostasis}$$

In the case of sulphanilamide $K = 6 \times 10^{-4}$, whilst for sulphathiazole $K = 3 \times 10^{-2}$. Thus it is possible to define the activity of a sulphonamide in terms of sulphanilamide. For example, the sulphanilamide coefficient of sulphathiazole=

$$\frac{K(\text{sulphathiazole})}{K(\text{sulphanilamide})} = \frac{3 \times 10^{-2}}{6 \times 10^{-4}} = 50$$

The sulphanilamide coefficient gives an indication of the relative *in vitro* activity of a sulphonamide, but does not necessarily indicate its clinical usefulness. Thus sulphathiazole is highly potent but particularly liable to cause clinical side effects and is now rarely prescribed alone.

The *in vivo* activity of sulphonamide compounds is usually tested in mice experimentally infected with an organism to which they are highly susceptible such as *Str. pyogenes* or *Str. pneumoniae*. Although there is often a close relationship between the results of such *in vivo* and *in vitro* tests, there are other factors which determine the therapeutic efficacy of a compound. These involve a consideration of its absorption, distribution, metabolism, protein binding and rate of clearance, as well as its liability to produce side effects.

Absorption, distribution and excretion of sulphonamides
Since the action of sulphonamides is bacteriostatic and not bactericidal the essential principle of sulphonamide therapy is to maintain an effective concentration in the blood for an adequate time.

When administered by mouth, most of the sulphonamides are fairly rapidly absorbed from the stomach and small intestine and peak concentrations in the blood are reached within four to six hours. An exception to this is the group of poorly absorbed compounds such as phthalylsulphathiazole which are mainly excreted unchanged in the faeces.

After absorption the sulphonamides are distributed throughout the body and the extent to which this occurs varies with the different compounds. An important factor which determines distribution to the tissues is the extent to which the compound is bound to plasma proteins. Only the proportion of diffusible drug is concerned in the antibacterial activity of these compounds, so that a comparison merely of blood concentration is not necessarily a measure of therapeutic efficacy. It is also relevant that concurrent administration of other drugs which are bound to plasma proteins may increase the diffusible proportion of sulphonamide. Sulphonamides also pass into pleural and other effusions and through the placenta into the foetal circulation. The diffusion of sulphonamide into the tissues of the foetus is an important point to appreciate when treating pregnant patients with sulphonamides.

Metabolism. These drugs are cleared in three ways; they are partly acetylated by the liver, partly oxidised in the body and partly excreted unchanged. The acetylated compound has no antibacterial activity and is generally less soluble than the unchanged drug and is therefore more liable to precipitate in the renal tubules. With the earlier sulphonamides this presented a serious toxic hazard to the patient, but the compounds in current use are much less likely to do so. The extent to which different sulphonamides are acetylated varies. The degree of acetylation of sulphonamides in individual subjects, as that of isoniazid (p. 28), appears to be genetically determined. Acetylation increases with time; hence differences in acetylation are due partly to differences in rate of excretion.

Excretion. With the exception of the poorly absorbed compounds, the main route of excretion of sulphonamides is by the kidneys. These drugs are filtered by the glomeruli and then partly reabsorbed by the renal tubules. Sulphathiazole is not readily reabsorbed so that its clearance is the same as the inulin clearance and it is rapidly excreted. Sulphadiazine and sulphadimidine have a renal clearance which is only about 20 to 30 per cent of the inulin clearance and are more slowly excreted. The long acting sulphonamides are excreted very slowly and are also slowly metabolised.

Toxic effects of sulphonamides

The undesirable side actions produced by sulphonamide drugs may be divided into mild, moderate and severe. Amongst the milder toxic effects are malaise, headache, loss of appetite and nausea. These are usually produced by full dosage of the drugs.

A common toxic effect is cyanosis, which is caused by the formation of methaemoglobin or sulphaemoglobin. Fortunately the cyanosis is much less dangerous than might be expected from the alarming appearance of the patient; it does not cause respiratory or cardiac distress, and it is not usually an indication for discontinuing treatment.

The haemoglobin metabolism is frequently deranged and there is increased production of porphyrins. These cause light sensitisation and may be responsible for some of the rashes that occur. It has been found that exposure to ultraviolet light during sulphonamide therapy produces undesirable effects.

Continuance of sulphonamide therapy may cause allergic reactions, the chief manifestations of which are skin rashes and drug fever. The most common skin reaction is an itching erythematous rash of variable distribution. Repeated application of sulphonamides to the skin often produces local and general sensitisation. For this reason sulphonamides should not be employed as local applications for the treatment of skin infections.

When hypersensitivity reactions occur it is necessary to discontinue the administration of the particular sulphonamide and it is usually not possible to continue treatment with another sulphonamide. Drug fever is difficult to diagnose because it may be mistaken for a sign of recrudescence of the original infection.

Sulphonamides are liable to give rise to kernicterus in premature and newborn babies.

The sulphonamide drugs are partly excreted as acetylated compounds some of which have a low solubility in acid or neutral fluids. Their deposition in the tubules may cause urinary irritation, haematuria, and in severe cases, anuria. This effect can be prevented by keeping the urine alkaline by administration of bicarbonates or citrates, and giving plenty of fluid. The most serious toxic action of these drugs is injury to the bone marrow. This may cause leucopenia or even agranulocytosis and occasionally aplastic anaemia. Fortunately these effects are rare, but with patients receiving full doses of these drugs a watch should be kept on the blood picture.

Mode of administration

The usual method of administration is to give the drug by mouth at frequent intervals. The sulphonamides are of chief value in the treatment of acute diseases and hence it is important to produce an adequate blood concentration as rapidly as possible. This can be produced by initial large doses and maintained by frequent smaller doses.

The following general principles apply. The amount of drug that can be given is limited by the toxic side actions that may occur and these depend on the maximum blood concentrations attained. All the available evidence indicates that the curative action of the drugs is a relatively slow one, and is dependent on the maintenance of an adequate concentration. Hence it is desirable to maintain as uniform a blood concentration as possible and since most of the drugs are rapidly excreted this can only be done by giving frequent doses. It therefore is preferable, when reducing the dosage, to reduce the size and not the number of the doses.

Relative merits of sulphonamide compounds

Of the many compounds investigated, only a few have been introduced into clinical practice and hence these are a highly selected group. Actually only three or four preparations need be used, one or two for general infections, one for gastrointestinal infections and one for infections of the eye.

Sulphadimidine (sulphamezathine) has relatively low *in vitro* activity but is one of the least toxic compounds and is often used in Great Britain as the drug of first choice in the treatment of systemic infections. It is rapidly absorbed and more slowly excreted than sulphadiazine; hence its concentration in the blood is relatively higher. In comparison with sulphadiazine, sulphadimidine and its acetyl derivative are more soluble in acid urine.

Sulphadiazine is highly active. It is readily bound to plasma proteins; it is liable to cause crystalluria.

Sulphafurazole (Gantrisin) is readily absorbed and rapidly excreted. It is highly soluble and this makes it a useful drug for the treatment of urinary infections.

Sulphamethoxypyridazine (Midicel, Lederkyn), *sulphadimethoxine* (Madribon) and other long acting sulphonamides are well absorbed but slowly excreted. After a single daily dose high plasma concentrations are maintained, but since these drugs are extensively bound to protein, the proportion which is diffusible and bacteriostatic is low; they are not likely to be as therapeutically effective for systemic infections as the shorter acting compounds and if toxic effects develop they may be more prolonged because of the slow rate of excretion. They are particularly liable to produce severe allergic reactions such as erythema multiforme, probably due to their strong protein binding.

Sulphacetamide (Albucid) yields an almost neutral sodium salt which, in solution, can be used as eye drops.

Therapeutic uses of sulphonamides
The therapeutic importance of these drugs was first realised in 1936 when Colebrook and Kenny reduced the mortality in a series of cases of puerperal fever to 5 per cent, whereas the previous mortality had been 24 per cent. Sulphonamides were originally employed against streptococcal, pneumococcal, gonococcal and staphylococcal infections, but have now been largely superseded by antibiotics in gonococcal, staphylococcal and streptococcal infections because of the frequent occurrence of sulphonamide resistance in many different bacterial strains. Many bacteria are already resistant to sulphonamides and many develop a high degree of resistance to the sulphonamides during treatment. Nevertheless, the sulphonamides are still used, because they are cheap and easy to administer, and because in a limited number of infections and in the absence of drug resistance they are as active or more active than the antibiotics available at present. One of their chief advantages is that they do not produce the troublesome disturbances of gut flora which frequently occur with broad spectrum antibiotics such as the tetracyclines.

Urinary tract infections. Sulphonamides are among the drugs of choice for treating acute, uncomplicated urinary tract infections. The majority of bacteria likely to be isolated from patients with symptomatic infections of the urinary tract in general practice, and from patients with bacteriuria in pregnancy are likely to respond to treatment, at least initially, with a sulphonamide such as sulphafurazole.

Although the sulphonamides are still widely used for the first line treatment of urinary infections, in chronic urinary infections they are less satisfactory than cotrimoxazole or antibiotics.

For patients who do not respond to sulphonamides or who suffer from recurrent urinary tract infections, fuller diagnostic investigation is often necessary. Depending on the sensitivity of the organisms responsible, effective therapy may be obtained with the use of a suitable antibiotic or other types of antibacterial drugs.

TRIMETHOPRIM AND CO-TRIMOXAZOLE

Trimethoprim is a diaminopyrimidine of the following structure:

Trimethoprim

It is chemically related to the antimalarial drug pyrimethamine (p. 440). In concentrations which can be achieved in the plasma, trimethoprim is active against all common pathogenic bacteria, with the exception of *mycobacteria* and *pseudomonas*. On its own it is bacteriostatic rather than bactericidal.

Clinically, trimethoprim is generally administered as a mixture with sulphamethoxazole; this is called *co-trimoxazole* (bactrim; septrin). The reason for this combination is that trimethoprim is not only a potent antibacterial agent in its own right but it acts on bacteria in the same metabolic sequence as sulphonamides so that when the two agents are given together they markedly potentiate each other. In addition to lowering the concentration of drug required to inhibit bacterial growth, it has been shown that whilst each drug alone is merely bacteriostatic, their mixture is bactericidal.

Mode of action of co-trimaxazole. The sequential effect of a mixture of sulphonamide and trimethoprim is illustrated below:

p-aminobenzoic acid ⟶ folic acid ⟶ folinic acid
↑ ↑
sulphonamide trimethoprim

The sulphonamide exerts its usual action of interfering with the role of *p*-aminobenzoic acid in the synthesis of folic acid whilst trimethoprim inhibits the enzyme dihydrofolate reductase which is involved in the conversion of folic acid to its reduced form, folinic acid. It is interesting that bacteria which synthesise folic acid cannot absorb it when it is preformed, whilst mammalian tissues can absorb preformed folic acid but cannot synthesise it.

Absorption and excretion. Trimethropim is rapidly and fully absorbed from the gut. Since it is a weak base its urinary elimination rises with falling pH.

Organisms can be made resistant to trimethoprim *in vitro*.

Clinical uses. Co-trimoxazole is considerably more active than the sulphonamides and has been used particularly in the control of acute and chronic urinary and respiratory infections. It is used in the treatment of gonorrhoea. It has also been successfully used in the treatment of severe enteric infections and of endocarditis.

Toxic effects include nausea, vomiting and skin rashes. An interesting toxic effect of trimethoprim is the induction of folate deficiency, which can be countered by feeding folate supplements. These do not interfere with its antibacterial activity, since, as has been explained, bacteria cannot absorb preformed folate.

NITROFURANTOIN (FURADANTIN)

Several nitrofuran compounds with different antibacterial activities have been synthesised, the most effective and least toxic of which is nitrofurantoin.

Nitrofurantoin

This drug is active against a range of Gram-positive and Gram-negative organisms but most strains of *Ps. pyocyanea* are resistant to it. It is well absorbed when given by mouth and concentrations of nitrofurantoin excreted in the urine are usually bactericidal to susceptible organisms, when daily doses of about 400 to 500 mg are administered. During treatment it may cause gastrointestinal disturbances such as anorexia or nausea, and hepatotoxicity from its use has been reported; peripheral neuropathy has been occasionally produced in patients with impaired renal function. Nitrofurantoin is mainly used for the treatment of urinary tract infections.

Nalidixic acid (Negram)

This is a synthetic antibacterial substance, effective particularly against Gram-negative organisms in the urinary tract. It is administered orally or by instillation into the bladder.

Nalidixic acid is rapidly absorbed and largely metabolised in the body. It is eliminated by the kidney, but only a fraction reaches the urine in an active bactericidal form. Resistance to the drug develops rapidly. It is used in the treatment of urinary tract infections but it may produce undesirable side effects which include visual disturbances, hallucinations and skin reactions, some of which are associated with photosensitisation.

ANTIVIRAL AGENTS

Although a number of substances have been found which are active against viruses on a laboratory scale, very few are clinically effective. One of the difficulties in dealing with virus infections is that viral multiplication often takes place before symptoms appear so that the treatment would have to be administered during the incubation period. Antiviral compounds would thus be expected to be effective as prophylactic rather than therapeutic agents. Amongst the few available antiviral agents are the following.

Methisazone

Methisazone belongs to the chemical class of thiosemicarbazones which are effective in the treatment of tuberculosis (p. 424). The antiviral acitivy of methisazone appears to be due to prevention of virus replication. Clinically methisazone has been shown to protect smallpox contacts from developing the disease. In a smallpox epidemic in Madras in which all contacts were vaccinated, 6 out of 2000 receiving methisazone contracted the disease whilst in an equal control sample 114 became infected. The drug was of no value in the established disease.

Methisazone is suitable for mass administration in the event of an epidemic of smallpox and conveys immediate protection. It gives better results than human vaccinia immunoglobulin, though smallpox vaccination is still the method of choice for longterm protection. It is irritant to the stomach but less so if taken after meals.

Methisazone is also given to prevent complications following vaccination and is used in the treatment of *eczema vaccinatum* in small children.

Idoxuridine

Idoxuridine is deoxy-iodourudine. It is an antiviral agent which blocks the uptake of thymidine into the DNA of the virus and inhibits replication of viruses such as adenovirus, cytomegalovirus, herpes simplex and vaccinia. It does not inhibit RNA viruses such as influenza virus or poliovirus.

It is mainly used in the treatment of superficial herpes simplex keratitis (dendritic keratitis) of recent origin in which it may produce healing in one or two weeks. Because idoxuridine inhibits the formation of DNA in the cornea as well as in the virus, prolonged administration may damage the cornea and prevent healing.

Idoxuridine is also used in the treatment of herpes zoster by application of a solution of idoxuridine, usually in dimethylsulphoxide, to the affected area. There is some evidence that local applications of idoxuridine may shorten the duration of recurrent herpes simplex lesions. It has been used in the treatment of encephalitis due to herpes virus, but is highly toxic when administered systemically.

Amantadine
This is a complex molecule which has been shown to be of some value in the treatment of Parkinsonism (p. 274) and to possess prophylactic antiviral activity in preventing infection with influenza type A2 virus, but not with other types of influenza virus. It may act by preventing penetration of the virus into host cells. It has no effect in herpes zoster.

Cytarabine (p. 381) is an important antineoplastic agent which inhibits the synthesis of DNA. It is also used in the treatment of herpesvirus infection.

Interferon
Interferon was discovered by Isaacs, at the National Institute for Medical Research London, who considered it to be an agent produced by cells which will enable the cell to withstand viral infections. It has been shown to be a low molecular weight protein produced in animal cells following exposure to a variety of agents. Viruses are powerful inducers of interferon but it is also produced after exposure to other micro-organisms, bacterial endotoxins, phytohaemagglutinin and to various synthetic copolymers such as pyran copolymer. Interferon has the property of interfering with the growth of a variety of viruses both within the cells in which it is produced and in surrounding cells.

Many different viruses can induce interferon production including influenza virus. Interferon can also be produced in tissue cultures. It appears that there exist a variety of species-specific interferons and that only human (or monkey) interferon is effective in man. Theoretically interferon could be used in virus infections either by administering it exogenously or by applying substances which stimulate the production of endogenous interferon.

In spite of great interest there has been little progress so far in the clinical use of interferon. Beneficial results have been obtained in dendritic keratitis by the topical application of solutions containing human interferon.

PREPARATIONS

Sulphonamides[130]
Short-acting
Sulphadiazine init 2–4 g, then 1 g every 4–6 h
Sulphamethizole (Methisul) 0.5–1 g 3–4x die
Sulphafurazole (Gantrisin) init 4 g, then 1–2 every 4–6 h
Intermediate acting
Sulphamethoxazole init 2 g then 1 g every 12 h
Cotrimazole (Bactrim, Septrin) = 5 sulphamethoxazole+1 trimethoprim 1 g 2–3x die
Long-acting
Sulfametopyrazine (Kelfizine) prol treat 1x weekly
Sulphamethodiazine (Sulfameter) init 1.5 g then 500 mg dl
Sulphamethoxypyridazine (Midicel) init 1 g then 500 mg dl
Sulphaphenazole (Orisulph) init 1 g every 12 h for 2 d then 500 mg every 12 h for 3 d
Antidiarrhoeal
Phthalylsulphathiazole (Thalidine) 5–10 g dl
Sulphasalazine (Rorasul) 1–2 g 4–6x die p.o.
Topical
Mafenide acet cream (burns)
Sulphacetamide sodium 10–15% (ophthalmic)

Drugs for urinary tract infections
Methenamine, Methenamine mandelate 1 g 4x die (req acid pH)
Nalidixic acid (Negram) 4 g dl
Nitrofurantoin (Furadantin) 50–100 mg 4x die
Oxolinic acid 750 mg 2x die

Antivirals
Amantadine hyd (Symmetrel) 200 mg dl
Cytarabine (Arabinosylcytosine) 2–4 mg/kg for 5 d (herpes)
Idoxuridine 0.1% (ophthalm)
Methisazone 3 g 2x die (smallpox proph)
Vidarabine (Adenine arabinoside) (herpes)

FURTHER READING

Bernstein L S, Salter A J (ed) 1973
  Trimethropim/sulphamethoxazole in bacterial infections. Churchill Livingstone, Edinburgh

32. Penicillin and cephalosporin antibiotics

Chemistry of penicillin 398; Mode of action 400; Antimicrobial action 400; Benzylpenicillin 400; Longacting preparations 402; Phenoxymethylpenicillin 402; Semisynthetic penicillins 403; Phenethicillin 403; Methicillin 404; Flucloxacillin 404; Carbenicillin 404; Ampicillin 404; Therapeutic uses 404; Penicillin prophylaxis 405; Toxicity 405; Allergy 405; Cephalosporins 406; Sodium fusidate 407.

Antibiotic substances are produced by a wide range of fungi, actinomycetes and bacteria. Amongst the chief antibiotics: penicillin, cephalosporin and the antifungal agent griseofulvin are derived from fungi; the tetracyclines, chloramphenicol, erythromycin, streptomycin and the antifungal agents nystatin and amphotericin are derived from actinomycetes; bacitracin, tyrothrycin and polymyxin are bacterial products. In this chapter the penicillin and cephalosporin groups of antibiotics are discussed.

PENICILLIN

Penicillin was the name given by Sir Alexander Fleming to an antibacterial substance produced by a mould of the genus *Penicillium*. Fleming had observed in 1928 that a culture plate containing colonies of staphylococci which had been contaminated by spores of a species of *Penicillium* showed signs of dissolution in the neighbourhood of the mould. He isolated the mould in pure culture and later showed that when different bacteria were planted near the mould culture, some of the bacteria grew right up to the area adjoining the mould whilst other bacteria were inhibited and failed to grow within a distance from the mould. This showed that the mould had produced an antibacterial substance which diffused in the culture medium and selectively inhibited certain organism (Fig. 32.1). Fleming later showed that the antibacterial substance not only inhibited the growth of many pathogenic bacteria, but also had bactericidal properties, and he was able to differentiate organisms which were sensitive from those which were insensitive to penicillin. A broth culture of the mould was three times more potent than phenol against staphylococci and, unlike this substance, was not toxic to human leucocytes. Penicillin was found to be a very unstable substance, easily destroyed and difficult to isolate from the mould.

Several attempts were made to produce purified penicillin and in 1940 Florey, Chain and their colleagues at Oxford succeeded in isolating a concentrated preparation of penicillin which, when dried, was relatively stable. They showed that in a dilution of 1 in 1 million it produced the bacteriostatic effects of the crude preparation and that these effects were not modified by the presence of blood or of pus. They also showed that the penicillin thus concentrated had powerful chemotherapeutic properties when tested on experimentally infected animals, that it did not injure leucocytes and that it had practically no toxic effects on the animals. The remarkable curative properties of penicillin in man were first reported by the Oxford workers in 1941 and vigorous attempts were then made in Britain and in America to produce penicillin on a commercial scale.

Chemistry of penicillin

Several strains of *Penicillium* and various culture media have been used for the production of penicillin and it was soon found that not one single substance but a number of penicillins were produced. Only two naturally occurring penicillins are used for clinical purposes, benzylpenicillin (penicillin G) produced by *Penicillium notatum*, and phenoxymethylpenicillin (penicillin V) which is obtained from *Penicillium chrysogenum*.

The general formula of a penicillin is shown below. All penicillins consist of a side chain, R, which is different in different penicillins and is attached by an amide linkage to a 6-amino-penicillanic (6-APA) residue; 6-APA consists of a 4-membered beta-lactam ring fused with a 5-membered thiazolidine ring (p. 406).

$$\underset{\text{6-APA}}{R.CO\underset{(1)}{\vdots}NH.CH\text{—}CH\underset{|}{\overset{S}{\diagup}}\underset{CH_3}{\overset{CH_3}{C\diagdown}}\ \ \ \atop CO\underset{(2)}{\vdots}N\text{——}CH.COOH}$$

Penicillins may be destroyed by chemical treatment or by enzymes. Enzymes which hydrolyse penicillin at site (1) to yield the free side chain and 6-APA are called amidases whilst enzymes which hydrolyse the beta-lactam ring in position (2) (p. 390) are called penicillinases.

Penicillinase is important because a number of strains of staphylococci produce this enzyme and are thus rendered resistant to penicillin. Destruction of the nucleus in position (2) also occurs during the degradation of penicillin in the body. The resultant penicilloic acid is able to react with protein and is believed to be largely responsible for the production of penicillin allergy.

Penicillin is normally produced from moulds but in 1957 a complete chemical synthesis of pheoxymethylpenicillin was achieved. However, the synthesis is

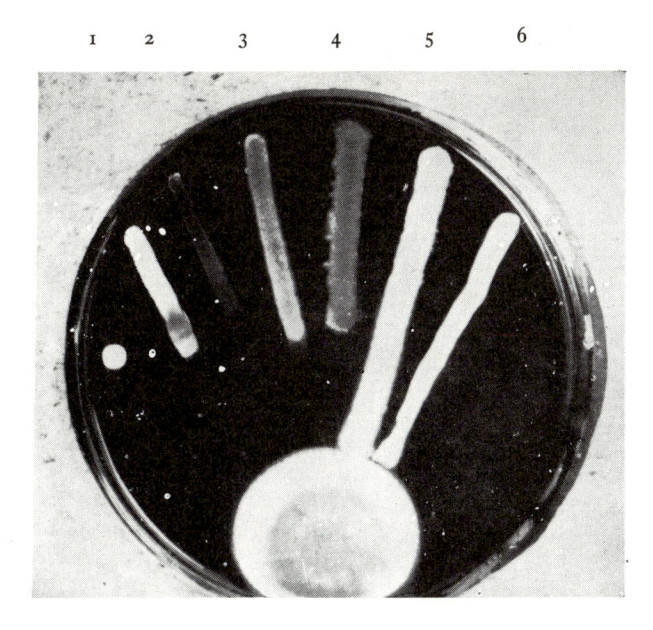

Fig. 32.1 Inhibiting action of *P. notatum* on different bacteria. 1. Staphylococcus. 2. Streptococcus. 3. Diphtheria bacillus. 4. Anthrax bacillus. 5. *E. coli*. 6. Typhoid bacillus. (After Fleming, 1945. *J. R. Inst. Publ. Hlth Hyg.*)

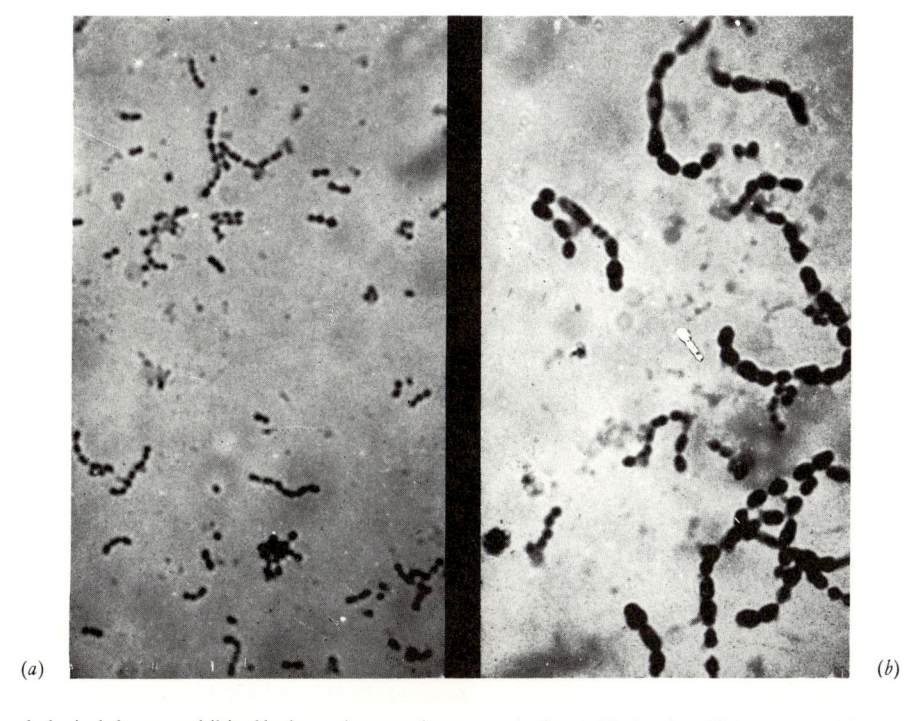

Fig. 32.2 Morphological changes exhibited by bacteria grown in a strength of penicillin just insufficient to stop all growth. (a) Normal streptococci (×1000). (b) Giant forms amongst penicillin-treated streptococci (×1000). (Chain and Florey, 1944. *Endeavour*.)

complex with a low yield and does not provide a practical means of producing penicillin. Penicillin is prepared by cultivating a mould which forms it in a suitable liquid medium. In the early stages it was found that several different penicillins were being formed of which benzylpenicillin (penicillin G) had the most desirable properties. The latter is almost exclusively formed if phenylacetic acid precursor is added to the medium.

Mode of action
Penicillin affects micro-organisms during growth but has little or no activity in the resting state. It not only stops growth, but kills the organisms when present in adequate concentrations; Figure 32.2 shows the morphological changes in bacteria grown in a low concentration of penicillin just insufficient to stop all growth. The formation of these giant forms is due to an interference by penicillin with the normal synthetic processes which are responsible for the formation of the bacterial cell wall. The mechanism of this interference has been discussed on page 389. Since the action of penicillin depends on interference with the building of the bacterial cell wall, it should not be administered simultaneously with bacteriostatic drugs which inhibit cell growth such as tetracyclines and sulphonamides.

Biological assay. Preparations of penicillin can be assayed biologically by comparing the quantity which inhibits the growth of a sensitive strain of *Bacillus subtilis* with inhibition by a standard preparation. The standard consists of the sodium salt of pure benzylpenicillin and the unit of penicillin is 0.6 μg of this preparation. Assay is carried out by one of two methods: (1) by measuring the distance through which the test organism is inhibited by penicillin solutions contained in a number of porcelain cylinders placed on the agar plate; (2) by noting the dilution of the penicillin solution which completely inhibits growth of the test organism in broth culture.

Benzylpenicillin (Penicillin G)
The sodium and potassium salts of benzylpenicillin are stable when dry. They are highly soluble in water, but aqueous solutions gradually lose activity even when stored in the refrigerator. Benzylpenicillin is destroyed by acids and alkalis and the optimum pH for stability in aqueous solution is about 6.5.

Antimicrobial activity
The distinction between bacteriostatic antibiotics which reversibly inhibit the growth of susceptible micro-organisms, and bactericidal antibiotics which kill the organism is based on determinations of their *in vitro* effects on certain strains of micro-organisms. Provided the results are obtained with concentrations of antibiotics attainable in serum and tissues by the administration of therapeutic doses, the distinction remains clinically valid. However, an antibiotic which is bactericidal in a certain concentration may be bacteriostatic at lower concentrations.

Benzylpenicillin is generally considered to be bactericidal, but it has bacteriostatic and bactericidal actions depending on its concentration. The antibacterial activity of benzylpenicillin measured in terms of the concentration usually required to inhibit bacterial growth *in vitro* varies over a wide range. Highly sensitive organisms include almost all the Gram-positive pathogens such as streptococci (including *Str. haemolyticus* and *pneumoniae* but less so *Str. faecalis and viridans*), most staphylococci, the bacilli of anthrax and tetanus and the fungus *Actinomyces israeli*. Amongst highly sensitive Gram-negative pathogens are gonococci and meningococci. Benzyl penicillin-sensitive Gram-negative organisms include *Haemophilus* and *Bacteroides* whilst *E. coli*, *Proteus* and *Salmonella* are relatively resistant. Fully resistant species include mycobacteria, rickettsias, mycoplasmas and viruses, but the treponemes of syphylis and yaws are penicillin-sensitive.

It is not always possible to draw a clear distinction between sensitive and insensitive organisms. In addition to the increasing incidence of penicillinase-forming resistant strains, certain strains of normally sensitive organisms are found to be much less sensitive and in this sense may be classified as insensitive. Similarly, among relatively insensitive organisms, wide variations in susceptibility occur and frequently the greatest differences are between strains of the same species. In other words, sensitivity is not always clearly related to bacteriological classification.

An overall classification by Garrod of the sensitivity of micro-organisms to benzylpenicillin is given in Table 32.1. The only reliable guide of the degree of sensitivity, however, is to determine this in organisms obtained from each patient.

Absorption and excretion. Benzylpenicillin, when given by mouth, is absorbed from the duodenum, but the extent of absorption is conditioned by the amount destroyed by gastric acid and the amount lost by adsorption on food. Absorption of benzylpenicillin is irregular and poor, even when the drug is administered on an empty stomach or combined with antacids.

An aqueous solution of benzylpenicillin administered intramuscularly is rapidly absorbed and reaches its maximum concentration in the blood within less than 15 minutes. The maximum concentration reached depends on the dose and on the method of injection, the effect being most rapid by intravenous and slowest by subcutaneous injection. About 35–60 per cent of benzylpenicillin is bound to plasma proteins but the protein-penicillin complex readily dissociates as the active free drug level is reduced. The blood level quickly falls, due to diffusion into the tissues and the rapid excretion of the drug by the kidneys. The duration of effect is a function of the dose,

Table 32.1 Sensitivity of micro-organisms to benzylpenicillin (after Garrod, 1950. *Br. med. J.*)

Fully sensitive (inhibited by 0.005–0.05 unit per ml)		Moderately resistant (inhibited by 1–10 units per ml)	
Gonococcus	*B. anthracis*	*H. influenzae*	
Meningococcus	*Actinomyces israeli*	*Str. faecalis*	
Pneumococcus	*Treponema pallidum*	*Proteus vulgaris*	
Str. pyogenes	*Vincent's organisms*	*Salm. typhi*	
Str. viridans	*Erysipelothrix rhusiopathiae*		
Staph. aureus			
Less sensitive (inhibited by 0.1–0.5 unit per ml)		**Highly resistant** (inhibited only by 50 units per ml)	
Clostridia		*Myco. tuberculosis*	*Ps. pyocanea*
C. diphtheriae		*Shig. dysenteriae*	*Bact. Friedländeri*
L. icterohaemorrhagiae		Most other Gram-negative bacilli. Yeast-like and some other fungi. Most viruses.	

and Figure 32.3 shows the length of time for which different doses will maintain an adequate level of penicillin in the blood.

The capacity of the normal kidney to excrete penicillin is practically unlimited, and a cumulative effect of the drug cannot be obtained. About 60 per cent of penicillin injected is excreted in the urine, the greater proportion of the dose being eliminated in the first hour. The drug is excreted by the renal tubules and in patients with impaired renal function the excretion is considerably retarded.

Since penicillin is rapidly excreted by the renal tubules, attempts have been made to inhibit the enzyme systems response for its tubular transport in order to raise the blood level of penicillin and prolong its duration of action. *Probenecid* (p. 154) has been used clinically to produce this effect.

Distribution. After absorption, penicillin is distributed in the body and can be detected in the bile and in the saliva. Diffusion also takes place in the serous cavities and through the placenta. The drug does not pass readily into

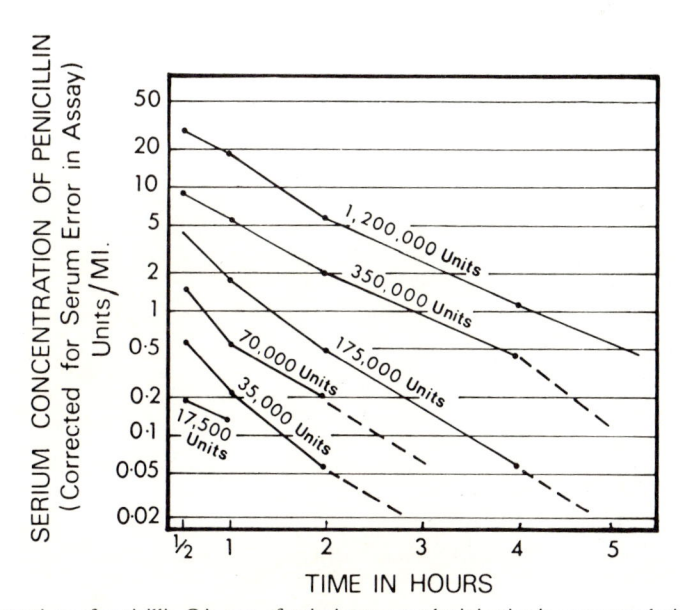

Fig. 32.3 The serum concentrations of penicillin G in man after its intramuscular injection in aqueous solution at varying dosage. The effect of doubling the dose is to prolong by about an hour the period during which an effective blood level of penicillin is maintained. (After Eagle, Fleischman and Musselman, 1949. *J. Bact.*)

the cerebrospinal fluid, and even after an intramuscular injection of 300 000 units, which produces a blood level of about 8 units per ml, only traces of penicillin are found in the cerebrospinal fluid. Nevertheless large doses of benzylpenicillin are administered intravenously in the treatment of bacterial meningitis caused by susceptible strains and this may be supplemented by the intrathecal injection of a solution of the drug. A single dose of 10 000 units (6 mg) will maintain an adequate level in the cerebrospinal fluid for 24 hours.

Long-acting preparations
Various attempts have been made to prolong the effects of a single dose of penicillin, either by delaying the absorption or by blocking excretion. The first attempts to delay absorption were made by suspending calcium penicillin in an oily base containing beeswax. This has been superseded by using a suspension of procaine benzylpenicillin in water.

Procaine penicillin has low solubility and is slowly absorbed; after an injection of 300 000 units of procaine benzylpenicillin the blood level slowly rises to a maximum in about four hours and detectable amounts are still present in the blood after twelve hours (Fig. 32.4). While these longer-acting preparations require to be injected only once every day they provide low blood levels of penicillin and cannot be used when a high blood concentration of penicillin is required.

Benzathine penicillin is obtained by the combination of two molecules of benzylpenicillin with one molecule of dibenzylethylenediamine. Its solubility in water is only 1 part in 5000 and it is quite stable in aqueous suspension. When this aqueous suspension is injected intramuscularly it is slowly absorbed, a single dose providing detectable concentrations of penicillin for at least 10 days.

Phenoxymethylpenicillin (Penicillin V)
This is a naturally occurring penicillin obtained when phenoxyacetic acid is added to the fermentation medium. Its main value is its acid stability; it is not destroyed in the stomach and can therefore be administered by mouth. It is, however, incompletely absorbed.

After oral administration, phenoxymethylpenicillin produces a slowly rising concentration of penicillin in the blood which reaches a maximum after about an hour. When the same dose of benzylpenicillin is injected intramuscularly it produces a higher blood level of penicillin initially, but after one hour the blood levels obtained by the two methods are about the same and they decline at the same rate (Fig. 32.4). About 25 per cent of an oral dose of phenoxymethylpenicillin is excreted in the urine compared with about 60 per cent of a dose of injected benzylpenicillin.

A satisfactory therapeutic blood concentration of penicillin can be maintained by oral administration of 250 mg of phenoxymethylpenicillin every four hours.

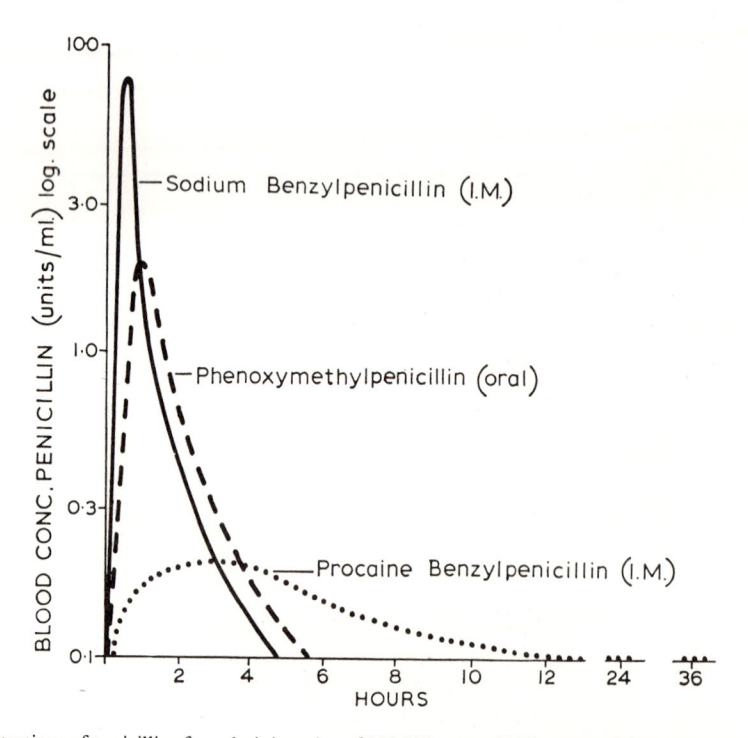

Fig. 32.4 Blood concentrations of penicillin after administration of 300 000 units of different penicillin preparations. (After Robson and Buttle, 1960. *Br. med. Bull.*)

Semisynthetic penicillins

An important advance has been the production of new semisynthetic penicillins starting from 6-APA. The first step was the isolation of crystalline 6-APA from mould cultures deprived of precursors required for the elaboration of complete penicillins. This was achieved by Batchelor and his colleagues in the Beecham laboratories in England in 1957. Another advance was the preparation of 6-APA from available penicillins by means of bacterial amidases. After the 6-APA nucleus became available new penicillins could be prepared by attaching to it a variety of side chains by a semisynthetic process.

A number of clinically important derivatives have been produced possessing one or more of the following advantages over benzylpenicillin: (1) resistance to acid, (2) resistance to penicillinase, (3) broader antibacterial spectrum.

The chemical structures of some important natural and semisynthetic penicillins are shown in Figure 32.5. The main features of the semisynthetic penicillins are as follows.

Acid resistance

Penicillin V is a naturally produced acid-resistant penicillin. Despite this property only about 25 per cent of the dose is absorbed and some semisynthetic acid-resistant penicillins such as *phenethicillin* and *propicillin* are better absorbed. The therapeutic effectiveness of these penicillins depends on three factors: antibacterial activity, efficiency of absorption and degree of protein binding in the blood. For general purposes each compound is suitable if administerd at 4-hourly intervals, but if they are used for a serious special indication the suitability of particular compounds should be ascertained by a test of the

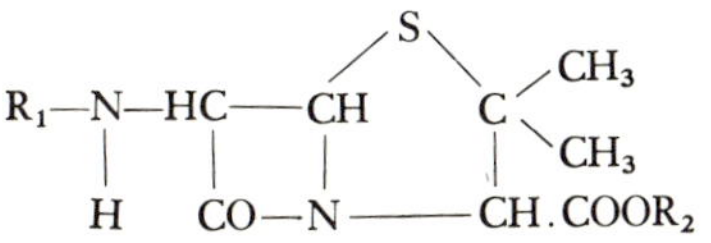

R_1	Name	R_2	Important Properties
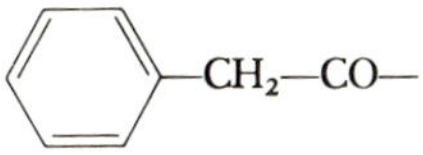 Phenyl–CH_2–CO–	Benzyl penicillin (Penicillin G) Procaine penicillin Benzathine penicillin	Na or K Procaine Benzathine	
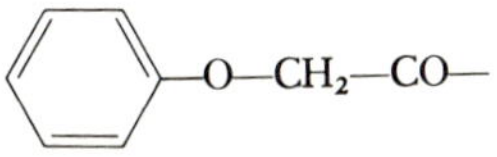 Phenyl–O–CH_2–CO–	Phenoxymethyl penicillin (Penicillin V)	H, K or Ca	Acid Resistant
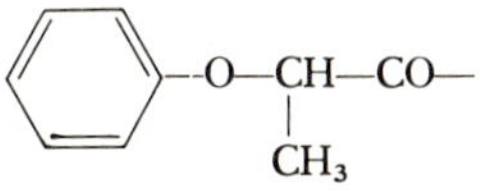 Phenyl–O–CH(CH$_3$)–CO–	Phenethicillin (Broxil)	K	Acid Resistant
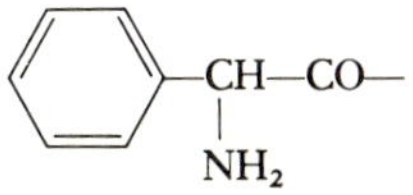 Phenyl–CH(NH$_2$)–CO–	Ampicillin (Penbritin)	H or Na	Acid Resistant Wider Range of Antibacterial Activity
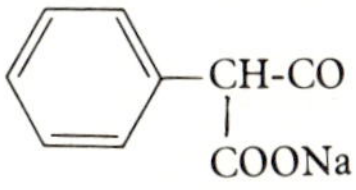 Phenyl–CH(COONa)–CO–	Carbenicillin (Pyopen)	Na	Activity against Pseudomonos, Proteus
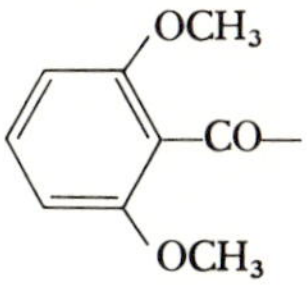 2,6-dimethoxyphenyl–CO–	Methicillin (Celbenin)	Na	Penicillinase Resistant
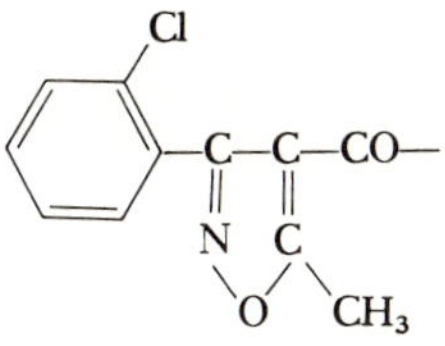 3-(2-chlorophenyl)-5-methylisoxazol-4-yl–CO–	Cloxacillin (Orbenin)	Na	Penicillinase Resistant Acid Resistant

Fig. 32.5

sensitivity of the organism to the penicillin which it is propsed to use.

Penicillinase resistance
Methicillin is highly resistant to staphylococcal penicillinase and is active against penicillin-sensitive strains of *Staph. aureus* whether they produce penicillinase or not. Since it is not acid resistant it has to be administered by intramuscular or intravenous injection and, being rapidly excreted, injections must be frequent. Peak plasma concentrations are attained within half to one hour of intramuscular injection and effective concentrations maintained for three to four hours.

Methicillin is used only in the treatment of infections due to penicillinase producing staphylococci. Strains of staphylococcus resistant to methicillin have recently been found. Some of these strains form large amounts of penicillinase but this is not the cause of the resistance since methicillin is not destroyed by penicillinase. Resistance in this case appears to be due to chromosomal mutation.

Penicillinase resistance and acid resistance
A series of isoxazole penicillins (Fig. 32.5) combine resistance to penicillinase with resistance to acid. They can therefore be administered by mouth. They should be given before meals since food interferes with their absorption which is in any case incomplete. Higher blood levels are produced by intramuscular injection.

The series includes *cloxacillin, dicloxacillin, oxacillin* and *flucloxacillin*. The latter is now widely used since it is well absorbed and produces high blood levels. It is used for infections due to staphylococci resistant to benzyl penicillin. It is also used for mixed streptococcal and staphylococcal infections when the staphylococci are penicillin G-resistant.

Broad spectrum
Carbenicillin (Fig. 32.5) is a semisynthetic penicillin which is clinically effective against species of *Pseudomonas* and *Proteus*. It is less active than benzylpenicillin against Gram-positive species but it is effective againt Gram-negative *E. coli* infections. Carbenicillin is frequently combined with gentamicin in *Pseudomonas* infections. It is much less toxic than the latter and the two drugs are believed to act synergistically. Combined administration may also prevent resistance formation. Probenecid enhances the blood level of the drug.

Carbenicillin is inactivated by penicillinase. It is not absorbed when given by mouth and must be administered intramuscularly or intravenously. It may cause pain at the site of injection.

Broad spectrum and acid resistance
The aminobenzyl side chain of *ampicillin* (Fig. 32.5) confers two distinct advantages over benzylpenicillin, namely a wider range of antibacterial activity and acid resistance.

Ampicillin, in contrast to the other penicillins, is only sparingly soluble in water. After oral administration it is relatively slowly absorbed and excreted in the urine and bile. Effective blood concentrations of the drug can be maintained by six-hourly dosage.

Against Gram-positive bacteria, ampicillin is slightly less active than benzylpenicillin but it is more active against some strains of *Streptococcus faecalis* and many species of Gram-negative bacilli. Ampicillin is also highly active against *H. influenzae* and *Salmonella* and *Shigella* species and has great value in the treatment of acute and chronic bronchitis and typhoid fever. It is inactivated by penicillinase; most strains of *Klebsiella aerogenes* and the *Proteus* group which produce this enzyme are resistant to ampicillin. However some strains of *E. coli* which secrete very small amounts of penicillinase are sensitive and because the drug is highly concentrated in urine, it is often effective in the treatment of urinary tract infections. Ampicillin is the most useful penicillin for this purpose when the organism is sensitive since it is much more active than benzylpenicillin in most urinary infections and can be given by mouth. In practice, ampicillin treatment is frequently instituted in these infections after treatment with the (cheaper) sulphonamides has failed.

A side effect of ampicillin is the occurrence of rashes which are decidedly commoner than with other penicillins; they occur particularly when ampicillin is given in glandular fever. Ampicillin rashes are maculopapular and differ from the urticarial rashes produced by benzylpenicillin.

Amoxycillin has a similar antibacterial spectrum to ampicillin but produces higher blood levels than the latter.

Therapeutic uses
The rational use of penicillin demands a knowledge not only of the disease to be treated, but also of the nature and extent of the infection. Bacteriological evidence of the nature of the infection should be available whenever possible, for no good purpose will be served by using penicillin against insensitive organisms. For most Gram-positive infections benzylpenicillin is the drug of choice because it has the highest activity against the majority of susceptible bacteria. According to the preparation used it can be injected intramuscularly or intravenously to give any desired blood concentration; the sodium or potassium salt can also be injected intrathecally. If an oral penicillin is chosen phenoxymethylpenicillin will serve most purposes. When an infection is known or suspected to be caused by a penicillin G resistant staphylococcus, cloxacillin or flucloxacillin can be given by mouth; in very severe infections it may be supplemented by injections of methicillin. Oral ampicillin has a special place in the treatment of infections due to organisms which are

resistant to benzylpenicillin but which do not produce penicillinase. It can be used in recurrent urinary tract infections including those caused by coliform organisms, proteus and *Str. faecalis* if the organism is sensitive. An important new synthetic penicillin is *carbenicillin* which is effective against many strains of *Pseudomonas* and indole-positive *Proteus*, particularly in urinary infections. It is important to appreciate that allergic hypersensitivity to benzylpenicillin implies probable cross sensitivity to all penicillins.

The duration of treatment depends on the intensity of the infection and the accessibility of the drug to the organisms. Severe acute infections may be adequately controlled within seven to nine days, whilst prolonged therapy for six to eight weeks may be required in the treatment of bacterial endocarditis.

Haemolytic streptococcal infection. The chief types are wound sepsis, puerperal fever and acute throat infections; these are all effectively treated with penicillin. Its chief advantage is that even the most severe infections can be quickly controlled and if necessary the dose of the drug may be increased 5- or 10-fold without risk of toxic effects. Indeed, fatal haemolytic streptococcal infections have practically disappeared due to the introduction of penicillin.

Penicillin is effective in the treatment of subacute bacterial endocarditis due to *Streptococcus viridans* if the organism is penicillin sensitive, but large doses (2 to 6 mega units ≈ 1.2 to 3.6 g) of benzylpenicillin must be injected daily for at least six weeks.

Staphylococcal infections. When penicillin was first introduced it was universally effective in the treatment of staphylococcal infections, but its usefulness has now become more limited due to the emergence of penicillinase producing penicillin-resistant strains. With sensitive strains of staphylococci the natural penicillins are generally most active. Frequently benzylpenicillin is combined with another drug, especially in the early stages of treatment.

A case in point is the treatment of acute osteomyelitis in which the infective organism is in most cases *Staph. aureus*. Specimens for bacteriological investigation should be taken and treatment started immediately afterwards without awaiting the test results. It is usual to start with a mixture of benzylpenicillin and a second drug such as flucloxacillin or a cephalosporin, effective against penicillinase-producing staphylococci. When the test results become available, treatment with penicillin alone is instituted if the organism is penicillin-sensitive. If on the other hand the organism is penicillin-resistant, treatment with penicillin G is discontinued and administration of the second drug continued.

Pneumococcal and gonococcal infections mostly respond to penicillin. A single injection of 1.2 mega units of procaine penicillin may be enough to eradicate an acute gonococcal urethritis.

Of all ordinary bacteria the gonococcus is most sensitive to penicillin, often disappearing from an infected lesion within two hours of a penicillin injection. Because of this rapid effect it was thought that the gonococcus would have no time to adapt to penicillin and would fail to develop resistance to it. Unfortunately there is now increasing evidence of penicillin resistance in gonococci, and this has become widespread, particularly in some countries.

In an attempt to deal with penicillin resistance the dose of benzylpenicillin used for treating acute gonorrhoea have been increased up to 5 mega units sometimes combined with probenecid to diminish penicillin excretion and raise its blood level. Alternatively, oral tetracyclines or ampicillin or co-trimazole or even parenteral kanamycin or cephaloridine have been used. More recently intramuscular *spectinomycin* has been used in gonorrhoeal infection when the penicillin group is contraindicated.

Penicillin is highly effective against *Treponema pallidum*, the organism responsible for syphilis (p. 435). All pneumococcal infections, including pneumococcal meningitis, respond well to penicillin. In the latter case large doses of benzylpenicillin, one mega unit several times daily, are given by intramuscular injection and 10 000 units daily by intrathecal injection.

The main drawback and most serious danger of all forms of penicillin treatment is penicillin allergy.

The prophylactic use of penicillin

When a dental extraction or tonsillectomy is carried out in a patient with rheumatic fever or otherwise predisposed, an antibiotic may be given prophylactically. If penicillin is used the drug should be given shortly before the operation so that its maximum concentration in the blood is reached at the time of operation. This is preferable to penicillin administration several days in advance since this may give rise to the appearance of resistant strains of streptococci.

Toxicity

One of the remarkable features of the penicillins is their relative freedom from toxic effects apart from hypersensitivity reactions. Despite the high concentration of the drug produced in the kidneys, no adverse renal effects due to penicillin have been reported. High concentrations of penicillin are, however, toxic to the central nervous system, and for this reason when penicillin is administered intrathecally the concentration should not exceed 1000 units per ml.

Penicillin allergy

The importance of the development of hypersensitivity to penicillin is becoming increasingly evident and it is now recognised that in some individuals penicillin may cause severe drug reactions. The allergy usually extends to all penicillin derivatives.

It is believed that either penicillin itself or one of its degradation products undergoes a combination with plasma proteins which renders it antigenic. The antibodies formed can be divided into two groups:

1. Non-sensitising antibodies can be readily detected by a haemagglutination method and are frequently found in patients receiving penicillin. Their detection has, however, little prognostic value since this type of antibody is probably not the cause of allergic reactions.

2. Sensitising antibodies or reagins. These may be detected by skin tests with penicillin or penicilloylpolylysine, or by means of Prausnitz-Kuester reactions. Alternatively they may be detected by passive sensitisation of human or monkey tissues *in vitro* with the patient's serum and measuring histamine release after adding penicilloylpolylysine as antigen (p. 101).

Another theoretical possibility is detection of serum IgE antibodies against penicillin by the serological radioimmunoabsorbent (RAST) test which is being increasingly employed in cases of pollen and dust sensitization. Unfortunately, none of these methods has so far produced a reliable method for detecting clinical penicillin hypersensitivity *in vitro* (p. 104).

Clinical manifestations. These may show themselves in three ways:

1. An immediate reaction of the anaphylactic type with circulatory collapse, oedema of the larynx and respiratory obstruction which may be rapidly fatal.

2. A less sudden response of the serum sickness type with fever, urticaria or other skin eruption and, in severe cases, multiple joint effusions and enlargement of lymph glands and spleen.

3. Contact dermatitis induced by local application of penicillin to skin or mucosa. Contact dermatitis is seen, for example, in nurses and other persons frequently exposed to penicillin.

Fatal anaphylaxis is fortunately rare, but difficult to protect against; most penicillin deaths have occurred without warning, often in persons who have had no history of allergy. Allergic reactions may occur after every form of administration of penicillin, including the intradermal administration of a minute test dose, and after oral administration. The severest manifestations of allergy, however, occur after parenteral administration. Topical administration is always undesirable.

Evidence of penicillin sensitization. No absolutely reliable test for penicillin hypersensitivity has yet been devised. Various *in vitro* tests have already been outlined. Intradermal injections of penicillin in patients may be dangerous, and they are far from infallible. Several cases of fatal reactions to penicillin have been reported in subjects in whom intradermal tests were negative. Skin tests are probably better able to predict serum sickness-type reactions than anaphylactic reactions.

Certain derivatives of penicillin have been used for skin tests and are said to be less dangerous than penicillin itself. Amongst these is penicilloylpolylysine and a material called 'minor determinant mixture' containing several penicillin degradation products. In clinical practice penicillin allergy may be suspected from the patient's history; if this is established some other antibiotic or synthetic drug must be used instead.

CEPHALOSPORINS

Cephaloridine (Ceporin)

Cultures of a Cephalosporium fungus, obtained from the sea near a sewage outfall in Sardinia were found to yield extracts which inhibited the growth of *Staph. aureus*. Subsequent work with other related species of this fungus resulted in the isolation of three distinct antibiotics; cephalosporin N and cephalosporin C which are closely related to penicillin, though much less active than benzylpenicillin against Gram-positive cocci, and cephalosporin P, a steroid antibiotic which resembles fucidin.

The nucleus of cephalosporin C has been isolated and named 7-aminocephalosporanic acid; its structural relation to the penicillin nucleus is shown below. In a similar way to the semi-synthetic penicillins, a number of different cephalosporin derivatives have been produced by the addition of sidechains to 7-aminocephalosporanic acid, amongst which is cephaloridine. Its mode of action is similar to that of the penicillins. It is bactericidal for rapidly multiplying bacteria and inhibits the synthesis of cell wall mucopeptides.

6-Aminopenicillanic acid

7-Amino-cephalosporanic acid

Cephaloridine has a spectrum of antibacterial activity resembling ampicillin. It is active against most strains of *Staph. aureus*, and although its structure contains the ß-lactam ring, it is less susceptible to penicillinase than ampicillin. Cross-sensitivity with penicillin has been shown to occur and it is generally unadvisable for patients who are penicillin-hypersensitive to take cephaloridine.

It is about as active against most species of streptococcus as benzylpenicillin but less so against *Str. faecalis*. Cephaloridine also resembles ampicillin in its activity against some *Salmonella* and *Shigella* species and many strains of *E. coli*, but is superior to the latter drug in that it inhibits nearly all strains of *Proteus mirabilis* including those which produce penicillinase.

Toxic effects of cephaloridine include skin rashes and urticaria. There is some evidence that large doses of cephaloridine may cause kidney damage and evidence of hyaline casts appearing in the urine has been seen during treatment with the drug.

Cephaloridine is poorly absorbed from the alimentary tract and must be administered by intramuscular or intravenous injection. It is distributed to most tissues other than the brain and cerebrospinal fluid. Like benzylpenicillin, it is rapidly excreted in the urine.

Cephalothin is less susceptible than cephaloridine to inactivation by penicillinase. It has the same spectrum of activity as cephaloridine and is given by intramuscular or intravenous injection.

Oral cephalosporins

Cephaloridine and cephalothin are poorly absorbed from the gastrointestinal tract and attempts have been made to find cephalosporins which are adequately absorbed when taken by mouth. *Cephalexin* is acid stable and well absorbed after oral administration. It is used in infections by susceptible bacteria found in the respiratory and urinary tracts. Long term use may result in the growth of resistant organisms such as *Pseudomonas*. *Cephadrine* may be administered both orally and parenterally.

Sodium fusidate (Fucidin)

This antibiotic has been isolated from strains of *Fusidium coccineum* and is chemically related to cephalosporin P. It is active against a wide range of Gram-positive bacteria and Gram-negative cocci, but the chief clinical interest lies in its activity against staphylococci including strains resistant to penicillins. Nearly all strains of *Staph. aureus* are inhibited by low concentrations of fucidin.

Fucidin is well absorbed after oral administration and slowly excreted as an inactive product in the urine. High blood concentrations can be maintained by eight-hourly doses of 500 mg. The therapeutic use of fucidin is mainly reserved for the treatment of staphylococcal infections in conjunction with other antibiotics such as erythromycin.

PREPARATIONS

Penicillins
Amoxycillin (Amoxil) 250 mg 3x die
Ampicillin (Penbritin) 1–6 g dl
Benzathine Penicillin (Penidural) proph 900 mg i.m. every 2–3 w
Benzylpenicillin (Penicillin G) i.m. 0.3–5 g dl, p.o. 0.5–3 g dl
Carbenicillin sod (Pyopen) 4–8 g i.m. dl
Cloxacillin sod (Orbenin) 1.5–3 g p.o. i.m. dl
Flucloxacillin sod (Floxapen) 250 mg p.o. i.m. 4x die
Methicillin sod (Celbenin) 3–12 g i.m. dl
Penamecillin (Havapen) 350 mg every 8 h
Phenethicillin pot (Broxil) 0.5–1.5 g p.o. dl
Phenoxymethylpenicillin (Penicillin V) 0.5–1 g p.o. dl
Pivampicillin hyd 350–700 mg p.o. 3–4x die
Procaine Penicillin 300–900 mg i.m. dl
Talampicillin hyd (phthalidyl ampicillin, Talpen) 250–500 mg 3x die

Antibiotics for penicillin-resistant strains
Fusidate sod 1–2 g dl
Spectinomycin dihyd 2 g for males, 4 g for fem (gonorrh)

Cephalosporins
Cefuroxime sod 500–750 mg dl i.m. i.v.
Cephalexin (Ceporex) 1–4 g dl p.o.
Cephaloridine (Ceporin) 0.5–1 g i.m. 2–3x die
Cephalothin (Keflin) 2–6 g dl i.m. or slow i.v.
Cephazolin sod (Kefzol) 1–4 g dl i.m. i.v.
Cephradine (Velosef) 1–4 g dl p.o.

FURTHER READING

Caterall R D, Nicol C S (ed) 1976 Sexually transmitted diseases. Academic Press, London
Fuerst R 1978 Microbiology in health and disease. Saunders, Philadelphia
Kucers A, Bennett N McK 1975 The use of antibiotics. Heinemann, London
Stewart G T, McGovern J P (ed) 1970 Penicillin allergy. Thomas, Springfield
Wilson David 1976 Penicillin in perspective. Faber & Faber, London

33. Other antibiotics for the chemotherapy of infections

Macrolides 408; Lincomycin and clindamycin 409; Tetracyclines 409; Clinical applications 410; Chloramphenicol 411; Aminoglycosides 411; Peptide antibiotics 412; Antifungal antibiotics 413; Flucytosine 414; Choice of antibiotic 414; Antibiotic prescribing chart 415.

A large number of antibiotics have been isolated from different strains of streptomycetes. They comprise some of the clinically most important antibacterial antibiotics including the chemical groups of macrolides, tetracyclines and amino-glycosides. These, as well as chemically unrelated antibiotics derived from streptomycetes, are discussed in this chapter. Some peptide antibiotics derived from bacteria and certain antifungal antibiotics will also be discussed.

MACROLIDES

The macrolides are so named because they possess a macrocyclic lactone ring (Fig. 33.1) to which different sugars are attached. Erythromycin was the first of this group to be discovered and it has been used most extensively.

Erythromycin

Erythromycin was isolated in 1952 from a strain of *Streptomyces erythreus* found in a soil sample from the Philippines.

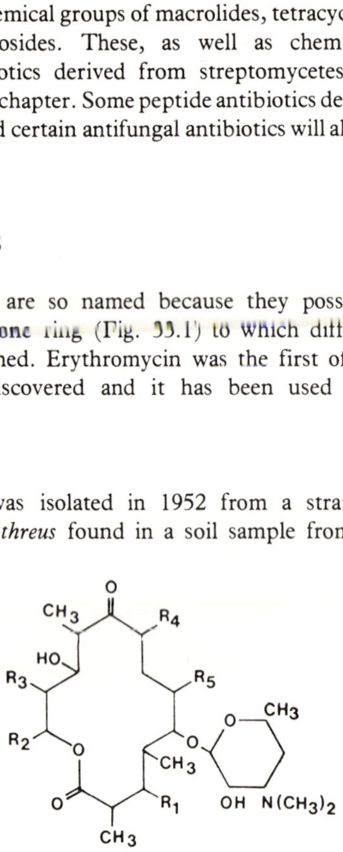

	Erythromycin A	Oleandomycin
R$_1$	L – cladinose	L – oleandrose
R$_2$	CH CH$_3$	CH$_3$
R$_3$	<CH$_3$ / OH	CH$_3$
R$_4$	CH$_3$	<CH$_2$ / O
R$_5$	<CH$_3$ / OH	CH$_3$

Fig. 33.1 Structure of macrolides. (After Garrod, Lambert and O'Grady, *Antibiotic and Chemotherapy*. Churchill Livingstone, 1973.)

Erythromycin is absorbed when taken by mouth, but is partly inactivated by gastric juice and is therefore administered in acid-resistant coated tablets. It diffuses freely into most tissues including the placenta, but does not pass readily into the cerebrospinal fluid; it is excreted largely in the bile.

Antibacterial activity. Like penicillin, erythromycin is active against Gram-positive bacteria and spirochaetes but, with the exception of *Neisseria* and to a less extent *Haemophilus influenzae*, the Gram-negative bacteria are resistant to it.

Therapeutic uses. Erythromycin can be used for the treatment of most infections which respond to penicillin and is particularly useful in patients who are allergic to penicillin. It can also be used to combat infections due to micro-organisms which have become resistant to penicillin, particularly penicillinase-producing staphylococci, especially where allergic reactions preclude the use of a penicillinase-resistant derivative such as flucloxacillin. The use of erythromycin for the treatment of syphilis in patients with penicillin allergy is discussed on page 436.

The development of bacterial resistance to erythromycin has been reported but there is no cross-resistance to other antibiotics except to those in the macrolide group. When treatment with erythromycin is needed for periods longer than about a week it may be combined with another unrelated antibiotic to which the pathogen is sensitive to prevent the emergence of a resistant strain. In the treatment of severely ill patients with staphylococcal enteritis resistant to tetracyclines, erythromycin may be given in conjunction with an isoxazole penicillin.

The toxicity of erythromycin is low and gastrointestinal disturbances are less frequent than with the tetracycline drugs.

Erythromycin estolate is an ester of erythromycin which has the advantages of acid resistance and tastelessness, but liver damage, possibly due to a hypersensitivity reaction, after this compound has been reported.

Spiramycin and *oleandomycin* are antibiotics which resemble erythromycin in their chemical structures, actions and uses. *Troleandomycin* is the triacetyl ester of oleandomycin.

Lincomycin and clindamycin

Lincomycin hydrochloride (Lincocin) differs chemically from the macrolides but has a similar range of antibacterial activity. Lincomycin is a natural product isolated from *Streptomyces lincolnensis* whilst clindamycin is a semi-synthetic modification of the original compound.

Clindamycin is better absorbed and more effective than lincomycin; it is a valuable drug especially against *Staph. aureus* infection. A serious side-effect of both clindamycin and lincomycin has been the occurrence of diarrhoea which may take the form of pseudomembranous colitis in some patients with chronic debilitating disease.

The antibiotics *Novobiocin* and *Vancomycin* have only limited uses because of their toxicity.

THE TETRACYCLINE DRUGS

Four important compounds isolated from cultures of streptomycetes are chemically closely related and are referred to as the tetracycline drugs (Fig. 33.2). Chlortetracycline (aureomycin) is obtained from cultures of *Streptomyces aureofaciens* and oxytetracycline (terramycin) from *Streptomyces rimosus*; tetracycline (achromycin, tetracyn) has also been isolated from soil cultures, but it is usually produced semi-synthetically by the catalytic hydrogenation of chlortetracycline. Demeclocycline (Demethylchlortetracycline, ledermycin) which lacks a methyl group in the R_1 position of chlortetracycline is formed by a strain of *Streptomyces aureofaciens* or produced semi-synthetically.

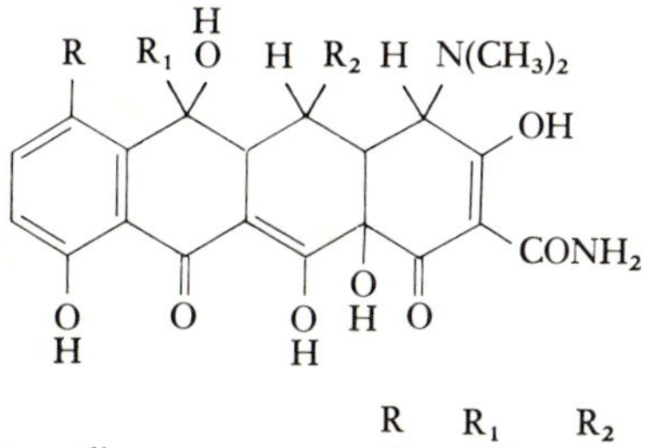

	R	R_1	R_2
Tetracycline	H	CH_3	H
Chlortetracycline	Cl	CH_3	H
Oxytetracycline	H	CH_3	OH
Demethylchlortetracycline	Cl	H	H

Fig. 33.2 Structural formulae of tetracycline drugs.

Chlortetracycline, tetracycline, oxytetracycline, demeclocycline

Chlortetracycline was the first of the tetracycline drugs to be isolated but it has now been superseded to some extent by the other related compounds. All tetracyclines are unstable in aqueous solution, chlortetracycline being the most and demeclocycline the least unstable. The tetracyclines are stable as dry powders. There are no important differences between the tetracyclines in antibacterial activity and only slight differences in their rates of absorption and excretion.

Mode of action. The basic action of tetracyclines is an interference with protein synthesis (p. 388). The tetracyclines are bacteriostatic agents that act by blocking the attachment of transfer RNA to ribosomes, thus interfering with protein synthesis. In contrast to penicillins and cephalosporins the tetracyclines do not affect synthesis of the bacterial cell wall and they are therefore effective against cell wall-deficient organisms such as *Mycoplasma pneumoniae*.

Antibiotic activity. In vitro studies indicate that as inhibitors of Gram-positive and Gram-negative organisms, the tetracyclines have a wider range of activity, but, on the whole, are less potent than penicillin. This also applies to the treatment of experimental infections in animals.

Micro-organisms susceptible to tetracyclines include not only those, mainly Gram-positive, species which are also sensitive to penicillin, but many Gram-negative species which do not respond to it. Species of *Proteus* and *Pseudomonas*, however, are normally resistant. Mycoplasmas and rickettsiae are very susceptible. Like penicillin, the tetracyclines are active against *T. pallidum* and they also have some slight activity against the tubercle bacillus. Fungal infections are normally resistant with the exception of actinomycosis, which responds well.

Bacterial resistance. Bacterial resistance to tetracyclines was initially believed to be rare but is now becoming increasingly identified. Resistance to tetracyclines is a slow process which is not often seen during the treatment of an individual patient, but, on an epidemiological basis, tetracycline-resistant strains of various organisms are often found. Cross resistance between all tetracyclines is common. Resistant strains of staphylococci and of coliform bacilli have become fairly frequent. Tetracycline resistance of haemolytic streptococci has been reported and is now appearing also in pneumococci. This is particularly ominous since respiratory tract infections have represented the largest field of use of tetracyclines.

Absorption, distribution and excretion. When given by mouth, all the tetracyclines are readily absorbed and peak concentrations in the blood usually occur within three to four hours. Demeclocycline is slightly better absorbed and more slowly excreted, so that effective blood levels of this drug can be maintained by six hourly doses of 150 mg compared with 250 mg of the others.

The tetracyclines are widely distributed in tissues; they diffuse into serous cavities and are present in bile and milk. They pass the blood-brain barrier and can be detected in the cerebrospinal fluid. The tetracyclines are partly destroyed in the body and partly excreted by the kidneys. About 10 to 20 per cent of an oral dose can be recovered from the urine.

Clinical applications
Due to their wide antibacterial activity, the tetracyclines can be used in a greater variety of infections than other antibiotics. They have been extensively used in cases where a bacteriological diagnosis is lacking but the justification for this usage has now become more doubtful with the occurrence of many drug-resistant strains. A further limitation of tetracyclines is the increasing recognition of their undesirable side effects, particularly superinfection. Since tetracyclines are bacteriostatic rather than bactericidal, they are contraindicated in conditions such as bacterial endocarditis when a bactericidal effect is required.

Tetracyclines were widely used in the treatment of infections of the respiratory tract, particularly in dealing with exacerbations of chronic bronchitis. In this indication, tetracyclines have to some extent been replaced by, or are alternated with, ampicillin, amoxycillin or co-trimazole. Acute infections of the respiratory tract are, however, frequently of viral origin when antibacterial drugs are ineffective. The tetracyclines are often used in the treatment of mixed infections of the urinary tract or in peritonitis but acquired resistance of various species of micro-organisms has restricted their value. The use of tetracyclines for acute throat infections is limited by frequent resistance of haemolytic streptococci.

Tetracyclines can be employed in place of penicillin for the treatment of syphilis, gonorrhoea, anthrax and actinomycosis. A fairly common, moderately effective, use of tetracyclines is for the long-term treatment of acne.

The tetracyclines may also be used by local application, for example in infections of the eye and the skin.

Administration. Tetracycline and oxytetracycline are usually given by mouth in doses of 250 mg every six hours; the daily dose should not normally exceed 2 g. Smaller doses (150 mg) of demeclocycline are equally effective and a total daily dose of 600 mg is seldom exceeded. Although a course of treatment with a tetracycline is usually limited to a few days because of the risk of superinfection, cases have been reported of patients with chronic bronchitis who have been treated continuously with up to 1 g daily for several months without untoward complications. If it is necessary to continue tetracycline treatment for longer periods, it is usual to give also vitamin B complex by mouth to prevent a vitamin deficiency arising from alterations in the bacterial flora of the intestine.

The tetracyclines are irritant in aqueous solution and parenteral administration is only justified in emergencies when the patient is unable to take the drug by mouth.

Toxic effects. The tetracycline drugs are relatively non-toxic but they are nevertheless liable to cause a number of disturbing side effects, partly because they are irritant drugs and also because, as a consequence of their wide antibacterial activity, they suppress the normal bacterial flora of the intestine.

Gastrointestinal disturbances such as nausea, vomiting and diarrhoea are fairly common. Lesions of the skin and mucous membranes may cause severe stomatitis and intense itching of the vulva and anorectal region. These lesions are often associated with proliferation of *Candida albicans*. Some of these lesions resemble those of riboflavin deficiency, but there is no convincing evidence that vitamin B deficiency occurs after short courses of tetracycline treatment.

The suppression of the normal bacterial flora makes the patient particularly susceptible to superinfection with tetracycline-resistant organisms, especially staphylococci. This is liable to occur in hospitals and may result in the invasion of the intestine by staphylococci which give rise to fulminating enterocolitis which can be fatal. Superinfection of the lungs with drug-resistant staphylococci may also occur during tetracycline treatment of pneumonia in hospitals. Another type of superinfection is the excessive growth of tetracycline-resistant *Proteus* and *Pseudomonas* during treatment of urinary tract infections, particularly where there is some anatomical abnormality or obstruction of the urinary tract. Severe superinfections are fortunately rare and indeed a remarkable feature of all the tetracycline drugs is their relative freedom from serious toxic effects.

High doses of tetracyclines especially after parenteral administration have been reported to produce liver damage. This is unlikely to occur after oral administration to patients with normal liver function, but implies cautious use of these drugs, in high doses or for prolonged periods, in patients with liver disease.

The tetracyclines act as chelating agents and when calcium is bound in this way in the body fluids, the tetracycline complex may be laid down in the bones or teeth. There is some evidence that this may result in retardment of growth of the foetus and young infant. Permanent staining of the teeth may also occur and after they have erupted and are exposed to light the yellow coloured stains become dark brown in colour. The deposits of tetracyclines in the teeth and bony structures fluoresce in ultraviolet light. Tetracyclines should not be administered after the fourth month of pregnancy and as far as possible their use should be avoided in infants and young children.

Although the tetracyclines are irritant when applied locally, true allergic reactions to the tetracycline drugs occur less frequently than to penicillin. Severe photosensitivity has been reported after treatment with demethylchlortetracycline.

Other tetracyclines. Several further tetracycline derivatives have been introduced with the general objective of increasing their rate of absorption and blood level. *Minocycline* has been reported to be particularly well absorbed and also to be effective against staphylococci resistant to other tetracyclines.

CHLORAMPHENICOL (CHLOROMYCETIN)

This antibiotic was isolated as a crystalline substance by Bartz in 1948 from cultures of *Streptomyces venezuelae*. The chemical structure of chloramphenicol was shown to be much simpler than that of other antibiotics, and it was later synthesised. The synthesis of an antibiotic on a commercial scale represented an important advance.

$$\begin{array}{c} NO_2 \\ | \\ \bigcirc \\ | \\ CHOH \\ | \\ HN-CH \\ | \quad | \\ CO \quad CH_2OH \\ | \\ CHCl_2 \end{array}$$

Chloramphenicol

Antibiotic activity. Like the tetracycline drugs, chloramphenicol has a wide range of activity against Gram-negative and Gram-positive organisms. It is highly effective against the rickettsiae of epidemic and scrub typhus, Rocky Mountain spotted fever, and *S. typhi* and paratyphoid infections. It is only slightly active against *M. tuberculosis*.

Fate. About 10 per cent of the drug is excreted in the urine as unchanged chloramphenicol, the remainder is inactivated in the liver either by conjugation with glucuronic acid or by reduction to inactive amines prior to renal excretion.

In infants and premature babies the capacity of the liver to conjugate chloramphenicol and the ability of the kidney to excrete it are poorly developed, so dangerously high blood levels of the drug may accumulate and produce severe circulatory collapse, abdominal distension and vomiting. This has been referred to as the 'grey syndrome' because of the ashen colour and fall in body temperature. The daily dose of chloramphenicol therefore should not exceed 25 mg per kg of body weight in infants under three months of age.

Therapeutic uses. The most important uses of chloramphenicol is in the treatment of typhoid and paratyphoid fever. The drug produces considerable symptomatic relief although it does not completely eliminate the organisms from the intestine; thus it does not prevent relapses nor does it prevent persistence of the carrier state.

Chloramphenicol is very effective against organisms of the haemophilus group (*H. influenzae* and *H. pertussis*) although ampicillin is generally as effective. Chloramphenicol is the most generally useful drug in meningitis due to *H. influenzae* and other organisms because of its good penetration into the c.s.f. If administered to a patient with whooping cough within the first week, it reduces the frequency and severity of paroxysms; however in this respect the tetracycline drugs are as effective and less liable to produce serious toxic effects.

Toxic effects. Chloramphenicol, like the tetracycline drugs, produces nausea, vomiting and diarrhoea and glossitis which is usually painful, by altering the bacterial flora of the intestine. Chloramphenicol depresses haematopoietic function and may cause blood dyscrasias, especially fatal aplastic anaemia.

Aplastic anaemia after chloramphenicol may occur not only after the administration of large doses for prolonged periods but also after small doses given for short periods. It is now considered, therefore, that chloramphenicol should be used only for severe infections or for the treatment of infections such as typhoid which do not respond to other antibiotics or where the results of bacteriological sensitivity tests preclude the use of others.

THE AMINOGLYCOSIDES

The aminoglycosides are a group of antibiotics of similar chemical structure of which the prototype is streptomycin (p. 420). A series of other aminoglycosides share with streptomycin the same general range of antibacterial activity and a similar absorption and distribution pattern. They all have a tendency to damage one or other branch of the eighth nerve and to produce kidney damage. The aminoglycosides are eliminated by the kidney and, because they are all oto- and nephrotoxic, their dosage must be reduced in patients with impaired renal function.

The aminoglycosides are all bases and they are usually employed as the sulphates. They are bactericidal in concentrations which are attainable in the blood stream.

Streptomycin

Streptomycin was discovered in the early searches for an antibiotic active against Gram-negative bacteria. The outstanding property of this drug is its high activity against *Mycobacterium tuberculosis*, an account of which is given in Chapter 34.

Apart from tuberculosis, streptomycin is also used for the treatment of plague and tularaemia in which it is highly effective. The combination of streptomycin and tetracycline provides an effective treatment of brucellosis.

Streptomycin is also active against certain Gram-negative penicillin-resistant organisms such as *H. influenzae*, *B. proteus*, *Ps. pyocyanea* and *E. coli* and can be used in the treatment of infections due to these organisms. The main drawback of streptomycin treatment is its toxic effect on the eighth nerve which causes vestibular disturbances, and the emergence of resistant organisms in the short-term treatment of non-tuberculous infections. In non-tuberculous infections, organisms may develop a 1000-fold resistance within a few days. Resistance to streptomycin and other aminoglycosides both *in vitro* and *in vivo* is acquired more rapidly than to any other of the antibiotics commonly used. In the treatment of urinary tract infections, large doses should be given for a short period and combined therapy should be considered since, unless the infective organisms are destroyed within a short time of the onset of treatment, drug-resistant strains are certain to appear. This resistance is permanent and a large proportion of bacteria from urinary tract infections of patients in hospital have become resistant to streptomycin. It is for this reason that the systemic use of this drug is now being restricted to the treatment of tuberculosis and a few infections which cannot be treated effectively with other antibiotics.

Streptomycin and penicillin are both bactericidal drugs which can act synergistically and their combined administration is often successful in the treatment of bacterial endocarditis, particularly that due to *Str. faecalis*.

Since streptomycin is not absorbed from the intestinal tract it can be given orally for its effect on the intestinal flora without risk of systemic toxicity.

Neomycin

This antibiotic, which is chemically related to streptomycin, was isolated from a culture of *Streptomyces fradiae*. The antibacterial activity of neomycin differs little from that of streptomycin. Resistance to it may develop and is usually accompanied by resistance to other aminoglycosides.

Due to the high ototoxicity of neomycin it is unsuitable for parenteral use. It has been used by local application for the treatment of superficial infections of the skin and eye with penicillin-resistant staphylococci and Gram-negative bacilli. To avoid the development of resistant strains, neomycin is often used in combination with another agent such as bacitracin or chlorhexidine. Sensitization to neomycin after topical application is rare but has occurred in some patients.

When administered orally, neomycin is not appreciably absorbed and may be used for the treatment of acute gastrointestinal infections or prior to abdominal surgery.

Kanamycin

This antibiotic was isolated in Japan from a strain of *Streptomyces kanamyceticus*. Its antibacterial activity against Gram-negative organisms including *B. proteus* is similar to that of neomycin but clinical evidence suggests that its ototoxicity is less. It is used parenterally for the treatment of urinary tract infections or septicaemias due to Gram-negative organisms such as *Proteus* resistant to other drugs.

Kanamycin is administered intramuscularly in a dose of 1 g daily for 7 days. This dose is near the toxic limit, and if renal function is impaired, may cause irreversible deafness. When kanamycin is used for the treatment of tuberculosis (p. 425) it can be administered at longer intervals, which diminishes the risk of toxic effects.

Paromomycin is an aminoglycoside which has been found particularly effective against *E. histolytica*.

Gentamicin

Gentamicin is derived from *Micromonospora purpurea*. It is the most active antibiotic of the aminoglycoside group, and in contrast to other members of the group has significant activity against *Ps. pyocyenea*, as well as other Gram-negative bacilli. It is also highly effective against *Staph. aureus*. Like the rest of this group, gentamicin is almost unabsorbed from the alimentary tract and, if used against systemic infections, must be administered intramuscularly. It readily traverses the placenta.

Gentamicin has considerable toxicity for the eighth nerve, vestibular function being particularly affected. It is more ototoxic than kanamycin. The safe upper limit of the blood level with each of these drugs is probably under 10 μg/ml.

Clinical uses. The main fields for gentamicin therapy are serious Gram-negative infections of the urinary tract or elsewhere, particularly *Ps. aeruginosa* infections. In systemic Gram-negative septicaemia it is often combined with large doses of carbenicillin.

Gentamicin may be used as a cream for burns and other surface infections, in view of its high activity against staphylococci. It can also be administered orally for pre-operative suppression of the bowel flora.

Tobramycin is closely related to gentamycin in its bacterial spectrum, degree of effectiveness and toxicity.

PEPTIDE ANTIBIOTICS

Several peptide antibiotics have been introduced, all derived from bacilli. They consist of peptide-linked amino acids, in some cases joined to non-amino acid moieties, such as the long-chain fatty acids of the polymyxins. The peptide antibiotics are mainly used for local application since they are toxic when administered systemically, but the polymyxins are also used systemically because of their effectiveness in *Pseudomonas* infections.

Polymyxins

Polymyxin is a general name given to a number of polypeptide antibiotics which have been isolated from

Bacillus polymyxa. Polymyxin B (aerosporin) is one of the least toxic of these compounds and is used clinically as the sulphate. It has a narrow range of activity, but is highly effective against many Gram-negative bacteria, particularly *Pseudomonas*. It is rapidly bactericidal to these organisms and resistance rarely develops.

Topical application. Polymyxin B is not absorbed from the gastrointestinal tract and can be used orally to treat *Pseudomonas* and *Shigella* infections of the intestine. It is also used locally to combat infections of the eye, ear and skin caused by Gram-negative bacteria. It can be applied locally in aqueous solution or as an ointment.

Systemic administration. Polymyxins are highly active against *Ps. aeruginosa* and are used systemically in infections involving these organisms; indeed until the recent advent of gentamicin and carbenicillin treatment, polymyxin was the drug of choice for infections due to *Ps. pyocyanea*. Polymyxin B sulphate is usually administered intravenously since it produces intense pain when injected intramuscularly.

Toxic effects. Polymyxin B and E produce similar neurotoxic and nephrotoxic effects.

When injected intravenously, polymyxin produces dizziness, drowsiness and paraesthesias. These neurotoxic effects disappear when the drug has been excreted and permanent after-effects have not been reported. Large doses, however, may produce respiratory arrest.

When a parenteral dose of polymyxin B is given daily for several days, patients frequently develop proteinuria, haematuria and urinary cylinders. In patients with normal renal function these effects are reversible and do not preclude the use of the drug. However, in patients with impaired kidney function great caution is needed in the use of polymyxin.

Colistin (colomycin) is polymyxin E and its antibacterial activity is very similar to that of polymyxin B. *Colistimethate* may be injected intramuscularly.

Bacitracin

This polypeptide antibiotic was first isolated from a culture of *Bacillus subtilis* obtained from a wound sustained by a child called Margaret Tracy. It was named bacitracin in honour of this patient. The range of antibiotic activity of bacitracin is similar to that of penicillin, but it is less liable to produce resistant organisms and is not destroyed by penicillinase.

Bacitracin is not readily absorbed from the gastrointestinal tract and when taken by mouth acts mainly on the intestine. The chief use of this drug is in the local treatment of infections of the mouth, nose, eye and skin where it is less liable than penicillin to produce sensitisation.

Although bacitracin was originally considered to be highly toxic to the renal tubules, it is now evident that some of these toxic effects were due to impurities. Nevertheless, even the purer preparations now available are sufficiently toxic to the kidneys to restrict the systemic use of this drug to the treatment of severe infections which cannot be treated otherwise.

Bacitracin can be applied locally in an ointment or aqueous solution.

ANTIFUNGAL ANTIBIOTICS

A number of antibiotics have been isolated from species of *Streptomyces* and of *Penicillium* which in general have little or no antibacterial action but are highly effective against fungal infections. They differ from each other in chemical structure and pharmacological properties and have different specificities against mycoses. Human fungus infections fall into three principal classes: (1) those due to dermatophytes affecting the skin, hair and nails; (2) local and usually superficial infections caused by *Candida albicans*; (3) systemic infections, which may also be caused by *Candida* species, of which other examples are aspergillosis, coccidiomycosis, cryptococcosis and histoplasmosis. The principal antibiotics available for their treatment are as follows:

Griseofulvin (p. 230)

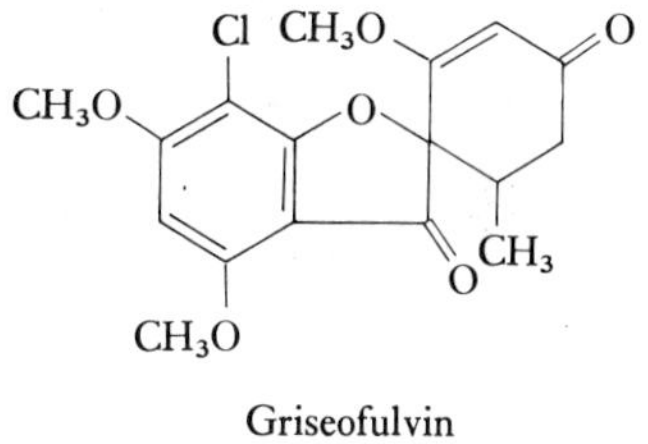

Griseofulvin

This antibiotic was isolated from cultures of *Penicillium griseofulvum* by Oxford, Raistrick and Simonart in 1939. It has also been obtained from other species of *Penicillium* and has the chemical structure shown above. In contrast to many topical antifungal preparations, griseofulvin is effective when taken by mouth. It is not effective when applied topically.

Antifungal activity. Griseofulvin has been shown by *in vitro* and *in vivo* experiments to decrease the rate of growth of some species of fungi. The highest activity of griseofulvin is against dermatophytes; griseofulvin is of no clinical value in infections due to *Candida albicans*.

Absorption and excretion. Griseofulvin is absorbed from the upper part of the gastrointestinal tract and the peak concentration in plasma is attained six hours after a dose. The drug is widely distributed in tissues and appears to be selectively taken up by the newly formed keratin of skin, hair and nails where it exerts its fungistatic effect.

Therapeutic uses. Griseofulvin is usually effective in the treatment of tinea (ringworm) of the hands, fingernails, beard, head, groin and soles of the feet, especially when the infection is caused by *Trichophyton rubrum*. Ringworm of the toe-nails responds slowly to treatment probably because of the slow formation of keratin and growth of the toe-nails.

Griseofulvin is given by mouth in doses of 0.5 to 1 g daily. For most fungal infections a course of treatment lasting from three to six weeks is required though more prolonged treatment may be necessary where the infection involves the finger-nails or toe-nails. The diagnosis and progress of treatment must be controlled by microscopic examination of scrapings or by culture.

Only minor side-effects such as headache, flatulence and nausea have been reported and these have not usually interfered with treatment.

Nystatin

This polyene antibiotic was isolated from cultures of *Streptomyces noursei* obtained from soil in Virginia and its name is derived from the New York State Department of Health whose members of staff were responsible for its isolation. The chemical structure of nystatin has not been fully elucidated.

Nystatin has been found to inhibit the growth of many species of fungi, the yeast-like fungi being most susceptible. It is particularly effective in controlling infections with *Candida albicans* and, to a lesser extent, in mice inoculated with certain strains of *Histoplasma*, *Cryptococcus* and *Coccidiosis*. It has no antibacterial activity.

Nystatin is poorly absorbed from the gastrointestinal tract. It is not absorbed through the skin or mucous membranes when applied locally. It is administered by mouth for the control of moniliasis (thrush) in the mouth and alimentary tract in doses of 500 000 to 1 million units, three times daily. For *Candida* infections of the skin and vulva, it can be applied locally in ointments or pessaries.

Natamycin is another polyene antifungal agent used for oral and vaginal candidiasis.

Amphotericin (Amphotericin B)

This antifungal antibiotic was obtained from a strain of *Streptomyces nodosus* found in a soil sample in Venezuela. It is a polyene, but its exact chemical nature has not been established.

Amphotericin is poorly absorbed when given by mouth or by intramuscular injection, and to be effective must be given by intravenous injection or intrathecally. Whilst nystatin is too toxic for parenteral use, amphotericin can be effectively used for the control of systemic moniliasis and various mycotic infections including histoplasmosis, cryptococcosis and penicillin-resistant actinomycosis.

The frequent and serious toxic effects of the drug limit its use. Solutions of amphotericin are irritant and liable to produce localised thrombophlebitis; generalised reactions include febrile reactions, anaphylactic shock, exfoliative dermatitis, anaemia and severe renal damage with nephrocalcinosis. Nevertheless it can be administered for the treatment of severe generalised fungal infections where the risks of toxicity are outweighed by the possible advantages of a satisfactory clinical cure.

Flucytosine is a synthetic antimetabolite lacking cytotoxic activity which has been found effective in fungus infections due to yeast-like fungi of *Cryptococcus* and *Candida* species. It is well absorbed when given by mouth and may be used in the treatment of severe systemic and urinary tract infections due to susceptible fungi. Resistance to flucytosine has been reported to occur during the course of treatment and this has led to the combined use of flucytosine and amphotericin in serious invasive fungal infections.

CHOICE OF ANTIBIOTIC

The selection of a drug for the treatment of an infection depends on several considerations. In the first place it is desirable to know the nature of the infecting organism and its sensitivity to various drugs. This information can sometimes be provided by the bacteriologist before treatment is commenced, but often it is necessary to start treatment without delay with an antibiotic or sulphonamide on the assumption that the organism is sensitive to it. Treatment can then be altered if there is no response within two days or the results of the laboratory tests show that the organism is more sensitive to another drug. Sometimes several different drugs may be effective against the same micro-organism and the choice of drug is determined by the ease with which it can be administered, its distribution in an effective concentration to the site of infection and the risk of producing undesirable side effects.

The sulphonamides can be given by mouth and are distributed in effective concentrations in all tissue fluids including the cerebrospinal fluid. The risk of severe toxic effects by modern sulphonamides is small, but their main disadvantage is the now common occurrence of sulphonamide resistant strains. For the treatment of urinary infections the nitrofurans are sometimes used. One of the most interesting developments has been the introduction of sulphonamide-trimethoprim mixtures with greatly enhanced effectiveness of both drugs.

The penicillins are extremely active when used against responsive organisms. Unfortunately their use is being limited by the emergence of drug resistant, particularly penicillinase-producing, strains. The natural penicillins are the most active and in order to obtain high concentrations in the tissues, benzylpenicillin must be given by injection. Semi-synthetic penicillins such as methicillin and cloxacillin are resistant to staphylococcal penicillinase, whilst another group of semi-synthetic penicillins, including ampicillin and carbenicillin, have a broad spectrum of antibacterial activity which makes them suitable for use in urinary tract infections. A serious drawback of all penicillins is the occurrence of drug allergy which can be a dangerous and sometimes fatal complication.

A wide variety of antibiotics are now available to take the place of penicillin where this is unsuitable because of the occurrence of resistance or allergy. They include the erythromycin group and lincomycin and its derivative clindamycin. The occurrence of *antibiotic-associated colitis* can be a serious drawback to clindamycin and related drugs. Cephaloridine may also be used in place of penicillin, but in this case some risk of allergic cross-sensitisation exists.

The broad-spectrum tetracycline drugs are all absorbed when given by mouth and pass freely into the placental circulation and cerebrospinal fluid. They can be used for a wide variety of infections but their most frequent application is probably for infections of the respiratory tract, although, since ampicillin became available, it is frequently prescribed in place of or alternating with the tetracyclines. The danger of these drugs is that by suppressing the normal bacterial flora, they are particularly liable to encourage the proliferation of fungi and the development of superinfection by drug-resistant organisms.

Progress has been made in combating *Pseudomonas* which may occur as a super-infecting agent after other micro-organisms have been eradicated. *Pseudomonas* infections can be treated by amphotericin B or by gentamicin together with carbenicillin. Although the first two drugs are toxic, their cautious use in these severe conditions is justified.

Interactions of antibiotics with other drugs. Several clearly undesirable interactions have been found. For example it has been shown that when cephaloridine is prescribed simultaneously with the diuretics frusemide or ethacrynic acid there is a risk of producing renal tubular damage. Both these loop diuretics are ototoxic and they should not be prescribed together with aminoglycosides all of which are ototoxic. The aminoglycosides have a neuromucular blocking action and they may potentiate the effects of neuromucular blocking agents during anaesthesia.

Combinations of antibiotics. It is a much debated subject whether more than one antibiotic should be administered at the same time. There are several theoretical reasons for combined treatment which have been summarised by Garrod as follows:

1. To achieve a synergistic effect when this is possible.
2. To deal with those mixed infections which are not susceptible to one antibiotic.
3. To delay the development of bacterial resistance.
4. To reduce the risks of toxic effects by giving smaller doses of each antibiotic.
5. To treat urgent cases before bacteriological diagnosis has been made.

Whilst these indications certainly apply in some instances, the use of combined antibiotics should be regarded as exceptional rather than routine therapy.

In vitro tests carried out by Jawetz and his colleagues suggest that in some instances antibiotics may act synergistically. They have shown that drugs which are mainly bactericidal such as penicillin, streptomycin, bacitracin, neomycin and polymyxin B when combined may potentiate each other. On the other hand when combined with drugs such as the tetracyclines and chloramphenicol which are mainly bacteriostatic they may antagonise their actions.

There are, however, only very few instances where synergism between antibiotics has been demonstrated clinically. An example of this kind of synergism is the greater effectiveness of a combination of penicillin and streptomycin compared with the use of each antibiotic alone in the treatment of endocarditis. In most cases, however, there is no evidence that the antibacterial activity produced by two or more antibiotics is greater than that of the most active component of the mixture.

Although there is ample evidence that in the treatment of tuberculosis combined antibiotic therapy greatly delays the emergence of drug resistant strains, it has not so far been clearly demonstrated that this applies to other infections. Since most of the antibiotics for systemic administration do not produce serious toxic effects the question of reducing toxicity by giving small doses of several antibiotics seldom arises.

In view of the confusion which results from the increasing number of mixtures of antibiotics now produced commercially, and the difficulty of assessing their relative merits, it would seem a sound general rule, unless there are clear reasons why more than one antibiotic should be used, to start treatment with a single antibiotic and to change to another only if the first choice proves to be unsuitable.

Antibiotic prescribing chart

Table 33.1 is a general *aide-memoire* in antibiotic prescribing. This authoritative summary represents Chairman's conclusions on the use of antibiotics in clinical practice from a recent British symposium. It is published by permission of Prescriber's Journal and is covered by Crown Copyright.

Table 33.1 Antibiotic prescribing chart. (Geddes A M 1977 In Prescriber's Journal, London. 17:no5.)

System	Infection	Commonest organism	Effective antibiotic	Comment
Ear, nose and throat	Tonsilitis	*Strep. pyogenes*	Penicillin i.m.→ pen V (erythromycin if pen-allergic)	Initial therapy with i.m. penicillin then change to oral penicillin V
		Virus	Antibiotic not indicated	
	Otitis media	*Strep. pyogenes* *Strep. pneumoniae* *H. influenzae**	Penicillin i.m.→ pen V or amoxycillin if under 5 (erythromycin if pen-allergic)	*under age of 5
	Sinusitis	*Strep. pyogenes* *Strep. pneumoniae* *H. influenzae*	Erythromycin or amoxycillin	
Respiratory tract	Exacerbations of chronic bronchitis	*H. influenzae* *Strep. pneumoniae*	(i) Tetracycline or (ii) amoxycillin or (iii) cotrimoxazole	Reserve co-trimoxazole for ill patients or if no response to (i) or (ii).
	Pneumonia (a) previously healthy	*Strep. pneumoniae* *Staph. aureus**	Flucloxacillin (clindamycin if penicillin allergic)	*Especially after viral infections e.g. influenza
	(b) previously unhealthy chest	*Strep. pneumoniae* *Staph. aureus** *H. influenzae*	Flucloxacillin and ampicillin or cotrimoxazole	*Especially after viral infections e.g. influenza
Skin and soft tissue	Impetigo	*Strep. pyogenes* *Staph. aureus*	Topical chlortetracycline + oral flucloxacillin if systemic toxicity	
	Erysipelas	*Strep. pyogenes*	Penicillin i.m.→ pen V	Initial therapy with i.m. penicillin if possible then change to oral penicillin V
	Cellulitis Wound infection	*Staph. aureus* *Strep. pyogenes*	Flucloxacillin (clindamycin if penicillin allergic)	
Gastrointestinal	Gastroenteritis	*Salmonella spp.* Viruses (Toxins)	Antibiotic not indicated	
	Bacillary dysentery	*Shigella spp.*	Antibiotic usually not indicated	
	Invasive salmonellosis	*Salmonella spp.*	Cotrimoxazole	
	Biliary tract infection	*Esch. coli* *Strep. faecalis* (Anaerobic bacilli)	Amoxycillin, or gentamicin, or a cephalosporin	
Eye	Purulent conjunctivitis	*Staph. aureus*	Chloramphenicol drops	
Bone and joint	Osteomyelitis Septic arthritis	*Staph. aureus* (*Strep. pyogenes*) *H. influenzae**	Clindamycin, or flucloxacillin, or fusidic acid (amoxycillin for *H. influenzae*)	*under age of 5. Treat acute disease for at least 6 weeks and chronic infection for at least 12 weeks

Table 33.1 *contd.*

System	Infection	Commonest organism	Effective antibiotic	Comment
Renal tract	Acute pyelonephritis/ prostatitis	*Esch. coli* *Proteus spp.*	Cotrimoxazole	not in pregnancy
	Lower urinary tract infection	*Esch. coli* or *Proteus spp.*	(i) Sulphonamide (ii) Ampicillin (iii) Cotrimoxazole	Select in order
	Recurrent urinary tract infection	*Esch. coli* *Proteus spp.* *Klebsiella* *Staph. albus*	Ampicillin, or cotrimoxazole, or a cephalosporin	For long-term therapy one tablet co-trim. or 500 mg of ampicillin or cephalexin at night.

PREPARATIONS

Aminoglycosides
Amikacin sulph (Amikin) 12 mg/kg dl i.m. i.v.
Framycetin sulph (Soframycin) 2–4 g dl p.o.
Gentamycin sulph (Cidomycin) 400–800 μg every 8 h i.m. i.v.
Kanamycin sulph (Kantrex) 15 mg/kg dl i.m.
Neomycin sulph (Neomin) topic eye skin; intest antisept 2–8 g p.o.
Streptomycin Ch. 34
Tobramycin sulph (Nebcin) 3–5 mg/kg dl i.m. i.v.

Macrolides and related antibiotics
Erythromycin 1–2 g dl p.o.
Lincomycin hyd 500 mg 3–4x die
Clindamycin (semis deriv of lincomycin) 150–450 mg every 6 h p.o.

Tetracyclines
Chlortetracycline hyd (Aureomycin) 250–500 mg 6-hourly p.o.
Clomocycline sod (Methylolchlortetracycline, Megaclor) 170 mg 4x die p.o.
Demeclocycline hyd (Demethylchlortetracycline, Ledermycin) 0.6–1.8 g dl p.o.
Doxycycline hyd (Vibramycin) init 200 mg, then 100 mg dl p.o.
Methacycline hyd (Rondomycin) 600 mg dl p.o.
Minocycline hyd (Minocin) init 200 mg, then 100 mg every 12 h p.o.
Oxytetracycline hyd (Terramycin) 250–500 mg every 6 h p.o.
Tetracycline hyd (Achromycin) 250–500 mg every 6 h p.o.

Chloramphenicol (Chloromycetin) 1.5–3 g dl p.o.

Polymyxins
Colistin sulph (Polymyxin E Sulphate) p.o. (gastroenteritis)
Polymyxin B sulph 15 000–25 000 u i.v. (pseudomonas)

Antifungal agents
Amphotericin B (Fungizone) 0.1 mg/ml slow i.v. inf (candidiasis)
Candicidin 0.06% (vaginal candidiasis)
Flucytosine (Ancobon) 150 mg/kg every 6 h (candida, cryptococcus) p.o.
Griseofulvin 0.5–1 g dl for 3–6 w p.o. (ringworm) p.o.
Nystatin (Fungicidin) 0.1–1 million u (candida of mucosa skin) topical.
Tolnafate (Tinactin) 1% cream
Undecynelic acid (Desenex) 10% (skin)

FURTHER READING

Garrod L P, Lambert H P, O'Grady F 1973 Antibiotic and chemotherapy. Churchill Livingstone, Edinburgh
Glashby J E 1979 Encyclopedia of antibiotics. John Willey,

Kagan B M (ed) 1974 Antimicrobial therapy. Saunders, Philadelphia
Smith, Hillas 1977 Antibiotics in clinical practice. Pitmans, London

34. Tuberculosis and leprosy

Properties of the tubercle bacillus 418; Assessment of tuberculostatis activity 419; Drugs for the treatment of pulmonary tuberculisis 420; Streptomycin 420; PAS 422; Isoniazid 422; Rifampicin 423; Ethambutol 424; Thiacetazone 424; Pyrazinamide 424; Ethionamide 425; Viomycin 425; Capreomycin 425; Kanamycin 425; Cycloserine 425; Therapeutic uses of antituberculosis drugs 425; Standard treatment 426; Intermittent chemotherapy 426; Resistance to antituberculosis drugs 427; Toxic and allergic reactions 427; Antileprotic drugs 427; Dapsone 428; Clofazimine 428; Thiambutosine 428; Antituberculosis drugs in leprosy 428.

TUBERCULOSIS

Properties of the tubercle bacillus

The chemotherapy of infections by *Mycobacterium tuberculosis*, the causative organism of tuberculosis, presents peculiar difficulties which are not encountered in the chemotherapy of other bacterial infections. They are due to the unusual chemical makeup of the organism, its slow growth and the complexity of the lesions it produces. The tubercle bacillus contains proteins, polysaccharides and lipids. Koch's old tuberculin is a water-soluble protein fraction of *M. tuberculosis* which, when injected into an animal which is already infected with tuberculosis, produces at the site of the injection a characteristic slowly developing inflammatory reaction called the tuberculin reaction. This reaction cannot be obtained in normal animals and is due to the presence of antibodies developed against the tuberculous infection. The antibodies responsible for the tuberculin reaction do not occur as such in the plasma. They are contained within circulating lymphoid cells to which they are firmly bound. When tuberculin is injected intracutaneously into an infected or otherwise sensitised animal, sensitised lymphoid cells accumulate at the site of injection and give rise to the tuberculin reaction. This is a typical example of a *delayed hypersensitivity reaction.*

Lipids are present mainly in the waxy capsule of the tubercle bacillus. It would seem that both the wax surrounding the organism and the protein fraction inside the organism are required for the production of hypersensitivity and immunity in tuberculosis. An animal may be sensitised towards tuberculin by injecting it with live or with dead tubercle bacilli or with a combination of old tuberculin and an extract of the waxy capsule, but not by injecting it with tuberculin alone. The polysaccharides are also essential constituents of the tubercle bacillus.

Five types of tubercle bacillus are known, but only the human and bovine type are found in clinical infections in man. Infection by the bovine type is almost exclusively by the alimentary tract whilst infection by the human type is mainly through the respiratory tract.

Tuberculosis rarely occurs in infants, but when it does it is often fatal. The incidence of tuberculosis increases steadily in childhood and can be demonstrated by the development of a tuberculin reaction when a small amount of tuberculin is applied to the scarified skin or injected intracutaneously (Mantoux reaction). It is generally considered that a previous symptomless tuberculous infection as revealed by a positive Mantoux reaction confers a degree of immunity.

Immunity of this nature can also be acquired by the injection of BCG (Bacillus Calmette Guerin) vaccine into a person who shows a negative Mantoux reaction. Vaccination by BCG is particularly desirable in medical students and nurses and other persons who are frequently in contact with tuberculous patients, but even in those who are not particularly exposed to the infection BCG vaccination has considerable prophylactic value. Thus in an investigation by the Medial Research Council on children about to leave secondary school, it was shown that the incidence of tuberculosis in the vaccinated group was less than half that in the control group.

Discovery of tuberculostatic drugs

It has long been suspected that the growth of *M. tuberculosis* might be arrested by other organisms and in 1885 Cantani claimed that cultures of various bacteria would cure tuberculosis. Prior to the isolation of streptomycin various antibiotics had been found which were active against tubercle bacilli *in vitro*, but they were either too toxic, or were inhibited by substances present in serum, and thus became inactive *in vivo*. Streptomycin was isolated in 1944 from a culture of the soil saprophyte *Actinomyces* (streptomyces) *griseus* by Schatz, Bougie and Waksman, who showed that it inhibited strongly the growth of tubercle bacilli and various other penicillin-resistant organisms. It was also shown to be relatively non-toxic, and capable of arresting, though not eradicating, experimental tuberculosis in guinea pigs. Within less than two years of the announcement of its discovery, streptomycin had been used successfully in the treatment of tuberculosis in man.

The discovery of isoniazid arose from the observation that nicotinamide inhibits the growth of the tubercle bacillus. Fox tried to combine derivatives of isonicotinic acid with thiosemicarbazone, another substance with tuberculostatic activity. Isoniazid was one of the intermediate products synthesised in the course of this work, and was found to have outstanding activity both *in vitro* and *in vivo*.

Assessment of tuberculostatic activity

In vitro tests
The first test for tuberculostatic activity of a drug usually consists in determining the minimum concentration at which it inhibits the growth of cultures of the microorganism. This information, however, is not sufficient to predict with any certainty the activity of the drug in the living animal, for many compounds which are tuberculostatic *in vitro* are inactive when tested *in vivo* either because they are inactivated by the body fluids or antagonised by certain cellular constituents or because they fail to reach the tuberculous lesion in a sufficiently high concentration.

In vivo tests
A variety of experimentally infected animals have been used for the evaluation of antituberculosis drugs including guinea-pigs, mice, rabbits and monkeys. The character of the infection varies in different species. In the guinea-pig even a mild infection tends to be progressive and ultimately fatal; in this species the tubercle bacilli occur mainly extracellularly and are found in great quantities in necrotic tissue. The mouse is much more resistant to tuberculosis than the guinea pig and tubercle bacilli frequently occur intracellularly. Man has a greater resistance to tuberculosis than the guinea-pig and the majority of such infections are controlled by the natural defences of the body; tubercle bacilli occur both extracellularly and intracellularly and large quantities are found in caseous lesions. Species differences in the character of the disease may make it difficult to predict from animal experiments the clinical effectiveness of new antituberculosis drugs.

Several types of experimental infections with tuberculosis in animals can be used for assaying the activity of tuberculostatic drugs. Either a localised lesion or a general infection may be produced. Rees and Robson used a method in which a tuberculous infection of the rabbit cornea is produced. Normally a tuberculous lesion develops within two weeks of inoculation, but if a tuberculostatic drug is injected into the vitreous humour it diffuses slowly into the anterior chamber and prevents the development of the lesion. A method used by Feldman and his colleagues consists in producing a generalised infection of guinea pigs by the intraperitoneal injection of tubercle bacilli. One half of the animals is treated for several months with a tuberculostatic drug and the other half used as an untreated control group. The survival rate and the severity of the lesions in the two groups can be used to assess the activity of the drug. In another widely used procedure mice are infected; treatment is started on the day of infection and the survival rate of the treated group is compared with a control group.

A particularly virulent infection can be produced by the intravenous injection of tubercle bacilli. In one such experiment Feldman found that all the control group died in less than one month, whereas in a group treated with streptomycin all the animals survived so long as the drug was administered. When the streptomycin was stopped, the animals died, showing that in doses which are tolerated *in vivo* this drug produces a tuberculostatic rather than a tuberculocidal effect.

The clinical assessment of tuberculostatic drugs presents a number of problems which cannot be solved, or even foreseen, by animal experiments. Thus when streptomycin was first tested in animals, toxic manifestations were produced only by extremely large doses, whereas in man relatively small doses were found to give rise to lesions of the eighth nerve. Another feature of these drugs which can only be assessed after extensive trials in large numbers of patients, is the incidence of drug resistance.

Combination of antituberculosis drugs
One of the chief difficulties in the clinical use of tuberculostatic drugs is the emergence of drug-resistant strains during treatment. It has been shown that the development of bacterial resistance can be greatly retarded by administering to patients a combination of two different tuberculostatic drugs. The reason for this is that resistance is due to a process of selection of a few resistant microorganisms which occur in normal strains. The distribution of resistant organisms within a population of bacilli may be regarded as random. Resistance to two different chemical substances usually involves two different mechanisms and the probability of these two mechanisms occuring by chance in any one micro-organism is very small since it is the product of the probabilities of each mechanism occurring separately. Thus when two drugs say, streptomycin and isoniazid are administered simultaneously, the streptomycin-resistant organisms are killed by the isoniazid and *vice versa*.

Desirable properties of antituberculosis drugs
Apart from the obvious requirements of efficacy and lack of toxicity, an acceptable new antituberculosis drug should be active when taken by mouth and, if it is to be used for mass treatment in under-developed countries, its cost should not be excessive. It would be an advantage for such a drug to be excreted slowly so that a high blood level persists for some time. The drug should be capable of penetrating cells, especially macrophages, and it should diffuse into caseous lesions; it should be capable of penetrating into the cerebrospinal fluid.

420 APPLIED PHARMACOLOGY

The drug should also be well tolerated and be capable of being combined with a standard drug such as isoniazid so as to delay the development of bacterial resistance.

Drugs for the treatment of pulmonary tuberculosis

It is now standard practice to administer two, and in some cases three, drugs concurrently for the treatment of pulmonary tuberculosis. For over 20 years the standard drug treatment of tuberculosis in Britain has been initial daily streptomycin, isoniazid and PAS followed by a period of 18–24 months of only two simultaneous drugs, usually isoniazid and PAS. This standard regimen has now been superseded by the introduction of the newer antituberculosis drugs rifampicin and ethambutol. They are used with isoniazid or streptomycin whilst the poorly tolerated PAS is much less employed. Other antituberculosis drugs are used chiefly as 'salvage drugs' because their therapeutic efficacy and patient acceptance is less and their potential toxicity is greater. They include, besides PAS, the synthetic compounds ethionamide, thiacetazone and pyrazinamide and the antibiotics capreomycin, viomycin, kanamycin and cycloserine.

Streptomycin

Streptomycin is a water-soluble aminoglycoside base (p. 411), the principal components of which are streptidine and the nitrogens disaccharide streptobiosamine. It is used as the sulphate. Solutions of streptomycin are much more stable than penicillin, and do not deteriorate readily at room temperature, neither are they destroyed by bacterial enzymes. Streptomycin was originally standardised biologically by methods similar to those used for penicillin. The dose is now expressed in terms of weight, 1 g corresponding to 1 million units.

Absorption and excretion

Streptomycin is usually administered intramuscularly. When given in this way, a dose of 0.5 g produces within 1 hour a maximum blood level of 15–30 μg/ml, which falls to 4–8 μg/ml in 6 hours and about 1 μg/ml in 12 hours. To maintain a continuous blood level, injections must be given every 4 to 6 hours; in tuberculosis, however, where the treatment usually lasts for many months, injections are given once daily or even less frequently. Streptomycin is excreted unchanged by the kidney; concentrations of 1000–2000 μg/ml of the drug may be obtained in urine. The mechanism of renal excretion is by glomerular filtration and there is no evidence of tubular secretion as with penicillin; thus the clearance rate of streptomycin is only about 50 ml per minute compared with 1000 ml per minute of penicillin. Figure 34.1 shows that the plasma level of streptomycin does not drop as rapidly after an intravenous injection as that of penicillin.

Streptomycin is distributed in the extracullular fluid; it does not penetrate cells. It penetrates poorly into the cerebrospinal fluid except when the meninges are inflamed, but it can be administered intrathecally in doses not exceeding 100 mg. When streptomycin is given by mouth it is not destroyed, nor is it appreciably absorbed, and it can therefore be used in the treatment of susceptible infections of the intestine.

Tuberculostatic activity

Although streptomycin is bactericidal in high concentrations, it is merely bacteriostatic in the tissue concentrations normally achieved during treatment of tuberculosis; it thus prevents the multiplication of tubercle bacilli without destroying them and it can be shown that after a fortnight's contact with the drug *in vitro* the organisms will still grow if the drug is washed away. It follows that the final destruction of tubercle bacilli in the

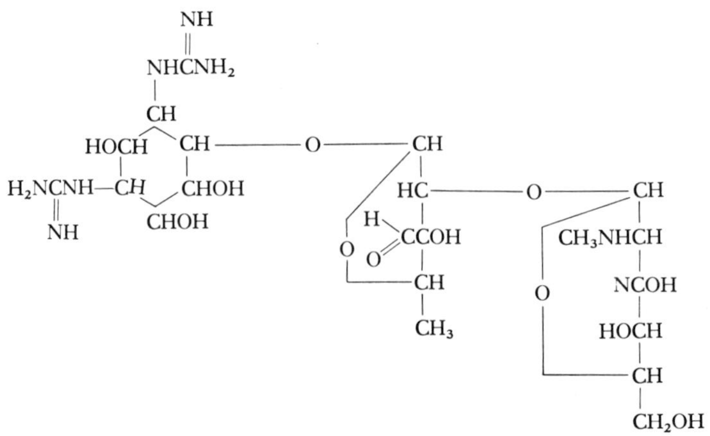

Streptomycin

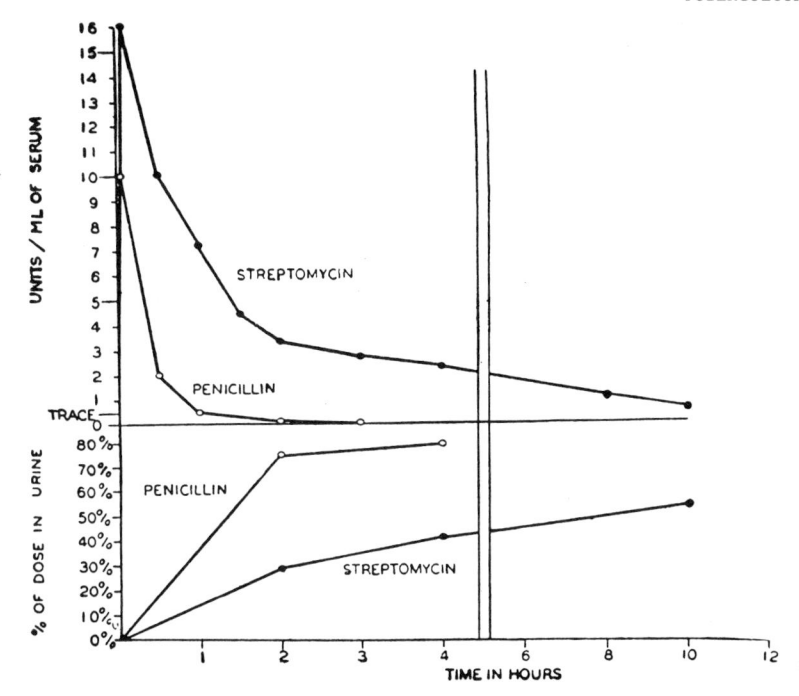

Fig. 34.1 Serum concentration and rate of urinary excretion after the intravenous administration of streptomycin (100 000 units) and of penicillin (100 000 units). (After Adcock and Hettig, 1946. *Arch. Intern. Med.*)

body must be achieved by the slow action of the defence mechanisms of the host. Histological investigations have shown that streptomycin treatment promotes repair and fibrosis in acute tuberculous lesions, but has little effect on caseating necrotic lesions which the drug presumably cannot penetrate.

Streptomycin resistance
During the treatment of a large group of patients with tuberculosis it was found that whereas 97 per cent of the strains of this organism were initially inhibited by streptomycin, 85 per cent were inhibited after one month and only 30 per cent after four months. Most naturally occurring strains of *M. tuberculosis* are inhibited by 1 µg/ml streptomycin, whilst resistant strains may grow in media containing 1000 µg/ml. Resistance is probably due to a process of selection of a few resistant micro-organisms which occur in normal strains. These resistant organisms are not detected by the usual bacteriological tests unless very large inocula are used, but when the fraction of resistant organisms exceeds about 1 in 10 000, the inoculum remains viable in the presence of streptomycin. Thus when resistance to the drug appears *in vitro* the majority of tubercle bacilli in the patient may still be susceptible to streptomycin. Nevertheless, patients whose tubercle bacilli are resistant *in vitro* to streptomycin usually fail to maintain their response to the drug, and probably remain resistant for the rest of their lives. The simultaneous administration of other tuberculostatic drugs greatly reduces the frequency with which strains of tubercle bacilli become resistant to streptomycin.

Mode of action of streptomycin
There is evidence that the fundamental action of streptomycin on sensitive bacteria is interference with protein synthesis. The initial action in sensitive cells may be to damage the cell membrane and permit penetration of streptomycin; within the cell streptomycin interferes with the ribosomal stage of protein synthesis and it has been suggested that it may prevent the normal attachment to messenger RNA (p. 388).

Ribosomes in resistant mutants are much less affected by streptomycin, and in certain streptomycin-dependent mutants they may actually require the antibiotic for normal functioning (p. 388).

Toxicity
When streptomycin is used for longer periods it may produce toxic effects of which vestibular disturbances are the most important. The principal symptom is giddiness, and when warm water is run into the external auditory meatus of the patient, nystagmus is not produced. Vestibular damage is often irreversible, but does not greatly harm the patient who eventually learns to compensate for the loss of vestibular function by visual and kinesthetic sensation. These patients usually remain unsteady in the dark and may feel giddy after a sudden rotation. It has been found that after 4 g streptomycin per

day, vestibular disturbances occur within a week in 98 per cent of patients, but with 1 g per day only 30 per cent of patients are affected after two months. Other toxic effects include fever, nausea and skin rashes which are seldom serious. Deafness occurs mainly in patients with tuberculous meningitis who have received the drug intrathecally.

Sodium aminosalicylate (PAS)

This compound is the sodium salt of *p*-amino-salicylic acid (PAS).

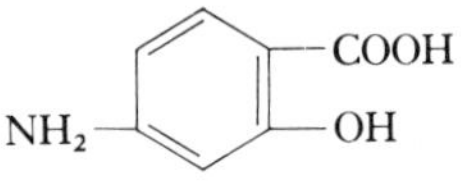

p-aminosalicylic acid

It has been found to protect guinea pigs experimentally infected with *M. tuberculosis*, but it is less active than streptomycin. Aminosalicylate is absorbed when given by mouth and is distributed throughout the body including the cerebrospinal fluid. Most of the drug is rapidly eliminated in the urine, partly in a conjugated form; excretion is chiefly by tubular secretion.

Clinical trials indicate that aminosalicylate is of limited value in the treatment of exudative forms of pulmonary tuberculosis, but its chief use is in conjunction with streptomycin or isoniazid. The drug has an unpleasant taste and its oral administration is often followed by anorexia, nausea, vomiting or diarrhoea. Although dangerous toxic reactions with sodium aminosalicylate are rare some patients are unable to continue to swallow the large daily amounts (10 to 20 g) required in the treatment of tuberculosis.

The prolonged administration of PAS occasionally produces goitre due to inhibition by the drug or organic binding of iodine in the synthesis of thyroid hormone. PAS, like salicylates, may interfere with the blood clotting mechanism and prolong the prothrombin time.

Isoniazid (Isonicotinic acid hydrazide, INH)

Isoniazid was introduced for the treatment of tuberculosis in 1952 although its synthesis was described in 1912. It is now the most important drug for the treatment of pulmonary tuberculosis because of its effectiveness, low cost and relative lack of toxicity. As shown in Figure 34.2 its chemical structure is relatively simple; it is readily soluble in water and produces a neutral solution.

Absorption and excretion

Isoniazid is readily absorbed from the gastrointestinal tract and freely distributed throughout the tissues including the cerebrospinal fluid. Isoniazid is excreted by the kidneys; the excretion products in man are the unchanged isoniazid, acetylisoniazid and other metabolites. It is now established that the metabolism of

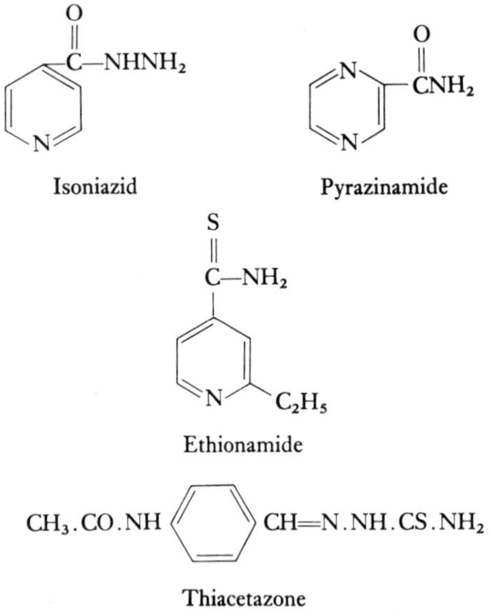

Isoniazid

Pyrazinamide

Ethionamide

Thiacetazone

Fig. 34.2

isoniazid is genetically controlled (Fig. 3.11). 'Slow inactivators' have high blood levels of the free compound and excrete a high proportion of the free drug in urine; 'rapid inactivators' have lower blood levels of the free compound and excrete a high proportion of acetylated drug. This has therapeutic implications and there is evidence that slow inactivators respond better to the drug and also show a higher incidence of toxic effects such as polyneuritis after prolonged administration.

Isoniazid and PAS are both acetylated in the body, hence if the two drugs are administered together they compete for the acetylating mechanisms and the concentration of free isoniazid in the blood is increased (Fig. 34.3).

Tuberculostatic activity

The antibacterial activity of isoniazid is limited almost entirely to mycobacteria against which it is extremely active. *In vitro* tests have shown that isoniazid inhibits the growth of *M. tuberculosis* at concentrations of about 0.05 μg/ml whereas to obtain the same inhibitory effect 0.5 μg/ml streptomycin are required. Isoniazid is also highly effective in suppressing experimentally produced tuberculous infections in animals.

One of the advantages of isoniazid is that, since it is freely diffusible, it can penetrate into caseous tuberculous lesions. Substantial concentrations of the drug are also found in the cerebrospinal fluid and in pleural effusions. It is as effective against intracellular tubercle bacilli as against extracellular organisms.

The mechanism of action of isoniazid has so far not been clarified. One suggestion is that it inhibits the synthesis of mycolic acid in *M. tuberculosis* by affecting an enzyme mycolic synthetase which is unique to mycobacteria.

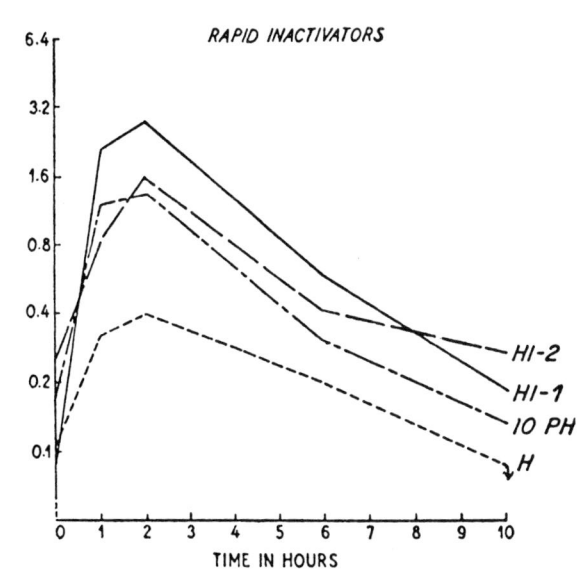

Fig. 34.3 Mean concentration of isoniazid in the serum of patients under treatment for pulmonary tuberculosis by four regimens: HI-1 = Isoniazid alone, 8.8 mg/kg daily, in one dose; HI-2 = Isoniazid alone, 8.8 mg/kg daily, divided into two doses; 10 PH = isoniazid 4.4 mg/kg plus PAS sodium 0.23 mg/kg daily, divided into two doses; H = Isoniazid alone 4.4 mg/kg divided into two doses. Note higher serum concentrations of isoniazid — 10 PH compared to H due presumably to competition for an inactivating (acetylation) system. HI-1 was therapeutically superior to H1-2 in spite of equality of total dose suggesting that achievement of a temporary high serum level of isoniazid is beneficial. (After Gangadharam, Devadatta, Fox, Narayna & Selkon, 1961. *Bull. World Health Org.* 25:793.)

Isoniazid is effective in the treatment of all clinical forms of tuberculosis, but the tubercle bacillus is very liable to become resistant to this drug. In a clinical trial conducted by the Medical Research Council, isoniazid when given alone was found as effective as a combination of streptomycin and aminosalicylate for the treatment of pulmonary tuberculosis, but after three months treatment, 70 per cent of the patients had developed strains of the organism resistant to isoniazid and their clinical response to the drug deteriorated. For this reason isoniazid is now used mainly in combination with other tuberculostatic drugs.

Toxicity
Although a wide variety of toxic effects have been recorded when large doses of isoniazid are administered the usual clinical daily dose of 200 to 300 mg seldom produces any disturbing side effects. Peripheral neuritis and psychotic disturbances have been reported after prolonged administration of large doses. These effects have been attributed to a deficiency of pyridoxine and can be prevented by the administration of this substance.

Rifampicin (Rifampin)
Rifampicin is a semisynthetic derivative of the antibiotic rifamycin obtained from *Streptomyces mediterranei*.

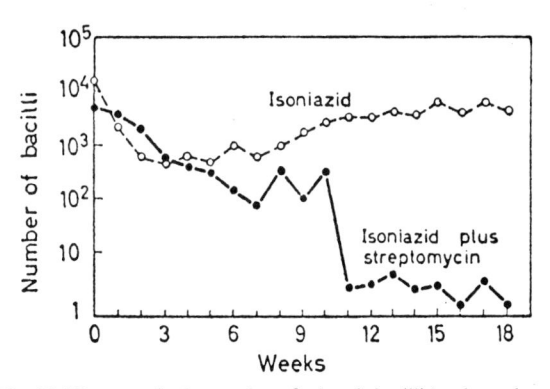

Fig. 34.4 Decrease in the number of tubercle bacilli (as shown by microscopical examination) in the sputum of 12 patients treated with isoniazid alone and 12 patients treated with isoniazid plus streptomycin. (After Joiner, MacLean, Pritchard, Anderson & Collard, 1952. *Lancet*, 2: 843.)

Rifampicin represents a remarkable advance over the original antibiotic in two respects, (1) it can be administered orally, attaining high blood levels; (2) it has much greater antibacterial activity, particularly against *M. tuberculosis*. It is one of the most active antituberculosis drugs known.

Pharmacology of rifampicin
The rifamicins are a group of antibiotics with similar chemical structures which act by inhibiting the RNA polymerase of bacteria. They are all rapidly excreted in the bile so that their serum concentrations are low. Rifampicin was produced by a synthetic modification of one of the rifamicins, leading to a compound which is secreted slowly by the bile and whose serum concentrations is maintained far longer than with other antibiotics of this group. After the administration of 450–600 mg rifampicin by mouth, peak serum concentrations of 5–10 μg/ml are found 2 hours later and the half-life of the drug is about 3 hours. An increase in dosage leads to a more than proportional increase in peak serum concentrations and to a lengthening of the half-life, because biliary excretion becomes saturated and more of the drug is excreted by the slower urinary route.

Rifampicin is highly bactericidal. Staphylococci and streptococci are inhibited by concentrations down to 0.002 μg/ml. The minimal inhibitory concentration against tubercle bacilli is 0.5–0.02 μg/ml. Resistance against rifampicin develops rapidly unless prevented by the simultaneous administration of another drug. Although rifampin is active against many bacteria and some viruses, its use is not generally recommended in infections other than tuberculosis and leprosy because of the rapid emergence of resistant strains.

Administration of rifampicin
Rifampicin is highly effective in experimental tuberculosis, particularly if combined with isoniazid and

the combination of rifampicin with ethambutol is almost as effective. If rifampicin is used alone, strains resistant to it develop rapidly.

Rifampicin is taken orally in single daily doses of 10 mg/kg (maximum 600 mg) in adults and of 10–20 mg/kg in children. It should be administered on an empty stomach to ensure a high plasma concentration. The urine, tears and sputum of patients taking the drug may be stained a brownish-red colour. Rifampicin is largely eliminated by the bile and may cause disturbances of liver function. Occasionally it may produce allergic symptoms including fever and itching. Rifampicin is an important drug but one of its main limitations is its high price.

Use in pulmonary tuberculosis

Rifampicin is increasingly used as a 'first-line' drug for the treatment of new patients with tuberculosis in regimens consisting of isoniazid and rifampicin, combined with either streptomycin or ethambutol for a period of three to six months, followed by maintenance therapy with isoniazid and rifampicin.

Rifampicin should not be used for long-term treatment in pulmonary tuberculosis unless prior laboratory tests have indicated that the invading strain of tubercle bacillus is susceptible to it; it is essential, when it is used, that one or more effective antituberculosis drugs be employed concomitantly. Periodic liver function tests should be performed to detect any indications of incipient hepatotoxicity.

Ethambutol

The chemical structure of ethambutol is as follows:

$$\begin{array}{ccc} CH_2OH & & C_2H_5 \\ | & & | \\ HC-NH-CH_2-CH_2-NH-CH \\ | & & | \\ C_2H_5 & & CH_2OH \end{array}$$

Ethambutol

Only the dextrorotatory isomer has tuberculostatic activity. Ethambutol inhibits the growth of tubercle bacilli *in vitro* in concentrations of 1 to 4 μg/ml and it is effective against isoniazid- and streptomycin-resistant strains. It is active in experimental tuberculosis of mice and guinea pigs as well as in human pulmonary tuberculosis. Resistance of tubercle bacilli to ethambutol is rapidly acquired and the drug should not be used alone, but in conjunction with another tuberculostatic drug. Ethambutol has been shown to be effective as a companion drug to isoniazid.

Toxicity

Ethambutol has low toxicity in animals and is well tolerated by patients but it may cause impairment of vision, and for this reason its use has until recently been restricted. The effect on vision is due to a retrobulbar neuritis, the incidence of which appears to be dose-related. Most workers consider that ethambutol is reasonably safe if administered orally in doses of 25 mg/kg for the first two months and thereafter 15 mg/kg.

The eyesight of patients receiving ethambutol should be watched and they should be instructed to report at once any reduction in visual acuity or colour discrimination. Ethambutol must then be stopped immediately, and this usually leads to complete restoration of vision. Ethambutol is much more pleasant to take than PAS and may be used in patients who are intolerant to the latter.

Thiacetazone

Thiacetazone (Thioparamizone) is one of a series of compounds investigated by Domagk in 1950. American workers who tested the drug, although impressed by its antituberculosis activity, were concerned by its toxicity when given in high dosage and the drug was discarded in most countries especially after the introduction of isoniazid. From 1960 onwards the Medical Research Council began a series of investigations in East Africa of thiacetazone as a companion drug to isoniazid. When used in this way and in moderate dosage, thiacetazone has been shown to be an effective, relatively non-toxic drug which has the further advantage of being cheap, small in bulk and suitable for oral administration. It is also used in the treatment of leprosy (p. 428).

The chemical structure of thiacetazone is shown in Figure 34.2. Its activity in experimental tuberculosis is intermediate between that of streptomycin and PAS.

Thiacetazone may produce toxic effects, the incidence and severity of which are markedly dependent on dosage. Toxic effects include anorexia and nausea, hepatitis, and skin reactions including exfoliative dermatitis.

In clinical trials in Africa combinations of 300 mg isoniazid with 150 mg thiacetazone daily were found to be as effective and not notably more toxic than the usual combination of isoniazid with PAS although when severe toxic effects occurred they tended to be more serious than with PAS. The highest success rate was obtained when this regime was supplemented by streptomycin 1 g a day for the first two months.

Pyrazinamide

This compound is related to isoniazid (Fig. 34.2) and has been shown to be effective in experimental tuberculosis in mice and guinea pigs. Clinically it appears to be intermediate in activity between aminosalicylate and streptomycin and it has been used to a limited extent in the treatment of pulmonary tuberculosis. Since strains of tubercle bacilli resistant to this compound develop rapidly, it is used mainly in conjunction with isoniazid.

Pyrazinamide has been shown to produce liver damage in a proportion of patients taking the drug over prolonged periods. The risk is related to the total daily dose. Early indication of liver damage may be obtained by carrying out regular determinations of glutamic oxalacetic transaminase in serum.

Ethionamide

This derivative of thio-isonicotinic acid (Fig. 34.2) has antituberculosis activity *in vitro* and *in vivo*. Its activity in the mouse and guinea pig is about one-tenth that of isoniazid.

Ethionamide is well absorbed when taken orally. Bacterial resistance to ethionamide develops rapidly if the drug is used alone. Strains of tubercle bacilli resistant to isoniazid, streptomycin and PAS are all sensitive to ethionamide but bacilli resistant to ethionamide may be resistant to thiacetazone.

Ethionamide may produce anorexia, nausea and vomiting but with a daily dose of 0.5 g these symptoms are only rarely seen. Larger doses may produce more severe effects including postural hypotension which may necessitate withdrawal of the drug.

Good clinical results have been reported in cases of pulmonary tuberculosis with bacteria resistant to other drugs but the usefulness of ethionamide in tuberculosis is limited because many patients cannot tolerate the drug in full therapeutic doses (1 g/day).

Viomycin

This is an antibiotic substance derived from a strain of *Streptomyces*. It is a strongly basic polypeptide which forms salts with organic and inorganic acids. Viomycin has a bacteriostatic effect on *M. tuberculosis* including streptomycin- and isoniazid-resistant strains. Resistance to viomycin may develop but is retarded by the simultaneous administration of another tuberculostatic drug.

Viomycin is poorly absorbed when given by mouth and is usually administered intramuscularly in doses of 1 g twice daily every third day for four to six months, in combination with isoniazid.

Viomycin is a toxic compound and is only used as a 'salvage' drug after resistance to the standard tuberculostatic drugs has developed. Viomycin produces renal damage and administration must be discontinued on the first appearance of albuminuria and renal casts. It also may cause vestibular disturbances and deafness and because of the similarity of their toxic effects on the eighth nerve, viomycin should not be used in conjunction with streptomycin.

Capreomycin

This is a polypeptide antibiotic chemically and pharmacologically related to viomycin. It must be given by deep intramuscular injection. It has a marked suppressive effect against *M. tuberculosis*; it is more active than viomycin, approaching streptomycin in effectiveness. Its main toxic effect is renal damage reflected by elevation of blood urea and decreased creatinine clearance.

Kanamycin

This is an aminoglycoside related to streptomycin. It has a similar *in vitro* action of *M. tuberculosis*, but some strains resistant to streptomycin are sensitive to it. Its drawback is ototoxicity as discussed on page 412.

Cycloserine (Seromycin)

This is a water-soluble antibiotic with a relatively simple chemical structure. It is effective against a wide range of micro-organisms including the tubercle bacillus and has been used to a limited extent in the treatment of pulmonary tuberculosis after the development of bacterial resistance to other drugs. Cycloserine produces toxic effects on the central nervous system including psychotic manifestations and convulsions.

Therapeutic uses of antituberculosis drugs

The introduction of streptomycin and isoniazid, and subsequently rifampicin and ethambutol, has completely changed the prognosis of many forms of tuberculosis.

Very remarkable successes have been achieved in the treatment of miliary tuberculosis and tuberculous meningitis. The mortality rate of these diseases was previously almost 100 per cent, whereas now there is a reasonable chance of recovery if treatment is instituted early. Even though many patients relapse after several months of apparently successful treatment, others become completely cured. The outlook for patients with tuberculosis of bone and joints and of the genito-urinary tract, where previously the mortality rate was high, is now greatly improved. Particularly favourable results have been obtained in the treatment of laryngeal, tracheobronchial and intestinal tuberculosis and in cutaneous sinuses and fistulae. Tuberculous ulcers of the mucous membranes of the mouth usually cease to be painful within a few days and heal within a few weeks. In general it has been found that lesions of mucous membranes yield more readily to treatment than do those of parenchymatous tissues.

The treatment of pulmonary tuberculosis by these drugs has been studied in a series of careful and extensive trials organised by the Medical Research Council in Great Britain and the Veterans Administration in the U.S.A.

In the first streptomycin trial organised in 1948 by the Therapeutic Trials Committee of the Medical Research Council, the following results were obtained (Table 34.1).

These results refer to a selected group of young adult patients with acute progressive bilateral pulmonary tuberculosis, all of whom were given the standard schedule of rest and dietetic treatment then available. In addition streptomycin treatment was allocated at random to half the patients. The radiological assessment was made by independent observers who did not know to which treatment group the radiographs belonged. This trial showed clearly the effectiveness of streptomycin in the treatment of tuberculosis. The main disadvantage of this treatment was the toxicity of the large doses of streptomycin and the rapid emergence of drug-resistant strains of tubercle bacilli.

Table 34.1 Assessment of radiological appearance at six months as compared with appearance on admission (after Br. med. J., 1948)

Radiological assessment	Streptomycin group		Control group	
		per cent		per cent
Considerable improvement	28	51	4	8
Moderate or slight improvement	10	18	13	25
No material change	2	4	3	6
Moderate or slight deterioration	5	9	12	23
Considerable deterioration	6	11	6	11
Deaths	4	7	14	27
Total	55	100	52	100

In later trials in which streptomycin was combined either with aminosalicylate or isoniazid it was found that smaller doses of streptomycin could be used whilst drug-resistant strains occurred much less frequently (Fig. 34.4).

Standard chemotherapy of tuberculosis
It is now considered that the most effective initial treatment of tuberculosis consists in a combination of isoniazid, rifampicin and ethambutol given simultaneously by daily administration. Ethambutol has been included in the initial treatment schedule in case the tubercle bacillus proves to be resistant to one of the two more powerful drugs. Such resistance is liable to occur in about 1 in every 20 newly diagnosed and previously untreated patients. If treatment is started with two drugs and the patient happens to be initially resistant to one of them, he would effectively be receiving only one drug to which resistance might then be rapidly established. Another reason for an initial triple regimen given for about two months is that it has a higher success rate, in the long run, than an initial double regimen. A further reason for starting with three drugs is that the patient may be unable to tolerate one of them.

After two to three months the reports of bacterial sensitivity will usually be available. If the organism is sensitive to all three drugs, one of them, frequently ethambutol, is omitted and treatment with two drugs continued. If no bacterial report is available it is usual to continue with the isoniazid, rifampicin combination. If bacteriological tests show that the organism is sensitive to only two drugs, treatment is continued with these two. If it is sensitive to only one, treatment must be continued with another drug combination including, if necessary, the use of one of the second line drugs.

Rifampicin is not universally advocated for initial treatment, partly because of its expense. Almost as good a therapeutic response is obtained with the combination of streptomycin, ethambutol and isoniazid; or of streptomycin, isoniazid and PAS; or even of isoniazid and ethambutol. Isoniazid and rifampicin are both powerful bactericidal agents and one reason for using them is that the total period of chemotherapy of tuberculosis might be reduced.

Duration of treatment
The course of treatment with tuberculostatic drugs is usually continued for at least 18–24 months in both pulmonary and extrapulmonary tuberculosis, during which assessment of the response to treatment by rest and drugs is made, and a decision taken as to whether surgical treatment should also be undertaken. It is conceivable that with the introduction of rifampicin the total duration of chemotherapy can be reduced to less than the standard two-year period but insufficient long-term evidence has as yet accumulated to decide on the optimum length of treatment with the newer antituberculosis drugs.

In the treatment of miliary tuberculosis and tuberculous meningitis it is usual to continue the administration of three drugs including the intrathecal injection of streptomycin.

Intermittent chemotherapy
Schemes of intermittent chemotherapy of tuberculosis have more recently been tried and shown to be as good and sometimes better than continuous treatment. Intermittent chemotherapy was first introduced following studies in Madras which showed that a dose of 400 mg isoniazid administered once a day was more effective than 200 mg given twice daily although the latter scheme produced continuous bactericidal levels of isoniazid in plasma while the former did not.

In spite of extensive investigations in places such as India and Africa in which tuberculosis continues to be one of the most serious health hazards, there exists no universal agreement as to the optimal way of treating pulmonary tuberculosis. Twice weekly streptomycin is now widely advocated because of the reduced risk of ototoxicity. There has been a tendency to combine twice weekly streptomycin with a high dose of isoniazid of up to 15 mg/kg, but higher doses have not been found practicable because of the risk of acute toxic effects. Trials of once-weekly streptomycin with a high dose of isoniazid have given clearly inferior results to the twice-weekly schemes, but when the findings were analysed in relation to isoniazid inactivation rates it became clear that the poor results of once weekly treatment were confined to rapid isoniazid inactivators.

Resistance to antituberculosis drugs

The development of resistance to antibacterial drugs is of great theoretical and practical importance, especially in relation to the treatment of tuberculosis. There has been much discussion on how resistance is brought about and the biochemical changes in resistant organisms have been partly elucidated. It is generally agreed that resistance is based on genetic mutation and selection (p. 390).

The development of resistance may be pictured as follows. If one normal tubercle bacillus which is sensitive to 0.05 μg/ml isoniazid is inoculated into a liquid medium it divides into two similar bacilli which in turn divide into four and so on. If the organisms are allowed to multiply until the culture contains about 1000 bacilli they may all be sensitive to 0.05 μg/ml isoniazid, but if they multiply to say 100 000 it would be most unusual if they had all remained equally sensitive; some descendants will have undergone mutation and become different from their parents. The cause of these spontaneous mutations is unknown. Some mutants may have become resistant to say 1 μg/ml isoniazid but are killed by 1000 μg/ml; they may then undergo a further mutation step so as to make them resistant to 1000 μg/ml; other mutants may become resistant to 1000 μg/ml by a single mutation step.

Although the chance that an organism may be resistant to both isoniazid and rifampicin or isoniazid and streptomycin is small it nevertheless exists, but clinically it may be possible to eliminate such doubly resistant organisms if they constitute only a small fraction of the bacterial population. Once the vast majority of organisms has been eliminated from a lesion the body's own defences may be able to destory the remaining resistant organisms.

Clearly the intensity and magnitude of the lesion matters; thus in a big cavity, containing many bacilli, the chances of finding resistant mutants is greater and resistance development is more probable. The magnitude of the drug dose also matters; thus isoniazid which can be given in doses which produce blood concentrations about fifty times higher than bactericidal is likely to eliminate also some of the resistant mutants, whereas the more toxic and less effective salvage drugs cannot be given in high doses and produce serum concentrations which are only just effective. Nevertheless it is essential that when two drugs are given in combination each should produce at least an effective serum level.

It follows from what has been said, that a triple drug regimen in tuberculosis should have a better chance of success than a double regimen and this is borne out by experience. Conversely single drug regimens, e.g. isoniazid alone, have a greater chance of resistance production. Nevertheless they are sometimes employed either for reasons of economy and acceptability or in individuals recovering, or those with small lesions.

Toxic and allergic reactions

Of the standard drugs, streptomycin is undoubtedly the most toxic. The risk of vestibular dysfunction depends on the age of the patient and becomes more serious in patients over 40, it also depends on the daily dose and the duration of administration. The risk is greater if renal function is impaired and concentrations of streptomycin in the serum are high. Dosage is often critical and it has been found that reduction of the dose from 1 g to 0.75 g considerably reduces the incidence of vertigo.

Isoniazid in doses up to 300 mg is practically non-toxic, but with larger doses peripheral neuritis occurs not infrequently, especially in slow inactivators. The neuritis is a manifestation of vitamin deficiency and can usually be prevented by the administration of pyridoxine. Whether pyridoxine also reduces the therapeutic activity of isoniazid is at present uncertain.

Rifampicin, in the standard single daily dose of 600 mg, is generally well tolerated. It sometimes causes an aching pain in muscles and joints. It may cause a reversible jaundice and some impairment of liver function shown by elevation of serum transaminase. If rifampicin is taken intermittently it may produce an allergic reaction characterised by a flu-like syndrome and dyspnoea. Severe reactions are rare.

The only serious adverse effect of ethambutol is ocular toxicity which is dose-related and reversible. The symtpoms of ethambutol toxicity are discussed on page 424. Ethambutol toxicity is rare in patients without ocular abnormalities receiving a single daily dose of 15–25 mg/kg body weight. If a patient complains of blurring or fading of vision, treatment with ethambutol should be stopped immediately.

Allergic reactions can occur with all of the commonly used drugs but they are more common with PAS and streptomycin. The manifestations are the same whichever drug is producing them; fever and rash are the commonest, but others are nausea, enlarged lymph nodes, jaundice and depression of the bone marrow. Most allergic reactions occur in the first few weeks of treatment and usually subside rapidly when the administration of the offending drug is stopped. Frequently patients can be desensitised by giving small and slowly increasing doses of the drug. When the allergic manifestations are mild, treatment with full doses may be continued, or combined with sufficient corticosteroid to suppress the hypersensitivity reactions.

LEPROSY

Antileprotic drugs

The leprosy bacillus is closely related to the tubercle bacillus and drugs effective in tuberculosis are usually also effective in leprosy. The testing of drugs for activity against *M. leprae* has been considerably impeded by the difficulty of *in vitro* cultivating *M. leprae* and of producing the characteristic features of the disease by inoculation of the organisms in experimental animals. More recently, a technique has been developed in which inoculation of the mouse foot-pad with suspension of bacilli from human leprotic lesions has made it possible to demonstrate the antimycobacterial properties of a number of compounds. The mouse footpad technique has been used to study the effects of different antileprotic drugs and to evaluate the degree of bacillary resistance to their action.

A number of drugs of different chemical structure have been found to be effective in the treatment of leprosy in so far as their use has been followed by a gradual reduction in the proportion and the concentration of viable *M. leprae* in the tissues. Streptomycin and isoniazid have antileprotic activity but the drugs most widely used in the treatment of leprosy are the sulphones such as dapsone and thiambutosine, a derivative of thiourea. Clofazimine, a phenazine derivative has also been shown in experimental animals to have considerable antileprotic activity.

Sulphones

Dapsone

Dapsone (diaphenylsulfone) is effective in all forms of leprosy, especially in lepromatous and tuberculoid leprosy. In most cases it produces clinical improvement and a decrease in the bacterial count of smears from lesions. Continuous treatment with dapsone produces a negative bacterial state in most patients with lepromatous leprosy, but five years or more may be required to achieve this condition. It is widely held that administration of dapsone should be continued for life in lepromatous leprosy. In other milder forms of the disease drug administration should be continued for 2–10 years.

A common side effect of dapsone and other sulphones is allergic dermatitis. A complication of treatment are lepra reactions which are not due to toxic effects of the sulphones but represent exacerbations of treated lepromatous leprosy. If severe lepra reactions occur, dapsone should be discontinued or reduced in dosage. When dapsone was administered to children contacts over a period of years it produces a slight lepra-prophylactic effect.

Acedapsone, *Solapsone* and *Sulfoxone* are sulphones with actions and uses similar to dapsone.

Other drugs used in leprosy

Clofazimine

This compound has antileprotic and anti-inflammatory activity. It is used in patients who are resistant or intolerant to dapsone. Its action is produced slowly and may take 8–12 weeks to become manifest. It is often combined with corticosteroids in the treatment of lepra reactions.

Clofazimine produces a long-lasting red pigmentation and discoloration of skin lesions.

Thiambutosine

Thiambutosine is used in the treatment of lepromatous and tuberculoid leprosy and in dermatitis herpetiformis. It is poorly absorbed from the gastrointestinal tract. It may be used in the treatment of leprosy alone or in conjunction with dapsone. It has a more rapid effect on lepra bacilli than dapsone. Bacterial resistance to thiambutosine develops after one to two years.

Antituberculosis drugs in leprosy

In accordance with the close species relationship between the mycobacteria of tuberculosis and leprosy many tuberculostatic drugs are clinically effective in leprosy.

Rifampicin given in single daily doses of 600 mg for several months to patients with lepromatous leprosy appears to be clinically as effective as dapsone and its bactericidal action is produced more rapidly than with dapsone.

Thiacetazone produces clinical improvement in leprosy comparable to that resulting from sulphones. It is on the whole better tolerated than the sulphones and continuous treatment with this drug is more often possible. Although toxic effects are infrequent after thiacetazone, when they occur they are severe (p. 424).

PREPARATIONS

Antituberculosis antibiotics
Capreomycin sulph (Capastat) 1 g dl for 2–4 w, then 1 g 2–3x weekly i.m.
Cycloserine (Seromycin) 250 mg 1–3x die p.o.
Kanamycin sulph 15 mg/kg 3–4x weekly deep i.m.
Rifampicin (Rifampin) 450–600 mg dl p.o. (single daily doses)
Streptomycin sulph init 1 g dl (single dose) for 2–3 w, then 3x and 2x weekly i.m.
Viomycin sulph (Viocin) 1–2 g dl for 2–4 w, then 2–3x weekly i.m.

Other antituberculosis drugs
Aminosalicylate sod 8–12 g dl p.o.
Ethambutol hyd (Myambutol) 15–25 mg/kg dl p.o.
Ethionamide (Trescatyl) 0.5–1 g dl p.o.
Isoniazid 300–600 mg dl p.o.
Prothionamide (Trevintix) 0.75–1 g dl p.o.
Pyrazinamide (Zinamide) 20–35 mg/kg dl p.o.
Thiocarlide 6–10 g p.o.

Antileprotics
Clofazimine (Lamprene) 200–600 mg/w p.o. (red skin pigm)
Dapsone (Avlosulfon) 25 mg 2–7x/w p.o.
Sulfoxone (Diasone) 1–3 g dl p.o.
Thiambutosine (Ciba 1906) 1–2 g dl p.o.

FURTHER READING

Cochrane R G, Davey T F 1964 Leprosy in theory and practice. Williams and Wilkins, Baltimore

Keers R Y 1978 Pulmonary tuberculosis. A journey down the centuries. Baillere Tindall, London

Robson J M, Sullivan F M 1963 Antituberculosis drugs. Pharmac. Rev. 15: 169

Waksman S A 1965 The conquest of tuberculosis. Robert Hale, London

Williams H 1973 Requiem for a great killer. The story of tuberculosis. Health Horizon, London

35. Trypanosomiasis, leishmaniasis and spirochaetal infections

Discovery of trypanocidal drugs 430; Discovery of antispirochaetal drugs 430; Drug resistance in trypanosomes 431; African and South American trypanosomiasis 432; Tryparsamide 433; Melarsoprol 433; Nitrofurazone 433; Pntamidine 433; Suramin 434; Leishmaniasis 434; Pentavalent antimony compounds 434; Nifurtimex 434; Spirochaetal infections 435; Penicillin 435; Bismuth 436; Oxophenarsine 437.

The discovery of trypanocidal drugs

At the beginning of this century a search for an effective trypanocidal drug was stimulated by the need to combat the *nagana* disease which killed domestic cattle in Africa. Bruce had shown that *nagana* was propagated by trypanosomes by way of a carrier, the tsetse fly, and Laveran and Mesnil (1902) found that trypanosomes could be maintained in mice by the inoculation of infected blood from one animal to the other. Although arsenious oxide was shown to produce a temporary improvement of trypanosome-infected animals it was also toxic and the animals eventually relapsed and died.

Thomas (1905) in Liverpool, prompted by the discovery that trypanosomes were also infectious in man and caused sleeping sickness, tested a less toxic arsenical, atoxyl, which had previously been used in clinical medicine for the treatment of skin diseases. He found that repeated doses of atoxyl would cure mice infected with trypanosomiasis and recommended its use against human sleeping sickness, after trying it first on himself in large intravenous doses.

Atoxyl proved to be an effective but toxic remedy for it caused optic nerve atrophy in some patients. At this juncture, Paul Ehrlich embarked on a systematic search for a more effective and less toxic trypanocidal compound. He varied the structure of atoxyl and with each new compound determined the minimum quantity required to cure an infected animal, and the maximum dose that could be administered without lethal effect. The ratio of tolerated dose to curative dose was named the curative ratio or chemotherapeutic index. Ehrlich believed that no substance could be administered safely to patients unless the curative ratio was at least three.

Atoxyl had presented a paradox since although it cured trypanosomiasis when injected into living animals it had no trypanocidal action when incubated with trypanosomes *in vitro*. Ehrlich and Bertheim established the structure of atoxyl and found it to be pentavalent (Fig. 35.1); they also showed that when atoxyl was reduced to the trivalent *p*-aminophenylarsenoxide (II) it acquired trypanocidal activity *in vitro*. This compound was toxic but further reduction to the corresponding arsenobenzol (III) gave a product which was inactive *in vitro*, active *in vivo* and relatively non-toxic. After studying many compounds the most favourable curative ratio against trypanosomiasis was given by compound 606 which Ehrlich called salvarsan (arsphenamine).

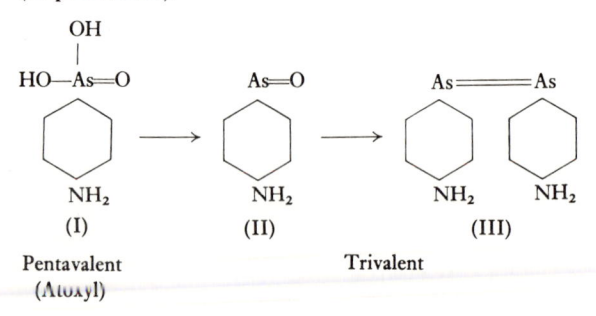

Fig. 35.1 Relation between pentavalent and trivalent arsenicals.

Discovery of antispirochaetal drugs

In view of Schaudinn's discovery that syphilis is caused by a spirochaete, *Treponema pallidum,* Ehrlich extended his investigations to animals infected by the spirochaetes of relapsing fever. He found that trypanosomes and spirochaetes reacted on the whole similarly to arsenicals and that compound 606 was also effective in spirochaetal infections. Salvarsan was shown in 1910 to cure human syphilis and subsequently three arsenicals: arsphenamine, neoarsphenamine and oxophenarsine (Fig. 35.2) became the mainstay of treatment of this disease. The discovery of salvarsan was for long the greatest practical achievement of chemotherapy until 1945 when arsenicals were largely replaced in the treatment of syphilis by the more effective and less toxic penicillin.

Mode of action of arsphenamines

Arsphenamine provides a good example of drug activation by the body. Voegtlin found that compounds of the type R—As=O acted immediately after intravenous injection, causing an immediate diminution of the number of trypanosomes in the blood; compounds of the type R—As=As—R had very little effect on the number of trypanosomes for at least one hour and pentavalent compounds acted even more slowly. Compounds of the type R—As=O also produced immediate toxic effects whilst the two others produced toxic effects only after a delay. If, however, R—As=As—R-type compounds were incubated at 37°C for three hours and then injected they became immediately toxic. Voegtlin concluded that

Fig. 35.2

arsphenamine was oxidised in the body to an active form and that only after activation did it produce its effects on either the parasite or the host. Pentavalent compounds, on the other hand, were reduced in the body to the trivalent form before they became active.

Drug resistance in trypanosomes
Ehrlich found that organic arsenicals would kill trypanosomes in an infected animal but that if sub-effective doses were given the trypanosomes acquired tolerance to the drug. In order to produce drug resistance, trypanosomes are exposed to a sub-effective dose of drug in an infected mouse, the strain is then passaged into fresh mice and exposed again and this is continued until highly or completely resistant trypanosomes are produced. The resistance is then usually permanent.

This power of the parasites to acquire resistance made it desirable to find a drug which could kill all the parasites before they had time to become tolerant. Ehrlich hoped to find a substance which would be so effective that a single dose would completely eradicate the parasites (*therapia sterilisans magna*).

He postulated that the effectiveness of chemotherapeutic drugs was due to their affinity for the parasite's chemoreceptors and the development of resistance in trypanosomes was due to a loss of affinity between the parasite's chemoreceptor and the drug. This view has since been confirmed by experiments such as that of Figure 35.3 which shows that a trypanocidal drug can be concentrated 100 times more in normal than in resistant trypanosomes.

Lack of attachment of chemotherapeutic drugs to receptors is not the only mechanism by which drug resistance of micro-organisms may be brought about. Thus, resistance to penicillin can be due to the production by micro-organisms of the enzyme penicillinase, which destroys penicillin; other mechanisms of resistance formation are discussed on page 390.

There is, however, a common factor in all types of resistance formation in that the production of drug-resistant organisms can be explained by the hypothesis that the drug selects out resistant individuals which then multiply. There is still controversy whether these resistant individuals are produced only by random mutation; or whether a limited but inheritable adaptation of the individuals may occur during the period between one cell division and the next. There is experimental evidence in

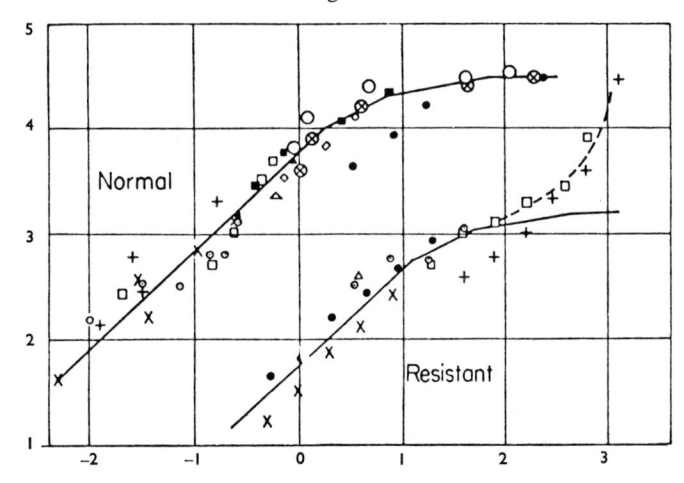

Fig. 35.3 The relation between the concentration of acriflavine inside normal and acriflavine-resistant trypanosomes and that in the surrounding medium. Temperature, 37°C. Horizontal scale, log concentration in medium, μg/ml. Vertical scale, log concentration in trypanosomes, μg/ml. The various signs refer to different experiments done on different days. (After F. Hawking, 1938, *Ann. Trop. Med. Parasitol.*)

support of both explanations but the random hypothesis is the most generally accepted.

Cross resistance. Ehrlich found that a strain of trypanosomes made resistant to one compound also became resistant to a whole series of related compounds; this phenomenon was called cross-resistance. Trypanosomes made resistant to compounds of one chemical type did not, however, usually become resistant to compounds of another chemical type. The chemotherapeutic drugs acting on trypanosomes could thus be grouped according to their cross-resistances and this was explained by assuming that different types of drugs attached to different chemoreceptors in the parasite, resistance being due to the absence of one type of specific receptor.

Ehrlich's early ideas of specific chemoreceptors for chemotherapeutic drugs had certain similarities to Langley's subsequent concept of specific cellular sites on which drugs such as adrenaline produce their effect, and out of which the modern drug receptor concept has evolved. It is interesting that Ehrlich tried to classify chemotherapeutic drugs in terms of the receptors on which they act in much the same way that modern pharmacologists classify drugs in terms of their specific receptors (p. 13). In this connection Ehrlich referred to resistant trypanosomes (i.e. trypanosomes which have lost their receptors) as 'therapeutic sieves' by which chemotherapeutic compounds acting on one type of receptor may be differentiated from those acting on another type.

AFRICAN AND SOUTH AMERICAN TRYPANOSOMIASIS

African trypanosomiasis is a disease produced by the parasites *Trypanosoma gambiense* transmitted by river haunting tsetse flies and *T. rhodesiense* transmitted by glossina flies in open woodlands. *T. gambiense* trypanosomiasis in man develops slowly over two to eight years and is characterised by infection of the blood stream and lymph nodes followed by infection of the c.n.s. In *T. rhodesiense* attacks, the infection of the blood stream is rapidly followed by c.n.s. infection and death may occur within a year or so if the disease is untreated.

Trypanosomiasis in man and in cattle presents a major problem in the economy of Africa. The steps taken to control the disease consist of:

1. The suppression and treatment of human trypanosomiasis by trypanocidal drugs.
2. The elimination of tsetse-fly breeding areas by bush-clearing and by insecticides, in order to reduce the chances of contact between the parasite and the host.
3. The eradication of the disease in cattle and other domestic animals by use of trypanocidal drugs.

Another form of trypanosomiasis (Chagas' disease) due to *Trypanosoma Cruzi* occurs in South America. This infection frequently brings about the destruction of the ganglion cells of the oesophagus, duodenum and rectum, causing achalasia and intestinal obstruction. Unfortunately the usual trypanocidal drugs appear to be generally less effective in Chagas' disease than in African trypanosomiasis but nifurtimox, a new drug (p. 434), is sometimes effective.

Measurement of activity of trypanocidal drugs

The activity of trypanocidal drugs may be measured *in vitro* and *in vivo*. Trypanosomes can be kept alive, but not multiplying, in a fluid medium consisting of serum, Ringer's solution and glucose. Various concentrations of a trypanocidal drug may be added to the medium and the number of live trypanosomes left after incubation counted. This technique detects compounds which are directly trypanocidal such as phenylarsenoxides, but it does not detect compounds which require chemical change in the body of the host such as pentavalent arsenicals, or those with a delayed action such as suramin.

Screening tests *in vivo* are usually carried out on mice which have been inoculated with blood containing trypanosomes. One or more days later the blood is examined for the presence of trypanosomes and when these are seen the mice are given the test compound. The blood is then examined at frequent intervals. If the trypanosomes disappear from the blood permanently, the animals are regarded as cured; if the trypanosomes disappear and then reappear during the period of observation the animals are classified as 'cleared'.

Animals may also be treated with a drug before being infected in order to test its prophylactic action. The chief drugs which are used as trypanocidal agents in man are arsenicals, nitrofurazone, suramin and aromatic diamidines. Other trypanocidal compounds are used mainly in cattle.

Arsenical compounds

Although the trivalent arsenicals are more effective in killing trypanosomes than the pentavalent compounds, they have been used less than the latter for the treatment of trypanosomiasis. The reason is that the pentavalent compound tryparsamide was found to penetrate the blood-brain barrier better than trivalent compounds and hence was believed to be more effective in destroying the parasites which, in the late stages of sleeping sickness, are in the central nervous system. Recent experience, however, has shown that trivalent arsenicals, although more toxic than the pentavalent compounds, are clinically highly effective against trypanosomiasis.

The arsenicals may kill trypanosomes by virtue of their interactions with SH groups in proteins. The integrity of SH groups is essential for enzymes involved in energy production and other cellular mechanisms in both parasite and host; it is thus not surprising that these compounds should be toxic to both, their selectivity depending on the concentration of drug present in the cells of the parasite or the host.

Tryparsamide
This compound (Fig. 35.4) is inactive *in vitro*. When it is injected into infected rats there is a delay of one to six hours before the trypanosomes begin to disappear from the blood, presumably due to the time required for the conversion of the pentavalent to the trivalent form. The value of tryparsamide in sleeping sickness lies in its ability to penetrate more readily into the central nervous system than the non-metallic compounds suramin and the diamidines.

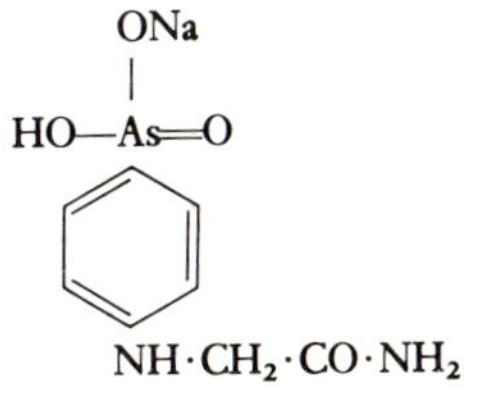

Fig. 35.4 Trypanocidal arsenical compounds

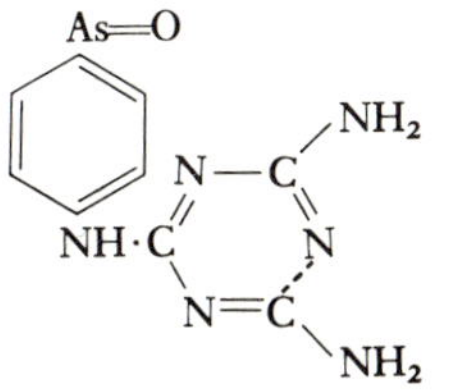

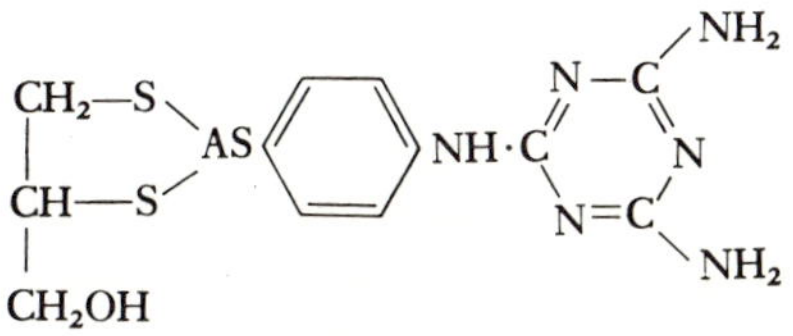

In the treatment of Gambian sleeping sickness tryparsamide is frequently useful in the intermediate and late stages of the disease but it may produce severe toxic reaction, particularly optic atrophy and blindness. A disadvantage of the drug is the long duration of the course of treatment.

Trivalent arsenicals
Melarsoprol (Mel B) is a condensation product of melarsen oxide with dimercaprol. It is highly effective in the treatment of all stages of *T. gambiense* infections and in *T. rhodesiense* infections involving the central nervous system. It is administered by intravenous injection.

Toxic reactions are common and are of two main types: (a) Jarisch-Herxheimer pyrexial reactions produced by the effect of the drug on trypanosomes, and (b) encephalopathy with sudden collapse and death. The incidence and severity of these reactions can be diminished by slow and careful injection of the solution and by prior administration of an antihistamine and a corticosteroid. Less serious gastrointestinal side-effects such as vomiting and abdominal colic also occur.

Melarsonyl Potassium (Trimelarsan, Mel W) is a water-soluble derivative of melarsoprol and can be given by subcutaneous or intramuscular injection in the treatment of *T. gambiense* infections.

Other trypanocidal drugs
Nitrofurazone (Furacin)

Nitrofurazone is chemically closely related to the urinary antiseptic nitrofurantoin (p. 396). Its most important use is for the oral treatment of patients with Gambian and Rhodesian sleeping sickness where the infection has failed to respond or has become resistant to treatment with melarsoprol or other related trypanocidal drugs.

Toxic effects. Severe polyneuropathy is a frequent complication and may occur during, or some weeks after, treatment.

Pentamidine isethionate (Fig. 35.5)
This drug is used in the treatment of the early stages of African trypanosomiasis, particularly in *T. gambiense* infections. It does not attain a sufficient concentration in the cerebrospinal fluid to be of value in the later stages involving the c.n.s., when treatment must be supplemented by tryparsamide or changed to melarsoprol. Pentamidine isethionate is also used as a prophylactic drug during outbreaks of *T. rhodesiense* sleeping sickness.

Pentamidine isethionate may also be employed in the treatment of leishmaniasis in patients who do not respond to antimonials.

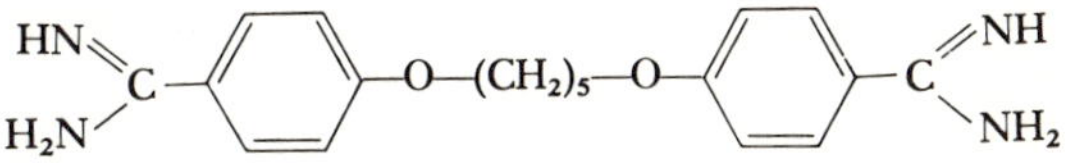

Fig. 35.5

Toxic effects. After administration of the aromatic diamidine compounds toxic effects may occur shortly after the injection or after a delay of several weeks. The immediate toxic reactions are rarely severe and consist of headache, nausea, vomiting and circulatory collapse. The delayed effects consist of neurological changes which involve the skin area supplied by the trigeminal nerve. The

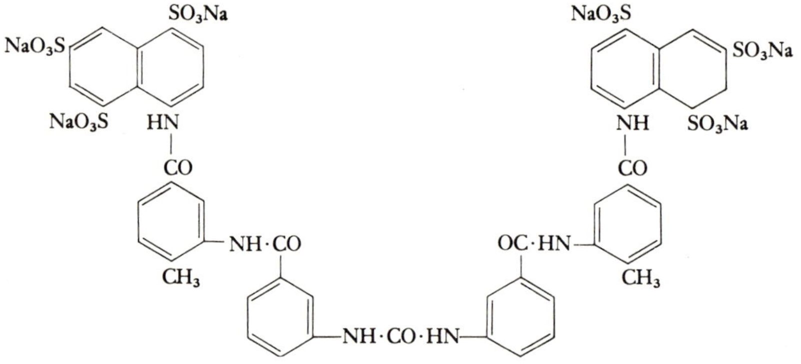

Fig. 35.6 Suramin

chief symptoms are numbness followed by hyperaesthesia and itching of the lips, face and forehead.

Suramin (Antrypol) (Fig. 35.6)
This substance is a derivative of trypan red, and was introduced as 'Bayer 205' in 1920. It is also called germanin. Suramin is very slowly excreted by the kidneys and after injection, the drug persists in the blood and tissues for several days due to its tight binding to plasma proteins. A single injection of suramin is capable of producing a complete cure in mice infected with *T. equiperdum*.

Suramin is an effective drug for the treatment of the early stages of African trypanosomiasis but it is ineffective in advanced disease when the c.n.s. becomes involved, since it does not reach the cerebrospinal fluid.

Toxic effects. Suramin has a toxic action on the kidneys so that after three or four injections the urine usually contains albumin and casts. Other toxic effects are conjunctivitis, and dermatitis.

Nifurtimox (Bayer 2502)
This drug has been shown to be of value in the treatment of acute and chronic South American trypanosomiasis (Chagas' disease) following infection by *T. cruzi*. The drug, though toxic, is better tolerated by children than by adults. It has been reported to produce a negative 'xenodiagnosis' test in patients with Chagas' disease.

LEISHMANIASIS

Leishmaniasis is the result of infection with protozoa belonging to the genus *Leishmania*. It is an insect-borne infection. The parasite which causes leishmaniasis in man is transmitted by the sand fly. Dogs or other mammals can provide a reservoir of infection and the control of leishmaniasis therefore presents problems which are more difficult to overcome than those met with in malaria.

In the mammalian host the parasites of leishmaniasis assume the shape of round or oval bodies about half the size of a red blood cell — Leishman Donovan (LD) bodies. In the insect vector they assume flagellate form with a long free flagellum at the anterior end.

The effectiveness of drugs in leishmaniasis is usually tested in infected animals; *in vitro* tests are of little value since many effective leishmanicidal drugs have negligible activity *in vitro*. The usual laboratory hosts are golden (Syrian) hamsters which are inoculated intraperitoneally with the parasite. The activity of drugs may be gauged by comparing the number of parasites in spleen or liver biopsies from treated and control groups of animals.

It is convenient on clinical grounds to subdivide the leishmaniases into three types: visceral, mucocutaneous and cutaneous. No morphological differences can be observed between one *Leishmania* and another but they can be distinguished serologically and complete immunity to the homologous *Leishmania* species is established after infection. Thus an attack of Kala-azar confers permanent immunity to *L. donovani* from any geographical area.

Visceral leishmaniasis
Visceral leishmaniasis, or kala-azar, is a condition due to infection of reticuloendothelial cells throughout the body with *Leishmania donovani*. There is an insidious onset with irregular fever and increasing enlargement of the spleen and liver. The mortality is high.

Pentavalent antimonials are the main drugs used for the systemic treatment of kala-azar and have now largely superseded the toxic trivalent antimonial tartar emetic.

Pentavalent antimony compounds
These are derivatives of phenylstibonic acid. The pentavalent compounds are concentrated in the liver and

spleen to a greater extent than are the trivalent compounds, and are chiefly excreted by the kidneys.

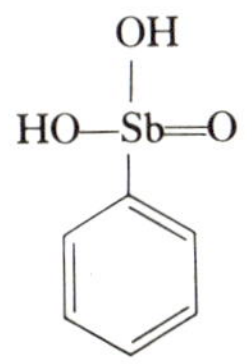

Fig. 35.7 Phenylstibonic acid

The action of pentavalent antimonials probably depends, as in the case of the pentavalent arsenicals, on their reduction to the corresponding trivalent compound. It has been found that after the injection of pentavalent compounds trivalent antimony is present in the liver of experimental animals and in human urine.

In the treatment of kala-azar the antimony compounds have a delayed effect, and the fall in fever, reduction in the size of the liver and spleen and gain in bodyweight usually occur about two weeks after beginning a course of treatment.

Sodium stibogluconate containing pentavalent antimony is used for the treatment of kala-azar. *Urea stibamine* which contains antimony in the pentavalent form has been widely used in the treatment of kala-azar in India. During treatment with pentavalent arsenicals a condition resembling anaphylactic shock sometimes occurs which may be treated by an intramuscular injection of adrenaline.

Diamidines. An effective alternative to the antimonials, in cases of visceral leishmaniasis refractory to antimony treatment, are the diamidines (p.433). They are effective in curing most forms of kala-azar but are not effective in the treatment of post-kala-azar dermal leishmaniasis. *Pentamidine isethionate* and *hydroxystilbamidine isethionate* may be employed.

Amphotericin. This antibiotic has been found effective in the treatment of some forms of advanced visceral leishmaniasis infections resistant to other drugs.

Mucocutaneous leishmaniasis, or espundia, is an infection of reticulo-endothelial cells, initially of the skin and subsequently of the mucosa, with *Leishmania braziliensis* prevalent in South America. The condition sometimes responds to pentavalent antimonials in full dosage. Alternatively it may respond to the antimalarial drug pyrimethamine or to the antibiotic amphotericin.

Cutaneous leishmaniasis. This is due to infection with *L. mexicana* or *L. tropica* (oriental sore). *Sodium stibogluconate* (Pentostam) may be effective in cutaneous leishmaniasis. *Cycloguanyl embonate,* the active metabolite of the antimalarial proguanil, is reported to be effective in the treatment of *L. braziliense* infections when given intramuscularly.

SPIROCHAETAL INFECTIONS

Spirochaetes are motile spiral micro-organisms which reproduce by transverse fission. The most important diseases of man caused by spirochaetes are associated with the genus *Treponema*, namely syphilis (*T. pallidum*) and the tropical diseases, yaws (*T. pertenue*) and pinta (*T. curateum*). These treponemes cannot be differentiated morphologically but they are nevertheless believed to be distinct because they cause different diseases. In each disease the serological Wassermann reaction is positive.

Other diseases caused by spirochaetes are Weil's disease, louse- and tick-borne relapsing fevers and rat-bite fever. Vincent's angina is a condition characterised by ulcerative lesions of the mouth in which spirochaetes are present although there is no general agreement that they cause the lesions.

Tests for spirochaeticidal drugs
These drugs may be tested *in vitro* and *in vivo*. Treponemes cannot be cultivated satisfactorily *in vitro* but if suspended in a suitable medium they retain their motility for some time and the effect of chemotherapeutic drugs upon them may be tested.

Experimental syphilis can be produced in rabbits and monkeys and antisyphilitic drugs tested in these animals. A period of several months is required for the adequate *in vivo* assay of an antisyphilitic drug.

Drug treatment of syphilis
Prior to the introduction of antibiotics, syphilis was treated with arsenical and bismuth compounds. In 1943 Lourie and Collier showed that penicillin cured infections in mice and in the same year it was reported that penicillin was effective in the treatment of early syphylis in man. Spirochaetes disappear from the primary lesion in about 12 hours and the lesions heal rapidly.

Although penicillin is the drug of choice in the treatment of syphilis, increasing numbers of allergic reactions to the drug have occurred. For this reason other antibiotics have been tested in syphilis and some of these, especially the tetracyclines, have been shown to have considerable antisyphilitic activity.

Penicillin
The aim of penicillin treatment of syphilis is to maintain a therapeutic level of the drug in the blood over a continuous period. An effective way of treating early infectious syphilis is to give intramuscular injections of a suspension of procaine benzyl penicillin of 600 mg daily for 10 days. Oral penicillin is less effective. Long-acting parenteral preparations such as 0.9 g of benzathine penicillin or benethamine penicillin may be given instead of procaine penicillin but single injections of these long-acting preparations tend to produce lower and less consistent blood levels.

A six month's follow-up examination of a patient who has been treated for early syphilis should include a serological test. If the titre is not appreciably decreased retreatment may be necessary.

Late latent syphilis, detectable only by a positive serological test, should also be treated with penicillin in dosage similar to that used in early syphilis, but further treatment may not be necessary even if the serological reactions after six months fail to revert to negative.

Late syphilis associated with gummas, cardiovascular lesions and neurological involvement should be treated with large doses of penicillin; 300 to 600 mg of procaine benzyl penicillin may be given daily or every other day for 10 to 15 injections. The object of treatment in these cases is the disappearance of a specific infectious process. Destructive changes such as occur in tabes or optic atrophy cannot be healed and the Wassermann reaction often fails to become negative.

Syphilis in pregnancy and congenital syphilis in the newborn must always be treated, but syphilitic interstitial keratitis of the newborn generally responds poorly to penicillin treatment.

U.S. Public Health Service recommendations. In view of the important public health problem involved, the following recommendations were issued by the public health service (U.S.) for the treatment of syphilis.

1. Primary, secondary and latent syphilis of less than one year's duration. Either aqueous procaine penicillin G 600 000 units daily intramuscularly for 8 days to a total of 4.8 mega-units; *or* benzathine penicillin G 2.4 mega-units intramuscularly (1.2 mega-units in each buttock) in a single dose. The latter is considered to provide effective treatment in a single visit.

2. Syphilis of more than one year's duration (latent, cardiovascular, late benign, or neourosyphilis). Either aqueous procaine penicillin G 600 000 units daily intramuscularly for 15 days to a total of 9 mega-units; *or* benzathine penicillin G 2.4 mega-units injected weekly, as for primary syphilis, for three successive weeks to a total of 7.2 mega-units.

3. Syphilis in pregnancy and congenital syphilis. Pregnant women with confirmed active syphilis are treated with penicillin unless they are allergic to it; otherwise they are treated with erythromycin. Infants with congenital syphilis should be given an intramuscular dose of benzathine penicillin G 50 000 units per kg body weight in a single dose, provided that their c.s.f. tests are normal.

The long-acting forms of penicillin are not suited for the treatment of gonorrhoea for which aqueous penicillin G or ampicillin should be used.

Reactions to penicillin. Two kinds of reactions may occur during treatment of syphilis by penicillin, Jarisch-Herxheimer reactions and allergic hypersensitivity reactions.

Jarisch-Herxheimer reactions are febrile reactions often accompanied by an exacerbation of a local syphilitic process and may occur in the initial stages of treatment by any effective antisyphilitic drug. This type of reaction is probably due to the abrupt massive destruction of treponemes in the syphilitic lesions and it usually subsides spontaneously within 24 or 36 hours. Jarisch-Herxheimer reactions are seldom dangerous.

Allergic reactions to penicillin on the other hand can be most dangerous and may necessitate the use of some other antibiotic.

Other antibiotics
In spite of the effectiveness of penicillin and the absence of resistance of treponemes towards it, other less active antibiotics may have to be used in the treatment of syphilis in patients who are allergic to penicillin.

The tetracyclines, although not as potent as penicillin have considerable activity both in experimental and clinical syphilis. When daily doses of 2 to 4 g of tetracycline or oxytetracycline are administered orally in early syphilis, spirochaetes disappear from the lesions within one or two days and the lesions heal in about one week. This treatment must be continued for 10–15 days. Others have used erythromycin, 500 mg 6 hourly for 10–15 days.

The use of bismuth and arsenicals for the treatment of syphilis is now mainly of historical interest although both are still employed in selected cases.

Bismuth
Soluble bismuth salts are directly spirochaeticidal *in vitro* and before the introduction of penicillin, bismuth salts were widely used in the treatment of syphilis because of their reliable action and lesser toxicity as compared to arsenicals.

After an adequate dose of penicillin, spirochaetes disappear from an early lesion within hours whilst after a dose of bismuth it takes about a week for the lesions to become sterile. This gradual action of bismuth is sometimes made use of in the treatment of late syphilis when treatment with penicillin is preceded by preliminary treatment with bismuth so that Jarisch-Herxheimer reactions are less likely to occur.

Arsenicals
The organic arsenicals are highly effective in syphilis but they have now been superseded because of their toxicity. The question nevertheless arises whether a combination of penicillin with arsenicals might not be more effective than penicillin alone.

Evidence from animal experiments is that the combined administration of the two drugs produces a greater proportion of cures then either drug alone but the clinical advantage of combined therapy is less obvious. Penicillin alone cures early syphilis in 80 to 90 per cent of cases, and although additional treatment with arsenicals slightly increases the proportion of patients serologically cured it also gives rise to the typical and often dangerous toxic effects of the arsenicals. For this reason most clinicians prefer to treat syphilis with penicillin alone.

Oxophenarsine (Mapharside)
This is a compound (Fig. 35.2) of constant composition, the purity of which can be determined by chemical methods.

Oxophenarsine is administered intravenously. The treatment of syphilis which involved the use of alternating courses of oxophenarsine and bismuth usually lasted about 18 months, but since the advent of penicillin, this method is seldom necessary.

The toxic effects of arsenicals are varied and include skin eruptions, jaundice and blood dyscrasias.

Iodides
These are sometimes used in the treatment of the later stages of syphilis. As far as is known they have no direct spirochaeticidal action, but they cause the absorption of newly-formed fibrous tissue and thus favour the destruction of spirochaetes that have produced gummata. This view of the mode of action of iodides is supported by their striking curative effects in actinomycosis, a condition due to a mould, which is also characterised by excessive formation of fibrous tissue. The usual dose of potassium iodide for this purpose is 1 to 2 g three times a day.

Treatment of other spirochaetal infections
Penicillin is highly effective in most spirochaetal infections.

Yaws (Framboesia), a disfiguring disease which is widely prevalent in the tropics, responds dramatically to penicillin. Procaine benzyl penicillin has been used by the World Health Organisation for the mass treatment of whole populations against this disease. Reports of yaws eradication campaigns emphasize the necessity for treating the entire population of an area since others may be incubating the disease or have it in a latent form. *Bejel* and *Pinta* are other treponematoses highly sensitive to penicillin.

In some types of spirochaetal disease other antibiotics are more effective. For example it has been shown that the tick-borne relapsing fever caused by *Spirochaeta persica* in Israel is resistant to penicillin and arsenicals, but responds to tetracycline and chlortetracycline.

PREPARATIONS

Trypanosomiasis
Melarsonyl potassium (Trimelarsan) 4 mg/kg s.c., i.m.
Melarsoprol (Melarsen oxide-BAL, Mel B) 3.6 mg/kg d.l. for 3 d i.v.
Nifurtimox (Lampit) init 5–7 mg/kg p.o. (Chagas' disease)
Nitrofurazone 1–2 g d.l. for 5–10 d p.o.
Pentamidine iseth 300 mg i.m.; ther for 3–7 d, proph every 3–6 m
Suramin (Germanin) init 200 mg i.v. then 1 g/w for 5 w
Tryparsamide 1–3 g s.c., i.m. i.v. every 5–7 d

Leishmaniasis

Antimonials
Stibogluconate iseth (Pentostam) 0.6–2g i.v. i.m.
Urea stibamine 100–200 mg/2 d i.v.

Amidines
Hydroxystilbamidine iseth 250 mg slow i.v. inj
Pentamidine (see above)

Syphilis
Benzathine penicillin 2.4 million u in single dose i.m.
or
Procaine penicillin (Procaine benzylpenicillin) 200 000 u/d for 8 d

Penicillin allergy
Tetracycline hyd 500 mg 4x/d for 15 d p.o.
Erythromycin 500 mg 4x/d for 15 d p.o.

FURTHER READING

Ciba Foundation Symposium 20 1974 Trypanosomiasis and leishmaniasis with special reference to Chagas's disease. Elsevier, Excerpta Medica
Ehrlich P 1909 On partial functions of the cell. Nobel Lecture. Collected Papers of Paul Ehrlich 1960: 3. Pergamon, London
Idsoe O, Guthe T, Willcox W R 1972 Penicillin in the treatment of syphilis. Bull. W.H.O.: 47, Supplement
Mulligan H W (ed) 1970 The African trypanosomiases. George Allen & Unwin, London
Maegraith B 1976 Clinical tropical diseases. Blackwell, Oxford
Smith C E G (ed) 1972 Research in diseases of the tropics. Br. med. Bull., 28: 1

36. Malaria and amoebiasis

Life cycle of the malaria parasite 438; Types of malaria parasites 439; Assessment of antiplasmodial activity 440; Aims of antimalarial treatment 440; Proguanil 440; Pyrimethamine 440; Chloroquine 440; Mepacrine 442; Quinine 442; Primaquine 443; Resistance to antimalarials 443; Immunity to malaria 443; Drugs used in amoebiasis 444; Metronidazole 444; Emetine 444; Iodinated 8-hydroxyquinolines 444; Aresenicals 445; Treatment of amoebic dysentery 446.

MALARIA

Malaria causes a greater economic loss than any other disease, for the total estimated annual incidence of cases in the world amounts to over a hundred million. The only disease with a greater incidence is hookworm infection, but this is much less lethal than malaria. The World Health Organisation, through its Expert Committee on Malaria, has instituted extensive programmes for the drug control and eradication of malaria.

The problem of controlling the disease requires the treatment of individuals suffering from malaria and the protection of those exposed to it. It is also necessary to eradicate systematically the larval and adult anopheline mosquitoes and to destroy their breeding places by drainage and insecticides. When this is effectively carried out in a well-organised and localised area, such as the island of Ceylon, it can virtually eradicate malaria. Nevertheless, in 1968, the combination of a rainfall pattern ideal for vector breeding with large-scale population movement, was responsible for an explosive epidemic there during which some two million cases of malaria occurred.

As a result of the extensive use of dicophane (DDT) (p. 467) sprays in countries such as Argentine, Greece and Italy, where malaria was a traditional scourge, it has now ceased to be a public health problem.

The widespread use of insecticides such as DDT and gamma benzene hexachloride (gammexane) to control the speed of the mosquito has, however, raised new problems. Apart from the economic difficulties of providing an efficient scheme, it has been found that many species of flies, ticks and anopheline mosquitoes have become resistant to DDT and certain birds and insects which are useful to the community are adversely affected by these insecticides.

The drug treatment of malaria has also made rapid strides. Cinchona bark and its alkaloids were for two centuries the only remedies for malaria, but a number of synthetic antimalarial compounds have been discovered and the chief difficulty now is to make them available to large poverty-stricken populations. Another problem, which has become more obvious during the last few years, is the appearance of resistance against antimalarial drugs in malaria parasites.

Life cycle of malaria parasite

The malaria parasite is introduced into the blood of animals and man by the bite of an infected anopheline mosquito. The life cycle of the malaria parasite consists of a sexual cycle which takes place in the mosquito and an asexual cycle which occurs in the vertebrate host (Fig. 36.1). When the mosquito probes the tissues in order to take a blood meal, sporozoites are directly injected along with the saliva and some are thus introduced into the peripheral blood and the asexual cycle begins. About half an hour later, the sporozoites disappear from the peripheral blood stream into the liver cells where they undergo an exo-erythrocytic stage of development during 10 to 14 days, giving rise to cryptozoites. At the end of this stage the liver cells rupture and liberate merozoites. Some of these may enter new liver cells, whilst others enter red cells where they grow and develop into asexual and sexual forms. The dividing asexual forms in the red blood cell are called schizonts which develop into merozoites. The red cells then disintegrate liberating asexual merozoites which infect other red cells, and male and female gametocytes which can only complete their development when taken up by the mosquito.

The further development of the sexual stage begins when the mosquito sucks blood from the infected vertebrate host. The asexual forms of the parasite which are present, disintegrate in the mosquito stomach and the male gametocytes undergo a further development, extruding several motile flagella one of which fertilises a female cell or gamete, developed from an ingested female gametocyte. The resultant zygote perforates the wall of the mosquito stomach and forms a sporocyst which finally ruptures into the body cavity of the mosquito, liberating sporozoites. These then migrate to the salivary glands of the mosquito which is now infective.

The periodic emission of the merozoites from red corpuscles produces the periodic attacks of fever. These asexual cycles are repeated as long as the conditions are favourable for the parasite and as long as they continue, the patient suffers from acute malaria. It is well recognised that when the fever subsides either spontaneously or as a result of the administration of antimalarial drugs, the parasite disappears from the general circulation. After an interval of weeks or months, however, the parasite may reappear in the peripheral blood and cause a clinical relapse. The sexual forms, or gametocytes, are particularly persistent and resistant to drugs, but they can only reproduce in the mosquito and not in man.

Immunity plays an important part in the course of malarial infection. A malaria carrier is an individual whose body has acquired sufficient resistance to prevent the rapid asexual multiplication of the parasites, but not sufficient to destroy the organisms completely. Many inhabitants in districts where malaria is endemic are carriers of this type and are highly infective to mosquitoes and hence encourage the spread of malaria.

plasmodia (*P. vivax*, *P. malariae* and *P. ovale*) is usually less severe and very rarely fatal. An important distinction between *P. falciparum* infections and the other types of malaria is that there are no persistent liver extra-erythrocitic phases in the former, so that true relapses do not occur. Hence, in patients who have left the endemic area, the *P. falciparum* parasites rarely persist for more than one year. In patients with other forms of malaria true relapses may occur after leaving the endemic area, particularly after incomplete treatment.

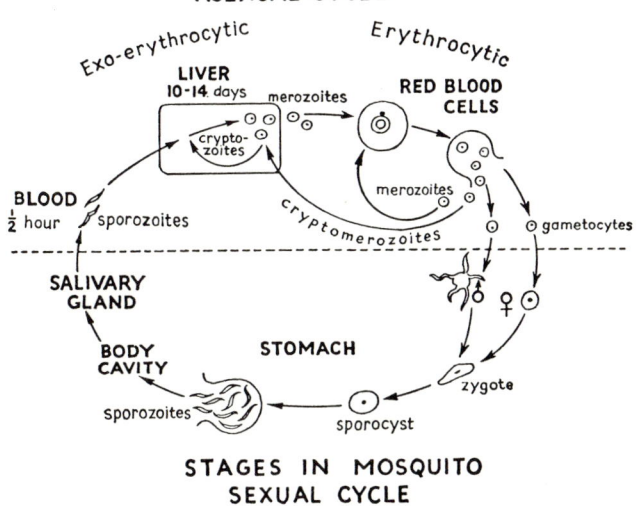

Fig. 36.1 Diagram of life cycle of malaria parasite in man.

Types of malaria parasite

The chief species of human malaria parasites are:

1. *Plasmodium vivax*, which has a cycle of 48 hours and produces benign tertian malaria. Acute attacks of malaria can be rapidly controlled by a number of different drugs but no single drug can be relied upon to eradicate all the parasites from the tissues. There is evidence that secondary exoerythrocytic forms persist for many years and, when they reinfect the red cells, cause a relapse.

2. *Plasmodium ovale* is the cause of ovale tertian malaria, a rarer form of malaria occurring mainly in Africa.

3. *Plasmodium falciparum* also has a cycle of 48 hours and produces malignant tertian or subtertian fever. The secondary exo-erythrocytic forms of *P. falciparum*, in contrast to those of *P. vivax*, rarely persist for longer than six months and infections due to the former are therefore more readily eliminated by antimalarial drugs or by removal from an endemic area.

4. *Plasmodium malariae* has a cycle of 72 hours and produces quartan fever.

The most severe clinical form of malaria is that caused by *P. falciparum* infection. Malaria caused by the other

Malaria parasites can multiply at an enormous rate by asexual reproduction. A single *P. vivax* parasite produces 16 new parasites in 48 hours, and at this rate of multiplication a single parasite in a case of benign tertian infection can produce 250 000 000 descendants in 14 days, a number which represents about 50 parasites per cubic millimetre of blood. This is a number which can be detected microscopically, but which will not produce fever; but the next generation will produce sufficient parasites to cause fever. This theoretical rate of multiplication is actually approached during the invasion stage of malarial infection since injection of malarial blood produces fever after an interval of 7–21 days. The fact that destruction of 94 per cent of the parasites every 48 hours will only maintain equilibrium and will not reduce their number indicates how powerful an action is needed if a drug is to cure the disease.

Asexual and sexual forms of the parasite differ as regards their susceptibility to drugs and the same is true of the different species of plasmodia. Furthermore, different strains of a species may vary widely both as regards virulence and response to drug therapy. The drug treatment of malaria is therefore a complex problem.

Assessment of antiplasmoidal activity

The antimalarial activity of a compound depends on the interaction of the parasite, the host and the drug. For the experimental investigation of antimalarial drugs the chief methods of infecting the host are: (a) injection of blood containing a definite number of parasites; (b) injection of ground-up salivary glands of infected mosquitoes; and (c) exposure of the host to the bite of infected mosquitoes.

The chief problem is to select a suitable host which can be infected with species of plasmodia which are pathogenic for that particular host. Avian malaria can be produced by infecting chicks, ducks, canaries or sparrows with a variety of non-human plasmodia; amongst mammalian hosts, the mouse and the Congo tree rat have been used, but none of these can be infected with human plasmodia. Only recently has it become possible to achieve infection with human malarial parasites in certain species of monkey. Various methods have been devised to test the curative and suppressive action of drugs on the infected host. A common method is to administer intravenously an inoculum of blood containing a definite number of infected cells, and to give the drug orally for three to four days. The activity of the drug is assessed by the fall in the parasite cell count. Attempts have been made to compare the activity of various drugs with that of a standard antimalarial. No species of avian parasite, or of avian host, is entirely satisfactory for the assessment of compounds suitable for use in human malaria; the same criticism holds for tests carried out in other vertebrate hosts.

The ideal method is to infect human volunteers with species of plasmodia which cause human malaria, using not only different species, but also different strains of the same species. This method, however, is expensive and time-consuming, and is only suitable for testing a limited number of drugs which have passed the preliminary screening tests in animals.

Aims of antimalarial treatment

Treatment with antimalarial drugs has three main aims:

1. *Propylaxis* which is the prevention of infection after the bite of an infected mosquito. To achieve this, an effective concentration of the drug must be maintained in the blood. It was formerly believed that '*causal prophylactic*' drugs such as proguanil and pyrimethamine act on sporozoites before they lodge in the liver cells, but it is now known that these drugs do not kill sporozoites but the early exoerythrocytic forms or cryptozoites.

2. *Suppression* or *clinical prophylaxis* which is the control of the fever and other symptoms of an acute attack of malaria. For this purpose the drug must be active against asexual schizonts which multiply inside the red cells. Such drugs are sometimes called schizonticides. An example is chloroquine which is widely used as a suppressant of malaria, sometimes by its addition to table salt.

3. *Radical cure* which means complete elimination of an established infection in the body. This may involve: (a) the eradication of the reservoir of exoerythrocytic parasites so as to prevent relapses, and (b) the inactivation of gametocytes so as to prevent the reinfection of mosquitoes. The 8-aminoquinolines are capable of destroying gametocytes.

In *P. falciparum* infection in man a radical cure can be obtained by drugs which have only a schizonticidal action, e.g. chloroquine, because in this infection the exoerythrocytic forms do not persist. In recent years chlorquine resistant strains of *P. falciparum* have developed and spread in South East Asia.

Prophylactic drugs

True prophylaxis is not at present possible in any form of malaria since no known drug is capable of destroying free sporozoites. Pyrimethamine and proguanil, however, have been shown to destroy the pre-erythrocytic liver forms of *P. falciparum* and may thus prevent the initiation of their erythrocytic cycle. This action has been referred to as 'causal prophylaxis'. Some causal prophylactic activity may also occur in *P. vivax* infections particularly with pyrimethamine.

Pyrimethamine (Daraprim)

This drug (Fig. 36.2) is a powerful dihydrofolate inhibitor used for the prophylaxis of malaria because of its slow action. It is also used in combination with sulphonamides or sulphones to treat chloroquine resistant strains of *P. falciparum*. Sulphonamides and folic acid antagonists are generally given together in the treatment of malaria, for their combined activity is many times greater than that of either drug alone (p. 395). Furthermore the number of malarial strains resistant to either agent is greatly decreased with the use of the combination.

The toxicity of small doses of pyrimethamine is small. Large doses may produce haematological abnormalities.

Clinical uses. Pyrimethamine is chiefly used as a prophylactic and is given by mouth in a dose of 25 to 50 mg once a week. The chief disadvantage of pyrimethamine is the development of resistance to its action.

Proguanil (Paludrine)

This drug is a biguanide (Fig. 36.2), which is chemically and pharmacologically related to pyrimethamine. Like the latter it is used for the prophylaxis of malaria. It is less potent than pyrimethamine.

Cycloguanil is the active metabolite of proguanil. An intramuscular injection of the embonate can produce a long-lasting prophylactic effect against susceptible strains.

Suppressive drugs

Chloroquine (Avloclor, Nivaquine)

The antimalarial properties of chloroquine were discovered in Germany in 1934 but the drug was rejected

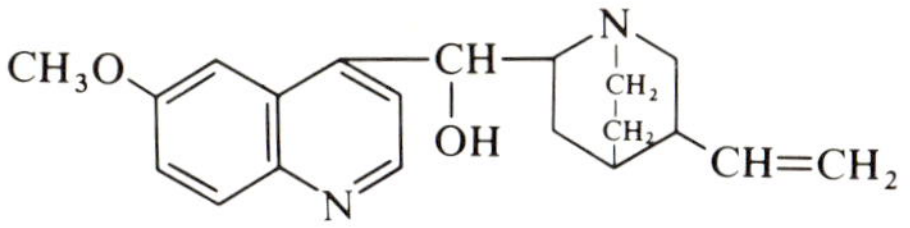

Fig. 36.2 Chemical structure of antimalarials.

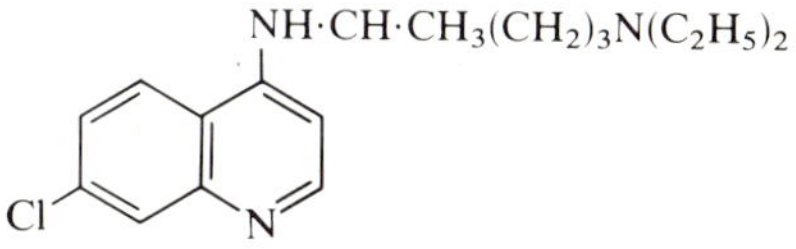

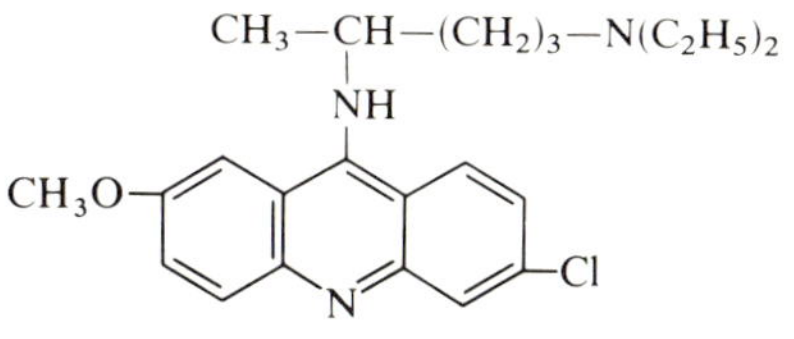

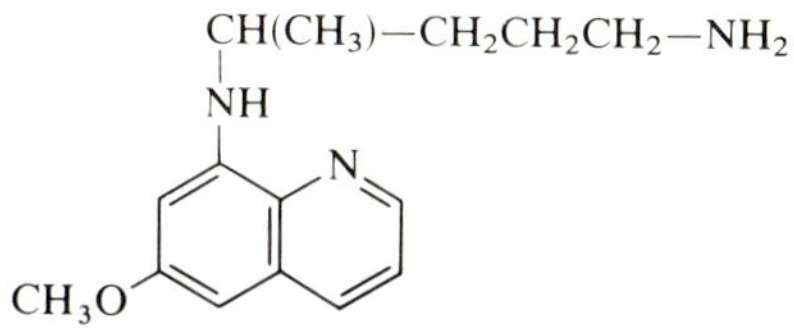

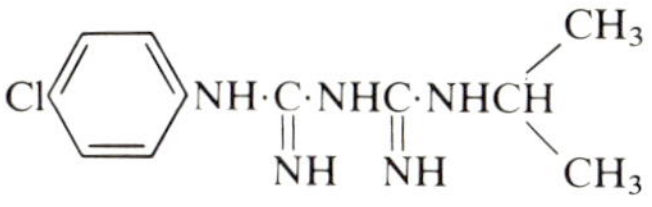

Chloroquine is a derivative of 4-aminoquinoline and has the structure shown in Figure 36.2.

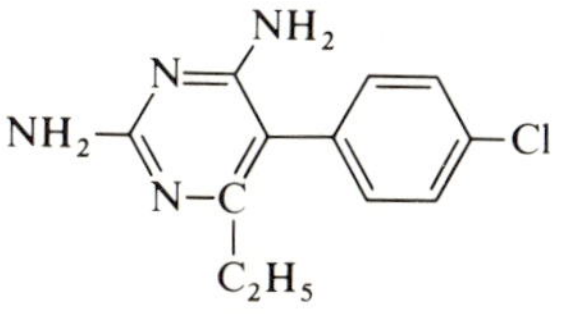

Antimalarial action. There is evidence that chloroquine can inhibit nucleic acid replication of the parasite by intercalating between the strands of double stranded DNA (p. 388). Chloroquine is very active against the schizonts in the red blood cells and suppresses acute attacks of all types of malarial parasites.

Chloroquine has a schizonticidal effect and kills the erythrocytic forms of malaria parasites at all stages of development. Chloroquine has no action on malarial sporozoites or on the tissue forms of plasmodia. Relapses may therefore occur in infections due to *P. vivax, P. ovale* and *P. malariae* during the year following the cessation of treatment. To prevent these relapses a single dose of 600 mg of chloroquine base is given by mouth to kill erythrocytic parasites and this is followed by a course of treatment with an 8-aminoquinoline derivative such as primaquine. Since the exo-erythrocitic forms of *P. falciparum* do not usually persist it is possible to eradicate this type of infection by means of chloroquine provided the organism is not chloroquine resistant.

It was formerly believed that resistance to chloroquine is rare, but it has now become obvious that resistance to it does occur, especially in *P. falciparum.* Some strains have become resistant not only to chloroquine but also to other standard antimalarial drugs such as mepacrine, proguanil and pyrimethamine, so that the only effective antimalarial against them is quinine.

Therapeutic uses. Chloroquine is rapidly absorbed from the alimentary tract and is therefore usually administered by mouth; it can also be given by intramuscular or intravenous injection. Chloroquine is fixed in the tissues and its concentration in the liver may be about 300 times that in the plasma. After a single oral dose appreciable concentrations of the drug are present in the plasma and tissues for several days.

Chloroquine is eliminated very slowly from the body and it may persist in tissues for a prolonged period. It is mainly excreted in the urine, either as unchanged drug or as metabolites.

Chloroquine has strong anti-inflammatory activity and this contributes to its antimalarial action.

Chloroquine has also been found to have a beneficial effect in certain connective tissue diseases such as *rheumatoid arthritis* and *lupus erythematosus* but this requires prolonged administration and its use for this purpose is limited by its toxic effects on the eye and pigment changes of the hair. Chloroquine is also used in the treatment of *hepatic amoebiasis.*

Toxic effects. The toxic effects of acute administration are relatively unimportant; blurring of vision, headache and dizziness occasionally occur. In contrast to mepacrine, chloroquine does not stain the skin but bleaching of the hair sometimes occurs.

in favour of mepacrine. It was rediscovered in the course of a large co-operative programme of antimalarial research carried out in the United States during the war. It is now agreed that chloroquine is less toxic and better tolerated in man than mepacrine and it is probably the most widely used suppressive antimalarial drug used for treatment of acute attacks of malaria.

Chronic administration of large doses, as in rheumatoid arthritis, causes two kinds of ocular effects: (1) corneal deposits which regress when the drug is discontinued; (2) a retinopathy which is progressive and may lead to blindness.

Amodiaquine (Camoquin) is closely related to chloroquine and is used for the same purposes.

Mepacrine (Quinacrine, Atebrin)
In 1933 Mauss and Mietzsch produced a number of compounds containing the same active side chain as pamaquin but attached to different heterocyclic nuclei. Mepacrine, whose structure is shown in Figure 36.2, has the same side chain as pamaquin, the first of the 8-aminoquinoline derivatives used for the treatment of malaria, but attached to a different nucleus.

Antimalarial action. The antimalarial action of mepacrine resembles that of chloroquine; it is a schizonticide acting on the asexual erythrocytic cycle of all parasites. It also has an action on gametocytes similar to that of chloroquine.

Mepacrine was formerly widely used for the suppression and treatment of malaria but it has now been largely superseded for these purposes by chloroquine and other more recently introduced antimalarials.

Both mepacrine and chloroquine are effective in the treatment of giardiasis, an infection due to *Gardia lamblia* which causes diarrhoea and steatorrhoea, especially in young children.

Quinine
Cinchona bark owes its name to the fact that soon after its discovery in Peru it was used to treat the Countess Cinchon, the wife of the Viceroy. It was introduced into Spain in 1640 by the Jesuits, and hence was also known as Jesuit's bark. The use of the bark was opposed by orthodox medicine because it was not in accordance with Galenic doctrines, and in Protestant countries it was viewed with suspicion because it had been introduced by the Jesuits. The value of the remedy was, however, so obvious that opposition soon subsided.

The alkaloid quinine was isolated in 1820. Over 20 other alkaloids have been isolated from various species of cinchona, but the 2 most important alkaloids are quinine and quinidine.

Quinine contains a quinoline and a quinuclidine group joined by a secondary alcohol group (Fig. 36.2). Quinine is laevo-rotatory, whilst its isomer quinidine is dextro-rotatory. The laevo-rotatory isomer has more antimalarial activity than the dextro-rotatory isomer.

Antimalarial action of quinine. Quinine is a highly active blood schizonticide with actions similar to chloroquine. Like the latter it has no action on the tissue forms of the malaria parasite and therefore does not prevent relapse of vivax, ovale and malariae infections. It was formerly widely used to control overt attacks of malaria but has been largely superseded by less toxic drugs. It has several disadvantages; high doses are required which frequently produce unpleasant side effects. It is also liable to produce blackwater fever especially in areas where *P. falciparum* infections are prevalent. Quinine has for long been mainly used in the treatment of cerebral malaria, for which quinine dihydrochloride can be administered intravenously. It is a curious fact that treatment with quinine has recently become important again, as a last resort for infections with strains of *P. falciparum* which have become resistant to all other antimalarial drugs.

Other actions of quinine. Quinine salts are very bitter in taste and are used as stomachic bitters in small doses, but when given continuously by mouth in large doses the bitter irritant salts are liable to produce digestive disturbance. Quinine produces an action similar to quinidine on the heart but the latter compound is used in the treatment of atrial fibrillation (p. 144).

Quinine decreases the excitability of the motor end plate. It can prevent nocturnal muscle cramps when taken at night in doses of 0.2 to 0.3 g; it is also effective in alleviating the muscle spasms which occur in *myotonia congenita* (Thomson's disease). By contrast the muscular fatigue in patients with myasthenia gravis is aggravated by administration of quinine and it is therefore sometimes used as a diagnostic aid in this disease.

Toxic actions of quinine. Quinine has a specific action on the special sense organs, and the first signs of an overdose are ringing and roaring in the ears accompanied by slight deafness (cinchonism); at the same time the eyes are affected, and there is diminution in the field of vision, and photophobia, and in some cases even temporary blindness.

When patients, infected with certain strains of *P. falciparum*, are treated with quinine, they may develop haemoglobinuria (blackwater fever). The mechanism of this haemolysis is discussed on page 29.

Toxic effects of quinine on the heart are only observed when the drug is given intravenously and can be detected by a fall in blood-pressure and a depression of the R-T segment and reduction or abolition of the T wave. The drug should be given slowly and in dilute solution, as fatal cases of ventricular fibrillation have occurred in patients who are ill-nourished and heavily infected with malaria.

Some individuals are hypersensitive to quinine, and develop urticarial eruptions when given small doses of the drug.

Drugs active against tissue stages and gametocytes

The destruction of the persistent liver infection by exo-erythrocytic parasites is achieved by only one group of drugs, the 8-aminoquinolines such as primaquine.

Primaquine

Primaquine has been the outcome of a large-scale research programme carried out in the U.S.A. during the war with the aim of finding better antimalarials. It was known that the 8-aminoquinoline derivative pamaquine had considerable activity against the tissue forms of parasites. Primaquine is the secondary amine corresponding to pamaquine and has been found to have similar antimalarial actions and to be the most useful and least toxic of the series.

Antimalarial action. Primaquine kills the primary exo-erythrocytic stages of all plasmodia active in man, it also kills gametocytes of all species, or renders them incapable of development in the mosquito. Primaquine has a powerful effect against the secondary tissue stage of *P. vivax* and is mainly used for the radical cure of *P. vivax* infections in people returning from malarious areas. For this purpose a short intensive course of treatment with a schizonticide such as chloroquine is given to kill any erythrocytic parasites and this is followed by a course of daily doses of primaquine.

Pentaquine is an 8-aminoquinoline with actions similar to primaquine.

Toxic effects of 8-aminoquinolines. The chief toxic effects of these drugs are methaemoglobinaemia and haemolytic anaemia. This is specially liable to occur in some races such as Indians and Sephardic Jews, due to a genetically transmitted lack of the enzyme glucose-6-phosphate dehydrogenase. The defect is determined by a sex-linked gene carried on the X-chromosome. Low levels or lack of the enzyme predispose the red corpuscles to acute haemolysis on contact with a variety of substances (p. 29).

Other toxic effects consist of anorexia, nausea, abdominal pain and muscular weakness.

Clinical malarial chemotherapy

Chemotherapy for persons entering endemic areas

Prevention of malaria whilst visiting malarious areas is termed clinical prophylaxis. This may be achieved by means of suppressive agents such as the 4-aminoquinolines chloroquine or amodiaquine. These drugs are given weekly, two weeks before, during and eight weeks after visiting the area. They have no action on sporozoites or on the tissues forms of plasmodia. Proguanil and pyrimethamine also exert prophylactic effects especially against falciparum malaria, less against vivax malaria. For radical cure of a malarial attack the most effective and least toxic drug is primaquine, which may be given for the first three days of an acute attack together with or following the administration of chloroquine.

Chemotherapy in drug-resistant areas

Proguanil and pyrimethamine resistant strains do not usually present major problems of treatment, since most of them respond either to chloroquine or to mepacrine or quinine. The treatment of chloroquine resistant strains, however, may present considerable difficulty and these have been classified according to the reaction of the parasite to the drug. Thus in grade I resistance, chloroquine may clear the blood of parasites but a recrudescence occurs within 28 days. Incomplete clearance of parasites from the blood (grade II resistance) and more rarely complete resistance to the drug (grade III) have been encountered in some areas. Fortunately many cases of grade I resistance respond to quinine. When patients cannot tolerate high doses of quinine or there is no satisfactory clinical response, an alternative method of treatment is a combination of pyrimethamine and a long-acting sulphonamide (sulphadoxine) or dapsone. This type of combined therapy is usually successful in semi-immune and in non-immune patients infected with strains of chloroquine resistant and proguanil or pyrimethamine resistant strains of *P. falciparum*.

Immunity to malaria

Inhabitants of malarial regions frequently acquire immunity to malaria; they may show no evidence of fever or ill health in spite of carrying malarial parasites in their blood. In such patients a degree of balance has developed between the immunity processes of the host and the tendency of the parasites to multiply. Nevertheless it is rare that a complete eradication of parasites is achieved without the aid of drugs; conversely the effectiveness of drugs depends greatly on the state of immunity of the patient.

Development of a malaria vaccine

It has been shown in several animal species that vaccination against malaria is both feasible and successful. The exo-erythrocytic stage has been controlled in rodent malaria by inoculation of sporozoites which gave complete protection lasting about three months in mice. Another type of vaccine has been produced by the isolation and injection into monkeys of blood stage merozoites. It has recently become possible to achieve continuous cultures of the erythrocytic stage of a human malaria parasite making feasible the provision of antigen for vaccination. The elaboration of a human malaria vaccine has thus become a realistic goal.

AMOEBIASIS

Amoebic dysentery is caused by *Entamoeba histolytica*, which burrows under the mucosa of the intestine, producing large ulcers. The parasite may also invade the liver, months or years after the original infection, or it may give rise to a large isolated ulcer or hyperplastic mass in the colon, resembling carcinoma.

The amoebae are present in the stools of infected individuals as clear greenish-tinted structures of about four times the diameter of a red corpuscle. Under adverse conditions they become encysted and the cysts normally carry the infection. The cysts can survive outside the body for about a week in moist and cool surroundings; heat and desiccation kills them. The infection may be transmitted by contamination from stools or by houseflies.

Measurement of chemotherapeutic effect. Amoebicidal drugs can be tested on cultures of *E. histolytica* or in animals infected with amoebiasis. For this purpose rats are laparotomised under anaesthesia and the parasites are injected into the lumen of the caecum. The animals are then allowed to recover and treated with the drug for several days. Finally the animals are killed and the progress of the local infection is assessed by microscopic and pathological examination.

Amoebicide drugs

The aim of amoebicidal treatment is to eliminate the causative agent from the body. *Entamoeba histolytica* generally attacks the intestinal wall and it may also invade the liver causing abscesses. Other tissues besides the liver may also be involved. A variety of drugs are used in the treatment of amoebiasis.

Metronidazole is effective against both intestinal and hepatic amoebiasis and has relatively low toxicity. The highly toxic drugs *emetine* and *dehydroemetine* are used in severe amoebiasis. Certain drugs, referred to as luminal amoebicides act primarily in the intestinal lumen. They include *diiodohydroxyquin* the relatively toxic arsenical *carbarsone* and the broad spectrum antibiotic *paromomycin*. Other antibiotics, notably the *tetracyclines*, act indirectly in the intestinal lumen by modifying the intestinal flora necessary for survival of the amoebae.

Metronidazole (Flagyl) (Fig. 36.4)

This nitroimidazole derivative has a wide range of antiprotozoal activity. It acts directly on *E. histolytica* and is effective in both amoebic dysentery and amoebic liver abscess. It is also effective against *Trichomonas vaginalis* and *Giarda intestinalis*.

Metronidazole is readily absorbed from the gastrointestinal tract and widely distributed in body tissues; it diffuses across the placenta and is present in the milk of nursing mothers. Peak concentrations in the serum occur within 2 hours and only trace amounts are detected after 24 hours. It is excreted in the urine partly unchanged and as unidentified metabolites.

Therapeutic uses. For the treatment of acute intestinal amoebiasis a 5 day course of 800 mg daily of metronidazole is usually effective; alternatively a higher dose schedule of 2.4 g daily may be given for 2 to 3 consecutive days.

In amoebic liver abscess metronidazole may be combined with chloroquine. Metronidazole is also extensively used in the treatment of *trichomoniasis* of the genitourinary tract in females and males in doses of 200 mg 3 times daily for 7 days. It is also used in similar doses for the treatment of *Vincent's* infection.

In *trichomonas vaginalis* infections vaginal discharge is the most common complaint. In the male, diagnosis is made by examination of urethral discharge or centrifuged urine. Metronidazole is generally effective and treatment of both female and male partners should be considered.

Toxic effects. Side effects of metronidazole are usually mild and infrequent. They include headache, nausea, dryness of the mouth and skin rashes; moderate but transient leucopenia has occasionally been reported.

Nimorazole and *Tinidazole* are drugs with similar actions and indications as metronidazole.

Emetine

Ipecacuanha was brought to Europe from Brazil in 1658 and has long been used in the treatment of amoebic dysentery. The alkaloid emetine contained in ipecacuanha was isolated in 1829. Emetine is an amoebicide acting principally in the bowel wall and the liver. In acute intestinal amoebiasis the symptoms are rapidly cleared by the first course of emetine injections and mobile amoebae and cysts disappear, but more than 50 per cent of patients later show cysts in their faeces and hence become carriers. Further treatment with emetine in these cases is of little value. For these reasons emetine is now used only in severe cases or acute exacerbation of amoebic dysentery, and only long enough to control the dysenteric symptoms.

Dehydroemetine (Mebadin) appears to be as active as emetine but less toxic, possibly because it is excreted more rapidly, and this compound is becoming established as a replacement for emetine.

Toxic effects. The chief objection to the use of emetine is that the effective therapeutic dose approaches the toxic dose. Not more than 600 mg emetine should be given in a course of treatment, after which a rest of some weeks should be allowed.

Emetine is specially harmful to the myocardium and in susceptible patients it causes characteristic electrocardiographic changes consisting of depression of the T wave and prolongation of the P—R interval; sometimes it causes acute congestive heart failure. Patients should therefore be kept at rest in bed during treatment with emetine.

Iodinated 8-hydroxyquinolines

These were amongst the earliest synthetic compounds tested, and found active, in amoebiasis. The most widely used are: *chiniofon* (Avlochin) *Clioquinol* (iodochlorhydroxyquin, (Vioform) and *diiodohydroxyquinoline* (Diodoquin) (Fig. 36.3). Clioquinol and diiodohydroxyquinoline are almost insoluble in water.

Therapeutic uses. In experimentally infected animals and in patients with amoebic dysentery, the hydroxyquinoline derivatives expel cystic forms of the parasite, but do not destroy amoebae which have penetrated into the gut wall.

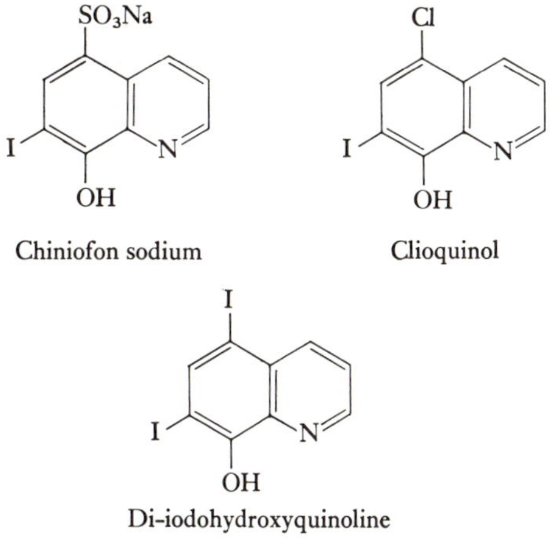

Chiniofon sodium

Clioquinol

Di-iodohydroxyquinoline

Fig. 36.3 Chemical structure of iodinated 8-hydroxyquinoline compounds.

Clioquinol in low dosage is frequently used as a preventive against amoebic infection in endemic areas.

Toxic effects. The development of a neurological syndrome associated with the use of hydroxyquinolines, notably clioquinol, was reported in 1965 by Japanese clinicians. The characteristic features of this neurological disease of unknown origin consist of sensory impairment of the lower limbs, disturbance of gait, visual impairment and psychic disorders. There was evidence of demyelination of the optic nerve, lateral and posterior columns of the spinal cord and peripheral nerves. The condition was named *subacute myelo-optico-neuropathy (SMON)* and was associated with the administration of daily doses of clioquinol for more than 14 days. In 1971 it was estimated that there were more than 10 000 patients with SMON in Japan.

Whilst there appears to be a causal relationship between the administration of this drug and these neurological disturbances, other aetiological factors, for example the role of infective agents, environmental pollutants and genetic and immunological features have been suggested. The widespread use of smaller and intermittent doses of clioquinol as a popular form of treatment for travellers' diarrhoea in Western countries has not been reported to give rise to these serious toxic effects. Self-medication should be limited to courses of treatment of not more than 7.5 g separated by intervals of at least four weeks.

Diloxanide furoate. This is one of a newer series of compounds (Fig. 36.4) found to have considerable amoebicidal activity *in vitro*. When tested clinically it produced a high percentage of cures in cyst-passing patients. It is also effective in acute amoebiasis. No serious effects have been reported so far.

Phanquone (Entobex). This is a phenanthridine derivative (Fig. 36.4) which is effective in acute and chronic amoebiasis. It is usually used in conjunction with other amoebicidal drugs, for example to supplement treatment with emetine hydrochloride.

The excretion of dark coloured urine during phanquone treatment is attributed to the presence of harmless excretory products of the drug.

Clefamide has been used in the treatment of acute and chronic intestinal amoebiasis.

Arsenicals

Organic arsenicals have been used with success in the treatment of amoebiasis. Although the trivalent arsenicals are the more effective, the pentavalent compounds are mainly used clinically because they are relatively less toxic.

The first pentavalent arsenical used for the treatment of amoebiasis was acetarsol; this became superseded by the

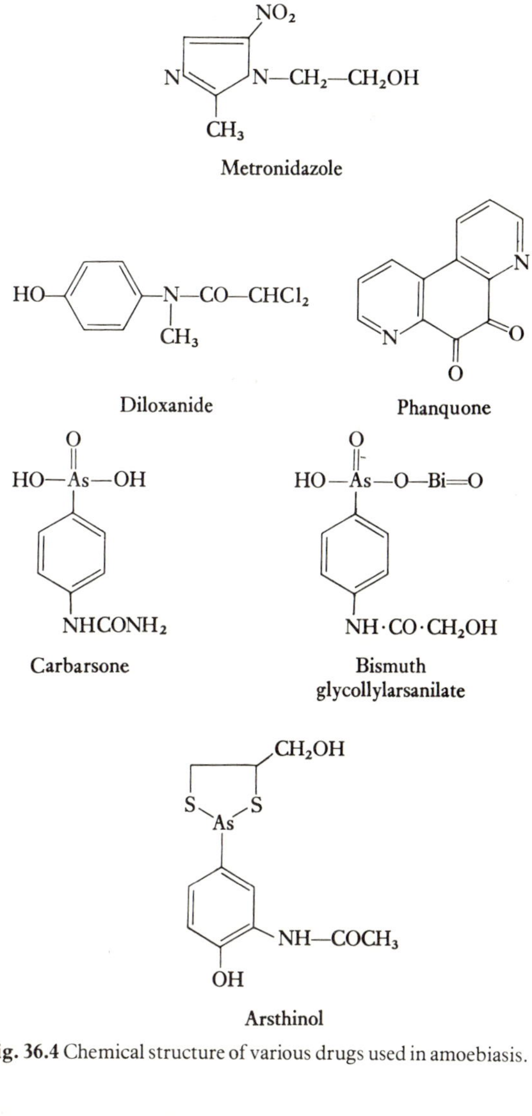

Metronidazole

Diloxanide

Phanquone

Carbarsone

Bismuth glycollylarsanilate

Arsthinol

Fig. 36.4 Chemical structure of various drugs used in amoebiasis.

more active and less toxic compound *carbarsone*. More recently a compound containing both arsenic and bismuth, *bismuth glycollylarsanilate* (Milibis, Glycobiarsol) and a trivalent thioarsenite, *arsthinol* (Balarsen) have been introduced (Fig. 36.4). These compounds are all relatively insoluble and they are incompletely absorbed from the gastrointestinal tract. Hence, whilst they occur in adequate concentrations in the lumen of the gut and relieve intestinal dysentery, they do not produce adequate concentrations at extraintestinal sites and are not effective in hepatic amoebiasis. They are used mainly in chronic intestinal amoebiasis, but their potential toxicity, including the rare occurrence of encephalitis, precludes their routine use.

Chloroquine
This antimalarial drug has only low activity against *Entamoeba histolytica* when tested *in vitro* and it has little or no activity when tested against experimental intestinal infections in animals. Chloroquine is, however, highly concentrated in the liver after repeated dosage and it has proved effective when tested against experimental hepatic infections.

Chloroquine has been found beneficial in patients with amoebic liver abscess and it can be used in this condition in place of emetine although it is probably somewhat less effective.

Antibiotics
The tetracyclines sometimes produce a rapid improvement of chronic intestinal amoebiasis, as shown by healing of the lesions and disappearance of the amoebae from the stools. Although these drugs have some direct effect on amoebae, their main action is probably produced indirectly by changing the bacterial flora of the gastrointestinal tract thereby reducing secondary infection. The tetracycline drugs are usually given for 10 to 20 days often in combination with other amoebicidal drugs and are particularly valuable in preventing relapses.

Other antibiotics have been found to produce beneficial effects in amoebiasis, for example, *paromomycin*.

Treatment of amoebic dysentery

For purposes of treatment it is necessary to distinguish between acute intestinal amoebiasis, chronic intestinal amoebiasis and amoebic liver abscess.

Acute intestinal amoebiasis, according to severity, may be treated in hospital outpatient or domiciliary practice. Patients with severe dysentery and confined to bed under medical supervision usually respond rapidly to oral treatment with metronidazole (800 gm daily) for 5 days. Alternatively a 10-day course of intramuscular injections of emetine hydrochloride (1 mg/kg) or twice this dose of dehydroemetine is effective but should be combined with a course of tetracycline, 250 mg every 6 hours and diloxanide furoate (Furamide), 500 mg 3 times daily. In view of the potential adverse cardiac effects of emetine drugs, bed rest is advisable; they must be used with caution in pregnant and elderly patients and are contra-indicated in patients with heart disease. Severe dehydration can often be adequately corrected by frequent oral administration of saline and fruit juice without resorting to parenteral therapy. For the management of ambulant patients, the choice of drugs includes metronidazole, paromomycin or a tetracycline, arsenicals such as carbarsone in conjunction with emetine bismuth iodide or a hydroxyquinoline derivative.

Chronic intestinal amoebiasis is characterised by the passage in the stools of cysts of *E. histolytica*. These patients respond to treatment with diloxanide or phanquone or to carbarsone or iodinated hydroxyquinolines.

For the treatment of hepatic amoebiasis the simplest form of treatment is a 5-day course of metronidazole. Treatment with parenteral emetine and oral chloroquine is also effective but necessitates bed rest and close medical supervision. In the management of amoebic dysentery it is important to ascertain the source of infection, particularly in patients in whom relapse and reinfection may be indistinguishable. Several successive stool examinations are desirable to establish the absence of amoebae and this should be repeated at least one month after completing treatment.

PREPARATIONS

Malaria

Schizontocidal agents
Amodiaquine hyd (Pasoquin) proph 400 mg/w, treatm 400–600 mg/d for 3 d p.o.
Chloroquine phosph (Resochin) proph 300 mg/w, treatm 600 mg then 300 mg to total 1.5 g p.o.
Chlorproguanil hyd (Lapudrine) proph 20 mg/w p.o.
Cycloguanil embonate (Camolar) proph 350 mg i.m.
Dapsone (for chloroq res falcip) Ch. 34
Mepacrine hyd (Quinacrine) 100 mg dl p.o. (giardiasis, obs for malaria)
Proguanil hyd (Chlorguanide, Paludrine) proph 100 mg dl p.o.
Pyrimethamine (Daraprim) proph 25 mg/w p.o.
Quinine sulph 650 mg every 8 h for 7 d p.o.
Sulfadoxine (Fanasil) 2 g then 1–1.5 g/w p.o. (for resist falcipar malar)

Causal prophylactic
Primaquine phosph 15 mg dl for 14 d

Amoebiasis

Luminal amoebicides
Carbarsone 250 mg 2–3x die for up to 10 d p.o. (toxic)
Diiodohydroxyquinoline (Diodoquin) 1–2 g for 20 d p.o.
Paromomycin (Humatin) 15–25 mg/d for 5–10 d p.o.

Amoebicidal by mod int flora
Tetracyclines Ch. 33

Tissue amoebicides
Chloroquine (see above)
Dehydroemetine dihyd
Emetine hyd 65 mg dl for 3-10 d i.m.
Universal amoebicide
Metronidazole (Flagyl) 500-750 mg 3x/d for 5-10 d

Trichomonas vaginalis infection
Metronidazole (see above)
Povidone iodine (Betadine) Ch. 38

FURTHER READING

Andersen H H, Hansen E L 1960 The chemotherapy of amoebiasis. Pharmac. Rev. 2: 399
Faust E C, Beaver P C, Jung R C 1975 Animal agents and vectors of human disease. Lea & Febiger, Philadelphia
Faust E C, Russell P F, Jung R C 1970 Clinical parasitology. Lea & Febiger, Philadelphia
Harrison Gordon 1978 Mosquitos, malaria and man. John Murray, London
Noble E R, Noble G A 1976 Parasitology. The biology of animal parasites. Lea & Febiger, Philadelphia
Peters W 1970 Chemotherapy and drug resistance in malaria. Academic Press, London
Piner R M 1973 Malaria. The design, use and mode of action of chemotherapeutic agents. Scientechnica, Bristol
Smith C E G (ed) 1972 Research in diseases of the tropics. Br. med. Bull. 28: 1
Thompson P E, Werbel L M 1972 Antimalarial agents. Chemistry and pharmacology. Academic Press, New York
W.H.O. Techn. Rep. 375 1967 Chloroquine resistance.

37. Anthelmintics

Types of worm infection 448; Action of anthelmintics 448; Tapeworm 448; Niclosamide 449; Dichlorophen 449; Mepacrine 449; Ascaris 449; Pyrantel 450; Piperazine 450; Trichuris 450; Mebendazole 451; Hookworm 451; Bephenium 451; Tetrachloroethylene 451; Enterobius 451; Viprynium 452; Strongyloides 452; Thiabendazole 452; Schistosomiasis 452; Antimonials 453; Niridazole 453; Lucanthone 453; Hycanthone 453; Oxamniquine 453; Metriphonate 453; Filariasis 454; Diethylcarbamazine 454; Suramin 454.

About half the human race is infected by worms of one species or another. In some cases these infections produce little injury to health, e.g. threadworms in children, but other infections, such as bilharziasis and hookworm disease, produce very serious dangers to health. In large areas of the world almost all the indigenous population is infected with these last mentioned parasites. The problem of the treatment of helminthiasis is, therefore, one of very great practical importance, although it is of much greater importance in tropical and subtropical than in temperate zones.

Infections with worms are of two types: those in which the worm lives in the alimentary canal, and those in which the worm lives in other tissues of the host,

The chief worms which infect the alimentary canal are:
Tapeworms (Cestodes): *Taenia saginata; Taenia solium; Hymenolepsis nana.*
Roundworms (Nematodes): *Ascaris lumbricoides; Enterobius vermicularis* (threadworm); *Trichuris trichiuria* (whipworm). *Strongyloides stercoralis. Necator americanus, Ancylo-stoma duodenale* (hookworms).

The chief worms which live in the tissues of the host are:
Schistosoma (Bilharzia). This is a trematode, or fluke, which is parasitic in man. The adult worm lives in the portal vein, and discharges ova which pass into the bladder and the gut and produce inflammation of these organs, with haematuria and loss of blood in the stools. Man is infected by penetration of the skin.

Filaria. The filariae are long thread-like nematodes. The adult worm lives in the lymphatics, connective tissues or mesentery of the host and produces live embryos or microfilariae which find their way into the blood stream where they may live for a long time without developing further. The chief filarial diseases are filariasis due to *Wuchereria* and *Brugia* which cause obstruction of lymphatic vessels producing elephantiasis; other related diseases are onchocerciasis, loiasis and dracontiasis.

Actions of anthelmintics
A large number of drugs have been shown to have an action on worms. To be an effective anthelmintic, a drug must have a deleterious action on the tissues of the worm and must be able to penetrate the cuticle or gain access to the alimentary tract of the worm.

An anthelmintic drug may act by causing narcosis or paralysis of worms, which may be temporary or permanent. Alternatively it may injure the cuticle leading to partial digestion of the worm. Anthelmintic drugs may also interfere with the metabolism of the worm and since the metabolic requirements of these parasites vary greatly from one species to another, this may be the reason why drugs which are highly effective against one type of worm are ineffective against others.

The effect of a drug may be observed after direct contact of the drug and the worm. Baldwin investigated the paralytic action of drugs on the neuromuscular apparatus of worms by using the isolated anterior fragments of ascaris. This method gives results which are specific for anthelmintic activity against ascaris. The test cannot be carried out on other species because ascaris has a cuticle of highly selective permeability, whereas earthworm and leech preparations of the kind previously employed for anthelmintic tests possess nothing analogous to the cuticular barrier present in ascaris.

A general criticism of *in vitro* tests is that they do not take into account the possibility that the action of the drug *in vivo* may depend upon its conversion by the host into a more active compound. Conversely a drug which is active by *in vitro* tests, may be inactivated by secretions in the alimentary tract of the host. For these reasons anthelmintic drugs are usually tested by measuring their ability to eliminate worms from infected animals. The clinical evaluation of drugs in intestinal helminth infections is usually based on the effect of the drug in reducing the number of eggs or worms in the stools. Control observations are concurrently made on untreated patients in order to take into account the occurrence of spontaneous cures.

TAPEWORM INFECTIONS

Tapeworms are segmented flat worms with a small head (scolex), a neck and a large number of segments (proglottids). The head of the parasite attaches itself to the small intestine of the host, whilst the proglottids carry out reproductive and nutritional functions. The proglottids can be regenerated from the head and neck, hence, to be effective, anthelmintic treatment must result in elimination of the head. The chief tapeworms infecting man are *Taenia saginata* present in 'measly beef' and *T. solium* which may occur in undercooked pork,

Diphyllobothrium latum (fish tapeworm) and *Hymenolepsis nana* (dwarf tapeworm). Although *T. saginata* may grow to a length of over 30 ft it cannot propagate in man because its fertilised eggs cannot form larvae except in the gastrointestinal tract of cattle. By contrast *T. solium* can propagate in man and the larvae which are hatched in the gastrointestinal tract are carried in the blood stream to the brain and muscles, where they become encysted and produce the condition of cysticercosis. Although cysticercosis is usually acquired by the ingestion of the eggs of *T. solium*, it is also possible that eggs may be released by an adult tapeworm into the small intestine. For this reason drugs that are prone to cause vomiting are undesirable for treating *T. solium* infection.

After any form of treatment for the removal of a tapeworm, the faeces must be examined carefully to see if the head of the worm has been passed. Large portions of the worm are certain to be passed, and indeed this effect may be produced by purgation alone without any form of specific treatment. Unless the head has been dislodged, no real benefit has been produced, because the worm will grow again rapidly if the head is left in position.

The anthelmintics chiefly used against tapeworms are niclosamide, dichlorophen and mepacrine.

Niclosamide (Yomesan)
This compound is active against most types of tapeworm including the dwarf tapeworm, *Hymenolepsis nana*, which is relatively refractory to other taenicidal drugs. Niclosamine is believed to act by inhibiting oxidative phosphorylation in cestode mitochondria. The scolex and proximal segments are killed by contact with the drug; the scolex separates from the intestinal wall and is evacuated. Since the dead worm is digested within the intestine, neither the scolex nor the proglottids can be identified in the stool, even after purging.

Niclosamide

Niclosamide is prepared as sweetened and flavoured tablets which are intended to be chewed before swallowing. No prior preparation or purgation of the patient is required. The drug is poorly absorbed from the gastrointestinal tract and is administered in a dose of 2 g on each of two successive days. Niclosamide is remarkably free from undesirable side effects other than occasional gastrointestinal upsets. Because of its high curative efficiency in tapeworm infections it is at present considered to be the drug of choice in these conditions.

Dichlorophen (Anthiphen)
This compound has been extensively used as a taenicide in dogs and more recently for the treatment of tapeworm infection in man. The drug is directly lethal to the worm, the segments of which are partially digested in the intestine. This may make it difficult to identify the passage of the scolex in the stools.

Dichlorophen can be administered without prior starvation or purging and is given by mouth before breakfast in a dose of 6 g on each of two successive days. It may cause nausea and intestinal colic. In *T. solium* infection the ova released from the segments may be regurgitated into the stomach and give rise to cysticercosis. This slight risk is lessened if a laxative is given after treatment to clear the colon.

Mepacrine
This antimalarial drug (Fig. 36.2) is an effective taenicide which is useful if it is desired to obtain the worm intact. The patient is starved for 48 hours and a duodenal tube is passed the night before treatment. A solution of the drug (1 g for an adult) is given through the tube, followed by 30 g magnesium sulphate in solution; the tube is then withdrawn. Purgation takes place within 2 hours and the worm is usually passed whole. In *T. solium* infestation mepacrine is preferred to dichlorophen or niclosamide which digest the segments and may thus liberate the eggs with the danger of causing cysticercosis.

Common side effects of a large dose of mepacrine are nausea, abdominal pain and gastrointestinal disturbances.

Paromomycin (Humatin)
This orally administered, broad spectrum antibiotic introduced for the treatment of intestinal amoebiasis (p. 446) has been found effective in *H. nana* infections.

Male fern (filix mas) is an effective anthelmintic for the expulsion of tapeworms but is now seldom used because of its toxic effects which may include amblyopia.

NEMATODES

Ascariasis
It has been estimated that over 600 million human beings are infected by *Ascaris lumbricoides*. Infection occurs by eating food, usually uncooked vegetables, contaminated with the eggs of the parasite from human faeces. The larvae hatch from the eggs in the small intestine and the adult worm reaches a length of 15 to 30 cm. The worms are not attached to the intestinal mucosa but tend to obstruct the lumen of the intestine (Fig. 36.1). The larvae may also enter the portal circulation and be carried to the lungs where they may cause pneumonitis.

A variety of drugs has been used in the past for the treatment of ascariasis including the toxic substances

450 APPLIED PHARMACOLOGY

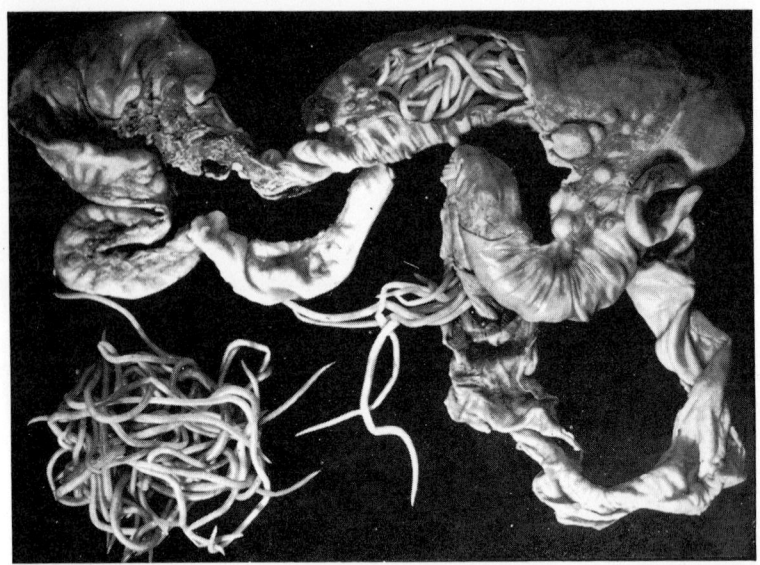

Fig. 37.1 Intestinal obstruction due to ascariasis. (From Manson Bahr, *Tropical Diseases*. Baillière, Tindall & Cassell, London, orig. from Cioni & Palazzi, *Atlas Path. Anat.*, Ambrosiana, Milano.)

santonin, oil of chenopodium and hexylresorcinol. These have now been superseded by the highly effective drug pyrantel pamoate or by treatment with piperazine which is safe and efficient.

Pyrantel pamoate
This is a new anthelmintic effective against roundworms (*Ascaris*), threadworms (*Enterobius*) and hookworms (*Ancylostoma*). It acts through neuromuscular blockade and subsequent immobilisation of *Ascaris*, which is then dislodged by peristaltic activity. The usual oral dose for *Ascaris* is the equivalent of 10 mg/kg body weight pyrantel to a maximum of 1 g. A single dose produces almost 100 per cent cure. It is well tolerated, on the whole, although it may produce some nausea, diarrhoea and drowsiness. Fasting before treatment is not necessary.

Piperazine (Antepar)
This drug is highly effective in the treatment of ascaris and threadworm infections. It is a basic compound and is used in the more stable form of one of its salts.

Piperazine (base)

The clinical effectiveness of piperazine in ascaris and threadworm infections was first reported in France. When its effect is tested on the movements of isolated ascarids suspended in Tyrode solution, it produces a slow paralysis of movement in the course of several hours (Fig. 37.2). When the drug is administered to a patient, paralysis of the worm leads to its expulsion. The paralysis is reversible and when ascarids thus expelled are placed in a piperazine-free medium they eventually recover their motility. Piperazine interferes with the metabolism of ascarids and it has been shown that it inhibits the formation of succinate.

Administration. Piperazine citrate 75 mg/kg will clear ascarids from 75 per cent of patients; this dose can be repeated the following day.

Adverse reactions. Piperazine is one of the safest anthelmintics known and may be used for the individual or mass treatment of ascariasis. Mild drug reactions include nausea, vomiting, abdominal discomfort and diarrhoea. Allergic reactions are occasionally seen and the drug should not be used in cases of liver disease or epilepsy.

Whipworm infections
The whipworm, *Trichuris trichiura*, is a common cause of intestinal infection in the tropics and a frequent cause of eosinophilia. It may also occur in temperate climates.

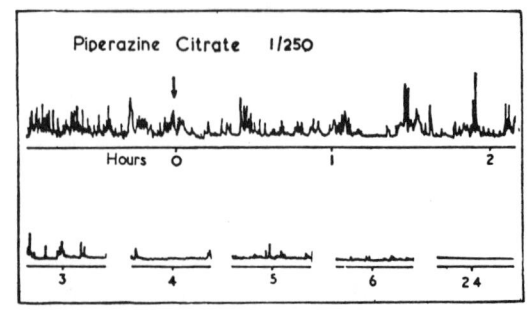

Fig. 37.2 Effect of piperazine citrate on *Ascaris lumbricoides* suspended in a bath of Tyrode solution. Piperazine caused a gradual decrease in activity. (After Goodwin, 1958. *Br. J. Pharmacol.*)

The worm is 3 to 5 cm long and lives embedded in the mucous membrane of the caecum; it may cause diarrhoea, blood-streaked stools and anaemia.

There are few satisfactory drugs at present available for the treatment of trichuriasis. Certain benzimidazole compounds are relatively effective.

Mebendazole. At a dose of 100 mg twice daily for 4 days, approximately two-thirds of whipworm infections will be cured; the remainder will exhibit a reduction in the egg count. The closely related drug *thiabendazole* is moderately effective but prone to produce a variety of unpleasant side effects.

Dichlorvos (Fig. 39.3, p. 468) is an organophosphorus insecticide of short persistence which has high activity in trichuris infestation.

Hookworm infections

Hookworm infection by *Ancylostoma duodenale* or *Necator americanus* is one of the most widespread causes of ill-health and it is estimated that about 500 million people are affected by the parasites. The infection is usually acquired through the skin; it is frequently acquired by plantation workers who tread barefooted in soil which is contaminated with human faeces. The larvae penetrate the skin, enter the circulation and finally reach the small intestine where they are attached to the mucosa and grow into adult worms of about 1 cm in length. The worms may cause severe anaemia by sucking blood from the intestinal villi.

Hookworm infections. Hookworm infection by *Ancylostoma duodenale* or *Necator americanus* is one of the most widespread causes of ill-health. The infection may cause persistent blood loss in women and children. The infection is usually acquired through the skin; it is frequently acquired by plantation workers who tread barefooted in soil which is contaminated with human faeces. The larvae penetrate the skin, enter the circulation and finally reach the small intestine where they are attached to the mucosa and grow into adult worms of about 1 cm in length. The worms may cause severe anaemia by sucking blood from the intestinal villi.

Hookworm infestation is present throughout hot and humid areas lying between latitudes 30° and 35°. Originally *Necator americanus* was confined to the New World and *Ancylostoma duodenale* to the Old World but this distinction has now ceased. The only important host of both parasites is man. Infection is due to insanitary conditions and indiscriminate defaecation.

Treatment

Anti-hookworm campaigns involve the treatment of tens of thousands of individuals and the choice of drug used depends on the efficiency, toxicity, ease of administration and cost of the preparation. Thymol was at one time extensively used but was replaced to some extent by carbon tetrachloride and later by tetrachloroethylene which is as effective but less toxic than carbon tetrachloride. At present the two principal drugs used to treat hookworm infections are pyrantel pamoate and bephenium hydroxynaphthoate.

Pyrantel pamoate

This drug is effective against *A. duodenale* and *N. americanus*. Three consecutive daily doses of 10 mg/kg are generally more effective than a single dose. Pyrantel is given orally as a suspension of the pamoate or embonate. Side effects include nausea and vomiting, abdominal pain and drowsiness.

Bephenium hydroxynaphthoate (Alcopar)

This is a sparingly soluble compound with a bitter taste. It has high activity against both human hookworms. *A. duodenale* and *N. americanus*, particularly against the former. It is also effective in ascariasis.

In man the optimal dose is 5 g bephenium hydroxynaphthoate containing 2.5 g of the base. Half this dose may be given to children. In severe infections daily treatment for several days may be necessary. More cures are effected against *A. duodenale* with one or two doses than against *N. americanus*.

The drug is remarkably non-toxic and may be given to the debilitated or very young, where tetrachloroethylene is contraindicated. Bephenium is administered by mouth on an empty stomach as a granular suspension in water or syrup. Owing to its bitter taste it may cause nausea.

Tetrachloroethylene (C_2Cl_4) was introduced as an anthelmintic in 1925. Its mode of action on hookworms has not been elucidated and when the parasites are expelled after treatment with tetrachloroethylene they maintain their motility. It is more active against *N. americanus* than against *A. duodenale* and is inactive against *Ascaris*.

Tetrachloroethylene is usually administered in the early morning after purgation on the preceding evening. The dose is 0.1 ml/kg up to a maximum total dose of 4 to 5 ml. A single dose of trichlorethylene has a low cure rate in hookworm disease, but repeated treatment at short intervals is effective.

Mebendazole is a broad spectrum anthelmintic which is effective against hookworm. It has a high cure rate after multiple administration and low toxicity; it is useful in treating mixed worm infections.

Threadworm infections

The threadworm or pinworm *Enterobius vermicularis* is about 1 cm long and inhabits the lumen of the large intestine without being attached to the intestinal wall. The female worm migrates to the perianal area where its eggs are deposited. The emergence of the gravid female worms from the anus on to the surrounding skin causes irritation. Scratching may result in severe dermatitis. The eggs are sticky and adhere to skin and clothing and in this way they form a reservoir for reinfection and spread of infection. Within a few days each fertile egg develops and if swallowed matures to an adult worm. This infection is the most prevalent form of worm infection in Great Britain and it occurs especially in children.

Concurrently with drug therapy, strict hygienic precautions are necessary to prevent reinfection of the patient by transfer of eggs to the mouth. Gloves should be worn at night-time and the anus should be smeared with a bland ointment or cream to diminish scratching.

A number of drugs including gentian violet, phenothiazine and diphenan have been used with varying success in the treatment of this infection. These drugs have now been largely replaced by more effective newer drugs. The aim has been to produce a high cure rate with the least untoward effects following if possible a single dose or very few doses. Mebendazole and pyrantel pamoate are usually effective after a single application. Viprynium embonate also produces cure rates approaching 100 per cent but must be given in two doses one week apart to be fully effective and has the disadvantage of staining the stool red. Piperazine is highly effective but requires a seven-day course for optimal action. Thiabendazole may be used but untoward effects occur relatively frequently.

Pyrantel. The embonate or pamoate are effective against *Enterobius*. Only a small proportion of a dose is absorbed from the gastrointestinal tract. A single dose of 10 mg/kg by mouth is curative in most children, with minimal side effects.

Mebendazole (Niclosamide). This drug is effective against threadworm (*Enterobius*). A single dose of 75 mg in children and 100 mg in adults is usually enough to eradicate the worm. Mebendazole is not significantly absorbed. Tablets must be chewed thoroughly before swallowing and washed down with a little water. The patient should abstain from solid food on the evening before treatment. Side effects are minimal.

Viprynium (Vanquin). This drug produces a high cure rate in threadworm infections. It should be given in two doses one week apart. The drug stains stools bright red and may stain clothing if vomited.

Piperazine salts are effective in threadworm infections. A course of treatment is continued for a week with doses ranging from 250 mg twice daily for children aged 1 year to 1 g twice daily for those over 13 years.

Strongyloides infections
Infection with *Strongyloides stercoralis* often occurs in association with other worm infections and is a common finding in stool examinations. *Strongyloides* infection is a potentially serious complaint which is common in parts of China, South East Asia, South America and Africa. Since eggs are seldom seen in faecal samples, diagnosis depends essentially on identification of the characteristic larvae of this parasite resembling those of the hookworm, for which various techniques have been devised. Of the various types of drugs which have been used for the treatment of mixed worm infections, thiabendazole has so far been shown to be most effective against *Strongyloides* infection.

Thiabendazole
This benzimidazole compound (Mintezol) has a wide range of anthelmintic activity in man and in domestic animals. In man it is particularly active against *Strongyloides*, but is also active against threadworm, hookworm and ascaris.

During the past ten years a number of clinical trials with thiabendazole have been reported from various countries including India, Iraq and Costa Rica. In general these relate to the treatment of mixed worm infections but the evidence suggests that this compound has been more effective than other drugs in reducing the prevalence of *Strongyloides* infection.

The recommended dose is 25 mg/kg twice daily for 2 days. Side effects are frequent but are usually mild and transient; they include anorexia, nausea, vomiting, vertigo and drowsiness.

Since about 90 per cent of a single oral dose of thiabendazole is excreted in the urine, partly as metabolites, due caution should be exercised in the treatment of patients with concurrent liver or renal disease.

SCHISTOSOMIASIS

Schistosomiasis or bilharziasis is a widespread and serious infection caused by three species of blood flukes, *Schistosoma haematobium, S. mansoni* and *S. japonicum*. Man becomes infected by exposure of the skin to water containing the larvae which are harboured by snails which act as intermediate hosts. The adult worm lives in the portal and mesenteric veins and produces eggs which pass out through the mucosa of the bladder and intestine and cause bleeding and inflammation of these tissues. The adults exist as males and females, the body of the male being rolled ventrally to form a kind of canal in which the thinner body of the female is enveloped (Fig. 37.3). The eggs of *S. haematobium* are excreted mainly in the urine whilst those of *S. mansoni* and *S. japonicum* are excreted in the faeces. Attempt to cure the disease have involved the use of many drugs.

The ideal objective of treating schistosomiasis is to eradicate the infection and so produce a cure, as a result of which all worms are destroyed and the laying of eggs permanently ceases. In practice it has been found that cure in this sense is difficult to achieve except in relatively light infections. It is usual therefore to define the action of a drug in terms of percentage reduction of egg excretion. Defined in this way, successful treatment can be obtained

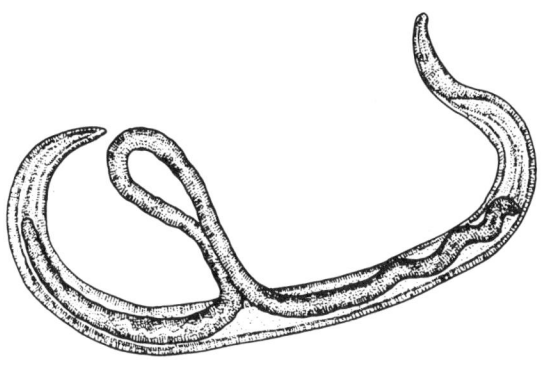

Schistosoma mansoni (blood fluke) copulating

Fig. 37.3 *Schistosoma mansoni* (blood fluke) copulating (after Philip Street. *Animal Partners and Parasites.*) Academic Press, London.

with various trivalent antimonial compounds and certain synthetic drugs such as niridazole and lucanthone.

Trivalent antimonials
Mode of action. The mode of action of trivalent antimonial compounds in schistosomiasis has been studied by Bueding who concluded that they produce their effects by inhibiting in the parasite the action of the enzyme phosphofructokinase which catalyses the phosphorylation of fructose monophosphate by adenosine triphosphate to fructose diphosphate and adenosine diphosphate according to the following reaction:

$$FMP + ATP \rightarrow FDP + ADP$$

Antimony sodium tartrate is toxic to the parasites of schisostomiasis. It inhibits their normal glucose metabolism and has been shown to cause *mansoni schistosomes* to migrate from the mesenteric veins into the liver where they are destroyed. It is given slowly intravenously and well diluted and great care must be taken to avoid leakage into the tissues which is followed by painful inflammation. It may produce severe side effects, nausea and vomiting. Despite these disadvantages antimony tartrate is still a widely used antischistosomal drug. It is used in treating infections caused by *S. japonicum*. It is not used to treat *S. mansoni* and *S. haematobium* infections because less toxic agents are effective.

Stibocaptate (antimony sodium dimercaptosuccinate) is regarded by many workers as a better and safer drug which has the advantage of being given, if desired, by the intramuscular route. It is used particularly against infection due to *Schistsoma haematobium*.

Stibophen is less toxic but also less effective than antimony sodium tartrate.

Other schistosomicidal drugs
Niridazole (Ambilhar). This nitrothiazole compound is particularly effective against infections due to *Schistosoma haematobium* but less so against *S. mansoni* and *S. japonicum*. It also has a strong amoebicidal action.

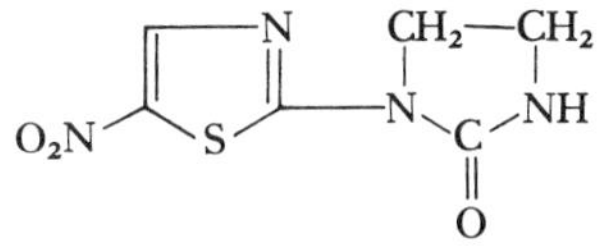

Niridazole

The mode of action of *niridazole* differs from that of the trivalent antimony compounds. It has a pronounced effect on the vitelline cells of female schistosomes which results in an arrest of egg shell formation and disappearance of most of the contents of the worm. In higher doses it also arrests spermatogenesis in the male worms.

When given by mouth the drug is well absorbed from the alimentary tract and is rapidly metabolised in the liver and mainly excreted by the kidneys. The metabolites colour the urine brown but have little schistosomicidal action.

Toxic effects of niridazole. The most common side effects are headache, anorexia, nausea and vomiting. Maculopapular and erythematous skin rashes have also been reported.

More serious toxic effects include mental depression, insomnia, nightmares and muscular tremors. These are usually associated with high concentrations of unchanged drug in the peripheral circulation, as a result of impairment of liver function and failure to metabolise the drug. Changes in e.c.g. pattern similar to those produced by trivalent antimony compounds have also been reported.

Lucanthone (Miracil D) is used in the treatment of schistosomiasis, especially *Schistosoma haematobium* infections. It is less effective against *S. mansoni* and of little value against *S. japonicum*. In *S. haematobium* infections it produces rapid clinical improvement with cessation of haematuria and disappearance of viable ova from the urine.

Lucanthone HCl may cause yellow discoloration of the skin and sclera. It should be used with caution in the presence of impaired renal function which may cause excessive blood concentrations of the drug. Nausea, vomiting and abdominal pains are common side effects.

Certain newer drugs are effective in single doses. They are invariably toxic and must be administered with care, but they have the great advantage that they can be used for the mass treatment of schistosomiasis. They include the following.

Hycanthone is related to lucanthone. It can be applied as a single intramuscular injection for the mass treatment of *S. haematobium* or *S. mansoni* infections.

Oxamniquine is a quinoline derivative active against *S. mansoni*. It is administered orally.

Metriphonate is an organophosphorus anticholinesterase active against *S. haematobium*.

FILARIASIS

This infection is produced by the parasitic roundworms, *Wuchereria* and *Brugia* in the lymphatics and by related species *Loa* and *Onchocerca* in the subcutaneous tissues. The adult filariae are long hair-like worms which are found coiled together in the larger lymphatic vessels. The female filariae give birth to embryos or microfilariae which escape from the lymphatics and appear in the peripheral blood. Filariasis is transmitted by several species of mosquitoes which become infected by sucking human blood containing microfilariae. The filarial infection is characterised by fever, lymphangitis and elephantiasis. Bancroftian and Malayan filariasis are both transmitted by mosquito vectors. The mosquito is more than a simple agent of transmission of the parasite; an essential developmental cycle take place within the body of the insect; measures directed against mosquitos and their larvae are therefore important in the control of the disease.

The effects of antifilarial drugs are usually tested on the cotton rat infected with filariasis.

Diethylcarbamazine (Hetrazan, Banocide)

This drug is a derivative of piperazine. Piperazine itself is ineffective in filariasis, but diethylcarbamazine is highly effective against the microfiliariae of *W. bancrofti* and *Loa loa*. The mode of action of diethylcarbamazine is not known, since whilst it rapidly removes the microfilariae from the circulating blood and also kills the adult worms, it has little action on microfilariae *in vitro*. It has been suggested that it modifies the parasite so that it becomes amenable to phagocytosis.

Diethylcarbamazine

In the treatment of filariasis due to *W. bancrofti* and *Loa loa* diethylcarbamazine citrate is administered by mouth. A report by WHO published in 1967 recommends a total dose of the citrate of 72 mg/kg given over a period of time. There is evidence that dosing once per month is more effective than dosing daily. This treatment will destroy most of the microfilariae and some of the adult worms, and it often reduces or completely stops the periodic attacks of fever and lymphangitis.

A course of treatment is usually continued for three to four weeks. The drug sometimes produces allergic reactions believed to be due to foreign proteins released from dead microfilariae; they include joint pains, swellings and rashes. These reactions are seldom severe enough to warrant discontinuing the drug.

Suramin (Antrypol)

This trypanocidal compound (p. 434) is the most effective agent in filarial infections due to *Onchocerca volvulus* (blinding filariasis); 0.5 to 1 g of suramin may be administered intravenously each week for seven weeks.

PREPARATIONS

Tapeworm
Niclosamide (Yomesan) 2x 1 g within 1 h
Mepacrine hyd (Quinacrine, Atabrine) 800 mg p.o., duod tube
Dichlorophen (Antiphen) 6 g (child 2–4 g)
Paromomycin Ch. 36

Roundworm, hookworm, threadworm, whipworm, strongyloidiasis

Ascaris
Pyrantel embonate (Antiminth) 11 mg/kg (max 1 g) p.o. single dose
Piperazine citr (or hydr) (Antepar) 3.5 g 1x dl on 2 consec days p.o.
Mebendazole q.v.
Thiabendazole q.v.
Viprinium Embonate q.v.
Bephenium hydroxynaphtoate q.v.

Hookworm (A. duodenale, N. americanus)
Bephenium hydroxynaphtoate (Alcopar) 5 g 2x die for 1–3 d p.o.
Pyrantel embonate q.v. for 3 consec days p.o.
Tetrachlorethylene 5 ml, no breakfast p.o.
Mebendazole q.v.

Threadworm (Enterobius)
Mebendazole (Vermox) 100 mg rep after week p.o.
Pyrantel embonate q.v.
Viprynium embonate (Vanquin) 350 mg (rep, stains) p.o.
Piperazine q.v.
Thiabendazole q.v.

Whipworm (Trichuris)
Mebendazole q.v. for 3–4 d

Strongyloides
Thiabendazole (Mintezol) 25 mg/kg 2x die for 1–2 d p.o.

Schistosomiasis
Hycanthone mesyl (Etrenol) 3mk/kg i.m. S. haemat, mans
Lucanthone hyd (MiracilD, Nilodin) 0.5–1g 2x die for 3 d p.o. S. heamat
Metriphonate 7.5mg/kg 1–3x p.o. S. haemat
Niridazole (Ambilhar) 25 mg/kg for 5–7 d, (S. haematobium) (also guinea worm) p.o.
Stibophen (Fuadin) (S. haematobium, S. mansoni) i.m.
Stibocaptate (Astiban) (S. haematobium, S. mansoni) i.m.
Antimony potassium tartrate (S. japonicum) very slow i.v.
Oxamniquine 7.5 mg/kg (S. mansoni) i.m.

Filariasis
Diethylcarbamazine citr 2 mg/kg 3x die for 7–21 days
Suramin Ch. 35 (onchocerciasis)

FURTHER READING

Bueding E, Schwartzfelder C 1957 Anthelmintics. Pharmacol. Rev. 9: 329

Davis A 1973 Drug treatment in intestinal helminthiases. World Health Organisation, Geneva

Gelfand M 1967 A clinical study of intestinal bilharziasis (*Schistosoma mansoni*) in Africa. Edward Arnold, London

Mansour T E 1964 The pharmacology and biochemistry of parasitic helminths. Advances in Pharmacology 3: 129

World Health Organisation Geneva 1965 Snail control in the prevention of bilharziasis. Monogr. 50

38. Disinfectants

Methods of disinfection 456; Phenol coefficient 456; Heat and irradiation 458; Detergents 458; Peroxides 458; Chlorine 458; Iodine 459; Silver 459; Boric acid 459; Organic disinfectants 459; Phenol 460; Acridines 460; Hexachlorophane 462; Chlorhexidine 462; Iodophors 462.

An enormous number of chemical substances can either kill or inhibit the growth of micro-organisms, and since the destruction of micro-organisms is required under many different conditions, it follows that a large number of agents are used as disinfectants.

The terms 'germicide' and 'disinfectant' are applied to substances which kill micro-organisms, while the term 'bacteriostatic' is applied to substances which inhibit the growth of micro-organisms but do not kill them. Surgical antiseptics are drugs which are applied locally to tissues to prevent or treat infection of tissues.

The number of disinfectants and antiseptics used is large, because there is no such thing as an allround ideal disinfectant. The properties required vary widely according to the manner in which the drug is intended to be used. The intensity and speed with which a drug kills bacteria can be measured in a test tube, and this information is of great value for determining, for example, the relative efficiency of disinfectants when applied to inorganic material. Such measurements give little indication of the relative values of disinfectants when applied to living tissues, because in this case the important problem is to find a substance that will kill or at least prevent the multiplication of bacteria without injuring the surrounding tissues. Indeed, some of the best antiseptics for the treatment of wounds are substances which have a relatively feeble and slow action *in vitro*.

The following is a list of the more important agents used for disinfection.

Physical methods

1. Heat, e.g. superheated steam in autoclaves.
2. Irradiation, e.g. sunlight and ultraviolet light.
3. Ultrasonic waves.
4. Osmotic pressure, e.g. concentrated solutions of salt and sugar to preserve foods.
5. Surface active agents, e.g. soaps and detergents.

Chemical methods

A Inorganic substances
 1. Oxidising agents and inorganic halogen compounds, e.g. hydrogen peroxide, potassium permanganate, hypochlorites and iodine.
 2. Heavy metals, e.g. mercury, silver.
B Organic substances
 3. Alcohol, formaldehyde, phenol and simple aromatic compounds, e.g. cresol and the organic halogenated compounds, povidone-iodine, chlorhexidine and hexachlorophane.
 4. Complex synthetic drugs, e.g. acridines.

The limits of this chapter prevent the consideration of all of the agents mentioned above. The action of some of the disinfectants of chief importance in medicine and surgery will be described. The chief agents used for the destruction of bacteria, spirochaetes, trypanosomes and protozoa within the body are described in other chapters.

Phenol-coefficient test

The activity of a disinfectant can be estimated either by the Rideal-Walker method or by some modification of this method. The essential point of these methods is that the disinfectant action of the drug is compared with the disinfectant action exerted by phenol under precisely similar conditions. The minimal concentration of phenol which will kill a micro-organism in a certain length of time, under a certain set of conditions, is first determined and then the concentration of the disinfectant of unknown potency which will produce the same effect under the same conditions is determined. The concentration of phenol thus obtained, divided by the concentration of the unknown disinfectant, gives a figure which is known as the phenol coefficient of the disinfectant tested.

The determination of the phenol coefficient of drugs is carried out under experimental conditions which are far simpler than those which occur in most pharmacological experiments, and it is of interest to note that the accurate determination of a phenol coefficient is a matter of considerable difficulty, and that quite small variations in technique may produce large variations in the result obtained. Chick and Martin studied the possible sources of error in determining the phenol coefficient, and found that in order to get accurate results it was necessary to keep all the conditions of the experiment absolutely constant. They showed that the activity of a disinfectant was modified by the following factors: (1) the temperature, (2) the length of time for which the disinfectant was allowed to act, (3) the species of bacteria upon which the test was performed, (4) the quantity of organisms used, (5) the nature of the culture medium, and (6) the presence of other organic material.

They found that different disinfectants were influenced in different degrees by the variation of any of these factors.

Alterations of temperature produced different effects with different drugs; for example, the velocity of action of mercuric chloride was increased threefold by a rise of temperature of 10°C, but the velocity of action of phenol was increased sevenfold by the same rise of temperature.

The length of time for which the drug was allowed to act was of very great importance, for the phenol coefficient of mercuric chloride was only 13.6 when the time allowed was 2½ minutes, but rose to 550 when the time was increased to 30 minutes.

The time required by the drug to produce its action is of great practical importance, and unless it is known, the phenol coefficient gives very little information. Such substances as the colloidal metals, which cannot produce a rapid action, and substances like the acridines, which only produce a rapid action in very high concentrations, appear to be almost devoid of disinfectant action when tested over a short period, and yet may be found to have a powerful action when tested over a longer period.

The species of bacteria on which the drugs are tested is naturally of great importance, since many drugs have a strong selective action upon certain micro-organisms. Chick and Martin found that the phenol coefficient of a coal-tar disinfectant was 4.5 when the test organism was *Staphylococcus aureus*, but rose to 40 when *B. pestis* was used. In the case of the more complex and powerful disinfectants an intense selective action is often observed, and even greater specificity is usually found in the natural antibacterial substances obtained from micro-organisms.

The presence of organic matter has only a slight effect upon the action of some drugs, but greatly reduces the action of others. The addition of 10 per cent of serum only reduces the activity of phenol by 10 per cent, but reduces the efficiency of mercuric chloride by 90 per cent.

The manner in which a weak disinfectant kills a population of bacteria is shown in Figure 38.1. The curve shows that a nearly equal proportion of the spores is killed in each equal interval of time, and hence a long time is needed for complete sterilisation even though the majority of the organisms are killed rapidly.

Destruction of bacterial spores
The action of disinfectants usually only refers to their action on the free living forms, and it must be remembered that bacterial spores possess amazing powers of resistance. For example, the spores of *B. tetani* survive for more than 10 days in the following solutions: ethyl alcohol (70 per cent), phenol (5 per cent), undiluted lysol, acriflavine (1 per cent) and perchloride of mercury (0.1 per cent). These spores are, however, killed in a few hours by hypochlorous acid (0.25 per cent), and iodine (1 per cent in 2 per cent KI), and they are killed in a few minutes by iodine trichloride (1 per cent). Formaldehyde in concentrations of 0.5 to 2.5 per cent will kill bacterial spores in about six hours.

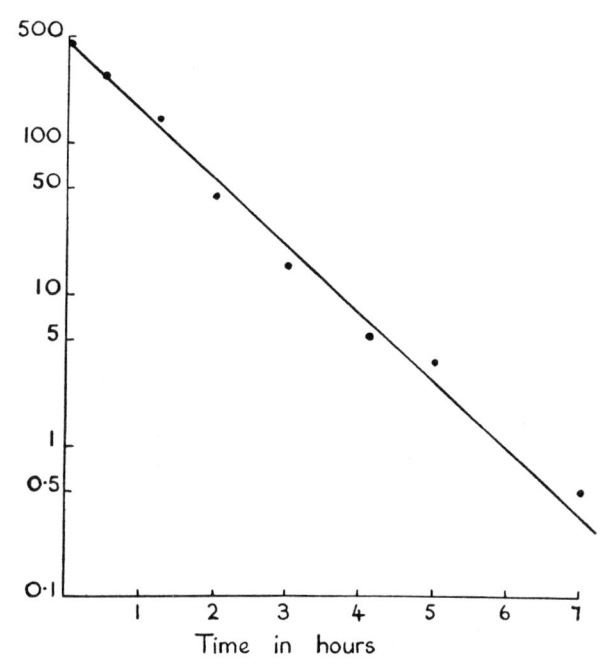

Fig. 38.1 Destruction of the anthrax spores by 5 per cent phenol at 33°C. The figures, representing the average number of surviving spores, are plotted on a logarithmic scale. Since the points lie on an approximately straight line it follows that a constant proportion of bacteria is killed in each equal interval of time. (After Chick, 1908. *J. Hygiene.*)

These results suggest that the ability of chemicals to destroy spores depends entirely on their power of penetration, and that very few chemicals can penetrate the surface membranes of the spores.

Tests of antiseptic activity. When it is desired to sterilise non-living material it is essential to produce complete sterilisation because if any bacteria are left alive they will multiply rapidly. The conditions are different in the case of living tissues because these possess considerable powers of resistance to bacterial invasion and the object of using antiseptics is to assist the natural defence mechanisms by checking the growth of bacteria rather than to attempt complete sterilisation. The important problem is to find drugs that will injure the bacteria without impairing the natural defence mechanisms.

In addition to the standard phenol-coefficient test a number of other methods are used to assess antiseptic activity. These tests are based on the effect of the drug in reducing the number of visible organisms rather than their complete eradication. They are generally designed to resemble as nearly as possible the actual conditions in which the antiseptic will be used. For example, one method consists in applying different concentrations of the drug to small marked areas of the skin. After an interval of time the areas are infected with a culture of *Staphylococcus aureus* and ten minutes later the presence of surviving organisms is assessed by swabbing and plating. Another method consists of washing the hands for a measured time with a dilution of the antiseptic then rinsing the hands in sterile water, which is subsequently plated to assess the surviving organisms.

Heat and irradiation

An organism may be considered dead when it has lost the power to reproduce. It is probable that a single quantum of ultraviolet rays, if absorbed at a specific location in the cell, destroys the capacity of the cell to reproduce. Sunlight is a powerful disinfectant. This property is due almost entirely to the ultraviolet radiations. Light of a wavelength more than 3500 A has little or no bactericidal effect, and the disinfectant action increases as the wavelength is decreased. The action of radiations of a wave-length of less than 2900 A is considerably greater than the action of radiations lying between 3000 and 3500 A.

Dry heat has a relatively feeble lethal action on bacteria, but moist heat has a powerful disinfectant action. This is due to the fact that the cause of death is different in the two cases. Death by dry heat is primarily an oxidation process, whilst death by moist heat is due to the coagulation of proteins. Most bacteria are killed almost instantaneously by exposure to moist heat at 100°C. Moist heat is the method of sterilisation usually employed for disinfection of instruments, surgical dressings and clothing. It is also used to sterilise many medicinal preparations for parenteral administration and for local application to traumatised tissues. The most effective agent is steam under pressure; this has great penetrative power.

Surface active agents

Soaps

Soaps are bactericidal to some organisms, and comparatively inert towards others; the action varies according to the type of soap used. For example, pneumococci are rapidly killed by soaps of the unsaturated fatty acids, whilst most of the pathogenic intestinal organisms are killed by soaps of the saturated fatty acids. Washing hands with a stiff lather of soap will destory many pathogenic micro-organisms, but *Staphylococcus aureus* is not affected. Hence, washing with soap alone cannot be relied upon to produce an efficient sterilisation of skin (p. 461).

Detergents

Long-chain molecules possessing a hydrophilic polar group and a hydrophobic non-polar group accumulate at interfaces and lower the surface tension. They can therefore be used as cleansing agents or detergents. The detergents are usually classified as anionic, cationic or amphoteric detergents, according to the charge on the hydrophilic portion of the molecule.

Cationic detergents, or inverted soaps were introduced by Domagk in 1935. He described *benzalkonium* (zephiran), which is a mixture of alkylammonium chlorides. Other cationic detergents are *cetyltrimethylammonium bromide* (cetrimide, cetavlon), *benzethonium chloride* (phemerol chloride) and *domiphen bromide* (bradosol). The main chemical feature of these compounds is that they are substituted quaternary ammonium derivatives containing a long non-polar side chain of about 16 carbon atoms. Owing to their positive charge they are incompatible with soaps or with anionic detergents.

The cationic detergents have a strong and rapid bacteriostatic action, especially in alkaline solution; their antibacterial activity is, however, greatly decreased by organic matter. For this reason they can only be used for skin sterilisation after gross organic matter has been removed by a preceding wash. It is generally agreed that complete skin sterilisation cannot be achieved in practice since the micro-organisms which are deeply situated in the crevices of the skin, in the hair follicles and sebaceous glands cannot be eradicated without producing severe tissue damage. The cationic detergents, however, penetrate deeply and produce an effective superficial sterilisation of skin which lasts for an hour or two. They have the further advantage that they are non-irritant, do not stain or crack the skin, and have very little smell or taste.

Inorganic agents

Potassium permanganate ($KMnO_4$)

This compound readily yields oxygen and is an effective disinfectant. It is irritant to mucosae and usually is employed in concentrations of less than 1 per 1000. It can oxidise and destroy organic poisons and has been used for gastric lavage in drug poisoning.

Hydrogen peroxide (H_2O_2)

This is generally used as a 3 or 6 per cent solution of H_2O_2 in water and yields 10 to 20 times respectively its volume of oxygen. The solution rapidly yields oxygen when it comes in contact with pus, or any organic matter containing catalase, and the nascent oxygen has a mild disinfectant action. The evolution of gas has a valuable mechanical cleaning effect, for it loosens pus or other organic matter. The solution is used extensively to clean septic wounds, to wash cavities that are difficult of access, and to loosen wax in ears.

Chlorine

Chlorine has a powerful bactericidal action. Chlorine gas is used to disinfect public water supplies. On a smaller scale the use of chlorine compounds is more convenient and sodium hypochlorite or chloramine may be used. For use in small swimming pools, *sodium hypochlorite* should be added daily to maintain a residual available chlorine concentration of 0.25 to 1 ppm. *Chloramine* (Chloramine-T) powder contains about 25 per cent chlorine. It is used as a wound disinfectant and a general surgical antiseptic.

The action of all the chlorine compounds is a simple chemical reaction; the available chlorine rapidly combines with all forms of protein and thus kills any micro-organisms with which it comes into contact, but when excess of protein is present all available chlorine is exhausted rapidly and the chlorine ceases to have any disinfectant or antiseptic action.

Iodine

Iodine precipitates proteins and has a strong disinfectant and irritant action. The use of iodine to prepare the skin for operations was introduced by Grossich in 1908. A 2 per cent solution of iodine in 70 per cent alcohol is a most efficient and rapidly acting skin disinfectant. The main drawback of iodine is its irritant action, especially when brought in contact with wound edges.

Alcohol (70 per cent) is, by itself, an efficient disinfectant capable of destroying most of the skin bacteria. Absolute alcohol is less bactericidal than 70 to 80 per cent alcohol, but since the skin is always moist, all concentrations above 70 per cent alcohol are highly bactericidal.

Silver compounds

Most of the heavy metals have some disinfectant action, but silver is the only other heavy metal much used in medicine for this purpose. Silver salts have about one-half the disinfectant activity of mercury salts, but they suffer from the great disadvantage that silver chloride is insoluble, and therefore all silver salts are precipitated as soon as they come in contact with any secretion of the body or with any tissue. The antiseptic action and the irritant properties of silver preparations are due to the presence of free silver ions.

Silver nitrate, when brought in contact with living tissue, coagulates proteins and forms a film of silver albuminate, which becomes black owing to reduction of the silver. Concentrated solutions of silver nitrate are caustic and can be used to remove warts; dilute solutions have an astringent action. An instillation of 1 per cent silver nitrate into the eyes of the new-born baby has been used for many years as a prophylactic against *ophthalmia neonatorum* caused by *gonococcal* infection during childbirth, but has now been largely replaced by silver proteinates. For application to mucous membranes, silver nitrate has the double disadvantage of being irritant, and of being precipitated by the chlorides in the secretions of mucous membranes, and the same objections apply to all silver preparations containing free silver ions.

There are various types of silver preparations which are relatively non-irritant because the greater part of the silver is in a non-ionised form, and are used as disinfectants of the eye, nasopharynx and urethra.

Colloidal preparations. These consist of silver or silver oxide in a state of colloidal dispersion, combined with some protective colloid such as casein or albumin. Collargol is an example of this class. These preparations contain a very low proportion of free silver ions and therefore are non-irritant, but they have a correspondingly slow disinfectant action.

Silver proteinates. These are of two types: (1) The argyrol type, which contain about 25 per cent of silver, very little of which is ionised. These preparations are non-irritant, and do not give a precipitate with chlorides. (2) The protargol type which contain about 10 per cent of silver, and are more irritant and yield a precipitate with chlorides.

Boric Acid (H_3BO_3)

This is freely soluble in boiling water (1 in 3), but much less soluble in cold water (1 in 25). Boric acid lotion is a saturated watery solution. It is non-irritant and has a feeble bacteriostatic action, and it was formerly one of the most widely and frequently used lotions. Boric acid was also used as an antiseptic dusting powder.

Boric lint (40 per cent boric acid) is commonly used as a fomentation. Boric acid dissolves freely in glycerine, and lint soaked in hot boroglycerine is another form of fomentation. Poultice of kaolin contains equal parts of kaolin and glycerine and 4 per cent boric acid.

Boric acid may produce severe toxic effects when absorbed into the circulation and a number of cases of fatal poisoning have been reported. They were usually due to the application of ointments or powders containing over 10 per cent boric acid to denuded areas of skin in infants. Paediatricians consider that there is no thereaputic justification for the continued use of boric acid and borax in infants.

A concentration of about 0.3 per cent boric acid added to foodstuffs checks putrefaction, and in the past this substance was used extensively as a food preservative. Its use for this purpose is now prohibited.

Organic disinfectants

Formaldehyde (H.CHO)

The pharmacopoeial solution contains 34–38 per cent w/v in water. Formaldehyde is a powerful disinfectant, but has an equally strong action on the body tissues. It is used to kill and fix tissues for pathological examination.

Formaldehyde is used chiefly to disinfect inorganic material, and particularly for disinfecting rooms. For this purpose tablets of the solid paraformaldehyde $(CH_2O)_3$ are used. These when heated liberate formaldehyde, and 20 g are needed to disinfect 1000 cu. ft. room space. Formaldehyde can be removed by ammonia, for the two gases combine to form the inert solid hexamine.

Formaldehyde vapour is a powerful irritant of mucous membranes and produces a characteristic effect on the eyes and nose. Symptoms of poisoning by formaldehyde include severe abdominal pain with vomiting, anuria, depression of the central nervous system and coma.

In sufficient concentrations, formaldehyde is an effective germicide against all organisms and it can be used to preserve surgical instruments in a sterile condition and free from rust. For this purpose an aqueous solution containing 2.5 per cent formalin, 1.3 per cent borax and 0.4 per cent phenol is used.

Phenol ($C_6H_5.OH$)
Phenol or carbolic acid is of historical importance because it was the chief disinfectant used by Lister. The fact that it is a relatively feeble disinfectant and has no marked selective actions makes it convenient for use as a standard.

The activity of phenol is not greatly reduced by the presence of organic matter, for the addition of serum or faeces to a solution of phenol only reduces its activity by about 10 per cent; the presence of organic matter produces a much greater effect than this upon the action of most other disinfectants.

Phenol was the first drug to be used extensively as an antiseptic, but it is seldom used today because of the following disadvantages. It acts indifferently on all living cells and will not kill bacteria in concentrations below those which kill the body cells, hence, when applied to wounds it kills the tissues, and when applied to the hands it injures the skin. Furthermore, it is toxic when taken internally, and hence is unsuitable for distribution to the public as a disinfectant.

Cresols
The acids derived from coal-tar consist of a mixture of cresols, $CH_3C_6H_4OH$, together with a number of other phenol derivatives. These substances are used in the form of emulsions, made by mixing cresol, soap, and water. These coal-tar acids are the basis of the majority of commercial disinfectants, such as Lysol, Izal, etc. Halogenated derivatives of phenol and cresol have a toxicity similar to that of the parent substance, but increased disinfectant activity. Chlorocresol is a compound with bactericidal properties which is added in concentrations of 0.05 to 0.1 per cent to preserve the sterility of aqueous solutions of drugs intended for use as eyedrops or parenteral administration.

Toxic action of phenol and cresols
Large quantities of phenol are occasionally taken by mouth either by accident, or with suicidal intent. Concentrated solutions (70 per cent or more) produce typical white scars on the skin, and rapidly produce death by their corrosive action on the gastric mucosa. Dilute solutions (7 per cent or less), if taken in large quantities, may also produce rapid death which probably is due to local corrosion.

Carbolic acid lotion (5 per cent) when applied to the skin produces tingling and warmth, and this is followed by a sense of numbness. If such solutions are applied to the skin for long periods the drug gradually penetrates and may produce an extensive dry gangrene.

Phenol absorption causes darkening of the urine due to excretion of its oxidation products; it also may produce renal irritation, and cause the excretion of albumin and casts. The drug has a typical toxic action on the central nervous system. At first there is weakness and lethargy, accompanied by muscular tremors and, later, by convulsions; the pulse and respiration are increased in frequency, but later on collapse occurs; the temperature falls, the respiration becomes slow, irregular and weak, and finally death occurs from respiratory failure.

Acridines

These compounds strongly inhibit bacteria in the presence of tissue fluids and are relatively innocuous to tissues and leucocytes.

Proflavine (2:8-diaminoacridine) was introduced by Browning in 1913. It is generally agreed that a buffered isotonic solution of proflavine is non-irritant to tissues but there is some evidence that proflavine when applied as a powder to open wounds is irritant and may cause necrosis.

Aminacrine. A number of acridines have been prepared by Albert and his co-workers, including the non-staining compounds aminacrine (5-amino-acridine) and 1:methyl-5-aminoacridine and the coloured compound 1:9-diethyl proflavine which is five times more active than proflavine.

Albert concluded that in this group of compounds only the cation possesses antibacterial activity whilst the undissociated base is inactive. He suggested that the mode of action of these 'cationic antiseptics' is as follows. The acridine cation competes with hydrogen ions for an acidic receptor on the surface of the bacterial cell forming a weakly dissociated complex with it. Hence when the hydrogen ion concentration of the test medium is increased there must be a proportionate increase in acridine ion concentration for bacteriostasis to occur. This is illustrated in Figure 38.2. It follows from this hypothesis that only those acridines which are sufficiently strong bases to be appreciably ionised at a neutral pH are bacteriostatic. The action of acridines at the molecular level is based on intercalation of DNA as discussed on page 388.

The acridines have a high degree of activity against Gram-positive bacteria. Their main disadvantage is that high concentrations are required to exert a bactericidal

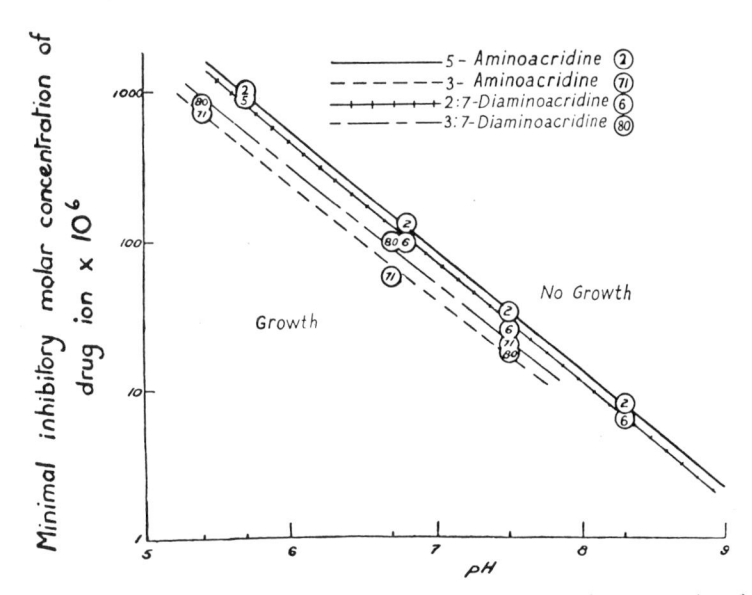

Fig. 38.2 Competition between hydrogen ions and acridine ions. Organism = *B. coli*. The ionic concentration of the drug was calculated from the total concentration and the pK value. The figure shows (a) that for bacteriostasis to occur an increase in the hydrogen ion concentration must be balanced by a similar increase in acridine ion concentration; (b) that equal numbers of ions of different acridines produce the same bacteriostatic effect, although the actual concentrations of compounds used may be quite different. (After Albert, Rubbo, Goldacre, Davey and Stone, 1945. *Br. J. exp. Path.*)

action in a short time, but on the other hand very low concentrations will inhibit bacterial growth and exert an eventual lethal effect if allowed to act for at least some hours.

The acridine derivatives are particularly suitable for the treatment of infected wounds, which after preliminary surgical cleansing may be swabbed or irrigated with a 0.1 per cent solution in normal saline. The acridine compounds are very good wound antiseptics, because they produce an antiseptic action in concentrations much lower than those required to inhibit phagocytosis or to produce irritation, and since their toxicity is fairly low they are not likely to produce toxic symptoms if absorbed.

Antiseptic preparations for preoperative scrubbing of skin

The microbial flora of the skin can be divided into 'resident' organisms which colonise the skin and 'transient' organisms which are present as contaminants. Many resident organisms are non-pathogenic although in some individuals *Staph. aureus* may be resident. The transient bacterial flora can be removed to a large extent by thorough scrubbing with soap but the resident flora cannot be so removed. Both types of microbial flora can be largely, if not completely, removed by the use of efficient antiseptics.

The following are the chief requirements in an antiseptic that is to be used to disinfect hands prior to operations. (1) The drug must sterilise the skin rapidly and with certainty. (2) It must penetrate and disinfect the ducts of the sweat glands and the hair follicles. (3) It must not stain the hands.

(4) It must not produce roughening or cracking of the epithelium even when used many times a day for long periods. Several organic halogen compounds (Fig. 38.3) are now available and are widely used as antiseptics for local application to skin and mucous membranes.

Fig. 38.3 Chemical structures of antiseptic organic halogen compounds.

Hexachlorophane (Hexachlorophene)
This chlorinated bis-phenol compound was introduced as a skin antiseptic in the United States in 1944. It is almost insoluble in water but readily soluble in alcohol; it is non-irritant and compatible with soap. Its antibacterial activity is greater against Gram-positive than against Gram-negative organisms; preparations containing hexachlorophane should have a pH between 5 and 6.

Hexachlorophane is frequently incorporated in medicated soaps or emulsions (1–3 per cent) which are used for scrubbing up before operations. Creams and ointments containing 1–3 per cent of hexachlorophane are used in the treatment of acne vulgaris and other pyogenic infections of the skin.

Toxic effects. Recent evidence has shown that systemic absorption of hexachlorophane can result in severe lesions of the central nervous system; histological evidence of status spongiosus of the white matter of the brain and spinal cord has been demonstrated in a number of different species given repeated oral doses of the compound.

Hexachlorophane must not be administered under conditions in which it can be absorbed systemically. Premature infants and young children should not be subjected to total body bathing with hexachlorophane and preparations containing it should not be applied to extensive wounds, lacerations or severe burns.

Chlorhexidine (Hibitane)
This compound has bactericidal activity against a wide range of organisms. A variety of preparations containing chlorhexidine hydrochloride are available for application to the skin and mucous membrane as antiseptic creams, burn and nasal creams and dusting powders. Aqueous solutions of chlorhexidine acetate (1 in 5000) are used for irrigation of the bladder and other body cavities; other antiseptic creams containing chlorhexidine gluconate are extensively used in general surgery and obstetrics. For pre-operative skin sterilisation a 5 per cent concentrate of this compound is diluted (1 in 10) with 70 per cent alcohol.

Chloroxylenol
Compounds of this type are the basis of many popular proprietary disinfectants such as *Dettol*. They are relatively non-irritant to tissues, particularly to the skin, and have a pleasant smell. Their bactericidal power is, however, not very great and they cannot be relied upon to destroy staphylococci on the skin.

Iodophors
The iodophors are mixtures of iodine with carriers, usually surface-active agents. They have a wide range of antibacterial activity and are effective skin antiseptics which do not stain or irritate the skin. *Povidone-Iodine*, a complex of iodine with polyvinylpyrrolidone, is used as a surgical scrub in concentrations equivalent to 0.5–3 per cent of available iodine; it has a more rapid effect than hexachlorophane in reducing the bacterial count in skin and is particularly active against *clostridial* infection.

Povidone-Iodine was reported to have been used for disinfecting the spacemen, the waiting raft and the frogmen in the Apollo 11 lunar mission of 1969.

PREPARATIONS

Detergents
Benzalkonium chl (Zephiran) 0.1–0.2%
Benzethonium chl (Phemerol) 0.1%
Cetrimide (Cetavlon) 0.1–1%
Domiphen brom (Bradosol) 0.02–0.05%

Various antiseptics
Chlorine releasing
Sodium hypochlorite sol
Iodine compounds
Povidone-Iodine (Polyvidone iodine, Betadine) (ionophore)
Weak Iodine Solution
Mercurial
Phenylmercuric nitrate 0.001–0.002%
Oxidising
Hydrogen peroxide 3%
Boron derivative
Boric acid 5–10%
Acridine
Proflavine sulph 0.1%
Chlorinated phenols
Chlorhexidine gluconate 0.5%
Chloroxylenol (Dettol) 1:80
Hexachlorophane 0.25–3%

FURTHER READING

Block S S (ed) 1977 Disinfection, sterilization and preservation. Lea & Febiger, Philadelphia
Lowsbury E J L 1966 Antiseptic soaps and detergent preparations. Prescribers' Journal 5: 78
Reddish G F (ed) 1957 Antiseptics, disinfectants, fungicides and sterilisation. Kimpton, London
Sykes G 1965 Disinfection and sterilisation. Spon, London

SECTION SEVEN

Environmental pharmacology

39. Ecology and environmental health

Current environmental problems 465; Protection of the environment 465; Air pollution 466; Lead 466; Carbon oxides 466; Nitrogen oxides 466; Pesticidies 467; Insecticides 467; Herbicides 469; Fungicides 470; Nematicids 470; Rodenticides 470; Antibiotics and food preservatives 470; Nutritional deficiencies 471; Carcinogens 472; Antidotes of heavy metal poisoning 473.

Current environmental problems

During recent years it has become increasingly apparent that the enhancement of man's welfare is accompanied by new risks to his environment. There is widespread concern about the physical and chemical hazards of air, water and soil pollution, for example the potential risks from the use of pesticides and antibiotics for the improvement of food production and its storage. The increasing occurrence of iatrogenic disease associated with the use of medicinal preparations for the prevention and treatment of minor and major illnesses and for the control of reproduction has given rise to new problems. There are social complexities which result from the misuse of drugs and manifest themselves in disturbance of behaviour and in serious errors of judgment including those in charge of motor vehicles and moving machinery.

In this and the following chapters, the ecological, and social aspects of these important areas of subject matter are discussed to illustrate that there is an enlarging scope for the application of pharmacological and toxicological skills and techniques in helping to resolve many important problems which were previously considered to be outwith the scope of pharmacology.*

Other aspects of environmental health discussed briefly in this chapter include 1) nutritional deficiency, in particular protein-calorie malnutrition; 2) occupational cancer; 3) antidotes of heavy metal poisoning.

Protection of the environment

Contamination or pollution of the physical environment has become a major subject of study. Whilst much has been done to safeguard the natural environment of a country such as Great Britain, as was pointed out in the report of the Royal Commission on Environmental Pollution (1970), much more could and must be done to improve the quality of the environment.

A basic principle in controlling the sources and causes of pollution is to appreciate that, even though these sources are not likely to be completely eliminated, it is important to ensure that pollution does not reach a level which would endanger the biological cycles on which all life, including that of man, depends. For example, micro-organisms and plankton are essential agents involved in recycling waste in soil and water and if these are overlooked or killed, the recycling of waste is endangered, as has already occurred in some rivers and inland lakes. More adequate means for dealing with domestic refuse and industrial waste are urgently needed; the long-term effects of disposal of toxic materials, radioactive waste and oil pollution of inshore waters and general dumping of unwanted materials in the sea are problems which require intensive study. They are all matters which involve the individual citizen and his influence on public opinion, as well as the concerted action of local authorities and central government in providing economic incentives supported by appropriate legislation and international agreements.

The development of the chemical industry has grown to a phenomenal extent and the output of chemicals, increasingly derived from petroleum, has reached an enormous figure. It has been estimated that from 1950 to 1970 the annual world production of organic chemicals (outside the Communist countries) has increased from 7 to 33 million tons. Whilst approximately 25 per cent of current production is used for the manufacture of medicinal chemicals, pesticides, food additives, detergents and solvents, the major output is used for the synthesis of plastics and resins, synthetic fibres and rubber. It has now become a major task to investigate and try to prevent the deleterious effects that these vast quantities of chemicals, in all their various forms, may have on the ecology. The disposal of discarded end products during manufacture and after consumer use has focused attention on the biological recycling processes involved in the biodegradation of chemicals and the important part they play in preserving the quality of the environment. Several types of substance such as plastics are not recycled by any biological process; polychlorinated biphenyl compounds (PCBs) used extensively in industry and some organochlorine pesticides such as DDT and dieldrin are very stable, slowly degraded and highly soluble in lipids so that they accumulate in the environment and are present in the tissues of most biological species, including man.

Increasing attention is now being directed to the study of preserving the quality of the air we breathe and the food and water we ingest not merely because it is beneficial to man but also because it is essential to maintain the quality of the environment for the survival of many other species.

---

*The ecological section was mainly contributed by the late Professor Andrew Wilson.

Air Pollution

Smoke and sulphur dioxide are major sources of pollution which result from the burning of coal and crude oil. In 1952, during a dense fog in London, air pollution reached an unusually high level and was responsible for the deaths of about 4000 people mainly from bronchitis and other diseases of the lungs and from heart disease (Fig. 39.1). The establishment of smokeless zones in towns and cities in Great Britain as a result of the Clean Air Act (1956) has substantially reduced the emission of smoke but less so of sulphur dioxide from domestic and industrial premises.

Lead. The extensive use of petrol and diesel engines is another source of air pollution. Incomplete combustion of these fuels results in the emission of black smoke; the addition of organic lead compounds as anti-knock agents gives rise to inorganic lead in the exhaust fumes but the air concentration of lead, even in heavy traffic conditions, is very small (3 $\mu g/m^3$). The absorption of lead by inhalation from this source appears to be well within the capacity of the body to excrete it; for example the American Industrial Hygiene Association considered in 1969 that an acceptable level of atmospheric lead in domestic premises should not exceed 10 $\mu g/m^3$.

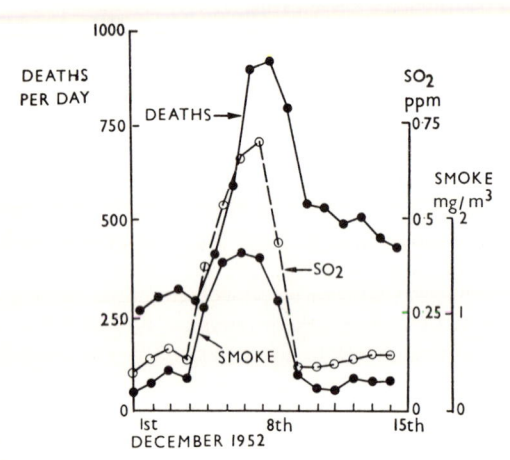

Fig. 39.1 Increase in death rate associated with increased air pollution with sulphur dioxide (SO_2) and smoke during a fog in London which lasted from 5th to 9th December 1952. (After *Air Pollution and Health in Report of the Royal College of Physicians of London* 1970, Pitman, London.)

A more serious cause of lead poisoning arises from the presence of lead in drinking water. The World Health Organisation in 1971 concluded that an upper limit of lead in drinking water of 100 $\mu g/l$ was acceptable. Several reports have shown that in Great Britain some supplies of domestic water, where plumbing systems consist of lead-lined storage tanks and lead piping, have a lead content from 100–1000 $\mu g/l$. This source of lead contamination has produced clinical or biochemical evidence of lead poisoning with blood levels exceeding the normal upper limit of 40 $\mu g/100$ ml.

There appears to be a close relation between increased lead concentration in blood and a decrease in the activity of delta-aminolaevulic acid dehydrase (ALA) in erythrocytes. In children, for example, depression of ALA dehydrase activity has been associated with blood lead concentrations of 25–30 $\mu g/100$ ml; it has been suggested that these findings may be connected with the well established fact that the central nervous system of infants and young children is more susceptible than that of adults to ingestion or inhalation of lead. Behavioural disturbances including hostility, aggression, destructiveness and rejection of educational and parental discipline have been associated with episodes of lead poisoning and in some children who survive an episode of lead encephalopathy, severe and permanent brain damage may result.

Carbon monoxide. The exhaust from petrol engines contains high concentrations of carbon monoxide which may be fatal if inhaled, for example when a car engine is left running in a closed garage. Exposure to heavy traffic, however, seldom gives rise to blood levels of carboxyhaemoglobin greater than those commonly found in cigarette smokers (about 4 per cent saturation). The eventual disposal of carbon monoxide is mainly by bacteria in the soil which use it as food.

Carbon dioxide is another byproduct of fuel combustion; it also enters the atmosphere as a waste product of plant and animal respiration. About 50 per cent of the CO_2 evolved is eventually dissolved in the oceans as magnesium and sodium carbonates and carbonic acid. It has been suggested that if the atmospheric CO_2 increases to twice its present level (320 ppm) this would interfere with the long-wave radiation emitted from the earth's surface into space and increase the temperature of the earth with consequent global effects such as increased thawing of polar ice and rises in sea levels. Estimates of atmospheric CO_2 have shown that since the 1890s the level has risen about 10 per cent, half of the rise taking place since 1945; projection of this trend for 30 years would result in a small temperature rise of 0.1 to 0.2°C.

Nitrogen oxides, chiefly NO and NO_2, are derived from the combustion of atmospheric nitrogen and contribute to the production of *photo-chemical smog.* This results from the action of ultra-violet light on nitrogen oxides which, in the presence of hydrocarbons emitted from motor exhausts, forms ozone which in turn reacts with hydrocarbons and other organic matter to produce compounds which are irritant to the eyes and respiratory tract. In cities such as Los Angeles, where there is strong sunlight and the air is still, the formation of photo-chemical smog is a particularly noxious form of air pollution; the climatic conditions in Great Britain do not give rise to this type of smog.

The influence of air pollution on the incidence of chronic infections of the middle ear and upper respiratory passages in children has been clearly established by surveys of schoolchildren in urban areas compared with those in rural areas.

Chemicals involved in food production

Many chemical compounds are now used for the purpose of food production; they include a wide range of pesticides used for agricultural, horticultural and food storage practices, antibiotics in animal husbandry and veterinary medicine, food additives such as colouring, flavouring and sweetening agents to improve the palatability and acceptability of processed foods, and antioxidants and stabilisers to ensure stability during storage and distribution to various parts of the world.

Pesticides

These substances are extensively used to control pests that destroy or endanger the production, transport and storage of food and to eradicate organisms involved in the transmission of human, plant and animal diseases.

It has been estimated that, without the use of pesticides, up to one-third of the world's food crops would be destroyed during growth, harvesting and storage. The introduction of effective pesticides has enabled large-scale eradication of the vectors of certain human diseases and substantially reduced the morbidity and mortality rates of malaria, typhus, yellow fever and filariasis.

Pesticides can be conveniently classifed according to the main purposes for which they are used; for example, insecticides, fungicides, herbicides, nematicides and rodenticides. Many of these compounds are potentially toxic to man and to various other important species such as fish, birds, other forms of wildlife and domestic animals.

Tolerance levels. An important aspect of national and international agreements on food production concerns the residue levels of the pesticide and its breakdown products which arise from the approved use of the pesticide in good agricultural practice. The Food and Agricultural Organisation (FAO) of the United Nations and the World Health Organisation (WHO) have jointly defined the maximum concentration of pesticide residue that should be permitted in or on food at a specified stage in the harvesting, storage, transport, marketing or preparation of the food up to the final point of consumption. The concentration is expressed in parts by weight of the pesticide residue per million parts by weight of the food (ppm). These tolerance levels are based on the results of chronic toxicity tests of each pesticide on at least two species of experimental animals and incorporate a large numerical safety factor, so that on the basis of all known facts there can be derived an *acceptable daily intake (ADI)* of the pesticide, which during the entire lifetime of an individual appears to be without appreciable risk to his health and welfare.

The techniques now used for determination of pesticide residues are extremely sensitive and are often capable of measuring amounts of 0.01 or even 0.001 ppm. In many cases the residue levels in foods are close to or even below the analytical limit of detection. The results of a recent survey in Britain of pesticide residues in the foods purchased in the market and prepared for consumption at the table showed that no samples contained residues above the safety margin and the estimated daily intake of some organochlorine compounds such as DDT was only 6 per cent of the official ADI level.

Nevertheless, there is evidence of contamination of the environment by the use of pesticides which has occasionally resulted in serious hazards to some wildlife species such as fish, bees, birds and some mammals. In most instances, these relate to substances such as organochlorine and mercury compounds which are slowly degraded and thereby accumulate in tissues with resultant toxic effects.

Insecticides

An extensive range of compounds is now available for the protection of crops against invasion by flies, caterpillars, moths, mites and similar pests. They consist of organochlorine and organophosphorus compounds, carbamates, substituted cresols and naturally occurring substances such as derris and nicotine. Many are also toxic to man and other mammals and when used in agriculture and horticulture, in public health campaigns for the eradication of malaria and in the control of nuisance pests such as cockroaches, ants and termites in and around domestic premises, protective clothing must be worn by workers who use them.

Organochlorine compounds are chlorinated hydrocarbons which are poorly soluble in water. Most are relatively stable and are slowly degraded and metabolised, so that they tend to persist and accumulate in tissues and in the environment. They consist of dicophane (DDT), gamma benzene hexachloride (BHC), lindane and cyclodiene compounds, such as aldrin, dieldrin (Fig. 39.2), heptachlor and endosulphan. They are used to prevent and treat infestations in man and animals, by pests which are sensitive to them, as well as for crop protection. *Aldrin, dieldrin* and *endrin* are long-lasting compounds and their accumulation in the tissues of animals such as sheep and cattle and of man, and in soil, has led to some restriction of their use. They are also extensively used in the preservation of timber and textiles such as carpets and clothes, and are incorporated in insulated cables.

Dicophane (DDT) was synthesised in 1874, but its insecticidal properties were not discovered until 1939. It kills mosquitoes, flies, lice and other insects by absorption from the feet and antennae and rapidly produces paralysis of the central nervous system. It is also toxic in much higher concentrations to most mammalian species, producing tremors, convulsions and death.

Gamma benzene hexachloride (Gammexane, gamma-BHC) has insecticidal properties similar to those of DDT but is about 20 times more active against lice and 10 times more active against mosquitoes. It is used mainly as a spray for the elimination of houseflies, mosquitoes and tsetse flies and for controlling infestation by lice. Its use in agriculture is limited because it is less persistent and is liable to impart an unacceptable taint to potatoes and other root crops.

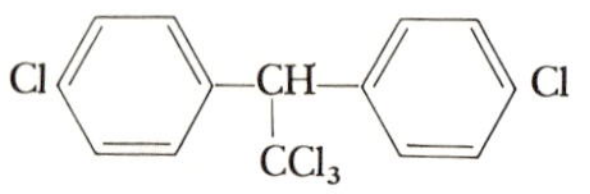

Dicophane (DDT)

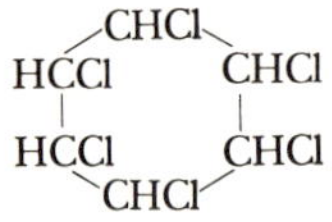

Gamma—BHC

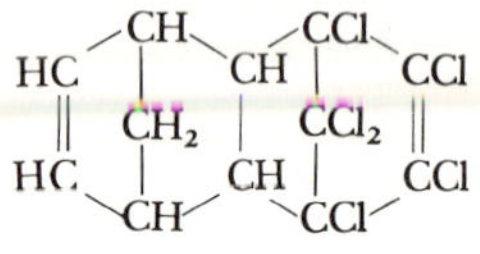

Aldrin

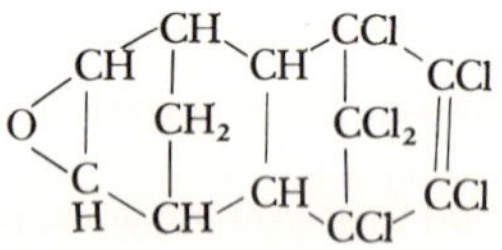

Dieldrin

Fig. 39.2 Chemical structure of some organochlorine pesticides.

Toxicity of DDT and Gammexane
Because of their world-wide use, the toxicity of these insecticides has received much attention. However, there is no evidence that the large scale use of DDT and Gammexane as delousing agents among military and civilian personnel in wartime and otherwise has resulted in significant toxicity. Their insecticidal effectiveness is very high. A single dusting of DDT on the clothing and body is effective in the treatment of body, head and pubic lice, but there are no proved cases of poisoning caused by DDT alone when used as a 10 per cent dusting powder for delousing. DDT produces no irritation of the skin. Gammexane 1 per cent used for scabies is irritating to the eyes, skin and mucosa and should not be applied to the eyelashes and urethral meatus. Gammexane can be absorbed through the intact skin and because it is excreted slowly (urinary half life 26 h) repeated applications may produce dangerously high blood levels.

With both agents systemic toxicity is generally manifested as central nervous system disturbances. With DDT paraesthesias and peripheral neuropathy has been described. Large scale absorption of both agents may lead to convulsions.

Organophosphorus compounds. The insecticidal properties of these compounds were discovered in Germany during World War II, when Allied and German authorities were engaged in a search for substances suitable for chemical warfare as so-called nerve gases. Whilst several compounds were synthesised and tested for this purpose, they were fortunately never used. Numerous organophosphorus compounds (p. 61) with widely different chemical structures are now available. An essential feature of these compounds is the variety of side chains that can be attached to one or more parts of the component nucleus.

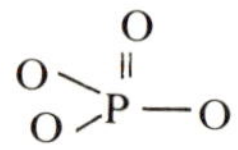

which itself may be varied by substitution of one or more of the oxygen atoms by C, S or N. The chemical structure of some typical compounds are shown in Figure 39.3.

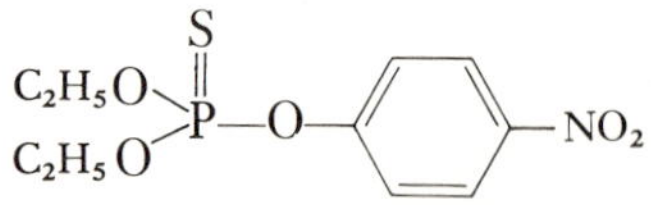

Parathion

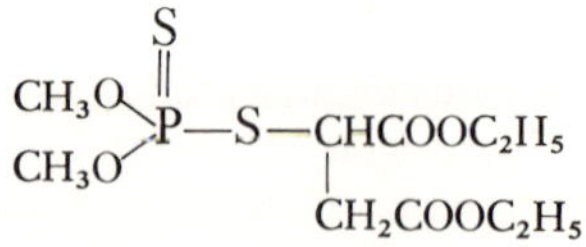

Malathion

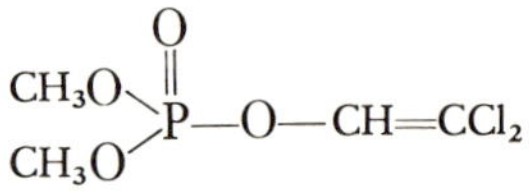

Dichlorvos

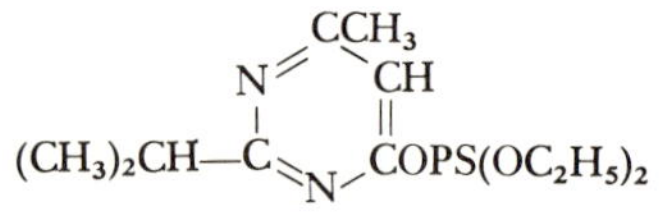

Diazinon

Fig. 39.3 Chemical structure of some organophosphorus pesticides.

Organophosphorus compounds are powerful inhibitors of cholinesterase and are effective against a wide range of insects and pests. They can be formulated as dusts and granules for soil application, as aqueous solutions or suspensions for spraying crops and buildings and as sheep dips; impregnated strips of plastic, from which the active compound is slowly released, are used indoors to eliminate household flies and other nuisance insects.

In comparison with most organochlorines, organophosphates are less stable and are more rapidly broken down in plants and animals; hence these are less likely to be distributed widely in the environment. There are considerable differences between organophosphates in their acute toxicity to mammals as shown in Table 39.1.

Table 39.1 The acute LD_{50} by oral administration and dermal application to rats of some typical organophosphorus compounds (after Ben-Dyke, Sanderson & Noakes, 1970, *World Review of Pest Control*)

Compound	LD_{50} mg/kg Oral	Dermal
Parathion	3–6	4–35
Dichlorvos	25–30	75–900
Dimethoate	200–300	700–1150
Malathion	1400–1900	More than 4000

Since they are absorbed through the skin and mucous membranes they are more hazardous to use than organochlorines, and the use of protective clothing is essential. Periodic determination of the blood cholinesterase activity of workers using anti-cholinesterase compounds is also necessary.

Acute poisoning by organophosphates is characterised by the onset of muscarinic and nicotinic effects similar to those of DFP (p. 61). The main principles of treatment are to maintain an adequate airway and respiration, the intravenous or intramuscular injection of atropine sulphate in doses of 2 mg, repeated at half-hourly intervals and the intramuscular injection of *pralidoxime* (P_2S) (p. 61). This substance is a specific reactivator of cholinesterase and reacts with the phosphorylated enzyme to free its active site; the reactivating effect of pralidoxime is particularly marked at the neuromuscular junctions of skeletal muscle.

Resistance to insecticides
Resistance to dicophane by arthropods, particularly by anopheline mosquitoes, has been reported since the 1950s. Resistance to dicophane has developed in many parts of the world and has extended progressively to increased numbers of species. Resistance has also developed to other chlorinated insecticides and resistance to organophosphorus insecticides, though less extensive, is also increasing.

The development of resistance to insecticides has prompted a search for other methods of insect control. Some success has attended the release into the normal fly population of large numbers of male flies which have been sterilised by gamma irradiation or by the use of chemical sterilants.

Insect repellents
Complete protection against biting insects requires the application of repellents to the skin and to clothing. *Dimethylphthalate* is effective against blackflies, mosquitos, midges, mites, ticks and fleas. When the drug is applied to the skin as a cream or lotion it is active for 3 to 5 hours, *Dibutylphthalate* and *Diethyltoluamide* have similar properties.

Herbicides
The control and eradication of weeds by the use of chemical substances is an important feature of modern agricultural and forestry practice. Substantial losses in crop yield can be avoided by eliminating both broadleaved and grassy weeds which compete with fruit, cereals and other crops for light, space, water and soil nutrients; they also act as hosts to fungi and bacteria which are harmful to food crops. Herbicides are also extensively used to clear unwanted vegetation which presents a fire hazard or causes damage to industrial sites, power lines, airways and railway tracks.

The work involved in the synthesis, biological and toxicity testing of herbicides constitutes an increasingly important part of the pesticides industry. In general herbicides can be classified according to their effects on plants, (a) by direct contact with the foliage, (b) by absorption through the roots and leaves and translocation through the plant, and (c) by sterilising the soil and preventing plant growth. They can be further categorised as selective or non-selective according to whether the intention is to suppress or kill the weeds without harming the crop, or to kill all vegetation. Examples of selective weedkillers which are translocated and affect mainly broadleaved plants but not crop grasses and cereals, include *phenoxyacetates* which are readily broken down and do not persist in the soil. The importance of using chemicals which are free from impurities was underlined when it was found in the U.S.A. that some supplies of a phenoxyacetate contained excessive amounts of tetrachlorodioxin, a highly toxic impurity which produces chromosome aberrations in plant tissues and teratogenic effects in mammals.

Contact herbicides such as *dinitro-orthocresol* (DNOC) interfere with phosphorylation processes in cells; in animals they cause a rapid increase in basal metabolic rate and body temperature. Since they are absorbed through the skin and by inhalation, full protective clothing must be worn by those who use them. In the early stages of their use, severe poisoning occurred in persons engaged in manufacturing and spraying them. An early symptom of absorption is a sense of wellbeing and abounding energy, which is presumably due to stimulation of metabolism. More prolonged exposure produces a yellow colouration of the skin, a rise in body temperature, sweating, fatigue and a pronounced loss in body weight. No specific antidote for this type of poison is known and symptomatic treatment consists of cooling, rehydration and the administration of oxygen if necessary.

Paraquat and diquat are bipyridylium compounds which are non-selective contact herbicides and act on both broad-leaved and grass weeds.

A number of cases of accidental and of intentional poisoning have resulted from swallowing paraquat or diquat concentrates; the immediate effects are nausea, vomiting, abdominal discomfort and diarrhoea with localised pain in the mouth and throat. Within two to three days evidence of severe renal and hepatic damage occurs and soon thereafter pulmonary function is severely impaired with resultant dyspnoea and pulmonary oedema. Paraquat is particularly dangerous, producing marked pulmonary fibrosis and severe respiratory failure.

The ultimate prognosis is grave, since no specific antidote is known; symptomatic treatment consists of initial attempts to evacuate the stomach contents and administration of an adsorbent such as a suspension of Fuller's Earth (B.P.). Excretion of the bipyridyl compound should be attempted by forced diuresis using oral and intravenous fluids.

Several other types of chemical compounds, which have relatively lower toxicity than these substances, are used as herbicides; they include triazine compounds, and inorganic and organic compounds of arsenic and mercury.

Fungicides

About 130 different chemical substances have been developed as fungicides; whilst some are fairly active compounds, they are much less toxic to mammals and other species than are insecticides. One of the basic problems in developing active fungicides is that the fungus itself has often a more intimate relationship with the plant host than is the case with insect pests. Most fungicides act as protective substances, preventing germinating fungus spores from entering plant tissues; they are mainly used as seed dressings and as sprays on developing fruit and food crops. Other compounds which are volatile are used as fumigants to protect harvested crops during storage and transport. Fungicides comprise a variety of inorganic or organic compounds of sulphur, arsenic, copper and mercury, and include a number of dithiocarbamates.

Whilst the hazards to man from the use of fungicides are relatively small, there have been reports of deaths in birds as a result of eating planted seeds treated with mercury compounds; incidents of fish kills and high contents of mercury in harvested fish, for example tinned tuna fish, have also been documented.

Mercury and its inorganic and organic compounds are used in industrial processes such as timber, paper and textile production to a much greater extent than in agriculture; any pollution of land surfaces and inshore waters that may occur is unlikely to be due to the agricultural use of these fungicides.

Nematicides

The successful eradication and control of nematodes or eelworms usually requires some form of fumigation of the soil by the use of a gaseous fumigant applied to the surface of the soil under gas-proof covers or the injection or implantation into the soil of volatile liquid or granular formulations from which the active substance is released. The chemical substances used include a variety of halogenated hydrocarbons such as methyl bromide, ethylene dibromide and chloropicrin and organophosphates. These compounds are also highly toxic to man and animals and during the relatively short periods of use, adequate precautions must be taken to exclude access to the treatment areas.

Rodenticides

The use of chemicals to eliminate rats, mice and moles depends on the extent to which the pests are brought into contact with the active substance. In enclosed premises such as industrial and farm buildings and ships' holds where all entrances and exits can be sealed off, the use of fumigants such as hydrogen cyanide, may be successful. In most instances, however, the method of treatment depends on devising an appropriate bait containing the rodenticide, which is acceptable to the rodents; this often requires several feedings because the bait does not usually carry a sufficiently lethal concentration of compound in the amount that is ingested on one occasion. Baits containing an anticoagulant of the coumarin type, for example *warfarin* (p. 213), are usually effective in controlling rats and house mice, but in some localised areas rat populations have become resistant to it. *Fluoroacetamide* and *sodium fluoroacetate* are highly toxic to all warm-blooded animals; they disrupt the normal energy exchanges in cells by blocking the tricarboxylic acid cycle and produce a rapid impairment of the heart and brain with resultant respiratory and cardiac failure. These compounds must be used only in specially authorised circumstances such as in sewers and ships' holds under the supervision of trained pest control operators. Other rodenticides include inorganic salts of arsenic, zinc and phosphorus; alphachloralose, a hypnotic closely related to chloral hydrate, produces its lethal effect by prolonged coma and reduction in body temperature.

Antibiotics

In addition to their importance in the prevention and treatment of human infections, antibiotics are also used in veterinary practice and by the livestock industry. The term 'feed' antibiotic includes a number of antibiotics, sulphonamides and nitrofurans which are added to animal feeding stuffs, in concentrations of 5–100 ppm, to promote growth in pigs, poultry and young calves. The extensive use of these substances in animal husbandry and veterinary medicine has considerable economic advantages in food production but it has also given rise to some concern about the potential risks to human and animal health. An important example is the occurrence in animals of strains of enterobacteria which are resistant to one or more antibiotics, and the ability of these resistant strain to transmit this resistance to other bacteria. Some of these organisms, particularly of the salmonella group cause disease in some species of farm livestock and also in man; *Salmonella typhimurium* may give rise to a generalised infection in persons who handle the animals and in consumers of inedaquately cooked meat and poultry. Antibiotic treatment of such patients is usually necessary and may be complicated if the strain of *S. typhimurium* shows multiple resistance to antibiotics. There is also evidence that some strains of *Escherichia coli* which do not normally cause disease in adults, may also become resistant to antibiotics and in the human intestine are capable of transferring antibiotic resistance to the typhoid bacillus (*Salmonella typhi*). Thus the use of chloramphenicol as a 'feed' antibiotic could lead to serious difficulties if chloramphenicol-resistant strains of the typhoid bacillus develop in man. There is also the possibility that antibiotic residues in meat and poultry and their products, such as milk and eggs, may create a potential risk of allergic reactions when the consumer is given antibiotic therapy; this risk applies also to workers who are frequently in contact with antibiotics during the preparation and mixing of animal feeding stuffs containing them.

Antibiotics are also used for the preservation of food. *Antibiotic-ice* containing oxytetracycline or chlortetracycline (up to 5 ppm) has been used in trawlers to extend the storage life of raw fish, between catching at sea and marketing. This has previously been justified on the grounds that any antibiotic residues tend to be destroyed during cooking but with the development of adequate deep-freezing facilities and current policy on antibiotic restriction there is no need to continue this practice. The use of *nystatin* (p. 414) to control fungal rot in bananas by dipping the fruit in solutions containing up to 400 ppm of nystatin prior to shipment has been permitted on the evidence that no antibiotic residues are present in the flesh of bananas. There is however a potential hazard to those engaged in dipping or handling dipped bananas, of harbouring nystatin-resistant *candida* organisms and this permitted use of nystatin is likely to be discontinued. *Thiabendazole*, an anthelmintic drug (p. 452) which has fungicidal properties is an alternative to nystatin for the preservation of citrus fruits and bananas.

Other food preservatives

The long established use of potassium nitrate (salt petre) in the curing and preserving of meat is based on the fact that nitrates occur naturally in many foods, especially in vegetables such as carrots, beans and spinach. Furthermore when nitrate is used to cure meat it is reduced to nitrite by micro-organisms on the meat; the subsequent interaction of nitrite with meat proteins, especially myoglobin and haemoglobin, imparts a red colour which adds to the attractive qualities of the cured meat. Nitrites inhibit the growth of *Clostridium botulinum*, the toxins of which, if present in canned meat products, can produce severe and sometimes lethal food poisoning. These advantages of nitrate as a food preservative have hitherto fully justified its use.

Recent evidence has shown, however, that nitrites in food can also react with any secondary amines that are present to form nitrosamines, some of which are known to cause severe liver damage in experimental animals; it has also been reported that malignant tumours can be induced experimentally in rats by the simultaneous feeding of nitrite and secondary amines. Several outbreaks of nitrite poisoning have been reported in children who developed methaemoglobinaemia as a result of drinking well-water containing nitrates and in others who were fed processed meat products.

Use of oestrogens in animal husbandry. The use of oestrogens is permitted to promote growth in poultry and young (veal) calves by the implantation of pellets of stilboestrol and other oestrogens in the neck or behind the ears, on the grounds that after slaughter, any oestrogen remaining in these parts of the animal are not used for human consumption, and that the amounts of oestrogen residue in consumed meat are small and not harmful. One of the possible delayed effects of oestrogen therapy has recently been highlighted by reports in the U.S. of adenocarcinoma of the vagina in adolescent girls whose mothers had been treated with stilboestrol during pregnancy (p. 477). With the widespread use of oral contraceptives a re-appraisal is now necessary of what were formerly acceptable as small and harmless oestrogen residues in meat, particularly for women who take contraceptive pills containing oestrogens.

There is increasing evidence of the need for continued research in the further development of toxicity standards and of sensitive methods for monitoring chemical residues and their long-term biological effects to ensure that the undoubted economic and social benefits of using chemical substances are not likely to affect adversely man and his environment. It must also be appreciated that highly toxic substances in food can arise from contamination with naturally occurring moulds and fungi, for example ergot in grain and aflotoxin in mouldy peanuts.

ENVIRONMENTAL HEALTH ASPECTS

Nutritional deficiencies

Deficiency diseases can be divided into two groups: those

which, although not completely eliminated, have become uncommon on a world scale compared with their previous prevalence and those which are still far from being prevented although their causes are known. To the first group belong the major vitamin deficiency diseases, beri-beri, pellagra, rickets and scurvy, discussed in Chapter 28. To the second group belong certain other deficiency diseases deserving the highest priority according to a report of the World Health Organisation. They are:

1. Protein-calorie malnutrition, because of its wide prevalence and high mortality rate and the irreversible physical and sometimes mental damage it may cause.

2. Xerophthalmia, which contributes to the mortality of malnourished children and may cause permanent blindness. This condition, due to vitamin A deficiency, is discussed on page 362.

3. Nutritional anaemias are widely distributed and contribute to the mortality of other disease conditions. They have important economic effects on working capacity.

4. Endemic goitre, discussed on page 332.

Figure 39.4 indicates in diagrammatic form the global extent of these conditions, their social significance and the feasibility of their prevention as it appeared in the year 1972.

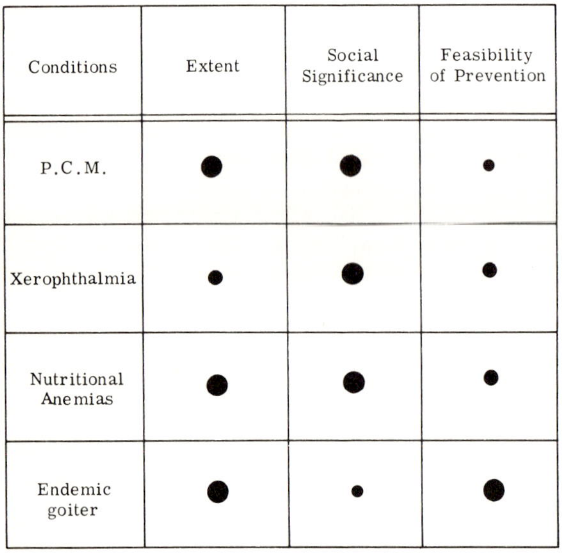

Conditions	Extent	Social Significance	Feasibility of Prevention
P.C.M.	●	●	•
Xerophthalmia	•	●	•
Nutritional Anemias	•	•	•
Endemic goiter	●	•	●

Fig. 39.4 Priorities among nutritional conditions: the circles give an indication of the magnitude in each case. (From Nutrition: A Review of the WHO Programme 1965-1971. World Health Organisation, Geneva, 1972).

Protein-calorie malnutrition (PCM)
This term is used for a range of pathological conditions arising from simultaneous deficiency of protein and calories and commonly associated with gastrointestinal and other infections occurring particularly in infants and very young children. When children become older they adapt to deficient diets and the incidence of nutritional marasmus becomes rarer. Nevertheless, the ill effects of protein-calorie deficiency in infancy persist into later life and may cause not only poor bodily development but also some degree of mental impairment.

PCM is the most important nutritional problem in the developing countries and at present affects between 0.1 and 10 per cent of infants in these countries in the severe form of marasmus and ultimately kwashiorkor and up to 50 per cent in a moderate form. The condition is produced by the interaction between infection and insufficient protein and calorie intake. It frequently starts after weaning with a bout of diarrhoea, which is always more frequent and serious in malnourished infants. In contrast, infants receiving sufficient breast milk are in no danger of protein-calorie malnutrition.

Prevention of protein-calorie malnutrition. The most important preventive measure is the provision of protein in the diet in the form of dried skimmed milk or other complete proteins. Proteins such as meat, fish, milk and eggs have high nutritional value due to their complete amino acid composition and good digestibility and are therefore ideal nutrients. Many vegetable proteins have a low content of such essential amino acids as lysine, tryptophan, threonine and methionine and are therefore less satisfactory if given by themselves. Recent studies have shown, however, that mixtures of vegetable proteins which together contain all the essential amino acids constitute diets on which children will thrive.

CARCINOGENS
Both genetic and environmental factors contribute to cancer. The diagnosis of environmental or occupational cancer in man may be difficult, requiring detailed epidemiological studies in comparison with the natural incidence of cancer in similar populations. Such studies may have to extend over many years, especially since occupational cancers generally develop slowly. Experimental cancer investigations in animals cannot substitute for epidemiological studies in man. Not only is the route of administration in man, which is usually by inhalation, difficult to simulate in animals but there is also considerable variation in the ability of an individual compound to give rise to tumours in different species. For example, ß-naphthylamine which causes bladder tumours in man did not produce bladder lesions in various experimental animals until the dog was used, in which the compound readily caused bladder tumours.

Compounds for which there is considerable evidence of carcinogenicity in man include the following:

ß-Naphthylamine. This compound is used in the production of azo dyes. It is also used in rubber vulcanisation. Its association with human bladder tumours has been demonstrated beyond doubt.

Chromium. Chromium is very extensively used in alloys, plating and corrosion inhibiting paints. There is strong evidence that chromates can produce lung cancer and this makes it necessary to apply stringent dust and vapour control in processes involving chromium.

Mineral-derived oils, coal tar and pitch. There is evidence that workers exposed to some of these products exhibit an increased incidence of cancer, for example, scrotal cancer. The carcinogenic activity of these materials is highly variable, depending upon source, content and method of preparation and distillation. Among specific compounds present in tar which are definitely carcinogenic, is 3,4-benzopyrene which is also found in tobacco smoke and is believed to be a contributory if not the main cause of lung cancer in cigarette smokers.

Asbestos. The dust of this fibrous material has been implicated not only in asbestosis but also in malignant endothelioma.

The prevention of carcinogenic risks in industry presents difficult problems of control. Short of absolute elimination of the offending agent, control is usually based on the idea that some *maximum allowable concentration* (MAC) of a carcinogen exists which must not be exceeded. Carcinogens are also discussed on page 376.

ANTIDOTES OF ARSENIC AND HEAVY METAL POISONING

Dimercaprol (British Anti-Lewisite, BAL)

This compound was developed as an antidote for vesicants which contain arsenic. Peters and his co-workers in Oxford believed that the vesicant action of chlorarsines, such as lewisite, on the skin was due to their lipid solubility which enabled them to penetrate the keratin layer and after hydrolysis to produce the general action of arsenoxides on living cells. Simple chemical substances containing reactive thiol (—SH) groups might be expected to react with arsenicals and in this way protect the cell.

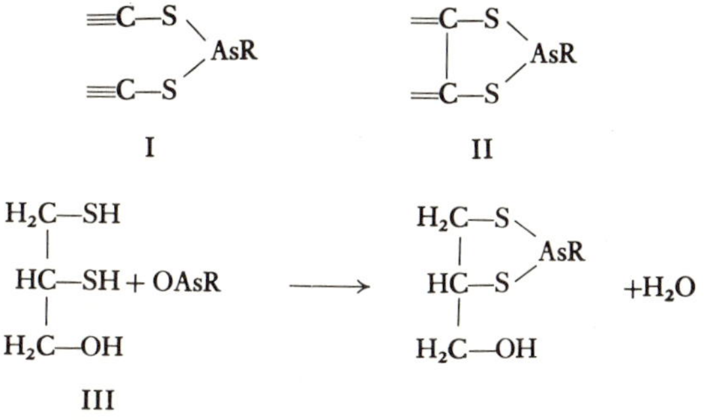

Fig. 39.5 Reaction of arsenic with thiol compounds.

They showed that arsenicals form more stable compounds with a dithiol (II) than with two molecules of a monothiol (I). The most effective dithiol compound was 2:3 dimercaptopropanol (III) to which the name BAL (British Anti-Lewisite) was given. The reaction of this compound with arsenoxide is shown in Figure 39.5.

Actions of dimercaprol

The effects of dimercaprol in arsenical poisoning are as follows:

1. Damage to the skin due to arsenical vesicants can be prevented by the previous application of BAL and can be arrested and probably reversed by applying BAL within two hours of contamination.

2. The systemic poisoning from oxophenarsine and other arsenicals can be prevented or counteracted by BAL.

Dimercaprol is also an effective antidote in poisoning by antimony, bismuth, mercury, gold, chromium and nickel but is relatively ineffective in lead poisoning.

Administration of dimercaprol

Dimercaprol is a colourless oil which is extremely irritant to mucous membranes. It is administered by intramuscular injection as a 5 or 10 per cent solution in arachis oil. It is rapidly metabolised and excreted in the urine in the form of a closely related compound. In doses of 2 to 3 mg/kg it produces no toxic effects but in higher doses it causes lachrimation, salivation, nausea, and a rise in blood pressure. These effects are greatest within 15 minutes of an injection and are transient.

Therapeutic uses

The prognosis of heavy metal poisoning especially with mercurial and arsenical compounds, has been considerably improved by the use of dimercaprol. Patients may recover from acute poisoning by mercuric chloride or mercurial diuretics after treatment with dimercaprol and a high proportion of patients with haemorrhagic encephalitis or exfoliative dermatitis due to organic arsenicals may respond to treatment with dimercaprol within two or three days.

In severe metallic poisoning intramuscular injections of 3 mg/kg are given at 4-hour intervals for 2 days; treatment is usually continued for about 10 days, the frequency of administration being gradually reduced to 2 injections daily.

Edetic acid (edathamil)

Ethylenediamine tetra-acetic acid forms water-soluble complexes with alkaline earths and heavy metals, the stability of which increases with the pH. This chelation process can become so complete that the cation loses its ionic characteristics. The order of binding preference of edetic acid increases from sodium and potassium to magnesium and calcium and to copper, nickel and lead. In sodium edetate two of the four valencies of edetic acid are occupied by sodium and this compound can be used to soften water by chelating calcium and magnesium; when sodium edetate is added to shed blood it prevents coagulation. When it is injected into an animal it combines with calcium to form a soluble stable complex; the calcium in consequence becomes unavailable to the tissues and hypocalcaemic tetany may result.

Sodium calcium edetate (Calcium disodium versenate)
In this compound two of the valencies of edetic acid are occupied by calcium. When sodium calcium edetate is administered it does not affect the serum calcium, but if lead or another heavy metal is present in the tissues, calcium is displaced from the compound and the corresponding heavy metal edetate is formed and excreted by the kideys (Fig. 39.7).

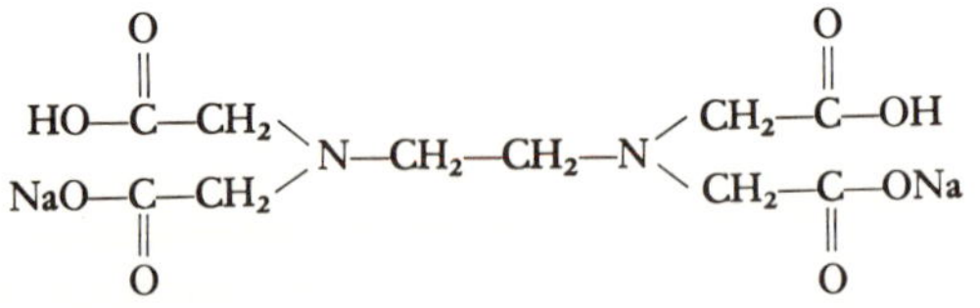

Fig. 39.6 Sodium edetate.

In lead poisoning sodium calcium edetate is administered intravenously in daily doses of 0.5 to 2 g, either as a slow intravenous drip or as injections every 6 hours. A course of treatment usually lasts 4 days and may be repeated after an interval of 2 days. This treatment produces rapid relief from colic and constipation, and an improvement in the central nervous symptoms of headache, irritability and tremors. This is accompanied by the excretion of several milligrams of lead each day in the urine and by a reduction in the punctate basophil count and urinary coproporphyrins.

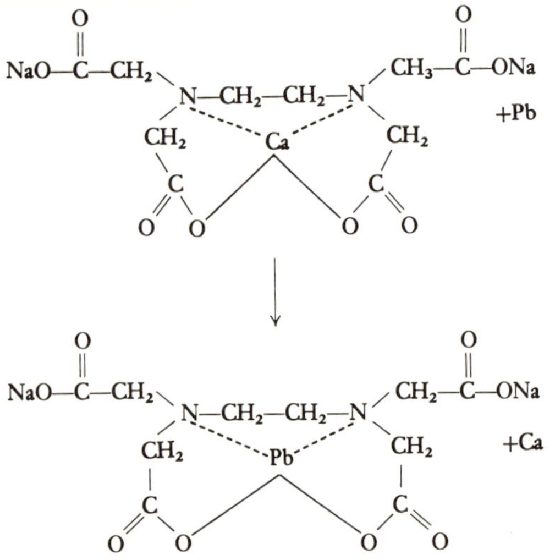

Fig. 39.7 Formation of disodium lead edetate from sodium calcium edetate.

Sodium calcium edetate can also be used for the treatment of poisoning by other metals such as plutonium and it has been used by local application to treat chrome ulceration of the skin. In arsenical and mercurial poisoning edetate is not as effective as dimercaprol.

Penicillamine
Penicillamine (dimethylcysteine) is a degradation product found in the urine of patients receiving penicillin.

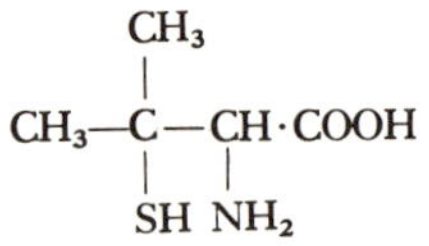

Fig. 39.8 D-Penicillamine.

As a thiol compound it chelates heavy metals. It has been shown to be a useful drug for the treatment of hepatolenticular degeneration (Wilson's disease), a genetically determined condition in which copper accumulates in the tissues, particularly in the brain and liver. After treatment with penicillamine there is a marked increase in the copper content of the urine and faeces of these patients.

Penicillamine is administered orally in doses of 300 mg, 3 or 4 times daily, and patients with Wilson's disease so treated usually begin to improve after about 3 months. It has also been administered in doses of 0.6–1 g daily, along with pyridoxine, for the treatment of cystinuria and of rheumatoid arthritis.

Its mode of action in the genetic condition of cystinuria is believed to be as follows. In this condition urinary calculi composed largely of cystine are formed. The D-penicillamine forms a penicillamine-cysteine disulphide that is about 50 times more soluble than cystine and can be excreted without forming calculi. D-penicillamine has been shown to benefit rheumatoid arthritis but its mode of action in this condition is not understood. In Wilson's disease D-penicillamine has advantages over dimercaprol and sodium calcium edetate since the former must be administered intramuscularly and often causes pain and discomfort whilst the latter, although useful when administered intravenously, is more toxic and less suitable than penicillamine for long term use. A disadvantage of penicillamine is that it occasionally causes an allergic sensitisation. D-penicillamine is used in preference to the L or DL forms as they inhibit pyridoxine and have caused optic neuritis.

Desferrioxamine
Desferrioxamine mesylate (Desferal) is a potent chelating agent which forms a soluble complex with iron. It is used in the treatment of acute iron poisoning (p. 205).

PREPARATIONS

Antidote to organophosphorus compounds
Pralidoxime mesylate 1 g slow i.v.

Chelating agents
Desferrioxamine mesylate (Desferal) 2 g i.m. 5 g p.o.
Penicillamine hyd (Cuprimine) 0.5–1 g p.o. d.l.
Sodium Calciumedetate (Ledclair) 4 g d.l. max

Insect repellents
Dibutyl phthalate
Diethyltoluamide (Metadelphene) 50–75% alc solution (mosquitoes, etc.)
Dimethylphthalate 40% cream (mosq repell)

Insecticides (pediculicides and scabicides) Ch. 21

FURTHER READING

Air Pollution and Health 1970 Report by Committee of Royal College of Physicians. Pitman, London
Deichmann W B (ed) 1973 Pesticides and the environment. Intercontinental Medical Book Corporation
Dinman B D 1974 The nature of occupational cancer. Thomas, Springfield
Fairchild E J (ed) 1978 Suspected carcinogens: A sourcebook of the toxic effects of chemical substances
Kahn M A, Haufe W O 1972 Toxicology, biodegradations and efficacy of livestock pesticides. Swets and Zeitlinger, Amsterdam
Further Review of Certain Persistent Organochlorine Pesticides used in Great Britain 1969 HMSO, London
Pesticides: benefits and dangers 1967 Proc. Roy. Soc. B. 761
World Health Organisation 1972 ARC Monographs on the evaluation of carcinogenic risks of chemical in man. 3 vols. WHO, Geneva

40. Control of population growth

Human populations and control of fertility 476; Hormonal contraceptives 476; Occlusive contraceptives 478; Intrauterine devices 478; Postcoital contraception 478; Medical and surgical methods of early termination 478; Contraceptives of the future 478; Immunisation against pregnancy 479; Male contraception 479.

Human populations and control of fertility

The size of the human population in any community or nation represents the balance between the death rate and the birth rate. In many countries in the western world the average annual death rate per 1000 inhabitants is approximately 10 and the corresponding figure for the birth rate 18, a net increase of 8, i.e. a rise in population of 0.8 per cent each year. In Great Britain the respective figures during recent years were 10 and 16 per thousand, which represents an annual population increase of 0.6 per cent. Very recently the population growth rate in Great Britain has been even lower. Similar low growth rates are found in several other countries of Western Europe; the growth rate in North America is 0.9 per cent. By contrast, several countries in South Asia, Africa and Latin America have growth rates around 2.6 per cent.

Since in many countries the annual death rate from malnutrition, infectious and other diseases has been consistently reduced because of improved food supplies and the use of effective drug therapy, an increase in population is inevitable, even if the birth rate remains the same. It has been estimated that, if present population trends continue, at the end of this century the total world population will be about 6500 millions, approximately double the size in 1970. There are, of course, considerable differences between countries in the annual rise in population but it is axiomatic that unless each country establishes an effective balance between its rise in population and the food supplies and other resources necessary for its maintenance, serious problems of famine, disease and destitution will inevitably follow. The most rational solution to the 'population explosion' is the development and use of appropriate methods for controlling the birth rate.

Family planning is a comprehensive term which includes the planning of pregnancies so that they occur at the desired time, the spacing of births for the optimum health of all family members and the prevention of further births when the family has reached the desirable total size. The general aim of family planning is to regulate fertility so as to promote the physical, mental and social well-being of the child, parents and other members of the family unit. This involves, in addition to the provision of information about different methods of fertility regulation, the integration of health education and general education services.

Hormonal contraceptives

Contraceptive steroids (p. 357) are currently available for oral administration (the 'pill') as combined formulations of oestrogen and progestogen or of progestogen alone (mini-pill). The daily administration of a progestogen in combination with a small dose of an oestrogen from the 5th to the 25th day of the cycle will prevent conception. Two to 4 days after completing the schedule of treatment, withdrawal bleeding occurs and the next cycle of treatment is begun on the 5th day after the beginning of bleeding. Sequential oral contraceptive methods in which oestrogen alone is administered in the beginning of the cycle followed by an oestrogen-progestogen combination at the end of the cycle are also effective but they are now considered to be less appropriate. They are slightly less effective than the oestrogen-progestogen method and there have been reports suggesting an increased incidence of endometrial pathology amongst users.

Progestogen-only products are taken daily continuously without interruption. The progestogen-only contraceptives make the cervical mucus thick and scanty during the whole cycle and may thus prevent the passage of the sperm and implantation of the ovum. Ovulation is often undisturbed. This method is not as effective as the combined method, but the absence of oestrogen diminishes the risk of thrombosis and the undesirable effects on metabolism.

Slow-release preparations of progestogens for subcutaneous implantation are currently under clinical trial.

In spite of the lessened risk of thromboembolic disease the progestogen-only preparations are less acceptable to some women. Menstrual patterns are often altered by the continuous use of these preparations. Unpredictable breakthrough bleeding and intermenstrual bleeding may occur throughout the duration of their use and short cycles are common.

Statistically it has been shown that if the combination contraceptive tablets are taken correctly without any omission the pregnancy rate is extremely low (about 0.1% i.e. 0.1 pregnancies per 100 women per year), whilst with progestogen alone it is significantly greater (about 2.5 pregnancies per 100 women per year).

Mode of action. The precise mechanism of action of these steroid contraceptives is not yet fully understood. The main factor is probably inhibition of ovulation by blocking the release of the luteinising hormone of the pituitary through an action on the hypothalamus. Other factors which may be involved are interference with the action of gonadotrophins on the ovarian follicle, alteration of the endometrium which prevents implantation and changes in the cervical mucus which impair penetration of the spermatozoa.

The successful use of steroid contraceptives depends on strict observance of the schedule of administration, particularly when the sequential method is used.

Benefits of oral contraceptives
The most important beneficial effect of 'the pill' is its remarkable efficacy which, coupled with a high degree of acceptability, has given many women a new freedom from anxiety about the risk of unplanned pregnancy. In addition, oral contraceptives have other well-documented beneficial effects. They tend to suppress some menstrual disorders such as menorrhagia and dysmenorrhoea. They have been shown to inhibit the development of benign lumps in the breast and ovarian cysts occur less frequently. Finally there is some evidence that oral contraceptives may diminish the risk of peptic ulceration.

Adverse reactions
During the initial stages of using oestrogen-progestogen hormonal contraceptives transient nausea often occurs but seldom persists. Other occasional side effects are headache, abdominal bloating, breast tenderness and a gain in body weight. Irregular slight vaginal bleeding may occur and if persistent must be investigated. More serious adverse effects are thromboembolic episodes, including cerebral and coronary thrombosis, pulmonary embolism and thrombophlebitis which have been reported in a small proportion of patients. Impairment of hepatic function has also been reported. Epidemiological studies have shown that a positive relationship exists between oestrogen dose of the pill and the risk of thromboembolism, and that contraceptives with a low oestrogen content are safer from that point of view than those with a high oestrogen content. For this reason the usual dose of oestrogen is now seldom greater than 50 μg daily.

There is no statistical evidence that the use of oral contraceptives increases the risk of cancer of the breast of the cervix or the uterus. The occurrence of vaginal carcinoma in young women, whose mothers had taken doses of at least 25 mg of stilboestrol daily during pregnancy has been reported in the United States. The Committee on Safety of Medicines have not received any reports of similar cases in the United Kingdom.

Contraindications
The results of many clinical trials and epidemiological studies on the immediate and long-term effect of hormonal contraceptives make it clear that in view of their side effects, these drugs should be prescribed with caution and their users should be kept under observation. The decision if an oestrogen-progestogen contraceptive or some other method should be used must be based on the medical history and social conditions of the individual. The decision to provide 'free contraception' in the National Health Service in Great Britain will require a detailed information service readily available to all potential users of contraceptive steroids about the possible risks, and the symptoms and side effects about which they should seek further medical attention. In general the decision is relatively straightforward for healthy women, but for growing adolescent girls the effects of continous administration of these steroids have not yet been fully assessed. For women with established illness or with a known or suspected predisposition to a particular disease, the balance of benefit and risk compared with other contraceptive methods may be difficult to decide. There is sufficient evidence, however, to show that in certain circumstances, combined steroid contraceptives should not be used. These include cholestatic jaundice of pregnancy, recurrent cholestasis and chronic familial jaundice; acute intermittent porphyria, pruritus of pregnancy and premenopausal cancer of the breast. Considerable caution must also be exercised in any decision to prescribe these drugs for patients with a history of venous or arterial thromboembolism, hypertension arising from different causes, congestive cardiac failure, liver disease or blood dyscrasias and diabetes mellitus whether established or potential. There is statistical evidence that thromboembolic complications are considerably more frequent in women taking oral contraceptives in the age group 35-49 than in the age group 20-34.

Since steroid contraceptives are known to influence carbohydrate and lipid metabolism, gain in weight is a common finding and must be taken into account; in obese individuals the use of these compounds may increase the potential hazards of diabetes, hypertension and occlusive vascular disease.

Migraine attacks and persistent headaches are associated with continued use of oral contraceptives and manifestations of latent epilepsy are an important indication for discontinuing this form of contraception.

Advantages and disadvantages of progestogen implants
The slow release progestogen implants have the advantage that as no synthetic oestrogens are used, the metabolic effects usually associated with oral contraceptives are avoided. Their main disadvantage is that they tend to produce unpredictable bleeding. The bleeding is generally light but the long periods of bleeding and spotting makes acceptance low in populations used to regular menstrual bleeding.

Other forms of contraception in the female

Occlusive contraceptives

Several types of physical methods are designed to prevent fertilisation in the female. They include the use of cervical caps or diaphragms; it is generally accepted that the contraceptive success rate is enhanced if they are used in conjunction with a contraceptive cream or jelly.

The diaphragm has few adverse or beneficial 'medical' effects of any importance although there is evidence that it may increase the risk of urinary tract infection and decrease the risk of cancer of the cervix, but its use is associated with an appreciable chance of unplanned pregnancy.

Intrauterine devices (IUD)

The antifertility effect of a foreign body in the uterus has long been recognised. Evidence from animal experiments and from human studies suggests that the principal mechanism of action of intrauterine foreign bodies is to stimulate leucocyte mobilisation in the uterus and prevent nidation of normal blastocytes. The antifertility effectiveness of an IUD seems to depend more on the nature of the material of which it is composed and the leucocyte responses it elicits in the uterus, than on its size and shape. Recent types consist of a slender T-shaped polyethylene strip with a surface area of about 200 mm^2, containing a thin copper wire around the vertical limb of the T. The daily release of metallic copper by ionisation in the uterine cavity is approximately 30 micrograms. During prolonged clinical trials no endometrial changes indicative of a carcinogenic action of the copper have been reported.

The antifertility success rate of the IUD is very good but statistically somewhat less than combined steroid contraceptives and the fact that the IUD requires insertion by a medical expert detracts from its utility in the developing world. Its acceptance has been increasing with the introduction of smaller devices. It has the advantage of maintenance of normal ovulatory patterns and of a prolonged action, although expulsion of the IUD, especially in teenagers, occurs fairly frequently.

Adverse IUD reactions

Uterine perforation which results in the translocation of part or all of the IUD into the abdominal cavity is fortunately rare. Prompt surgical removal from the abdominal cavity is essential.

Bleeding and pain. Although women with IUDs have normal ovulatory patterns they generally exhibit an increased loss of blood during menstruation. Pain frequently occurs especially during the first few weeks after insertion. Both are common reasons for removal of the device.

Infections. Pelvic inflammatory disease due to deposition of bacteria during insertion of the IUD may occur.

Ectopic pregnancy. The IUDs have little or no protective effect against extrauterine pregnancies. There is a relatively high incidence of ectopic gestation among women using an intrauterine device.

Postcoital contraception.

The reliability of stilboestrol as a 'morning after' pill to prevent pregnancy after sexual intercourse, has been investigated. The results of two trials have recently been reported in which women of child-bearing age were instructed to take within 72 hours of sexual intercourse, a course of treatment with 25 mg of stiboestrol twice daily for 5 days. No pregnancies occurred in 1000 patients who followed these instructions but 50 per cent had transient typical side-effects of the drug.

The mechanism of this antifertility action is not fully understood but is probably due to an inhibition of endometrial implantation or to an increase in the speed of ovum transport through the genital tract. This use of stilboestrol should be regarded as an emergency type of treatment and not as a routine method of contraception.

Medical and surgical methods of early termination of pregnancy

Evaluating abortion techniques has made it abundantly clear that the earlier in pregnancy an abortion is performed the better, as both the mental and physical complications are substantially reduced. Besides the usual method of uterine curettage two newer methods have been used.

Prostaglandins. Naturally occurring prostaglandins and their analogues administered by the intrauterine route are effective in producing an early termination of pregnancy (p. 222). The method is associated with a high incidence of side effects, it requires premedication and medical supervision is essential.

Suction evacuation. This method, if carried out at up to six weeks of amenorrhoea, is referred to as menstrual extraction. Under local anaesthesia a curette attached to a syringe is introduced through the cervical canal into the uterus. The uterus is then evacuated by withdrawing the plunger of the syringe.

Sterilisation

Voluntary sterilisation has emerged as a viable alternative method of birth control.

Contraceptives of the future

This was the title of a Royal Society discussion held in London in 1976. In spite of the remarkable contraceptive success rate of the pill, if properly used, it has certain serious health risks mentioned earlier. Furthermore it is not an ideally simple method of family planning suitable for the needs of the developing world. Considered below are two possible new developments in the field of contraception which were discussed at the Royal Society discussion.

I. *Immunisation against pregnancy*
Experimental immunisation against pregnancy has been achieved in primates through the production of antibodies against the ß subunit of chorionic gonadotrophin. As discussed on page 325, gonadotrophins consist of α and ß subunits. The α subunit is immunologically similar in luteinising hormone (LH), follicle stimulating hormone (FSH), thyroid stimulating hormone (TSH) and human chorionic gonadotrophin (HCG), whilst the ß subunit is immunologically specific to each hormone. Chorionic gonadotrophin is essential for the maintenance of pregnancy in primates. It probably acts as part of the luteotrophic stimulus maintaining the production of progesterone by the corpus luteum during the first few weeks until the placenta itself secretes sufficient progesterone to support pregnancy.

Specific antibodies have been produced that are capable of reacting with HCG without cross-reacting with LH and FSH. They have been employed for active and passive immunisation in marmoset monkeys. Marmosets actively immunised against the ß-HCG subunit in early pregnancy, aborted within 25 days and then resumed apparently normal ovarian cycles, indicating that the circulating antibodies were not cross-reacting with endogenous LH or FSH. Passive immunisation of marmosets with anti-HCG-ß antiserum during early pregnancy caused abortion within hours or days.

It has not been possible, so far, to use these immunological methods for the control of human pregnancy. They may, however, represent a possible means of contraception in the future.

II. *Male contraception*
The development of an effective contraceptive technique for men, other than the condom and the potentially irreversible vasectomy, presents another future possibility for contraception. There are several potential sites for contraceptive action in males. Male fertility may be temporarily interrupted by: (1) interference with the hormonal control of the testis, (2) a direct action of agents on spermatogenesis and (3) interference with the acquisition of fertilising ability once the sperm leaves the testis.

Interference with hormonal control of the testis
The spermatogenic process is dependent on hormonal stimulation by the pituitary gland via FSH and LH. FSH is believed to be necessary for the spermatogenic process, whilst LH is responsible for the control of steroidogenesis by the interstitial cells of the testis, the testosterone thus produced supporting the spermatogenic process.

The secretion of FSH and LH by the pituitary is in turn controlled by the testis through a feedback mechanism. It seems likely that complete separation of the feedback control of FSH and LH is not possible. Whether the negative feedback action on the pituitary gland is direct, or indirect via the hypothalamus and its gonadotrophic releasing hormone (LHRH) remains unknown. There is no doubt, however, that the decapeptide LHRH can stimulate the pituitary gland to produce both LH and FSH.

The principal attempts to disrupt spermatogenesis by hormonal mechanisms have rested on interfering with the secretion of gonadotrophic hormones by the pituitary gland. From a clinical point of view it is essential to achieve this without the loss of libido and potency.

Androgens. The action of testosterone in suppressing the secretion of LH and FSH by the pituitary is well documented by radioimmunoassay. Figure 40.1 shows that testosterone proprionate injected intramuscularly in a dose of 25 mg daily in male volunteers produced azoospermia within 60 days in all 7 men treated. In all volunteers no loss of libido and potency occurred and sperm counts returned to normal by 150 days. These effects were achieved by intramuscular injection of testosterone and no detailed studies are available whether similar effects can be produced by oral preparations which are considerably less active as androgens.

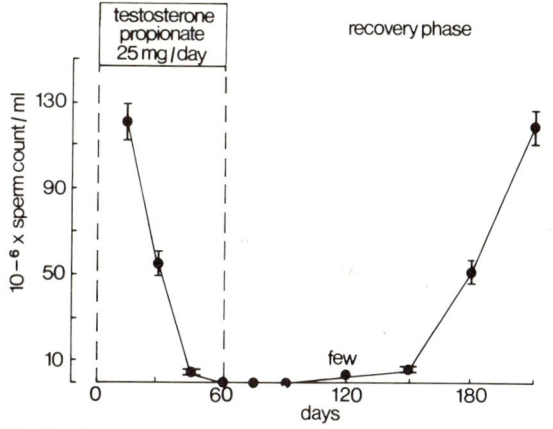

Fig. 40.1 Mean sperm count in seven volunteers treated with 25 mg testosterone proprionate daily. (After de Kretzer, Proc. R. Soc. B. 1976. Data by Reddy & Rao.)

Oestrogens and progestogens. Both produce reversible azoospermia but this is generally accompanied by a loss of male sexual function unless these drugs are combined with testosterone administration. Oestrogens may also produce gynaecomastia and thromboembolic complications.

Spermatogenic disruption by agents affecting the testis directly
Cytotoxic agents such as the alkylating agents interfere with spermatogenesis but they have effects on other tissues such as bone marrow which preclude their use as male contraceptives. Their application may damage the spermatogenic compartment irreversibly.

The compound *5-thio-D-glucose* has been shown to inhibit spermatogenesis in male mice which recovers after cessation of the drug. The compound has not, so far, been used clinically in man.

Interference with sperm maturation
Spermatozoa released from the seminiferous epithelium do not have the ability to fertilise ova, but acquire this capability during passage through the epididymis. Sperm collected in the caput epididymis are therefore unable to fertilise ova, but those collected from the caudal region have this capability. The possibility of interrupting the process of epididymal sperm *maturation* and thus preventing the development of the fertilising ability of sperm presents a theoretical method of male contraception. No compound has so far been definitely shown to operate by this mechanism, however.

A simple monochloroderivative of glycerol α-*chlorhydrin* which is capable of inducing temporary sterility in various animals, including monkeys may possibly work by this mechanism. But it has been found to produce bone marrow lesions in monkeys.

In conclusion it appears that the best prospect of an oral contraceptive for men in the near future is through the interruption of spermatogenesis by hormonal mechanisms using androgens either alone or in combination with progestogens and oestrogens, but the method of androgen administration and the type of androgen replacement remain unsatisfactory at present.

FURTHER READING

Contraceptives of the future (A discussion meeting.) 1976 Proc. R. Soc. B.
Hawkins D F, Elder M G 1979 Human fertility control. Butterworths, London
Swyer G I M (ed) 1970 Control of human fertility. Br. med. Bull. 26:1

PREPARATIONS

Oral contraceptives

Preparations containing only progestogens

Trade name	Progestogen	
Femulen	Ethynodiol Diacetate	500 μg
Micronor	Norethisterone	350 μg
Microval	Levonorgestrel	30 μg
Neogest	Norgestrel	75 μg
Noriday	Norethisterone	350 μg

Preparations containing less than 50 μg of Oestrogen

Trade name	Oestrogen		Progestogen	
Brevinor	Ethinyloestradiol	35 μg	Norethisterone	500 μg
Conova 30	Ethinyloestradiol	30 μg	Ethynodiol Diacetate	2 mg
Eugynon 30	Ethinyloestradiol	30 μg	Levonorgestrel	250 μg
Loestrin 20	Ethinyloestradiol	20 μg	Norethisterone Acetate	1 mg
Microgynon 30	Ethinyloestradiol	30 μg	Levonorgestrel	150 μg
Norimin	Ethinyloestradiol	35 μg	Norethisterone	1 mg
Ovran 30	Ethinyloestradiol	30 μg	Levonorgestrel	250 μg
Ovranette	Ethinyloestradiol	30 μg	Levonorgestrel	150 μg
Ovysmen	Ethinyloestradiol	35 μg	Norethisterone	500 μg

Preparations containing 50 μg of Oestrogen

Trade name	Oestrogen		Progestogen	
Anovlar 21	Ethinyloestradiol	50 μg	Norethisterone Acetate	4 mg
Demulen 50	Ethinyloestradiol	50 μg	Ethynodiol Diacetate	500 μg
Eugynon 50	Ethinyloestradiol	50 μg	Norgestrel	500 μg
Gynovlar 21	Ethinyloestradiol	50 μg	Norethisterone Acetate	3 mg
Minilyn	Ethinyloestradiol	50 μg	Lynoestrenol	2.5 mg
Minovlar	Ethinyloestradiol	50 μg	Norethisterone Acetate	1 mg
Minovlar ED*	Ethinyloestradiol	50 μg	Norethisterone Acetate	1 mg
Norinyl-1	Mestranol	50 μg	Norethisterone	1 mg
Norinyl-1/28*	Mestranol	50 μg	Norethisterone	1 mg
Norlestrin	Ethinyloestradiol	50 μg	Norethisterone Acetate	5 mg
Orlest 21	Ethinyloestradiol	50 μg	Norethisterone Acetate	1 mg
Ortho-Novin 1/50	Mestranol	50 μg	Norethisterone	1 mg
Ovran	Ethinyloestradiol	50 μg	Norgestrel	500 μg
Ovulen 50	Ethinyloestradiol	50 μg	Ethynodiol Diacetate	1 mg

*These brands include some inert tablets in the packs for use during part of the menstrual cycle.

41. Drug dependence

Addiction and habituation 481; Social aspects of drug dependence 481; Types of drug dependence 481; Mechanism of drug dependence 482; Opiates 482; Amphetamine 483; Cocaine 484; General c.n.s. depressants 484; Absorption and metabolism of ethyl alcohol 484; Actions of alcohol on c.n.s. 485; Medicolegal aspects 486; Chronic alcoholism 487; Disulfiram 487; Methanol 488; Barbiturate dependence 488; LSD 488; Cannabis 489; Tobacco dependence 490; Treatment and prevention of drug dependence 491.

Addiction and habituation

Man has displayed a remarkable ingenuity in finding drugs which produce actions on the central nervous system. Primitive tribes have discovered independently the most varied methods for producing alcohol by fermentation, and most racial groups have also discovered some source from which they can produce drinks containing caffeine and related compounds. The uses of hashish, coca leaves, opium and tobacco to provide pleasurable relief of pain, hunger and fatigue were all discovered by primitive people, who also recognised the addictive properties of these substances. As civilisation has increased in complexity, drug addiction has become a serious problem.

Drug addiction has been defined as a state of chronic intoxication which is produced by the repeated administration of a drug and which is detrimental to the individual and to society. The addict is under a compulsion to continue taking the drug and to increase the dose. This leads to psychological and sometimes physical dependence on the effects of the drug so that the life of the addict eventually becomes dominated by the need to secure continued supplies of the drug.

Three factors may be involved in drug addiction: (1) *tolerance* whereby increasing amounts of the drug are required to produce the same effect; (2) *physical dependence* whereby the body adapts to the drug and various abnormal reactions, termed withdrawal symptoms, occur when administration of the drug is abruptly stopped; and (3) *psychic dependence* whereby the drug produces a feeling of satisfaction and pleasure such as to require its periodic or continuous administration to maintain the sense of pleasure or to avoid discomfort.

The term 'drug addiction' itself has given rise to considerable discussion, and the WHO Expert Committee on the subject has suggested abandoning it altogether as well as the term 'habituation' in favour of 'drug dependence'.

The term 'drug abuse' is frequently used in relation to addictive drugs, especially in the American literature. Important drugs that are frequently abused and may produce dependence include morphine and related derivatives, whether natural, semisynthetic or wholly synthetic; the c.n.s. depressants such as barbiturates and other sedative-hypnotics, and to a lesser extent the minor tranquillisers, and, most importantly, alcohol; stimulants of the c.n.s. including amphetamines and cocaine, and hallucinogenic drugs including LSD and cannabis.

The characteristic features of drug dependence vary with the type of drug involved. For example caffeine and related compounds which are present in tea and coffee are capable of producing drug dependence but in most societies this is not regarded as harmful. On the other hand other types of drugs, such as those described above, can produce substantial stimulation or depression of the central nervous system which result in a disturbance of perception, mood, behaviour and motor function such as to cause serious problems for the individual and the community in which he lives.

Types of drug dependence

A convenient method of classifying dependence-producing drugs according to various prototype agents is listed in Table 41.1.

Table 41.1 Types of dependence-producing drugs (from Youth and Drugs, WHO Report No. 516 (1973))

Type	Compounds
Alcohol-barbiturate	Ethanol, barbiturates and other hypnotics and sedatives, e.g. benzodiazepines
Amphetamine	Amphetamine, dexamphetamine, methylamphetamine, methylphenidate and phenmetrazine
Cannabis	Preparations of *Cannabis sativa*, e.g. marihuana and hashish
Opiates	Opium, morphine, heroin, methadone, pethidine, etc.
Cocaine	Cocaine and coca leaves
Hallucinogens	Lysergic acid diethylamide (LSD), mescaline and psilocybin
Volatile compounds	Acetone, carbon tetrachloride and other solvents, e.g. 'glue sniffing'.
Nicotine	Tobacco, snuffs

Social aspects of drug dependence

Throughout the world, drug dependence has long been associated with the use of drugs for ritual, recreational and social purposes and to a much less extent for medical practice. At one time drugs were traditionally taken in certain geographical regions, for example cannabis in parts of the Indian and African continents, coca leaves in South America, opium in South East Asia and some Eastern Mediterranean countries, and alcohol and tobacco smoking in the western hemisphere and Europe. Their pattern of use was often associated with middle and older age groups and sometimes with poor social and economic conditions. In more recent years, however, substantial changes have taken place in the mobility of populations, their standard of living and their attitude to traditional habits and customs. There is now a greater variety of both naturally occurring and synthetic drugs in different countries and a much greater participation in their use by younger age groups. Moreover there has been an increasing trend to use several types of drugs either concurrently or sequentially. In European and North American countries and Japan the natural curiosity of young people has been stimulated by various sources of information and propaganda to experiment more freely in the use of many of these substances. Although the drugs most likely to be tried first are tobacco, alcohol and cannabis, their smell and ready detection is often regarded by many young persons and older ones as a serious disadvantage to continued experimentation in their use and they may then try amphetamine and barbiturates or mixtures of these and alcohol.

It has become clear that such experimentation does not necessarily lead to the development of clearly established evidence of psychic or physical dependence. The episodic use of alcohol for a few hours or several days is well known and a similar 'spree' use of amphetamines, cannabis and barbiturates occurs. These occasions do not inevitably lead to a consistent pattern of established use.

One of the more disturbing features of episodic use, however, is the possibility of a lasting impression on persons who may later become the subject of psychic or physical stresses. The pharmacological reaction between the drug and the drug-taker and the interaction between the drug-taker and his environment may have unpredictable end-results which may later involve the individual in seeking recourse to more frequent self-treatment with drugs to combat depression, frustration and other forms of social and economic stress.

Mechanism of drug dependence

In spite of much research and theoretical speculation, the basic mechanisms of drug dependence remain unclear. Most speculation has dealt with morphine tolerance and dependence and the morphine abstinence syndrome. Morphine is known to inhibit the release of the cholinergic transmitter in guinea pig gut and it has been suggested that morphine may also reduce transmitter release within the c.n.s. The inhibition of transmitter release by morphine may cause a form of denervation supersensitivity which is normally counterbalanced by a reduced transmitter output, but if morphine is suddenly withdrawn and the normal output of transmitter is restored this acts on a supersensitive receptor system causing the abstinence syndrome.

According to Way, serotonin (5HT) may be involved in the development of morphine tolerance and dependence. A reduction of serotonin synthesis by p-chlorophenylalanine which blocks its metabolic formation, interferes with the development of tolerance to morphine, whereas stimulation of serotonin synthesis by administering its precursor 5-hydroxytryptophan, promotes the development of morphine tolerance and physical dependence.

PATTERNS OF HUMAN DRUG DEPENDENCE
Opiates

The pharmacology of opiates is discussed on page 279, and the concept of opiate receptors on page 241.

Dependence on opium, morphine and related compounds such as heroin and other synthetic analgesics for example pethidine and methadone may be acquired in various ways which differ according to different national or regional customs. The traditional pattern of opiate use in Britain until the early 1960s involved about 400 adults of mature years who became dependent in the course of medical treatment or as a result of their professional access to these drugs as members of the medical, dental and nursing professions. A similar situation obtained also in other European countries and in the U.S.A., though the number of addicted persons was greater. In South East Asia and in some countries east of the Mediterranean, where there was extensive cultivation of poppies, the non-medical use of opium was widespread. For example in Iran with a population of about 30 million people, it has been estimated that there are about 85 000 registered opium users and from 150 000 to 500 000 unregistered users mostly middle-aged and older men, who consume the drug orally or by smoking.

Since then new trends have been observed in most countries in the use of opiates; heroin, for example, is now being increasingly taken by persons in the younger age groups in most countries of the world, seldom as a result of medical treatment, usually after initial experimentation with one or several types of other dependence-producing drugs.

Tolerance to opiates is rapidly produced; for example if morphine is given several times daily to a patient to produce a specific effect, such as relief of pain, the dose has to be increased after a week or two in order to produce the original effect. At about the same time both psychic and physical dependence is established and if the drug is abruptly withheld the patient feels distressed. The longer the administration continues the greater becomes the tolerance and the more severe the dependence. A similar condition results, but much more rapidly, when heroin is used intravenously for non-medical reasons. After dependence is acquired, a compulsion to continue taking the drug arises, not so much because it produces pleasure but because lack of it results in acute misery. Opiates produce a feeling of relaxation and contentment in dependent individuals who have no particular wish for the company of others but desire to be left alone.

Prolonged administration either to animals or human individuals can produce an extraordinary tolerance to opiates, for example many times the usual lethal dose can be given parenterally without producing any immediate serious adverse effects. It is quite common for addicts to take 4 g morphine daily or intravenous injections of 10-20 mg of heroin every 2 or 3 hours. An interesting feature of this tolerance is the fact that some parts of the central nervous system respond to the drug in the usual way, whilst others do not. Thus morphine in the dog produces, normally, slowing of the pulse, vomiting and sleep. When a dog is made tolerant to morphine, a dose 100 times greater than the original effective dose will not produce vomiting or sleep, but the original dose will still cause slowing of the pulse. Tolerance is also associated with an increased ability of the tissues to metabolise this drug to less active compounds.

The heroin or morphine addict suffers a general degradation of character and will power. He loses his sense of moral responsibility, and will do anything in order to obtain the drug. His general health suffers considerably; he is often emaciated and suffers particularly from gastric and intestinal disorders. The effects of opium smoking and opium eating are much less catastrophic than addiction to morphine or heroin. There is no doubt that opium smoking and eating are serious social evils, but it cannot be said that in all cases they cause rapid degeneration.

Withdrawal syndrome. If heroin or morphine is abruptly withdrawn from an addict, a charcteristic abstinence syndrome develops. This has been described by Isbell and White, as follows. During the first 12 to 14 hours of abstinence there are no obvious symptoms or signs; then occasional yawning, light perspiration, rhinorrhoea and mild lacrimation are likely to appear. The addict usually goes into an abnormal tossing, restless sleep (the 'yen'). After 18 to 24 hours of abstinence the patient awakens and, thereafter, has insomnia. Yawning, rhinorrhoea, lacrimation and perspiration become much more marked; dilatation of the pupils and recurring waves of gooseflesh are seen. Twitching of various muscle groups occurs. The patient complains bitterly of severe aches in the back and legs and of hot and cold 'flashes'. The addict usually curls up in bed, his knees drawn up to his abdomen and covers himself with as many blankets as he can find, even though the weather may be hot. He continuously twitches his feet.

After about 36 hours restlessness becomes extreme; the addict moves from side to side in the bed, gets in and out of bed and is constantly in motion. Frequently this hyperactivity leads to chafing of the skin on the elbows and knees. The patient begins to retch, vomit and have diarrhoea. Concomitantly, the intensity of all the other signs increases and the addict is unable to sleep. Relentless insomnia may persist for as long as a week. He eats and drinks very little and loses weight rapidly, sometimes as much as 10 lb in 24 hours. He becomes dishevelled, unkempt, unshaven, dirty and extremely miserable. Respiration usually increases, particularly in depth, blood pressure rises 15-30 mmHg and body temperature is elevated about 1°C. Symptoms reach peak intensity 48 hours after the last dose of morphine is administered, remain intense until the 72nd hour of abstinence and then begin to decline. After 7 to 10 days all objective signs of abstinence have disappeared, although the patient may still complain of insomnia, weakness, nervousness and muscle aches and pains for several weeks.

Dependence on related analgesic drugs. The general picture of dependence on these drugs resembles that of morphine. The differences depend mainly on the potency and duration of action of the drugs. Heroin is more powerful but its duration of action is less than that of morphine, hence the number of doses required each day is greater and the duration of the abstinence syndrome is shorter. Drugs with a longer duration of action such as levorphanol produce a more prolonged abstinence syndrome. Tolerance to methadone develops more slowly than that to morphine and the abstinence syndrome is less severe. Dependence on pethidine also occurs, especially in doctors and nurses. It causes more dizziness and a greater degree of elation than morphine.

The use of methadone to support morphine withdrawal. Since methadone can prevent or relieve acute withdrawal symptoms of morphine and morphine-like drugs it has been used orally in the detoxification treatment of morphine or heroin-dependent patients. The withdrawal of methadone itself produces symptoms which are less intense but more prolonged than those produced by withdrawal of morphine. Methadone is also used orally in the maintenance treatment of some morphine addicts (p. 491).

c.n.s. stimulants

Amphetamine

Amphetamine and related drugs (p. 262) were introduced into medical practice for the relief of fatigue and mental depression and as appetite suppressants in the treatment of obesity. Unfortunately abuse of amphetamine-like drugs often occurs in neurotic and depressed housewives who begin using the drug on medical prescription; the abuse is seen even more extensively in teenagers who seek the excitement and euphoric effects of these substances by obtaining them illegally. The desire to continue taking the drug leads to psychic dependence and the consumption of increasing amounts to obtain greater excitatory and euphoric effects leads to tolerance, such that amphetamine dependence has now become an increasingly important social phenomenon.

The high degree of tolerance developed to these drugs by some individuals leads to the daily consumption of several hundred milligrams by mouth and to the more serious and hazardous practice of intravenous injection of preparations intended only for oral administration. Severe overdosage and deaths have resulted from this use and also from intravenous methylamphetamine by addicts seeking rapid effects ('speed'). Another danger of amphetamine dependence is that to obtain the large doses necessary to satisfy their needs, addicts may resort to thieving and other antisocial behaviour.

Violent behaviour and the onset of a psychotic state are the two most common untoward effects of amphetamine action. Of all drug-induced psychotic states, amphetamine psychosis most closely resembles endogenous paranoid schizophrenia. Compulsive behaviour and visual and auditory hallucinations have been reported in amphetamine abusers and the rate of disappearance of delusions closely parallels the rate of urinary excretion of the amphetamines. About 10 per cent of those who develop an amphetamine psychosis fail to recover completely and continue to exhibit psychotic traits such as extreme suspicion towards everyone even after many months.

Rapid withdrawal can cause abnormalities in the e.e.g. and a state of profound lassitude and depression leading to suicide.

Cocaine

For several centuries the chewing of coca leaves has been a traditional custom in certain Andean regions of South America and it is estimated that about six million inhabitants in these areas follow this practice without serious harmful effects. About 1880 the alkaloid cocaine was introduced as a cure for morphine dependence in America and Europe but it was soon discovered that the cure was worse than the disease. Cocaine abuse became a serious problem, users either sniffing the powder or injecting it intravenously for greater effect; in recent years there has been an extension of this abuse to many parts of the western hemisphere.

The behavioural effects of cocaine resemble those produced by amphetamine, but they persist for a shorter period. Frequent use of cocaine as a snuff produces irritation of the nasal mucous membrane and because of its local anaesthetic action perforation of the nasal septum may result from unrestrained nose picking.

General depressants of the c.n.s.

Alcohol (ethyl alcohol), sedatives and hypnotics all produce sedation and sleep and they also all show a common pattern of dependence and abstinence. The similarity of the abstinence syndrome, which follows the abuse of barbiturates and that following alcohol abuse, was first clearly demonstrated in a clinical study by Isbell and colleagues carried out in 1950. These workers administered large daily doses of barbiturates to human subjects during three to four months. Sudden cessation of barbiturate administration in these subjects provoked a withdrawal syndrome closely similar to abstinence in severe alcoholism including the production of delirium tremens. It is now realised that similar patterns of withdrawal may occur in abusers of other sedative-hypnotic drugs including those taking excessive doses of 'minor tranquillisers'. All these drugs exhibit the following common features of dependence and abstinence:

1. Whilst these drugs are all potentially addicting their daily intake must be prolonged and exceed a certain threshold value for physical dependence to develop. For example with pentobarbitone, severe withdrawal symptoms are seen only after doses of at least 600 mg per day. If withdrawal symptoms occur they are often severe and may even lead to death.

2. Some degree of tolerance develops to these drugs but is not nearly as great as tolerance to opiates. Chronic alcoholics show less behavioural disturbance when they can consume alcohol and they also develop patterns of behaviour which help to hide the signs of intoxication. Some metabolic tolerance develops both to alcohol and barbiturates but there has been no evidence that the lethal doses producing respiratory paralysis are different in alcoholics and normals.

3. It is now widely agreed that physical dependence on the effects of alcohol, barbiturates and other sedative-hypnotics can develop and that the craving for these drugs may become overwhelming. A barbiturate addict will persistently demand more drug even when he is so intoxicated that he cannot walk.

The typical withdrawal syndrome for this type of drug has been most clearly established for alcohol. It can be divided into three stages. In the first stage (the 'shakes') the patient is trembling, sweating and complaining of anxiety. He may also begin to 'see' and 'hear' things (acute alcoholic hallucinosis). In the second stage, occurring only in some subjects, seizures resembling *grand mal* may occur. The third stage is one of agitated delirium (delirium tremens) in which all insight is lost. The patient is extremely agitated and may describe bizarre delusions. This is a serious and potentially fatal stage often accompanied by peripheral vascular collapse.

Central pharamacology of alcohol

Absorption and metabolism of ethyl alcohol

Alcohol is absorbed more rapidly than most substances from the alimentary canal and it is absorbed in considerable quantities from the stomach. When an ordinary dose of alcohol is given by mouth, about one-quarter is absorbed in the stomach and the rest in the upper part of the small intestine, and no alcohol reaches the colon.

Alcohol appears in the blood five minutes after it has been taken by mouth, and the concentration in the blood reaches a maximum in about an hour. The rate of absorption varies considerably. It is most rapid when alcohol in moderate concentration (10–15 per cent) is taken on an empty stomach. More concentrated solutions irritate the duodenum and delay the emptying of the stomach and large quantities of concentrated alcohol may remain in the stomach for hours. This delays absorption because, although alcohol can be absorbed from the stomach, it is absorbed much more rapidly from the duodenum. Beer is absorbed more slowly than alcohol diluted with water. The presence of food in the stomach delays the absorption of alcohol and the maximum blood concentration may not be reached until four or five hours.

Nearly the whole of the alcohol taken is broken down in the body; small amounts are excreted in the breath and in the urine, but usually only about 2 per cent of the dose taken is excreted in this manner, and never more than 10 per cent.

Alcohol is distributed throughout the whole of the body water, that is to say throughout about two-thirds of the body volume. The fat and bones contain little alcohol, but the concentration in the rest of the body is fairly uniform. The amount of alcohol present in the body can therefore be calculated from the blood concentration. Moreover, since the kidneys cannot concentrate alcohol, the alcohol concentration in the urine is nearly the same as the blood concentration.

Alcohol is oxidised in the body to acetaldehyde and then to carbon dioxide and water. The amount of alcohol oxidised per minute by an individual is nearly constant, and is but little affected by the concentration. This fact is indicated by the curves in Figure 41.1. The oxidation factor varies in different individuals, but an average value in a man of 70 kg is 10 g or 12.5 ml per hour.

The fate of alcohol in the body is therefore relatively simple, namely diffusion throughout the body water and oxidation at a constant rate. No other drug is dealt with in such a simple manner. This simplicity implies, however, that the body has very little control over the fate of alcohol; since the amount oxidised is constant it cannot be adjusted to meet the metabolic requirements of the body and because no tissue can concentrate alcohol it cannot be stored by the body like other foodstuffs.

Actions of ethyl alcohol on the central nervous system

The actions of alcohol on the functions of the brain have been tested by a variety of methods. In most cases it has been found that alcohol causes a decrease in the speed and accuracy of reflex responses. Alcohol has no stimulant action on the brain, but acts as a mild hypnotic, and makes the brain less rapid and less accurate in its action. The most marked effect is to make the subject less critical of himself and more easily satisfied with imperfect performance.

This picture of the purely depressant action of alcohol on the brain is of course completely at variance with the

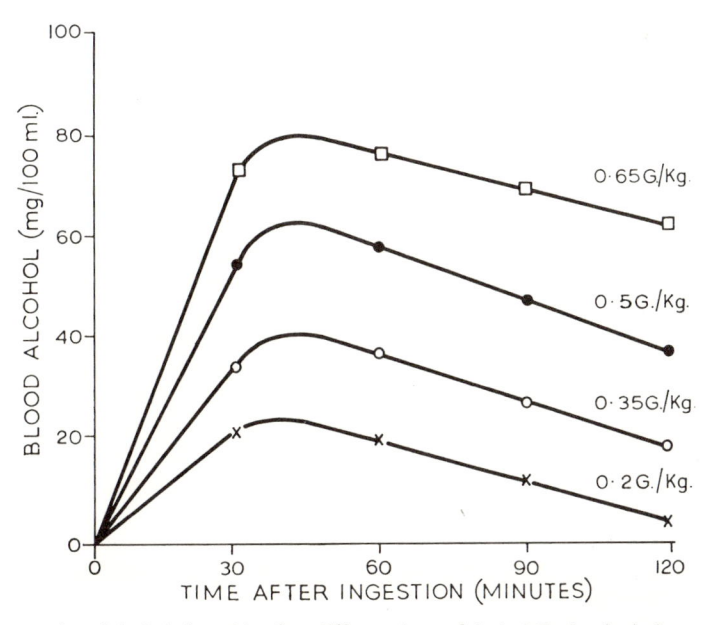

Fig. 41.1 The blood concentration of alcohol after taking four different doses of alcohol. Each point is the mean of 40 subjects. The lowest dose is equivalent to about ¾ pint of beer or 1½ whiskies and the largest dose to 3 pints of beer or 6 whiskies. (After Drew, Colquhoun and Long, 1958. *Br. med. J.*)

popular idea that alcohol is a stimulant to mental processes. This belief is explained by the fact that the highest and most easily deranged functions are chiefly inhibitory and hence the first action of alcohol is to diminish such characteristics as hesitation, caution, and self-criticism. Alcohol may actually assist in the performance of a task in which these characteristics are a hindrance rather than a help, as for instance in the making of an after-dinner speech. A moderate dose of alcohol often makes the individual appear more extraverted, hence it increases the desire for self-expression, and both the subject and uncritical observers may mistake this effect for increased mental activity.

The effects produced by alcohol on the brain when given in increasing doses may be summarised as follows:

Stage 1. Euphoria and minor disorders of conduct. The subject may appear to be uninfluenced by the drug, but adequate tests will show that the speed and accuracy of all reflexes are impaired. The power of restraining the emotions is impaired; the sociable individual becomes more talkative, and the reserved individual often becomes morose.

Behaviour in this stage depends partly upon the nature of the individual and partly upon his surroundings. A man who in quiet surroundings would go quietly to sleep may, in exciting surroundings, become excited.

Stage 2. Obvious symptoms of impaired functions. Speech becomes careless and the gait slightly unsteady, and movements are performed less accurately. Self-control is greatly impaired, but, as in the first stage, the effects observed depend on the nature of the individual and the character of his surroundings.

Stage 3. Deep sleep passing into coma. The stage of 'dead-drunk'. Blood alcohol about 300 mg/100 ml. Still larger quantities of alcohol produce impairment of the medullary centres, and may lead to death from respiratory failure. Blood alcohol about 400–500 mg/100 ml.

Even in the same subject the degree of intoxication is not strictly proportional to the content of alcohol in the blood. A large dose of alcohol produces a rapid rise in concentration to a maximum followed by a slow decline. Maximum intoxication may precede the maximum blood concentration, and recovery may be well marked before any significant fall in the alcohol concentration in the blood has occurred. At a given blood concentration impairment of performance tends to be greater if the blood alcohol concentration is rising than if it is falling.

Alcohol has the same general pharmacological action on the central nervous system as have the general anaesthetics such as ether, but differs in certain important respects. Consciousness persists relatively longer in alcoholic intoxication than it does during the induction of anaesthesia, and consequently the excitement or intoxication stage is much longer in alcoholic poisoning than in anaesthesia. This difference is partly due to the mode of administration, since ether when it is drunk produces an intoxication which is transient and violent. On the other hand, there is very little interval between loss of consciousness and dangerous depression of the vital centres in alcoholic poisoning, whereas with anaesthetics this stage of anaesthesia can be maintained for several hours.

Medicolegal aspects

The later stage of intoxication, or obvious drunkenness, is a condition that does not demand any exact test for its demonstrations or measurement. The advent of motor vehicles has forced the law to take cognisance of the earlier stages of drunkenness, because a man who is not sufficiently affected to be a nuisance under ordinary conditions may be a public danger if he is in charge of a motor car. This offence has been defined as being 'under the influence of drink or a drug to such an extent as to be incapable of having proper control of the vehicle'. This law defines a particular condition of intoxication instead of using the hopelessly vague term 'drunk', but this increased severity of the law regarding alcoholism in motorists has made it necessary to estimate as accurately as possible minor degrees of intoxication. Two forms of tests are available, namely, tests of behaviour and chemical tests.

1. *Behaviour tests.* The general appearance of the subject is important. Dilated pupils and rapid pulse may be signs of alcoholism, but they also may be due to excitement caused by such events as an accident and consequent arrest. The classical tests are such performances as standing with the eyes shut, walking along a straight line or pronouncing difficult words such as 'mixed biscuits'. Before applying such tests it is well to consider whether the individual would be likely to be able to perform them when completely sober.

The more thoroughly any performance has been practised the less easily is it impaired by intoxication. It is indeed very difficult to devise any form of behaviour test which can be satisfactorily applied unless the normal performance of the subject is known. One important precaution is to allow an adequate time for any test, so that the effects of initial excitement and confusion may subside and also in order to take into account the ability of many drunk persons to pull themselves together and appear normal for a short time. When examining subjects suspected of drunkenness it is important to exclude such possibilities as confusion due to metabolic diseases for example diabetes mellitus and the effects of hypoglycaemic drugs, head injuries, hypertension and the effect of antihypertensive drugs, neurological disorders, ataxia and tremor. Other possibilities include prodromata of cardiovascular emergencies, e.g. myocardial ischaemia or of cerebrovascular features such as confusional states, amnesia, aphasia or vertigo. Absorption of carbon monoxide from within the vehicle may give rise to severe hypoxia.

2. *Chemical tests.* Blood-alcohol estimations are recognised as legal evidence in several European countries. Widmark has perfected a delicate method for the estimation of alcohol in small quantities of blood. The carrying out of this test is a task for a specialist, but as regards the taking of blood samples it may be pointed out that alcohol must not be used either to cleanse the skin or the syringe. Failure to observe this elementary precaution produces spurious results. The test provides direct objective evidence regarding the amount of alcohol in the subject, although it does not provide any certain evidence concerning the effect produced by the drug on his conduct.

The alcohol level in blood can be determined indirectly by urine or breath analysis. Their advantage lies in the simplicity of collecting samples. The alcohol concentration in urine is somewhat higher than in blood and reaches its peak later; these differences are not large and can be allowed for. The distribution of alcohol between alveolar air and blood obeys Henry's Law and estimations of the blood alcohol levels by breath analysis (breathalyser or alcotest) are in close agreement with estimates made by direct analysis of the blood.

Tests made by Halcombe in the United States are particularly convincing. He tested a random sample of 1750 motor drivers and found that only 2 per cent of these showed a blood-alcohol of over 100 mg/100 ml. On the other hand of 270 drivers involved in accidents, 23 per cent had a blood-alcohol above this level. These results indicate that a blood-alcohol concentration above 100 mg/100 ml greatly increases the chance of an accident.

This direct evidence regarding the correlation between blood-alcohol and incidence of accidents supports the contention that in Great Britain a person with a blood-alcohol concentration in excess of 80 mg/100 ml or urine alcohol concentration in excess of 107 mg/100 ml is probably not fit to be in charge of a motor vehicle.

It is a continuing and important responsibility of medical practitioners to warn patients for whom they prescribe particular types of medicines, of the interaction between such drugs and alcohol. This applies especially to those drugs which may accentuate or potentiate the effects of alcohol taken during normal social occasions. Amongst the drugs of special importance are barbiturates and tranquillizers and antihypertensive drugs. There is a clear obligation on the prescriber to warn patients of the danger of taking other drugs or alcohol when they are likely to be in charge of a motor vehicle or moving machinery.

Chronic alcoholism

Excessive drinking of ethyl alcohol-containing beverages often produces a state of dependence on alcohol which results in a disturbance of physical and mental health and the impairment of personal relationships between the individual, his family and the society in which he lives. Early diagnosis of alcoholism is often difficult because of the alcoholic's skill in covering up his methods of satisfying the compulsive need for alcohol; the economic and other social stresses which arise, are for some time at least, contained within his immediate family circle. The situation may be brought to light when the individual is involved in police investigation of a motoring offence or when he is found to be drunk and incapable, or disorderly, in a street or public place. The prevalence of alcoholism is thus difficult to ascertain but the results of several surveys suggest that in England and Wales there are at least 300 000 alcoholics. There is also recent evidence of an increasing incidence of alcoholism in women and in younger age groups.

Regular drinkers acquire considerable tolerance to alcohol, and some individuals take as much as two bottles of whisky daily; this corresponds to 500 or 600 ml of absolute alcohol. Such a quantity would produce coma, or even death, in a person unaccustomed to alcohol.

Bernhard and Goldberg found that the blood-alcohol curve following ingestion of alcohol was nearly the same in alcoholics and in abstainers. The alcoholics absorbed the alcohol more rapidly and the maximum attained in the blood was higher in their case. The rate of disappearance of alcohol from the blood was, however, nearly identical in the two groups. Tolerance to alcohol observed in alcoholics must therefore be due to an actual tolerance of their central nervous system to alcohol in the blood. The gastric mucosa and the liver, however, do not acquire tolerance, but undergo progressive degeneration in heavy drinkers. Alcoholic cirrhosis of the liver does not appear to be due only to the direct action of alcohol but is related also to a reduction in the daily intake of wholesome food.

Disulfiram (Antabuse)

The effects of this compound on the metabolism of ethanol were described by Hald and Jacobsen in 1948.

$$(C_2H_5)_2-N-\underset{\underset{S}{\|}}{C}-S-S-\underset{\underset{S}{\|}}{C}-N-(C_2H_5)_2$$

Disulfiram

When taken by mouth disulfiram produces no effects but if alcohol is subsequently taken, even in small amounts, characteristic unpleasant symptoms develop. These consist of a feeling of heat and intense flushing in the face which often spreads to the neck and upper chest; the conjunctival vessels are dilated and the subject looks 'bull-eyed'. Palpitations with a pulse rate of 120–140 per minute are usually accompanied by headache and slight dyspnoea without any particular effect on the blood pressure; intense nausea and vomiting occur if larger amounts of alcohol are consumed. These effects last for a few hours, making the patient sleepy and tired, but after a short rest he usually recovers without any symptoms.

Disulfiram blocks the further oxidation of acetaldehyde from alcohol; these symptoms can be reproduced by intravenous injection of acetaldehyde. Small amounts of acetaldehyde are usually found in the blood of normal persons taking alcohol, but if disulfiram is taken, the blood acetaldehyde level rises to about 10 times and the aldehyrde content of the breath to about 10 times that which occurs after the same dose of alcohol without disulfiram. Disulfiram is slowly absorbed from the gastrointestinal tract and the action of a single dose of 0.5 gm lasts about 3 or 4 days.

The role of disulfiram in the treatment of alcoholism is entirely ancillary to the more important psychiatric management and social rehabilitation of the patient.

Methyl alcohol (Methanol). The fate of methyl alcohol in the body is quite different from that of ethyl alcohol; whereas the latter is oxidised rapidly to carbon dioxide and water, methyl alcohol is oxidised very slowly, and a large part is converted to formic acid and excreted as formates which are toxic (p. 43).

Severe poisoning with methanol arises from the drinking of varnishes and methylated spirit which contain various amounts of methanol and pyridine; cheap alcoholic wines are often adulterated with the former. The management of the solitary or vagrant alcoholic is complicated by the acidosis and mental confusion resulting from ingestion of these toxic substances; visual disturbances arising from bilateral inflammation of the optic nerve and retina may lead to permanent blindness. An important feature of immediate treatment is the effective restoration of the alkali reserve by intravenous injection of a 5 per cent solution of sodium bicarbonate. Since ethanol prevents the oxidation and conversion of methanol to formic acid, another effective method of treatment (and prevention) is to produce and maintain a blood alcohol concentration of about 100 mg/100 ml.

Barbiturate dependence

Prolonged administration of barbiturates can produce psychic and physical dependence as has been discussed. The symptoms of barbiturate dependence resemble those of chronic alcoholism except that the barbiturate addict maintains a better state of nutrition. There is usually a marked deterioration of social behaviour and impairment of mental ability. The addict is slovenly in dress and appearance and is incapable of regular work. He is emotionally unstable and may become aggressive or very depressed. The neurological signs are predominantly motor and resemble those of a cerebellar lesion and include tremor, ataxia and depression of the abdominal reflexes.

Patients who take an ordinary hypnotic dose of a barbiturate for several weeks do not, as a rule, show withdrawal symptoms after discontinuing the drug, but it is important, especially in elderly patients, to avoid abrupt cessation of treatment. Dependence on barbiturates is particularly evident, however, in individuals who take a mixture of barbiturates and amphetamine (purple hearts) since in these conditions the unpleasant depressant effects of the barbiturate are masked by the stimulating effects of amphetamine.

Dependence on volatile solvents

Various volatile solvents are attractive to some pre-adolescent and adolescent subjects who obtain a 'kick' from inhaling or 'sniffing' a variety of commonly available products such as glue, boot and furniture-polishes and dry cleaning fluids, which contain toluene, benzene, acetone or carbon tetrachloride. These experiences may then encourage experimentation with other types of dependence-producing substances. Anaesthetists or surgical-theatre personnel may become dependent on volatile anaesthetic agents such as nitrous oxide, the effect of which may disastrously impair their professional skill and judgment.

Hallucinogens

The history and pharmacology of some hallucinogens is discussed on page 265. Their mode of action is not understood but some of these drugs, e.g. LSD and mescaline, exhibit cross-tolerance which may indicate that they share a common mechanism of action. Physical dependence on drugs such as LSD has not been demonstrated but they frequently exert a powerful psychological attraction which leads to their abuse. The chemical structures of some hallucinogenic drugs are shown in Figure 41.2.

Lysergic acid diethylamide (LSD) (p. 265)

Subcutaneous injections of LSD in doses of 35 μg or less are hallucinogenic in man. LSD, which in Great Britain may not be supplied except to medical practitioners for professional purposes, is frequently abused by addicts. Probably very few users take LSD at regular intervals. More frequently it is taken intermittently, generally in company, with the intention of 'seeking out feelings of greater insight and sensory stimulation' and 'to make life more meaningful, and facilitate interpersonal relationships'. Occasionally LSD takers experience highly unpleasant reactions to the drug ('bad trip') in which they are seized by uncontrollable panic to the point of attempting to jump out of the window.

Attempts have been made to use LSD clinically to treat psychiatric conditions but such uses are now seldom advocated because of the danger of initiating a long-lasting toxic psychosis with LSD.

Other hallucinogens which are liable to abuse include the following:

Peyote or mescal buttons contains mescaline (p. 266) a sympathomimetic compound with hallucinogenic activity. Peyote is widely used by North American Indians for cult purposes.

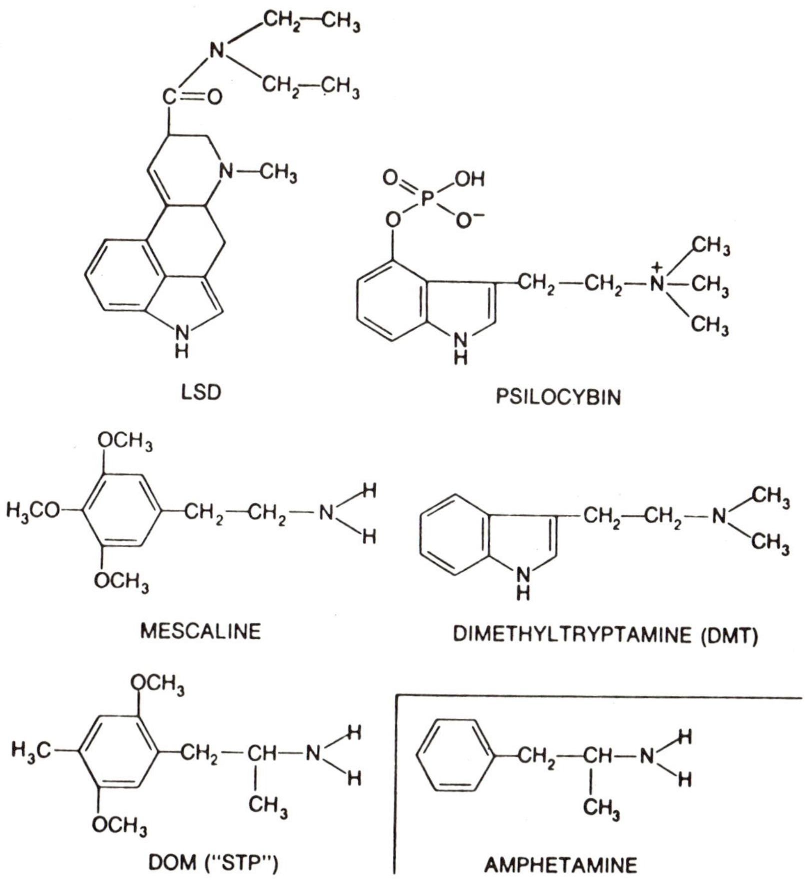

Fig. 41.2 Chemical structure of hallucinogens.

Dimethoxy-methyl amphetamine (DOM) is a synthetic compound with structural resemblance and actions resembling both amphetamine and mescaline.

Psylocybin was isolated from the Mexican 'sacred mushroom' by the Swiss biochemist Hofmann. It is structurally related to 5HT (serotonin). Psylocibin is the only naturally occurring hallucinogen known to contain phosphorus.

Dimethyltryptamine (DMT) is another tryptamine derivative related to serotonin. It is present in hallucinogenic snuffs used by American Indians.

These compounds all produce psychic effects resembling LSD but they are generally less active, weight for weight.

Cannabis

The cultivation of *Cannabis sativa* L. as a source of fibre (hemp) and for the psychoactive substances contained in its leaves and flowering tops has a long history and was well known to the Assyrians in the seventh century B.C. The plant produces in the flowering tops and upper leaves a resinous substance which contains the major proportion of the psychoactive and intoxicating ingredients. Preparations of cannabis are known by different names in different countries; *hashish* consists primarily of the resin, *marihuana* refers to a mixture of leaves and flowering tops and *ganja* to preparations of flowering tops but no leaves. Other names include charas, kif, dagga and pot.

Cannabis contains a number of pharmacologically active principles, called cannabinoids, of which the two most active are Δ^9- and Δ^8-*trans*-tetra-hydro-cannabinol (Δ^9-THC and Δ^8-THC). These compounds volatilise readily when smoked and are rapidly absorbed from the lungs; they are also absorbed more slowly from the alimentary tract when cannabis products are ingested. They are metabolised to 11-hydroxy derivatives which are also active and have been shown to persist in the tissues of experimental animals for long periods of time. The content of Δ^9-THC in different preparations of cannabis varies widely according to the country of origin and the conditions of storage; the average content in hashish is about 5 per cent.

When hashish is smoked its effects occur rapidly and last for a short time; when it is ingested they may last for several hours. The main effect of small doses is to produce a dream-like state with alterations of consciousness and perception often accompanied by a feeling of rather foolish well-being marked by uncontrollable laughter and giggling. The excitement produced is described as being 'high'. But the effects of the drug depend on disposition and circumstances and some persons become drowsy and withdrawn. Larger doses may produce hallucinations and even simulate a psychosis.

Although a certain amount of tolerance to hashish develops, physical dependence to the drug does not occur. There is no evidence that hashish can produce lasting mental disturbances but in predisposed persons its prolonged use may cause personal neglect and a loss of social responsibility. Rarely it may cause a temporary toxic psychosis.

There is widespread agreement that cannabis products have no useful therapeutic properties and that there are no indications for their use in current medical practice. The social and recreational use of cannabis has spread extensively throughout the world, especially amongst young people of all social classes, and its illegal possession and use has presented a considerable challenge to national and international regulatory authorities.

Tobacco dependence

This is probably the most widespread form of drug dependence. The smoking of tobacco is today the most popular drug habit in the world. The chief active constituent of tobacco is nicotine. The effect produced by smoking tobacco depends, however, not upon the content of nicotine in the tobacco, but upon the amount of nicotine that is absorbed from the smoke. This absorption depends upon a large number of factors. More nicotine passes into the smoke from a damp than a dry tobacco. A large proportion of the nicotine condenses in the stump of a cigar or cigarette and in the bottom of a pipe, and hence the amount inhaled depends upon how large a stump is left unsmoked, and upon whether a pipe is clean or dirty. The practice of inhalation greatly increases the absorption of nicotine. It is these factors which determine whether a tobacco is strong or mild rather than the nicotine content which is relatively uniform. For instance, Virginian cigarettes, medium pipe tobacco and both strong and mild cigars, all contain about 2 per cent nicotine.

Nicotine produces actions on all the ganglia of the autonomic nervous system and also on the central nervous system. It also causes a release of vasopressin from the posterior pituitary gland. The effects it produces are therefore very complex.

The effects of smoking on a novice are as follows: fall of blood pressure, slowing of pulse, nausea accompanied by cold sweat and pallor, followed by vomiting. These central effects are not seen in a habitual smoker in whom the effects of nicotine are mainly vasoconstrictor due to stimulation of sympathetic ganglia and release of vasopressin. There is a slight rise in blood pressure, a quickening of the pulse and increased intestinal activity.

None of these effects explains the pleasure derived from smoking, nor why a habit is formed. Nicotine also appears to exert a slight depressant effect on the higher centres of the brain, and thus to allay irritability and excitement. The tobacco habit is one of the strongest drug habits, for even moderate smokers usually find great difficulty in abandoning the habit, and if they stop smoking they may experience certain physical reactions, such as intermittent transient bouts of dizziness, fine tremors or jerking movements of the limbs and changes in eating habits.

Tobacco smoking and health

The effects of smoking on the health and welfare of the individual depend on his general environment, whether rural or urban and on the extent and method of smoking tobacco. During the past 20 years cigarette smoking has been shown to play an important part in the development of several diseases such as chronic bronchitis and emphysema, ischaemic heart disease and lung cancer. The annual death rate from lung cancer in Great Britain rose from 2286 in 1931 to 26 398 in 1965 of whom 84 per cent were males. The delayed effects of smoking are particularly evident in men aged 40 to 64 years where the mortality rates from lung cancer increased from 4500 in 1949 to 10 800 in 1969. There is now well-documented evidence from several countries that this disease occurs 20 times more frequently in heavy smokers than in non-smokers and that it is related to the amount and method of smoking. The risk of developing lung cancer is greater in cigarette smokers than in pipe and cigar smokers; but some protection seems to be provided by cigarette holders or filter tips. If a heavy cigarette smoker stops smoking in middle-age the probability that he will die from lung cancer is reduced. Certain other forms of cancer appear to be related to smoking; for example there is an abnormally high incidence of cancer of the larynx in pipe and cigar smokers. Although statistical evidence suggests that smoking is one of the factors associated with the increase in lung cancer it is unlikely to be the only one. Lung cancer occurs more frequently in town dwellers than in those living in the country and it has been suggested therefore that air pollution, particularly by exhaust gases from diesel engines, may be a contributing factor.

MANAGEMENT OF DRUG DEPENDENCE

The problems associated with drug dependence involve the interaction of many different factors relating to the individual and the type of drugs on which he has become dependent. Whereas formerly the predominant pattern of abuse has been to one type of drug such as opiate or alcohol, there has been a universal trend towards multiple drug use with resultant dependence on more than one drug. This has complicated the management of drug dependence so that more comprehensive methods have been necessary to deal adequately with the treatment of the individual and to control by legislation and international agreement the availability of drugs which are specially liable to be abused.

Treatment

The treatment of a drug-dependent patient usually involves a therapeutic programme for the gradual withdrawal of the drugs, appropriate attention to malnutrition and bacterial or virus infections and the use of other supportive measures to promote the individual's rehabilitation within the community. Several different methods have been devised to achieve these aims. In some localities integrated hospital and community services provide appropriate medical, social and educational facilities; in others various types of 'therapeutic community' have been developed, where the main aim is to encourage self-discipline and restructuring of character and no drug-taking or physical violence are allowed. Various forms of compulsory treatment for alcoholism and other types of drug dependence have been practised, with or without detention, on the grounds that this form of illness necessitates the care of the individual and the protection of the community analogous to quarantine treatment for patients with certain infectious diseases or committal procedures for some types of mental illness. There is, as yet, no general consensus of opinion on the overall success of these different methods of treatment, but it is widely accepted that various forms of counselling and follow-up services are necessary to avoid relapse to drug abuse.

Withdrawal and maintenance therapy. Sudden withdrawal of most dependence-producing drugs can have disastrous effects. Abrupt withdrawal of heroin or morphine causes a severe physical reaction and in the presence of complications such as malnutrition, infections and hepatitis, dangerous collapse may occur. Likewise sudden withdrawal of alcohol and barbiturates may be followed by serious effects, such as psychosis, cardiovascular failure and epileptiform seizures; severe depression and apathy resulting in suicidal attempts may follow abrupt withdrawal of amphetamine, cocaine and other stimulant drugs. For similar reasons considerable caution must be exercised in the use of specific antagonists, such as nalorphine, naloxone and cyclazocine for opiate dependence and of disulfiram (Antabuse) in the treatment of alcoholism.

The concept of maintenance therapy with a drug of dependence such as heroin, morphine or cocaine which involves a gradual reduction in daily intake of the drug, is designed to reduce the chances of sudden collapse and to curtail the channels of illegal supplies of these drugs. In Great Britain, although not in the U.S.A., heroin is available for normal medical therapeutic purposes and can be so prescribed by medical practitioners. A dramatic increase, however, in the number of known heroin and cocaine users from about 400 in 1964 to 1500 in 1967 necessitated a change in the arrangements for prescribing heroin and cocaine for dependent persons in Britain whose names must now be notified to the Home Office and be supervised only by physicians specially licensed to do so. Maintenance therapy with orally administered *methadone* can be used as an alternative to heroin or morphine maintenance or to supplement it. Dependence on methadone is less severe than on other morphine-like drugs and this enables gradual reduction in the daily dosage and finally complete withdrawal of the drug.

Prevention of drug dependence

In addition to educational and social measures designed to provide information about the dangers of drug abuse to the individual and to the community, legal controls restricting the supply and possession of such drugs have been advocated by international agreements since 1931. The extent to which they have been implemented by different nations has varied according to social attitudes and customs and the extent to which the various substances are considered to be essential for medical, dental and veterinary practice.

In Britain the supply, distribution and use of most dependence-producing drugs, with the exception of alcohol has been controlled by a number of Statutes and Regulations which include the Dangerous Drugs Act, 1965, the Pharmacy and Poisons Act 1933 and the Drugs (Prevention of Misuse) Act 1964, each with various subsequent modifications. Considerable further changes have been enacted in the Medicines Act 1968 and the Misuse of Drugs Act 1971 which provides for much stricter control on the supply distribution, use and possession of 'controlled drugs'; these are defined as Class A, B, and C drugs and comprise almost every dependence producing drug except alcohol and tobacco. An important feature of this new legislation is the establishment of an Advisory Council on the Misuse of Drugs which is required to keep under review any misuses of drugs in the United Kingdom which are capable of having harmful effects sufficient to constitute a social problem and to advise on appropriate methods for preventing such misuses and for dealing with the social problems created by them.

PREPARATIONS

Treatment of alcoholism
Citrated calcium carbimide (Abstem) 50–100 mg dl p.o.
Disulfiram (Antabuse) init dose 800 mg, then 100–200 mg dl p.o.

Narcotic antagonists (Ch. 21)

FURTHER READING

Blum K (ed) 1977 Alcohol and opiates. Neurochemical and behavioural mechanisms. Academic Press, New York

Bourne F G, Fox Ruth (ed) 1973 Alcoholism. Progress in research and treatment. Academic Press, New York

Harris R T, McIsaac W H, Schuster C R (ed) 1970 Drug dependence. University of Texas Press, Austin

Landstreet B F 1977 The drinking driver. Charles Thomas, Springfield

Ludwig A M, Levine J, Stark L H 1970 LSD and Alcoholism. Charles Thomas, Springfield

Martin W R (ed) 1977 Drug addiction. I Morphine, sedative-hypnotic and alcohol dependence. II Amphetamine and psychotogen dependence. Marihuana dependence. Handb exp pharmac. Springer, Berlin

Neumann R G 1977 Methadone treatment in narcotic addiction. Academic Press, New York

Paton W D M, Crown June 1972 Cannabis and its derivatives. Pharmacology and experimental psychology. Oxford University Press, London

Pradhan S N, Dutta S N (ed) 1977 Drug abuse. Clinical and basic aspects. Mosby, St Louis

Index

Abortion
  early, medical, 478
  threatened and habitual, use of progestogens, 356-357
Absorption of drugs, 34-39
  active transport, 35
  bioavailability, 38-39
  delayed, 39
  facilitated diffusion, 35
  filtration through pores, 35
  from intestine, 36-38
  from mouth, 36
  glyceryl trinitrate, 123
  physico-chemical factors controlling, 36-38
  pinocytosis, 35-36
  rate, 36
  from stomach, 36
  from subcutaneous and intramuscular injection sites, 38-39
  through alimentary canal, 35-39
  through lipid phase of cell membrane, 34-35
Acebutolol, 116, 130
Acedapsone, 428
Acetanilide, 291
Acetazolamide, 164, 166, 393
  in epilepsy, 273
  in glaucoma, 87
Acetohexamide, 349
Acetophenetidine, 291
Acetoxyl (benzoyl peroxide gel) in skin fungal infections, 231
Acetyl-ß-methylcholine, 59
Acetylcholine, 57-60
  and atropine, competitive antagonism, 11, 12
  chloride, 89
  drugs mimicking, 71
  early work, 57-58
  interference with ganglionic transmission, 63-64
  muscarine and nicotine actions, 58
  in neuromuscular transmission, 65-66
  pharmacological chemistry, 59
  receptors, 11, 12, 13
    identification, 17-18
    membrane noise, 17, 18
  synthesis, storage and release in nerves, 66
  transmitter role in CNS, 63, 235
Acetylcysteine spray (mucolytic) 183
Acetylsalicylic acid, 287, 288
  see also Aspirin
ACH, see Acetylcholine

Achlorhydria, management, 188-189
Achromycin, 417
Acne vulgaris, treatment, 230
  preparations, 231
  use of oestrogens, 355
Acridines as disinfectants, 460-461, 462
ACTH, 346, 347, 348, 349
  actions and release, 327
    on adrenal cortex, 327
  chemical structure, 327
  clinical uses, 327
  function test, 349
  side effects, 328
  supplementary therapy, 347
  tetracosactrin, 328
Acthar, 336
Actidil, 104
Actinomycin D
  as antitumour agent, 382, 384
  in leukaemia, 383
Actrapid insulin, 340
Adalat, 130
Adalin as hypnotic, 247
  preparation, 256
Addison's disease, corticosteroids, 343, 347
Adenine arabinoside, 397
Adenosine
  antagonist of ADP-induced platelet aggregation, 209
  monophosphate, cyclic, see Cyclic AMP
Adenylcyclase, 79
  mode of action, 319-320
  hormones affecting, 320
Adenylic acid, structure, 380
ADH see Vasopressin
Adrenal cortex, 343-346
  corticosteroids, 343
  structure, 344
  see also Corticosteroids
Adrenal cortical insufficiency, 155
Adrenal glands, 343-349
Adrenaline
  action on
    circulation, 79-81
    eyes, 88
    heart, 81
    skeletal muscle, 81-82
    smooth muscle, 81
  biological assay, 73
  in bronchial asthma, 176, 177-178
  as cardiac stimulant, 149
  central effects, 82
  chemical assay, 73-74

Adrenaline, cont'd
  content of tissues, 73
  enzymic degradation, 76-77
  formation, 74
  inactivation and fate, 76-79
  intermediate stages, 75
  in local anaesthesia, 313
  in local haemorrhage, 215
  metabolic effects, 82
  metabolic pathways, 76
  oxidation products, 74
  piloerection, 82
  preparations, 85, 130
  storage and release, 75
  structure, 74
  sweating, 82
  effect on uterus, 218
  as vasoconstrictor, 125
Adrenergic
  mechanisms, 73-85
    action on eyes, 88
    drugs modifying, 82-84
    formation on adrenergic transmitters, 74
    inactivation and fate, 76-79
    see also Catecholamines
  neurone blocking drugs, 83-84, 130
    assessment, 84
    differentiation, 84
    false transmitters, 84
    in hypertension, 115-116, 118-119, 120-121
    see also Alpha blockers: Beta blockers
  receptors, characteristics, 78-79
  receptor blocking drugs, 82-83
    alpha, 83
    beta, 83
    postsynaptic, 82-83
    presynaptic, 82
    structural requirements of drugs which act on, 79
Adrenoceptors, see Adrenergic receptors
Adrenochrome, 73, 74
Adrenolutin, 73, 74
Adriamycin as antitumour agent, 382, 384
Advertisements, drug, 8
Aerosporin, 413
Agar, 197
Agarol, 197
Agranulocytosis
  drug-induced, 208
  following H_2-histamine antagonists, 188
Air pollution, 466-467
Ajmaline, action on heart, 147

494 APPLIED PHARMACOLOGY

Akathisia, major tranquillisers, 254
Alcofenac, anti-inflammatory drug, 293
Alcohol
  dependence, 484-488
    absorption and metabolism of ethyl alcohol, 484-485
    actions on CNS, 485-486
    behaviour tests, 486
    blood concentrations, 485
    central pharmacology, 484
    chemical tests, 487
    chronic alcoholism, 487
    effect of disulfiram, 487
    effect of methyl alcohol, 488
    medicolegal aspects, 486
    stages, 486
    withdrawal symptoms, 484
    use of benzodiazepines, 251
  as disinfectant, 459
  unspecific depressant action, 296
Alcoholism, chronic, 487
Alcopar, 454, 451
Alcuronium chloride in anaesthesia, 306
Aldcorten, 350
Aldomet, 130
  in hypertension, 117
Aldosterone, 111-112, 114, 344, 345-346, 350
Aldosteronism, primary, 111-112
Aldrin structure, 468
Aleudrine in bronchial asthma, 183
Alimentary canal, 184-201
  action of drugs on gastric secretion, 185-191
  chief functions, 184-185
Alkavervir, 130
  in hypertension, 120
Alkeran, in neoplastic disease, 379, 384
Alkylating agents in neoplastic disease, 378-379
  choice, 379
  pharmacological actions, 278
  preparations, 384
  side effects, 378
Allegron, 258
Allergy, 98-104
  anaphylaxis, 100-102
    mechanism, 102-103
  antibodies, 98
  antigens, 98
  to aspirin, 289
  formation of antigen by drug, 104
  hypersensitivity to drugs, 31, 103-104
  hypersensitivity reactions, types, 99-100
    see also Hypersensitivity
  to penicillin, 405-406
    clinical manifestations, 406
  to phenothiazines, 255-256
Allobarbitone (Dial), dosage and duration of action, 245
Alloferin in anaesthesia, 306
Allopathy, 3-6
Allopurinol in gout, 293
  preparation, 293
Aloes, as purgative, 198

Alpha blockers, 83
  in hypertension, 120-121
  in obstetrics, 218
  preparations, 85
  see also Adrenergic, and specific drugs
Alpha receptors for catecholamines, 14
Alphadolone acetate, and Alphaxalone anaesthesia, 306
Althesin anaesthesia, 305, 306
Aluminium hydoxide gel,
  action, 191
  neutralising powers, 190
  preparation, 200
Alupent, in bronchial asthma, 180
Alytesin, 91
Amantadine, antiviral agent, 397
  in Parkinsonism, 274, 277
Ambilhar, in schistosomiasis, 453, 454
Amenorrhoea, oestrogen treatment, 355
Ametazole, 104
Amethocaine,
  local anaesthetic, 311, 312, 315
    eyes, 313
  spinal anaesthesia, 314
Amethopterin, in neoplastic disease, 380, 384
Amidopyrine, 291
  causing agranulocytosis, 208
Amikacin (Amikin), 417
Amiloride, 164, 166
Aminacrinel
  as disinfectant, 460
  structure, 460
Amine neurotransmitters, and mental disease, 240-241
Amino acid transmitters in CNS, 235-236
Aminocaproic acid, antifibrinolytic agent, 211, 216
7-Amino-cephalosporanic acid, structure, 406
Aminoglycosides, 411-412
  preparations, 417
6-Amino-penicillanic acid, structure, 406
Aminophylline, 130
  in bronchial asthma, 182, 183
  as cardiac stimulant, 149
  as respiratory stimulant, 175, 183
8-Aminoquinolines, in malaria, 443
  toxicity, 443
Aminosalicylate sodium (PAS), 428
  tuberculostatic activity, 422
Amitriptyline
  mode of action, 259
  in depression, 258, 260
  preparation, 266
  structure, 258
Ammonia formation, urinary, 157
Ammonium carbonate as expectorant, 175, 176
Amodiaquine in malaria, 442, 446
Amoebiasis, 443-446
  amoebicide drugs, 444-446
  dysentery, treatment, 446
  measurement of chemotherapeutic effect, 444
  preparations, 446-447
Amoxil, 407

Amoxycillin, 404, 407
Amphetamine and related drugs in depression, 262-265
  absorption, distribution and fate, 263
  action, 262
  amphetamine-barbiturate mixtures, 264
  anorexia, 264
  central stimulation, 262, 263
  dependence, 264-265, 483-484
  effects in man, 262-263
  preparations, 267
  psychosis, 240, 264
  structure, 262
  therapeutic uses, 263-264
  toxic effects, 264
  as vasoconstrictor, 126
Amphetamine sulphate
  in depression, 263
  effects in man, 262
  in hyperkinesis, 264
  preparation, 267
  in weight reduction, 263
Amphotericin, 414, 417
  cream (Fungilin) in fungal infections, skin, 231
  in leishmaniasis, 435
Amphotericin B, 388
Ampicillin
  half-life, 46
  preparation, 407
  properties, 403, 404
  side effects, 404
  skin reactions, 231
  therapeutic use, 404-405, 405, 415, 416, 417
Amyl nitrite, 130
  in angina, 122-123
  in biliary spasm, 195
  in cyanide poisoning, 171
Amylobarbitone, human assay, 24, 25
  dosage and duration of action, 245
  preparation, 256
  sodium (Sodium amytal), dosage and duration of action, 245
  preparation, 256
Amytal
  dosage and duration of action, 245
  individual variation in response, 27
  preparation, 256
Anabolic steroids, 358-359
  side effects, 358
  structures, 358
  therapeutic uses, 359
Anaemias
  macrocytic, 205-208
  pernicious, 206
    cobalamins, 206-207
  types, 202
Anaesthesia
  althesin, 305
  atropine and other anticholinergic drugs, 71
  barbiturates, 303-304, 306
  choice, 306
  ether, 296-298
  inhalation, 298-302

INDEX

Anaesthesia, *cont'd*
    distribution, 299
    methods of administration, 300
    solubility, 299
    uptake, 299-300
  in labour, 224
  local, 308-315
    caudal, 313
    conduction, 313, 311, 312
    dangers, 315
    dental, 313
    epidural, 311, 313
    infiltration, 312
    methods of producing, 308
    mode of action, 309
    mucous membranes, 312
    nerve impulse, 308-309
    specific agents, 309-311
    spinal, 312, 313-315
    surface, 311, 312
    terminal, 313
    testing and applying, 311-312
    therapeutic index, 312
    toxicity tests, 312
    uses, 312-315
  neuroleptanalgesia, 305
  neuromuscular-blocking drugs, 305-306
  postoperative complications, 301
  premedication, 305
  preparations, 306-307
  stages, 296-298
  intravenous, 303-305
Anaesthetics, 295-307
  choice, 306
  development, 298
  gases, 302-303
  intravenous, 303, 305
  mode of action, 295-296
  neuromuscular-blocking drugs, 305
  premedication, 305
  preparations, 306-307
  stages of anaesthesia, 296-298
  volatile liquids, 300-302
Analeptic drugs, as respiratory stimulants, 171-172
Analgesic drugs, 278-294
  antipyretic, 285-291
  classification, 278
  in gout, 292-293
  in labour, 223-224
  measure of activity, 278-279
  opioid, 279-285
  drug dependence, 279, 481
Anaphylaxis, 100-102
  clinical allergy, 100
  desensitisation, 100
  mechanisms of histamine release, 101-102
  reactions in man, 100
  reaginic antibodies, 100-101
  tests, 101
Anapolon, 359
Ancolan in travel sickness, 193, 201
Ancrod, 211, 216

Androgens, 357-358
  actions, 357
  control of prostatic cancer, 382
  effects on fetus, 225
  in mammary cancer, 382
  receptors, 321
  synthetic, 358
  testosterone *see* Testosterone
  therapeutic uses, 358
Androsterone structure, 357
Anectine in anaesthesia, 307
Aneurine *see* Thiamine
Angina pectoris
  nitrites, 122-123
  vasodilators, 122-123
Angiotensin, 111
  amide, 130
    chemical derivation, 127
    composition, 127
    effects on blood vessels, 127
Anorexia, amphetamine, 238, 264
Anquil as tranquilliser, 256
Antabuse in alcoholism, 488
Antacids, 190-191
Antagonism, drug, 19, 11-16
Antepar, 450
Anthelmintics, 448-455
  actions, 448
  filariasis, 454
  nematodes, 449-452
  preparations, 454-455
  schistosomiasis, 452-453
  tapeworm infections, 448-449
Anthisan, 104
Anthracene purgatives, 198, 201
Anthralin in psoriasis, 228, 231
Antianginal drugs, 121-129, 130
Antiarrhythmic agents, 144-148, 149
  clinical uses, 147-148
Antibacterial chemotherapy, basic aspects, 385-391
  antibiotic development, 385-386
  bacterial resistance, mechanism, 390-391
  targets for attack in cells, 386-390
Antibiotics, 408-417
  in acne, 230
  aminoglycosides, 411-412, 418
  antifungal, 413-414, 418
  bacterial infections of skin, 229, 231
  choice, 414-415
  classification according to mechanism, 386, 387
  combinations, 415
  development, 385-386
  in eczema, 230
  interactions with other drugs, 415
  macrolides, 408-409, 418
  peptide, 412-413
  preparations, 407, 418
  prescribing chart, 415-417
  synergistic action, 415
  tetracyclines, 409-411, 418
  transplacental transmission, 225
  see also Penicillin and other specific names

Antibiotics, *cont'd*
  in veterinary practice, 470-471
    antibiotic-ice, 471
    in livestock industry, 470-471
    in preservation of food, 471
Antibodies, 98-99
  in penicillin allergy, 406
Anticancer drugs, 375-384
  see also Cytotoxic drugs
Anticholinergic agents
  action on eyes, 88
  as antispasmodics, 200
  in Parkinsonism, 274-275, 277
    adverse effects, 274
    indications, 274
Anticholinesterases, 60-62
  action on eyes, 87-88
    side effects, 87-88
  irreversible inhibitors, 60-62
  mode of action, 60-62
  effect on myasthenia gravis, 62
  preparations, 71
  reversible inhibitors, 60
Anticoagulants, 211-215
  causing haemorrhage, use of vitamin K, 366
  drugs used *in vitro*, 211
  drugs used *in vivo*, 211
  heparin, 212
  local haemorrhage, control, 215
  oral, 212-215
  therapeutic uses, 214
Anticonvulsants
  effects of benzodiazepines, 250
  in epilepsy, 268-273, 276
    methods of assessing, 268
    mode of action, 268
    see also Epilepsy
Antidepressants, 257-267
Antidiuretic hormone *see* Vasopressin
Antiemetic effects of haloperiodol, 255
Antiemetics
  fluphenazine, 254
  haloperidol, 255
  perphenazine, 254
  see also Vomiting
Antifungal antibiotics, 413-414
Antigens, 98
  complete, formation by drug, 104
Antihistamines, 97-98, 189
  in allergy, actions, 102
  assessment, 97
  in bronchial asthma, 181
  in travel sickness, 193
  H_1 action 96-97
    pharmacological, 96, 97-98
    chemical structures, 96
    preparations, 104
    see also specific names
    simultaneous occurence with H_2, 97
    therapeutic uses, 98
    toxic effects, 98
  H_2 action chemical, 96-97
    action on gastric secretion, 187
    clinical uses, 187-188
    side effects, 188

Antihypertensive drugs, 112-121, 130
Antileprotic drugs, 427-428
Antimalarials, 440-443
Antimetabolites in neoplastic disease, 379-381
    preparations, 384
Antimigraine drugs, 130
    see also Migraine
Antimonials in schistosomiasis, 453, 454
Antimony sodium tartrate in schistosomiasis, 453
Antiphen in tapeworm infections, 449, 454
Antipyretic analgesics, 285-291
    analgesic action, 286
    antiflammatory effect, 286
    antirheumatic drugs, 289, 290
    classification, 285
    non-steroidal, 289
    para-aminophenol analgesics, 290-291
    preparations, 293
    pyrazole derivatives, 291
    salicylates, 286-289
Antirheumatic drugs, 289, 290-291, 293
Antiseptics see Disinfectants and specific names
Antisialagogue drugs, 71
Antispasmodic drugs, 200-201
Antispirochaetal drugs, discovery, 130
Antithyroid drugs, 333-334
    and beta-blockers, 334
    chemical structure, 334
    clinical effects, 334
    dosage and duration of treatment, 334
    mode of action, 333
    and potassium perchlorate, 334
    toxic effects, 334
Antituberculosis drugs, 418-427
    see Tuberculosis chemotherapy
Antiviral agents, 396-397
Antrenyl in hyperchlorhydria and peptic ulcer, 190
Antrypol, 434, 454
Anturan in gout, 292
    platelet aggregation inhibition, 209, 216
Apocrine glands, 227-228
Apomorphine, 201
    as emetic, 192-193
    dopaminergic activity, 193
Appetite reducing drugs, 264
Approved names for drugs, 8
Apresoline in hypertension, 114
Aprindine, action on heart, 147, 149
Aprinox, 166
Aqueous humour, origin and fate, 87
Arabinosylcytosine, 397
Aramine as vasoconstrictor, 126
Arfonad, 130
    in hypertension, 121
Aristocort, 347
Arrhythmias, cardiac, 134-135
Arsenic poisoning, antidotes, 473-474
Arsenicals
    in amoebiasis, 445
    in syphilis, 436-437

Arsenicals, cont'd
    in trypanosomiasis, 432-433
    toxic reactions, 433
Arsphenamines
    mode of action, 428-429
    structure, 431
Arsthinol in amoebiasis structure, 445
Artane, in Parkinsonism, 274, 277
Arterio-venous anastomoses, 109
Arthus reactions, 99
Artificial ventilation, 169
Arvin, 211, 216
Asbestos, as carcinogen, 473
Ascariasis, drugs for, 449-450, 454
Ascorbic acid, 369-370
    clinical effects, 370
    daily requirements, 370, 371
    deficiency, 370
    natural sources, 369
    preparations, 371
    therapeutic uses, 370
Asparaginase as antitumour agent, 382, 384
Aspartate, transmitter role in CNS, 235
Aspirin, 286-289, 293
    absorption, 287
    allergy, 289
    as antirheumatic drug, 289
    compound tablets, 291, 293
    fate in body, 287-288
    and gastrointestinal bleeding, mechanism, 209
    half-life, 46
    pharmacological actions, 288
    poisoning, 288
        treatment, 289
    possible teratogenic effects, 225
    prevention of post-operative thrombosis, 209
    toxic effects, 288
    treatment, 289
Assays, biological, see Biological assays
Asthma, bronchial, see Bronchial asthma
Astringent drugs in local haemorrhage, 215
Atabrine, 454
Atarax, as sedative hypnotic, 252, 256
Atebrin in malaria, 442
Atenolol, 116, 130
    in angina, 124
Atoxyl, 430
Atromid-S, as lipid lowering agent, 196
    preparation, 201
Atrophic rhinitis, use of oestrogens, 355
Atropine, 69-71
    actions, 69-70
        central, 71
        on eyes, 88
            preparations, 89
        on gastric secretion, 189
        peripheral, 70
    and acetylcholine, competitive antagonism, 11, 12
    in anaesthesia, 71
    as antispasmodic, 200
    in bronchial asthma, 181
    chemical features, 70

Atropine, cont'd
    and histamine, antagonism, 11-12
    methonitrate, 71
    poisoning, 71
    structure, 70
    substitutes, 71
    sulphate in travel sickness, 193
Aureomycin, 417
Auricular
    fibrillation, 134-135
        cardioversion, 147
        effect of drugs, 135
    tachycardia, paroxysmal, management, 148
Aurothiomalate sodium in rheumatoid arthritis, 290
Autonomic nervous system, physiology, 53-55
    central control, 54
    chief functions, 54-55
    humoral transmission of nerve impulse, 55-57
    peripheral nervous system, chemical organisation, 56-57
    schematic representations, 53, 56
Autopharmacology, see Cholinergic transmission
Aventyl, 258
Avlochin, 444
Avloclor in malaria, 440
Avlosulfon, 428
Azapropazone, anti-inflammatory drug, 293
Azathioprine in tissue transplantation, 381, 384
6-Azauridine in leukaemia, 381

Bacillus Calmette Guérin, 418
Bacitracin, 413
    inhibition of bacterial cell wall synthesis, 390
Baclofen as muscle relaxant, 276, 277
Bacterial cell, targets for chemotherapy, 386-390
    competition for an essential metabolite, 386-387
    control of microbial enzymes, 387
    impairment of bacterial cell wall, 389
    increased permeability of cytoplasmic membrane, 388
    inhibition of ribosome function, 388
    interference with DNA function, 388
Bacterial cell wall, impairment, 389-390
Bacterial endocarditis, penicillin, 405
Bacterial resistance, mechanism, 390-391
    biochemical basis, 390
    importance of extrachromosomal resistance factors, 391
    plasmid location of resistance genes, 390-391
Bactrim, 395, 397
Balarsen, in amoebiasis, 446
Banocide, 454
Barbitone, dose and duration of action, 245
    sodium, dose and duration of action, 245

Barbiturates, 243-246
   absorption and fate, 243-244
   in anaesthesia, 303-304, 306
      dangers, 304
   analgesia, 246
   biochemical effects, 244-245
   in bronchial asthma, 182
   dependence, 484, 488
      withdrawal symptoms, 484
   duration of action, 244, 245
   effect on rapid eye movement, 237
   effect on reticular activating system, 238
   electrophysiological effects, 246
   hypnotic dose, 245
   intravenous anaesthesia, 246
   long-acting, 246
   pharmacological actions, 246
   poisoning, 248
      treatment, 248
   possible teratogenic effect, 225
   in psychotherapy, 246
   and related compounds in epilepsy, 269-270, 277
      chemical structure, 270
   short-acting, 246
   and thiobarbiturates, chemical relationships, 245
Barbituric acid, structure, 243
Bateman function, 47
Baycaron, 166
BCG vaccine, 418
Beclamide as anticonvulsant, 276
Beclomethasone diproprionate, 349
   aerosol in bronchial asthma, 182, 183
Bejel, penicillin in, 437
Benadryl in travel sickness, 98, 193
Bendrofluazide, 166
Benemid in gout, 292, 293
   preparation, 293
Benorylate, anti-inflammatory drug, 293
Benoxinate in local anaesthesia, eyes, 313
   preparation, 315
Benperidol as tranquilliser, 256
Benserazide in Parkinsonism, 274, 277
Benuride as anticonvulsant, 276
Benzalkonium as disinfectant, 458, 462
Benzathine penicillin, 402, 407
   properties, 403
   structure, 403
   in syphilis, 435, 437
Benzedrine, 263
Benzedrex, 130
   as vasoconstrictor, 126
Benzene causing blood dyscrasias, 208
Benzethonium chloride as disinfectant, 458, 462
Benzhexol in Parkinsonism, 274, 277
Benzodiazepines, 248-252
   alcohol withdrawal symptoms, management, 251
   anti-anxiety effect, 250
   anticonvulsant activity, 250
   chemical structures, 249
   hypnotic effects, 250-251
   in labour, 223
   muscle relaxant property, 249

Benzodiazepines, *cont'd*
   other clinical applications, 251
   sedative effects, 250-251
   taming effect, 249-250
   toxic effects, 251
Benzoic acid compound ointment in fungal infections, 231
Benzothiadiazine diuretics, 160-161, 166
   action, 160-161
   chemical structure, 160
   choice, 165
   undesirable effects, 161
Benzoyl peroxide gel in skin fungal infections, 231
Benztropine in Parkinsonism, 274, 277
Benzyl benzoate in scabies, 230, 231
Benzylpenicillin (Penicillin G), 400-402, 407
   absorption and excretion, 400-401
   acid resistance, 403
   antimicrobial activity, 400-402
   blood concentrations, 402
   distribution in body, 401-402
   in erysipelas, 229
   long-acting preparations, 401
   procaine, 402
   properties, 403
   sensitivity of micro organisms, 401
   serum concentrations, 401
   structure, 403
   in syphilis, 436
   therapeutic uses, 404-405
Bephenium hydroxynaphthoate in hookworm infection, 451, 454
Beri-beri, 360, 367
Beta-blockers, 83, 130
   in angina, 123-124
   antiarrhythmic effect, 147
   cardioselectivity, 124
   in hypertension, 115-117
   in hyperthyroidism, 334
   in obstetrics, 218
   stimulant activity, 124
   see also Adrenergic receptor blocking drugs: and specific drugs
Beta receptors for catecholamines, 14
Betacardone, 130
Betadine, 462
Betahistine, 104
Betamethasone, 349
   relative potency, 345
   side effects, 231
Betazole, effect on gastric secretion, 187
Bethanechol, action on gastric juice, 185
Bethanidine, 83, 130
   in hypertension, 119
Betnesol, 349
Bile, pharmacology, 194-196
   bile flow, 194
   biliary spasm, 195
   cholelithiasis, 195
   formation and excretion, 194
   organic constituents, 195
Bilharziasis, 452-453
   preparations, 454
Biligrafin, 195
Bioavailability of drugs, 38

Biological assay, 19-28
   analgesic drugs, 24
   analytical, 22-23
   ceiling effects, 28
   comparative in man, 23-25
   definition, 19
   design, 21-22
   histamine, 23
   indirect, 21-22
   oxytocic drugs, 24
   quantal, 21-22
      ceiling effects, 26
   quantitative, 21
   radioimmunoassay, 19-20
   sedative drugs, 24
Biological standardisation, 20-21
Biotin (Vitamin H), 369
Biperiden in Parkinsonism, 277
Bisacodyl as purgative, 199
Bishydroxycoumarin, *see* Dicoumarol
Bismuth
   glycollylarsanilate in amoebiasis, 446
      structure, 445
   oxycarbonate, as antacid, 191
   in syphilis, 436
'Black tongue', 368
Blood
   brain barrier, functions, 42-43
   coagulation, 210-215
      anticoagulants, 211-215
      factors, 210-211
         pathway, schematic approach, 210
      fibrinolysis, 211
   dyscrasias, caused by chlorpromazine and other phenothiazines, 255
   flow, measurement, 110
      through lungs, rate, 167
   letting, 3, 4
   pressure, arterial, 109-110
      measurement, 110-111
Body
   fluid compartments, and drug distribution, 40-41
   water, drug distribution, 40
Bombesin, 91
Bone marrow, depression, and anaemia, 202
Boric acid as disinfectant, 459, 462
   toxicity, 459
Bradosol, 458, 462
Bradykinin, 90-91
   as bronchoconstrictor, 176
   related polypeptides, 91
Bran as laxative, 197, 201
Breast cancer, oestrogen and androgen treatment, 382, 384
Bretylium
   antiarrhythmic effect, 147
   in hypertension, 118
Brevidil M (Suxameth. br.), 306
Brevital sodium dosage and duration of action, 245
Brietal in anaesthesia, 306
British anti-lewisite, 473
Bromides in epilepsy, 273
Bromism, 273
Bromocriptine in Parkinsonism, 274, 277

Brompheniramine maleate, 104
Bronchi, functions, 176
Bronchial asthma
　assessing severity, 177
　pharmacology, 176-183
　preparations, 183
　symptoms, 176-177
Bronchial musculature, 176
Broxil, 403, 407
Brufen, anti-inflammatory drug, 289-290, 293
Bumetamide, 162, 166
Bupivacaine, as local anaesthetic, 311, 315
Burimamide, 187, 188
Burinex, 162, 166
Burkitt's lymphoma, 383
Busulphan in neoplastic disease, 379, 383, 384
Butacaine, local anaesthetic, 311, 315
Butazolidin, anti-inflammatory drug, 293, 291
Butobarbitone dosage and duration of action, 245
　preparation, 256
Butriptyline hyd., 266
Butyn, 311, 315

Caerulein, 91
Caffeine, 265
　as diuretic, 164
　toxic effects, 265
Calcifediol, 371, 363
Calciferol, 363, 371
Calcitonin (thyrocalcitonin), 336
Calcium
　absorption and vitamin D, 363-364
　carbonate
　　action, 191
　　neutralising power, 190
　　preparation, 201
　current, heart, 130
　disodium versenate, 474
　requirements, 364
Calcynar, 336
Calomel, 3, 4
Camolar in malaria, 440, 446
Camoquin, 442
Cancer
　cell, genetic make-up, 375
　　cycle and anticancer drugs, 377
　　tumour-specific antigens, 375
　　see also Cytotoxic drugs
　chemical induction, 376, 472
　chemotherapy, general principles, 376-378
　drugs used, 378-384
　cytotoxic drugs, see Cytotoxic drugs: and names of specific drugs
Candicidin, 417
　intravaginal, 231
Candida infections, 229-231
　nystatin, 414
Canestan in skin fungal infections, 231
Cannabis, 266
　dependence, 489-490
　pharmacological effects, 266

Capastat, 428
Capreomycin in tuberculosis, 425, 428
Caramiphen in Parkinsonism, 274
Carbachol, 59
　action on gastric juice, 185
　eye preparation, 89
Carbamazepine in epilepsy, 272, 276
Carbamoylcholine, 59
Carbamylmethylcholine, action on gastric juice, 185
Carbarsone in amoebiasis, 446
　structure, 445
Carbenicillin, preparation, 407
　properties, 403, 404
Carbenoxolone sodium effect on gastric mucus, 190
Carbidopa in Parkinsonism, 274, 277
Carbimazole
　dosage, 334
　preparation, 336
　structure, 333, 334
　toxic effects, 336
Carbocaine, 315
Carbon dioxide
　influence on respiratory centre, 168
　as respiratory stimulant, 171
　　with oxygen, 171
　as source of air pollution, 466
　tension, alveolar, 167-168
Carbon monoxide
　poisoning, 170
　treatment, 170
　as source of air pollution, 466
Carbromal (Adalin) as hypnotic, 247
　preparation, 256
Carcinogenic chemicals, action in man, 376
Carcinogens, genetic and environmental factors, 472-473
Carcinogenicity of drugs, tests, 30-31
Cardiac
　action potential, 131-132
　glycosides, action on heart, 135-144
　　action of digitalis on vagus and on conduction, 137-140
　　chemistry, 135-136
　　effect on contractility and output, 136-137
　　effect on oxygen consumption, 137
　　mode of action, 140-143
　　preparations, 149
　　radioimmunoassay, 120, 141
　　see also Digitalis
　　structure, 135
　output, 133
　stimulants, 148-149
Cardiazol, 172
Cardioversion, 147
Carisoma (Carisoprodol)
Carisoprodol as muscle relaxant, 276, 277
Cascara as purgative, 198, 201
Castor oil as purgative, 198, 201
Catecholamines, 73-85
　actions, 79-82
　alpha and beta receptors, 14
　content of tissues, 73
　and cyclic AMP, 79

Catecholamines, cont'd
　formation, 74-75
　measurement in tissues, 73-74
　metabolism, interference in hypertension, 117
　receptors, 78-79
　regulation of turnover, 75
　storage and release, 75-76
　tissue uptake, 77
　urinary secretion, 77
　see also Adrenaline: Dopamine: Isoprenaline: Noradrenaline
Catechol-O-methyl-transferase, 76, 77
Catapres, 130
　in hypertension, 117
　as migraine prophylactic, 129
Caudal anaesthesia, 313
Cedinalid, 149
Cefuroxime, 407
Celbenin, 403, 407
Celevac, 197, 201
Cell membrane, absorption of drugs through, 34-35
Central depressants, 243-256
　effects of morphine, 280
　dependence on
　　hypnotics, 243-248
　motor function, 268-277
　tranquillisers, 248-256
Central nervous system
　effect of morphine, 280
　synaptic transmission, 235-242
　see also Specific drugs
Central venous pressure, measurement, 111
Cephalexin, 407
Cephaloridine, 406-407
　preparation, 407
　structure, 406
Cephalosporins, 406-407
　inhibition of bacterial cell wall synthesis, 39
　preparations, 407
Cephalothin, 407
Cephazolin, 407
Cephradine, 407
Ceporex, 407
Ceporin, 406-407
Cerebrospinal fluid, and drug distribution, 40
Cetavlon as disinfectant, 458, 462
Cetrimide
　in bacterial infections of skin, 231
　as disinfectant, 458, 462
Cetyltrimethylammonium bromide as disinfectant, 458
Chagas' disease, 432, 434
Chelating agents, 473-474, 475
Chemical industry, development, environmental aspects, 465
Chemotherapy, development, 385-386
　see also Antibacterial: Cytotoxic drugs
Chenodeoxycholic acid, 195
　gallstone dissolving, 201
Chiniofon, 444
　structure, 445
Chloral betain as hypnotic, 247

INDEX

Chloral hydrate
  as anaesthetic, 298
  as hypnotic, 247, 256
  structure, 247
Chlorambucil, in neoplastic disease, 378, 384
  structure, 379
Chloramine, as disinfectant, 459
Chloramphenicol, 411, 415, 417
  antibiotic activity, 411
  causing blood dyscrasias, 208
  fate, 411
  as 'feed' antibiotic, 471
  side effects, 411
  structure, 411
  therapeutic use, 411
  toxicity, 411
Chlorates causing methaemoglobinaemia, 208
Chlordiazepoxide, 250
  assay in man, 24, 25
  as muscle relaxant drug, 276, 277
  preparation, 256
Chlorethylamine, derivatives, 83
Chlorguanide in malaria, 440, 446
Chlorhexidine
  as disinfectant, 462
  gluconate solution in bacterial infections of skin, 231
  structure, 461
Chlorimipramine in depression, 256, 266
Chlorine as disinfectant, 458-459
Chlormethiazole edisylate as tranquilliser, 256
Chloroform anaesthesia, 301
  toxicity, 301
Chloromycetin, 417
Chloroproguanil in malaria, 446
Chloroquine in malaria, 440-442
  antimalarial action, 441
  preparations, 446
  properties, 440-441
  structure, 441
Chloroquine in malaria,
  sulphate, 293
  therapeutic uses, 441
  toxicity, 441
Chlorothiazide, 166, 393
Chlorotrianisene, 354
Chloroxylenol as disinfectant, 462
  structure, 461
Chlorpheniramine, structure, 96
Chlorphenoxamine in Parkinsonism, 277
Chlorpromazine as major tranquilliser, 252-255
  administration and fate, 254
  allergic sideeffects, 255
  alterations in animal behaviour, 253
  as antiemetic, 193-94, 254
  assay, 26
  effects in man, 253
  effect on reticular activating system, 238
  in intractable hiccough, 254
  pharmacological effects, 252-253
  related phenothiazines, 254
  in senile agitation and mania, 254

Chlorpromazine, *cont'd*
  structure, 255
  tardive dyskinesia, 255-256
  in tetanus, 254
  treatment of schizophrenic psychoses, 254
  untoward effects, 254-255
Chlorpropamide, 340, 341, 349
  chemical structure, 341
Chlortetracycline, 409, 416, 417
  bacterial resistance, 409
  in bacterial skin infections, 231
  clinical application, 410
  as 'feed' antibiotic, 471
  mode of action, 409
  in spirochaetal infections, 437
  structure, 409
  toxicity, 410
Chlorthalidone, diuretic action, 161, 166
Cholecalciferol, 363, 371
Cholecystokinin-pancreozymin, 194
Cholelithiasis, 195-196
Cholestyramine, as lipid lowering agent, 196
  preparation, 201
Choline, 369
  theophyllinate in bronchial asthma, 182
Cholinergic transmission, 53-72
  acetylcholine, 57-59
  anticholinesterases, 60-62
  drugs stimulating cholinergic receptors, 57-62
  drugs which block cholinergic receptors, 62-71
  eyes, 87-88
  ganglion blocking drugs, 62-64
  humoral transmission, theory, 55-56
  interference with neuromuscular transmission, 64
  muscarinic receptor blocking drugs, 69
  neuromuscular blocking drugs, 65
  peripheral nervous system, chemical organisation, 56-57
  physiology of the autonomic system, 53-56
Cholinesterase, mode of action, 60
Chorionic gonadotrophin, 325-326
Chromium, 473
Ciba, 1906, 428
Cidomycin, 417
Cimetidine, effect on gastric secretion, 187, 188
  preparation (Tagamet), 200
Cinchocaine, as local anaesthetic, 311, 315
  relative efficiency, 312
  spinal anaesthesia, 314
Cinchona bark, 3
Cinnarizine as antiemetic, 194
Circulation
  action of drugs, 110-130
  adrenaline, 79-81
  coronary vasodilator and antianginal drugs, 121-124
  hypertension and antihypertensive drugs, 111-121
  peripheral, 109
  vasoconstrictor drugs, 124-129

Circulatory collapse, treatment, 129
  drugs, 129
  transfusions, 129
Citanest, 311, 315
Clefamide in amoebiasis, 445
Clindamycin, 409, 415, 416, 417
Clinoril, anti-inflammatory drug, 293
Clioquinol, 444
  structure, 445
Clobetasol propionate, 350
Clofazimine, 428
Clofibrate
  as lipid lowering agent, 196
  preparation, 201
Clomiphene, 354, 359
  citrate, structure, 354
Clomocycline, 417
Clonazepam in epilepsy, 272, 276
Clonidine, 130
  in hypertension, 117
  in migraine, 118
    prophylactic, 129
  side effects, 118
Clorevan in Parkinsonism, 277
Clotrimazole in skin fungal infections, 231
Clotting factors, 210, 213
  deficiencies, 210-211
Clorexolone, diuretic action, 161, 166
Cloxacillin preparations, 407
  properties, 403, 404
Clozapine as tranquilliser, 256
Coagulant drugs, 215
Coal tar, as carcinogen, 473
Cobalamins, 206-207
  preparations, 216
Cobalt edetate in cyanide poisoning, 171, 183
Cocaine, 265, 309-310
  sympathomimetic action, 309
  central stimulant action, 310
  dependence, 484
  hydrochloride, 309-310
  as local anaesthetic, 309
  preparation, 315
  relative efficiency, 312
  structure, 310
  toxicity, 310
Codeine, analgesic activity, 279
  biological assay, 25
  as cough depressant, 175, 183
  pharmacological actions, 282
  preparation, 293
  structure, 281
Cogentin in Parkinsonism, 274, 277
Colaspase as antitumour agent, 382, 384
Colchicine
  as antitumour agent, 382, 384
  in gout, 292, 293
Colistimethate, 413
Colistin, 413, 417
Collagen diseases, corticosteroids, 347
Colloidal preparations as disinfectants, 459
Colofac, as antispasmodic, 200, 201
Cologel, 197
Colomycin, 413

Competitive neuromuscular block and depolarising block, differences, 68
  blocking agents, 66
Concordin, 267
Conduction anaesthesia, 311, 312, 313
Conn's syndrome *see* Aldosteronism, primary
Constipation, causes, 199
  see also Purgatives, and specific names
Contact sensitization, 230
Contraceptives
  future, 478
  hormonal, 476-480
    adverse reactions, 477
    benefits, 477
    contraindications, 477
    male, 479-480
    mode of action, 476-477
    oral, 476-477
    postcoital, 478
    preparations, 480
    properties, 476
    progestogen implants, 477
  immunisation against pregnancy, 479
  occlusive, 478
Copper sulphate
  as emetic, 192
  preparation, 201
Cordilox action on heart, 146, 149
Coronary insufficiency, 122
Corticosteroids, 343-349
  administration, 347
  in bronchial asthma, 182, 183
  causing hypertension, 111-112
  complications of therapy, 349
  control of secretion, 344
  in eczema, 230-231
  empirical use, 349
  glucocorticoids, 346
  in leukaemia and allied disorders, 382, 383-384
  mineralocorticoids, 345-346
  preparations, 349-350
  replacement therapy, 347
  in rheumatic diseases, 289
  in status asthmaticus, 183
  supplementary therapy, 347
  synthetic, 343
  therapeutic uses, 347-349
  topical, in psoriasis, 229
    side effects, 231
Corticotrophin, 336
  in bronchial asthma, 182, 183
  releasing factor, 323
  see also ACTH
Cortisol, 346-348
  half-life, 46
  see also Hydrocortisone
Cortisone, 343, 349
  relative potency, 345
Corticosterone, 343
Cortrosyn, 328
Co-trimoxazole, 395-396, 415, 417
  clinical uses, 396
  effect on PABA, 396
  mode of action, 395

Co-trimoxazole, *cont'd*
  possible teratogenic effect, 225
  preparation, 397
  toxic effects, 396
Cough
  depressants, 173-176, 183
  reflex, 173-174
Coumarin, 211-216
  anticoagulants, antagonise vitamin K, 365, 366
  contraindications, 215
  preparations, 216
  structures, 213
Cresol as disinfectant, 460
  toxicity, 460
Cretinism, 333
CRF, *see* Corticotrophin releasing factor
Cromolyn sodium in bronchial asthma, 181-182, 183
Crotamiton in scabies, 230, 231
Cumulation of drugs, 47-48
Cyanide poisoning, 170-171
  treatment, 170-171
Cyanocobalamin, 206, 216, 369, 371
Cyclazocine, 293
Cyclic AMP
  and catecholamines, 79
  formation and metabolism, 319
  hormones affecting levels, 320
  second messenger concept, 320
  structure, 79
Cyclic GMP, 320-321
Cyclic nucleotides and hormone action, 319
Cyclizine
  preparation, 201
  in travel sickness, 193
Cyclobarbitone
  effect on PGR, 25
  dosage and duration of action, 245
  preparation, 256
Cycloguanyl embonate in leishmaniasis, 435
  in malaria, 440, 446
Cyclopenthiazide, 166
Cyclopentolate
  action on eye, 88
  preparations, 89
Cyclophosphamide
  in neoplastic disease, 378, 383, 384
  structure, 379
  in psoriasis, 229
  structure, 379
Cycloplegics, 88
Cyclopropane anaesthesia, 303, 306
Cycloserine
  inhibition of bacterial cell wall synthesis, 390
  in tuberculosis, 425, 428
Cyproterone, 321
  acetate, 359
Cytamen (cyanocobalamin) 206, 216
Cytarabine, 397
  in leukaemia and virus diseases, 381, 383, 384
Cytochrome P450, 43

Cytoplasmic membrane, increased permeability by antibiotics, 388
Cytosine arabinoside, in leukaemia and virus diseases, 381, 384
Cytotoxic drugs
  in cancer treatment, 375-384
    administration, 384
    agents of natural origin, 381-382
    alkylating agents, 378-379
    antimetabolites, 379-381
    and cell cycle, 377
    dose-response curve, 383
    drug resistance, 377
    drugs used, 378-384
    hormones, 382-383
    immunosuppressive effects, 376
    preparations, 384
    testing, 377
    two-stage sequential procedure, 378
    unwanted effects, 383
  causing blood dyscrasias, 208
  in psoriasis, 229

Dacarbazine in neoplastic disease, 379, 383, 384
Dactinomycin as antitumour agent, 382, 384
Daktarin (miconazole) in skin fungal infections, 231
Danazol, 359
Danthron as purgative, 198, 201
Dantrium as muscle relaxant, 276, 277
Dantrolene as muscle relaxant, 276, 277
Daonil, 349
Dapsone, 393
  in leprosy, 428
  in malaria, 446
Daranide, 166
Daraprim in malaria, 440, 446
Daricon, in hyperchlorhydria, 190
Dartalan (thiopropazate) as tranquilliser, 256
Daunorubicin
  as antitumour agent, 382, 384
  in leukaemia, 383
DDAVP (desmopressin), 336
DDT, 467
Debrisoquine, 130
  sulphate, 130
Decadron, 349
Decamethonium, 66
  structure and action, 67-68
Declinax, 130
7-Dehydrocholesterol, 363, 371
Dehydroemetine in amoebiasis, 444, 447
Demecarium, action on eyes, 87
  preparation, 89
  side effects, 87-88
Demeclocycline, 417
  bacterial resistance, 409
  clinical application, 410
  mode of action, 409
  structure, 409
  toxicity, 410
Demecolcine as antitumour agent, 382

Demethylchlortetracycline, 409, 417
  structure, 409
Dental anaesthesia, 313
Deoxycortone acetate, 345, 346, 350
Depolarisation block, 66
  and competitive blocks, differences, 68
Depolarising blocking agents in anaesthesia, 306, 307
Depressants, central, 243-256
  dependence, 248
Depression, amine mechanism, 240
  drugs for, 257-265
    amphetamine and related drugs, 262-265
    imipramine and related antidepressants, 257-260
    lithium, 261-262
    monoamine oxidase inhibitors, 260-261
Derbac in lice infections, 230, 231
Dermovate, 350
D-receptors, effect of 5-HT, 93
Desenex, 417
Deseril, 130
  as migraine prophylactic, 128-129
Deserpidine, 130
Desferal, 474, 475
  as chelating agent, 205, 216
Desferrioxamine in iron poisoning, 474, 475
  mesylate, as chelating agent, 205, 216
Desipramine
  chemical properties, 258
  preparation, 266
  structure, 258
Deslanoside, action on heart, 149
Desmopressin, 130, 336
Desonide, 350
Detergents as disinfectants, 458, 462
Dettol as disinfectant, 462
Dexamethasone, 343, 349
  relative potency, 345
Dexamphetamine sulphate
  in depression, 263, 267
  in hyperkinesis, 264
Dexedrine in depression, 263
  preparation, 267
Dextrans in circulatory collapse, 129
Dextroamphetamine sulphate, 263
Dextromethorphan as cough depressant, 175, 183
Dextromoramide as analgesic, 284
  preparation, 293
Dextropropoxyphene as analgesic, 284, 293
Dextrothyroxine in hyperlipidaemia, 196
  preparation, 201
DFP, see Diisopropylfluorophosphonate
Diabetes insipidus, 155-156
Diabetes mellitus
  coma, 342
  experimental, 337
  human, 337
  insulin in, 337-8, 341
    insulin preparations, 339-340, 349
    see also insulin
  oral hyperglycaemic drugs, 349

Diabinese, 340, 349
Dial dosage duration of action, 245
Diamidines in leishmaniasis, 435, 437
Diamorphine
  as analgesic, 293
  as cough depressant, 175
  pharmacological action, 282
Diamox, 87, 164, 166
Diaphragm as contraceptive, 478
Diarrhoea, drugs affecting, 200, 201
Diasone, 428
Diazepam
  in anaesthesia, 304, 305
  anticonvulsant activity, 250
  as muscle relaxant, 276, 277
  pharmacological effects, 24, 249
  in premedication, children, 251
  sedative and hypnotic effects, 250-251
  preparation, 256
  in status asthmaticus, 183
  in status epilepticus, 273
Diazinon structure, 468
Diazoxide, 130, 349
  in hypertension, 121
Dibenzocycloheptene derivatives, 258
Dibotin, 340, 349
Dibutylphthalate, 469
Dichloralphenazone, as hypnotic, 247
  preparation, 256
Dichloroisoprenaline, 78, 83
Dichlorphenamide, 87
Dichlorvos, 469
  structure, 468
Dichlorophen in tapeworm infections, 449, 454
Dichlorphenamide, 166
Dichlorvos, in whipworm infections, 451
Diclofenac sodium anti-inflammatory drug, 293
Dicloxacillin, properties, 404
Dicophane(DDT), 467
  in lice infections, 230, 231
  resistance, 469
  structure, 468
  toxicity, 468
Dicoumarol, 211, 212, 213, 216
  dosage, 213
  half-life, 46
  structure, 213
Dicyclomine, 71
Dienoestrol, 354, 355, 359
  clinical potency, 355
  clinical uses, 355
Dietary therapy in diabetes, 341-342
Diethazine in Parkinsonism, 274
Diethylcarbamazine in filariasis, 454
Diethylether, 306
Diethylpropion in appetite reduction, 264
  preparation, 267
Diethylstilboestrol, 359
Diethyltoluamide, 469, 475
Diflucortolone valerate, 350
Digitalis, 135-144
  action on conduction, 138-139
  action, onset and duration, 141
  action on vagus, 137-138
  administration, principles, 142-143

Digitalis, cont'd
  clinical use, 143
  effect on excitability of heart muscle, 139
  effect on oxygen consumption, 137
  mode of action, 140-143
  receptor, 140-141
  side effects, 139
  toxic action, 143-144
  in treatment of congestive heart failure, 143
Digitoxin
  pharmacokinetics, 141-142
  preparation, 149
Digoxin
  pharmacokinetics, 141-142
  preparation, 149
  radioimmunoassay, 141
  structure and chemistry, 135-136
Dihydroergotamine, 83
  tartrate, 130
Dihydroergotoxine mesylate, dosage, 85
Dihydrohydroxymorphinone, 282
1, 25-Dihydroxycholecalciferol, 363, 371
Diiodohydroxyquinoline, 444, 446
  structure, 445
Diisopropylfluorophosphonate (DFP), action, 61, 61-62
  action on eye, 87
  side effects, 87-88
Dilators, see Vasodilators
Diloxanide
  in amoebiasis, 446
  turoate, 445
  structure, 445
Dimelor, 349
Dimenhydrinate, as antiemetic, 201
Dimercaprol, 473
  actions, 473
  administration, 473
  therapeutic uses, 473
Dimethindene maleate, 104
Dimethoate, 469
Dimethothiazine mesylate, 104
Dimethoxy-methyl amphetamine (DOM) chemical structure, 489
Dimethylaminopropyl derivatives, 254
Dimethylphthalate, 469, 475
Dimethyltryptamine (DMT) dependence, 489
Dimethyl tubocurarine, 307
Dimotane, 104
Dindevan, 214, 216
Dinitro-orthocresol (DNOC), 469
Dinoprost trometamol (prostaglandin $F_{2\alpha}$), 225
Dinoprostone (prostaglandin E_2), 225
Dioctyl sodium sulphosuccinate, 197, 201
Diodone, 166
Diodoquin, 444, 446
Diodrast, 166
Diparcol in Parkinsonism, 274
Diphenhydramine, 98, 104, 193
  structure, 96
  in travel sickness, 193

Diphenoxylate, as antispasmodic, 200, 201
Diphenpyraline, 104
Dipipanone as analgesic, 284
Diprophylline in bronchial asthma, 182
Dipropylacetate in epilepsy, 272
Dipyridamole, 130
   as coronary vasodilator, 123
   and platelet aggregation, 209, 216
Diquat, 470
Disinfectants, 456-462
   heat, 458
   inorganic agents, 458-459
   irradiation, 459
   methods, 456
   organic agents, 459-462
   phenol-coefficient test, 456-458
   for pre-operative scrubbing of skin, 461-462
   preparations, 462
   surface active agents, 458
Disipal in Parkinsonism, 275, 277
   Disodium cromoglycate in bronchial asthma, 181-182, 183
   Disodium edetate, inhibition of blood coagulation, 211
Disopyramide, action on heart, 147, 149
Distal tubules, and drug excretion, 44
Distalgesic as analgesic, 201
Disulfiram in alcoholism, 488
Dithranol in psoriasis, 228, 231
Diuresis, forced alkaline, 164-165
Diuretic drugs, 158-166
   choice, 165-166
   classification, 160
   clinical use, 160
   evaluation, 158
   forced alkaline, 164
   hypertension, 113-114
   loop, 161-163
   mercurial, 161
   obsolete, 164-165
   potassium sparing, 163-164
   preparations, 166
   reabsorption and excretion, 158-160
   sodium, potassium and water, 158-159
   thiazides, 160-161
Divinyl ether anaesthesia, 301
Dixarit as migraine prophylactic, 129
DNA function, drug interference, 388
Dobutamine, as cardiac stimulant, 149
Doca, 345, 350
DOM *see* Dimethoxy-methyl amphetamine
Domiphen bromide as disinfectant, 458, 462
Dopa decarboxylase, 74
Dopamine
   action, 125
   blood-brain barrier, 41
   content of tissues, 73
   formation, 74
   hypothesis of schizophrenia, 240-241
   as neurotransmitter, 82
   in Parkinsonism, 273
   preparation, 85

Dopamine, *cont'd*
   receptors, central, 239
      extrapyramidal control, 239
      tardive dyskinesia, 239
   stimulation in hypertension, 120
   transmitter role in CNS, 235
Dopaminergic activity of apomorphine, 192
Doriden as hypnotic, 247
   preparation, 256
Dothiepin hyd, 266
Doxapram, as respiratory stimulant, 173, 183
Doxepin in depression, 258, 266
Doxorubicin as antitumour agent, 382, 384
Doxycycline, 417
Droleptan as tranquilliser, 256
Dromoran as analgesic, 283, 293
Droperidol
   as analgesic, 293
   as tranquilliser, 256
Droperidol-fentanyl mixture in neuroleptanalgesia, 305
Drostanolone, 384
Drugs
   absorption, *see* Absorption of drugs
   action, and chemical composition, 9-10
      assessment of toxicity, 30-31
      biological assay, 19-28
      measurement, 19-33
      structural specificity, 12
     on circulation, 110-130
     on cough, 174-176
       assessment, 174-175
       on cough centre, 175-176
     on the eye, 87-88
     on the fetus, 224-225
     on gastric secretion, 185-191
     on heart, 135-149
     on intestinal movements, 197-200
       smooth muscle, 200-201
     on respiration, 170-183
     pharmacogenetics, 28-29
     specific and non-specific, 16-17
     therapeutic index, 29-30
   administration, frequency, 48-49
   adverse effects, 31
      classification, 31
   advertisements, 8
   affecting peripheral cholinergic mechanisms, 57
   allergic reactions, 31
   antagonism, chemical, 16
      competitive, 11-15
      non-equilibrium, 16
      physiological, 16
      true non-competitive, 16
      unsurmountable, 15-16
   approved names, 8
   binding to plasma proteins, 41-42
      competition for sites, 42
   clearance, 42
   commercial influences, 7-8
   control, mandatory scheme, 7
      voluntary schemes, 6-7

Drugs, coronary vasodilator, 121-124
   cumulation, 47-48
   dependence, 481-491
      addiction and habituation, 481-482
      alcohol, 481, 484-488
      analgesics, tests, 279
      barbiturate, 488, 481
      cannabis, 489-490, 481
      CNS depressants, 484
      CNS stimulants, 483-484
      hallucinogen, 488-489, 481
      maintenance therapy, 491
      management, 490-491
      mechanism, 482
      opiates, 482, 481
      patterns, 482-490
      prevention, 491
      social aspects, 481-482
      tobacco, 490, 481
      treatment, 491
      types and compounds, 481
      withdrawal syndrome, 483, 484
        management, 491
   distribution in body, 39-40
   diuretic action on kidneys, 158-166
   excretion, by kidney, 44-45, 154
      secretory mechanisms, 45
   half-life, 46
   hypersensitivity, 31, 103-104
   induced blood dyscrasias, 208-209
      treatment, 208-209
   idiosyncracy, 31
   in circulatory collapse, 129
   intolerance, 31
   metabolism, 42-46
      see also Metabolism
   mode of action, 9
   mimicking acetylcholine, 71
   modifying adrenergic activity, 82-84
   and monoamine oxidase inhibitors, interaction, 44
   nephrotoxic effects, 154-155
   penetration into fat depots, 41
   pharmacokinetics
      see also Pharmocokinetics
   physico-chemical activity, 10
   proprietary names, 7-8
   reactions of skin, 231
   receptors, 10-18
      concept, 10
      interactions, 9-18
      see also Receptors, drug
   secondary effects, 31
   side effects, 31
      and plasma concentration, 48, 49
   stimulating cholinergic receptors, 57-62
      see also Acetylcholine: Methacholine: Muscarine: Pilocarpine: Anticholinesterases
   teratogenicity, assessment, 31
      effects, 225
   therapeutic trials, 32-33
      statistical methods, 32
   toxicity, assessment, 30-31
   variation in response, individual, 26-28
   vasoconstrictor, 124-129

DTIC in cancer, 384
Dulcolax, as purgative, 199, 201
Duodenal hormones, 194
Duphalac, 201
Durabolin, 358, 359
Dydrogesterone, 359
Dyflos, see Diisopropylfluorphosphonate
Dysmenorrhoea, use of progestogens, 357
Dytax, 163-164, 166

Eccrine glands, 227
Ecology, 465-471
Ecothiopate, see Phospholine iodide
Ectopic pregnancies, and IUDs, 478
Eczema, 230-231
    treatment, 230-231
Edathamil, 473-474
Edecrin, 162, 163, 165, 166
    actions, 163
    clinical effects and toxicity, 163
Edetic acid, 473-474
Edrophonium chloride, action, 61
Efcortelan, 349
Elamol, 267
Electroconvulsive therapy, 257
Electrocortin, 350
Electroencephalogram and sleep, 236-238
    rapid eye movement, 237
    reticular activating system, 237-238
Electrolytes, intestinal absorption, 36-37
    weak, excretion by kidney, 43-44
Eledoisin, 91
Eltroxin, 336
Emeside in epilepsy, 276
Emetics, 192-193
    central, 192-193
    early use, 3
    local, 192
Endoxana, in neoplastic disease, 378-379, 384
Enduron, 166
Enflurane, 302
Enkephalins, role, 241
Entamoeba histolytica, 444
Entobex, in amoebiasis, 445
Envacar, 130
Environment
    current problems, 465
        air pollution, 466
        chemical industry, 465
        health aspects, 471-473
        protection, 465
            carcinogens, 472
            nutritional deficiencies, 471-472
            protein-calorie malnutrition, 472
Enzymes
    microbial, control, 387
    microsomal, hepatic, and drug metabolism, 43-44
        interaction of drugs, 44
    see also specific names
Epanutin, action on heart, 146, 149
    in epilepsy, 270, 271
    toxic effects, 270
Ephedrine, 130
    in bronchial asthma, 180-181, 183
    as cough depressant, 175

Ephedrine, *cont'd*
    hydrochloride in depression, 263
    as vasoconstrictor, 126
Epidural anaesthesia, 311, 313
Epilepsy, 268-273
    anticonvulsant drugs, 268-273, 276
        assessment, 268
        barbiturates and related compounds, 269-270, 277
        bromides, 273
        carbamazepine, 272, 276
        hydantoin derivatives, 270-271
        mode of action, 268
        oxazolidinediones, 271-272
        sodium valproate, 272-273
        status epilepticus, 273
        succinimides, 271
Epilim in epilepsy, 277
Epinephrine in bronchial asthma, 177-178, 183
Epodyl, 384
Epontol, 306
Epsom salts, 197, 201
Equanil as muscle relaxant, 276, 277
Eraldin, 130
Ergocalciferol, 363, 371
Ergot alkaloids, 83
    clinical uses, 220, 225
    toxicity, 220-221
Ergometrine, 221-222
    action on uterus, 221
    assay, 24
    chemical structure, 221
    preparation, 225
    in prevention of postpartum haemorrhage, 223
Ergonovine, 225
Ergotamine, 127-128
Erysipelas, treatment, 229
Erythromycin, 408, 415, 417
    antibacterial activity, 408
    estolate, 408
    half-life, 46
    in syphilis, 437
Esbatal, 130
Eserine, see Physostigmine
Estramustine phosphate (Estracyt), 384
Ethacrynic acid, 162, 165, 166
    in hypertension, 114
Ethambutol in tuberculosis, 424, 426, 428
    structure, 424
    toxicity, 424
Ethamivan, as respiratory stimulant, 173, 183
Ether anaesthesia, 296-298
    method of administration, 300
    pharmacological effects, 300
    preparation, 306
    stages, 296-298
Ethinyl oestradiol, 353, 359
    clinical potency, 355
    in menopausal disorders, 355
Ethionamide, in tuberculosis, 425
    structure, 422
Ethisterone, 356
Ethoglucid, 384
Ethopropazine in Parkinsonism, 275

Ethosuximide in epilepsy, 271
Ethotoin as anticonvulsant, 276
Ethrane, 302
Ethyl alcohol, dependence, 484
    absorption and excretion, 484-485
    action on CNS, 485
Ethyl biscoumacetate, 213
    half-life, 46
Ethyl chloride, 298
Ethyloestrenol, 359
Etomidate sulphate in anaesthesia, 306
Etrenol, 454
Eudemine, 130
Eumydrine, see Atropine methonitrate
Eutonyl, 130
Evadyne, 266
Eve's rocking method of resuscitation, 169
Evipan, 298
    sodium dosage and duration of action, 245
Exophthalmos, 332
Expectorants, 175-176
Extracellular fluid, and drug distribution, 40
Extrachromosomal resistance factors, importance, 391
Extrapyramidal system, 239-240
    central dopamine receptors, 239
    haloperidol, 256
    Parkinsonism, 239
    phenothiazines, 254-255
    tardive dyskinesia, 239-240
Eyes
    anaesthetics for, 313
    autonomic control of intrinsic muscles, 86-89
    diseases, corticosteroids, 348
    drops, 89
    drugs acting on, 87-88
        side effects, 87-88

Fabahistin, 104
Factor VIII antihaemophilic factor, 211, 216
Fanasil, 446
Family planning, 476
False transmitters, 84
Fat depots, penetration of drugs, 41
Fazadininium bromide (Fazadon) in anaesthesia, 306
Felypressin, 329, 336
Femergin, 130
Fenfluramine in appetite reduction, 264
    preparation, 267
Fenoprofen, anti-inflammatory drug, 289, 293
Fenoterol bromide, 183
Fentanyl
    as analgesic, 283-284, 293
    in neuroleptanalgesia, 305
Fentazin as tranquilliser, 256
Feprazone anti-inflammatory drug, 293
Ferric ammonium citrate in iron deficiency, 205, 216

Ferrous fumarate in iron deficiency, 205, 216
Ferrous gluconate in iron deficiency, 205, 216
Ferrous glycine sulphate complex in iron deficiency, 205, 216
Ferrous salts in iron deficiency, 204, 216
Ferrous sulphate in iron deficiency, 204, 216
Fertility control, 476
Fetus, effects of drugs on, 224-225
Fibrin foam, 215
Fibrinogen, substances which clot, 215
Fibrinolysis, 211
   aminocaproic acid, 211
   ancrod, 211
   enhancement, 211
   therapy, 211, 214-215
Fick principle in measuring cardiac output, 133
Filariasis, anthelmintics, 454
Filix mas in tapeworm infection, 449
Flagyl, 444, 447
Flazedil in anaesthesia, 306
Floxapen, 407
Fluanxol as tranquilliser, 256
Flubiprofen anti-inflammatory drug, 293
Flucinolone, side effects, 231
Flucloxacillin, 415
   preparation, 407
   properties, 404
Flucytosine, 414, 417
Fludrocortisone, 345
   preparation, 350
   structure, 345
Fluocinolone acetate, 343, 347, 349
Fluocinonide, 350
Fluomar, 306
Fluopromazine major tranquilliser, 254
   structure, 255
Fluorouracil in cancer, 381, 384
Fluothane anaesthesia, 301, 306
Fluoxymesterone, 358, 359
   structure, 357
Flupenthixol as tranquilliser, 256
Fluphenazine
   as antiemetic, 254
   in schizophrenia, 254
   structures, 255
Fluprednidene acetate, 350
Flurandrenolone, 350
Flurazepam
   preparation, 256
   as sedative and hypnotic, 251
Fluroxene anaesthesia, 306
Folate deficiency induced by trimethoprim, 396
Folic acid, 207-208, 216, 369
   analogues in neoplastic disease, 380
   antagonists, possible teratogenic effects, 225
   deficiency, 369
   requirements, 369, 371
Follicle-stimulating hormone, 322, 325, 336
   influence on ovarian cycle, 351
Follitropin, 336

Food
   interaction with monoamine oxidase inhibitors, 44
   preservatives, 471
   production, chemicals involved, 467
Forane, 302
Forced alkaline diuresis, 164-165
Formaldehyde as disinfectant, 459-460
Fortral as analgesic, 283
Framboesia, drug treatment, 437
Framycetin, 417
Froben, 293
Frusemide
   as diuretic, 162, 165, 166
   in hypertension, 114
Fuadin in schistosomiasis, 454
Fucidin, 407
Fuller's earth, 470
Fungicides, 470
Fungicidin, 417
Fungilin, in fungal infections, skin, 231
Fungizone, 417
Fungus infections of skin, 229-230
Furacin, 433
Furadantin, 396, 397
Furamide, 446
Fusidate sodium, 407
Fusidic acid, 415
Fybranta, 201

GABA, transmitter role in CNS, 235-236
Gallamine triethiodide in anaesthesia, 306
   structure and action, 67
Gallstone
   dissolving chenodeoxycholic acid, 196, 201
   formation, 195-196
Gamma-aminobutyric acid, see GABA
Gamma benzene hexachloride insecticide, 467-468
   in scabies, and pediculosis, 230
   structure, 468
   toxicity, 468
Gammexane, 467
   toxicity, 468
Ganglion blocking agents, 62-64, 130
   and gastric secretion, 190
   in hypertension, 120
Gantrisin, 395, 397
Gardenal, and Gardenal sodium, dosage and duration of action, 256
Gases
   anaesthetic, 302-303
      isonarcotic concentrations, 295
   respiratory, interchange, 167-168
Gastric juice, secretion, 184-185
   and histamine, 95
   H_2 receptor antagonists, 187-188
   phases, 184-185
   mucus, drugs affecting, 190
   secretion, drugs acting on, 185-191
      inhibition, 189
Gastrins
   assay, 186
   chemical structure, 186
   pentagastrin, 186

Gastrins, *cont'd*
   pepsin secretion, 187
   properties, 185-187
Gastro-intestinal hormones, radioimmunoassays, 20
Gaussian curve, 22, 30
Gelatin, 130
   sponge in local haemorrhage, 215
Gelofusine, 130
Gentamycin, 412, 415, 417
   cream in impetigo, 229, 231
Germanin, 437
Gestronol hexan, 384
GH, see Growth hormone
Gitalin, 135
Gitaloxin, 135
Gitoxin, 135
Glibenclamide, 341, 349
Glibenese, 349
Glibornuride, 349
Glipizide, 349
Globin Zinc insulin injection, 349
Glomerular filtration of drugs, 44
Glucagon (HGF), 342-343, 349
   action, 342
   clinical uses, 343
Glucocorticoids, 343, 346-349
   administration, 347
   complications of therapy, 349
   cortisol (hydrocortisone), 346-348
      see also Hydrocortisone
   metyrapone (Metopirone) 349, 350
   preparations, 349
   relative potencies, 345
   therapeutic uses, 347-348
Glucophage, 340, 349
Glutamic acid hydrochloride, in hypochlorhydria, 189
Glutamine, transmitter role in CNS, 236
Glutethimide
   half-life, 46
   as hypnotic, 247
   preparation, 256
Glutril, 349
Glyceryl trinitrate, 130
   in angina, 122, 123
   in biliary spasm, 195
Glycine, transmitter role in CNS, 235, 236
Glycobiarsol, 446
Glycosides, cardiac, see Cardiac glycoside: digitalis
Glymidine, 349
Glyotoxin, 385
Goitre, 330
   endemic, 332-333
Gold compounds in arthritis, 290
Goldblatt kidney, 111
Gonadorelin, 323
Gonadotrophins, menopausal, 354
Gondafon, 349
Gonadotrophic hormones, 325-326
   chorionic, 325
   preparations, 336
   see also Follicle stimulating hormone: Luteinising hormone

Gonococcal infections, treatment with penicillin, 405
Gout, drugs used in, 292-293
Gram-negative penicillin-resistant organisms, streptomycin use, 411
Gram-positive infections, penicillin, 404
Graves' disease, 332
Griseofulvin, 230, 231, 413-414, 417
  absorption and excretion, 413-414
  antifungal activity, 413
  structure, 413
  therapeutic uses, 414
Growth hormone, 322, 336
  releasing factor, 323
  release-inhibiting hormone (GHRIH), 322, 323
Guanethidine, 83
  in hypertension, 118
  monosulphate, 130
Guanine monophosphate, cyclic, *see* Cyclic GMP
Guanoclor sulphate, 130
Guanoxan sulphate, 130

Haelan, 350
Haemolytic anaemia, drug-induced, 208
Haemolytic streptococcal infections, penicillin treatment, 405
Haemophilia, 211
Haemopoietic system, 202-216
Haemorrhage
  due to anticoagulant drugs, use of vitamin K, 366
  local, control, 215
  postpartum, ergometrine in preparation, 223
Halciderm, 350
Halcinonide, 350
Half-life of drugs, 46
Hallucinations, drug-induced, 265-266
Hallucinogenic drugs
  dependence, 488-489
  and schizophrenia, 241
  structure, 489
Haloperidol
  in neuroleptanalgesia, 305
  in psychoses, 256
    preparations, 256
    side effects, 256
  causing tardive dyskinesia, 239
Halothane anaesthesia, 301, 306
Hansch analysis, 12
Harmonyl, 130
Havapen, 407
Heart, 131-150
  action of catecholamines, 81
  activity, reflex mechanisms controlling, 133
  antiarrhythmic agents, 144-148, 149
  calcium current, 132
  cardiac action potential, 131-132
  cardiac output, 133
  cardiac stimulants, 148-149
  cardioversion, 147
  contractions, interval, 131
  disordered rhythms, 134-135

Heart, *cont'd*
  effect of oxygen lack, 121-122
  failure, congestive, digitalis in, 143
  muscle, properties, 133
  transmission of wave of excitation, 131
Heat as disinfectant, 458
Heavy metal poisoning, antidotes, 473-474
  salts, as emetics, 192
Helium and oxygen in bronchial asthma, 182
Heminevrin (chlormethiazole) as sedative hypnotic, 256
Hemofil, 216
Henderson-Hasselbalch equation, 34
Heparin, 211, 212, 216
  administration in man, 212
  low-dose, prophylactic use, 212
  protamine sulphate, 212, 216
  structure and action, 212
Hepatic microsomal enzymes, and drug metabolism, 43-44
Herbicides, 469-470
  functions, 469
Heroin, as cough depressant, 175
Heroin dependence, 482-483
  pharmacological action, 293
  preparation, 293
  structure, 281
Herpes infections, idoxuridine, 396-397
Herpes simplex, treatment, 229
Herpes zoster, treatment, 229
Hetrazan, 454
Hexachlorophane (Hexachlorophene) as disinfectant, 462
  structure, 461
  toxicity, 462
Hexafluorenium bromide, 307
Hexamethonium, ganglion blocking action, 64-65
  in hypertension, 113, 120
Hexobarbitone, 245, 298
  sodium dosage and duration of action, 245
Hexoestrol, 355, 359
  clinical potency, 355
HGF *see* Glucagon
HGH *see* Growth hormone
Histalog, effect on gastric secretion, 187
Histaminase, 95
Histamine, 94-98
  acid phosphate injection, 104
  and analogues preparations, 104
  antagonists, 96
  effect on gastric secretion, 187
  H_1 antagonists, 96-98
    biological assays, 23
    preparations, 104
    in travel sickness, 193
  H_2 receptor antagonists, 96-97
    action on gastric secretion, 187-189
    clinical uses, 187-188
    side effects, 188
  as bronchoconstrictor, 176
  effect on pulsations in migraine, 128
  formation and destruction, 94-95

Histamine, *cont'd*
  forming capacity, (HFC), 95
  and gastric acid secretion, 95, 187-188
  log-dose response curves, 11-14
  and mepyramine, competitive antagonism, 12
  pharmacological actions, 95-96
  receptors, 11-14
    H_1, H_2, 96-97
  structure, 94
Histantin *see* Chlorcyclizine
Hodgkin's disease, 378, 379, 383
Homatropine
  action, 71
  on eyes, 88
  hydrobromide, 88
    eye preparation, 89
  structure, 70
Homeopathy, 24
Hookworm infections, treatment, 451
  preparations, 454
Hormone
  action, 319-323
  control of the kidney, 155-156
  control of testis and male contraception, 479
  cyclic nucleotides, 319-321
  duodenal, 194
  hypothalamic control of anterior pituitary, 322-323
  local, 90
  oestrogen receptors, 321
  in treatment of cancer, 382, 384
  true, 90
  see also names of specific hormones
Human chorionic hormone *see* Chorionic hormone
Human growth hormone, *see* Growth hormone
Humatin, 449
Hycanthone in schistosomiasis, 453, 454
Hydantoin
  derivatives in epilepsy, 270-271
  structures, 270
Hydrallazine, 130
  in hypertension, 114
Hydrea, 384
Hydrenox, 166
Hydrochlorothiazide, 166
Hydrocortisone, 343, 346, 349
  acetate, 347, 348, 350
  actions, 346-347
  administration, 347
  binding and measurement, 346
  in eczema, 230-231
    side effects, 231
  relative potency, 345
  sodium succinate in status asthmaticus, 183
  therapeutic uses, 347-348
Hydroflumethiazide, 166
Hydrogen peroxide as disinfectant, 458
Hydrosaluric, 166
Hydroxocobalamin, 206, 207, 216, 369, 371
Hydroxychloroquine anti-inflammatory drug, 293

25-Hydroxycholecalciferol, 363, 371
Hydroxyprogesterone caproate, 356
8-Hydroxyquinolines, in malaria, 444-445
Hydroxystilbamidine in leishmaniasis, 435, 437
5-Hydroxytryptamine (serotonin), 93-94
  actions, 93
  clinical implications, 93
  formation, 93
  involvement in migraine, 127
  possible functions, 93
  receptors, D and M, 93
  structure, 93
  transmitter role in CNS, 235, 260
Hydroxyurea, 384
  in psoriasis, 229
Hydroxyprogesterone hexanoate, 359
  structure, 356
Hydroxyzine, as sedative-hypnotic, 252, 256
Hygroton, diuretic action, 161, 166
Hyoscine
  as antiemetic, 201
  antisialogogic action, 71
  methobromide, 71
  structure, 70
  in travel sickness, 193
Hypercapnia, clinical evidence, 171
Hyperchlorhydria
  antacids, 190
  control by drugs, 189-190
Hyperkinetic syndrome
  amphetamines in, 263-264
  methylphenidate, 265
Hyperlipidaemia, lipid lowering agents, 196
Hyperproteinaemia, clofibrate in, 196
Hypersensitivity to drugs, 31, 103-104
  penicillin, 405-406
  reactions, skin, 230
    delayed, 230
    types, 99-100
      Arthus reaction, 99
      delayed, 100
      due to cell-fixed antibodies, 99
      due to circulatory antibodies, 99
      mediated by sensitised cells, 99-100
      T and B lymphocytes, 100
      tuberculin reaction, 99, 100
Hypertensin, 130
  chemical aspects, 127
  composition, 127
  effects on blood vessels, 127
Hypertension, 111-121
  drugs, 112-121
    adrenergic neurone-blocking drugs, 118-119
    alpha-blockers, 121
    beta-blockers, 115-117
    central action, 117-118
    combined, 121
    diazoxide, 121
    diuretics, 113-114
    emergencies, 121
    ganglion-blocking drugs, 120

Hypertension, *cont'd*
    interference with catecholamine metabolism, 117
    mechanisms, 113
    postural, 117
    properties required, 113
    reflex hypotension, 120
    reserpine, 119-120
    sodium nitroprusside, 121
    vasodilators, 114-115
  experimental, 111-112
    due to corticosteroids, 111-112
    due to neurological and psychological factors, 112
    following renal artery constriction, 111
  preparations, 130
  reduction of blood pressure, 112-121
    general measures, 112
Hyperthyroidism, 334
  see also Thyroid gland
Hypnotics, 243-248
  barbiturates, 243-246
    see also Barbiturates; and specific names
  carbromal (adalin), 247
  chloral hydrate, 247
  glutethimide (Doriden), 247
  others, 247
  paraldehyde, 246
  preparations, 256
  relative merits, 248
Hypochlorhydria, 188-189
Hypoglycaemic drugs, oral, 340-341, 349
  mode of action, 341
  place, 341
  structures, 341
  therapeutic uses, 341
  toxic effects, 341
Hypogonadism, use of androgens, 358
Hypoparathyroidism, 335
Hyposensitisation, clinical, 101
Hypotension
  reflex, 120
  severe, angiotensin in, 126
Hypothalamus
  control of anterior pituitary, 322-323
  control over 'vital centres', 53
  function, 238
  hypophysiotropic hormones, 322-323
    significance, 323
  neurosecretory pathways, 328
Hypovase, 130
5-HT, *see* 5-Hydroxytryptamine

Ibuprofen, anti-inflammatory drug, 289-290, 293
Idoxuridine
  antiviral agent, 396, 397
  in herpes viruses, 229
Imferon in iron deficiency, 205, 216
Iminodibenzyl derivatives, 258
Imipramine and related antidepressants, 240, 242, 257-260
  actions, 257, 258-259
  adverse effects, 259
  chemistry, 258

Imipramine, *cont'd*
  clinical effectiveness, 259
  effects in man, 259
  half-life, 46
  pharmacological action, 258
  preparations, 266
  structures, 258
Immunisation against pregnancy, 479
Immunosuppression and cancer, 376
Immunosuppressive effects of cytotoxic drugs, 376
Imodium as antispasmodic, 200, 201
Impetigo, treatment, 229
Imuran in tissue transplantation, 381, 384
Inderal, 130
  antiarrhythmic effect, 147
Indomethacin anti-inflammatory drug, 290, 293
  clinical use, 290
  toxicity, 290
Indoramin in hypertension, 115, 120
Infections, chemotherapy, synthetic compounds, 392-397
Infertility, use of progestogens, 357
Infiltration local anaesthesia, 312
Inositol, 369
Insect repellents, 469, 475
Insecticides, 467-469
  organochlorine compounds, 467-468
  organophosphorous compounds, 468-469
    antidote to, 469, 475
  poisoning by, 469
  resistance to, 469
Insidon, 267
Insulin, 337-342
  actions, 337-338
  administration, 339-340
  allergy to, 340
  chemistry, 339
  coma, 342
  dietary therapy, 341-342
  discovery, 5
  half-life, 46
  immunological responses to, 340
  novo-, 340
  preparations, 339-340, 349
  purified pro-insulin free preparations, 340
  receptors, 339
  slow-acting, 339-340
  soluble, 339
  structure, 338
  standardisation, 340
Intal in bronchial asthma, 181-182, 183
Interferon, 397
Intestine, absorption of drugs from, 36-38
  bioavailability, 40
  electrolytes, 37
  inorganic salts and water, 37
  particle size, 37-38
Intolerance of drugs, 31
Intraocular fluid, drainage, 87
  intraocular pressure, 87
Intrauterine devices, 478
  adverse reactions, 478
  ectopic pregnancies, 478

INDEX 507

Intravenous anaesthesia, 303-305
Intrinsic factor, 206, 216
Instrinsic muscles, eye, autonomic control, 86-89
Inversine, 130
Iodides, 334, 336
　in syphilis, 437
Iodinated 8-hydroxyquinolines in malaria, 444-445
　in subacute myelo-optico-neuropathy, 445
　therapeutic uses, 444-445
Iodine,
　action, 334
　allergy, management, 166
　deficiency, 330
　as disinfectant, 459, 462
　metabolism 332-333
　preparations, 336
　radioactive, 334-335
　　diagnostic use, 334-335
　　therapeutic use, 335
Iodipamide methylglucamine, 195
Iodochlorhydroxyquin, 444
Iodophors as disinfectants, 462
Iodopyracet, 166
Ionophore, 462
Iopanoic acid, 195
Ipatropium, preparation, 183
Ipecacuanha
　as emetic, 192
　as expectorant, 175, 176
　preparation, 201
Iprindole, 266
Iproniazid in depression, 260, 261
　preparation, 267
　structure, 261
Iron
　absorption, 203
　deficiency, causes, 203-204
　dextran injection, in iron deficiency, 205, 216
　poisoning, chelating agent, 205, 216
　sorbitol injection, in iron deficiency, 205, 216
　therapeutic uses, 204-205
　transport and storage, 203
　turnover, 202-203
Irradiation as disinfectant, 458
Ismelin, 130
Isocarboxazid, 267
　in depression, 261
　structure, 261
Isoetharine in bronchial asthma, 180
Isoflurane, 302
Isoniazid (Isonicotinic acid hydrazide) discovery, 418
Isoniazid
　absorption, 422
　excretion, 422
　half-life, 46
　preparation, 428
　serum concentration, 423
　sputum count, 423
　structure, 422
　toxicity, 423
　tuberculostatic activity, 422-421

Isophane insulin injection, 349
Isoprenaline, 73
　in bronchial asthma, 178-179, 183
　as cardiac stimulant, 81, 149
　central effects, 82
　clinical features, 81
　metabolic effects, 82
　metabolism, 179
　preparation, 85
　smooth muscle, 81
Isoproterenol in bronchial asthma, 178
Isoxsuprine in obstetrics, 218

Jaundice
　and anabolic steroids, 358
　post-halothane, 301-302
Jectofer in iron deficiency, 205, 206

Kallikrein-Kinin system, 90
Kanamycin, 412, 417
　in tuberculosis, 425, 428
Keflin, 407
Kefzol, 407
Kemadrin in Parkinsonism, 277
Ketamine in anaesthesia, 304-305, 306
Kidneys, 151-166
　diuretic drugs, 158-166
　drug excretion, 44-45, 154
　functions, 151
　nephrotoxic effects of drugs, 154-155
　pH of urine, 156-158
　radioscopy, drugs used in, 166
　renal tubular function, 153
　structure, 151
　urinary clearance, 153-154
Kininases, 91
Kininogen, 90
Kininogenase, 90
Kinins, 90-91
　action and possible roles, 91

Labetalol, 116-117, 130
　in hypertension, 120
Labour
　analgesia in, 223-224
　clinical course, 222
　use of drugs, 222-223
Lachesine chloride
　action on eye, 88
　structure, 70
Lactation, inhibition, use of oestrogens, 355
　by bromocriptine, 323
Lactogenic hormone see Prolactin
Lactulose, 201
　as purgative, 199, 201
Laevohyoscyamine hydrobromide in travel sickness, 193
Lampit, 437
Lamprene, 428
Lanatoside, action on heart, 149
Lanitop, action on heart, 149
Lanvis in cancer, 384
Lapudrine in malaria, 446
Largactil see Chlorpromazine
Laroxyl, 258

Lasix, as diuretic, 162, 165, 166
LATS, see Long-acting thyroid stimulator
Laxatives, 197-199
　see also Purgatives
Lead
　poisoning antidote, 474
　as source of air pollution, 466
Lederkyn, 395
Ledermycin, 417
Leeches, 4
Leishmaniasis, drugs in, 434-435
　cutaneous, 435
　mucocutaneous, 435
　visceral, 434, 435
Lentard insulin, 340, 349
Leponex, 256
Leprosy, drugs in, 427-428
　antituberculosis drugs in, 428
　clofazimine, 428
　preparations, 428
　sulfones, 428
　thiambutosine, 428
Leptazol, analeptic drug, 172
Lethidrone as morphine antagonist, 285, 293
Leucine-enkephalin, 241
Leukaemias, cytotoxic drug treatment, 382, 383-384
Leukeran, in neoplastic disease, 378, 384
Levallorphan as morphine antagonist, 285, 293
Levodopa in Parkinsonism, 273-274, 277
　adverse effects, 274
　clinical effects, 274
Levophed, 130
Levorphanol
　as analgesic, 283, 293
　structure, 281
Levothyroxine, 336
Librium
　as muscle relaxant, 276, 277
　as sedative, 250, 251
　　preparation, 256
Lice infections, 230
　preparations, 231
Lidocaine (lignocaine)
Lignocaine, 311, 312
　action on heart, 145-146, 149
　activity, 312
　antiarrhythmic agent, 315
　dental anaesthesia, 313
　as local anaesthetic, 311
　preparation, 315
　spinal anaesthesia, 314
　structure, 310
Limbic system, 238-239
Lincomycin, 409, 417
Lioresal as muscle relaxant, 276, 277
Liothyronine, 331-332, 336
Lipid lowering agents, 196-197
　cholestyramine, 196
　clofibrate, 196
　dextrothyroxine, 197
　niacin, 196
Lipoatrophy, 340
Liquid paraffin, 197, 201

Lithium, 261-262
　blood levels and toxic effects, 262
　clinical uses, 261-262
　mode of action, 261
　preparations, 267
Loewi's theory of chemical transmission of nerve impulse, 55-57
Log-dose-response curves, competitive antagonism, 12, 13
Lomotil as antispasmodic, 200, 201
Lomustine, 384
Long-acting thyroid stimulator, 327
Loop diuretics, 161-163, 166
Loperamide as antispasmodic, 200, 201
Lopressor, 130
Lorazepam, 256
Lorfan as morphine antagonist, 285, 293
LRH, see Luteinising hormone-releasing hormone
LSD see Lysergic acid diethylamide
Lucanthone in schistosomiasis, 453, 454
Ludiomil, 266
Luminal
　dosage and duration of action, 245
　in epilepsy, 269-270, 277
　preparation, 256
Lung
　spirometry, 178
　see also Respiration
Lupus vulgaris, vitamin D treatment, 364
Luteinising hormone, 325, 336
　influence on ovarian cycle, 351
Luteinising hormone-releasing hormone, 322, 322-323, 325
Lutotropin, 336
Lymphocyte
　transformation test, 104
　T and B, and hypersensitivity, 100
Lysergic acid diethylamide (LSD), 265-266
　action on CNS, 235
　chemical structure, 221, 489
　dependence, 488
　hallucinations, 265-266
　mode of action, 265-266
Lysivane in Parkinsonism, 275

M-receptors, effect of 5-HT, 93
Marcoumar, 214, 216
Macrocytic anaemias, 205-208
Macrolide antibiotics, 408-409
　preparations
　　structure, 408
　　therapeutic uses, 408, 409
Madribon, 395
Mafenide acetate, 397
Magnesium citrate, as purgative, 198, 201
Magnesium hydroxide, 198, 201
Magnesium oxide, 190
　action, 190
　neutralising power, 190
　preparation, 201
Magnesium sulphate, 197
Magnesium trisilicate
　action, 191

Magnesium, cont'd
　neutralising power, 190
　preparation, 201
Malaria, 438-443
　assessment of anti-plasmodial activity, 440
　control, 438, 439
　drug-resistant areas, chemotherapy, 443
　early treatment, 3, 4
　immunity, 443, 439
　insecticides, 438
　life cycle of parasite, 438-439
　Plasmodium falciparum, 439, 440
　preparations, 446
　treatment, 440-443
　　aims, 440
　　clinical chemotherapy, 443
　　drugs active against tissue stages and gametocytes, 442-443
　　prophylaxis, 440
　　resistance, 438
　　suppressive drugs, 440-442
　　types of parasites, 439
　vaccine, 443
Malathion, 469
　in lice infections, 230, 231
　structure, 468
Male fern in tapeworm infection, 449
Mandrax, as hypnotic, 247
Mania, use of lithium, 261-262
Manic-depressive disease, amine mechanism, 240
Mannitol, as diuretic, 166
Mapharside
　structure, 431
　in syphilis, 437
Maprotiline hyd., 266
Marcaine, 315
Marcoumar, 214, 216
Marihuana, 266
Marplan, 261, 267
Marsilid, 266
Mazindol
　in appetite reduction, 264
　preparation, 267
Marzine in travel sickness, 193
Mebadin, 444
Mebendazole
　in hookworm infection, 451, 454
　in threadworm infection, 452
　in whipworm infections, 451
Mebeverine as antispasmodic, 200, 201
Mebhydrolin, 104
Mecamylamine, 130
　ganglion blocking action, 65
　in hypertension, 120
Mechlorethamine, in neoplastic disease, 384
Mecholyl, 59
Meclozine
　possible teratogenic effects, 225
　in travel sickness, 193, 201
Medazepam, 256
Medicine
　experimental, 4
　systems, 3-5

Medicines Act 1968, 7
Medicines Commission, 7
Medigoxin, action on heart, 149
Medinal, dose and duration of action, 245
Medroxyprogesterone, 384
　acetate, 359
Mefenamic acid, anti-inflammatory drug, 290, 293
Mefruside, 166
Megaclor, 417
Megestrol acetate, 359
Mel B, 433, 437
Mel W, 433, 437
Melanoma, 383
Melarsen oxide-BAL
　structure, 433
　in trypanosomiasis, 437
Melarsonyl potassium in trypansomiasis, 433, 437
Melarsoprol in trypanosmiasis, 433, 437
　structure, 433
Melatonin, 93
Melleril major tranquilliser, 254, 256
　structure, 255
Melphalan, in neoplastic disease, 383, 379, 384
Membrane noise, and drug-receptor interaction, 17-18
Menadiol, 365, 366
　sodium diphosphate, 216
Menadione, 365
Menopausal
　disorders, oestrogens, 355
　gonadotrophin, 336
Menotropins, 336, 354
Menstrual cycle, 351
Mental activity, development of drugs which affect, 242
Mepacrine
　in malaria, 442, 446
　structure, 441
　in tapeworm infections, 449, 454
Meperidine as analgesic, 283
Mephentermine as vasoconstrictor, 126
Mepivacaine hyd., 315
Meprobamate
　in anxiety states, 251, 251-252
　　additive effect with alcohol, 252
　　clinical effects, 251-252
　　pharmacological effects, 251
　　undesirable effects, 252
　as muscle relaxant, 276, 277
Mepyramine, 104
　and histamine specific antagonism, 12
　maleate, 104
　structure, 96
Mephenesin as muscle relaxant, 275-276, 277
Meratran in depression, 265
Merbentyl, see Dicyclomine
Mercaptopurine
　in cancer, 381, 384
　in leukaemia, 383
Mercurial diuretics, 161-162, 166
　clinical effects, 162
　mode of action, 162

Merital, 266
Mersalyl, 161, 166
Mescaline, 266
   dependence, 488
   hallucinations, 266
   mode of action, 266
   structure, 489
Mesontoin in epilepsy, 271, 276
Mesterolone, 359
Mestinon, see Pyridostigmine bromide
Mestranol, 353
Metabolism of drugs, 42-46
   catalysed by hepatic microsomal enzymes, 43-44
   conjugation, 42
   inactivation, 42
   transformation, 42-43
Metadelphene, 475
Metaraminol, 130
   as vasoconstrictor, 126
Metformin, 340, 349
Methacholine, 59-60
Methacycline, 417
Methadone
   as analgesic, 283, 284
      clinical trials, 284
      preparation, 293
      structure, 283
   as cough depressant, 175, 183
   to support withdrawal syndrome, 483, 284
Methaemoglobinaemia, drug-induced, 208
Methallenoestril, 359
Methamphetamine as vasoconstrictor, 126
Methanol poisoning, 488
Methaqualone as hypnotic, 247
Methedrine, 263
Methicillin
   preparation, 407
   properties, 403, 404
Methimazole, 336
   dosage, 334
   structure, 333, 334
Methiodal, 166
Methionine-enkephalin, 241
Methisazone, antiviral agent, 396, 397
Methisul, 397
Methixene hyd., in Parkinsonism, 277
Methocarbamol as muscle relaxant, 277
Methohexitone sodium in anaesthesia, 304, 306
   dosage and duration of action, 245
Methoin in epilepsy, 271, 276
Methotrexate
   in neoplastic disease, 380, 383, 384
   possible teratogenic effect, 225
   in psoriasis, 229
Methotrimeprazine as tranquilliser, 256
Methoxamine, 130
   as vasodilator, 126
3-Methoxy-4-hydroxyphenol glycol, 259
Methoxyflurane anaesthesia, 302, 306
   in labour, 224
Methoxyphenamine, 183
Methrazone anti-inflammatory drug, 293

Methyclothiazide, 166
Methylalcohol poisoning, 488
Methylamphetamine hydrochloride in depression, 263
   central stimulation, 263
   in hyperkinesis, 264
   preparation, 267
   structure, 262
Methylcellulose, 197, 201
Methyldopa, 130
   in hypertension, 117
   metabolic conversion, 84
Methylergometrine, 222, 225
   assay, 24
   in labour, 223
Methylolchlortetracycline, 417
Methylpentynol as hypnotic, 247
   preparation, 256
Methylphenidate in hyperkinetic syndrome, 265
   preparation, 267
Methylphenobarbitone
   dosage and duration of action, 245
   in epilepsy, 270, 276
Methylprednisolone, 349
   relative potency, 345
Methyltestosterone, 358
   structure, 357
Methyl thiouracil, 336
   structure, 333
Methyprylone as hypnotic, 247
   preparation, 256
Methysergide, 93, 94, 130
   as migraine prophylactic, 128-129
Metiamide, 187, 188
Metoclopramide as antiemetic, 194
Metocurine iodide in anaesthesia, 307
Metopirone, 349, 350
Metoprol, 130
   in hypertension, 116
Metozalone, 166
Metriphonate in schistosomiasis, 453, 454
Metronidazole in amoebiasis, 444, 446, 447
Metubine in anaesthesia, 307
Mexiletine, action on heart, 147, 149
Mianserin, 260, 266
   5-HT antagonist, 260
Miconazole in skin fungal infections, 231
Microcirculation, 109
Midamor, 166
Midicel, 395, 397
Migraine
   clonidine, 118
   ergotamine in, 127-128
   and 5-HT, 94
   preparations for, 130
   prophylactic drugs, 128-129
Milibis, 446
Milk, neutralising power, 190
Miltown as muscle relaxant, 276, 277
Mineralocorticoids, 345-346
   preparations, 350
Minocycline, 410
Mintezol, 452, 454
Miochol see Acetylcholine chloride
Miracil D in schistosomiasis, 453, 454

Mitobronitol, 384
Moditen
   as antiemetic, 254
   in schizophrenia, 254
Monoamines, transmitter role in CNS, 235
Monoamine oxidase, 76, 77
Monoamine oxidase inhibitors, 260-261
   actions in man, 260
   chemical structure, 261
   fundamental action, 260
   in hypertension, 120, 260
   interaction with food and drugs, 44
   preparations, 267
   specific drugs, 261
   toxic effects, 260-261
Monotard monocomponent insulins, 340, 349
Morphine, 279-285
   action on respiratory centre, 173
   analgesic effect, 280
   antagonists, 284-285
   biological assay in man, 25
   dependence, 482-483
   derivatives, 282-283
   effects on CNS, 280
   effects on skin, 281
   effects on smooth muscle, 280-281
   as emetic, 192
   fate in body, 281
   mode of action, 281
   pharmacological actions, 279-280
   poisoning, 280
   preparations, 293
   structure, 281
   sulphate, 293
   therapeutic uses, 281-282
Motor function, central depressants, 268-277
Mouth, absorption of drugs, 36
Mucous membranes, anaesthesia, 312
Muscarine, 60
   actions of acetylcholine, 58
Muscarinic receptor blocking drugs, 69-70
   intestinal activity, 200
   preparations, 71
Mustine
   in neoplastic disease, 378, 384
   structure, 379
Mutagenicity of drugs, tests, 30-31
Myambutol, 428
Myanesin as muscle relaxant, 275-276, 277
Myasthenia gravis
   neostigmine, 61, 62
   neuromuscular function, 69
Mycobacterium tuberculosis, properties, 418
   see also Tuberculosis
Mycosis fungoides, 380
Mydriacil see Tropicamide
Mydriatics, 89, 88
Myelobrom 384
Mylaxen, 307
Myotonia congenita, quinine in, 442

Mysoline in epilepsy, 270, 277
Myxoedema, 333

Nacton in hyperchlorhydria and peptic ulcer, 190
Nadolol, 130
Nalidixic acid, 396, 397
    skin reactions to, 231
Nalorphine as morphine antagonist, 285, 293
Naloxone, 241
    as morphine antagonist, 285, 293
Nandrolone phenyproprionate, 358, 359
    structure, 358
Naphazoline, 130
    as vasoconstrictor, 126
ß-Naphthylamine, 472
Naproxen, anti-inflammatory drug, 293
Narcan as morphine antagonist, 293
Nardil, 261, 267
Narex, 130
Narphen as analgesic, 283
Natamycin, 414
    in skin fungal infections, 231
Natulan, in neoplastic disease, 379, 384
Navane as tranquilliser, 256
Navidrex, 166
Nebcin, 417
Nefrolan, diuretic action, 161, 166
Negram, 396, 397
Nematicides, 470
Nembutal
    dosage and duration of action, 245
        preparation, 256
    sodium, dosage and duration of action, 245
        preparation, 256
Nematode infections, 449-452, 454
Neoarsphenamine, structure, 431
Neocytamen, 206, 207, 216
Neomercazole, 336
Neomycin, 412, 417
    in bacterial skin infections, 231
    toxicity, 412
Neosalvarsan, structure, 431
Neostigmine
    action, 60
        on gastric juice, 185
    characteristics and action, 61
    eye preparation, 89
    structure, 61
Nephril, 166
Nerisone, 350
Nerve impulse
    nature of, 308
    humoral transmission, theory, 55-57
Neulactil major tranquilliser, 256
Neuroblastoma, 383
Neurophysin, 218
Neuroleptic drugs causing tardive dyskinesia, 240
Neuromuscular block
Neuromuscular blocking drugs, 65-69
    in anaesthesia, 305-306
    evaluation, 68

Neuromuscular transmission
    interference, 66-69
        postsynaptic, 66
        presynaptic, 68-69
    in myasthenia gravis, 69
Neutral insulin injection, 349
Niacin *see* Nicotinic acid
Niamid (nialamide)
    in depression, 261
    preparation, 267
    structure, 261
Niclosamide, 452
    in tapeworm infections, 449, 454
Nicotinamide, possible teratogenic effect, 225
Nicotine actions of acetylcholine, 58
Nicotinic acid (niacin), 368-369, 371
    deficiency, 368
    in hyperlipidaemia, 197
    requirements, 371
    therapeutic use, 368
Nicoumalone, 216
Nifedipine, 130
Nifurtimox in trypanosomiasis, 432, 434, 437
Nikethamide
    as respiratory stimulant, 173, 183
Nilevar, 358
Nilodin, 454
Nimorazole in amoebiasis, 444
Nipride, 130
    in hypertension, 121
Niridazole in schistosomiasis, 453, 454
Nitrazepam as tranquilliser, 256
Nitrites
    in biliary spasm, 195
    causing methaemoglobinaemia, 208
    tolerance, 123
    as vasodilators, 122-123
Nitrofurantoin, 396, 397
    structure, 396
Nitrofurazone, in trypanosomiasis, 433, 437
    toxicity, 433
Nitrogen mustards in cancer, 378, 384
Nitrogen oxides as source of air pollution, 466
Nitroglycerin, in angina, 122, 123
Nitroprusside in hypertension, 121
Nitrous oxide
    anaesthesia, 302-303
    and oxygen in labour, 223
    untoward effects, 303
Nivaquine in malaria, 440
Nobrium, 256
Noise analysis and drug receptors, 18
Noludar as hypnotic, 247
    preparation, 256
Nolvadex, 384
Nomifensine, 260, 266
Noradrenaline
    actions, 79-82
    action on eyes, 88
    action on heart, 80, 81
        smooth muscle, 81
    central effects, 82
    chemical assay, 73-74

Noradrenaline, *cont'd*
    content of tissues, 73
    distribution in dog's brain, 74
    effect on labour, 218
    enzymic degradation, 76-77
    inactivation and fate, 76-79
    injection, 130
    in local haemorrhage, 215
    metabolic effects, 82
    metabolic pathways, 76
    preparation, 85
    regulation of turnover, 75
    slow intravenous infusion, 125
    storage and release, 75
    sweating, 82
    tissue uptake, 77
Noradrenergic neurones and depression, 240
Norethandrolone, 358
    structure, 358
Norethindrone in hyperlipoproteinaemia, 197
Norethisterone, 356
    in uterine bleeding, 357
Norethisterone acetate, 359
Norethynodrel, 356
    in uterine bleeding, 357
Normacol, 197, 201
Nortriptyline in depression, 258
    structure, 258
Noveril, 266
Novo insulins, 340, 349
Novocaine, 315
Numorphan, analgesic action, 282
Nupercaine, 311, 315
Nutritional deficiencies
    environmental aspects, 471-472
    priorities, 472
Nydrane as anticonvulsant, 276
Nystatin, 414, 417
    to control fungal rot in bananas, 471
    in skin fungal infections, 231

Oblivon as hypnotic, 247
    preparation, 247, 256
Obtetrics
    analgesic drugs, 223-224
    oxytocic drugs, 220-223
Octapressin, 329, 336
Octyl nitrite, 130
Ocuserts, 89
Oestradiol, 321, 353, 359
    acetate, 359
Oestrogens
    in acne, 230
    actions, 353
    in cancer control, 382, 384
    clinical uses, 355
    comparative activity, 354
    effects on fetus, 225
    influence on conception, 352
    in mammary cancer, 382
    as oral contraceptives, 479
    preparations, 359
    receptors, 321
    structures, 356

INDEX 511

Oestrogens, *cont'd*
  synthetic, 353
  toxic effects, 354-355
Oestrone, 359
  clinical potency, 355
Oils, mineral as carcinogens, 473
Oleandomycin, 408
Oncovin, antitumour agent, 381, 384
Opiates
  constipating effect, 200
  dependence, 482-483
    effects, 483
    related analgesic drugs, 483
    tolerance, 482-483
    withdrawal syndrome, 483
  receptors, 241-242
Opioid analgesics, 279-285
  preparations, 293
Opipramol hyd., 267
Orabolin, 359
Oral contraceptives, 477-479
  preparations, 480
  see also Contraceptives, hormonal (oral)
Orbenin, 403, 407
Orciprenaline in bronchial asthma, 180, 183
Organochlorine compounds, 467-468
Organophosphorous compounds, 468-469
Orisulph, 397
Orphenadrine in Parkinsonism, 275, 277
Orthoxine, 183
Ospolot in epilepsy, 273
Osteomyelitis, acute, penicillin treatment, 405
Osteoporosis, use of anabolic steroids, 359
Otrivine, 130
  as vasoconstrictor, 126
Ovarian cycle, hormonal control, 351-353
  menstrual cycle, 351
  pregnancy, 351-353
  regulation, 351
  see also Pregnancy
Overdosage of drugs, 31
Ovulation induction, clomiphene, 354, 359
Oxacillin, properties, 404
Oxalic acid, 211
Oxamniquine in schistosomiasis, 453, 454
Oxandrolone, in hyperlipoproteinaemia, 197
Oxazepam as tranquilliser, 256
Oxazolidinediones in epilepsy, 271-272
  structures, 270
Oxedrine tartrate, 130
Oxidised cellulose (Oxycel), 215, 216
Oxolinic acid, 397
Oxophenarsine
  structure, 431
  in syphilis, 437
Oxprenolol, 130
Oxybuprocaine (benoxinate) in local anaesthesia, eyes, 313
  preparation, 315
Oxycel, 215, 216
Oxycodone pectinate, analgesic, 283

Oxygen
  administration in respiratory failure, 168-169
  with carbon dioxide as respiratory stimulant, 171
    evidence of hypercapnia, 171
  consumption, and digitalis, 137
  and helium in bronchial asthma, 182
  influence on respiratory centre, 168
  lack, effect on heart, 121-122
  poisoning, 169-170
Oxymetazoline, 130
Oxymetholone, 359
Oxymorphone
  analgesic action, 282
  structure, 281
Oxyphenbutazone, anti-inflammatory drug, 290, 293
Oxyphenisatin, as purgative, 199, 201
Oxyphenonium, in hyperchlorhydria, 190
Oxyphencyclimine in hyperchlorhydria and peptic ulcer, 190
Oxytetracycline, 409, 417
  in acne, 230
  bacterial resistance, 409
  clinical application, 410
  as 'feed' antibiotic, 471
  mode of action, 409
  structure, 409
  in syphilis, 436
  toxicity, 410
Oxytocic drugs
  human biological assays, 24
  clinical uses, 220, 222, 225
  see also Oxytocin: Prostaglandin: Ergometrine
Oxytocin, action, 220
  clinical use, 220
  first stage of labour, 223
  preparations, 225
  release, 218-219
  role of suckling, 218, 219
  structure, 329
  in uterine inertia, 222

P₂S *see* Pralidoxime: Pyridine-2-aldoxime mesylate
Palfium as analgesic, 293
Paludrine in malaria, 440, 446
Pamine, *see* Hyoscine methobromide
Panadol, 291
Pancuronium in anaesthesia, 306
Pantothenic acid, 369
Papaverine, as coronary vasodilator, 123
Paracetamol as analgesic, 284
Para-aminobenzoic acid, 369
  as essential metabolite, 387
Para-aminophenol analgesics, 290-291
Para-amino-salicylic acid *see* PAS
Paracetamol, 291, 293
  advantage over aspirin, 291
  toxicity, 291
Paradione in epilepsy, 271, 276
Paraldehyde, as hypnotic, 246-247, 256
  structure, 247

Paramethadione
  in epilepsy, 271, 276
  structure, 270
Paramethasone acetate, 349
Paraquat, 470
Parasites, skin, 230
Parasympathetic nerves, effects of stimulation, 54-55
Parasympathomimetic drugs causing increased gastric juice flow, 185
Parathion, 469
  structure, 468
Parathyroid glands, 335-336
  calcitonin, 336
  hormone, 335
  hypoparathyroidism, 335
Parathyroid injection, 336
Pargyline, 130
  in hypertension, 120
Parkinsonism
  drugs in, 273-275
  effect of antihistamines, 98
  extrapyramidal disturbances, 239
  levodopa in, 273
  major tranquillisers, 254
Parlodel in Parkinsonism, 277
Parnate, 261, 267
Paromomycin, 412
  in tapeworm infection, 449
Paroxysmal auricular tachycardia, management, 148
Parpanit in Parkinsonism, 274
PAS (aminosalicylate sodium) 428
  half-life, 46
  structure, 422
  tuberculostatic activity, 422, 426
Pasoquin in malaria, 446
Pavulon in anaesthesia, 307
Peganone as anticonvulsant, 276
Pellagra, 368
Pemoline, 267
Pempidine in hypertension, 120
Penamecillin, 407
Penbritin, 403, 407
Penicillamine, 474, 475
  anti-inflammatory drug, 293
Penicillin, 398-406
  acid resistance, 403-404
  allergy, 104, 405-406
  in bejel, 437
  benzathine, 402, 403
  biological assay, 400
  blood concentrations, 402
  broad spectrum, 404
  chemistry, 398-400
  choice, 415
  derivatives, for skin tests, 406
  in erysipelas, 229
  G, 400-402, 403, 407
  half-life, 46
  mode of action, 390-400
  penicillinase resistance, 404
  in pinta, 437
  preparations, 407
  prescribing chart, 415-417
  prophylactic use, 405

Penicillin, *cont'd*
  properties, 398
  semi-synthetic, 403-404
  sensitization, 406
  structures, 398, 403
  in syphilis, 435-436
  therapeutic uses, 404-405
  toxicity, 405
  transplacental transmission, 225
  types, 400-404
  U.S. Public Health Service
      recommendations, 436
  V, 402, 403, 407
  in yaws, 437
  see also specific types
Penicillinase, 398
  resistance, 403, 404
Penicilloylpolylysine, 406
Penidural, 407
Pentaerythritol tetranitrate, 130
Pentagastrin, 186
Pentamidine isethionate in
      trypanosomiasis, 433-434, 437
  in leishmaniasis, 435, 437
  toxicity, 433
Pentaquine, 443
Pentavalent antimony compounds in
      leishmaniasis, 434-435
Pentazocine as analgesic, 283, 293
Pentobarbitone, 246
  dosage and duration of action, 245
  in premedication, 305
      preparation, 256
  sodium dosage and duration of action,
      245
      preparation, 256
Pentostam in leishmaniasis, 435, 437
Pentothal in anaesthesia, 303-304, 306
  sodium dosage and duration of action,
      245
Penthrane anaesthesia, 302, 306
Pepsin secretion, 187
Peptide antibiotics, 412-413, 417
  preparations, 417
Peptidoglycan structure in *Staph. aureus*,
      389
Pergonal, 336
Pernicious anaemia, 206
  cobalamins, 206-207
Peripheral nervous system, chemical
      organisation, 56-57
Perphenazine, as antiemetic, 201, 254
  in schizophrenia, 254
  structure, 255
  as tranquilliser, 256
Perhexiline maleate, 130
Persantin, 130
Pericyazine as tranquilliser, 256
Pertofran, 258, 266
Pesticides, 467
  residues, determination, 467
  tolerance levels, 467
  toxicity, 467
Pethidine as analgesic, 283, 293
  structure, 283
  hydrochloride, as cough depressant, 175
  in labour, 223

Peyote, dependence, 488
Phaeochromocytoma
  effects of phentolamine, 83
  3-methoxy-4-hydroxymandelic acid
      excretion, 77
Phanodorm dosage and duration of
      action, 245
  preparation, 256
Phanquone
  in amoebiasis, 445
  structure, 445
Pharmacogenetics, 28-29
Pharmacokinetics, 45-47
  Bateman function, 47
  compartmental analysis and
      computers, 47
  exponential elimination rate, 46-47
Pharmacology
  applied, definition, 3
  development, 5
Pharmacopoeias, history, 5-6
Phemerol, 462
Phemitone
  dosage and duration of action, 245
  in epilepsy, 270
Phenacetin, 291
Phenazocine
  as analgesic, 283, 293
  structure, 281
Phenelzine
  in depression, 261
  preparation, 267
  structure, 261
Phenergan, 104
  as hypnotic, 247
  preparation, 256
  structure, 96
  in travel sickness, 193
Phenethicillin
  preparation, 407
  properties, 403
Pheneturide as anticonvulsant, 276
Phenformin, 340, 341, 349
  structure, 341
Phenindamine, 98
  tartrate, 104
Phenindione, 213, 214, 216
Phenmetrazine in appetite reduction, 264
Phenobarbitone, effect on eye
      movements, 244
  dosage and duration of action, 245
  in epilepsy, 269-270, 277
  toxic effects, 269
  pharmacological action, 246, 249
  preparation, 256
  sodium, 245, 246
  in status asthmaticus, 183
Phenol
  coefficient test, 456-458
      destruction of bacterial spores, 457
      methods, 456-457
      tests of antiseptic activity, 457-458
  as disinfectant, 460, 462
  toxicity, 460
Phenolphthalein as purgative, 198, 201
Phenoperidine as analgesic, 283-284, 293

Phenothiazines
  allergic effects, 255-256
  blood dyscrasias caused by, 255
  causing tardive dyskinesia, 239
  chemical structures, 255
  as major tranquillisers, 252-255
    administration and fate, 254
    alterations in animal behaviour, 254
    effects in man, 253
    in mania, 254
    pharmacological effects, 252-253
    in schizophrenic psychoses, 254
    in senile agitation, 254
    specific, 254
    untoward effects, 254-255
Phenoxybenzamine, 83
  dosage, 85
Phenoxymethyl penicillin (penicillin V),
      402, 407
  blood concentrations, 402
  properties, 403
  structure, 403
  in erysipelas, 229
Phenprocoumon, 214, 216
Phensuximide in epilepsy, 271
  chemical structure, 270
Phentermine, 267
Phentolamine, 83
  preparation, 85
Phenylbutazone, anti-inflammatory
      drug, 290, 291, 293
  clinical uses, 290
  metabolism 290
  toxicity, 290
Phenylephrine, 130
  action on eyes, 88
  eye preparation, 89
  as vasoconstrictor, 125-126
Phenylstibonic acid, structure, 435
Phenytoin
  action on heart, 146, 149
  possible teratogenic effect, 225
  sodium, in epilepsy, 270-271
  toxic effects, 270
Pholcodeine as cough depressant, 175,
      183
Phosphate buffer system, urinary, 157
Pholcoline iodide
  action on eyes, 87
  side effects, 87-88
  eye preparation, 89
Phthalidyl ampicillin, 407
Phthalylsulphathiazole, 393
  preparation, 397
  structure, 392
Physalaemin, 91
Physeptone as analgesic, 284, 293
Physostigmine, action, 60
  action on eye, 87
  preparation, 89
  side effects, 87-88
  characteristics, 61
Phytomenadione, 213, 216
Picrotoxin, analeptic drug, 172
Pilocarpine, 60
  action on eyes, 88

Pilocarpine, *cont'd*
  eye preparation, 89
  ocusert action on eye, 88, 89
Piloerection, action of catecholamines, 82
Pimafucin in skin fungal infections, 231
Pindolol, 130
Pinocytosis, 35-36
Pinta, penicillin in, 437
Piperazine
  in ascariasis, 450
  derivatives, 254
  in threadworm, 452, 454
Pipradrol in depression, 265
  action, 265
Piriton, 104
Pitch as carcinogen, 473
Pituitary gland, 324-330
  adrenocorticotrophic hormone, 327-328
  anterior, hypothalamic control, 322, 323
    hormones, 322-323, 324-326
  function test, 349, 350
  gonadotrophic hormones, 325-326
  growth hormone, 324-325
  hormones, 324
    anterior, 324-326, 322-323
Pituitary gland, 324-330
  hypothalamic-hypophysiotropic hormones, 323
  lactogenic hormone (prolactin), 325
  posterior, 328-330
    biological assay, 330
    hormones, 329-330, 220
    hormones, release, 328
      physiological stimuli causing, 328-329
    neurosecretory pathways, 328
    oxytocin, action, 329-330
    preparations, 336
    vasopressin, action, 329
    preparations, 336
  thyrotrophic hormone, 326-327
  see also specific headings
Pizotifen malate, 130
Platelet aggregation, 209-210
  drugs inhibiting, 209-210
Placenta, drugs crossing, 224-225
Placental lactogen, 325
Plaquenil, 293
Plasma
  concentration of standard drugs, 48, 49
  individual variation, 48-49
  proteins, binding of drugs, 41-42
    competition for sites, 42
    and drug distribution, 40
  substitutes, 130
    see also Dextran
Pneumococcal infections, penicillin treatment, 405
Poldine methylsulphate, in hyperchlorhydria and peptic ulcer, 190
Polymyxins, 412-413, 417
  B, 413
Polythiazide, 166
Polyvidone iodine, 462

Polyvinylpyrrolidone (PVP) in circulatory collapse, 129
Ponderax, 267
Ponstan, anti-inflammatory drug, 293
Population growth, control, 476-480
Pores, absorption of drugs through, 35
Postcapillary venules and veins, 109
Postsynaptic interference of neuromuscular transmission, 66
Potassium iodide as expectorant, 175, 176, 183
Potassium nitrate as food preservative, 471
Potassium perchlorate, 336
  in hyperthyroidism, 334
Potassium permanganate as disinfectant, 458
Potassium-sparing diuretics, 163-164
  preparations, 166
Potassium reabsorption and excretion, 158-160
Povidone-Iodine as disinfectant, 462
Practolol, 116, 130
  in angina, 124
  skin reactions to, 231
Pralidoxime, antidote to organophosphorous compounds, 61, 469, 475
Prausnitz-Kuestner reaction, 101
Prazosin, 120, 130
  in hypertension, 115
Prednisolone, 343, 349
  half-life, 46
  relative potency, 345
  in status asthmaticus, 183
Prednisone, 343, 349
  in bronchial asthma, 182
  in leukaemia, 383
  relative potency, 350
Pregnancy
  ectopic, and IUDs, 478
  hormonal control, 351-352
    factors influencing conception, 352
  tests for, 352-353
  and syphilis, management, 436
  termination, 478
Pregnyl, 336
Preludin, 264
Prenylamine lactate, 130
Prescribing chart, antibiotics, 415-417
Presynaptic receptors, 56, 82
PRIF, *see* Prolactin release inhibitory factor
Prilocaine as local anaesthetic, 311, 315
Primaquine in malaria, 443, 446
  structure, 441
Primidone in epilepsy, 270, 277
  structure, 270
Priscol *see* Tolazoline
Privine, 130
  as vasoconstrictor, 126
PRL, *see* Prolactin
Prinalgin, anti-inflammatory drug, 293
Probanthine in hyperchlorhydria and peptic ulcer, 190

Probenecid in gout, 292-293
  preparation, 293
Probit, 28
Procainamide, action on heart, 145, 149
Procaine, 310-311
  activity, 312
  antiarrhythmic agent, 315
  dental anaesthesia, 313
  as local anaesthetic, 310
  preparation, 315
  relative efficiency, 313
  safe use, 310
  spinal anaesthesia, 313-314
  structure, 310
  toxicity, 310
Procaine benzylpenicillin, 402
  preparation, 407
  properties, 403
  in syphilis, 435, 437
  in yaws, 437
Procarbazine in cancer, 379, 384
Prochlorperazine as tranquilliser, 256
Procyclidine in Parkinsonism, 277
Proflavine as disinfectant, 460, 462
  structure, 460
Progesterone, structure, 356
Progestogens
  effects on fetus, 225
  influence on conception, 352
    actions, 355-356
    assay, 356
    clinical uses, 356-357
    as oral contraceptive, 357, 479, 480
    preparations, 359
    structures, 356
    synthetic, 356
    toxic effects, 357
Proguanil in malaria, 440, 446
  structure, 441
Prolactin, 322, 325, 336
  action, 325
  blood level, 325
  chemistry, 325
  function, 351
  release inhibitory factor, 323
Promazine, major tranquilliser, 254, 256
Promethazine
  in bronchial asthma, 182
  as hypnotic, 247
    preparation, 256
  structure, 96
  in travel sickness, 193
Prominal in epilepsy, 270, 276
Prondol, 266
Pronestyl, action on heart, 145, 149
Pronethalol, 83
Prontosil
  structure, 392
Propaderm, 349
Propanidid anaesthesia, 305, 306
Propantheline
  bromide, structure, 70
  in hyperchlorhydria and peptic ulcer, 190
Propicillin, 403

Propranolol, 83, 130
  in angina, 123-124
  antiarrhythmic effect, 147
  in hypertension, 115-116
    membrane stabilising activity, 116
    potency, 115
    selectivity, 115
    side-effects, 115
    structure, 116
Proprietary names, for drugs, 7-8
Propylhexedrine, 130
  as vasoconstrictor, 126
Propylthiouracil, 336
  dosage, 336
  structure, 333
Prostaglandins, 91-92
  action on uterus, 222
    preparations, 225
  as bronchoconstrictor, 176
  E_1 inhibition of platelet aggregation, 209
  E_2, structure, 91
  in early abortion, 478
  $F_2\alpha$, 92
  metabolism, 92
Prostatic cancer, androgen control, 382
  oestrogen control, 355
Prostigmine, see Neostigmine
Protamine sulphate, 212, 216
Protein-calorie malnutrition, 472
Prothionamide, 428
Protirelin, 323
Protriptyline hyd., 267
Proviron, 359
Proximal tubules
  compounds secreted by, 45
  and drug excretion, 44
Pseudoephedrine, 183
Pseudomonas infections, carbenicillin, 404
  treatment, 405, 415
Psoriasis, 228-229, 380
  drug treatment, 228-229, 231
  nature and mechanism, 228
Psychogalvanic reflex, 24, 25
  chlordiazepoxide, 250
Psychotropic drugs, development, 242
Psylocybe mexicana, 266
Psylocybin, 266
  dependence, 489
Pteroylglutamic acid *see* Folic acid
PTH, (parathyroid hormone), 335
Pupil, nervous control, 86-87
  drainage of intraocular fluid, 87
  mechanism of accommodation, 86-87
Purgatives, 3, 197-199
  abuse, 199
  bulk laxatives, 197
  irritant purgatives, 198-199
  saline purgatives, 197-198
  therapeutic use, 199
Puri-nethol in cancer, 381, 384
Purine analogues, in neoplastic disease, 380-381
PVY, *see* Polyvinylpyrrolidone
Pyopen, 403, 407
Pyramidon, 291

Pyrantel embonate, in hookworm infection, 451, 454
Pyrantel pamoate, antihelmintic, 450
  in hookworm infection, 451
Pyrazinamide, in tuberculosis, 424-425
  preparation, 428
  structure, 422
Pyrazole derivatives, 291
  structures, 291
Pyridine-2-aldoxime mesylate, 61
  see also Pralidoxime
Pyridoxine, 368-369, 371
  deficiency, 368
  requirements, 369, 371
Pyridostigmine bromide
  action, 61
  structure, 61
Pyrimethamine in malaria, 440, 446
  structure, 441
Pyrimidine analogues in neoplastic disease, 380-381

Quaternary ammonium compounds in neuromuscular block, 66
Quinacrine, 454
  in malaria, 442, 446
Quinalbarbitone
  effect on eye movements, 244
  in premedication, 305
  preparation, 256
Quinethazone, 166
Quinidine
  actions, 145, 149
  causing blood dyscrasias, 208
  effect on cardiac action potential, 144-145
Quinine in malaria, 442, 446
  antimalarial action, 442
  causing blood dyscrasias, 208
  early use, 3
  structure, 441
  toxicity, 442

Rapid eye movement, 237
  and barbiturates, 246
Radioimmunoabsorbent test, 406
Radioimmunoassays, 19-20, 141
  clinical application, 19-20
  types, 20
Radioscopy, kidney, drugs used in, 166
Ranatensin, 91
Rapitard insulin, 340, 349
Rastinon, 340, 349
Raynaud's disease, 83
Receptors
  androgen, 321
  D and M, effect of 5-HT, 93
  drug, affinity theory, 15
    characteristic properties, 10-11
    classification, 13-15
    competitive antagonism, 11-13
    efficacy theory, 15
    equations, 13
    general principles, 11-15
    isolation and identification, 17-18
    membrane noise, 17-18
    rate (Paton) theory, 15

Receptors, *cont'd*
  specific drug
    α adrenergic, 78
    ß adrenergic, 79, 115-116
    $ß_2$ adrenergic, 179-180
    Ach muscarine, 57-60, 61-63
    Ach nicotine gangl, 63-65
    Ach nicotine neuromusc, 65-68
    dopamine, 79, 239
    H_1 histamine, 13, 96-98
    H_2 histamine, 13, 189
    5-HT, 93
    opiate, 241
    theories, 15
  oestrogen, 321
  thyroid stimulating hormone, 326-327
Reflex hypotension, 120
Renal tubular function, 153
Renin, 111
Renin-angiotensin system, 111
Repressor genes, 387
Reserpine, 130
  and depression, 240
  in hypertension, 119-120
  in psychiatry, 256
Resochin in malaria, 446
Respiration, normal, mechanism, 167
  artificial ventilation, 169
  emergency resuscitation, 169
  influence of carbon dioxide and of oxygen, 168
  interchange of respiratory gases, 167-168
  oxygen administration, 168-169
  oxygen poisoning, 169-170
  respiratory failure, 168
Respiratory
  centre, influence of carbon dioxide and oxygen, 168
  depressant drugs, 173-176, 183
  failure, 168
    oxygen administration, 168-169
  gases interchange, 167-168
  stimulants, 171, 183
    carbon dioxide, 171
    clinically used, 172-173, 183
    with oxygen, 171
Resuscitation, respiratory emergency, 169
Reticular activating system, drugs affecting, 237-238
Retinoic acid in acne, 230, 231
Retinol
  structure, 361
  see also Vitamin A
Rheumatic diseases, corticosteroids, 347-348
  drugs in, 289, 290, 293
  fever, effect of cortisone, 348
Rheumatoid arthritis
  corticosteroids, 347-348
  drugs in, 289, 290, 293
Rhubarb as purgative, 198
Riboflavin (vitamin B_2), 367, 371
  deficiency, 367
  requirements, 367, 371

Ribosome function, inhibition by antibiotics, 388
Rifampicin
  in leprosy, 428
  in tuberculosis, 423-424, 428
    administration, 423-424, 426
    pharmacology, 423
    pulmonary, 424
Rimiterol hydroxide aerosol, 183
Ringworm
  griseofulvin for, 414, 417
  treatment, 229-230
Ritalin in hyperkinesis, 265
  preparation, 267
Rivotril in epilepsy, 272
Robaxin as muscle relaxant, 277
Rodenticides, 470
Rogitine, *see* Phentolamine
Romilar as cough depressant, 175, 183
Rondomycin, 417
Ronyl, 267
Rorasul, 397
Rubidomycin as antitumour agent, 382, 384
Russell's viper venom, 215
Rynacrom in bronchial asthma, 182
Rythmodan action on heart, 147, 149

Safety of Drugs Committee, 6-7
Salbutamol, 126
  in bronchial asthma, 179-180
Salcatonin, 336
Salicylates, 286-289
  absorption of aspirin, 287
  allergy, 289
  fate in body, 287-288
  individual variation, 26, 27
  pharmacological actions, 288
  structures, 286
  toxic effects, 288
Salivary secretion, 184
Salt diet, high, and corticosteroids, causing hypertension, 111
Saluric, 166
Salvarsan, structure, 431
Salyrgan, 161, 166
Scabies, drugs in, 230, 231
Schistosomiasis, 452-453
  preparations, 454
Schizophrenia
  dopamine hypothesis, 240-241
  and hallucinogenic drugs, 241
Schizophrenic psychoses, treatment, 253-254
Scopolamine, *see* Hyoscine
Scurvy, 370
Sebaceous glands, 228
Seborrhoea, use of oestrogens, 355
Secretory mechanisms, and drug excretion, 45
Sectral, 130
Sedative-hypnotics, 246-248
  drug dependence, 248
  preparations, 256
Semitard insulin, 340, 349
Senega, as expectorant, 176
Senna as purgative, 198, 201

Septrin, 395, 397
  possible teratogenic effect, 225
Serenid-D as tranquilliser, 256
Seromycin, 428
Serotonin, *see* 5-Hydroxytryptamine
Serpasil, 130
Sex hormones, 351-359
  anabolic steroids, 358-359
  androgens, 357-358
  control of ovarian cycle, 351
  oestrogens, 353-355
    see also Oestrogens
  preparations, 359
  progestogens, 355-357
Shingles, treatment, 229
Shock, 129
  see also Circulatory collapse
Side effects of drugs, 31
  and plasma concentration, 49
  see also Drugs
Silver compounds as disinfectants, 459
Sinequan, 258
Sinus
  bradycardia, management, 147
  tachycardia, management, 147
Skeletal muscle, action of catecholamines, 81
Skeletal muscle relaxants, centrally acting
  clinical usefulness, 276
  control of muscle tone, 275
  effects, 275
  preparations, 277
  specific drugs, 275-276
Skidan, 166
Skin
  diseases, corticosteroids, 348
  drug reactions, 231
  hypersensitivity reactions, 100, 230-231
  pharmacology, 228-231
  pre-operative scrubbing, disinfectants, 461-462
  preparations, 231
  structure and function, 227-228
Sleep, use of tranquillisers to promote, 248
  see also Barbiturates
Smallpox, methisazone, 396
Smog, 466
Smoking and health, 490
Smooth muscle
  action of catecholamines, 81
  effects of morphine, 280
Soaps as disinfectants, 458
Sodium amytal
  dosage and duration of action, 245
  individual variation in response, 27
  preparation, 256
Sodium bicarbonate
  action, 191
  neutralising power, 190
  preparation, 201
  reabsorption, urinary, 157
Sodium calcium edetate in heavy metal poisoning, 474, 475

Sodium citrate in coagulation prevention, 211
Sodium cromoglycate in bronchial asthma, 181-182, 183
Sodium diatrizoate (hypaque), 166
Sodium hypochlorite as disinfectant, 459
Sodium nitrite in cyanide poisoning, 171, 183
Sodium nitroprusside, 130
  as coronary vasodilator, 123
  in hypertension, 121
Sodium reabsorption, and excretion, 158-160
Sodium salicylate individual variation in response, 26-27
Sodium sulphate, 198, 201
Sodium thiosulphate in cyanide poisoning, 171
Sodium valproate in epilepsy, 272, 277
Soframycin, 417
Solapsone, 428
Somatostatin, 323
Soneryl (butobarbitone), dosage and duration of action, 245
  preparation, 256
Sorbide nitrate, 130
Sotalol, 130
Sparine major tranquilliser, 254, 256
Spectinomycin, 407
Spermatogenic disruption as male contraceptive, 479
Spinal anaesthesia, 312, 313-315
  anaesthetic agents, 314
  dangers, 314-315
  onset and duration, 314
Spiramycin, 408
Spirochaetal infections, 435-437
  diseases, 435
  drug treatment, 435-437
  preparations, 437
  tests for spirochaeticidal drugs, 435
Spironolactone, 163, 165, 166
  in essential hypertension, 111, 114
Squill, as expectorant, 175
SRS-A, 92
  as bronchoconstrictor, 176
Staphylococcal infections, penicillin treatment, 405, 404
  cephaloridine, 406
Status asthmaticus, management, 183
Status epilepticus, drugs in, 273
Stelazine as tranquilliser, 256
Stemetil as tranquilliser, 256
Sterculia, 197, 201
Sterilisation, voluntary, 476
Steroids
  anabolic, *see* Anabolic steroids
  mode of action, 321
  radioimmunoassays, 20
  see also individual names
Stibocaptate in schistosomiasis, 453, 454
Stibogluconate in leishmaniasis, 435, 437
Stibophen in schistosomiasis, 453, 454

Stilboestrol, 353, 359
  clinical potency, 355
  in lactation inhibition, 355
  in menopausal disorders, 355
  as post-coital contraceptive, 478
  in prostatic cancer, 382, 384
  teratogenic properties, 353
Stomach, absorption of drugs, 36
'STP', 489
Streptokinase, 211, 216
Streptomycin, 420-422, 427, 411-412
  absorption, 420
  clinical use, 411
  discovery, 418
  effect on fetus, 225
  excretion, 420, 421
  half-life, 46
  mode of action, 421, 388
  preparation, 427
  resistance, 421
  serum concentration, 421
  toxicity, 411-412, 421-422
  transplacental transmission, 225
  tuberculostatic activity, 420, 426
Strongyloides infections, drugs for, 452, 454
Strophanthin frog assay, 21
Strophanthus gratus, 136
Strychnine
  as analeptic, 172
  poisoning, 172
Stugeron, as antiemetic, 194
Subacute myelo-optico-neuropathy associated with hydroxyquinolines, 445
Substance P, 91
  transmitter role in CNS, 236
Succinimides
  in epilepsy, 271, 276
  structures, 270
Suckling and release of oxytocin, 218-219
Sulfadoxine in malaria, 446
Sulindac anti-inflammatory drug, 293
Sulphacetamide, 395, 397
Sulfoxone, 428
Sulphadiazine, 393
  preparation, 397
  relative merits, 395
  structure, 392
Sulphadimethoxine, 395
  half-life, 46
Sulphadimidine, 393
  half-life, 46
  relative merits, 395
  structure, 392
Sulphafurazole, 393
  preparation, 397
  relative merits, 395
  structure, 392
Sulphamethizole, 397
Sulphamethoxazole, 397
Sulphamethoxypyridazine, 395, 397
Sulfametopyrazine, 397
Sulphamezathine, 395

Sulphanilamide
  antibacterial activity, 393
  inhibition by yeasts, 386-387
  structure, 392
Sulphaphenazole, 397
Sulphasalazine, 397
Sulphathiazole, 394
  antibacterial activity, 393
Sulphinpyrazone
  in gout, 292
  platelet survival inhibition, 209
Sulphonamides, 392-395, 416
  absorption, distribution and excretion, 393
  antibacterial activity, 393
    comparative, 393
  chemistry, 392-393
  discovery, 5
  excretion, 394
  metabolism, 394
  mode of administration, 394
  preparations, 397
  related compounds, 393
  relative merits of compounds, 394-395
  structure-activity relations in, 387
  structures, 392
  therapeutic uses, 395
  transplacental transmission, 225
  toxic effects, 394
  urinary tract infections, 395
Sulphones in leprosy, 428
Sulphonylureas, 340-341
  preparations, 349
Sulthiame in epilepsy, 273
Suramin
  in filariasis, 454
  structure, 434
  in trypanosomiasis, 434
Surface
  active agents as disinfectants, 458
  anaesthesia, 311, 312
Surital in anaesthesia, 306
Suxamethonium, 66
  action, 68
  bromide in anaesthesia, 306, 307
  chloride in anaesthesia, 306, 307
  structure, 67
Sweat glands, 227-228
  apocrine, 227-228
  eccrine, 227
Sweating action of catecholamines, 82
Symmetrel, 397
  in Parkinsonism, 274, 277
Sympathetic nerves, effects of stimulation, 54-55
Sympathomimetic drugs, 124-126
  in bronchial asthma, 177-181, 183
  relative potencies, 173
  structure and actions, 125
  see also specific names
Sympatol, 130
Synacthen, 328, 336
Synalar, 343, 347, 349
Synaptic transmission in CNS, 235-240
Synkavit, 216, 365, 366
Syphilis, drug treatment, 435-437

TACE, 354
Tagamet (see Cimetidine)
Talampicillin, 407
Talpen, 407
Tamoxifen, 384
Tandacote, anti-inflammatory drug, 293
Tapazole, 336
Tapeworm infections, 448-449
Tar in psoriasis, 228
Tardive dyskinesia, drug-induced, 239-240, 255
Tavegil, 104
TEA, *see* Tetraethylammonium
Tegretol, in epilepsy, 272, 276
Telepaque, 195
TEM, in neoplastic disease, 379
Tenormin, 130
Tensilon, *see* Edrophonium chloride
TEPP, *see* Tetraethylpyrophosphate
Teprotide, 127
Teratogenicity, drug, assessment, 31
Terbutaline sulphate preparation, 183
Terminal anaesthesia, 313
Terramycin, 417
Tertroxin, 336
Testosterone, 321
  action, 357-358
  contraindication, 338
  enanthate, 359
  preparations, 359
  therapeutic, 359
Tetracaine, 311, 315
Tetrachloroethylene in hookworm infection, 451, 454
Tetracosactrin, 328, 336
  in bronchial asthma, 182, 183
  long- and short-acting, 328
Tetracyclines, 409-410, 415, 417
  absorption, distribution and excretion, 409
  in acne, 230
  administration, 410
  antibiotic activity, 409
  bacterial resistance, 409
  chemical features and structures, 409
  clinical applications, 410
  effects on fetus, 225
  half-life, 46
  mode of action, 409, 388
  preparations, 417
  in spirochaetal infection, 437
  in syphilis, 436, 437
  toxic effects, 410
  transplacental transmission, 225
Tetraethylammonium, ganglion blocking action, 64
Tetraethylpyrophosphate (TEPP), action, 61
Tetramethylammonium, 59
Thalidine, 397
Theophylline
  in bronchial asthma, 182
  as diuretic, 164, 165
  ethylenediamine, as cardiac stimulant, 149
  structure, 165
Thephorin, 104

Therapeutic(s)
  commercial influences, 7-8
  index, 29-30
  nihilism, 4-5
  range of drugs, and plasma concentration, 49
  trials of drugs, 32-33
    statistical methods, 32
Thiabendazole in Strongyloides infection, 452, 454
Thiadiazines, 393
Thiambutosine, 428
Thiamine, 366-367, 371
  daily requirements, 367, 371
  deficiency, 366-367
    partial, 367
  half-life, 46
  therapeutic uses, 367
Thiamylal sodium in anaesthesia, 304
Thiazides, 160-161, 166
  chemical structure, 160
  choice, 165
  diuretic action, 160-161
  hypertension, 113-114
  undesirable effects, 161
Thiocarlide, 428
Thiacetazone
  in leprosy, 428
  structure, 422
  in tuberculosis, 424
Thioguanine in cancer, 381
  in leukaemia, 382
Thioparamizone, in tuberculosis, 424
Thiopentone sodium in anaesthesia, 303-304, 306
  dosage and duration of action, 245
Thiopropazate as tranquilliser, 256
Thioridazine major tranquilliser, 254, 256
  structure, 255
Thiotepa, in neoplastic disease, 379, 384
Thiothixene as tranquilliser, 256
Thiouracil
  compounds causing agranulocytosis, 208
  dosage, 334
  preparation, 336
  structure, 333
Threadworm infections, drugs for, 451, 454
Thrombin preparations, 215, 216
Thrombocytopenic purpura, drug-induced, 208
Thromboplastin, 216
Thrombosis
  pharmacology, 209-215
  postoperative, aspirin in prevention, 209
  see also Anticoagulant drugs
Thymoxamine, preparation, 85
Thyrocalcitonin, 336
Thyroid gland, 330-335
  antithyroid drugs, 333-334
  cretinism, 333
  function tests, 332
  goitre, 330
  hormones, 331-335

Thyroid, cont'd
  iodine, 330
  metabolism, 332-333
  radioactive, 334-335
  myxoedema, 333
  potassium perchlorate, 334
  preparations, 336
  radioimmunoassays, 20
  secretion, 332
  thyroxine, 331-332
  triiodothyronine, 331
Thyroid stimulating hormone (TSH), 326-327, 336
  receptor, 326
Thyrotoxicosis, 333, 334
Thyrotrophic hormone, 326-327, 336
  long-acting thyroid stimulator, 327
Thyrotrophin-releasing hormone, 322
Thyroxine, (T$_4$), 331-332
  action, 331
  chemical features, 331
  dosage, 331-332
  overdosage, 332
  preparation, 336
  structure, 331
  toxic effects, 332
Tigloidine hyd. in Parkinsonism, 277
Timolol, 130
Tinactin, 417
Tinaderm in skin fungal infections, 231
Tinidazole in amoebiasis, 444
TMA, see Tretramethylammonium
Tobacco dependence, 490
  smoking and health
Tobramycin, 412, 417
Tocopherol, 364-365, 371
Tofenacin hyd., 267
Tofranil, 258
Tolamolol, in angina, 124
  in hypertension, 116
Tolanade, 349
Tolazamide, 349
Tolazoline, 83
  preparation, 85
Tolbutamide, 340, 341, 349
  chemical structure, 341
Tolnaftate, 417
  in skin fungal infections, 231
Tosmilen, 87, 89
Toxaemia of pregnancy, and 5-HT, 94
Trandate, 130
Tranexamic acid, 216
Tranquillisers
  in labour, 223
  major, 252-256
  preparations, 256
  minor, preparation, 256
  see also Hypnotics
Transfusion in circulatory collapse, 129
Transglutaminase, 210
Tranylcypromine
  in depression, 261
  preparation, 267
  structure, 261
Trasicor, 130
Travel sickness, prevention, 193

Treponema pallidum, penicillin treatment, 405
Trescatyl, 428
Tretamine, in neoplastic disease, 379
Tretinoin in acne, 230, 231
Trevintix, 428
TRH, see Thyrotrophin-releasing hormone, 322
Trials, therapeutic, of drugs, 32-33
  statistical methods, 32
Triamcinolone, 343, 347, 349
  acetonide, 350
  relative potency, 345
Triamterene, 114, 163, 165, 166
Trichlorethylene anaesthesia, 302, 306
  in labour, 223
Triclofos, as hypnotic, 247, 256
Tricyclic antidepressants, 257-260
  actions, 257, 258-259
  adverse effects, 259
  chemistry, 258
  clinical effectiveness, 259
  effects in man, 259
  effect on REM sleep, 237
  pharmacological action, 258
  preparations, 266
  structures, 258
  see also Imipramine and specific names
Tridione in epilepsy, 271, 277
Triethylene thiophosphoramide in neoplastic disease, 379
Triethylenemelamine in neoplastic disease, 379
Trifluoperazine as tranquilliser, 256
Triflupromazine, major tranquilliser, 254
  structure, 255
Triiodothyronine (T$_3$), 331-332
  action, 331
  dosage, 332
  function tests, 332
  preparations, 336
  structure, 332
Trilene anaesthesia, 302, 306
  in labour, 223
Trimelarsan, 433, 437
Trimetaphan camsylate, 130
Trimethadione in epilepsy, 271, 277
Trimethaphan, 120, 130
Trimethoprim, 395-396
  absorption and excretion, 396
  clinical uses, 396
  possible teratogenic effects, 225
  structure, 395
  toxic effects, 396
Trimethylene (Cyclopropane) anaesthesia, 303, 306
Trimipramine maleate, 367
Triprolidine, 104
Triseldon, 350
Tropicamide, action on eyes, 88
  eye preparation, 88
Troleandomycin, 408
Troxidone in epilepsy, 271, 277

Trypanosomiasis, 430-434
  African, 432-434
    arsenical compounds, 432-433
    control, 432
    measurement of activity of drugs, 432
    preparations, 437
    trypanocidal drugs, 432-434
  cross resistance, 432
  discovery of trypanocidal drugs, 430-432
  drug resistance, 431-432
  preparations, 437
  South American (Chagas' disease), 432, 434
    drugs in, 432, 434
    preparations, 437
Tryparsamide
  structure, 433
  in trypanosomiasis, 433
Tryptizol, 258, 266
TSH, see Thyroid stimulating hormone
Tuberculin reaction, 99, 100
Tuberculosis, chemotherapy, 418-427
  allergy, 427
  assessment of tuberculostatic activity, 419-420, 426
  bacilli, properties, 418
  BCG vaccine, 418
  combination of drugs, 419
  desirable properties, 419
  discovery, 418-419
  duration of treatment, 426
  intermittent chemotherapy, 426-427
  preparations, 428
  pulmonary, drugs, 420
  radiological appearances after treatment, 426
  resistance, 427
  specific drugs, 420-427
  standard chemotherapy, 426
  therapeutic uses, 425
  toxic and allergic reactions, 427
  toxicity, 427
Tubocurarine
  action, and structure, 66-67
  chloride in anaesthesia, 305, 307
  half-life, 46
  structure, 67
  two postsynaptic actions, 18
Tubules, proximal, and distal, and drug excretion, 44
  compounds secreted by, 45
Tumour-specific antigens, 375
Tyglissin in Parkinsonism, 277
Typhoid fever, chloramphenicol, 411
Tyrosine hydroxylase, 74

Ultandren, 359
Ultracortenol, 349
Ultratard insulin, 340, 349
Ultraviolet light in acne, 230
Undecylenic acid, 417
Urea stibamine in leishmaniasis, 435, 437
Urinary clearance by kidney, 153-154

Urinary tract infections, drugs for, 395, 397
Urine
  ammonia formation, 157
  change, 157-158
  clearance, 153-155
  excretion, hormonal control, 155-156
  pH, 156-158
  phosphate buffer system, 157
  sodium bicarbonate reabsorption, 157
Urokinase, 211
Urticaria, symptoms, 231
  treatment, 231
U.S. Public Health recommendations for treatment of syphilis, 436
Uterus, 217-226
  analgesia in labour, 223-224
  bleeding, control by progestogens, 357
  clinical course of labour, 222
    use of drugs, 222-223
    see also Oxytocin
  clinical uses of oxytocic drugs, 220-222
  contractions, 221, 217-218
  inertia, 222
  innervation, 218-220
  movements, 217-218
  postpartum haemorrhage, 223
  preparations, 225
  role of neurosecretion, 218-220

Vagal secretory activity, drug stimulation, 189
Valium
  as muscle relaxant, 276, 277
  in status epilepticus, 273
  see also Diazepam
Vallestril, 359
Valproate sodium in epilepsy, 272, 277
Vanquin, 452
Vapours, anaesthetic
  isonarcotic concentrations, 295
Variation, individual, 48-49
Vasoactive intestinal peptide, 194
Vasoconstrictor drugs, 124-129, 130
  angiotensin amide, 127
  centrally acting, 124
  ergotamine, 127-128
  local application, 126
  in local haemorrhage, 215
  migraine prophylaxis, 128-129
  peripheral, 124-126
Vasodilators, 130
  coronary, 121-124
  effect in angina, 122
  in hypertension, 114-115
Vasopressin, 130
  actions, 130, 329
  clinical uses, 329
  preparation, 336
  structure, 329
  as vasoconstrictor, 127
Vasoxine, 130, 126
Vatensol, 130
Velbe, antitumour agent, 381, 384

Velosef, 407
Ventolin in bronchial asthma, 179, 183
Veractil as tranquilliser, 256
Verapamil, action on heart, 146, 149
Veratrum alkaloids in hypertension, 120
Veriloid, 130
Vibramycin, 417
Vidarabine, 397
Viloxazine hyd., 267
Vinblastine, antitumour agent, 381, 383, 384
Vinca alkaloids, use in cancer, 381-382, 383
Vincristine, antitumour agent, 381, 383, 384
Vinyl ether anaesthesia, 301
Vioform, 444
Viomycin in tuberculosis, 425
Viprynium in threadworm infection, 452, 454
Virus infections
  antiviral agents, 396-397
  skin, treatment, 229
Visken, 130
Vitamin(s), 360-372
  deficiency, causes, 360-361
  diet content, 370-371
  discovery, 5, 360
  fat-soluble, 361
  nomenclature, 361
  preparations, 371
  recommended daily allowances, 371
  requirements, 361
  water-soluble, 366-370
Vitamin A, 361-362, 371
  acid, in acne, 230, 231
  activity, 362
  deficiency, 362
    clinical effects, 362
    effects in animals, 362, 371
  food sources, 361-362
  preparation, 371
  requirements, 362
  structure, 361
  therapeutic use, 362
Vitamin A_1, 361
Vitamin B complex, 366-369, 371
  see also Thiamine (aneurine): Riboflavine: Nicotinic acid (niacin): Pyridoxine, Folic acid (pteroylglutamic acid): Cyanocobalamin (Vitamin B_{12}): Pantothenic acid (Vitamin B_5): Biotin: Choline: Para-aminobenzoic acid: Inositol
Vitamin B_{12}, deficiency, and pernicious anaemia, 206
Vitamin C see Ascorbic acid
Vitamin D, 362-364, 371
  and calcium absorption, 363-364
  chemical features, 363
  deficiency, 363
  food sources, 364
  half-life, 46
  metabolites, 362, 371
  physiological function, 363

Vitamin D, *cont'd*
    preparations, 371
    requirements, 371
    sunlight, 364
    therapeutic uses, 364
    toxic effects, 364
Vitamin D$_2$, 363, 371
Vitamin D$_3$, 363, 371
Vitamin E, 364-365, 371
    deficiency, 365
    natural source, 364
    therapeutic use, 365
Vitamin H, 369
Vitamin K, 213, 216, 365-366
    chemistry, 365
    deficiency, 366
    dependent clotting factors, 210, 211, 213, 216
    functions, 366
    K$_1$ (phytomenadione), 365, 366, 371
        in haemorrhage, 366
    K$_3$ (menadione), 365
    occurrence and metabolism, 365
    therapeutic uses, 366
Vivàlan, 276
Voltaren, anti-inflammatory drug, 293

Vomiting, 191-194
    act, 191
    centre, 191
        production of emesis, 192
        drugs, 192-193
    function, 191
    in pregnancy, 193
    prevention, 193

Warfarin, anticoagulant, 213-214
    chemical structure, 213
    preparation, 216
Water reabsorption and excretion, 158-160
Wave of excitation, transmission in heart, 131
Weight reduction and amphetamine, 263
Welldorm (dichloralphenazone), as hypnotic, 247
    preparation, 256
Wheal and flare reaction, 101
Whipworm infections, drugs for, 450-451, 454
Whitfield's ointment in skin fungal infections, 231

Wilms's tumour, 383
Wilson's disease, penicillamine in, 474
Withdrawal syndromes
    alcohol, 484
    amphetamine, 484
    barbiturates, 484
    management, 491
    opiates, 483

Xanthine derivatives, as coronary vasodilators, 123
Xylocaine, 311, 315
Xylometazole as vasoconstrictor, 126

Yaws, drug treatment, 437
Yomesan in tapeworm infections, 449, 454

Zephiran, 462
Zinamide, 428
Zinc sulphate as emetic, 192
Zollinger-Ellison syndrome, 188
Zyloric in gout, 293
    preparation, 293